PASS PCCN!®

Robin Donohoe Dennison, DNP, APRN, CCNS, CNE
Consultant and President
Robin Dennison Presents, Inc.
Winchester, Kentucky

Kathleen Farrell, DNSc, APRN, ACNP
Professor
Murray State University
Murray, Kentucky

ELSEVIER

ELSEVIER

3251 Riverport Lane
St. Louis, Missouri 63043

PASS PCCN®!   ISBN: 978-0-323-07727-9

Notices

Knowledge and best practice in this field are constantly changing. As new research and experience broaden our understanding, changes in research methods, professional practices, or medical treatment may become necessary.

Practitioners and researchers must always rely on their own experience and knowledge in evaluating and using any information, methods, compounds, or experiments described herein. In using such information or methods they should be mindful of their own safety and the safety of others, including parties for whom they have a professional responsibility.

With respect to any drug or pharmaceutical products identified, readers are advised to check the most current information provided (i) on procedures featured or (ii) by the manufacturer of each product to be administered, to verify the recommended dose or formula, the method and duration of administration, and contraindications. It is the responsibility of practitioners, relying on their own experience and knowledge of their patients, to make diagnoses, to determine dosages and the best treatment for each individual patient, and to take all appropriate safety precautions.

To the fullest extent of the law, neither the Publisher nor the authors, contributors, or editors assume any liability for any injury and/or damage to persons or property as a matter of products liability, negligence or otherwise, or from any use or operation of any methods, products, instructions, or ideas contained in the material herein.

Library of Congress Cataloging-in-Publication Data

Dennison, Robin, author.
 Pass PCCN! / Robin Donohoe Dennison, Kathleen Farrell.
   p. ; cm.
 Includes bibliographical references and index.
 ISBN 978-0-323-07727-9 (pbk. : alk. paper)
 I. Farrell, Kathleen (Professor of nursing), author. II. Title.
 [DNLM: 1. Critical Illness--nursing--Examination Questions. 2. Critical Care Nursing--methods--Examination Questions. WY 18.2]
 RT120.I5
 616.02'8076--dc23
                                                                            2015035367

Executive Content Strategist: Lee Henderson
Content Development Manager: Jean Sims Fornango
Senior Content Development Specialist: Tina Kaemmerer
Publishing Services Manager: Catherine Jackson
Project Manager: Clay S. Broeker
Design Direction: Paula Catalano

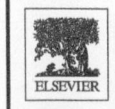 

Working together
to grow libraries in
developing countries

www.elsevier.com • www.bookaid.org

Printed in the United States of America

Last digit is the print number: 9 8 7 6 5 4 3

Clinical Consultants

Lori A. Catalano, JD, MSN, RN, CCNS, PCCN
Assistant Professor of Clinical Nursing
College of Nursing
University of Cincinnati
Academic Health Center
Cincinnati, Ohio

Barbara Pope, MSN, RN
Critical Care and Progressive Care Nurse Educator Consultant
Willow Grove, Pennsylvania

Reviewers

Katherine Alford, MSN, CCRN, PCCN
Quality Management Clinician
South Texas Veterans Health Care System
San Antonio, Texas

Lori A. Catalano, JD, MSN, RN, CCNS, PCCN
Assistant Professor of Clinical Nursing
College of Nursing
University of Cincinnati
Academic Health Center
Cincinnati, Ohio

Jeanine M. Goodin, MSN, RN-BC, CNRN
Associate Professor of Clinical Nursing
College of Nursing
University of Cincinnati
Cincinnati, Ohio

Sheryl E. Leary, PhD, RN, CNS, CCRN, PCCN
Nurse Manager
VA San Diego Healthcare System
San Diego, California

Kathleen M. Stacy, PhD, RN, CNS, CCRN, PCCN, CCNS
Critical Care CNS
Clinical Associate Professor
Hahn School of Nursing and Health Science
University of San Diego
San Diego, California

Amanda Maxwell Swedhin, RN, BSN
Clinical Nurse Educator, MS PCU
University of Colorado Health
Aurora, Colorado

Tamekia L. Thomas, MSN, APRN, PCCN, ACNS-BC
Critical Care Education Coordinator
Christiana Care Health System
Newark, Delaware

This book is dedicated to my mother, Violet Donohoe. She has always been the type of parent who expected excellence and did not feel compelled to praise. As the years have passed, I realize how much I am my mother's daughter. My strength, persistence, and focus on producing work that I can be proud of comes from her. She has always been quietly proud of my accomplishments, and I do hear about her sharing copies of my books with the healthcare providers in the nursing home where she now resides. I am proud that I have made her proud.

Robin Donohoe Dennison

This book is dedicated to my father, Frank X. Murphy, and my co-author and mentor, Robin Dennison. From an early age, through role modeling and setting expectations, my father instilled the values of a strong work ethic, accountability, and responsibility. These character traits, along with my innate desire to constantly learn and explore, has enabled me to strive for excellence in any endeavor. The process of publishing a book was a new experience, and I have learned a tremendous amount through the act of doing. I express my profound gratitude to my co-author and mentor, Robin Dennison. Prior to this endeavor, my knowledge base on the subject, clinical expertise, and nursing faculty teaching experience was strong; however, the interaction, guidance, and honest and constructive critique Robin provided enabled me to meet this new challenge. I am profoundly grateful for my father's influence on my life and to have a mentor such as Robin, and I dedicate this book to them.

Kathleen Farrell

Preface

Welcome to *Pass PCCN*®! And congratulations—you have chosen the most up-to-date, comprehensive review of progressive care nursing available on the market today. If you are a registered nurse planning to take the PCCN® examination for certified progressive care practice offered by the American Association of Critical-Care Nurses (AACN) Certification Corporation, this book is the tool that you need to prepare for the examination with confidence.

Information in this text is organized according to the latest PCCN® examination blueprint, which is summarized inside the back cover for quick reference. This test plan, issued by the AACN Certification Corporation, identifies the content areas tested and the percentage of the examination devoted to each. Only content included in the test blueprint is included in this book, eliminating extraneous information that can be distracting. The book also offers an array of learning activities to help you understand and retain key concepts. These are integrated throughout each chapter, with synthesis activities at the end of the chapter. Answers for these learning activities are located at the end of the book. In addition to the learning activities, there are more than 900 additional multiple-choice questions provided on the Evolve website. By practicing your test-taking skills at a computer, it will simulate the examination itself.

We have written this book for nurses who are preparing to take the PCCN® examination. We have both taught acute and critical care nursing for many years. We have also been involved in exam preparations for many certification exams. Our goal is to provide a pertinent content review, fun but challenging learning activities, realistic practice questions, and comprehensive mock examinations that reflect the content and complexity of the PCCN® examination.

CONTENT REVIEW

Pass PCCN®! uses a narrative format with integrated learning activities. The information is well organized and easy to read, understand, and remember. Illustrations and tables further explicate and clarify content, highlight key concepts, and enhance written explanations. This book also includes many concept maps to illustrate the pathophysiology of conditions to aid understanding of the linkage between pathophysiology and clinical presentation. Pharmacology is integrated throughout the book.

Coverage of each body system begins with a brief review of anatomy and physiology. This refresher lays the foundation for introducing more complex topics in the areas of assessment, intervention, and evaluation. Assessment includes health history, physical examination, diagnostic studies, and system-specific assessment methods. For example, the cardiovascular chapter

discusses electrocardiography, and the pulmonary chapter covers interpretation of arterial blood gases. The format varies for the Multisystem, Professional Caring and Ethical Practice, and the Behavioral/Psychosocial chapters due to the nature of the content in those sections.

Pathologic conditions listed on the PCCN® blueprint are included in the content review. Each condition is first defined, followed by discussions of etiology, pathophysiology, clinical presentation, and collaborative management, which includes medical and nursing management.

LEARNING ACTIVITIES

Sometimes we learn best when information is organized and accessed in unfamiliar ways, and that's the principle at work behind the diverse learning activities in this book. Every chapter features a range of activity styles, including matching, fill-in-the-blank, comparison, case studies, and crossword puzzles to test comprehension and improve recall for readers with a variety of learning styles.

You won't be asked to complete a crossword puzzle or a matching exercise when you take the PCCN® examination, of course, but these learning activities will help you learn and retain an astonishing amount of information. This also makes your study sessions more enjoyable, encouraging you to stick to the timetable that you have set for yourself. We hope that working through these activities will be a pleasurable way to review crucial content.

PRACTICE QUESTIONS AND EXAMINATIONS ON THE EVOLVE WEBSITE

Another great way to study is to use the practice questions and examinations on the Evolve website. It contains more than 900 review questions written in a format that represents the actual PCCN® examination. The practice examinations have been thoroughly updated to reflect the percentages set forth for each content area on the most recent test blueprint and current practice.

The Evolve website offers two modes: a quiz mode in which practice questions are arranged by body system, and a test mode that offers realistic practice PCCN® examinations. The quiz mode allows you to select topic areas in which you need additional review and create quizzes that target those areas. The test mode, on the other hand, replicates the actual PCCN® exam as closely as possible. This timed mode draws questions from all content areas in the number and proportion called for in the latest PCCN® exam blueprint. The program will reshuffle the questions randomly (retaining the correct percentages in each content area) to create as many practice tests as you like. Both modes are self-scoring. Instant rationales are given to explain which answer is correct and why it is the best answer among the possible choices. Test-taking strategy tips are provided as appropriate to show you how to think through the questions if you are not sure of how to approach the question. Both of these features will boost your confidence and make you a better test taker on the important day of the PCCN® examination. Analyzing your performance on several practice exams will help you focus your final preparation on your weakest areas.

OTHER HELPFUL FEATURES

Appendix A is a table describing etiology, ECG criteria, significance, and treatment of common dysrhythmias. This is very important content to master prior to the PCCN® examination. Appendix B is a table describing hemodynamic parameters, including how they are either measured or calculated and the normal value for the parameter. Although hemodynamic monitoring is performed in a higher-acuity level of care, it is important to understand the concepts because a major role of progressive care nursing is the early identification of a need to facilitate transfers and/or care for patients who received hemodynamic monitoring once stabilized. Appendix C is a list of abbreviations and acronyms used in this book and common in progressive care. Each term is always spelled out in the text the first time it is used, but this appendix will help you identify these abbreviations or acronymns later if you don't remember them. Appendix D lists laboratory studies important in the care of acutely ill adults, including the normal range of values for each. We recommend that you study this list just before taking the exam because

you are expected to know common normal laboratory values. Appendix E is a list of formulae commonly used in the evaluation of acutely ill patients.

This book is not a comprehensive progressive care textbook, nor is it intended to be. Instead, we've focused selectively on the information likely to be tested on the PCCN® examination. We believe *Pass PCCN®!* is the only book you need to prepare for the examination. Progressive care nursing has never been more exciting. For those of us who thrive on this challenge, keeping up with new research and clinical developments is a continual test of our mettle. PCCN® certification is a prestigious credential for those of us who specialize in progressive care nursing. We are confident that if you study this book and use the Evolve website to practice your test-taking skills, you will pass the examination.

We would love to hear from you about your success with the examination, how this book helped you, and how you feel it could be even more useful. E-mail us at *rddennison@aol.com* or *kfarrell@murraystate.edu* or write us at the following address:

Robin Donohoe Dennison, DNP, APRN, CCNS, CNE
Kathleen Farrell, DNSc, APRN, ACNP
c/o Content Education
Elsevier
3251 Riverport Drive
Maryland Heights, MO 63043

We believe that this book will be your most valuable resource in preparing for the PCCN® examination. Good luck!

Robin Donohoe Dennison and Kathleen Farrell

Acknowledgments

We want to thank our editors Tamara Myers, Lee Henderson, Tina Kaemmerer, and Clay Broeker. We are so pleased to be associated with Elsevier and with this talented and dedicated team.

We also thank the clinical consultants who critically reviewed each chapter and made suggestions for changes. We also appreciate the clinical consultants who critically reviewed every practice question and suggested revisions and rewrites to make this current and consistent with the PCCN® examination.

Finally, once again, we thank our husbands and the loves of our lives, R. Russell Dennison, Jr. and Ray Farrell. Their love and support have helped us realize personal and professional goals, and this edition is yet another manifestation of their encouragement. We are truly blessed.

Contents

Preparing for and Performing on the PCCN Examination

Congratulations on taking this first step to obtain your certification in progressive care nursing! This chapter will describe certification, preparing for certification, and performing on the examination to allow you to pass the Progressive Care Certified Nurse (PCCN)® examination.

CERTIFICATION

Licensure indicates a minimum level of knowledge and is granted by a governmental agency, such as state boards of nursing, whereas certification indicates an advanced level of knowledge and is granted by a nongovernmental agency. Certification validates a nurse's qualifications and knowledge for practice within either a functional role, such as educator or nurse administrator; an advanced practice role, such as nurse practitioner or clinical nurse specialist; or a clinical specialty, such as critical care, progressive care, or oncology. The validation process is based on predetermined standards of practice (AACN, 2010). These standards of practice are determined by role delineation studies that are conducted periodically to determine the role requirements and the knowledge and skills required of a nurse in the functional or clinical area of nursing.

The certifying body determines the requirements to obtain certification. Certification is offered by a specialty organization, such as the American Association of Critical-Care Nurses (AACN), which offers the PCCN® certification for progressive care nurses, or the American Nurses Credentialing Center (ANCC), the credentialing arm of the American Nurses Association. The requirements for certification include education, practice, and documentation of knowledge, usually in the form of an examination, though portfolios are now being used for this purpose for some certifications.

There are many benefits to obtaining professional certification. The most important benefit for nurses is the self-satisfaction of becoming certified, which validates their knowledge and clinical judgment in their chosen role and/or specialty. Many nurses report that the scheduled examination provides them with a professional challenge and motivation to update their knowledge base.

Certified nurses earn recognition and respect, and they are more likely to feel empowered (Fitzpatrick, Campo, Graham, & Lavandero, 2010). They also enjoy improved career mobility because this is a national credential and many hospitals and other health care institutions prefer certified nurses. Most nurse managers encourage their nursing staff to become certified, and the majority of managers prefer to hire certified nurses over non-certified nurses when other qualifications are equal (Stromborg

et al., 2005). Some hospitals actually require certification in the specialty to work on a specialty unit.

Many health care institutions offer a bonus or a differential for certification. This extra remuneration aids in supporting the cost of continuing education to maintain certification. Most health care institutions do reimburse the nurse for the expense of taking the examination if he or she obtains certification. Certification is often recommended or required for promotion up a clinical career ladder, which provides an additional financial incentive.

There are also benefits to the health care institution. Having certified nurses provides evidence of excellence for marketing as well as for awards such as the Magnet Recognition Program by the ANCC, AACN Beacon Award for Critical Care Excellence, or Malcolm Baldrige National Quality Award. In addition, Fitzpatrick, Campo, Graham, and Lavandero (2010) found that having certified nurses improved retention of nurses, which would reduce recruitment and orientation costs to the institution.

The benefits to patients and their families include assurance that certified nurses are competent and knowledgeable regarding their specialties. Certification improves patient safety (Kendall-Gallagher & Blegen, 2009) and improves competence in detecting signs and symptoms of complications and initiating prompt intervention (Cary, 2001).

Several perceived barriers to certification exist (Teal, 2011; Altman, 2011). These include the following:
- Cost of the examination
- Fear of testing and/or failure
- Lack of institutional support
- Lack of rewards
- Lack of time for preparation and maintenance of renewal requirements
- Lack of experience

PCCN® CERTIFICATION

This certification is offered by the AACN Certification Corporation, which also offers CCRN for critical care nurses, CCNS for critical care clinical nurse specialists, and CNML for nurse managers and leaders.

AACN describes progressive care as the care of the acutely ill adult with a variety of medical diagnoses and comorbidities. It is considered part of the continuum of critical care. Patients in progressive care units can easily become unstable; require intensive resources including staffing, resources, equipment, and supplies; and require persistent nursing vigilance (AACN, 2013a).

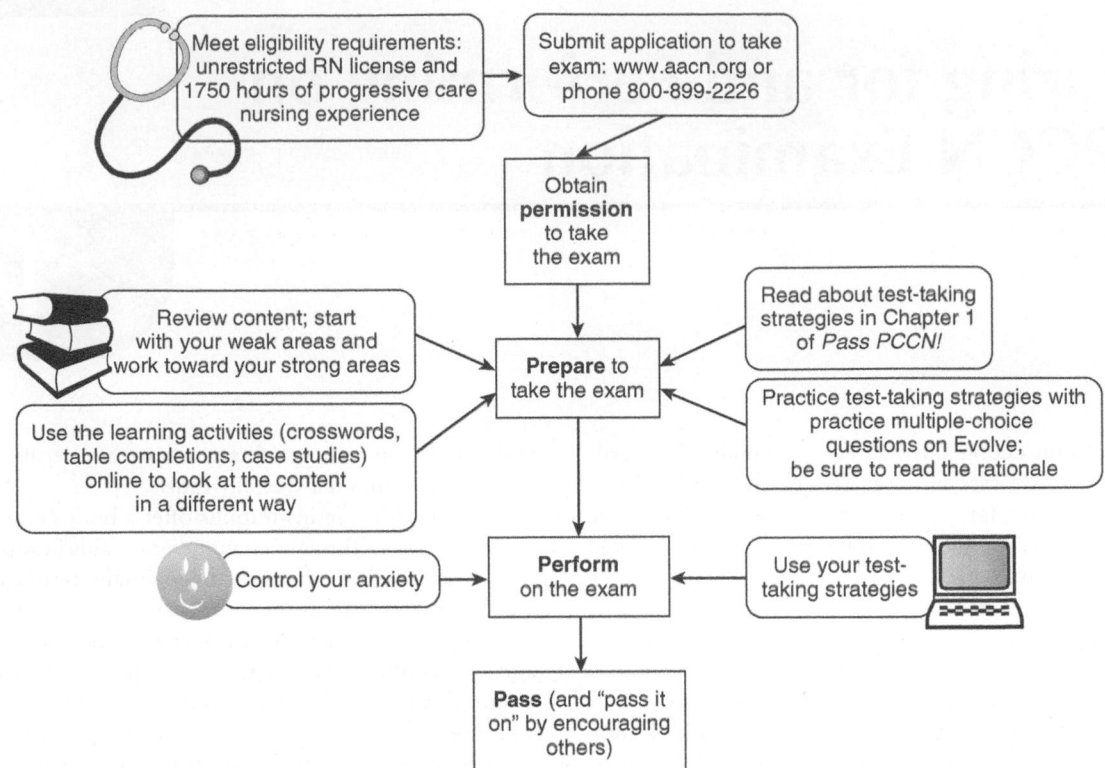

FIGURE 1-1 Plan for passing the PCCN® examination.

The plan for obtaining PCCN® certification (Figure 1-1) begins with obtaining *permission* to take the examination, diligently *preparing* to take the examination, and *performing* well on the examination to *pass* and obtain this important credential.

Permission to Take the Examination

As part of the plan for becoming certified as a PCCN®, permission must be granted to take the examination. The requirements to be approved to take the examination include a current unrestricted RN license in the United States or in any of its territories that use the NCLEX for RN licensure, clinical practice in progressive care, and completion and submission of the application with the appropriate fee.

The clinical practice in progressive care requirement is 1750 hours within the previous 2-year period with 875 of the hours accrued in the most recent year preceding application. Because PCCN® certification is a clinical credential, you must maintain a clinical practice to maintain your certification. Eligible hours are those spent caring for adult patients in a progressive care setting, including intermediate care units, direct observation units, step-down units, telemetry units, and transitional care units. Other settings may also be considered "progressive care" depending on the characteristics of the patient population cared for in the setting; the AACN Certification Corporation can assist you in determining your eligibility to take the examination. To obtain an application, contact the AACN Certification Corporation by phone (800-899-2226) or email (certcorp@aacn.org) or visit the website at http://www.aacn.org/DM/Certifications/CertificationCenter.aspx?type=certificationcenter. After completion of the application process, approval to take the examination is received by mail. You will be sent an authorization letter indicating that you meet the requirements to take the examination, along with instructions on how to

schedule the examination. The test must be scheduled within 90 days. Computer-based testing is available most weekdays year-round, whereas a pencil-and-paper version is available only once a year at the location of the AACN National Teaching Institute. Applied Measurement Professionals (AMP) administers the computerized form of the test at its testing centers nationwide.

Schedule the examination so that you have a target date; you can reschedule up to 4 business days before the scheduled test day if something unforeseen occurs. Schedule the time of the examination according to when you do your best thinking or when you are most productive: Schedule for morning if you are a lark or afternoon if you are an owl.

Preparation for the Examination
Know about the Examination

The PCCN® examination is designed to evaluate your understanding of the common body of knowledge needed to function effectively in a progressive care setting. The test consists of 125 multiple-choice questions to be completed within 2.5 hours; 25 of these items are not scored but are test items for the development of future examinations. The questions relate to patient problems common to progressive care and to nationally recognized practice with the focus being on clinical decision making rather than memorization and recall.

As described earlier, certification examinations are based on role delineation studies so that the examination is reflective of practice. The most current study conducted by AACN to identify tasks, knowledge, and experiences required of a registered nurse practicing in a progressive care setting was conducted in 2012, and the current PCCN® test plan (Table 1-1) was revised for use beginning in June 2013. The test plan identifies the categories tested and the percentage of questions in each category as well as what disease entities are on the examination.

TABLE 1-1	Test Plan for the PCCN® Examination	
Clinical Judgment		**80%**
Cardiovascular		33%
Pulmonary		14%
Endocrine/Hematology/ Gastrointestinal/Renal		18%
Neurology/Multisystem/ Behavioral		15%
Professional Caring and Ethical Practice		**20%**

From American Association of Critical-Care Nurses (AACN). (2013). *PCCN test plan.* Retrieved from www.aacn.org/wd/certifications/docs/pccn-test-plan.pdf.

Questions on the examination may be categorized using Bloom's taxonomy for the cognitive domain:

- Knowledge questions require you to remember previously learned information.
- Comprehension questions require you to understand the information.
- Application questions require you to use information.
- Analysis questions require you to break down information into its component parts and recognize commonalities, differences, and interrelationships.
- Evaluation questions require you to judge the value of information.
- Synthesis questions require you to put parts of information together to form a new conclusion.

Questions on the examination are distributed across these cognitive levels, but the majority of the questions are at the application and analysis levels (AACN, 2010). Also, all phases of the nursing process are included on the examination.

The passing score for the PCCN examination is 68 of the 100 scored items (AACN, 2013a). About two-thirds of nurses pass the PCCN® examination on their first try (AACN, 2013b); nurses retaking the test for recertification have a higher passing rate. For more specific information about the examination, the application and application process, and the testing process, download the Certification Examination Handbook at http://www.aacn.org/WD/Certifications/Docs/certexamhandbook.pdf.

Be Positive!

Avoid negative self-talk since "I'll never pass this examination" can be a self-fulfilling prophecy. Practice positive self-talk by using affirmations (i.e., positive statements). Write down some affirmations related to your preparation and performance on this examination; suggested affirmations are listed in Box 1-1.

Say these and other affirmations that you have written over and over again throughout your preparation time; say them like you believe them and you will! Also consider recording your affirmations and play them often; play them in the car, while you walk or do dishes, or any other time when you can listen and repeat them.

Prepare for the Examination

Establish a realistic schedule for your preparation; 1- to 2-hour time slots are probably the most helpful. Plan to review one system per day or weekend, depending on how much time you have left before the examination.

BOX 1-1
Affirmations
I understand the information important for this examination. I am a knowledgeable progressive care nurse. I feel prepared for this examination. I am an excellent test-taker. I will pass this examination.

There are two ways to view priorities: study your weak areas first or review the high-percentage content areas first, even if you feel confident about those areas. Because the cardiovascular and pulmonary systems together are 47% of the examination, you should feel very confident about those content areas.

Review content using this book. Highlight areas that you do not feel confident about; you may need to refer to more comprehensive textbooks or articles when you need additional clarification. Complete the learning activities integrated throughout or at the end of each chapter to consolidate your knowledge by looking at the information in another way. Practice your test-taking skills by completing practice questions on the Elsevier Evolve website. In addition to looking at the answer, read the rationale; remember that a test question may not be written exactly the same as a practice question, but the concept may be on the examination. If, after reading the rationale, you still do not understand why you missed the question, refer back to the section in this book or a textbook to understand why the correct answer is better than your answer. In addition to looking at the answer and the rationale, read the test-taking strategy; this information will help you identify how to approach a similar question to which you do not know the answer.

For each question that you get incorrect, analyze why you missed a question. Consider the following:

- Did you not know the content? Study this content again.
- Did you misread the question? Slow down and read the question more thoroughly.
- Did you misread the options? Slow down and read all of the options and select the best one.
- Did you miss an important element, such as age, diagnosis, or parameter? Again, slow down and read the question carefully; mentally highlight the critical points in the case study that you feel are important.
- Did you read into the question? Do not assume information that is not given; take the question at face value. Also, do not assume that the question is intended to "trick" you; there are no "trick" questions on the practice examination on the Evolve website or on the PCCN® examination

When you study, select a quiet place with minimal distractions. Turn off the television and radio, and let the answering machine or voice mail pick up phone calls. You should also avoid getting too comfortable—don't study in a bed or recliner; sit upright at a desk or table so that you can spread out your study materials. Also, ensure you have adequate lighting.

Reading, repeating, and writing are methods that improve memory. Use the book margins to write down memory joggers or additional thoughts. Voice-record key points on your smartphone to play back later.

If you like study groups, consider organizing a study group of nurses who are also preparing for the PCCN® examination.

Choose your members wisely because you want to include only members who will fulfill their obligation to participate. Meet to discuss the following:

- Guidelines for the group.
- Expectations of the group.
- When you will meet.
- What you will do at the meetings. For example, you may have members present essential content related to their specific area of interest, have members collect resource materials related to the specified content area and distribute them to fellow members, or plan to discuss review questions related to the specified content area.

Use and create memory joggers. Almost everyone knows "On Old Olympus' Towering Tops A Fin And German Viewed Some Hops" to remember the 12 cranial nerves, but perhaps you can establish others that help you identify things that you have trouble remembering. Also remember specific patients from your clinical experience to recall conditions or treatments.

Take a practice test on the Evolve website 1 week before the examination; use this test to identify weak areas for final study time:

- Analyze which categories (i.e., systems) are your weakest and strongest.
- Analyze which cognitive level question is the most difficult for you.
- Analyze which component of the nursing process is most difficult for you.

Don't cram the night before the examination; cramming usually just decreases your self-confidence and increases your anxiety. Go to bed at your usual time because if you go to bed early, you probably won't go to sleep anyway and will just worry about the test. Don't consume alcohol or other sedating drugs the night before or the day of the examination.

In dressing for the examination, choose comfortable clothes that allow layering so you can remove or add clothing in response to the room temperature. Consider wearing bright colors to project a more optimistic image. Take a watch, tissues, and hard candy. Don't forget your reading glasses. You will need two forms of identification, one of which should be a government-issued photo identification that contains a signature.

The morning of the examination you should eat a healthy but light meal before the examination. Avoid simple carbohydrates, such as doughnuts. Eat protein-rich foods, such as peanut butter on whole wheat toast or an egg sandwich, to sustain you through the examination.

Make sure that you know where the testing site is located and how long it will take you to get there in traffic to arrive at your scheduled test time. Getting lost or just having to rush to arrive on time causes anxiety and may affect your performance. Plan to arrive 15 minutes before your scheduled appointment. If you arrive later than 15 minutes after the scheduled testing time, you may not be admitted. You should also take the time to visit the restroom before you check in.

Performance during the Examination
Control of Anxiety

Remember that some anxiety increases your performance; however, panic decreases your performance. Because feeling adequately prepared decreases anxiety, take the time to prepare for this examination, including practicing your test-taking strategies.

Use visualization to see yourself receiving a passing score. Deep breathing and progressive muscle relaxation are also helpful. Deep breathing is performed by putting your hand below your costal margin and breathing deeply enough to raise your hand; focus on your breathing. Use this method at any time during the examination when you feel frustrated or stressed. Progressive muscle relaxation is performed by contracting a group of muscles and then relaxing them in a top-down or bottom-up order: for example, contract and relax your right leg, left leg, right arm, left arm, stomach, chest, and face. Use this technique in the car before you go in to take the examination and at any time during the examination when you feel tense. Also, consider using meditation or prayer depending on your religious beliefs.

Don't let a memory lapse or a difficult question affect your attitude or throw you into panic mode. Move on to the next question rather than let it affect your performance on the entire examination.

Test-taking Strategies

Instructions are given at the beginning of the examination. Take the time to read the instructions carefully. You can mark items to go back to so if you do not feel confident about your answer, you can view that item again and give it more thought before you submit your examination.

Always read all questions thoroughly including the stem and all options. Though you can't highlight or mark through items on a computer monitor, you can mentally highlight key points as you read the question. Note the following:

- Age and gender of the patient
- Setting: prehospital, emergency, progressive care, home care
- Medical diagnosis and other coexisting diagnoses
- Timeframe in relation to admission, trauma, surgery, pain, medication, visitation
   Also look for qualifying words such as:
- All, most, some, few, none
- Always, usually, frequently, seldom, never
- First, last
- Best, worst
- Most, least
- Smallest, largest
- Acute, chronic
- Partial, total
- Early, late

Remember that options that include global answers such as *all, always, never,* or *none* are rarely correct.

Though negatively stated questions are not recommended, it is possible that you could see this type of question. It is very important to look for negative words such as *no, not,* or *except* because missing one of those words changes the question from having one right answer to having three right answers. Also, look for terms that denote an exception such as *contraindicated* or *inappropriate.*

After you read the stem, try answering the question without looking at the options. If your answer is there, it is probably correct. However, still go ahead and read all options because there may be an option that is better than your answer.

When reading the stem, consider that included information is probably important. Extraneous information is not usually included, so if the case study or question gives you information that you feel is extraneous or superfluous, ask yourself why this information was given and how it is important to this situation.

A common testing error is to assume information that is not given. Remember that all important information is included, so do not read into the question with thoughts such as "maybe she's a diabetic" or "maybe he has COPD." If this was true and the information was important to the question, it would be included.

When choosing the correct answer, it is important that you understand what the question really is; answer *the* question, not just *a* question. Always choose the best answer; even if there are two answers that you consider correct, choose the one that best answers the question asked. If more than one option appears correct, look for the most comprehensive option.

When selecting the best answer, consider the following:

- Answer questions according to national standards of care and national guidelines rather than regional, local, or specific physicians' practices.
- Select options that are therapeutic based on current best evidence and that show respect and acceptance for the patient and the family.
- Eliminate options that are based on tradition rather than science, and options that are inappropriate, disrespectful, or punitive.
- Look for repetition of a word or a synonym of a word in the stem and in one of the options; that option is likely the correct answer.
- Choose a middle number or number range when the options are numbers or number ranges if you are not sure of the correct answer; the extremes are less likely to be the correct option.
- Remember that no one specific option is more likely than the others; because the examination is computerized and answers are random, c is no more likely to be the correct answer than a, b, or d, and there are no patterns to the correct answers.

Priority questions are common and can be difficult. Consider the following:

- Priority one is always whatever must be done to prevent death.
- Priority two is whatever must be done to prevent disability or serious complication.
- Priority three is pain or discomfort; if nothing in the case study or question could cause death or disability, pain should be considered the priority.

Actual problems always take precedence over potential problems; for example, actual hypoxemia takes precedence over potential oxygen toxicity. If there are two potential problems, the priority is the one that is more likely to cause death or disability.

If the option has more than one answer (such as x and y, or even w, x, y, and z), all of the answers must be correct for the option to be correct. Elimination works well with this type of question because if there is one answer in the option that is incorrect, that option may be immediately eliminated.

You are not penalized for guessing on this examination, so answer every question even if you must guess. Don't leave any question blank; unanswered questions are counted as incorrect. Even though you are not penalized for guessing, it should be used only as a last resort. Start by eliminating any choices that you can because it is better to guess between two choices than to guess among four. Eliminate the following:

- Clearly wrong answers
- Any response that has no relationship to the question
- Similar options that say essentially the same thing because they cannot both be correct

If you cannot reduce your choices to two answers, then look for the option that is different from the others; for example:

- If there are three antibiotics and an antifungal, choose the antifungal option.
- If there are three beta-blockers and a calcium channel blocker, choose the calcium channel blocker.
- If there are three specific options and one comprehensive option, choose the comprehensive option.

If you are unsure of your answer and want to look at it again, go ahead and answer it with your first impression. Click on "mark" at the bottom of the screen so that you can go back to it at the end of the examination. At the end of the examination, the computer allows you to go back to these marked items and review them. Examine the question again during this review process and see if there is something in the question that changes your mind about the correct answer. Once you are set on the correct answer you want to submit for that question, click on "unmark" and then continue to the end of the examination.

You may have been told to never change answers, and you should not change an answer unless you have a good reason for changing it. One good reason is that you missed a negative qualifier, such as *not, except,* or *contraindicated,* when you read it the first time.

When you are doing a practice examination, keep track of the items that you changed. After the examination, assess how many you changed from wrong to right and how many you changed from right to wrong. If you change more from wrong to right, you most likely miss questions because you don't read them thoroughly, so when you realize that you misread a question, then by all means change your answer. On the other hand, if you change more from right to wrong, don't change your initial answer (unless you realize in this case that you had misread the question) because first impressions tend to be correct more often.

The test may have math questions, which are usually drug calculations. You are provided with scratch paper and pencil. Always recheck your math if you have time.

Sometimes it is difficult to maintain concentration, especially toward the end of the examination. You should start the examination by writing down important formulas, normal values, toxic levels, etc., on your scratch paper. When you are physically tired or mentally anxious, or if you hit a particularly difficult question, try to change your normal process of reading the case study, the stem, and then the options. Instead, try reading the options in reverse order from option d to option a. Rephrase the question rather than rereading the same question over and over. Take three slow, deep breaths to regroup and get refocused at any time. You may also sign out and go to the restroom and splash water on your face if you are losing your ability to concentrate, but remember that the clock does not stop during this time.

If you are a slow test-taker, you may run short on time but more likely you will run out of mental energy because concentrating for a 2- to 3-hour period is very difficult. You should try to be at least halfway through the examination in 60 minutes; this halfway point will leave you some time to recheck your math and go back to the marked items. One helpful technique to save time is to first read the question at the end of the case study and then go back and read the case study, because we frequently read the case study, then the question, and then need to reread the case study. This technique saves you time by knowing what you are looking for in the case study. Do not be distressed by people finishing before you; everyone takes examinations at different speeds, and the others may not even be taking the PCCN® because several examinations are given at the same place and same time.

Passing the PCCN® Examination and Passing It On

You will be given your examination results at the completion of computerized testing or within 6 to 8 weeks by mail for pencil-and-paper testing. If you pass, do the following:

- Use your new credential proudly by displaying it on your name badge.
- Write it after RN when you sign your name; PCCN is not written with periods so, for example, it is written as Your Name, RN, PCCN.
- Pass it on by encouraging others to become certified; offer to tutor, mentor, and share study materials to assist your colleagues in becoming certified too.

Common reasons for failing the examination include the following:

- Knowledge deficit
- Testing errors
- Test anxiety and negative thinking

To avoid failing due to knowledge deficit, you must prepare to take the examination even if you feel that you are an experienced progressive care nurse because everyone has chosen areas of interest and weak areas. Use this book to review the content for the examination and complete the integrated learning activities of each chapter. Take a practice examination on the Evolve website 1 week before the examination to identify your weak areas and use your final study time to focus on those weak areas.

To avoid failing due to testing errors, practice using your test-taking skills with the sample questions included with this book. Pay close attention to both the rationale and the test-taking strategy included with each question. Use the learned test-taking strategies during the PCCN® examination.

To avoid failing due to test anxiety and negative thinking, believe in your ability to pass the examination and control your anxiety with prayer, meditation, deep breathing, and/or progressive relaxation.

If you fail, try again! You will likely do better the next time because the fear of the unknown is now gone and you can clearly identify your weak areas from the score breakdown provided to you upon leaving the testing site. Prepare by focusing on your weak areas and then reapply to take the test again.

Certification as a PCCN® is for a 3-year period. Recertification is achieved by providing evidence of continued practice (432 hours over the 3-year period with 144 of those hours accrued in the year before recertification) and either retaking the examination or submitting evidence of appropriate information about your continuing education and professional activities for review for renewal.

Once again, congratulations on beginning this journey! As Ralph Waldo Emerson said, "Life is a journey, not a destination."

Learning Activities

1. What are your personal reasons for becoming PCCN® certified?
   a.
   b.
   c.
2. List your top five life priorities for the next year. Is PCCN® certification on this list? What is the ranking for PCCN certification?
   1st
   2nd
   3rd
   4th
   5th
3. Prioritize this list from 1 (least comfortable) to 10 (most comfortable). Use this list to schedule your preparation with 1 being first and 10 being last.

Knowledge Area	Comfort Level
Cardiovascular	
Pulmonary	
Neurology	
Multisystem	
Gastrointestinal	
Renal	
Endocrine	
Behavioral/Psychosocial	
Hematology/Immunology	
Professional Caring and Ethical Practice	

4. Describe your plan to prepare for the PCCN® examination.
   a. Identify how many study days you have until your examination date.
   b. Decide if content review, case studies, or practice questions are the most effective method for you.
   c. Set up a schedule for your study with your weakest content areas scheduled early.
5. Explore the AACN website (www.aacn.org), focusing on the Certification tab.
6. List three new test-taking strategies that you have learned from this chapter and will use while taking the PCCN® examination.
   a.
   b.
   c.

Professional Caring and Ethical Practice

PROGRESSIVE CARE NURSING: GENERAL CONCEPTS

Nursing

The American Nurses Association (ANA) defines nursing as the "protection, promotion, and optimizations of health and abilities, prevention of illness and injury, alleviation of suffering through the diagnosis and treatment of human responses, and advocacy in the care of individuals, families, communities and populations" (2012a, paragraph 1). When providing care, a nurse uses the nursing process of assessment, diagnosis, planning, implementation, and evaluation to effect healing through treatment of the illness, continued assessment, and knowledgeable and skillful interventions while establishing caring relationships (ANA, 2012b).

Progressive Care Nursing

Progressive care nursing is a challenging nursing specialty that deals with human responses of potential life-threatening problems in high-acuity patients. The mission, vision, and values of the American Association of Critical-Care Nurses (AACN, 2010) emanate from the needs of patients and families cared for by nurses. The 2012 job analysis study defined progressive care nursing and determined the roles and responsibilities of nurses caring for this high-acuity patient population. The findings of this study were used to develop the Progressive Care Certified Nurse (PCCN)® examination blueprint (AACN Certification Corporation, 2013).

The scope of practice of a progressive care nurse includes caring for patients across the lifespan and requires active collaboration and interaction among the patient, families, critical and progressive care nursing staff, and interdisciplinary health team members within the environment. A certified progressive care nurse has clinical expertise; specialized knowledge and skills; strong, ethical decision-making skills; and commitment to interprofessional collaboration, and he or she integrates the AACN Synergy Model for Patient Care into practice (AACN, 2010).

The progressive care nurse provides stability to vulnerable patients across the lifespan by using the supportive framework of clinical expertise and knowledge, teamwork, and the AACN Synergy Model. This framework assists the nurse to integrate and prioritize data to take immediate and decisive patient-focused action. The progressive care nurse responds with confidence and adapts to dynamic patient conditions. The unique needs of patients and families coping with unanticipated treatment, quality-of-life, and end-of-life decisions are responded to in a therapeutic manner (Chuly & Burns, 2010).

Technology used in the treatment of high-acuity patient environments may be invasive, complex, and threatening to a patient and family; therefore, the progressive care nurse needs to allay fears and explain the equipment. The nurse needs to create a safe, healing, and caring environment where respect and humane health care interventions restore, rehabilitate, cure, maintain, or palliate the patient. Establishing trust with patients and families in this resource-intensive environment is crucial during the monitoring and allocation of progressive care services (AACN, 2010).

Progressive Care Environment

The spectrum of care that a progressive care patient requires includes moderate to complex assessment and interventions, monitoring, vigilance, education, and rehabilitation. It is important for the progressive care nurse to work with available intraprofessional team members to create a healing environment. An organizational model for health and healing containing five elements is utilized in progressive care environments to establish the required type of environment. The elements of the organizational model place emphasis on common values of health as a function of mind-body-spirit interrelationships, patient- and family-centered philosophy, and a supportive physical environment (O'Grady & Malloch, 2011). In addition, the model states that the organization needs to support professional growth of the progressive care nurse to provide a wide range of complementary, alternative, and traditional therapies. The progressive care nurse provides patients and families with consistency in an ever-changing environment and therefore is the ideal agent to create an organizational culture that supports the unit's community of interest: patients and families along with the nursing, medical, and ancillary staff (Chuly & Burns, 2010).

The progressive care nurse demonstrates professionalism that drives quality health care delivery within the selected environment. The progressive care nurse is culturally sensitive, values diversity, and advocates for patients and families to make sure the individual patient's values and preferences drive care decisions. The progressive care nurse promotes ethical decision making while utilizing evidence-based practice to facilitate a professional, caring, healing, and humane environment. The progressive care nurse maintains responsibility for professional growth through lifelong learning, leadership development, collegiality, and collaboration. Effective communication, appropriate human resource utilization, creativity, and recognition of practice excellence are hallmarks of a certified progressive care nurse (Bell, 2015).

AACN SYNERGY MODEL

The development of AACN's vision of a health care system in 1992 was based on the needs of patients and their families. Based on this vision, the AACN Synergy Model provides the basis for clinical practice and is the driving force for patient-centered care and ethical practice. Synergy develops when individuals work together conjointly toward a common goal (AACN, 2010). Synergy in clinical practice results when the needs and characteristics of the patient are matched with a nurse's competency. Clinical assignment needs to be based on patient diagnoses and important components of the nurse's role and clinical setting. The best clinical outcomes occur with optimal nursing care driven by the patient and family needs; therefore, the organizational framework for the AACN Certification Corporation PCCN® examination is the Synergy Model (AACN, 2010). Review the complete AACN Synergy Model for Patient Care (2003) and detailed explanations on the assumptions, patient characteristics, and nurse dimensions on the AACN website (http://www.aacn.org).

Core Concept

The characteristics of patients and families guide and determine the characteristics and competencies of nurses. Nursing practice should be centered on the needs of the patient and family. Patients have similar needs at varying levels across the wide spectrum of health to illness. Patients with more complex health care needs require nurses with advanced knowledge and expertise. Levels of complexity are dependent on the multifaceted problems present and the degree of patient compromise. The nurse's practice is driven by the needs of the patient and family; therefore, a certified nurse is expected to be proficient in multiple dimensions. The application of the Synergy Model produces optimum outcomes for the patient, family, nurse, and health care system.

Assumptions

When using the model, the patient, family, and nurse characteristics must be viewed in context. The assumptions that guide the Synergy Model are that patients are biological, psychological, social, and spiritual entities who present at a particular developmental stage and the patient, family, and community all contribute to providing a context for the nurse-patient relationship.

Patient Characteristics and Nurse Dimensions

Patients can be described by a number of interconnected characteristics. These characteristics are to be viewed in totality, not isolation. These include resiliency, vulnerability, stability, complexity, resource availability, participation in care, participation in decision making, and predictability (Table 2-1). The nurse can be described by interrelated dimensions that outline competencies used to restore a patient to an optimal level of wellness as defined by the patient. The dimensions include clinical judgment, advocacy/moral agency, collaboration, systems thinking, response to diversity, clinical inquiry, and facilitation of learning (Table 2-2).

Outcomes

Progressive care nursing is based on the AACN vision and the Synergy Model, making patients' needs and outcomes the concentrated focus of certification and practice. The outcomes derived from the model can be categorized into three areas: patient, nurse, and system. Patient outcomes center on functional change,

TABLE 2-1 | **Patient Characteristics of Synergy Model**

Characteristic	Definition
Resiliency	Capacity to return to a restorative level of functioning using coping strategies. In essence, it is the ability to bounce back quickly after an insult.
Vulnerability	Susceptibility to actual or potential stressors that may adversely affect patient outcomes.
Stability	Ability to maintain a steady balance of health care status.
Complexity	Multifaceted involvement of two or more problems or systems (e.g., body, family, therapies).
Resource availability	Extent of support (e.g., technical, fiscal, personal, psychological, social).
Participation in care	Extent to which the patient and family can and are willing to participate in portions of care to be delivered.
Participation in decision making	Extent to which the patient and family get involved in making health care decisions.
Predictability	Expected prognosis and trajectory of illness.

From American Association of Critical-Care Nurses. (2003). *The AACN Synergy Model for Patient Care.* Retrieved from http://www.aacn.org/wd/certifications/content/synmodel.pcms.

quality of life, perceptions, behavioral change, satisfaction ratings, and comfort ratings. Nurse outcomes include expected physiologic changes to monitoring and treatments, presence or absence of preventable complications, and extent to which care and treatment goals were actualized. System outcomes include reduction in cost due to a decrease in readmissions or length of stay, and improved resource utilization.

Application of the Synergy Model

Several applications exist for the Synergy Model in system operations, clinical practice, education, and research. Institutional leadership uses the model to develop the organizational structure required to achieve and maintain Magnet status (refer to application examples at www.aacn.org). The model is used to develop patient care standards, integrate technology into patient care, and establish staff mentoring program evaluation. The model is also used to enhance clinical practice delivery in a variety of progressive care settings. Educational use of the model has been effective in preceptor and orientation programs. The model has been used to guide online learning programs and simulation activities in progressive care courses. Research on the model has been used to validate progressive care practice, patient characteristics, outcomes, and nurse indicators such as staffing and productivity measures.

The certification examination categories for professional and caring ethical practice include a focus on the Synergy Model's patient and nurse characteristics (Figure 2-1). The patient characteristics determine the needed nursing characteristics or

TABLE 2-2	Nurse Dimensions of Synergy Model
Competency	**Definition**
Clinical judgment	Clinical reasoning inclusive of critical thinking, decision making, and a global grasp of the situation, coupled with nursing skills acquired through the process of integrated formal and experiential knowledge.
Advocacy/moral agency	Ability to work on another's behalf and representing the concerns of the patient, family, and community. To serve as a moral agent in identifying and helping to resolve ethical and clinical concerns within the clinical setting, the nurse needs to be knowledgeable of and observe the American Nurses Association Code of Ethics (available at http://nursingworld.org/ethics/code/protected_nwcoe629.htm).
Caring practices	Collection of nursing activities that are responsive to the distinct patient and family preferences and that create a compassionate and therapeutic environment with the aim of promoting comfort and preventing suffering.
Collaboration	Interprofessional teamwork that promotes and encourages each person's contributions toward achieving optimal and realistic patient goals.
Systems thinking	Expertise that allows the nurse to appreciate the care environment from a perspective that recognizes the holistic interrelationship that exists within the health care system.
Response to diversity	Sensitivity to recognize, appreciate, and incorporate all inclusive differences into the provision of care.
Clinical inquiry	Ongoing process of questioning and evaluating practice and providing informed practice and innovation through research and experiential learning.
Facilitator of learning	Ability to facilitate formal and informal learning for patients and families, nursing staff, other members of the health care team, and the community.

From American Association of Critical-Care Nurses. (2003). *The AACN Synergy Model for Patient Care.* Retrieved from www.aacn.org/wd/certifications/content/synmodel.pcms.

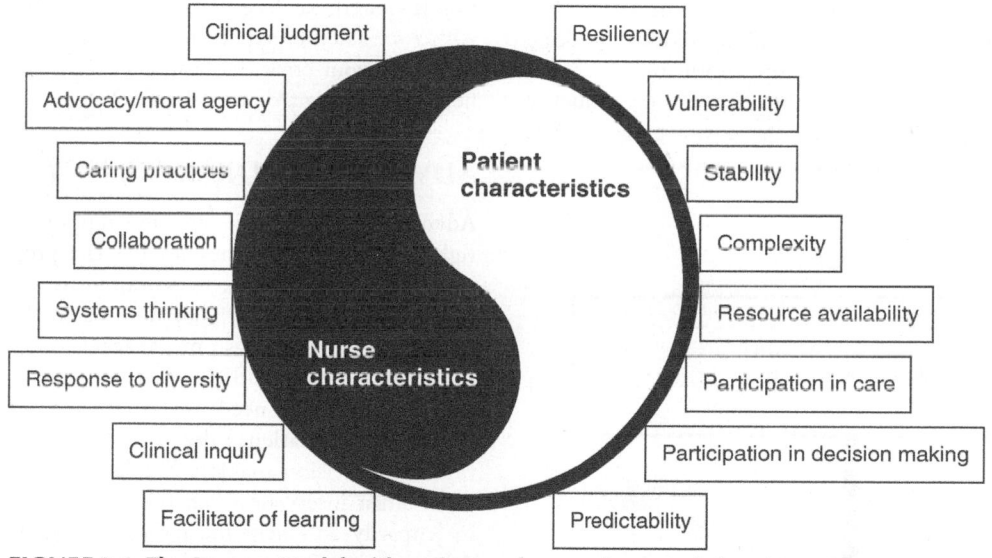

FIGURE 2-1 The Synergy Model with patient and nurse characteristics. (From Dennison, R. D. [2013]. *Pass CCRN!* [4th ed.]. St. Louis, MO: Elsevier.)

competencies: moral advocacy, caring practices, collaboration, systems thinking, response to diversity, clinical inquiry, and facilitation of learning. Although this model serves as the theoretical model for the PCCN® examination, you are not tested regarding knowledge of the Synergy Model or terminology; you are tested on application of the model.

CLINICAL JUDGMENT

Application of the Synergy Model in progressive care nursing requires varied levels of clinical judgment dependent on the needs and characteristics of the patient. Clinical judgment is based on an individual nurse's clinical reasoning, which includes decision making, critical thinking, and an overall grasp of the situation's context, along with nursing skills and knowledge acquired through the education, experience, and current evidence-based guidelines (AACN, 2012b). Clinical knowledge and skills by system will be explored in Chapters 3 to 11. The descriptions of each level of nursing expertise range from competent to expert (levels 1-5) based on the nurse's clinical judgment competency and are outlined in the nurse characteristics of the Synergy Model.

Decision Making

Clinical decision making involves a number of steps by which information is assimilated, integrated, weighed, and valued to arrive at the selection of a course of action from a number of possible alternatives. The decision-making process includes several steps. First, collect information, and then identify the problem. After the problem is identified, and the next step is to brainstorm the possible solutions or actions. Each solution or action then needs to be analyzed for all possible consequences. The best possible solution or action is implemented and, finally, the results are evaluated.

2.1   Learning Activity

List the six steps of the decision-making process.

1. _____
2. _____
3. _____
4. _____
5. _____
6. _____

Answers to this activity can be found in the Answer Key.

Critical Thinking, Clinical Reasoning, and Clinical Judgment

There is a relationship between critical thinking, clinical reasoning, and clinical judgment (Figure 2-2). The process of critical thinking and clinical reasoning influences clinical judgment and patient outcomes (Alfaro-LeFevre, 2013). Critical thinking is a well-organized process that requires information retrieved to be validated, including any assumptions that may influence the decisions. Careful reflection on the entire process while evaluating the effectiveness of necessary actions should be done.

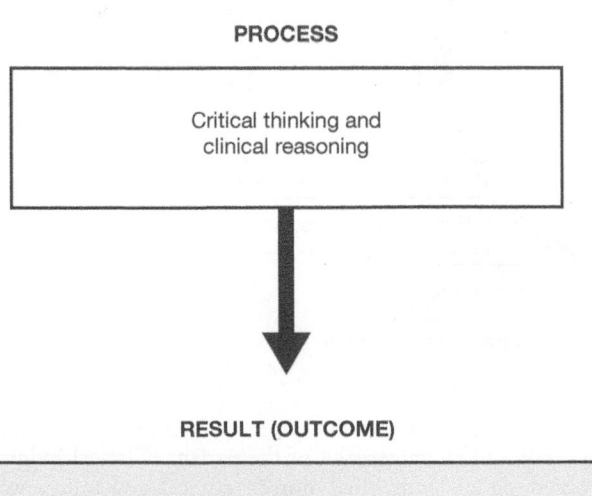

FIGURE 2-2 Relationship between clinical judgment, clinical reasoning, and critical thinking. (From Alfaro-LeFevre, R. [2013]. *Critical thinking, clinical reasoning, and clinical judgment: A practical approach* [5th ed.]. St Louis, MO: Saunders.)

Clinical reasoning is the use of clinically specific data regarding specific populations or disease processes and making evaluations regarding their meaning (Braude, 2012). Astute critical thinking and clinical reasoning lead to sound clinical judgment to guide clinical decisions. Clinical judgment is defined as the development of opinions in the clinical practice setting, based on experience and knowledge, to guide the decisions made regarding the care of the patient.

Alfaro-LeFevre (2013) identified nine key questions of clinical judgment. There is a need to figure out what outcomes are expected in the patient, family, or group when the plan of care is terminated. Careful analysis and reflection determine what problems or issues must be addressed to achieve these outcomes. Further reflection needs to assess what the circumstances are and what knowledge is required. Evaluating the potential hazards, clinical judgment also involves knowing the safety margin, how much room there is for error, and the available resources and timeframe. Additionally, clinical judgment must consider all necessary perspectives and be aware of what influenced the thinking process.

Critical thinking can be enhanced by several strategies. Develop good inquiry skills and an inquisitive nature. Anticipate the questions others might ask. Ask the "W" questions such as "why?", "what else?", and "what if?". Evaluate data retrieved by paraphrasing information, comparing and contrasting data, and reorganizing the information. Look for flaws in thinking and ask others to look for flaws as well. Revisit the information and repeat the processes periodically. Most importantly, to improve critical thinking, reframe the philosophic way information is viewed. Replace the phrases *I don't know* and *I'm not sure* with *I need to find out.* Turn errors into learning opportunities and share your errors with others because they are valuable to help others learn (Alfaro-LeFevre, 2013).

ADVOCACY/MORAL AGENCY

Advocacy refers to respecting and supporting the basic values, rights, and beliefs of the patient. The progressive care nurse must become confident in working on another's behalf and representing the concerns of the patient, family, and nursing staff as well as serving as a moral agent in identifying and helping resolve ethical and clinical concerns in practice (AACN, 2012b). The nurse needs to respect and support the right of the patient or patient's designated surrogate to autonomous informed decision making. While caring for the patient, the nurse must intervene when the best interest of the patient is in jeopardy and help the patient obtain the necessary care. Advocacy requires the nurse to render support and respect the values, beliefs, and rights of the patient even when they do not align with the nurse's own personal values. In order to help the patient or surrogate make decisions, the nurse must provide support and education. The nurse represents the patient in accordance with the patient's choices, intercedes for patients who cannot speak for themselves in situations that require immediate action, and supports the decisions of the patient or surrogate. The nurse is required to transfer care to an equally qualified nurse if this cannot be done due to personal beliefs. The nurse monitors and safeguards the quality of care provided and acts as a liaison between the patient, family, and health care professionals (Dennison, 2013).

Moral agency is the ability to serve as a moral agent in identifying and resolving ethical and clinical concerns (Curley, 2012) and to be accountable for actions. To be a moral agent requires an understanding of ethics. Ethics is a system of valued behaviors and beliefs that govern proper conduct to ensure the protection of an individual's rights, which involves judgments that help to differentiate right from wrong or indicate how things ought to be (Guido, 2010). Values are personal beliefs about the truth and worth of thoughts, objects, and behaviors. Accountability refers to the answerability or responsibility for personal and public ethical behaviors. Personal accountability is to oneself or the patient. Public accountability is to the employer, community, and society.

Ethics

Deontology provides the theoretical basis for ethical progressive care nursing practice and ethical decisions. Deontology, the duty-based ethic theory associated with Immanuel Kant, guides the practice of health care providers to believe that they have a duty to care for patients. Actions are right or wrong based on a set of morals or rules (Guido, 2010). Deontology emphasizes duty or obligation to another person and is the only acceptable ethical theory for decision making in health care. Teleologic ethics is a theory of morality that derives duty or moral obligation from what is good or desirable as an end to be achieved. It focuses on positive outcome results. Also known as consequentialist ethics, it is opposed to deontological ethics, which holds that the basic standards for an action's being morally right are independent of the good or evil generated. The theory of utilitarianism is the belief that actions are morally evaluated on how they facilitate or promote happiness or well-being, producing the greatest good for the greatest number (Guido, 2010). Progressive care nurses intervene daily with patients to bring about desired outcomes; therefore, this theory has an effect on nursing. Ethical egoism takes the position that moral agents ought to do what is in their own self-interest and has no place in clinical care. Natural law is a system of law that is purportedly determined in the accord of human nature and refers to the use of reason to analyze both social and personal human nature and deduce binding rules of moral behavior from it. Social contract theory is the view that a person's moral and/or political obligations are dependent on a contract or agreement among them to form the society in which they live.

The ethical principles of autonomy, beneficence, nonmaleficence, veracity, and justice guide behaviors and actions of the progressive health care team's application of the Synergy Model in clinical practice. A competent adult patient has the right to patient autonomy and self-determination regarding health care decisions. Individuals have an obligation to respect and support a person's right to make his or her own informed decisions. Paternalism occurs when health care providers make decisions for the patient based on the rationale that it is in the patient's best interest. The practice of paternalism denies the patient the autonomy to make his or her own decisions and should be avoided unless the rights of one person interfere with another individual's rights, health, or well-being, or there is a high probability that a person may injure himself or herself or others (e.g., smoking).

2.2 Learning Activity

Match the ethical approach to the statement that best describes a "right" decision using the approach.

__ 1. Utilitarianism
__ 2. Egoism
__ 3. Deontology
__ 4. Paternalism
__ 5. Social contract
__ 6. Natural law
__ 7. Teleology

a. When it results in the most good for the most people
b. When it results in a positive outcome
c. When it is the best thing in the opinion of the decision maker
d. When it provides significant benefit to the decision maker
e. When it is in accordance with human nature
f. When it is inherently right morally
g. When some rights must be lost for the greater good of society

Answers to this activity can be found in the Answer Key.

The principle of beneficence refers to an individual's obligation to do "good" and is a source of common ethical conflicts. Health care providers face the dilemma between perceived obligations to do good and obligations to respect the patient's autonomy. Differences in opinion occur between health care providers, patients, and health care surrogates on what is best for the patient, who should make the decision, and long-term or short-term benefits (Guido, 2010).

The principle of nonmaleficence is an individual's obligation to do no intentional or unintentional harm. A large component of this principle is that the health care provider is responsible to protect those unable to protect themselves including the mentally incompetent patient, nonresponsive patient, and children. This principle is not unconditional; sometimes it is necessary to cause harm to enact a cure or improvement in a patient's condition (i.e., surgery).

The principle of veracity is an individual's obligation to tell the truth and to not intentionally deceive or mislead a patient or family. This principle is not absolute. Consider cultural beliefs because in some cultures the principle conflicts with held values. Conflicts related to veracity can also occur when harm may occur when telling the truth (e.g., attempted suicide when given a certain diagnosis).

The principle of justice is an individual's obligation to treat everyone fairly. People deserve respect and to be treated fairly and equally regardless of race, sex, marital status, medical diagnosis, social standing, economic level, or religious belief. On a broader scale, the principle of justice also supports social health policy such as resource allocation and health care access. The principle of justice is examined when trying to determine things like the distribution of scarce organs, availability and allocation of critical care/progressive care beds and clinical staff, cost-benefit ratio of treatments, limiting access to expensive treatments, and futility of care versus patient autonomy. The allocation decisions are categorized as macro and micro events. The macro category is handled by public health policy, whereas the micro category addresses events such as wartime triage, critical bed triage, and clinical staff assignment (Dennison, 2013).

Confidentiality is an individual's responsibility to respect privileged information. Access to patient information is limited to those individuals with a "need to know." Patients have the right to access their own records. A nurse should be available to provide explanations to questions the patient may ask regarding his or her health records. Anyone else wishing access to patient data must have the patient's permission. The status and even the known presence of an individual in the health care setting are limited to those people whom the patient has identified.

The implementation of computerized patient records has created new challenges to keeping patient data safe and secure. Strategies to meet this challenge include keeping passwords secret, logging off when needing to leave the computer terminal unattended, ensuring screen view protection when looking at patient data, and avoiding viewing things that are not relevant to the care you render.

2.3   Learning Activity

Match the situation with the ethical concept demonstrated.

___ 1. Veracity
___ 2. Confidentiality
___ 3. Autonomy
___ 4. Nonmaleficence
___ 5. Fidelity
___ 6. Justice
___ 7. Advocacy

a. The new surgical resident has made three attempts to place a central venous catheter in an elderly patient. The nurse insists that no more attempts be made until the attending physician is present.

b. The nurse makes a medical error but the patient suffers no harm. She reports the error and completes an incident report.

c. The patient has decided that he does not want to be intubated again. You ensure that his wishes are recorded and honored.

d. The nurse explains to the patient that care will still be provided despite the fact that he has no health insurance.

e. The nurse's next-door neighbor is in the hospital. She visits him, but she does not read his chart.

f. The nurse begins on time, takes only the allotted time for lunch, and leaves after completion of work and report.

g. The confused patient keeps reaching for and pulling on his central line. The nurse applies soft restraints to prevent self-injury.

Answers to this activity can be found in the Answer Key.

Moral Distress

Nurses have reported that a major stressor in the profession is moral distress. Moral distress occurs when one knows the right thing to do but cannot do the right thing due to internal and external obstacles. Moral distress contributes to nurses' dissatisfaction, resulting in burnout and actual loss of nurses to the profession (AACN, 2012c). A strategy called the Four As (i.e., Ask, Affirm, Assess, Act) provides nurses with steps to confront and rise above moral distress (Epstein & Delgado, 2010). Step one, Ask, determines whether the nurse is experiencing moral distress. Nurses need to evaluate whether they are feeling angry, resentful, or frustrated by reflection and paying attention to "why" statements. Suffering from physical symptoms such as a change in weight, sleep patterns, and depression can also be an expression of moral distress. Step two, Affirm, actually acknowledges the distress. During this step, the nurse affirms the professional obligation to act as described in the ANA Code of Ethics for Nurses. Step three, Assess, identifies the sources and severity of the moral distress. During this time, the nurse also assesses the readiness to act by analyzing the risks and benefits. Step four, Act, prepares the nurse to personally and professionally act. The nurse takes action based on self-exploration regarding obligations, responsibilities, and risks. At that time, the nurse needs to anticipate setbacks, then manage them and seek support with other professionals suffering distress over the same or similar issues (Epstein & Delgado, 2010).

Common Ethical Distinctions

Four common distinctions used in clinical ethics discussions are active versus passive means to an end, ordinary versus extraordinary means, killing versus letting die, and withholding versus withdrawing. According to Burke, Evans, and Jarvik (2014), it is important to determine whether these group distinctions are logically valid, morally relevant, and morally justifiable. The validity of active versus passive means to an end, often associated with euthanasia, is questioned because even the decision involves active behaviors (e.g., meeting to discuss options). This distinction involves serious moral issues and is not recommended for use in clinical ethics assessments. In the distinction of ordinary versus extraordinary means, attempts are made to identify interventions related to a standard of practice. Practice standards are a reflection of what is done, not necessarily what should or should not be done based on scientific evidence. The main question is, however, should a patient be required to consent to standard means of extending life even if grounded in evidence? This distinction is not recommended as part of a clinical ethics assessment unless the patient adheres to a religious belief that prohibits a specific intervention. In the distinction of killing versus letting die, *killing* is defined as a deliberate, active process such as giving a lethal injection. *Letting die* refers to a more passive process of allowing the disease process to take its course. No one has a moral obligation to rescue a person if the attempt would not prolong life or would put the person attempting the rescue at risk for harm. The killing versus letting die distinction appears to be valid and morally relevant but creates serious ethical dilemmas, especially related to assisted suicide. In the final distinction to be considered, withholding versus withdrawing, logical validity is questionable because there are few instances in which the distinction is clear, leaving no legal basis for the distinction. There is also no clear distinction in terms of moral relevance. For example, is it more justifiable to not intubate a patient than it is to extubate a patient when the outcome may be similar in both situations? Despite the lack of logical validity and moral relevance, this distinction is commonly applied in clinical ethics (Jonson, Siegler & Winslade, 2010).

Informed Consent and Patient Self-Determination

There is a professional and legal duty to provide needed information to a patient so that an informed decision about treatment can be made. The right to treat a patient is based on a contractual relationship based on mutual consent (Guido, 2010). An informed consent includes an explanation of the treatment or procedure, the name of the person and assistants performing the procedure, and the significant risks. In addition, alternative therapies including no treatment and the right to refuse treatment without consequences of rendering alternative care are required to be discussed. Patients may refuse treatment at any time prior to or during therapy. Exceptions to patient informed consent include patient-initiated waiver, prior established knowledge for repeat procedures, and implied consent during medical situations.

Physicians or independent licensed practitioners have full accountability for obtaining informed consent. The nurse's role in obtaining informed consent varies with the situation, institution, and state law. Nurses should explain all nursing care procedures to patients and families. If a patient refuses the procedure or care, this must be honored. In some cases, a physician may delegate the obtaining of informed consent to nurses, but due to liability, most institutions do not recommend this practice. If done, the nurse must ensure that all aspects of an informed consent are disclosed. Nurses usually witness the patient signature, but if the nurse has knowledge that an already signed consent does not meet the criteria for informed consent or the patient revokes the consent, the nursing supervisor and physician must be notified.

Even if a patient withholds consent, law enforcement may request blood sampling. Five conditions must be met for law enforcement to request blood sampling when the patient withholds consent. These conditions must be documented in the medical record. The five conditions to be met include:

- Suspect must be under arrest.
- Blood sample will produce evidence.
- Delay of blood sampling would lead to destruction of evidence.
- Blood test needs to be reasonable and not medically contraindicated.
- Blood sample needs to be performed in a logical manner.

A blanket consent form is usually required before admission and covers routine and customary care. A specific consent form contains the following elements:

- Signature of competent patient or legally authorized representative
  - Signature cannot be coerced
  - Patient cannot be impaired because of medications
- Name and description of procedure in lay language
- Descriptions of risks and alternatives to treatment
- Description of probable consequences of proposed procedure
- Signatures of witnesses attesting that the patient signed the form

Informed consent forms are also used in human research. Institutional review boards must approve protocols for the protection of human participants. Special precautions are in place for vulnerable populations such as minors, mentally disabled persons, students, and prisoners. A research consent form must include the purpose of research, routine medical care and experimental procedures, alternative treatment, foreseeable risks, benefits, voluntary participation, confidentiality, explanation of any compensation, and right to withdraw. Language used in the consent needs to be easy to understand and should omit any reference to the researcher's lack of liability for patient outcomes. A disclosure statement about any additional costs and notification of findings to participants is also recommended.

Advance Directives

The Patient Self-Determination Act of 1990 mandated patient education about advance directives and provides assistance in executing them. An advance directive is a document in which a patient gives directions or identifies a designee to make medical decisions if mental capacity to do so is lost. A durable power of attorney for health care allows competent adults to designate someone to make health care decisions for them if they cannot. *Living will* is a generic term for an advance directive. Some states do not recognize living wills; therefore, they are not binding for medical practitioners and do not protect them from criminal or civil liability.

Natural death acts have been enacted by several states to protect practitioners from civil and criminal liability while ensuring patients' wishes are followed. A legally recognized living will may be developed by a competent adult (age 18 or older), but it must be witnessed by two persons. In some states, restrictions are placed on who can witness. This legal living will becomes effective only when the person becomes qualified by having a terminal illness or by having an irreversible condition with loss of decision-making capacity. Two physicians must certify that procedures or treatments will not prevent death but merely prolong it. This document does not apply to medications and therapies given to prevent suffering and provide comfort. A more detailed medical directive, allowed in some states, may list a variety of treatments and procedures the patient wants.

Do-not-resuscitate (DNR) orders are institutional-based policies that allow patients to direct physicians to not resuscitate in the event of cardiopulmonary arrest. Some states have out-of-hospital DNR laws that allow an individual to request not to be resuscitated by emergency personnel, which remain in effect for outpatient treatment and emergency department care. DNR directives may not be acceptable in some states during surgery. If state law allows DNRs during surgery, clarification of the decision needs to be clearly documented in the medical record before surgery.

Declaration of Death

Confusion and controversy over the term *brain death* and the relation of such death to organ donation persist despite guidelines of the World Medical Association Declaration of Death and the President's Commission for the Study of Ethical Problems in Medicine and in Biomedical and Behavioral Research. Determination of death by the cardiopulmonary criteria is recognized in all states. When the physician determines the patient has experienced an irreversible cessation of cardiopulmonary function, patient death is declared. Consent of family or surrogate is not required. Determination of brain death requires family or surrogate consent and a request for a second opinion is an option. Procedural guidelines for the declaration of death include a neurologic evaluation, an obligation to declare death (i.e., cardiopulmonary or brain death criteria), and immediate cessation of treatment unless the patient is pregnant. Also, efforts must be made to save the fetus or organs that are to be donated per the Uniform Anatomical Gift Act (UAGA). In organ donation cases, the declaration of death should not be by health care professionals who are members of the organ transplant team or the patient's family, or who have malpractice charges pending against them related to the case or other special interests.

Organ Donation

The need for organs far surpasses resources available, and initiatives are in place to increase tissue and organ availability (i.e., license designation). A study by Exley, White, and Martin (2002) indicated the following characteristics influenced the likelihood of families to make the decision to donate tissues and organs:

- Anglo-American ethnicity
- Any religious affiliation
- Discussion of donation initiated by family, physician, or a member of an organ procurement team
- Death caused by gunshot or suicide
- Timing of request: before or during declaration of death process
- Presence of signed donor card

Organ donation includes both tissue and living organs. Donors may be alive (e.g., bone marrow) or deceased (e.g., cornea). Due to increased risks to donors' lives, organ donation by living donors provides special concerns (Benner, 2002). In brain death, the heart may still be beating but respiratory function is maintained by mechanical ventilation. In non-heart-beating donors, organs are procured immediately after cessation of cardiopulmonary function.

Emergency Medical Treatment and Labor Act

The Emergency Medical Treatment and Labor Act (EMTALA) was enacted in 1986 to require hospitals participating in Medicare to screen and stabilize patients or to provide protected transfers for medical reasons (Centers for Medicare and Medicaid Services, 2004; Frank, 2011). This prevented institutions from refusing care for any reason. Failure to comply resulted in large fines or loss of funding from Medicare. In some cases, EMTALA has had a negative impact on organ donation where minutes could make a difference. Revisions to the UAGA were implemented in 2006 to facilitate organ donations and permit deviation from the EMTALA regulations. The UAGA provides clarity and enhances the rights of individuals to donate gifts.

Ethical Dilemmas

An ethical dilemma is a situation that requires a choice between two or more equally undesirable alternatives. Curtin (1982)

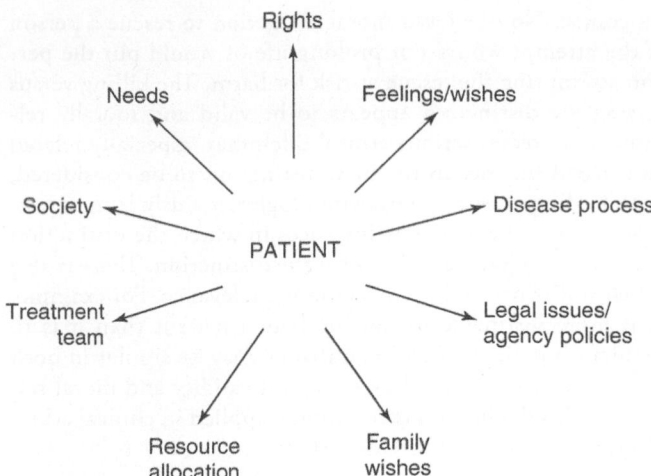

FIGURE 2-3 Factors affecting ethical issues and ethical decision making in nursing. (From Kinney, M. et al. [1998]. *AACN's clinical reference for critical care nursing* [4th ed.]. St Louis, MO: Mosby.)

described an ethical dilemma as being a problem that cannot be solved using only empirical data, one that is so perplexing it is difficult to decide what facts and data should be used to make the decision, and there are far-reaching effects to the decision. Some common ethical dilemmas faced by progressive care nurses include conflicts related to patient rights of autonomy versus paternalism, resource allocations, and personal versus professional beliefs.

The common conflicts involving patient autonomy versus paternalism include issues with informed consent, technology versus quality of life, resuscitation versus DNR, and behavior control such as misuse of restraints and sedation to suppress freedom in contrast to the obligations to maintain societal order.

Conflicts involving the principles of justice versus utilitarianism are demonstrated with resource allocation issues such as triage decisions; quality-of-life decisions; fiscal restraints such as lack of insurance or inability to pay for care; and organ transplant decisions that involve the rights of donors, recipients, families, and society. Issues such as the potential for elitism when choosing the transplant recipient, utilizations of health care resources due to tremendous cost of transplantation, and decisions on the designation of death and when an organ can be removed are common dilemmas.

A nurse may deal with personal conflicts related to his or her professional role. Veracity is an individual's obligation to tell the truth and not deceive or mislead. Fidelity is an obligation to be loyal to agreements and responsibilities that an individual has accepted. Fidelity is one of the key elements of accountability. Conflicts related to fidelity may occur between fidelity to patients and fidelity to employer, government, or society. Dilemmas occur with these principles when faced with withholding therapy and advocating for the patient's right to die whether by positive (assisted suicide) or negative (DNRs) euthanasia. In addition, conflicts occur that are related to professional integrity and personal values, morals, and beliefs such as abortion or domestic violence. Many patient factors affect ethical issues and decision making (Figure 2-3).

General Legal Issues

Each state writes statutory laws on the scope of nursing practice. The purpose of State Nurse Practice Acts is to protect the public. The Board of Nursing governs nursing practice through regulations or administrative law. The Scope of Practice sets a standard and guides acceptable nursing practice, roles, and responsibilities in each state. Nurses are expected to practice within their defined scope and follow the Nurse Practice Act and the American Nurses Association (ANA) Ethical Code for Nurses (http://www.nursingworld.org/mainmenucategories/ethicsstandards/codeofethicsfornurses), which outline the nurse's responsibility to the employer, and to society.

The expanded roles for nurses beyond the general nursing scope of practice are termed *advanced practice* and are also governed by the state. The advanced practice roles include nurse practitioner (NP), clinical nurse specialist (CNS), certified nurse midwife (CNM), and certified registered nurse anesthetist (CRNA). These roles require additional graduate education (master's or doctorate degrees) and clinical practice hours beyond the basic nurse's education. The general title of advanced practice registered nurse (APRN) has been assigned to these four roles by a regulation in 2008 called the Consensus Model (Consensus Work Group and the National Council of State Boards, 2008).

Standards of Care

An established measure of quality, quantity, or value for performance and clinical expertise and excellence determines a standard of care. Standards are set based on usual and customary practice and include standards of care, standards of practice, policies, procedures, and performance criteria to establish acceptable performance. Several professional organizations have relevant standards (Box 2-1) applicable to progressive care nursing.

Certification is a process by which a nongovernmental agency (e.g., American Association of Critical-Care Nurses) validates an individual nurse's qualification and knowledge for practice in a defined functional or clinical area of nursing; this validation is based on predetermined standards of practice (AACN, 2010). These examinations (Table 2-3) are developed and governed by the AACN Certification Corporation, which is certified by the National Commission for Certifying Agencies, the accreditation arm of the National Organization for Competency Assurance. The purpose of certification is to promote consumer protection and higher standards of practice. Licensure indicates a minimum level of knowledge, whereas certification indicates an expert level of knowledge. The certified nurse may be held to a higher standard of practice in the specialty. Certification validates the nurse's knowledge and experience in a specialty area and is an assurance of continued competence because renewal of certification occurs every 3 to 5 years. Competence is defined as "the application of knowledge and the interpersonal, decision-making, and psychomotor skills expected for the nurse's practice role, within the context of public health, welfare, and safety" (National Council of State Boards of Nursing, 1996, page 5). Continued competence refers to the maintenance of adequate knowledge and skills for safe ongoing practice that occurs after the initial demonstration of competence (National Council of State Boards of Nursing, 1996).

PROFESSIONAL LIABILITY

Malpractice is a specific type of negligence that takes into account the status of the caregiver, as well as the standard

---

BOX 2-1

Relevant Organizational Standards for Progressive Care Nursing

- AACN Scope and Standards for Acute and Critical Care Nursing Practice (Bell, 2008)
- ANA Standards: Generic and Specialty
- Scope and Standards of Professional Performance for the Acute and Critical Care Clinical Nurse Specialist (Bell, 2002)
- Scope and Standards of Practice for the Acute Care Nurse Practitioner (Bell, 2006)
- National Facility Standards: Joint Commission, National Committee for Quality Assurance (NCQA), Institute for Healthcare Improvement (IHI), and the National Quality Forum (NQF)
- Community and regional standards
- Hospital and medical center standards
- Unit practice standards, policies, and protocols (e.g., insulin protocols)
- Other professional nursing and interdisciplinary specialty organizations (American Heart Association [AHA], Society of Critical Care Medicine, and Association of Perioperative Registered Nurses)

TABLE 2-3 **Acute and Critical Care Specialty Certifications Awarded by the AACN Certification Corporation**

Credential	Nursing Specialty
PCCN	Certification process for nurses practicing in progressive care
CCRN	Certification process for critical care nurses practicing with neonatal, pediatric, or adult populations
CCNS	Advanced practice certification for clinical nurse specialists who practice in acute, progressive, and critical care
ACNP	Advanced practice certification for acute care nurse practitioners who practice in acute, progressive, and critical care

---

of care. Professional negligence is when failure to do what a reasonable, prudent nurse would do under similar circumstances (or doing something that a reasonable, prudent professional would not do under similar circumstances) results in injury to another person. Malpractice includes professional misconduct, improper discharge of duties, failure to meet the standard of care, and failure to foresee consequences that a professional person who has the necessary skills and education would see.

The most common types of malpractice or negligence in progressive care settings include medication errors, failure to prevent patient falls, failure to assess change in patient status, and failure to notify the primary care provider of changes in patient status. The four elements of duty, breach of duty, causation,

TABLE 2-4	**Professional Malpractice and Negligence**
Elements	**Definition**
Duty	The nurse has a duty to provide care and follow an acceptable standard of care.
Breach of duty	Failure by nurse to do what a reasonable, prudent nurse would do in the same or similar situation. Failure to perform within a given standard of care. The standard defines the nurse's duty to the patient.
Causation	Failure to meet standard of care must have caused injury to patient.
Damages	Proof of actual loss, damage, pain, or suffering caused by the nurse's conduct.

TABLE 2-5	**Five Rights of Delegation and Examples**
Right	**Description**
Right task	RN ensures that the task that is to be delegated is appropriate for that specific patient. Example: delegating suctioning for a patient to a licensed practical nurse is appropriate, but if the patient suffers from intracranial hypertension and becomes hypotensive during the treatment, it would not be appropriate.
Right circumstances	RN ensures the setting is appropriate and that resources are available for successful completion of the delegated task. Example: transporting a patient to radiology with a monitor and a staff member with the authority and competency to initiate Advanced Cardiac Life Support (ACLS).
Right person	RN delegates the right task to the right person to be performed on the right patient. Example: UAP to obtain routine ordered AC & HS blood glucose levels on a patient with diabetes and notify RN if value > 180 mg/dl.
Right direction	RN must provide clear explanations of tasks and expected outcomes. Example: Obtain vital signs, TPR, & BP every 4 hours on postoperative patients and record.
Right supervision	RN appropriately monitors, evaluates, and intervenes as needed. RN sets parameters and provides feedback to designee. Example: Administers insulin to a patient based on blood glucose before lunch and informs designee to recheck blood glucose 2 hours after lunch.

and damages must be established to bring suit of professional malpractice and negligence (Table 2-4).

Good Samaritan Laws

Good Samaritan Laws were enacted to allow health care personnel and citizens trained in first aid to deliver needed emergency care without fear of incurring criminal and civil liability. Most of these laws require that care be given in good faith and that it be gratuitous, but the laws do vary from state to state; therefore, nurses should be familiar with the state law where care was rendered. There is no legal duty to render care to strangers in distress.

Delegation and Supervision

Delegation refers to sharing the activities you are accountable and responsible for with other staff who have the proper authority, knowledge, and skill to accomplish the work. Direct delegation is the result of the RN actively deciding what to delegate. Indirect delegation occurs when the decision to delegate is the result of organizational protocols that designate a specific task as appropriate for another to perform. It is important to remember that the nurse retains accountability for the delegation; therefore, the "five rights" of delegation should be followed (Table 2-5). Base the delegation of nursing tasks on appropriate assessment, planning, implementation, and evaluation. Review the Joint Statement on Delegation by the American Nurses Association (ANA) and the National Council of State Boards of Nursing (NCSBN), which can be found on the website www.ncsbn.org/Delegation_joint_statement_NCSBN-ANA.pdf.

In the progressive care environment, delegation of care often occurs with unlicensed assistive personnel (UAP), licensed practical nurses (LPNs), and other professional nurses. Clearly define job descriptions and scope of practice for personnel in roles with various levels of expertise. Job descriptions for UAPs do not include responsibilities for which a license is required. Provide adequate training and consistent orientation, and a mechanism should be in place for regular evaluation. Additional

training and experience are required for nurses because of the many complex therapies needed by the vulnerable, acute, and complex patients in the progressive care environment. The nurse managers must ensure the policies and procedures concerning supervision and delegation are in place and consistent with the Nurse Practice Act. Assignment of care is guided by the available nurse competencies and the patient characteristics and care procedures required.

Staffing

Progressive care unit (PCU) nurses care for patients with high-acuity needs that require greater surveillance because they have the potential to become unstable. Staffing PCUs by matching the patient's needs with the competencies and experience of the PCU nurse is optimal care. Patient- and family-centered care requires the right caregiver be assigned to each patient and an institutional system that provides support to deliver optimal care, incorporating legal and

TABLE 2-6 Elements to Address Critical Staffing Shortages	
Elements	Rationale
Hospital staffing policies	Grounded in ethical principles and support the professional obligation of nurses to provide high-quality care.
Nurse participation	Organizational phases of staffing process from education-planning-evaluation and includes matching nurse competencies with patients' assessed needs.
Staffing evaluation process	Formal processes in place to evaluate the effect of staffing decisions on patient and system outcomes. This evaluation includes analysis of when patient needs and nurse competencies are mismatched and how often contingency plans are implemented.
Staffing and outcome data	Organization facilitates team members' use of staffing and outcomes data to develop more effective staffing models.
Support services	Organization provides support services at every level of activity to ensure nurses can optimally focus on the priorities and requirements of patient and family care.
Technology	Organization adopts technologies that increase the effectiveness of nursing care delivery. Nurses are engaged in the selection, adaptation, and evaluation of these technologies.

From Barden, L. ed. (2005). *AACN standards for establishing and sustaining healthy work environments: A journey to excellence.* Aliso Viejo, CA: American Association of Critical-Care Nurses.

regulatory considerations and measuring the outcomes of care. In Standard 4, adequate staffing is addressed in AACN's *Standards for Establishing and Sustaining Healthy Work Environments* (Barden, 2005). Recommendations (Table 2-6) call for six elements to be put in place to address critical staffing shortages.

Documentation

Regulatory agencies mandate some types of documentation of patient care. Laws regarding narcotics, controlled substances, and organ transplantation fall under the federal jurisdiction. There are also national voluntary requirements such as the Joint Commission requirements related to quality improvement activities. Documentation in relationship to minors and guardianship are state requirements. In some areas, community regulations may exist for things such as epidural medications and sedation. Hospitals, medical centers, and health maintenance organizations (HMOs) also have regulations on documentation.

Regardless of regulatory mandates, the purpose of nursing care documentation is to provide clear and concise communication between providers. Good documentation facilitates the planning and evaluation of care while demonstrating the use of the nursing process. The documentation shows the progress of the patient's treatment, changes in condition, and continuity of care as it records a patient's status, appearance, and behavior. The medical record may be used in litigation both to protect the patient and to reduce the risk of possible litigation for the health care professionals and institution.

CARING PRACTICES

Caring practices are nursing activities that are responsive to the uniqueness of the patient and family and that create a compassionate and therapeutic environment with the aim of promoting comfort and preventing suffering (AACN, 2012b). Caring practices relevant to progressive care nursing include issues related to death and dying, pain management, complementary therapies, rest, and family stress.

TABLE 2-7 Stages of Death and Dying	
Stage	The Patient May Say
Shock and disbelief	"I can't be dying; you're wrong"; "No, not me."
Denial	"Most people with this disease die but not me."
Anger	"Me? What have I done to deserve this?"
Bargaining	"If I do this…? Let me live until…"
Depression	"What's the use?"
Acceptance	"I'm ready to die."

From Kübler-Ross, E. (1969). *On death and dying.* New York: Macmillan.

Death and Dying

Dying is a psychophysiologic process that ultimately terminates in death for an individual and grieving for significant others. During this process each patient and family progress through defined stages of death and dying (Kübler-Ross, 1969) (Table 2-7).

It is necessary for progressive care nurses to develop a personal philosophy of death in order to deal effectively with dying patients and living families. A very important aspect of this is that the nurse must not eliminate hope. Hope is the expectation that a desire will be fulfilled and aids in the tolerance of pain and suffering throughout the dying process. Nursing interventions include encouraging the patient and family to discuss their fears and concerns. The nurse must listen attentively and provide a presence with compassion, along with comfort measures and analgesia. Assist the family as needed during this time. Allow the family to be with the patient and encourage participation in patient care. Reassure the family of the patient's comfort and the provision of analgesia. Provide information about the patient's status frequently. Encourage ventilation of anxiety, fears, and concerns. Ensure a private, comfortable area for the family and refer the family to other sources of support, such as the chaplain, the social worker, or a support group. When death is imminent, ensure that someone stays with the family.

Pain Management

Nurses are responsible to assess, evaluate, and manage pain. Pain is a subjective experience and is anything the patient says it is; it occurs whenever the patient says it does (McCaffery, 1968). Categories of pain include acute, chronic, and neuropathic. Acute pain follows an insult or injury and ends when healing occurs. An example of acute pain is postsurgical incision discomfort. Chronic pain lasts longer than the normal healing period. An example of chronic pain is low back pain. Neuropathic pain is a type of chronic pain caused by nerve damage. An example of neuropathic pain is diabetic neuropathy.

Patients are encouraged to report pain by using some type of pain scale: numerical, Wong-Baker FACES™, verbal, or graphic. McCaffery (2002) provided nurses with recommended guidelines for teaching a patient how to use a pain rating scale. Topics to explain include the purpose of the scale, increments of the scale, and what is meant by "pain." In addition, it is recommended to ask the patient to give an example of pain to practice using the scale and have the patient practice using the scale to rate the pain. Finally, the nurse is to assist the patient to set a goal for an acceptable level of pain.

The nurse evaluates signs and symptoms of pain by observing verbal cues, such as moaning and crying, and nonverbal cues, such as rubbing, splinting, and guarding. Facial expressions of grimacing and frowning indicate pain. Physiologic signs such as tachycardia, elevated blood pressure, and tachypnea may also signify the presence of pain, but it is important to remember that physiologic signs are not evident when the pain is of a chronic nature. The Behavioral Pain Scale (Table 2-8) assesses pain beyond the patient's self-report or if the patient is unable to self-report due to being ventilator dependent or sedated. The scale examines facial expressions, upper limb movement, and compliance with ventilation.

Pharmacologic agents used in the pain management of progressive care patients include opioids, nonsteroidal antiinflammatory agents (NSAIDs), and local anesthetics. The drugs are administered by several delivery methods: sustained release tablets and patches, orally, and intravenous continuous infusions and intermittent injections. Patient-controlled analgesia (PCA) usually consists of a continuous infusion with patient-controlled injection for breakthrough pain.

Nurses also provide nonpharmacologic pain control measures (Table 2-9). The application of heat or cold, relaxation techniques, and distraction such as music, television, reading, needlepoint, coloring, drawing, writing, and visitors are effective nursing interventions for pain. In addition, complementary therapies in conjunction with conventional therapies augment pain management by enhancing the patient's ability to cope, producing feelings of well-being, and decreasing tension in difficult situations. These therapies cause relaxation and decrease stress and anxiety. Many of these therapies augment pain relief by causing a release of endorphins; altering mood; reducing inflammation, edema, congestion, and muscle tension and spasm; improving circulation and ventilation; and improving the quantity and quality of sleep. They also help to communicate a physical presence through encouragement, support, or empathy.

2.4 Learning Activity

List eight complementary therapies that are helpful to patients with stress, anxiety, or pain.

a. _____
b. _____
c. _____
d. _____
e. _____
f. _____
g. _____
h. _____

Answers to this activity can be found in the Answer Key.

Rest

A common problem in hospitalized patients is sleep deprivation. Patients have minimal daily activity and spend long periods in bed in a supine position. Uncontrolled physical symptoms such as pain, discomfort, and dyspnea disturb rest. Many pharmacologic agents can cause agitation or wakefulness. Even with the sedatives, hypnotics, and analgesia that cause the appearance of sleep, it is unclear as to whether this "sleep" has the same restorative qualities as normal physiologic sleep. Frequent interruptions for assessments and treatments prevent both the quantity and quality of sleep. Also, there is little to no light variation within the 24-hour day.

Recommendations to improve sleep quality and to promote rest are to promote wakefulness during the day, to keep the patient up in a chair and ambulating as tolerated, and to use sedatives judiciously during waking hours. During the night, the noise and light should be decreased and staff must minimize disruptions and avoid awakening the patient (Holley, 2010; Matthews, 2011).

Noise Control

Noise can produce serious physical and psychological stress and may impair the healing process. The Environmental Protection Agency (1974) recommends that daytime noise levels in a

TABLE 2-8	Behavioral Pain Scale		
Item	**Description**		**Score**
Facial expression	Relaxed		1
	Partially tightened (e.g., brow lowering)		2
	Fully tightened (e.g., eyelid closing)		3
	Grimacing		4
Upper limbs	No movement		1
	Partially bent		2
	Fully bent with finger flexion		3
	Permanently retracted		4
Compliance with ventilation	Tolerating movement		1
	Coughing but tolerating		2
	Fighting ventilator		3
	Unable to control ventilation		4
Total Score			**3-12**

From Payen, J. F., Bru, O., Bosson, J. L., Lagrasta, A., Novel, E., Deschaux, I., et al. (2001). Assessing pain in critically ill sedated patients using a behavioral pain scale. *Critical Care Medicine, 29*(12), 2258-2263.

hospital not exceed 45 decibels (dB) and that nighttime levels not exceed 35 dB. In 2005, the average daytime noise level in hospitals was 72 dB and the average nighttime noise level was 60 dB. Hospital units need to be designed or upgraded with improved sound acoustics, decentralized nurses' stations, and single-patient rooms. Half of hospital sound peaks are directly related to human behavior with staff conversations being the most disturbing noise to patients.

Staff should be educated and encouraged to reduce volume of conversation and to close patient doors. Equipment carts, meal tray carts, and transport stretchers need to be maintained to prevent excess squeaking noises. The volume ring on equipment alarms needs to be lowered and activated alarms should be checked on immediately. Overhead pages should be eliminated in a hospital setting and phone ringers and beepers need to be placed on vibrate only. Television and music volume need to be kept low or individual headphones and ear plugs can be encouraged and provided as needed (Choiniere, 2010).

Family Support

Family consists of the individuals who are relatives or significant others with whom the patient shares an established relationship. It is important for the progressive care nurse to assess family availability, structure, and communication patterns; the role of the patient within the family, as well as the roles of the primary decision maker and family spokesperson; and any actual or potential conflicts within the family. The nurse determines the family perceptions and understanding of the current situation to display empathy, which comes as the result of a close identification and connection with another person (Dracup & Bryan-Brown, 1999). Determine whether the family has knowledge of the patient's condition and the progressive care environment and has past experience with similar health situations. Identifying the family's previous responses to crisis, their effective coping patterns, and their resources will help the nurse develop strategies to deal with family maintenance needs during this time. The nurse investigates family needs such as transportation, lodging, finances, and spirituality and encourages the family to maintain dietary, hygiene, sleep/rest, and medication regimens during their loved one's illness.

It is very stressful to observe a loved one in a life-threatening acute situation. Fear of death, pain, and discomfort of their loved one cause anxiety. Temporary or permanent role reversal of the patient and other members of the family may be frightening. Health care costs and actual or potential loss of income create a negative impact on financial situations. The technology, equipment, and required medical regimens can be emotionally overwhelming along with issues of family separation, role reversal, and financial burdens. Progressive care staff may observe a variety of emotions and behaviors due to these stresses, from mild anxiety and nervousness to severe dysfunction. Severe dysfunction may result in argumentativeness, aggression, intoxication, guilt, blame, and verbal or physical abuse directed toward the health care workers.

The most important family need is to have questions answered honestly and be assured the best care possible is rendered to their

TABLE 2-9	Complementary Pain Management Techniques
Technique	Description
Progressive muscle relaxation	Progressive tensing and relaxing of successive muscle groups.
Breathing techniques	Instruction, practice, and encouragement in the use of diaphragmatic breathing or pursed-lip breathing.
Meditation	Intentional concentration and repetition of a special word, phrase, or muscular activity.
Comeditation	Concentrates on certain sounds, images, or words of a script spoken in the rhythm of the patient's exhalations.
Guided imagery	Guiding the patient's thoughts to a self-identified concept of a relaxing location or situation through the use of specific words and suggestions.
Massage	Controlled touch to manipulate soft tissue by pressure exerted by the hands, fingers, thumbs, or special instrument.
Hypnosis	Suggestion to enable a person to experience the imaginary as real, allowing deep relaxation.
Biofeedback	Conscious mental effort to control involuntary body functions, such as blood pressure, heart rate, and respiratory rate triggered by a biofeedback instrument to alert the patient to the cues.
Therapeutic touch	Transfer of energy to help restore the balance of the energy field from the practitioner's hands.
Purposeful touch	Creating a safe, caring physical presence by a comforting, empathetic touch.
Music therapy	Use of simple, repetitive, low-pitched music of patient's preference to soothe and relax.
Aromatherapy	Use of essential oils extracted from flowers, leaves, stalks, fruits, and roots may be used in massage, baths, compresses, or inhalation.
Pet therapy	Visits by the patient's own pet or trained, approved pet-visitation animals.
Humor	Using appropriate words and images to elicit laughter after determining the type of humor the patient appreciates, depending on receptiveness and proper timing.
Acupuncture	Insertion of needles into specific areas of the body. May also use heat (moxibustion), pressure (acupressure), or electromagnetic energy to stimulate acupuncture points.

loved one. The patient's family needs to be given clear explanations of what is being done and why. Patients and their families need to see each other frequently and feel that the health care team cares about the patient and that there is some kind of hope. Speaking with the doctor and nurses daily; understanding the diagnosis, medical treatment, and prognosis; and being updated about changes in the patient's condition, including any transfer or discharge plans, are very important for the family (Leske, 1991).

The nursing staff needs to be available during family visitation to answer questions and provide explanations and information about the status of the patient. Introduce yourself and ask names and relationships of family members. Use touch therapeutically as indicated and allowed by the family members. Encourage family members to make notes regarding information that the physicians or other nurses have given or questions that they would like to ask during the next interaction with the other nurse or physician. Also, encourage the designation of one family member to phone or be phoned who will then communicate to the other family members. A brochure describing the unit, usual activities, visitation policies, and other useful information is often helpful.

Visiting times should be individualized based on the needs and response of the patient and the family. In a recent AACN practice alert, it is stated that "evidence shows that the unrestricted presence and participation of a support person can enhance patient and family satisfaction, because it improves the safety of care" (AACN, 2011). Previously cited concerns about unrestricted visiting hours resulting in physiologic stress, barriers to care provision, family exhaustion, and risk of infection have not been supported through research (AACN, 2011). Flexible visitation for the patient has decreased length of stays, reduced cardiovascular complications, and been found to decrease anxiety, confusion, and agitation while increasing quality, safety, and patient satisfaction (AACN, 2011). The benefits of flexible visitation to the family members includes improved communication, increased satisfaction, and decreased anxiety resulting in improved understanding of the patient situation and more opportunities for participation in care.

The progressive care nurse's role and responsibility in regards to family visitation has several components. The nurse may need to explain why visitation is interrupted or postponed by a procedure or crisis; or the nurse may need to warn the family about a patient's unusual behavior (e.g., confusion) and explain why their loved one is acting this way. The nurse should encourage family members to talk to and touch the patient, hold the patient's hand, and express their feelings and participate in care if they desire. The family needs to be given the opportunity to be involved in decision making. The nurse needs to identify, respect, and accommodate the cultural beliefs and rituals of the family.

2.5   Learning Activity

List five of the most important needs of families as identified by the classic work of Leske.

a. _____
b. _____
c. _____
d. _____
e. _____

Answers to this activity can be found in the Answer Key.

COLLABORATION

Collaboration is the process where the health care team works with others in a way that promotes and encourages each person's contributions toward achieving optimal and realistic patient and family goals. Collaboration teams involve intradisciplinary and interdisciplinary work with colleagues and the community (AACN, 2012b). To create synergy teams, establish a clear purpose and commit to a resolution. Effective teams create respectful working environments that are informal, comfortable, and relaxed, facilitating focused and shared group discussions.

Functioning teams listen to one another, handle conflict with open discussion, and reach decisions by consensus. The working dynamics of an effective team keep ideas and discussions flowing. Accomplishment of this task is dependent on clearly stated, accepted assignments and strong rotational leadership that imparts frequent, frank, and constructive criticism while giving dissenters the freedom to voice opinions. Freely expressed feelings open discussions. Frequent and ongoing self-regulation will keep the team focused on solutions (Yoder-Wise, 2011).

Collaborative practice occurs when members of the medical and nursing professions, together with members of other related health care disciplines such as respiratory therapists, physical therapists, social workers, clergy, and case managers, work together to ensure quality patient and family care. This type of partnered practice includes a sharing of the planning, decision making, problem solving, goal setting, and responsibility. The partners actively consult with each other and communicate openly and respectfully while coordinating care. Recognizing and accepting the separate and interrelated spheres of practice, everyone cooperates, resulting in quality health care delivery.

Essential elements of effective collaboration include administrative support to set high expectations for communication, trust, respect, understanding of roles, competence, shared responsibility and accountability, shared goal setting, and flexibility. The governance components of a collaborative practice include a practice committee with physician and nurse codirectors that has the autonomy for clinical decision making, uses integrated patient records, and conducts regularly scheduled multidisciplinary reviews of care.

Although collaboration is ideal and essential for quality care, blocks to collaboration exist in health care. These blocks stem mainly from nonassertive nurses, authoritative physicians, and traditional hierarchy. There may be ineffective, or lack of, communication between the professions and lack of administrative support, as well as systems issues that nursing leaders and team members have to work toward resolving, both inside and outside the profession.

Misunderstanding or lack of understanding regarding the role and practice of professional nursing is problematic. Nurses have their own license and do not practice under the license of the physician. Physicians cannot discipline or fire nurses employed by the hospital. Nursing is not medicine; these are two separate and interrelated professions. If an umbrella term is needed, it should be *health care*, which encompasses both medicine and nursing. Nurses have independent functions as well as dependent functions, and they can perform these independent functions without a physician's order. In fact, the term *physician's order* conveys an attitude of patriarchal obedience and should be changed to *physician prescription*. Nursing research has established a unique body of scientific knowledge. Nursing practice is controlled by nurses through State Nurse Practice Acts, not by physicians. The nursing profession must continue to work on self-identity and a clear understanding of our place in health care and demand respect for true collaboration to occur.

Progressive care nurses have a responsibility to establish a professional nursing environment. Assurance of competency, knowledge of and ability to articulate the unique role of nursing, and encouragement of professional development of nursing staff creates a professional nursing environment. Moving forward, nurses can then set strategies in place to begin to evaluate the current interdisciplinary relationships on the unit and establish a multidisciplinary critical care committee cochaired by a nurse and a physician. The committee should handle issues related to practice, communication, and improving the effectiveness or efficiency of clinical care. Disciplines have equal representation and decision-making authority. Multidisciplinary professional activities such as rounds, integrated patient records, orientation and education programs, quality and safety improvement initiatives, problem-solving task forces, and research will facilitate the development and continued practice of intraprofessional collaboration.

2.6 Learning Activity

List five of the essential elements of collaboration.

a. _____
b. _____
c. _____
d. _____
e. _____

Answers to this activity can be found in the Answer Key.

Communication

Communication skills are vital to quality clinical practice. Nurses utilize and must perfect all types of communication: oral, written, and nonverbal skills; symbolic gestures; visual images; and multimedia. Effective communication helps develop and maintain patient-nurse, family-nurse, nurse-nurse, and nurse-team relationships to provide a good work environment. Good communication requires a person to be clear as to what is to be communicated, to deliver the message succinctly, and to request feedback to verify the message has been clearly and correctly understood. Avoid the common pitfalls of communication: advice giving, defensiveness, patronizing, blaming and accusing others, giving false reassurance, and asking "why" questions (Yoder-Wise, 2011).

Leonard, Graham, and Bonacum (2004) developed a communication tool referred to as *SBAR* (i.e., Situation, Background, Assessment, Recommendation), that is an effective and efficient way to communicate important information. SBAR offers a simple way to help standardize communication and allows parties to have common expectations related to what is to be communicated and how the communication is structured.

S = Situation (a concise statement of the problem)
B = Background (pertinent and brief information related to the situation)

A = Assessment (analysis and considerations of options— what you found/think)
R = Recommendation (action requested/recommended— what you want)

SYSTEMS THINKING

Systems thinking is defined as the body of knowledge and tools that allow the nurse to appreciate the care environment and resources from a perspective that recognizes the holistic interrelationship that exists within and across health care systems. A system is a group of interdependent components that work together to achieve a common goal. Nursing is just one aspect to patient care; therefore, nurses must work together with other members of the health care team and understand the organizational structure of the institution. AACN is committed to fostering work and care environments that are "safe, healing, humane, and respectful of the rights, responsibilities, needs, and contributions of all people — including patients, their families, and nurses" (AACN, 2005, page 5) (Box 2-2).

Organizational Structures

Various types of organizational structures exist in health care. Traditionally, bureaucracy is most common, but the newer paradigms for health care recommend shared governance and self-governance. Bureaucracy is a formal, centralized, hierarchical structure where communication and decisions flow from top to bottom with limited employee input. The bureaucratic organization utilizes rules, policies, and procedures that ensure consistency and promote efficiency and productivity. Shared governance is an organizational structure with governance shared by staff and management. Authority, responsibility, and accountability are decided with input from both staff and administration. A shared governance structure is often referred to as a professional practice model and creates a desirable working environment; therefore it is an essential criterion for Magnet status designation.

Patient Care Delivery

Recommended guidelines for progressive care nursing include both patient-centered and family-centered care. In

---

BOX 2-2

AACN Standards for Establishing and Sustaining Healthy Work Environments

- Nurses must be as proficient in communication skills as they are in clinical skills.
- Nurses must be valued and committed partners in making policy, directing and evaluating clinical care, and leading organizational operations.
- Staffing must ensure the effective match between patient needs and nurse competencies.
- Nurses must be recognized and must recognize others for the value each brings to the work of the organization.
- Nurse leaders must fully embrace the imperative of a healthy work environment, authentically live it, and engage others in its achievement.

patient-centered care, the focus is meeting the needs of the patient to provide a seamless health care experience and to decrease fragmentation of care. Family-centered care allows the patient and family members to maintain their normal roles as much as possible, including communication between the interdisciplinary team and patient and family members. This model of delivery considers the nurse, patient, and family as partners in the care of the patient and the effect of the patient's illness on the family unit. Key components of patient-family–centered care are RN or case manager coordination, cross-trained staff, adequate ancillary personnel, and a team approach between licensed and unlicensed staff that brings care closer to the patient.

Everyone benefits with this model of care. The patients and families benefit from the need to interact with fewer health care providers along with improved coordination and quality of care, and this increases patient satisfaction. The hospital benefits by reducing management layers with the emphasis on shared governance and self-directed work teams. Society benefits from a reduction of health care costs.

Change Process

Change is one constant in health care organizations. Change can be a reactive process to adjustments that were not planned or an active process with intentional, predetermined mutual goals. Progressive care nursing requires nursing staff and leadership to be effective change agents. With knowledge of group dynamics and a supportive and perceptive nature about political issues, effective change agents utilize excellent communication and observational skills to bring about the change. These agents have the ability to establish trusting relationships and to identify facilitators and barriers. To effectively lead change, Kotter (1995) recommended development of a detailed plan that remains fluid and flexible. Effective change agents involve all stakeholders in a shared vision, create goals, and select an appropriate model to guide the process. The planned change determines the selection of one of the many models of planned change (Table 2-10).

2.7   Learning Activity

Describe a change model and how you might use it to make changes that you feel are needed on your unit.

_____

_____

_____

Answers to this activity can be found in the Answer Key.

RESPONSE TO DIVERSITY

Progressive care nurses need to have the sensitivity to recognize, appreciate, and incorporate differences into the provision of care. Diversity is defined as those differences that make each person unique. Diversity includes national origin, religion, age, gender, sexual orientation, race, ethnicity, education, socioeconomic status, and abilities/disabilities. Culture is the learned, shared, and transmitted values, beliefs, and practices of a particular group that guide thinking, actions, behaviors, interactions with others, emotional reactions to daily living, and one's world view.

TABLE 2-10   Selected Planned Change Models

Model	Planned Change
Lewin (1951) Model of Change	Status quo (diagnosis of problem) Unfreezing (develop the solution) Disequilibrium (overcome resistance) Moving (implement change) Refreezing (reestablishing balance) Equilibrium
Lippitt, Watson, and Westley (1958) Seven Phases of Planned Change	Aware of need for change Development of relationship between client system and change agent Definition of the change problem Establishment of change goals and exploration of options for achievement Implementation of the plan for change Acceptance and stabilization of the change Redefinition of the relationships of the change entities
Havelock (1973) Six Phases of Planned Change	Building a relationship Diagnosing the problem Acquiring relevant resources Choosing a solution Gaining acceptance Stabilizing the innovation and generating self-renewal
Rogers (1995) Diffusion of Innovation Model	Knowledge Persuasion Decision Implementation Confirmation
Prochaska (2000) Prochaska et al. (2001) Transtheoretical Model	Precontemplation: the individual is not thinking of change Contemplation: the individual is thinking of but not committed to change in the near future Preparation: the individual intends to change in the near future Action: the individual actively attempts to change Maintenance: the individual sustains the change over time
Kotter (1995) Process for Leading Change	Establish a sense of urgency Form a powerful guiding coalition Create a vision Communicate a vision Empower others to act on the vision Plan for and create short-term wins Consolidate improvements and produce still more change Institutionalize new approaches
Berwick (2003) From Description to Prescription	Find sound innovations Find and support innovators Invest in early adopters Make early adopter activity observable Trust and enable reinvention Create slack for change Lead by change

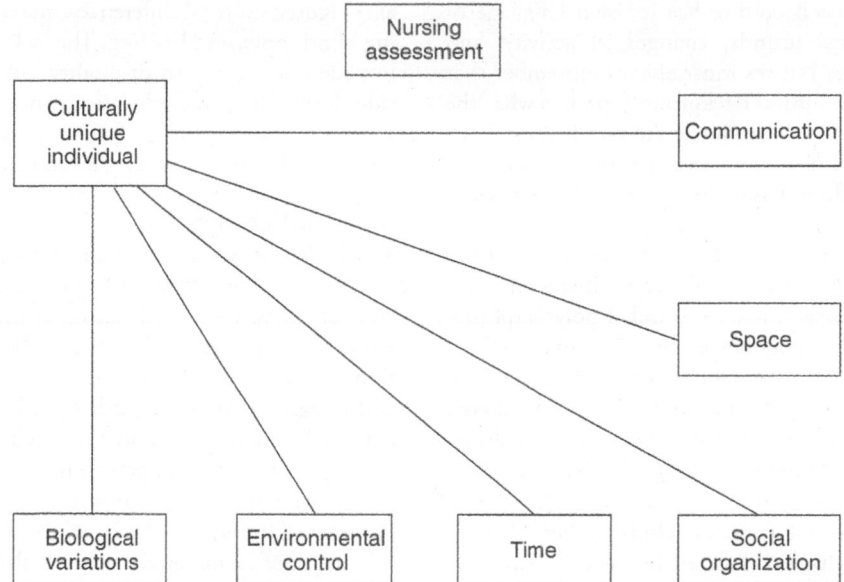

FIGURE 2-4 Application of cultural phenomena to nursing care and nursing practice. (From Giger, J., & Davidhizer, R. [2013]. *Transcultural nursing: Assessment and intervention* [6th ed.]. St. Louis, MO: Mosby.)

Subcultures also exist and are a recognizable segment of a larger cultural group that shares some characteristics of the larger group but with unique features of its own.

Cultural sensitivity is a learned skill in which a person has an awareness of and appreciation for another's cultural uniqueness. Cultural competence is a "set of congruent behaviors, attitudes, and policies that come together in a system, agency, or among professionals that enables effective work in cross-cultural situations" (HRSA, 2001). Culturally congruent nursing care employs cognitively based nursing techniques that incorporate an individual's cultural values, beliefs, and lifestyle. These techniques facilitate, assist, support, and/or enable an individual toward health and well-being or to face illness or death in culturally meaningful ways.

Of the developed countries in the world, the United States has the greatest increase in population and diversity of inhabitants. Immigration accounts for at least one-third of the increase. The percentage of whites of European origin, the dominant culture in the United States, will continue to decline, creating a more multicultural power base. The U.S. Census Bureau population projections indicate that non-Hispanic whites will no longer compose the majority of the population in 2042 (U.S. Census Bureau, 2011).

Nurses must be aware that issues of culture, race, gender, and socioeconomics strongly influence health status and utilization of the health care system. Culturally inappropriate care and inattention to cultural differences in care may negatively affect health outcomes.

A progressive care nurse must first become culturally sensitive by examination of personal cultural beliefs and values and respect of the unfamiliar. Acknowledge that cultural diversity exists and appreciate that cultural values are ingrained and difficult to change. The nurse must avoid stereotypes and appreciate the uniqueness of each patient. The nurse must modify care to include interventions consistent with the patient's culture. Recognize that the patient's health practices may be very different from yours, but that each cultural group has health practices that attempt to improve health and temper illness. Finally, and most importantly, realize that diversity within cultures exists. All people within a cultural group are not the same and do not respond to illness the same.

A vital part of the nursing assessment process is a cultural assessment. Many cultural phenomena (Figure 2-4) affect nursing care. These phenomena include individual uniqueness, communication patterns, orientation to time and space, social organizations, environmental controls, and biological variations. The nurse needs to encourage the patient to discuss cultural beliefs and practices, especially in relation to the origin and treatment of health/illness. The degree of acculturation — how the patient has acclimated to Western culture — should be determined. Important information to obtain includes English language skills, language spoken in the home, length of time in the country, and food preferences. Make efforts to respect and understand different communication styles and orientation to time and space. Provide privacy according to individual needs and be aware that in many cultures, it is extremely important for family members to be present during assessments. Identify the decision maker within the family because it may be someone other than the patient.

The progressive care nurse examines the cultural phenomena affecting nursing care (see Figure 2-4). The nurse should recognize that biological variations and responses to disease processes and treatments exist. Be aware of biological variations among cultures, such as body structure, skin/hair color, population-specific diseases, and psychological coping characteristics. Recognize that dietary and religious practices and cultural taboos have important implications related to nursing care. Patients' reactions to pain are sometimes culturally driven. Note cultural practices and modify care as necessary.

Pain is not purely a neurophysiologic response; cultural, social, and psychological denominators influence pain. Culture influences pain intensity, expression, tolerance, and expected responses from caretakers and determines a patient's attitude and beliefs about pain. Each culture has its own language of distress: facial expressions, sounds, changes in activity, and words to describe feelings. Nurses must always remember that regardless of the patient's cultural background, pain is what the patient says it is and it occurs when he or she says it does. Consider and treat all pain as "real" and treat compassionately. Be aware that patients who do not verbally express the presence of pain may not be pain-free.

Age, drug, gender, body size, and body composition affect individual responses to drugs. A variation in the DNA that is too common to be due merely to new mutation is called polymorphism. Factors that influence drug polymorphism vary among ethnic groups and can be categorized as environmental, genetic, and cultural; these do not include all the aspects that affect a patient's response to drugs but raise awareness regarding possible differences in response. Drug metabolism is genetically determined.

Race may also affect drug response; this is called *genetic polymorphism*. Environmental factors including diet, alcohol, smoking, malnutrition, vitamin deficiencies, stress, fever, and physiologic rhythms can affect drug absorption. Cultural factors include values, beliefs, compliance, family influence, and prior drug experience; patients may be taking herbal or homeopathic remedies that can alter response to drug absorption. Nurses must become familiar with the different effects drugs can have on patients of different ethnicity.

2.8 Learning Activity

Note whether the following statements are True (T) or False (F).

___ a. The nurse's own values and beliefs affect his or her sensitivities with patients

___ b. Pain is influenced by culture

___ c. Race is not a factor in drug absorption and action

___ d. It is never appropriate for a nurse to pray with a patient; a chaplain should be called

___ e. Physical care should always take precedence over psychosocial and spiritual care

Answers to this activity can be found in the Answer Key.

Cultural Diversity

Progressive care nurses must respect and embrace diversity among the patient and health care team members. The unit should have cultural reference material available and have a list of employees who speak another language and are willing to assist with translation. Phone translation services should also be available.

Nurses face a number of problems in providing culturally congruent health care (Table 2-11). Each of the following problems and issues can lead to inadequate culturally congruent health care that leads to poor health outcomes: personal biases and bigotry, cultural differences, stereotyping, prejudice, ignoring blind spots, and labeling. The lack of the following resources impedes the provision of quality culturally congruent patient care: interpreters and educational materials in the patient's language, diverse nursing staff, time to listen to patient and family, and flexibility with teaching methods.

Spiritual Diversity

Spirituality is a basic human phenomenon that helps create meaning in the world and encompasses a person's ideology, view of the world, and meaning of life. It gives an individual a sense of inner peace and harmony. Spiritual distress is a disruption in the life principle that pervades a person's entire being and integrates and transcends one's biological and psychosocial nature. Many factors contribute to a person's spirituality, such as religion, meditation, prayer, hope, and faith.

An individual's religion is a system of beliefs in and reverence for a supernatural power. Beliefs may not be based on logical proof or material evidence. Religious symbols are often used in the expression of faith (e.g., rosary beads, prayer cloth, prayer rug, medicine bundles, red ribbon, charms, "the garment"). Patients use meditation as a devotional exercise of reflection. Some patients use prayer, an intimate conversation between an individual and God or other Higher Being, for comfort. Maintaining a sense of hope is necessary for patients and family to cope. They need to wish for something with an expectation of its fulfillment. Faith, a confident belief in the truth of a person, idea, or thing (e.g., God), sustains people through trying times.

Exclusion of the important role of spirituality for patients and families can impact recovery and health. Care of the whole person enhances healing and health. Spiritual beliefs of providers may be an important consideration for many patients when selecting a health care provider. A nurse needs to explore personal values and beliefs. Acknowledge that agreement with every aspect of the patient's spiritual beliefs and practices is not possible, but the nurse must be nonjudgmental and respect the patient's right to worship the Supreme Being of his or her choice. Develop good listening skills and encourage the patient to discuss spiritual concerns. Know your limits. If you are uncomfortable discussing spiritual needs with the patient or praying with the patient, contact the patient's personal spiritual advisor or consult the hospital chaplain service as requested by the patient or family.

Schedule physical care to allow religious rituals and practices and respect the patient's rights and privacy. Increase your knowledge regarding different faiths and how to perform a spiritual needs assessment (Table 2-12). Determine whether there are religious or spiritual practices (e.g., communion) that the patient wishes to participate in during hospitalization and identify specific religious concerns such as dietary needs or refusal of blood administration. Provide care that is sensitive to the patient's spiritual/religious needs.

Generational Diversity

Each generation has a peer personality that lends itself to a collective mind-set (Table 2-13), referred to as the generation gap. It is important not to avoid overgeneralizing because not everyone in each age group fits the description or every aspect of the description of an age group. Generational diversity can affect communication with patients, families, peers, and intraprofessional teams (Johnson & Romanello, 2005).

TABLE 2-11 Relevant Cultural Behaviors to Nursing Care

Cultural Group	Cultural Variations (Common Belief/Practice)	Nursing Implications
African Americans	• Dialect and slang terms require careful communication to prevent error (e.g., "bad" may mean "good").	• Question the patient's meaning or intent.
Mexican Americans	• Eye behavior is important. An individual who looks at and admires a child without touching the child has given the child the "evil eye."	• Always touch the child you are examining or admiring.
American Indians	• Eye contact is considered a sign of disrespect and is thus avoided.	• Recognize that the patient may be attentive and interested even though eye contact is avoided.
Appalachians	• Eye contact is considered impolite or a sign of hostility. • Verbal patter may be confusing.	• Clarify statements.
American Eskimos	• Body language is important. • The individual seldom disagrees publicly with others. • Patient may nod yes to be polite, even if not in agreement.	• Monitor own body language closely, as well as patient's, to detect meaning.
Chinese Americans	• Individual may nod head to indicate yes or shake head to indicate no. • Excessive eye contact indicates rudeness. • Excessive touch is offensive.	• Ask questions carefully and clarify responses. • Avoid excessive eye contact and touch.
Filipino Americans	• Offending people is to be avoided at all cost. • Nonverbal behavior is important.	• Monitor nonverbal behaviors of self and client, being sensitive to physical and emotional discomfort or concerns of the patient.
Haitian Americans	• Touch is used in conversation. • Direct eye contact is used to gain attention and respect during communication.	• Use direct eye contact when communicating.
East Indian Hindu Americans	• Be aware that men may view eye contact by women as offensive. • Avoid eye contact.	• Women avoid eye contact as a sign of respect.
Vietnamese Americans	• Avoidance of eye contact is a sign of respect. • The head is considered sacred; it is not polite to pat the head. • An upturned palm is offensive in communication.	• Limit eye contact. • Touch the head only when mandated and explain clearly before proceeding to do so. • Avoid hand gesturing.

From Giger, J. (2013). *Transcultural nursing: Assessment and intervention* (6th ed.). St. Louis: Mosby.

2.9 Learning Activity

Match the religion with the implication.

___ 1. Islam (Muslim)
___ 2. Catholicism
___ 3. Judaism
___ 4. Hinduism
___ 5. Christian Scientist
___ 6. Seventh-Day Adventist
___ 7. Jehovah's Witness

a. Provide kosher diet as required
b. Opposed to blood transfusion
c. Provide same-sex caregivers
d. Medical care may be refused; prayer is used as the primary treatment of illness
e. The patient must be baptized before death
f. Procedures may be refused between dusk on Friday and dusk on Saturday
g. The patient's head is turned to the right after death

Answers to this activity can be found in the Answer Key.

CLINICAL INQUIRY OR INNOVATOR/EVALUATOR

The Synergy Model describes clinical inquiry as the ongoing process of questioning and evaluating practice, providing informed practice, creating changes and innovation through evidence-based practice, utilizing research or best evidence, and learning through experience. Clinical inquiry competence varies depending on the nurse's practice level. For example, at a minimum, the competent progressive care nurse follows policies, procedures, standards, and guidelines without deviation, while the expert nurse would use experience or published outcome data to improve, modify, or individualize policies, procedures, standards, and guidelines.

Evidence-based practice (EBP) is the conscious integration of best research evidence, clinician expertise, patient values, and circumstances. EBP is a problem-solving approach to clinical practice that uses five steps (Straus, Glasziou, Richardson, & Haynes, 2011). Clinicians ask the best questions and are actively seeking answers to questions when using evidence-based practice. Clinicians ask the questions; collect evidence;

TABLE 2-12   Appropriate Nursing Interventions for Religious Beliefs

Religion	Belief	Interventions
Catholicism	• God does not cause suffering, but allows it for furthering human growth • Baptism is necessary for salvation	• Inform patient that Holy Communion is available • Have Catholic priest/deacon available to perform Anointing of the Sick • If patient is close to death and a Catholic religious representative is not available, any Christian may perform the baptism and then notify the priest immediately • Make all efforts to leave religious symbols (e.g., rosary) in place
Christian Scientist	• Sin, sickness, and death can be overcome by a full understanding of the divine principle of Jesus's teaching and healing • Disease and illness are delusions of the nonspiritual mind and can be overcome by prayer	• Be aware that medical care may be refused • May utilize the services of physicians for the purpose of setting bones, treatment of malignancies, and delivering babies • Pain medications may be accepted for severe pain only • There is no clergy or priesthood
Hinduism	• Illness may result from misuse of the body or sins from a previous lifetime • Meditation and prayer must be done at specific times throughout the day • Females cannot be left in the presence of an unfamiliar male	• Plan care around religious practices • Provide same-sex caregivers • Provide vegetarian meals as requested • May refuse medication by capsule because many capsules are made from beef • Allow the family to wash the patient's body after death; do not remove any sacred threads that are placed on the body
Islam (Muslim)	• Submit to Allah's will in matters of health • Prayer and washing required five times a day • The left hand is considered unclean; food will not be handled with the left hand	• Provide privacy and plan care to accommodate prayer times • Educate regarding pain-reducing techniques • Provide diet with dietary restrictions as requested • Pork and some other foods prohibited • May refuse to take capsules because many are made from pork • Follow patient and family wishes regarding therapies; prolonging life by life-support machinery is often seen as unacceptable • Allow family to stay with relative during process of dying • Allow family to wash patient's body after death • Turn deceased person's face toward the right
Jehovah's Witness	• Opposed to transfusions of blood obtained from a blood bank and some blood products (the source of the soul is believed to be in the blood) • Opposed to eating foods to which blood has been added • Do not celebrate national holidays (including Christmas) or birthdays or salute flags; it is believed that violators will spend an eternity in nothingness	• Assess the patient's religious beliefs and practices before administering blood or blood products • Most Witnesses carry cards indicating types of acceptable transfusions • "Mature minors" may refuse blood transfusions • Be aware that the patient may refuse surgical or medical interventions that will require blood transfusion • Consider the use of volume expanders such as saline, lactated Ringer's solution, and hetastarch (Hespan) • Implement blood-conservation strategies, especially in children • Consult hematologist and/or medical centers familiar with bloodless medicine and surgery management, if needed • Respect patient and family decisions to refuse blood products • Avoid foods to which blood has been added (e.g., certain sausages, lunch meats) • Avoid attempts to involve the patient in preparations for celebrations of national holidays

Continued

TABLE 2-12	**Appropriate Nursing Interventions for Religious Beliefs—cont'd**	
Religion	**Belief**	**Interventions**
Judaism	• Sabbath begins at sundown on Friday and ends at sundown on Saturday • There is hope for recovery until death is imminent • May not eat nonkosher foods • Orthodox Jews: work of any kind is prohibited on the Sabbath, including driving or using the telephone • Orthodox Jews: prayer is required three times a day • A person must stay with a critically ill or dying family member until death so that the soul will not feel alone	• Provide kosher diet as requested • Provide privacy and plan care considering prayer times • Allow a relative to stay with the dying patient • Notify rabbi/rebbe according to family's wishes • Caregivers should leave the body untouched for approximately one-half hour after death to allow the soul to depart • After death, by Judaic law, the body cannot be left alone • Autopsies generally are not allowed unless required by law • Assist and respect practices of the Sabbath • Do not shave body hair of Hasidic Jews • Hasidic/Orthodox: provide same-sex caregivers
Seventh-Day Adventist	• Sabbath is recognized as dusk on Friday to dusk on Saturday • The body is a temple of God and should be kept healthy	• Provide diet with dietary restrictions as requested • The church encourages a vegetarian diet • Be aware that the patient may avoid seafood, meat, caffeine, alcohol, drugs, and tobacco • Protein and iodine deficiency may occur • Be aware that the patient may refuse procedures (medical or surgical) that occur on the Sabbath

TABLE 2-13	**Characteristics of Today's Generations**	
Generation	**Born Between**	**Characteristics**
Silent Generation (AKA Veteran Generation) ~10% of today's workforce	1925-1942	• Tend to be hard working, thrifty, disciplined • Value traditions • Appreciate conformity, consistency, and uniformity at work and value the system over the individual • Tend to work at large corporations that offer security and reward longevity • Prefer direct orders • Prefer assignments that are structured and task oriented
Baby Boomer ~45% of today's workforce	1943-1960	• Tend to be rebellious and questioning of the status quo • Equate work with self-worth • Are driven and dedicated; willing to work overtime • May be resistant to technology • Prefer facilitation • Prefer assignments that require flexibility, independent thinking, and creativity
Generation X ~30% of today's workforce	1961-1981	• Tend to be ironic, cynical, and resourceful • Balance work and leisure time; less likely to work overtime • Are more independent; do not belong to any group • Are comfortable with technology • Embrace diversity • Adapt well to change • Attempt to attain several goals at once • Prefer coaching with feedback and credit for accomplishments • Prefer assignments that allow self-direction
Millennial (AKA Nexters or Generation Y) ~15% of today's workforce	1982-2002	• Tend to be optimistic, assertive, self-confident, and friendly • Accept authority and prefer to be led • Are cooperative team players; prefer to work in groups and teams • Have difficulty focusing on one task; prefer to multitask • Are very technology-savvy • Prefer collegiality and mentoring • Prefer assignments that challenge and stretch their capabilities

appraise the data; integrate the evidence with clinical expertise, patient preferences, and values; and then evaluate the decisions.

Clinical questions begin with a background of an issue and ask the common questions of who, what, where, when, how, and why. To seek specific causal knowledge, questions use the PICOT process to assist in clinical decisions or actions (Table 2-14). PICOT is a mnemonic frequently used for ensuring clinical decisions based on the best evidence (Melnyk & Fineout-Overholt, 2015).

Seek evidence through published research reports using search engines such as CINAHL, Pub Med/MEDLINE, the Cochrane database, and Google scholar. Review bibliographies of the helpful studies and unpublished research reports, and consult with known researchers. Critically appraise the evidence for validity and usefulness. The traditional hierarchy of evidence based on study designs starting at the top is double-blinded randomized controlled trials, nonblinded randomized clinical trials, nonrandomized clinical trials, prospective cohort studies, case-control studies, case reports, and expert opinion including consensus groups. Randomized controlled trials are considered the *gold standard*, but many nursing questions are not answered using quantitative techniques due to sample size and inability to control extraneous variables. Due to these limitations, factors such as quantity, consistency, and relevance are given due consideration. Quantity supports the strength of the evidence and refers to the magnitude of effect, numbers of studies, and sample size or power. Consistency is the extent to which similar findings are reported using similar and different study designs, and relevance is the study question's similarity to the clinical question and the extent to which the findings from the study can be applied in other clinical settings to different patients.

There are many grading scales used to grade sources of evidence. The recently modified AACN system integrates findings with clinical expertise, patient values, and circumstances and, if appropriate, applying these findings (Table 2-15). The system evaluates performance and the outcomes of the clinical practice based on evidence.

The primary goal of nursing research is to develop a specialized, scientifically based body of nursing knowledge to facilitate improvement in patient care. The scientific method is a systematic approach to solving problems that controls variables and biases. To provide quality care, progressive care nurses need to have an understanding of how to translate research into practice. Basic research advances knowledge and helps in understanding relationships to phenomena. Applied research has a purpose to solve a particular problem. This type of research helps in making decisions or evaluating techniques. The progressive care nurse must have an understanding of relevant definitions, types of studies, process steps, and nursing responsibilities related to research.

An understanding of a hypothesis and types of variables are important research definitions for the progressive care nurse to comprehend. A hypothesis is a statement that predicts a relationship among two or more variables. The hypothesis may be simple, complex, directional, nondirectional, or null. A variable is a measureable concept that varies among the subjects in a research study. An independent variable is referred to as the treatment variable because it is the concept that is being observed, introduced, and/or manipulated. The dependent

TABLE 2-14	Five-Step PICOT Process
P	Population/problem
I	Intervention
C	Comparison intervention
O	Outcome
T	Time

From Melnyk, B., & Fineout-Overholt, E. (2015). *Evidence-based practice in nursing and healthcare: A guide to best practice* (ed 3). Philadelphia: Wolters Kluwer.

TABLE 2-15	AACN Levels of Evidence
Level	**Description**
A	Meta-analysis of multiple controlled studies or meta-analysis of qualitative studies with results that consistently support a specific action, intervention, or treatment
B	Well-designed controlled studies, both randomized and nonrandomized, with results that consistently support a specific action, intervention, or treatment
C	Qualitative studies, descriptive or correlational studies, integrative reviews, systematic reviews, or randomized controlled trials with inconsistent results
D	Peer-reviewed professional organizational standards with clinical studies to support recommendations
E	Theory-based evidence from expert opinion or multiple case reports
M	Manufacturers' recommendations only

From Armola, R. et al. (2009). AACN levels of evidence: What's new? *Critical Care Nurse, 29*(4), 70-73.

variable is the concept that is observed for a change after the intervention. Although not studied, an extraneous variable may or may not be relevant to the results of the study. This variable can affect the dependent variable and interfere with research results.

Quantitative research is one type of study design. Quantitative research is a deductive process that tests hypotheses and examines cause-and-effect relationships to examine specific phenomena. The emphasis is on facts and data to validate or extend existing knowledge. Several types of quantitative designs are used. Experimental design uses randomization and a control group to test the effects of an intervention. Quasi-experimental design involves manipulation of variables but lacks a comparison group or randomization. Nonexperimental designs include descriptive or ex post facto studies. Experiences and phenomena are described as they exist in descriptive studies. Ex post facto studies are correlational studies that describe the relationship between variables.

Qualitative research uses an inductive process to understand phenomena in a defined context. Qualitative research emphasizes development of new insights, theory, and knowledge. Techniques used in qualitative research include case studies, open-ended questions, field studies, and participant observation. Qualitative research relies less on numbers and measurements and more on nursing strategies, interpersonal communication techniques, intuition, and collaboration between nurse and patient to discover underlying relationships. The research process for both qualitative and quantitative studies includes the following steps:

- Formulate the research problem
- Review related literature
- Formulate the hypothesis
- Select the research design
- Identify the population to be studied
- Specify the methods of data collection
- Design the study
- Conduct the study
- Analyze the data
- Interpret the results
- Communicate the findings
- Utilize the findings to improve patient care

The progressive care nurse has ethical responsibilities related to research studies. Protect the rights of the research subjects and ensure that the potential benefits of the study outweigh any potential risk to the subjects. Submit all proposed studies to the institutional review board (IRB) for approval.

In addition to ethical responsibilities related to research, progressive care nurses need to recognize the need for active participation and utilization of research in nursing practice. Progressive care nurses may design and conduct nursing research, but it is also important that nurses actively identify problem areas and research questions for investigation. They should assist in the collection of data as requested. The progressive care nurse has a responsibility to read, interpret, assess the quality and applicability of the research, and incorporate findings into clinical practice. Use research findings to change clinical practice and improve patient care, and share these results with peers. The cycle of knowledge transformation involves the steps of discovery, summary, translation, integration, and evaluation described in the Cycle of Knowledge Transformation Using the ACE Star Model (Stevens, 2012).

The ACE Star Model demonstrates the processes of knowledge transformation (Figure 2-5). The five steps of the model include discovery, evidence summary, translation, integration, and evaluation. The primary goal of nursing research is to discover a specialized scientific body of knowledge to improve patient care. Evidence summaries or systematic reviews provide a summary of all evidence related to a specific research question using vigorous methods of analysis. Translation into practice is facilitated by the clinical practice guidelines (CPGs). Then, using EBP models, integration into practice occurs. Finally, both formative and summative evaluation of the EBP effect is completed.

Research discovers information. Nurses identify problem areas and research questions for investigation, assist in data collection, query and interpret reports, critique the practice applicability, and apply research findings to change clinical practice and improve patient care. The professional nurse also shares research findings with peers and may design and conduct nursing research.

Evidence summary refers to the use of systematic reviews, which use a rigorous method to summarize all the evidence

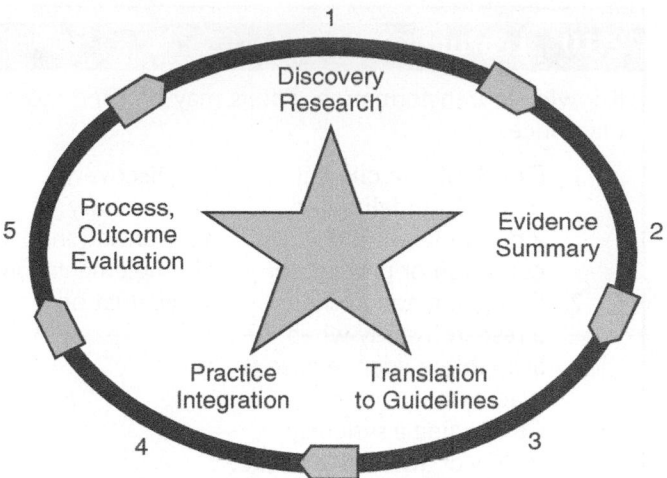

FIGURE 2-5 Stevens Star Model of Knowledge Transformation. (From Stevens, K. R. [2015]. *Stevens Star Model of Knowledge Transformation*. Retrieved from www.acestar.uthscsa.edu.)

TABLE 2-16	Finding Systematic Reviews	
Source	**Website**
Agency for Healthcare Research and Quality	www.ahrq.gov
The Cochrane Collaboration	www.cochrane.org
The Campbell Collaboration	www.campbellcollaboration.org
The Joanna Briggs Institute	www.joannabriggs.edu.au/

related to a specific research question. The advantage of using systematic reviews is that they provide critically appraised high-quality studies to help make decisions for clinicians, administrators, policy makers, and researchers. Various agencies conduct systematic reviews (Table 2-16) and bring together large quantities of information into a manageable form with a recommendation for clinical practice that shortens the time between research and clinical implementation.

Translation of the best scientific evidence into practice recommendations results in CPGs. CPGs are statements based on the best scientific evidence designed to assist clinical decision making about appropriate health care for specific clinical circumstances; Stevens (2012) states that CPGs explicitly articulate the link between the clinical recommendation and the strength of supporting evidence. CPGs published as clinical application documents help to surmount research utilization barriers because they reduce journal searches, overcome nurses' fear of limited critical analysis skills, and minimize the impact of research jargon and unfamiliar terminology (Ciliska, Pinelli, DiCenso, & Cullum, 2001). Standards of care, patient care pathways or multidisciplinary action plans (MAPs), policies and procedures, and protocols incorporate CPGs. They can be developed based on a condition (e.g., MI), symptom (e.g., chest pain), or clinical procedure (e.g., cardiac catheterization).

2.10   Learning Activity

Knowledge transformation. Points may be used more than once.

___ 1. Developing a clinical practice guideline for a common clinical condition or procedure.

___ 2. Designing and conducting a research study when the available evidence base is inadequate.

___ 3. Conducting a systematic review of available evidence related to a clinical issue.

___ 4. Initiation of an evidence-based clinical change.

___ 5. Appraisal of the effect of an evidence-based clinical change.

___ 6. Conducting a literature search for available evidence related to a clinical question.

a. Discovery
b. Summary
c. Translation
d. Implementation
e. Evaluation

Answers to this activity can be found in the Answer Key.

TABLE 2-17   Clinical Practice Guidelines, Sources, and Evaluation Toolkits

Organization	Guideline
Governmental agencies	• National Guideline Clearinghouse: www.guidelines.gov • Scottish Intercollegiate Guideline Network (SIGN): www.sign.ac.uk/guidelines/index.html
Professional associations	• Sigma Theta Tau International (STTI): www.nursingknowledge.org • American Association of Critical-Care Nurses: www.aacn.org • Registered Nurses' Association of Ontario: www.rnao.org/bestpractices • Emergency Nurses Association: www.ena.org
EBP centers	• Joanna Briggs Institute: www.joannabriggs.edu.au
Implementation and evaluation toolkits	• Registered Nurses' Association of Ontario Toolkit for Implementation of CPG: http://rnao.ca/sites/rnao-ca/files/BPG_Toolkit.pdf • Appraisal of Guidelines for Research and Evaluation (AGREE) Instrument: www.agreetrust.org

CPGs encourage treatment that offers patients maximum likelihood of benefit and minimum harm and is acceptable in terms of cost. The guidelines reduce inappropriate variations in practice related to clinical decision making, differing approaches to problem solving, varied routines and standards, access to resources, and lack of consensus related to appropriate treatment for given conditions. In essence, CPGs promote the delivery of evidence-based health care. Common sources are available to provide ready evaluation criteria by which health care professionals are held accountable for clinical performance and reduction of health care expenditures (Table 2-17).

Integration of research into practice involves the use of a change model and consideration of organizational barriers and strategies to facilitate EBP. Four recommended EBP change models include the Iowa Model of EBP to Promote Quality Care, the Stetler Model of Research Utilization, the Rosswurm-Larrabee Model of EBP, and the Johns Hopkins EBP Conceptual Model. The organization can foster an environment that values inquiry and critical thinking by using the following strategies:

• Encouragement of formal education
• Provision of time to read research and evaluate applicability to setting
• Provision of access to the Internet, e-journals, library, and photocopying
• Provision of opportunities to attend conferences, continuing education, and in-service education, including education regarding critical appraisal of research
• Addition of scholarship to the nurse's role so that dissemination through local, regional, and national presentations and publication is encouraged and expected

• Establishment of nursing leadership to spearhead EBP activities, such as a nurse researcher, clinical nurse specialist, or nurse practitioner
• Encouragement of the questioning of the status quo and nursing rituals
• Development of intraprofessional collaborative teams

The institution needs to establish and communicate the expectation of EBP. Make EBP a requirement of changes and revision of policies, procedures, and protocols. EBP activities incorporated into job descriptions, performance appraisals, merit raises, and career ladder promotions clearly articulate the expectations of EBP to all constituents. Consistently, formal and informal nursing leaders need to ask the question: what is the evidence? Strategy recommendations for EBP implementation will increase nurse autonomy over practice and help eliminate the approximately 10-year gap between research and practice. EBP implementation includes the following:

• Development of unit-level EBP committees
• Establishment of joint appointments between academic and practice settings
• Appointment of a nurse researcher on staff
• Utilization of expert consultants as necessary
• Provision of support for EBP committees and research activities
• Development of research presentations (e.g., Nursing Research Grand Rounds)
• Establishment of journal clubs
• Publication of a monthly research newsletter
• Utilization of resources appropriately with commitment of expertise, money, and time to EBP activities, including having adequate staffing
• Utilization of systematic reviews and implementation of clinical practice guidelines

Evaluate the effect of EBP by both formative and summative methods. Formative evaluation involves the assessment during the change process to ensure that the change has actually occurred and its preliminary effects. Summative evaluation involves the assessment at the completion of the change process to evaluate the effect of the change. Evaluation criteria should include patient health outcomes such as length of stay, quality of life, patient satisfaction, staff satisfaction, and cost-benefit impact.

2.11 Learning Activity

List five ways to share research findings with colleagues.

a. _____
b. _____
c. _____
d. _____
e. _____

Answers to this activity can be found in the Answer Key.

Continuous Quality Improvement

Quality improvement (QI) emphasizes progressive improvement through innovation that is customer and system outcome focused (Yoder-Wise, 2011). The QI process identifies needs, assembles a multidisciplinary team, and collects data to measure current status. Emphasis is on improving systems and processes based on data rather than assigning blame, and requires commitment from administration and staff. Customers ultimately define quality, but others involved in the definition of quality include governmental agencies, accreditation agencies, and third-party payers.

QI processes include structure, process, and outcome evaluation. Structure evaluation examines the components of services, such as the setting and environment that affect quality of care. Process evaluation examines activities and behaviors of the health care provider. Outcome evaluation measures changes in patients. Elinson (1987) identified the Five Ds to measure patient outcomes: death, disease, disability, discomfort, and dissatisfaction. Other indicators used currently include functional status and quality of life.

Clinical indicators should reflect desired outcomes and represent high-quality care delivery. Patient outcomes make a comparison of observed practice with expectations established from benchmarks, standards, policies and procedures, nurse practice acts, accrediting and governmental agencies (Joint Commission, AHRQ), professional associations (ANA, AACN), award criteria (Magnet, Beacon & Baldwin), and other comparable hospitals or units.

A National Database of Nursing Quality Indicators (NDNQI) developed by the ANA promotes and facilitates the standardization of information submitted by hospitals across the United States on nursing quality and patient outcomes. The database provides comparison data (e.g., teaching status, number of beds, and type of patient care unit) from similar hospitals and units.

Nursing-Sensitive Indicators capture nursing care or its outcomes most affected by nursing care (Box 2-3) (ANA, 2012d). The progressive nurse manager and staff should select and implement a plan to reconcile discrepancies between observations and expectations on the unit, and evaluate the implementation of the plan and the achievement of outcomes.

BOX 2-3
Common Nurse and Patient Indicators

Nurse Indicators
- Mix of RNs, LPNs, and unlicensed staff caring for patients in acute care settings
- Total nursing care hours provided per patient day
- Nurse staff satisfaction
- Nursing turnover

Patient Indicators
- Pressure ulcer rate
- Patient falls
- Restraints
- Patient satisfaction with pain management
- Patient satisfaction with educational information
- Patient satisfaction with overall care
- Patient satisfaction with nursing care
- Nosocomial infection rate

The Institute for Healthcare Improvement (IHI, 2011) advocates the Model for Improvement (Table 2-18) for accelerating improvement. Members of the improvement team should be multidisciplinary and are critical to a successful improvement effort. The model asks three fundamental questions and uses the Plan-Do-Study-Act (PDSA) cycle to test and implement changes in real work settings. The three fundamental questions address how to set the aims, establish measures, and plan changes and can be addressed in any order.

Patient Safety

Quality and safety are emphasized in today's world of health care delivery. The Institute of Medicine's (IOM) report *Keeping Patients Safe: Transforming the Work Environment for Nurses* (2008) spearheaded the implementation of safety recommendations and initiatives into clinical practice to create effective safe cultures. The IOM report examined the culture of organizations where there was evidence of low error and accidents, and concluded that there needed to be environmental structures and processes in organizations to promote safety. Placing an emphasis on developing strong attitudes and perceptions of safety for the workers will eventually translate into safe behaviors exhibited by individuals within an organization.

Standards and National Patient Safety Goals (NPSGs) are reviewed and developed annually by the Joint Commission's Accreditation Organization (JCAHO) for specific clinical areas. The hospital and critical access hospital NPSGs (2014) address significant implications relative to the moderate-to-high acuity of patients in progressive nursing care. These NPSGs include identifying patients and their safety risks correctly, using medications and alarms safely, preventing infections and mistakes in surgery, and improving staff communications. Of particular importance in the progressive care environment is safety goal number 2, which focuses on communication safety. Progressive care units tend to have high traffic control situations. A high number of patients require handing off due to diagnostic procedures, admissions, transfers, and discharges. The mnemonic SBAR, which stands for **S**ituation, **B**ackground, **A**ssessment, and **R**ecommendation, is an effective handoff technique to use during report to facilitate staff interaction and safe health care delivery (Haig, Sutton, & Whittington, 2006; Leonard, Bonacum, & Graham, 2004). The safety goal for the procedural time-out requirement for preoperative and

TABLE 2-18	IHI Model for Improvement	
	IHI Model	**PDSA Cycle**
Aims	What are we trying to accomplish?	
Measures	How will we know that the change is an improvement?	
Changes	What changes can we make that will result in improvement?	

Act → Plan → Do → Study → Act (PDSA Cycle diagram)

postoperative care can also apply to several procedures commonly done in progressive care, such as cardioversion and chest tube insertion. Safe medication delivery, medication reconciliation, and limitation of drug concentrations (e.g., heparin) in an organization are other applicable safety considerations implemented in progressive care.

In recent years, safety concerns regarding alarm fatigue have been recognized and strategies have been implemented to address the issue. The reliance on physiologic monitors to alert the nurse when a serious problem occurs is standard practice on monitored units. Alarms alert the nurse about individual patient deviations from a predetermined baseline status. However, alarm fatigue may occur when the sheer number of monitor alarms overwhelms the nurses, possibly leading to alarms being disabled, silenced, or ignored. Excessive numbers of monitor alarms and fear that nurses have become desensitized to these alarms were the impetus for quality improvement initiatives (Graham and Cvach, 2010). In this alarm fatigue initiative, it was determined that nurses need to individualize patients' alarm parameter limits and levels and adjust monitor alarm defaults. Careful assessment and customization of parameter limits and levels can reduce the number of audible alarms. Alarms are important and sometimes life-saving, and they can compromise patients' safety if ignored.

Experts say the disturbance caused by hospitals' increased use of monitoring devices can desensitize nurses to alarms and raise the likelihood that a true safety event will go unnoticed. In addition, noisy environments increase patient anxiety and make rest and healing difficult. Safety advocates are increasingly concerned about the damage done by alarm fatigue. In April 2013, the Joint Commission, the nation's largest hospital accreditation organization, issued a sentinel event alert warning of the dangers of alarm desensitization and urging hospitals to beef up alarm management protocols and alarm setting guidelines. Just 2 months later, the Joint Commission raised the stakes even higher when it announced a newly drafted National Patient Safety Goal on clinical alarm safety. As of January 2014, hospitals are required to demonstrate that they have made alarms an organizational priority and identify the types of alarms they plan to target. By 2016, hospitals must develop and implement specific protocols aimed at curbing unnecessary alarms (McKinney, 2014).

The mindfulness of safety is a paradigm within health care delivery organizations that has gained momentum in the last decade. Creating a culture of safety requires changing attitudes and behaviors. AACN's *Standards for Establishing and Sustaining Healthy Work Environments* (Barden, 2005) facilitates the development of safe environments. Using the standards that address skilled communication, true collaboration, effective decision making, appropriate staffing, and meaningful recognition and authentic leadership, the progressive care nurse and unit-based council can create a culture of safety. This culture involves the bedside nurse in practice decisions, quality improvement activities, research, and staff recruitment and retention, and it improves collaboration and communication between nursing and the intraprofessional team (Lewis & Vickers, 2008). Staff can also be involved in outcome measurement of the implemented standards. Schmalenberg and Kramer (2008) developed the Essentials of Magnetism tool to evaluate the magnitude and status of the implementation strategies of the standards in the progressive care unit.

Quality and Safety Education for Nurses

The Quality and Safety Education for Nurses (QSEN, 2012) established competencies for nursing and has proposed targets for knowledge, skills, and attitudes (KSAs). Organized into six categories, the KSAs include patient-centered care, teamwork and collaboration, evidence-based practice, quality improvement, safety, and informatics. Each of the competencies is incorporated into program curricula and are applicable for clinical practice as well.

Nurses are most likely to be involved in medication errors than any other form of medical errors. Safety focus is on the prevention of medication errors (Dennison, 2005). The nurse has the responsibility to include the 10 rights of medication administration (Box 2-4). Errors and near-hits (also referred to as near-misses) need to be reported so that system analysis can occur and prevent future errors. Systems thinking should focus on a nonpunitive culture and the development and adherence of safe policies, procedures, and protocols. These safety measures should include policies dictating the avoidance of unapproved abbreviations, trailing zeroes, avoidance of verbal orders, and proper drug labeling. Up-to-date medication electronic references (e.g., Micromedex, Epocrates) and drug books need to be available to staff.

Technology such as electronic medical records (EMRs), automated medication dispensing devices, bar code point of care (BPOC), computerized provider order entry (CPOE), and "smart" pumps with imbedded safety devices to alert the nurse of a too high or too low dose of medication have been found to reduce errors. Standardization such as formulary restriction, lower infusion concentrations, and infusion equipment are also beneficial safety initiatives.

> ### BOX 2-4
> #### Ten Rights of Safe Medication Administration
>
> - Right patient: Use two patient identifiers (not room and bed number)
> - Right drug
> - Right dose
> - Right time
> - Right route
> - Right reason
> - Patient's right to education
> - Patient's right to refuse
> - Patient evaluation: Clarify titration parameters
> - Right documentation

> ### BOX 2-5
> #### Characteristics of the Adult Learner
>
> - Goal-oriented
> - Less flexible
> - Requires longer time in learning task performance
> - Impatient in the pursuit of objectives
> - Finds little use for isolated facts
> - Strives for recognition and success
> - Has multiple responsibilities, which draw upon his or her time
> - Experienced in the "school of life"
> - Requires a more constant and ideal learning environment
> - Usually comes to the teaching program on a voluntary basis
> - Wishes to be involved in mutual planning of learning experiences
> - Likes to participate in diagnosing needs for learning, formulating learning objectives, and evaluating learning
> - Expects a climate of mutual respect, trust, and collaboration that supports learning

Safe medication practice requires a pharmacist to review all prescriptions and dispense medications. The pharmacist's presence on the unit and during rounds reduces medication errors. Controlling the environment by providing adequate lighting, noise reduction, distraction avoidance, and a clean, clutter-free, organized space for medication preparation is vital to promote medication safety. Medication reconciliation policies and teamwork also decrease error. Nurses need to clarify any unclear prescription and perform medication reconciliation procedures during admission, transfers, and discharges. Relying on teamwork to complete independent double-checks of drug, dose, calculation, patient identity, infusion rate, and appropriate line for all high-alert medications reduces error along with a use of time-out if there is a question about the safety of the drug. Finally, documenting and communicating changes in patient response or adverse drug events ensures safe medication administration.

TEACHING THE PATIENT AND FAMILY

The ability to facilitate patient and family learning is a measure of the nurse's Synergy Model competence. Teaching is the process of facilitating learning and is defined as a two-way interaction designed to help a person learn to do something that he or she is currently unable to do. Learning is the process by which a person becomes capable of doing something he or she could not do before; this includes anything from motor skills to intellectual skills. Learning is an emotional experience that can be negative or positive, traumatic or pleasant. Patient education is the process of teaching patients and their families about an illness, treatment, and other health-related matters, including how to adhere to the regimen and helping to change behavior.

Patient education is a regulatory requirement. Multiple reasons exist for this regulation. The patient has a need and a right to know those things that are relevant to his or her condition, disease, or situation to produce changes in knowledge, skills, attitudes, appreciation, and understanding that will promote and improve health. Patient education encourages the patient to assume responsibility for disease management, to prevent illness and complications, and aids in coping with illness and adaptation to change. In addition, education promotes compliance with the therapeutic regimen and reduces patient and family anxiety. Patient education reduces the number of visits to the physician's office, emergency department, hospitalizations, and length of stay, thereby reducing health care costs.

Principles of Adult Education

The adult learner is a self-directed independent person who becomes ready to learn when the need to know or need to perform is experienced. Consider that adult learners have specific characteristics when developing a teaching plan (Box 2-5).

Pacing is an educational concept useful with adults. Tasks or methods involving significant time pressure are likely to be difficult for adults. Some degree of anxiety arousal is necessary for learning; however, older adults make up the majority of progressive care patients and may become too anxious in this type of learning situation. Minimize the role of competition and evaluation for adult patients. If possible, allow adults to set their own pace and allow individuals an opportunity to become familiar with a situation. A problem likely to affect older adults is that some tasks may produce considerable mental or physical fatigue; therefore, shorten the instruction sessions or provide frequent rest breaks.

Arrange materials from the simple to the complex in order to build the individual's confidence and skills. Structure the tasks so errors are avoided and do not have to be unlearned. Provide an opportunity for practice on similar but different tasks to develop generalizable skills. Provide information on the adequacy of previous responses and give the patient cues during the teaching process. Present materials to compensate for any potential sensory problems of older adults. Direct attention toward the relevant aspects of the task and keep the level of irrelevant information to a minimum. Organize the information appropriately because learning and remembering often require that information be grouped or related in some way. To elaborate or organize the material, better instruct individuals in the use of various mnemonic techniques (e.g., mental images, verbal associations). People learn and remember what is important to them. Attempt to make the task relevant to the individual's concerns and experience. When the individuals are able to integrate the new information with known information, improved performance results.

TABLE 2-19	Teaching Plan Components
Components	**Descriptions**
Objectives	What behavior should the learner be able to do? • Cognitive • Affective • Psychomotor
Criteria	How well should the learner be able to do it?
Condition	Under what conditions should the learner be able to do it?
Content	What information should be taught? • Language and terminology • Health care system: personnel, organization and structure, routines and procedures, norms and expectations, immediate environment • Basic anatomy and physiology of affected body system • Diagnosis and disease process • Therapy: treatments, medication, diet, activity, and personal health habits • Prevention of complications • Skills (e.g., insulin administration, taking pulse)
Community resources	Support groups Indigent medication programs Transportation services
Methods	Individual Group

The teaching process begins with an assessment and requires a teaching plan (Table 2-19). Conduct an assessment to determine readiness and desire to learn. The patient's education level and reading ability and how he or she learns best help the nurse develop individual, group, formal, and informal teaching plans. This information will also influence teaching supplies such as print materials, pictures and videos, auditory tapes, and/or tactile manipulatives.

2.12   Learning Activity

List five qualities of an adult learner.

a. _____

b. _____

c. _____

d. _____

e. _____

Answers to this activity can be found in the Answer Key.

Finally, assess the environment to avoid distractions, assess the patient's current health status, and consider how to compensate for any patient sensory or motor deficits. The patient needs to have adequate energy and be free of acute distress, such as pain or dyspnea. Barriers to teaching and learning include nurse, physician, and patient factors (Table 2-20). Remove or compensate for barriers before initiating a teaching plan.

TABLE 2-20	Barriers to Teaching and Learning
Barrier	**Rationale**
Nurse	• Lacks time and knowledge • Low care priority
Physician	Does not want patient/family taught
Patient • Physiologic • Availability • Psychological • Sensory/motor deficits • Attitude/beliefs	 Instability, sedation, pain Procedures, e.g., physical therapy Anxiety, pain Vision, hearing, dexterity Cultural conflicts with teaching

Conduct patient teaching individually or in groups. Combinations may be helpful to meet some patients' individual needs. Use the individual method when you are assessing a patient's knowledge, when family members or friends try to dominate teaching sessions, and when the information being conveyed provokes anxiety or is considered a topic not generally discussed in public. Individual methods include programmed instruction, reading materials, audio-visual aids, and one-to-one instruction. Group sessions lessen feelings of alienation and being "different," and patients can learn from each other during sessions. Patient-operated groups and self-help groups offer the benefit of encouraging patients to share coping techniques and useful hints. Group teaching saves the organization time and money. Family members gain support from health care professionals, other patients, and family members.

Teaching methods include lecture, discussion, audio-visual aids, printed materials, demonstration/return demonstration, role-playing, and so on. The teacher of adults is a facilitator more than a teacher, and uses various teaching methods. Consider your presentation style and remember to keep the presentations short. Place key points up front, use verbal headings, and summarize. Obtain feedback and request questions. Remember that successful learning takes time and reinforcement. Provide a means for the patient to learn more, such as written information for reading and review, resource groups, and an outpatient program. Coordinate education through written teaching plans and patient care conferences and document results. Determine if the patient met objectives or if the patient needs reinforcement or repeated instruction. Teaching by the lecture method may be done in group sessions, on videotape, or on closed-circuit TV, and sessions usually last no longer than 20 minutes. Lecture should include an introduction to establish the need to know, the content, and a summary to review what was covered. Discussion helps the patient to ask any questions and guides the nurse to assess what the patient needs to know. Audio-visual aids include visual and auditory stimulation to teach content.

When the patient must learn a new skill, demonstration and return demonstration is the best method. The nurse describes what he or she is going to do, and then the nurse demonstrates the skill while the patient observes. The next step involves the nurse talking the patient through the process while the patient performs the skill. Finally, the patient performs the skill while telling the nurse what he or she is doing.

When used as a teaching method and/or as a supplement, printed material should always include a discussion with the nurses after reading for clarification of content. Prepare printed material in the patient's language but at no higher than a sixth-grade reading level, and lower if possible (Institute for Healthcare Advancement, 2012) since individuals reading at a fifth-grade level are considered literate.

The nurse should assess the literacy level. Hand-printing instructions and asking the patient to read them back to you is a nonthreatening way to assess reading ability. Incongruent behavior may signal a literacy problem, so be alert for behavior that does not match the reported level of understanding. Identify and eliminate or minimize stress, anxiety, or other distractions before teaching, and correct misconceptions that affect reading and learning. Personalize the health message and explain the need for the written information. Relate information to the patient's past experiences and actively involve the patient and family in discussions. Several teaching strategies exist that can help poor readers (Table 2-21).

TABLE 2-21   Appropriate Teaching Strategies for Poor Readers

Qualities of Poor Readers	Teaching Strategies
Take words literally	Explain the meaning of all words
Read slowly; miss meaning	Use common words and examples
Skip over uncommon words	Use examples, review content frequently
Miss content	Describe content first, use verbal heading and visuals
Tire quickly	Use short segments

2.13   Synthesis Learning Activity: Clinical Vignette

A 70-year-old white male is scheduled for triple coronary artery bypass on Monday following a diagnostic cardiac catheterization today (Friday) that revealed extensive three-vessel disease. Risk factors include a family history of cardiac disease, history of hypertension, gastroesophageal reflux disease (GERD), iliac aneurysm, hyperlipidemia, prostate cancer, and a history of smoking. Family reports that the patient complained of sharp, time-limited episodes of occasional chest pain that the patient thought was from GERD, but was relieved with rest. The patient's family physician referred the patient to a cardiologist following a stress test that showed right coronary artery (RCA) ischemia. The patient has strong family support — a wife and three married daughters and five grandchildren. The wife still works and teaches nursing at a local university. Two daughters live locally, and the youngest lives a few states away. All immediate family members are present at the hospital, are very helpful, and have good relationships with their parents. The patient is retired, but a very physically active male used to doing what he wishes. He reports no previous limitations, but realizes he is slowing down due to age. The patient expected and agreed to the cardiac catheterization and even a possible stent, but now he has expressed shock at the diagnosis and need for surgery. The patient keeps stating, "I was fine 'til I came in here for this catheterization. I was chopping wood yesterday. I cannot need a bypass." The patient's current clinical presentation is stable. Blood pressure is 130/80 mm Hg, heart rate is 68 beats per minute (BPM), respiratory rate is 16 breaths per minute, and temperature is 98.6 degrees Fahrenheit. The cardiac monitor shows sinus rhythm with a rate between 60 and 70 per minute. The lungs are clear. There is no peripheral edema. The patient's weight is 172 pounds and height is 5'11". He says he has a good appetite and denies chest pain at present. He says he was told by the cardiac surgeon, "Congratulations, you are no longer a smoker." The patient said, "We will see" but states he has been compliant so far.

To apply the Synergy Model, circle the patient's characteristics and nurse dimension levels that best describe how to provide synergy and competent care during the next 48 hours.

A. Patient's Characteristics
Resiliency: Level 1 2 3 4 5
Vulnerability: Level 1 2 3 4 5
Stability: Level 1 2 3 4 5
Complexity: Level 1 2 3 4 5
Predictability: Level 1 2 3 4 5
Resource Availability: Level 1 2 3 4 5
Participation in Care: Level 1 2 3 4 5
Participation in Decision Making: Level 1 2 3 4 5

B. Nurse Dimensions
Clinical Judgment: Level 1 2 3 4 5
Advocacy/Moral Agency: Level 1 2 3 4 5
Caring Practices: Level 1 2 3 4 5
Collaboration: Level 1 2 3 4 5
Systems Thinking: Level 1 2 3 4 5
Response to Diversity: Level 1 2 3 4 5
Clinical Inquiry: Level 1 2 3 4 5
Facilitator of Learning: Level 1 2 3 4 5

Answers to this activity can be found in the Answer Key.

2.14   Synthesis Learning Activity: Crossword Puzzle

Complete the following crossword puzzle.

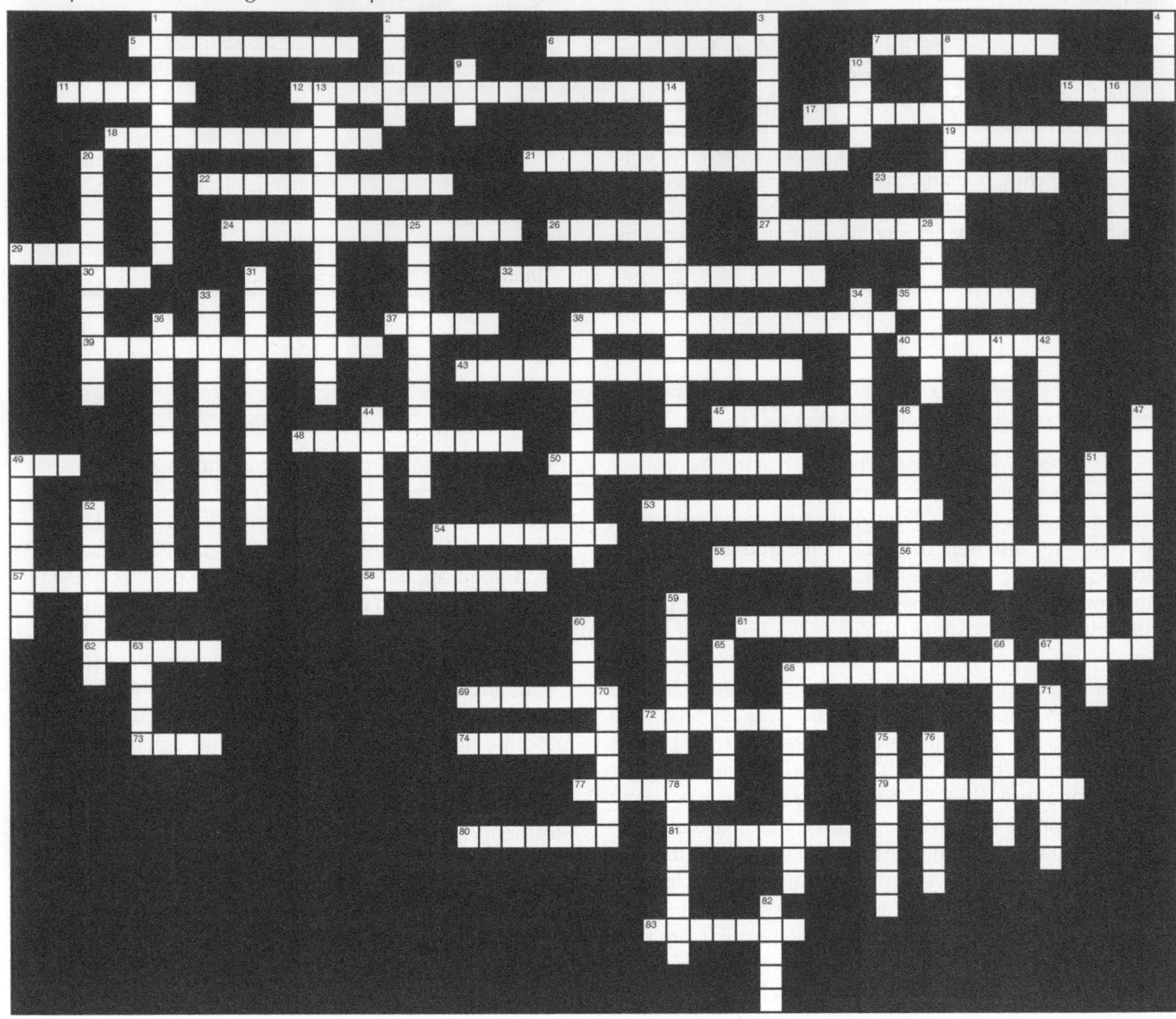

Answers to this activity can be found in the Answer Key.

ACROSS

5. A nurse who was born in 1950 would be in this generational group
6. Ethical approach that asserts that actions are right or wrong based on a set of morals or rules
7. Working on another's behalf
11. A collection of interdependent elements that interact to achieve a common purpose
12. The quantitative research design that does not utilize a control group or randomization

15. A common format for posing clinical questions (abbrev)
17. The obligation to be fair to all people
18. The process of seeking, giving, and receiving help
19. This type of thinking is controlled, purposeful, and goal-directed reasoning
21. The obligation to do no harm
22. The obligation to do good
23. A concept examined in a research study
24. Working together

26. An intimate conversation between an individual and God or other Higher Being
27. Nursing _____ indicators are those indicators that capture care or the outcomes most affected by nursing care
29. To wish for something with the expectation of its fulfillment
30. The integration of best evidence, clinician expertise, patient values, and circumstances (abbrev)
32. Answerability or responsibility

35. Personal beliefs about the truth and the worth of thoughts, objects, and behaviors
37. Belief not based on logical proof or material evidence
38. The fourth point on the ACE Star Model
39. The process by which an individual or group takes on the behaviors and practices of the dominant culture
40. Culturally prescribed codes of behavior
43 The obligation to respect privileged information

45 This type of consent applies when the patient cannot give consent but treatment is needed immediately

48. Achieving performance of care outcomes for which you are accountable and responsible by sharing activities with other individuals

49. The "gold standard" of evidence (abbrev)

50. Assault, battery, and defamation are all examples of this type of tort

53. M level on the AACN Level of Evidence scale includes recommendations from _____

54. This type of report is completed for errors or other unusual occurrences

55. Patterns and practices within a cultural group that encompass collective learned behaviors

56. Failing to do something that a reasonable and prudent professional would do or doing something that a reasonable and prudent professional would not do

57. The type of consent that must be obtained prior to inclusion as a subject in a study

58. The kind of evidence that is "best" if it is available

61. The third point on the ACE Star Model

62. Systems of valued behaviors and beliefs that govern proper conduct

67. One way to eliminate the gap between research and practice is to establish _____ appointments between academic and clinical facilities

68. A statutory right of a defined group

69. The nursing _____ is assess, diagnose, plan, implement, and evaluate

72. The type of charges that would be filed if a nurse intentionally caused a patient's death

73. A group of people related by common descent of heredity who have similar physical characteristics

74. An ethical _____ is a situation that requires a choice between two undesirable alternatives

77. The second point on the ACE Star Model is the _____ of evidence

79. The type of variable that is the response or outcome the researcher would like to explain or predict

80. The type of evaluation or review that might look at a physiologic parameter

81. The process of facilitating learning

83. Focusing and directing the imagination through the use of specific words and suggestions

DOWN

1. To assist an individual to make a decision when he or she does not have the data or expertise

2. The type of charges that could be filed if a nurse intentionally causes a patient's death

3. A statement that predicts a relationship among two or more variables

4. A legal wrong committed against a person or property

8. A(n) _____ includes behavior, criteria, and condition

9. A statement designed to assist the clinician in making decisions about the appropriate health care for specific clinical situations (abbrev)

10. The process for rapid cycle change (abbrev)

13. The ethical approach that asserts that actions are right or wrong based on the greatest good for the greatest number

14. Progressive care nurses deal with human responses to acute and potentially _____ problems (two words)

16. Learned, shared, and transmitted values, beliefs, and practices of a particular group that guide thinking

20. This involves use of conscious mental effort to control involuntary body function, such as blood pressure, heart rate, and respiratory rate

25. Use of scents for therapeutic purposes

28. The obligation to tell the truth

31. A basic human phenomenon that helps create meaning in the world

33. The statistical technique for conducting quantitative systematic reviews; yields a summary statistic

34. When one knows the right thing to do but cannot pursue the right action (two words)

36. The type of research that controls study variables as much as possible and has objective and measurable data collection; results in numbers

38. The type of variable that is the presumed cause of the change in the dependent variable

41. The insertion of needles into specific points in the body for therapeutic purposes

42. This method is a systematic approach to solving problems that controls variables and biases

44. A reference point against which performance can be compared

46. The type of research that uses randomization and a control group to test the effects of an intervention

47. Quality _____ emphasizes innovation

49. Specific unified system of an expression of the belief in and reverence for a supernatural power accepted as the creator and governor of the universe

51. Type of research that takes place in the individual's natural setting, with emphasis on understanding human experience; results in words or phrases

52. This type of consent is voluntarily given after the patient has been given required information

59. A goal for fostering EBP is to create a spirit of _____

60. A collection of essential nursing information for comparison across patient populations (abbrev)

63. The use of words and images to elicit laughter

65. The nursing care delivery system in which one nurse has accountability for the patient's care during the entire hospitalization

66. The fifth point on the ACE Star Model

68. Systems of valued behaviors and beliefs that govern proper conduct

70. A nurse practice act is an example of a _____

71. The process by which a person becomes capable of doing something he or she could not previously do

75. The obligation to be faithful to agreements and responsibilities accepted

76. A type of research to solve a particular problem

78. The right to self-determination

82. Quality, quantity, and consistency are used to _____ the evidence

The Cardiovascular System

ANATOMY AND PHYSIOLOGY

The cardiovascular system is a continuous, fluid-filled elastic circuit that functions as a pump, providing communication between all body parts through the transportation of oxygen, nutrients, hormones, water, enzymes, vitamins, minerals, buffers, leukocytes, antibodies, and wastes. All of these elements help the body maintain homeostasis by ensuring a dynamic equilibrium. The cardiovascular system consists of the heart and vascular system.

Heart

The heart is a bioelectrically driven, muscular, four-chamber organ that provides forward propulsion of the blood into the vascular system. The heart is about the size of a closed fist, approximately 9 cm wide and 12 cm long and weighs about 4 g/kg of a person's ideal body weight. The heart lies in the mediastinum between the sternum (anterior) and the spine (posterior) (Figure 3-1). Two thirds of the heart rests to the left of the midline and one third of the heart rests to the right of the midline.

The heart is a cone-shaped muscular pump located in the mediastinal cavity of the thorax between the lungs and beneath the sternum. The cone-shaped heart lies on its side on top of the diaphragm, with its base (the widest part) upward and leaning toward the right shoulder, and its apex pointing down and to the left. The apex at the level of the fifth left intercostal space (LICS) at the midclavicular line (MCL) on the upper surface of the diaphragm. The base is at the level of the second intercostal space.

The cardiac wall (Figure 3-2) has several layers. Each layer serves a different function. The pericardium, a double-layered membrane (outer and inner), maintains the heart in a stationary position. A loose-fitting, white fibrous outer layer acts as a barrier against infection and neoplastic invasion. The serous pericardium has two layers termed the parietal layer and the visceral layer. The parietal layer lines the inner surface of the fibrous pericardium and the visceral layer lines the external surface of the heart. Between the parietal and visceral layers of the serous pericardium lies the pericardial space (also known as the pericardial cavity). This cavity holds 10 to 30 mL of lubricating fluid that protects the heart against friction and erosion as it moves during contraction.

The *epicardium* is synonymous with the visceral layer of the serous pericardium. Epicardial fat, a thin layer of adipose tissue found between the visceral pericardium and the epicardium, increases in obese individuals, possibly contributing to their increased risk of coronary artery disease. The *myocardium* is the largest portion of the cardiac wall and consists of specialized conduction fibers and interlacing cardiac muscle fibers. The *endocardium* is the innermost layer of heart tissue. This layer consists of connective tissue, elastic fibers, and endothelial cells that form a smooth surface for blood contact, thus deterring clot formation. The endocardium is contiguous with the lining of the great vessels and lines the heart chambers and valves.

The *cardiac skeleton* is composed of continuous dense connective tissue located at the base of the heart and in the interventricular septum. It serves as the point of origin and insertion for cardiac muscle fibers and supports the heart valves, including the four valve rings (annuli).

There are four cardiac chambers (Figure 3-3), which are called the right and left atria and the right and left ventricles. The atria are located posterior, superior, and to the right of the corresponding ventricles. The interatrial septum divides the left and right atria and trabeculae divide the atria and ventricles. The atria are thin-walled, low-pressure chambers. The right atria is 2 mm thick, exerting 2 to 6 mm Hg of pressure, and the left atria are 3 mm thick, exerting 8 to 12 mm Hg of pressure. They act as reservoirs and booster pumps for the ventricles. Approximately 70% to 75% of ventricular filling is passive as blood falls through the atrium into the ventricle, whereas 25% to 30% of ventricular filling is active (i.e., atrial kick) as the atrium contracts at the end of ventricular diastole.

The inflow tracts of the right atrium include the superior vena cava, the inferior vena cava, the coronary sinus, and the thebesian veins. Outflow from the right atrium occurs through the tricuspid valve to the right ventricle. The inflow tracts of the left atrium occur through four pulmonary veins. This is the only case when veins carry oxygenated blood. Outflow from the left atrium occurs through the mitral valve to the left ventricle.

The ventricles are located anterior, inferior, and to the left of the corresponding atrium. They contain the interventricular septum, which divides the left and right ventricles, and the trabeculae, which divide the atria and the ventricles. The ventricles are contiguous with the lining of the great vessels and serve as pumps receiving blood from the atria and pumping blood out into the great vessels.

The right ventricle is thin-walled, only 3 to 5 mm thick, and pumps at a low pressure, approximately 25/5 mm Hg. The inflow tract is from the right atrium through the tricuspid valve and the thebesian veins. Outflow occurs through the pulmonic valve and into the pulmonary artery. This is the only case where an artery carries deoxygenated blood. Unlike the right ventricle, the left ventricle is thick-walled, approximately 8 to 15 mm thick. Left ventricular pressure is approximately 120/5 mm Hg.

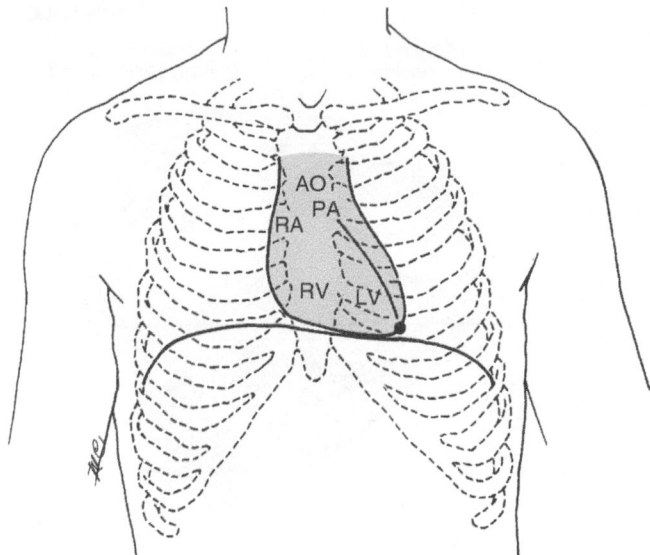

FIGURE 3-1 Location and orientation of the heart chambers and great vessels within the thorax. *AO,* Aorta; *PA,* pulmonary artery; *RA,* right atrium; *RV,* right ventricle; *LV,* left ventricle. (From Price, S., & Wilson, L. [2003]. *Pathophysiology: Clinical concepts of disease processes* [6th ed.]. St. Louis, MO: Mosby.)

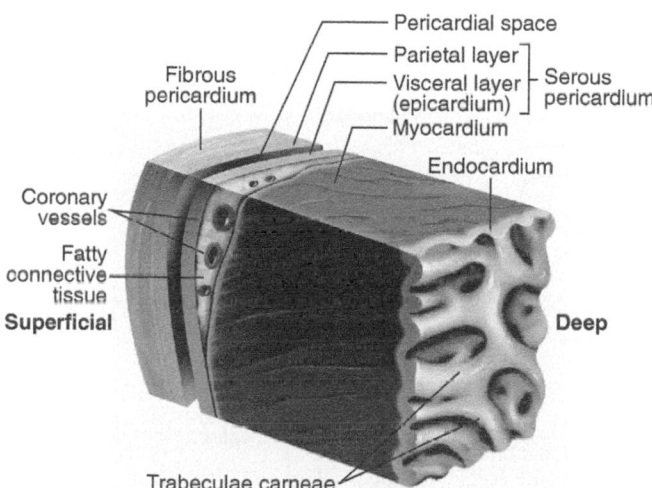

FIGURE 3-2 Layers of the cardiac wall. Note the fibrous pericardium, the parietal and visceral layers of the serous pericardium, the pericardial space between the two layers of the serous pericardium, the myocardium, and the endocardium. The visceral layer of the serous pericardium is also referred to as the epicardium. (From Patton, K. T., & Thibodeau, G. A. [2016]. *Anatomy & physiology* [9th ed.]. St. Louis, MO: Mosby.)

The inflow tract is from the left atrium through the mitral valve and the thebesian veins. The outflow tract is through the aortic valve and into the aorta.

Cardiac Valves

The cardiac valves (Figure 3-4) are located between the heart chambers and great vessels. The aortic, pulmonary, mitral and tricuspid valves serve to maintain a unidirectional flow. The valves permit antegrade flow and prevent retrograde flow. *Stenosis* is the narrowing of the valvular orifice that prevents antegrade flow. Valve *regurgitation, incompetence,* or *insufficiency* is the inadequate closure of the valvular orifice allowing retrograde flow.

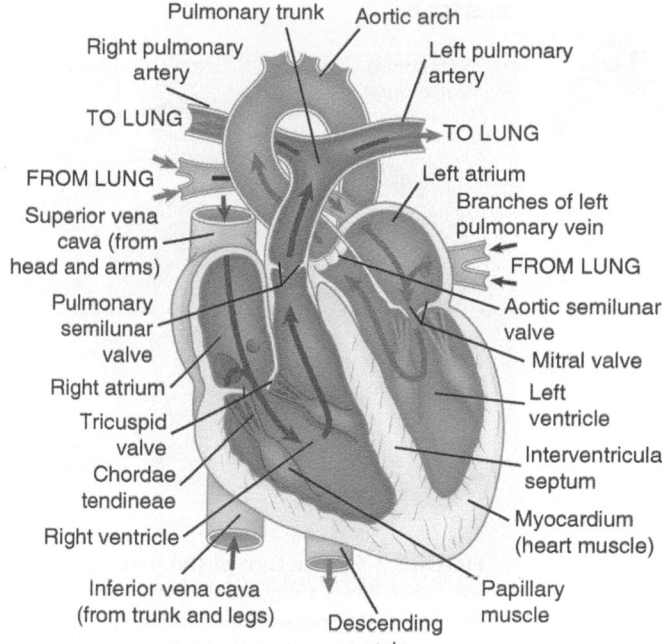

FIGURE 3-3 Cardiac chambers and the structures that direct blood flow through the heart. Arrows indicate path of blood flow through chambers, valves, and major vessels. (From McCance, K. L., & Huether, S. E. [2014]. *Pathophysiology: The biologic basis for disease in adults and children* [7th ed.]. St. Louis, MO: Mosby.)

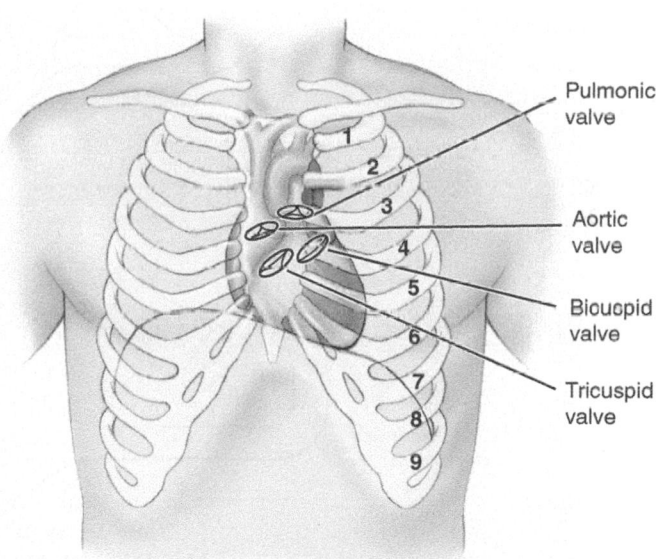

FIGURE 3-4 Location of the cardiac valves. (From Herlihy, B. [2011]. *The human body in health and illness* [4th ed.]. St. Louis, MO: Saunders.)

The cardiac valves (Figure 3-5) are flexible and fibrous and supported by rings of connective tissue. The tricuspid valve and the mitral valve are atrioventricular (AV) valves located between the atria and the ventricles. The tricuspid valve lies between the right atrium and the right ventricle. The mitral valve lies between the left atrium and the left ventricle. The AV valves consist of a fibrous supporting ring called the annulus, cusps (two for the mitral, three for the tricuspid), and papillary muscles that attach to the valve cusps by cord-like structures called

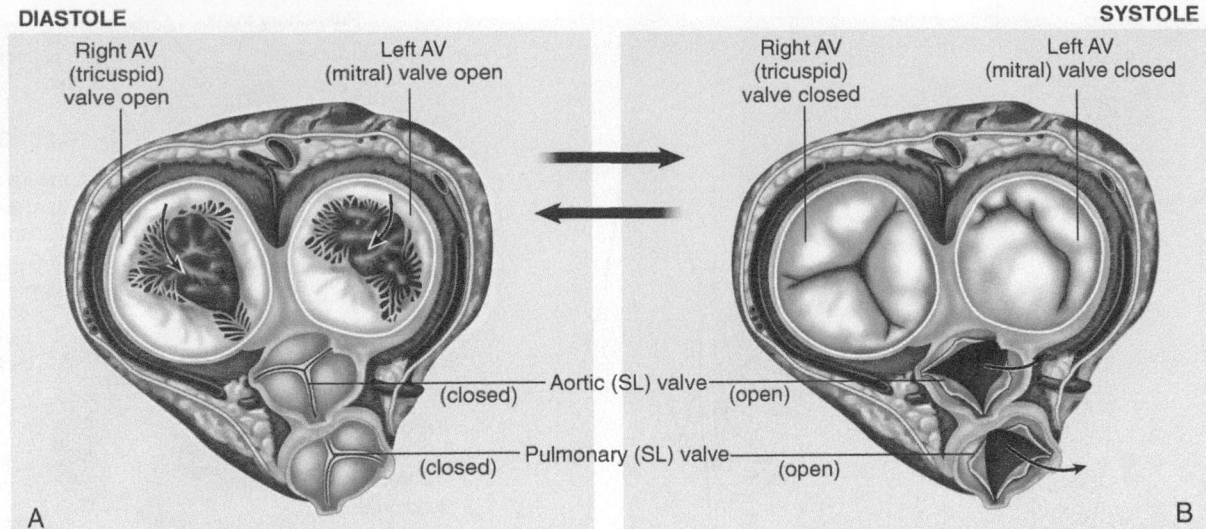

DIASTOLE   SYSTOLE

Right AV   Left AV   Right AV   Left AV
(tricuspid)   (mitral) valve open   (tricuspid)   (mitral) valve closed
valve open   valve closed

Aortic (SL) valve
(closed)   (open)

Pulmonary (SL) valve
(closed)   (open)

A   B

FIGURE 3-5 Structure of the cardiac valves, viewed from above. A, Ventricular diastole when semilunar valves are closed and atrioventricular valves are open. **B,** Ventricular systole when atrioventricular valves are closed and semilunar valves are open. (From Patton, K. T., & Thibodeau, G. A. [2016]. *Anatomy & physiology* [9th ed.]. St. Louis, MO: Mosby.)

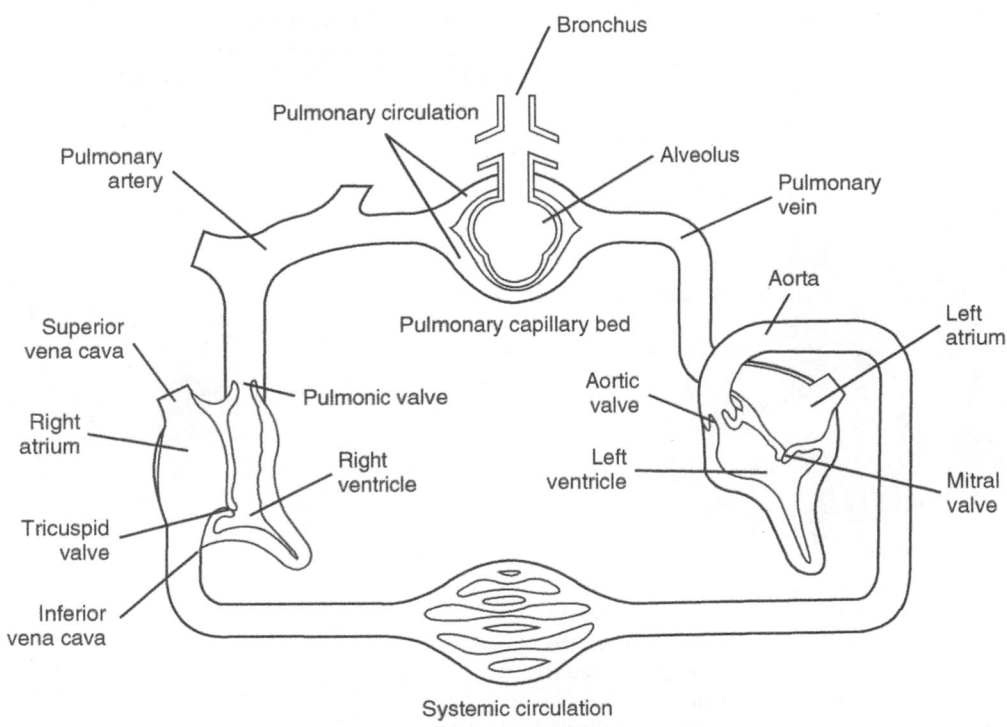

Bronchus

Pulmonary circulation

Pulmonary
artery   Alveolus

Pulmonary
vein

Aorta

Pulmonary capillary bed

Left
atrium

Superior
vena cava

Aortic
valve

Pulmonic valve

Right
atrium

Right
ventricle

Left
ventricle

Mitral
valve

Tricuspid
valve

Inferior
vena cava

Systemic circulation

FIGURE 3-6 Pathway of blood through the heart and the vascular system. (Courtesy Edwards Lifesciences, Irvine, CA.)

chordae tendineae. The commissure is the 0.5 to 1.0 cm area at the annulus where the cusps are joined together. They open passively during diastole and close when the papillary muscles contract during systole. Vibrations set in motion by the closing of the mitral and tricuspid valves cause the first heart sound, S_1. There are two components of the S_1 heart sound: the mitral valve component (M_1) and the tricuspid valve component (T_1). M_1 is first and loudest.

The aortic and pulmonic semilunar valves are located between each ventricle and the corresponding great vessel. The pulmonic valve is located between the right ventricle and the pulmonary artery. The aortic valve is located between the left ventricle and the aorta. The valves consist of an annulus and three cusps. Pressure gradients control the semilunar valves' function. The pressure pushes the valves open during systole and closes the valves during diastole. Vibrations set in motion by closure of the semilunar valves cause the second heart sound (S_2). There are two components of the S_2 heart sound: the aortic valve component (A_2) and the pulmonic valve component (P_2). A_2 is first and loudest.

The blood follows a specific pathway (Figure 3-6) through the heart and the vascular system. Blood flows through a

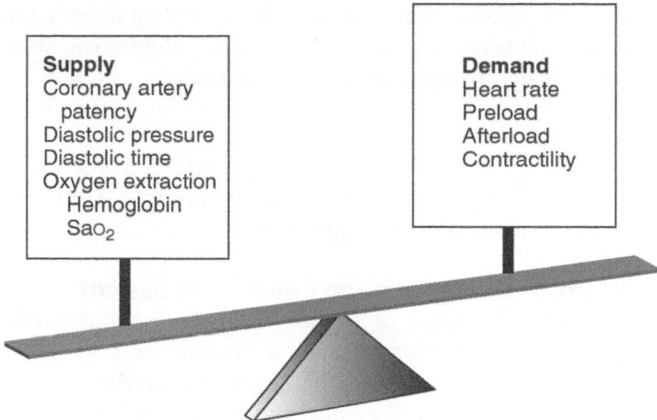

FIGURE 3-7 Factors affecting myocardial oxygen supply and myocardial oxygen demand.

continuous "closed" circuit from the superior and inferior venae cava → right atrium → tricuspid valve → right ventricle → pulmonic valve → pulmonary artery → pulmonary capillary bed → pulmonary veins → left atrium → mitral valve → left ventricle → aortic valve → aorta → arteries → arterioles → capillaries → venules → veins → venae cavae.

Coronary Vasculature

The coronary arteries are the first branch of arteries off the aorta located immediately outside the aortic valve. They lie on the epicardium, but the branches penetrate through to the myocardium and subendocardium. The aortic root pressure is the pressure in the aorta immediately outside the aortic valve and it is a significant component in coronary artery filling pressure. The normal coronary artery perfusion pressure (CAPP) is 60 to 80 mm Hg. Coronary blood flow is about 70 to 90 mL/min. The myocardium receives 5% of cardiac output and extracts 65% to 80% of oxygen in the blood at the basal rate. Because the heart uses most of the oxygen available in the coronary circulation, there is little oxygen reserve.

In response to the metabolic needs of the myocardium, local autoregulation determines blood flow through the coronary arteries. The coronary circulation has the ability to increase flow to meet added needs up to approximately six times the normal flow. Dilation of the coronary arteries increases myocardial blood flow. Coronary artery perfusion occurs as an effect of the cardiac cycle. Perfusion of the left ventricle occurs primarily during diastole because there is significant compression of musculature around intramuscular vessels during systole. Perfusion of the right ventricle occurs throughout the cardiac cycle, but perfusion is greatest during diastole. Hypotension and tachycardia, which induces a decrease in LV diastolic filling time and mechanical obstruction from coronary artery obstruction caused by clot, atherosclerotic plaque, or spasm, reduce coronary blood flow.

Heart rate and stroke volume determine myocardial oxygen demand (Figure 3-7). Preload, afterload, and contractility determine the stroke volume. Therefore, heart rate, preload, afterload, and contractility determine myocardial oxygen consumption. The patency of the coronary arteries, diastolic pressure, diastolic time, and oxygen content determine myocardial oxygen supply. Hemoglobin (Hgb)

and arterial oxygen saturation (SaO_2) determine oxygen content in the arterial blood. Imbalances between supply and demand determinants cause ischemia while prolonged imbalance causes infarction. Several conditions alter the myocardial oxygen supply and demand balance. Both cardiac (e.g., MI, HF) and noncardiac (e.g., COPD, pulmonary embolism) conditions create such an imbalance.

<table>
<tr><td colspan="2">**3.1   Learning Activity**</td></tr>
<tr><td colspan="2">Identify the determinants of myocardial oxygen supply and myocardial oxygen demand.</td></tr>
<tr><td>**Myocardial Oxygen Supply**</td><td>**Myocardial Oxygen Demand**</td></tr>
<tr><td></td><td></td></tr>
<tr><td></td><td></td></tr>
<tr><td></td><td></td></tr>
<tr><td></td><td></td></tr>
</table>

Answers to this activity can be found in the Answer Key.

Coronary Arteries

The distribution of coronary arteries (Figure 3-8) supplies oxygenated blood to all areas of the heart. The coronary arteries are end (i.e., terminal) arteries that supply a specific area of myocardium. Partial or temporary blockage of one of these arteries results in ischemia while complete or permanent occlusion causes infarction. The left coronary artery before bifurcation is referred to as the *left main coronary artery*. The left main coronary artery divides into the left anterior descending (LAD) and the left circumflex arteries (LCA). The LAD supplies the anterior left ventricle, the anterior two thirds of the interventricular septum, the apex of the left ventricle, and the bundle of His and bundle branches. The LCA supplies the left atrium, the SA node in 45% of hearts, and the AV node in 10% of hearts. The marginal (or obtuse marginal) branch supplies the lateral left ventricle and posterior left ventricle. The right coronary artery (RCA) supplies the right atrium, the SA node in 55% of hearts, the left posterior hemibundle (note the dual blood supply of the LAD and RCA), and the AV node in 90% of hearts. The marginal branch supplies the lateral right ventricle and inferior right ventricle. In RCA-dominant hearts (approximately 80% of hearts), a branch of the RCA referred to as the *posterior descending artery* supplies the anterior right ventricle, the inferior wall of the left ventricle, the posterior left ventricle, and the posterior third of the septum.

Collateral circulation consists of interarterial vessels that connect, or anastomose, with each other. The conditions of anemia, hypoxemia, and gradual coronary artery occlusion, such as those caused by arteriosclerosis, foster the development of collateral flow. Development of collateral circulation provides potential vascular connections to supply blood from another artery if stenosis of one of the coronary arteries exists; however, the collateral circulation cannot augment flow to meet acute requirements for increased flow.

3.2   Learning Activity

Identify the coronary artery that usually supplies the following structures. Identify the coronary artery as LAD (left anterior descending), LCA (left circumflex artery), or RCA (right coronary artery).

Structure	Coronary Artery
Anterior left ventricle	
AV node	
Bundle branches	
Inferior left ventricle	
Lateral left ventricle	
Left atrium	
Posterior left ventricle	
Right atrium	
Right ventricle	
SA node	
Septum	

Answers to this activity can be found in the Answer Key.

Coronary Veins

Most coronary veins empty into the coronary sinus, which empties into the right atrium. The thebesian veins drain some venous blood from the myocardium directly into the right atrium, right ventricle, and left ventricle rather than through the coronary sinus. This venous blood emptying directly into the left ventricle accounts for a normal physiologic shunt because it slightly decreases oxygen saturation.

Lymph Vessels

The main lymphatic cardiac channel empties into the pretracheal node and then into the right lymphatic duct. Cardiac contraction facilitates the drainage of lymph.

Electrophysiology and the Conduction System

There are three types of cardiac cells: (1) pacemaker cells, (2) electrical conducting cells, and (3) myocardial muscle cells. Certain cardiac cells have specific characteristics. Among these is *automaticity*, that is, the ability to initiate impulses regularly and spontaneously. Another is *excitability*, or the ability of the cardiac cells to respond to a stimulus. *Conductivity* is the ability of cardiac cells to respond to a cardiac impulse by transmitting the impulse along cell membranes. *Contractility* is the ability of the cardiac cells to respond to an impulse by muscle contraction. Finally, *rhythmicity* allows spontaneously generation of an action potential at a regular rate.

Stimulation of myocardial cells may be chemical, electrical, or mechanical. When the cell is stimulated, the electrical charge inside the cell becomes less negative and a depolarization occurs. Changes occur in the membrane when the cell reaches the threshold potential. The cell membrane's permeability is altered, and specialized channels in the membrane open, which allows the entry of sodium and calcium ions into the cell. Depolarization of cardiac chambers occurs from endocardium to epicardium. Repolarization of cardiac chambers occurs from epicardium to endocardium.

The action potential of myocardial cells (Figure 3-9) has phases delineated as phase 0 through phase 4. **Phase 4**, the resting membrane potential, coincides with the isoelectric line between T wave and QRS complex. The electrical charge within the cell is –80 to –95 mV. The sodium-potassium pump maintains the negativity. The sodium-potassium pump is an active transport system that

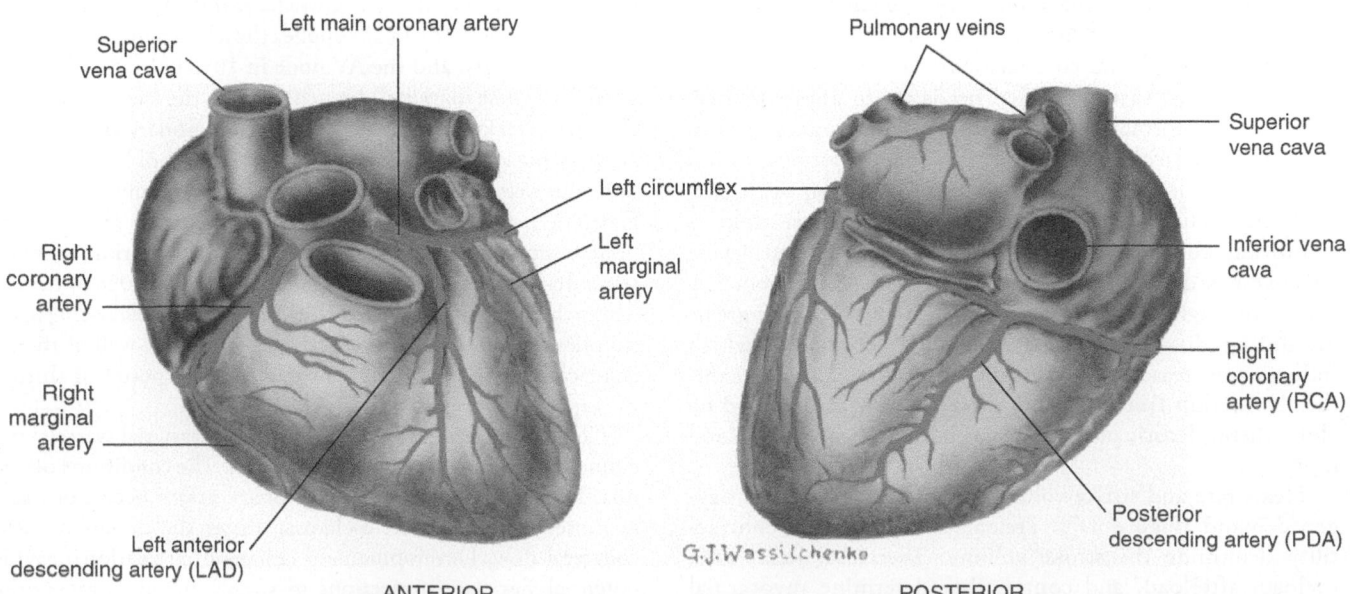

FIGURE 3-8 Anterior and posterior views of the coronary artery circulation and major vessels.
(From Urden, L., Stacy, K., & Lough, M. [2010]. *Critical care nursing: Diagnosis and management* [6th ed.]. St. Louis, MO: Mosby.)

requires energy to pump sodium out of the cell and potassium into the cell. When cellular energy (i.e., adenosine triphosphate [ATP]) supplies are low, such as during shock, failure to maintain this resting membrane potential occurs and irritability occurs.

During **phase 0**, rapid depolarization of the cell occurs. This phase coincides with the QRS complex and occurs when a stimulus is applied to the cell. Cell membrane permeability to sodium increases significantly so that sodium rushes into the cell (i.e., influx) and potassium begins to move out (i.e., efflux). If the stimulus is strong enough to reach a critical level known as the *threshold potential* (approximately –60 to –70 mV), then the cell responds entirely and depolarization occurs. This phase is referred to as the *sodium* (or *fast*) *channel*. Class I antidysrhythmic agents (e.g., procainamide, quinidine, lidocaine) block the influx of sodium into the cell, thereby preventing the achievement of threshold potential and depolarization.

Phase 1 involves brief, partial repolarization during which sodium channels close and potassium efflux continues. During **phase 2**, repolarization slows down causing a plateau. This phase coincides with the ST segment. Calcium influx keeps the cell isoelectric, but still depolarized, as potassium efflux occurs at approximately the same rate. This plateau allows a more sustained contraction and is referred to as the *calcium* (or *slow*) *channel*. Class IV antidysrhythmics (calcium channel blockers [e.g., verapamil, diltiazem]) block the movement of calcium and prolong repolarization and refractoriness.

During **phase 3**, the rate of repolarization accelerates suddenly. Potassium movement accelerates with the potassium efflux occurring at the beginning of phase 3 and exceeding the influx of calcium and potassium influx at the end of phase 3. At this point, repolarization is complete. Class III antidysrhythmics

(e.g., amiodarone, ibutilide, dofetilide) block the movement of potassium during this phase and prolong refractoriness.

The action potential of pacemaker cells (Figure 3-10) occurs because the pacemaker cells have the property of *automaticity*. They demonstrate slow diastolic depolarization due to a time-dependent leak of sodium into the cell. When enough sodium has entered the cell to reach the threshold potential, spontaneous depolarization occurs. The rate of diastolic depolarization determines the intrinsic rate of pacemaker cells. In the sinoatrial (SA) node, the rate is 60 to 100 times per minute. In the AV junction, the rate is 40 to 60 times per minute, while in the Purkinje fibers in the ventricles, the rate is 20 to 40 times per minute.

During what is called the *absolute refractory period* (Figure 3-11), a cell cannot be depolarized, no matter how strong the impulse is. This period correlates with the period from phase 0 through mid-phase 3 on the action potential and from the QRS complex to the peak of the T wave on the electrocardiogram (ECG). During the *relative refractory period*, the cell may respond provided the impulse is strong enough, but it may respond abnormally (e.g., R-on-T may cause ventricular tachycardia or ventricular fibrillation). This period correlates with late phase 3 of the action potential and the descending limb of the T wave on the ECG. The absolute refractory period plus the relative refractory period is referred to as the *effective refractory period*.

The Conduction System

The conduction system (Figure 3-12) begins with the SA node, which functions as the natural pacemaker of the heart because it has the fastest intrinsic rate (60 to 100 times per minute). The SA node is located in the right atrial wall near the opening of the superior vena cava. There are three internodal pathways

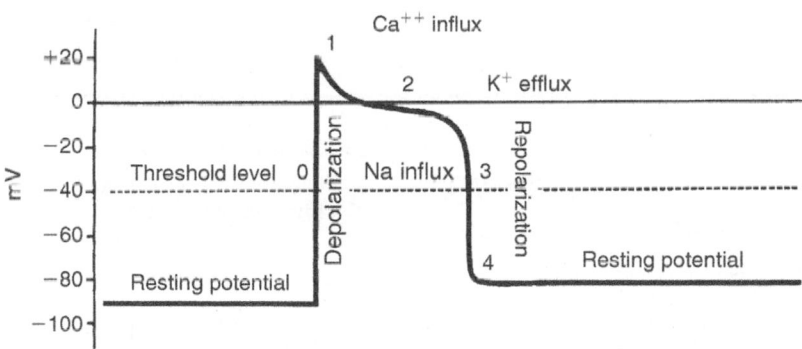

FIGURE 3-9 Action potential of a nonpacemaker cell. (From Thompson, J. M., et al. [2002]. *Mosby's clinical nursing* [5th ed.]. St. Louis, MO: Mosby.)

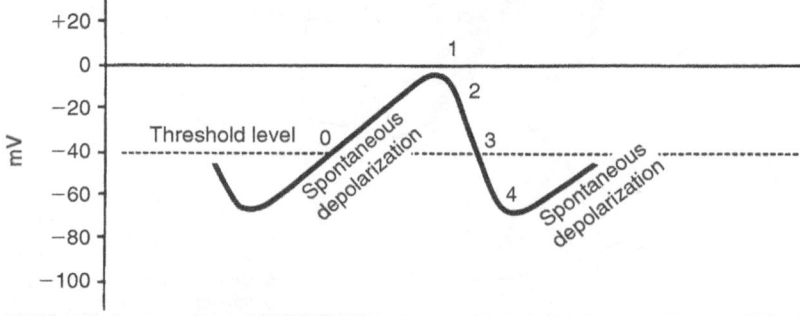

FIGURE 3-10 Action potential of a pacemaker cell. (From Thompson, J. M., et al. [2002]. *Mosby's clinical nursing* [5th ed.]. St. Louis, MO: Mosby.)

between the SA node and the AV node: the anterior tract (i.e., Bachmann's), the middle tract (i.e., Wenckebach's), and the posterior tract (i.e., Thorel's). Bachmann's bundle (the interatrial pathway) takes the impulse from the right atrium to the left atrium. The AV node, located at the base of the right atrium at the top of the interventricular septum, accounts for the physiologic delay of 0.08 to 0.12 seconds to allow the atria to depolarize completely, contract, and finish filling the ventricles before

the ventricles are stimulated. There are no pacemaker cells in the AV node. Its primary function is to slow down the impulse. The AV junction (the tissue surrounding the AV node and bundle of His that contains pacemaker cells) functions as a secondary pacemaker at an intrinsic rate of 40 to 60 times per minute.

The first portion of the intraventricular conduction system is the bundle of His. The bundle of His bifurcates into the right bundle branch (RBB), which takes the impulse to the right ventricular myocardium, and the left bundle branch (LBB), which takes the impulse into three hemibundles. The septal hemibundle depolarizes the interventricular septum in a left-to-right direction. The left anterior hemibundle (LAH) depolarizes the anterior and superior left ventricle and the left posterior hemibundle (LPH) depolarizes the posterior and inferior left ventricle. A block of the septal hemibundle does not cause a clinically identifiable situation, while blocks of the other two hemibundles are referred to as hemiblocks. The posterior hemibundle is thicker than the anterior hemibundle and has a dual blood supply, making it less susceptible to block than the anterior hemibundle. The three major branches of the intraventricular conduction system (i.e., RBB, LAH, LPH) are referred to as *fascicles* as in *unifascicular, bifascicular,* and *trifascicular block*.

The fascicles divide into the Purkinje fibers, which continue to divide and take the impulse through the ventricular walls to terminate in the subendocardial surface of the ventricles. These fibers act as a final tertiary pacemaker at the inherent rate of 20 to 40 times per minute if the upper pacemakers fail. Depolarization of cardiac chambers occurs from endocardium to epicardium. Repolarization of cardiac chambers occurs from epicardium to endocardium.

Muscle Mechanics
The cardiac muscle is similar to the skeletal muscle except that it contains more mitochondria than skeletal muscle. The cardiac

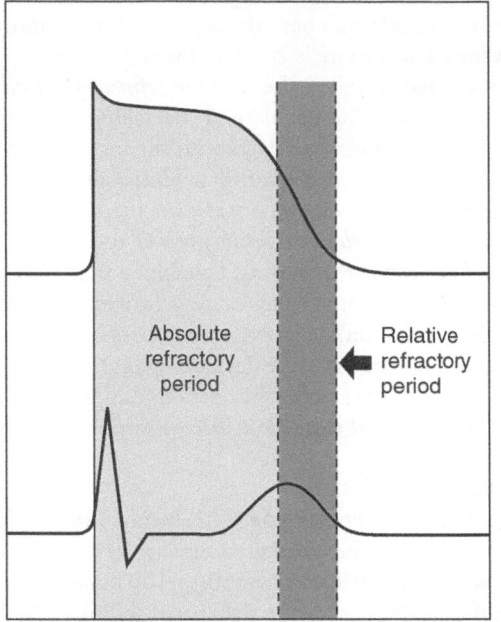

FIGURE 3-11 Absolute and relative refractory periods correlated with the myocardial cell action potential and with ECG tracing. (From Urden, L., Stacy, K., & Lough, M. [2016]. *Priorities in critical care nursing: Diagnosis and management* [7th ed.]. St. Louis, MO: Mosby.)

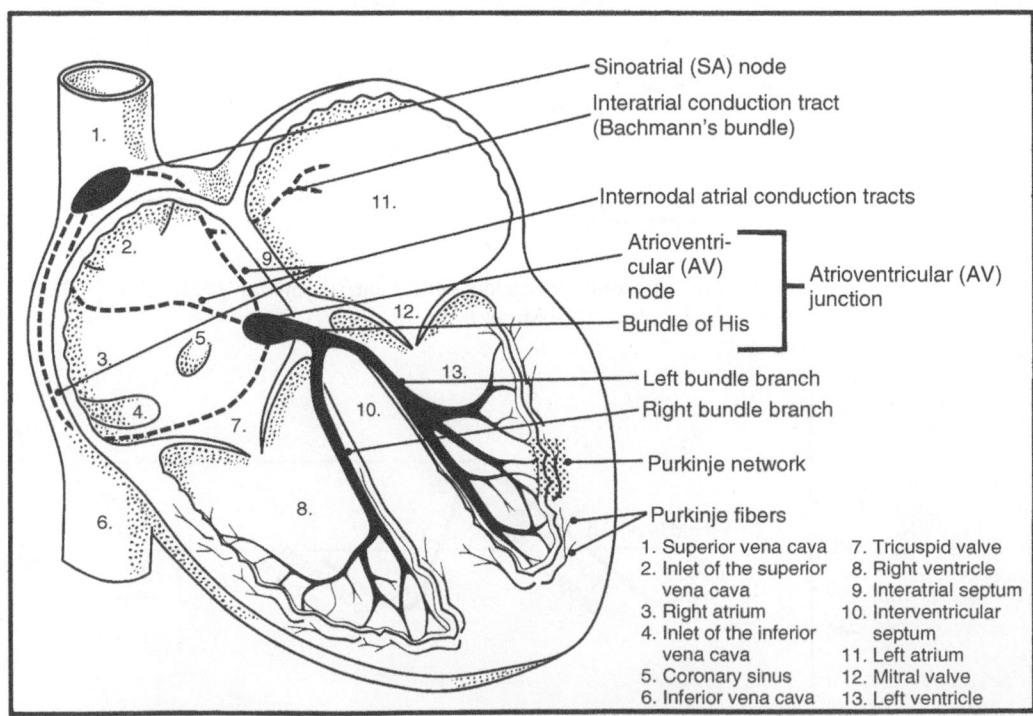

FIGURE 3-12 The conduction system. (From Huszar, R. J. [1994]. *Basic dysrhythmias: Interpretation and management* [2nd ed.]. St. Louis, MO: Mosby.)

muscle has greater ATP requirements because of the high energy requirements of the repetitive muscular action of the heart. The cardiac muscle remains contracted 150 to 300 times longer than the skeletal muscle. Intercalated disks lie between myocardial cells, offering low electrical impedance and allowing electrical stimuli to pass with ease from cell to cell. Stimulation of any muscle fiber results in stimulation of the entire muscle mass (an all-or-none response). The heart acts as if it were one muscle (i.e., a functional syncytium).

The ultrastructure of the cardiac muscle (Figure 3-13) contains a sarcomere, the basic contractile unit of the myocardium. The sarcomere measures between 1.6 and 2.2 μm and contains a centrally placed nucleus surrounded by intracellular protein fluid called sarcoplasm surrounded by a membrane called a sarcolemma. The sarcomere comprises two sets of overlapping myofilaments, including the thick myosin myofilament and the thin actin myofilament. Troponin and tropomyosin are regulatory proteins in the sarcomere that form a troponin-tropomyosin complex to cover the myosin binding sites and inhibit crossbridging of actin and myosin when the muscle is in a resting state. The sarcoplasmic reticulum, a continuation of the sarcolemma, penetrates the cell to form a complex tubular (T tubule) system surrounding each fibril. Calcium, necessary for the crossbridging of actin and myosin, is stored in the sarcoplasmic reticulum.

The excitation-contraction process involves the wave of depolarization that spreads through the conduction system to the myocardial muscle cell. This action potential reaches the sarcoplasmic reticulum, and the T tubules transmit the action potential from the sarcolemma to the interior of the cell. Calcium then enters the cell during phase 2 of the action potential through calcium channels in the sarcolemma and the T tubules, where the intracellular stores in the sarcoplasmic reticulum release more calcium.

Calcium binds with troponin to move the troponin and tropomyosin out of the way of the myosin binding sites. Actin and myosin myofilaments interact to form crossbridges that slide these overlapping myofilaments past one another, initiating shortening of the sarcomere. Multiple sarcomere shortening, muscle contraction, and ejection of blood from the chamber occur. The calcium pumped back into the sarcoplasmic reticulum dissociates the actin-myosin crossbridges. Without the antagonist effect of calcium, troponin and tropomyosin form a troponin-tropomyosin complex, inhibiting the crossbridging of actin and myosin and resulting in muscle relaxation.

The cardiac cycle (Figure 3-14) begins with systole, which is also called the contraction phase. During subphase 1, isovolumetric contraction occurs during which the pressure increases in the ventricle. No change in volume occurs because the AV valves are closed and the semilunar valves have not yet opened. For the semilunar valves to open, the ventricular pressure must exceed the pressure in the great vessel. This subphase accounts for two thirds of the oxygen consumption of the ventricle and follows the QRS complex.

Maximal ejection occurs during subphase 2. When the pressure in the ventricle exceeds the pressure in the great vessel, the semilunar valve opens and the heart rapidly ejects blood into

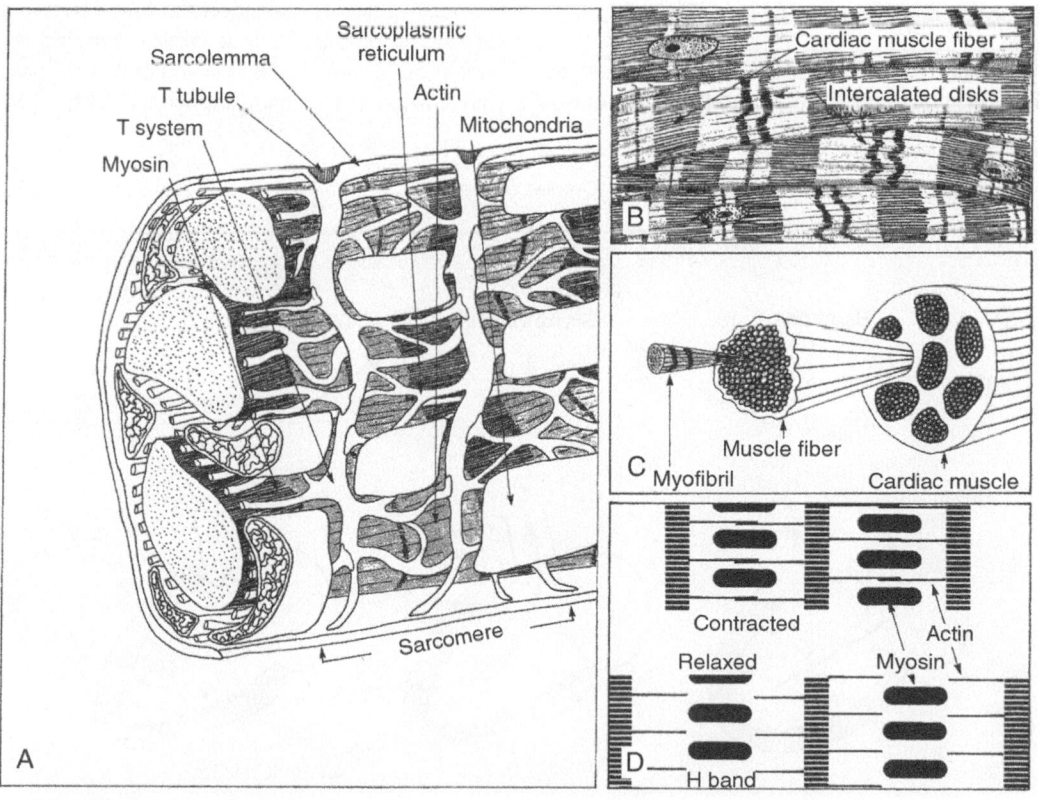

FIGURE 3-13 Cardiac muscle. A, The ultrastructure. **B,** Intercalated disks lie between muscle cells. **C,** Myofibrils form muscle fibers, which form cardiac muscle. **D,** Actin and myosin are myofilaments, which interlace in the presence of calcium to cause muscle contraction and shortening. (From Guzzetta C. E., & Dossey, B. M. [1992]. *Cardiovascular nursing: Holistic practice.* St. Louis, MO: Mosby.)

the great vessel. Aortic and pulmonary artery pressures increase rapidly and ventricular volume decreases sharply. This subphase occurs during the ST segment.

Reduced ejection (also referred to as *protodiastole*) occurs during subphase 3, when the heart slowly ejects blood from the ventricle to the great vessel, decreasing ventricular pressure and volume. When the pressure in the great vessel is greater than the pressure in the ventricle, the semilunar valve closes and systole ends. This subphase occurs during the T wave.

Diastole is the relaxation phase. During subphase 1, isovolumetric relaxation occurs and ventricular pressure decreases, but volume does not change because the semilunar valves have closed and the AV valves have not yet opened. This subphase occurs after the T wave. Rapid filling occurs during subphase 2, and the AV valves open and blood rushes into the ventricles. Atrial and ventricular pressures decrease and ventricular volume increases. Ventricular pressure is less than atrial pressure. This subphase occurs during the TP interval.

During subphase 3, there is reduced filling (also referred to as *diastasis*). Atrial and ventricular pressures slowly increase and ventricular volumes increase with slow filling of the ventricles. Coronary artery blood flow is optimal. This subphase occurs during the TP interval.

During subphase 4, atrial contraction, also known as *atrial kick*, occurs. This final push of blood into the ventricle usually accounts for 15% to 30% of diastolic filling volume but may be as high as 50% when left ventricular filling is impeded (e.g., by mitral stenosis). Atrial pressure decreases, while ventricular volume and pressure increase during subphase 4. This subphase occurs after P wave.

Regulation of Cardiac Function
Intrinsic Control of the Heart

The heart rate (HR) and stroke volume (SV) determine the cardiac output (Figure 3-15). The HR is the number of times per minute that the ventricles contract. The stroke volume is the volume of blood pumped by the heart with each beat. Preload, afterload, and contractility determine the stroke volume.

Various factors may affect the four determinants (Table 3-1) of cardiac output. Various clinical conditions and treatments can increase or decrease each of the defined parameters of heart rate, preload, afterload, and contractility. The hemodynamic

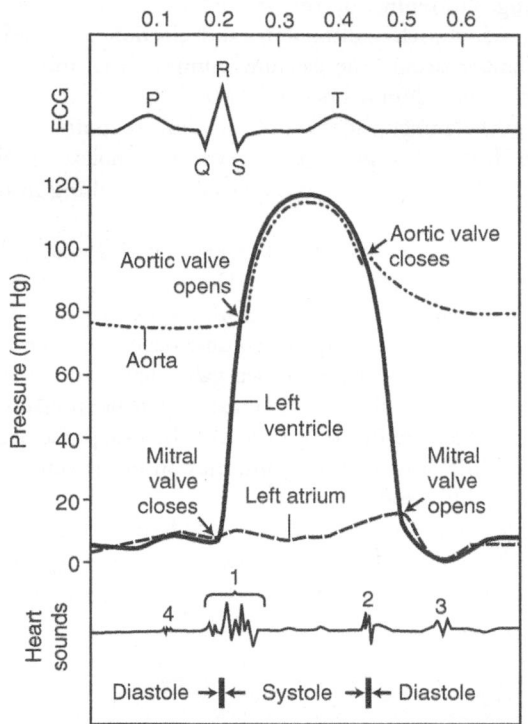

FIGURE 3-14 Wiggers diagram demonstrates the cardiac cycle, showing ECG events, heart sounds, and pressure curves.

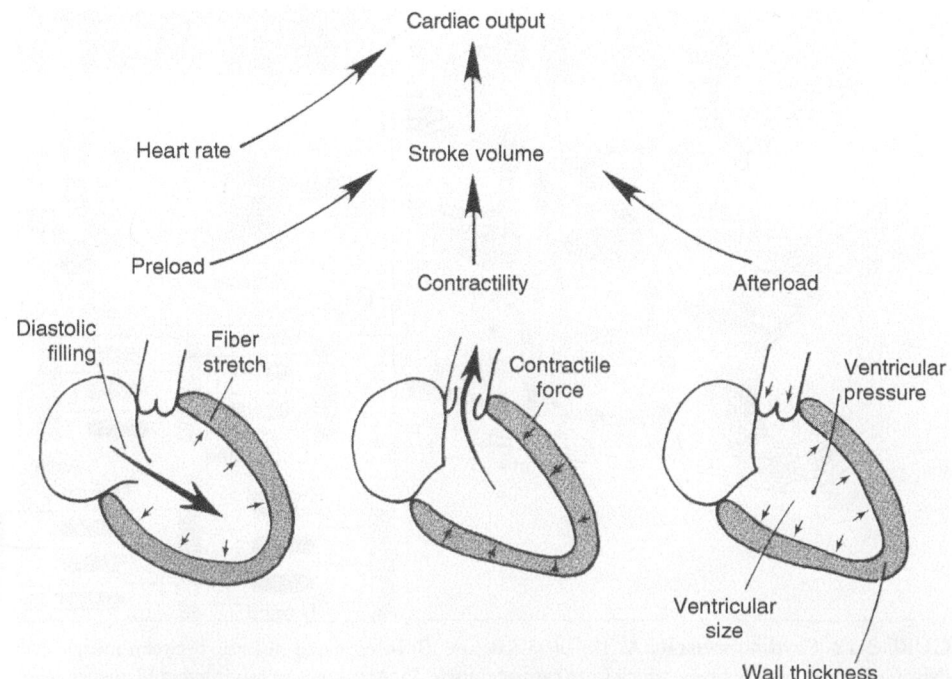

FIGURE 3-15 Determinants of cardiac output. (From Price, S., & Wilson, L. [2003]. *Pathophysiology: Clinical concepts of disease processes* [6th ed.]. St. Louis, MO: Mosby.)

| TABLE 3-1 | Determinants of Cardiac Output |

Parameter	Conditions		Treatments	
	Increased	**Decreased**	**To Increase**	**To Decrease**

Heart rate: evaluated by palpation of pulse	• SNS stimulation (e.g., exercise, fever, infection, pain, anxiety, hypovolemia or hypervolemia, most physiologic or psychologic stressors)
	• Drug effects (e.g., epinephrine, dopamine)
		• PNS (vagal) stimulation (e.g., Valsalva maneuver, coughing, suctioning, vomiting, carotid stimulation)
		• Conduction abnormalities (e.g., sinus arrest or block, second- or third-degree AV blocks) caused by ischemia, infarction, or inflammation
		• Drug effects (e.g., beta-blockers, digoxin)
			• Treatment of cause (e.g., reperfusion therapies for myocardial infarction, antiemetics for vomiting)
			• Parasympatholytic drugs (e.g., atropine)
			• Sympathomimetic drugs (e.g., epinephrine)
			• Pacemaker
				• Treatment of cause (e.g., antipyretics for fever, analgesics for pain, anxiolytics for anxiety)
				• Dependent on rhythm:
				  • Cardiac glycosides (e.g., digoxin)
				  • Beta-blockers (e.g., propranolol, esmolol)
				  • Calcium channel blockers (e.g., verapamil, diltiazem)
				  • Other antidysrhythmic drugs dependent on rhythm
				• Vagal maneuvers
				  • Overdrive pacemaker
				  • Ablation
				• Cardioversion or defibrillation

Preload: evaluated by PAOP (LV) and RAP (RV)	• HF • Hypervolemia • Bradydysrhythmias	• Hypovolemia • Excessive vasodilation (e.g., vasogenic shock) • Increased intrathoracic pressure (e.g., positive pressure mechanical ventilation) • Cardiac tamponade • Right ventricular failure or infarction (LV) • Tachydysrhythmias • Loss of atrial contraction (e.g., atrial fibrillation)	• Fluids • Isotonic crystalloids (e.g., normal [0.9%] saline, lactated Ringer's) • Colloids (e.g., albumin, plasma protein fraction [PPF], dextran, hetastarch) • Blood and/or blood products • Adjustment of vasodilator dosage	• Diuretics (e.g., furosemide) • Venous vasodilators (e.g., nitroglycerin, morphine sulfate, nitroprusside, calcium channel blockers [e.g., nifedipine]) • ACE inhibitors (e.g., captopril, enalapril) or angiotensin receptor blockers (ARBs) (e.g., losartan, valsartan) • Nesiritide (Natrecor)
Afterload: evaluated by calculation of SVR and SVRI (LV), and PVR and PVRI (RV)	• Vasoconstriction as from SNS stimulation or vasopressors • Hypertension • Aortic stenosis • Hypercoagulability • Pulmonary hypertension (RV)	• Hypotension • Vasodilation (e.g., vasogenic shock such as septic shock, neurogenic shock, or anaphylactic shock)	• Adjustment of vasodilator dosage • Vasopressors (e.g., phenylephrine, norepinephrine, epinephrine, dopamine, vasopressin)	• Arterial vasodilators (e.g., nitroprusside, nitroglycerin >1 mcg/kg/min, hydralazine, calcium channel blockers [e.g., nifedipine], alpha blockers [e.g., phentolamine, labetalol]) • ACE inhibitors (e.g., captopril, enalapril) or angiotensin receptor blockers (ARBs) (e.g., losartan, valsartan), phosphodiesterase (PDE) inhibitors (e.g., milrinone, inamrinone) • Intraaortic balloon pump • Right ventricle specifically: oxygen, pulmonary vasodilators (e.g., aminophylline, nitric oxide, epoprostenol [Flolan], bosentan [Tracleer])

Continued

TABLE 3-1   **Determinants of Cardiac Output—cont'd**

Parameter	Conditions		Treatments	
	Increased	Decreased	To Increase	To Decrease
Contractility: evaluated by calculation of stroke volume and LVSWI (LV) and RVSWI (RV)	• SNS stimulation (see heart rate for selected factors that stimulate SNS) • Sympathomimetic drugs (e.g., epinephrine)	• Myocardial ischemia or infarction • Cardiomyopathy • Hypoxemia • Acidosis • Shock (i.e., myocardial depressant factor) • Drug adverse effects (e.g., barbiturates, anesthetics, beta-blockers, calcium channel blockers, most antidysrhythmics)	• Cardiac glycosides (e.g., digoxin) • Sympathomimetics (e.g., dobutamine, dopamine at medium [~5 mcg/kg/min] dose) • PDE inhibitors (e.g., milrinone, inamrinone) • Glucagon	• Beta-blockers (e.g., propranolol, metoprolol, esmolol) • Calcium channel blockers (e.g., diltiazem, verapamil)

parameters may also be evaluated invasively using a pulmonary artery catheter. Understanding the hemodynamic concepts (see Appendix B) related to invasive evaluation is important to rendering quality patient care to a patient in the progressive care unit even though the actual hemodynamic procedures used to obtain these parameters are not considered typical assessment methods done at this acuity level. Hemodynamic monitoring is a procedure performed in a critical care unit, operating room, or catheterization laboratory. Use of invasive monitoring may be required for early detection of physiologic changes and responses to pharmacologic agents, fluids, and other therapeutic modalities.

SIDEBAR 3-1

Definitions Related to Cardiac Function

Cardiac output (CO) is the amount of blood ejected by the ventricle in 1 minute.

Cardiac index (CI) is the cardiac output indexed for differences in body size by dividing by body surface area.

Stroke volume (SV) is the amount of blood ejected by the ventricle with each contraction; also defined as the difference between the end-diastolic volume and the end-systolic volume.

Stroke index (SI) is the stroke volume indexed for differences in body size by dividing by body surface area.

Ejection fraction (EF) is the percentage of blood in the ventricle ejected during systole; normal this is 55% to 75%. EF is a good reflection of left ventricle performance.

Afterload is the pressure against which the ventricle must pump; the pressure required to open the semilunar valve.

Preload is the volume of blood in the ventricle at the end of diastole; it determines the stretch on the myofibrils and the subsequent force of the next contraction (according to Starling's Law of the Heart).

To determine the heart rate, count the number of pulses palpable in 1 minute. The radial, brachial, femoral, or carotid pulse is most often used. When auscultating the apical or if

an ECG monitor is used to evaluate the HR, it is important to confirm a palpable pulse with each audible heart sound or QRS. If the heart rate is less than 50 beats/min or greater than 150 beats/min, the cardiac output often falls and increases the tendency for dysrhythmias. Although an increase in heart rate may increase cardiac output, an increase in the heart rate greater than 120 beats/min has two significant disadvantages. First, the time allowed for diastole is reduced, which reduces diastolic filling volume and therefore stroke volume. In addition, this heart rate tends to increase myocardial oxygen demand more than the increase in coronary blood flow, potentially causing ischemia, especially in patients with coronary artery disease.

Preload is the stretch on the myofibrils at the end of diastole. The ventricular volume affects the degree of myofibril stretch. While preload is a volume concept, traditionally it has been evaluated by the pressure in the ventricle at the end of diastole. The compliance of the ventricle influences the relationship between volume and pressure. In a normally compliant ventricle, there is a linear relationship between volume and pressure. In a noncompliant ventricle, there is a disproportionate increase in pressure with changes in volume, referred to as *diastolic dysfunction*. Some causes of noncompliance of the ventricle include myocardial ischemia or infarction, ventricular hypertrophy, hypertrophic cardiomyopathy, restrictive pericarditis, and cardiac tamponade.

The clinical findings of jugular venous distention (JVD), hepatomegaly, and peripheral edema indicate high RV preload. Flat neck veins when the patient is flat and oliguria indicate low RV preload. Auscultation of an S_3 over the apex and crackles over the lung bases along with dyspnea indicate high LV preload. Clinical indications of hypoperfusion (Table 3-2) may indicate low LV preload, though they may also indicate poor contractility.

Atrial pressure correlates to end-diastolic pressure for the respective ventricle so RV preload correlates to central venous pressure (CVP) or right atrial pressure (RAP) if there is no tricuspid valve disease. A catheter in the superior vena cava, usually a multilumen catheter, measures CVP in centimeters of H_2O pressure. Normal CVP is 3 to 8 cm/H_2O. The effect

TABLE 3-2	Clinical Indications of Hypoperfusion			
Normal	**Subclinical Hypoperfusion**	**Clinical Hypoperfusion**	**Shock**
CI 2.5-4.0 L/min/m²	CI 2.2-2.5 L/min/m²	CI 2.0-2.2 L/min/m²	CI <2.0 L/min/m²
Normal	• No clinical indications of hypoperfusion though an expert nurse may detect subtle changes in the patient • Hypoperfusion at this stage is detected by hemodynamic monitoring	• Tachycardia • Narrowed pulse pressure • Tachypnea • Cool skin • Oliguria • Diminished bowel sounds • Restlessness → confusion	• Dysrhythmias • Hypotension • Tachypnea • Cold, clammy skin • Anuria • Absent bowel sounds • Lethargy → coma

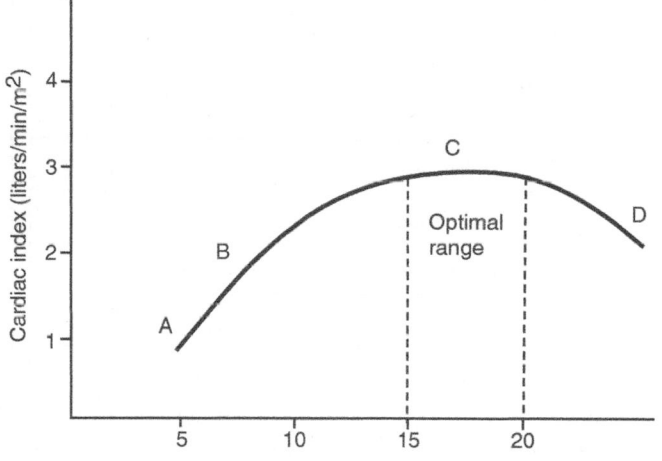

FIGURE 3-16 Relationship between PAOP and cardiac index. A, Understretched myofibrils resulting in decreased contractility and cardiac index. **B,** Normal stretched myofibrils resulting in normal (but suboptimal) cardiac index. **C,** Optimally stretched myofibrils resulting in optimal cardiac index. **D,** Overstretched myofibrils resulting in decreased contractility and cardiac index. (From Dennison, R. D. [2013]. *Pass CCRN!* [4th ed]. St. Louis, MO: Elsevier.)

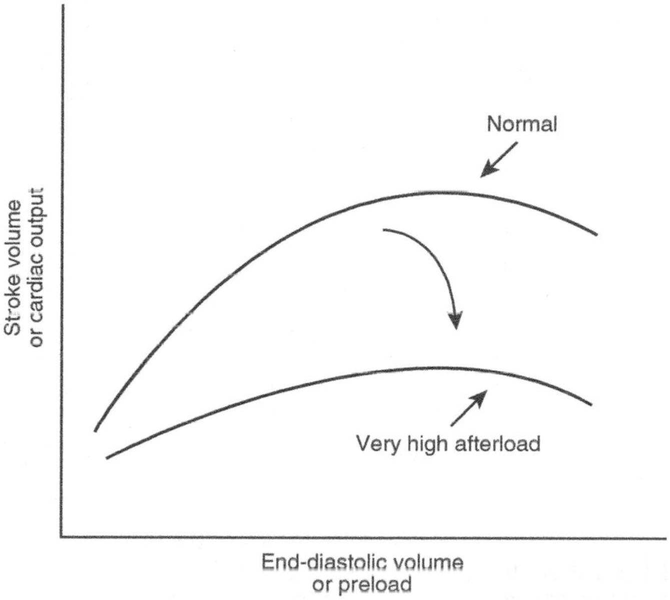

FIGURE 3-17 Relationship between afterload and stroke volume. (From Hicks, G. H. [2000]. *Cardiopulmonary anatomy and physiology.* Philadelphia, PA: Saunders.)

of preload on stroke volume and cardiac output is understood through Starling's Law of the Heart and the Frank-Starling mechanism: *Within physiologic limits, the greater the stretch on the myofibrils, the greater the force of the subsequent contraction* (Figure 3-16). Both understretching and overstretching of the myofibrils result in a less than optimal contraction. Preload also affects myocardial oxygen consumption: as preload increases, myocardial oxygen consumption increases.

Afterload describes the pressure against which the ventricle must pump to open the semilunar valve. Vascular resistance, ventricular diameter, and the mass and viscosity of blood influence afterload. Afterload affects stroke volume (Figure 3-17); as afterload increases, stroke volume decreases. The effect of afterload on stroke volume is due to the fact that the maximum pressure that the heart can develop is lower at lesser ventricular volumes. Therefore if the systolic pressure is lower, the heart will be able to contract to a smaller volume at the end of systole. This will result in an improved stroke volume. Conversely, if the systolic pressure is higher, the heart will be unable to contract to as small a volume at the end of systole and will decrease the

stroke volume index. Afterload also affects myocardial oxygen consumption; as afterload increases, myocardial oxygen consumption increases.

A loud P_2 may indicate high RV afterload. A loud A_2 plus cool, pale extremities, and high systemic arterial diastolic pressure indicate high LV afterload. A low systemic arterial diastolic pressure indicates low LV afterload, which affects stroke volume and cardiac output. *Contractility* is the force and velocity of the ejection of blood from the ventricle independent of preload and afterload. Contractility affects stroke volume and cardiac output (Figure 3-18) according to Laplace's law, which states that the contractile force generated within a chamber depends on the radius of the chamber and the thickness of its walls; therefore, the smaller the radius and the thicker the wall, the greater the force of contraction. Endogenous catecholamines (e.g., epinephrine) or other inotropic agents (e.g., digoxin, dobutamine) also significantly affect contractility. As contractility increases, myocardial oxygen consumption increases. Because myocardial oxygen consumption decreases with decreased contractility, patients with coronary artery disease and myocardial ischemia receive treatment with drugs to decrease contractility, such as beta-blockers. Clinical indicators of hypoperfusion (see Table 3-2) are evident in patients with decreased contractility. Multiple gated acquisition (MUGA) scan or Doppler echocardiograph assesses the ejection fraction. In the progressive care unit, nurses use the clinical indicators to assess the patient's heart rate, preload, afterload, and contractility.

3.3   Learning Activity

Identify the *primary* factor or factors affected in each condition and the primary effect or effects of each treatment; indicate increase or decrease of heart rate, preload, afterload, or contractility by appropriate arrows (↑ or ↓). (**Note:** Secondary sympathetic nervous system responses may occur in any of these conditions.)

Conditions

Condition				
Aortic stenosis	___Heart Rate	___Preload	___Afterload	___Contractility
Bradydysrhythmias	___Heart Rate	___Preload	___Afterload	___Contractility
Cardiac tamponade	___Heart Rate	___Preload	___Afterload	___Contractility
Cardiogenic shock	___Heart Rate	___Preload	___Afterload	___Contractility
Cardiomyopathy	___Heart Rate	___Preload	___Afterload	___Contractility
HF	___Heart Rate	___Preload	___Afterload	___Contractility
Hypertension	___Heart Rate	___Preload	___Afterload	___Contractility
Hypovolemia	___Heart Rate	___Preload	___Afterload	___Contractility
Left ventricular MI	___Heart Rate	___Preload	___Afterload	___Contractility
Neurogenic shock	___Heart Rate	___Preload	___Afterload	___Contractility
Pulmonary hypertension	___Heart Rate	___Preload	___Afterload	___Contractility
Right ventricular MI	___Heart Rate	___Preload	___Afterload	___Contractility
Septic shock—early	___Heart Rate	___Preload	___Afterload	___Contractility
Septic shock—late	___Heart Rate	___Preload	___Afterload	___Contractility
Tachydysrhythmias	___Heart Rate	___Preload	___Afterload	___Contractility

Treatments

Treatment				
Aminophylline	___Heart Rate	___Preload	___Afterload	___Contractility
Digoxin (Lanoxin)	___Heart Rate	___Preload	___Afterload	___Contractility
Dobutamine (Dobutrex)	___Heart Rate	___Preload	___Afterload	___Contractility
Dopamine (3-5 mcg/kg/min)	___Heart Rate	___Preload	___Afterload	___Contractility
Dopamine (5-10 mcg/kg/min)	___Heart Rate	___Preload	___Afterload	___Contractility
Dopamine (>10 mcg/kg/min)	___Heart Rate	___Preload	___Afterload	___Contractility
Fluid challenge	___Heart Rate	___Preload	___Afterload	___Contractility
Furosemide (Lasix)	___Heart Rate	___Preload	___Afterload	___Contractility

3.3 Learning Activity—cont'd

Treatments

Intraaortic balloon pump	___Heart Rate	___Preload	___Afterload	___Contractility
Isoproterenol (Isuprel)	___Heart Rate	___Preload	___Afterload	___Contractility
Milrinone (Primacor)	___Heart Rate	___Preload	___Afterload	___Contractility
Nesiritide (Natrecor)	___Heart Rate	___Preload	___Afterload	___Contractility
Nitroglycerin	___Heart Rate	___Preload	___Afterload	___Contractility
Nitroprusside (Nipride)	___Heart Rate	___Preload	___Afterload	___Contractility
Phenylephrine (Neo-Synephrine)	___Heart Rate	___Preload	___Afterload	___Contractility
Propranolol (Inderal)	___Heart Rate	___Preload	___Afterload	___Contractility
Vasopressin (Pitressin)	___Heart Rate	___Preload	___Afterload	___Contractility

Answers to this activity can be found in the Answer Key.

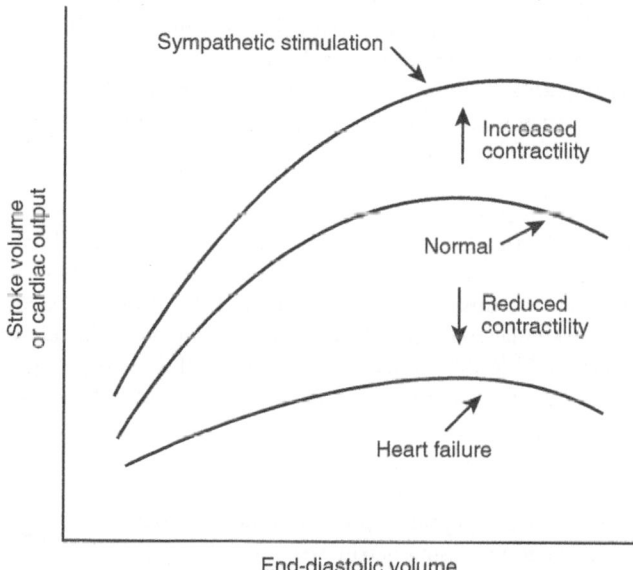

FIGURE 3-18 Relationship between contractility and stroke volume. (From Hicks, G. H. [2000]. *Cardiopulmonary anatomy and physiology*. Philadelphia, PA: Saunders.)

TABLE 3-3 **Sympathetic Nervous System (Adrenergic) Receptors and Effects**

Receptor	Location of Receptors	Effects
Alpha$_1$	Vessels	Vasoconstriction of most vessels, especially the arterioles
Beta$_1$	Heart	Increase in heart rate (chronotropic effect), contractility (inotropic effect), and conductivity (dromotropic effect)
Beta$_2$	Bronchial and vascular smooth muscle	Bronchodilation, vasodilation
Dopaminergic	Renal and mesenteric artery bed	Dilation of renal and mesenteric arteries

Neurologic Control of the Heart

The autonomic nervous system (ANS) influences heart rate, contractility, and the rate of conductivity. The ANS consists of the sympathetic nervous system (SNS) and parasympathetic nervous system (PNS) branches. The SNS is frequently referred to as "fight or flight." Physiologic or psychological stress stimulates this branch. During these times, the SNS releases chemicals called neurotransmitters, such as epinephrine and norepinephrine, from the adrenal gland. The neurotransmitters stimulate the adrenergic receptors (Table 3-3). Stimulation of these receptors causes positive chronotropic, inotropic, and dromotropic effects. Adrenergic drugs (Table 3-4) also stimulate these receptors. These drugs are used in situations such as cardiac arrest, shock, or to open the airways during an asthma attack or allergic reaction.

The PNS maintains a steady state. The PNS causes negative chronotropic, inotropic, and dromotropic effects. Although the cardiovascular effects of the PNS are generally undesirable in acutely ill patients, they may decrease the myocardial oxygen consumption by up to 50%. Parasympatholytic (i.e., vagolytic) agents, such as atropine, block these effects.

Chemoreceptors are located in the carotic and aortic bodies. They are sensitive to Pao$_2$, Paco$_2$, and pH so hypoxia,

TABLE 3-4	Sympathomimetic Agents and Receptor Stimulation		
Drug	**Alpha$_1$**	**Beta$_1$**	**Beta$_2$**
Phenyleph-rine	++++	0	0
Norepi-nephrine	++++	++	0
Epinephrine	++++	++++	++
Dopamine	++ >5 mcg/kg/min; +++ >10 mcg/kg/min	++++ <10 mcg/kg/min	+
Dobutamine	+	++++	++
Isoproterenol	0	++++	++++

hypercapnia, and acidosis cause changes in heart rate and ventilatory rate.

Baroreceptors located in the carotid sinus and aortic arch stimulate the baroreceptor reflex (i.e., the aortic reflex). They are sensitive to increased arterial pressure. Medullary discharge causes vagal stimulation, which results in a decrease in heart rate and contractility, with decreases in cardiac output and arterial pressure.

The Bainbridge reflex (i.e., the atrial reflex) occurs when the heart responds to an increase in atrial pressure. Baroreceptors located in the right atrium are sensitive to increased venous pressure and right atrial pressure. Medullary discharge decreases vagal stimulation. Decreased parasympathetic tone causes an increase in heart rate and cardiac output, which decreases venous pressure and right atrial pressure.

Inspiration decreases intrathoracic pressure, increasing venous return to the right side of the heart, which causes the respiratory reflex. When the increased venous return reaches the left side of the heart, left ventricular cardiac output increases. The increase in cardiac output in turn increases arterial blood pressure and decreases the heart rate through stimulation of the baroreceptors. This process is at least partly responsible for sinus dysrhythmia. Another contributor is the interaction between the respiratory and cardiac centers in the medulla.

3.4   Learning Activity

Match the receptor of the sympathetic nervous system with its physiologic effect.

_____ 1. Increase in heart rate, contractility, conductivity
_____ 2. Dilation of the renal and mesenteric arteries
_____ 3. Vasoconstriction
_____ 4. Vasodilation and bronchodilation

a. Alpha$_1$
b. Beta$_1$
c. Beta$_2$
d. Dopaminergic

Answers to this activity can be found in the Answer Key.

3.5   Learning Activity

Identify which sympathomimetic (adrenergic) drug causes the most powerful stimulation of each of these receptors.

_____ 1. Alpha$_1$
_____ 2. Beta$_1$
_____ 3. Beta$_2$
_____ 4. Dopaminergic

a. Albuterol (Proventil)
b. Fenoldopam (Corlopam)
c. Phenylephrine (Neo-Synephrine)
d. Dobutamine (Dobutrex)

Answers to this activity can be found in the Answer Key.

Endocrine Function of the Heart
Atrial Natriuretic Peptide
Specialized atrial muscle cells produce, store, and release atrial natriuretic peptide (ANP). The primary cause of ANP release is increased atrial stretch. Other causes of ANP release include an acute increase in intravascular volume, exercise, and endogenous or exogenous vasopressors. ANP is an important regulator of blood volume and BP. It inhibits sodium transport in the collecting ducts of the kidney, resulting in increased urine output, and acts as an antagonist to angiotensin II, epinephrine, and endothelin, resulting in a decrease in heart rate and vasodilation. ANP also blocks the renin-angiotensin-aldosterone system (RAAS), resulting in sodium and water excretion, and decreases proliferation of cardiac fibroblasts and smooth muscle cells, resulting in the prevention of ventricular remodeling.

Brain Natriuretic Peptide
Brain natriuretic peptide (BNP) was first discovered in animal brain tissue, but it is produced by ventricular muscle tissue. Intravascular volume triggers the release of BNP. Its actions and effects are similar to those of ANP with dilation of both arteries and veins. Clinically, the measurement of BNP is a diagnostic study used for HF. The hormone is also a therapeutic pharmacologic agent (i.e., nesiritide [Natrecor]) for HF.

C-type Natriuretic Peptide
C-type natriuretic peptide is present in the lowest concentration of the circulating plasma natriuretic peptides. Distributed predominantly in the central nervous system (CNS), kidneys, and endothelial cells, the peptide has marked vasodilation effects, but no natriuretic effect.

Endothelin
Endothelin is a potent vasoconstrictive peptide produced by endothelial cells. It causes an increase in renin, aldosterone, antidiuretic hormone, and SNS, which all contribute to an increase in systemic vascular resistance.

The Vascular System
The vascular system serves to supply blood, nutrients, and hormones to the tissues while removing metabolic wastes from the tissues. Resistance to flow (i.e., Poiseuille formula) is dependent on several factors: the length of the vessel, the radius of the vessel, and the viscosity of the blood. Neurologic stimulation,

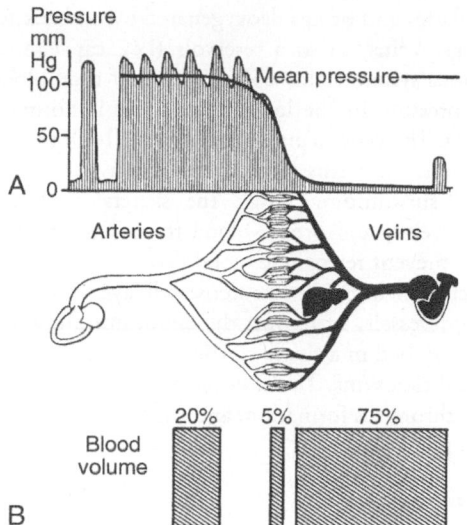

FIGURE 3-19 Components of the vascular system. A, Mean pressure in components of vascular system. **B,** Volume in components of vascular system. (From Rushmer, R. [1976]. *Cardiovascular dynamics* [4th ed.]. Philadelphia, PA: Saunders.)

which affects vascular tone, and features that cause turbulence within the vascular lumen, such as bifurcations or protrusions from the vessel wall into the vessel lumen (e.g., atherosclerosis), also influence blood flow through the body.

There are approximately 5 L of total circulating blood volume in the adult body moving through the vascular system. Components of the vascular system (Figure 3-19) include the arteries, arterioles, and capillaries. The arteries are the delivery system that distributes and regulates the amount of oxygenated blood flow to various tissue beds. Arteries are able to stretch during systole and recoil during diastole. The arterial system is a high-pressure circuit.

The layers of the arterial wall (Figure 3-20) consist of the intima, the media, and the adventitia. The intima is a thin lining of endothelium and a small amount of elastic tissue. It decreases resistance to flow and minimizes the chance of platelet aggregation. The media consists of smooth muscle and elastic tissue and changes the lumen diameter as needed. The adventitia is composed of connective tissue that strengthens and shapes the vessels. The arteries are a strong, compliant, high-pressure circuit. The elastic-walled arterial vessels that branch off the aorta are able to stretch during systole and recoil during diastole.

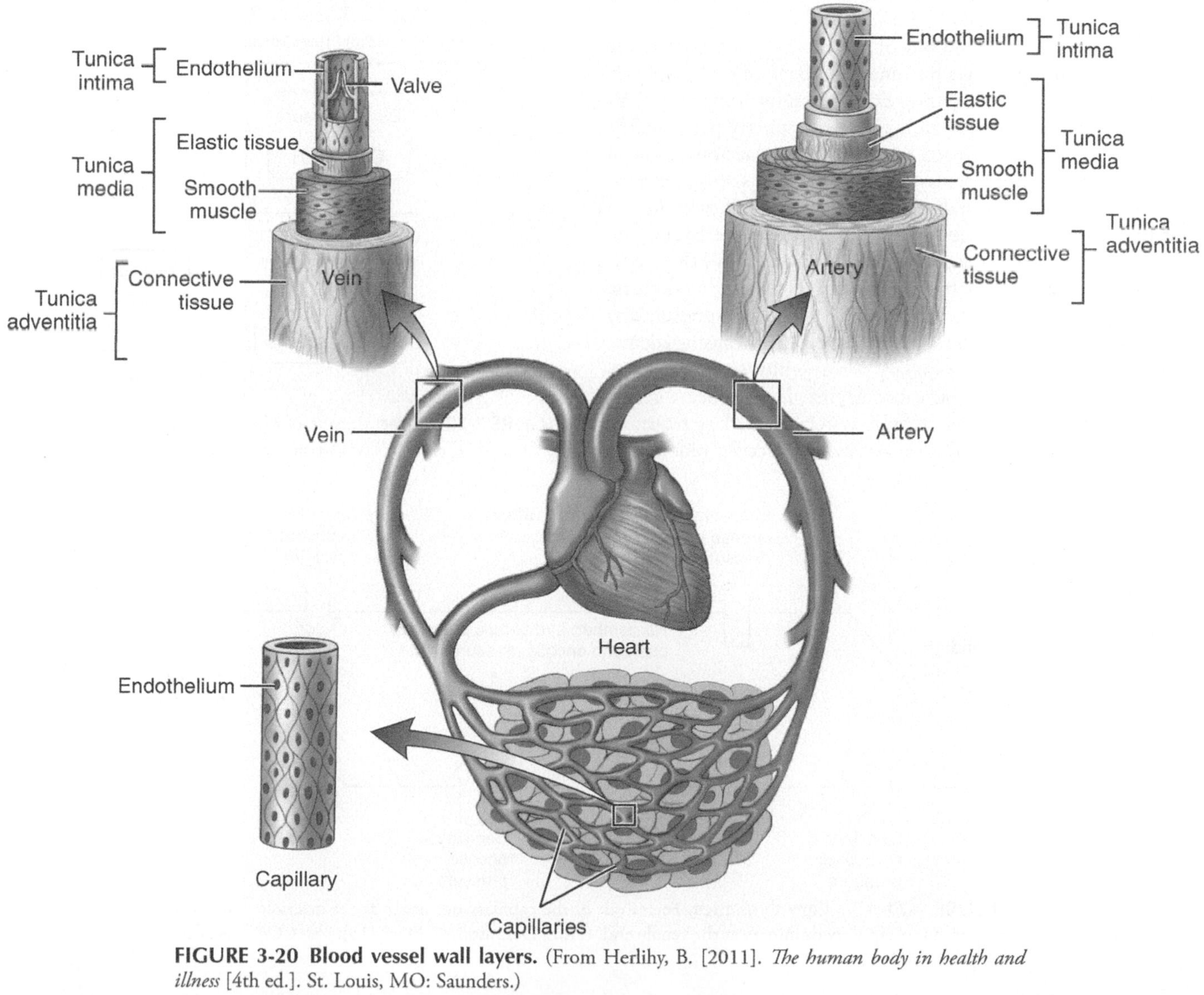

FIGURE 3-20 Blood vessel wall layers. (From Herlihy, B. [2011]. *The human body in health and illness* [4th ed.]. St. Louis, MO: Saunders.)

They carry blood away from the heart and distribute blood to the capillary beds throughout the body.

The arterioles are vital to the maintenance of arterial blood pressure and systemic vascular resistance. The arterioles have strong smooth muscle walls stimulated by the ANS. The arterioles lead to either capillaries, metarterioles, or precapillary sphincters, which control the blood flow into the capillary bed.

The capillary bed is a nutrient bed where the exchange of gases, nutrients, and metabolites takes place by the process of diffusion. Diffusion of a substance occurs from an area of higher concentration to an area of lower concentration until reaching an equilibrium. Capillaries contain no smooth muscle, and their diameter depends on changes in precapillary and postcapillary tone. Capillary dynamics (Figure 3-21) are influenced by four pressures: capillary hydrostatic, interstitial hydrostatic, colloidal oncotic, and interstitial colloidal oncotic. Capillary hydrostatic pressure pushes fluid out of the capillary and into the interstitium. Interstitial hydrostatic pressure pushes fluid out of the interstitium and into the capillary. Colloidal oncotic pressures pull and hold fluid in the capillary. Finally, interstitial colloidal oncotic pressure pulls and holds fluid in the interstitium. The plasma protein concentration in the capillaries provides the oncotic gradient, retains fluid in the intravascular space, and prevents edema formation. Albumin accounts for 75% of the total plasma osmotic pressure. A serum albumin level is a good indicator of a patient's colloid oncotic pressure.

Pressures pushing fluid out of the capillary dominate at the arterial end and pressures pushing fluid back into the capillary dominate at the venous end. Edema results from an imbalance in these pressures or an increase in capillary permeability. *Third spacing* is a term used to describe fluid accumulation in any space that is not intravascular or intracellular (e.g., interstitial edema, ascites, pleural effusion, pericardial effusion, lumen of the intestine). Venous congestion and excessive hydrostatic pressure at the venous end cause the edema seen in HF. Conditions such as protein malnutrition or liver disease that decrease plasma proteins decrease capillary colloidal oncotic pressure and allow excessive fluid to leak out of the capillary causing edema. Conditions that increase capillary permeability, such as anaphylaxis and angioedema, also cause edema. Lymphedema occurs when fluids remain in the lymph system instead of returning to the vascular system. The venous system receives blood from

the capillaries and brings deoxygenated blood back to the heart and lungs. Veins act as a reservoir (i.e., capacitance vessels). The venous system holds 65% to 75% of total blood volume. Venous pressure in the lower extremities is normally 20 mm Hg or less. The venous pump sends blood back to the right side of the heart. The veins have no muscle layer. Skeletal muscles compress surrounding veins. The skeletal muscles contract, compress veins, and propel blood toward the heart. Valves in the veins prevent retrograde blood flow.

The endothelium is an immense cell layer that lines the heart and blood vessels, surrounds the endocardium, and makes up the capillary bed in a single continuous layer. The endothelium has several functions. The endothelium regulates vascular tone, prevents thrombus formation, and contributes to the regulation of blood pressure.

Blood Pressure

Systemic vascular resistance (SVR) and CO (Figure 3-22) determine blood pressure. Vessel length, vessel diameter, and blood viscosity affect SVR. As discussed previously, CO is affected by heart rate, preload, afterload, and contractility.

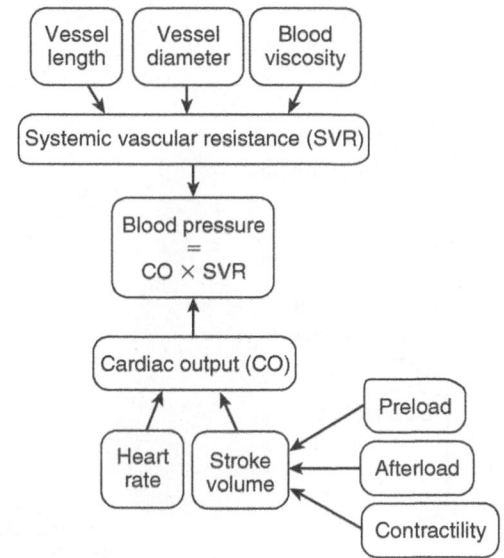

FIGURE 3-22 Determinants of blood pressure. (From Dennison, R. D. [2013]. *Pass CCRN!* [4th ed]. St. Louis, MO: Elsevier.)

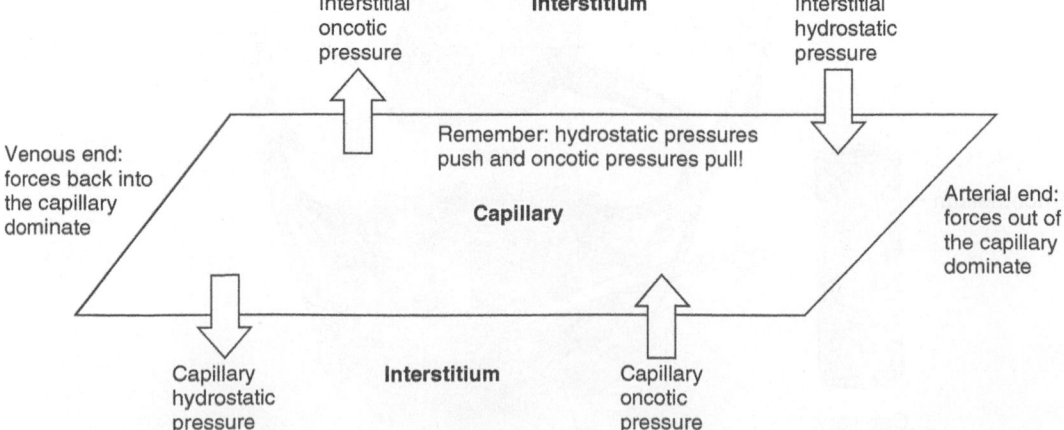

FIGURE 3-21 Capillary dynamics. Forces out of the capillary dominate at the arteriole end; forces back into the capillary dominate at the venule end. (From Dennison, R. D. [2013]. *Pass CCRN!* [4th ed]. St. Louis, MO: Elsevier.)

Measurements to consider include systolic pressure, diastolic pressure, pulse pressure, and mean arterial pressure (MAP) (Figure 3-23). Systolic pressure is the maximal pressure in the aorta during contraction of the left ventricle. The diastolic pressure is the pressure in the aorta during ventricular relaxation. The pulse pressure is the difference between systolic and diastolic pressures. Stroke volume and distensibility of the arterial system influence the pulse pressure. Normal pulse pressure is 30 to 40 mm Hg. MAP is the average pressure in the aorta and its major branches during cardiac cycle. CO and SVR influence the MAP. Its normal range is between 70 and 105 mm Hg. Calculate the MAP with either of two formulas.

SIDEBAR 3-2

MAP Calculation Formulas

- BP systolic + (BP diastolic × 2)] ÷ 3
- BP diastolic + 1/3 pulse pressure

Regulation of Arterial Pressure

Regulation of blood pressure is primarily through the ANS and the RAAS. Baroreceptors in the aortic arch, carotid sinus, pulmonary arteries, and atria keep MAP constant. When increased pressure is present, the receptor responds to the stretching of the arterial walls. The aortic arch via the vagus nerve transmits an impulse to the medulla. The PNS is stimulated and the SNS is inhibited, which results in a decreased heart rate and contractility, dilation of peripheral vessels, decreased SVR, and decreased BP. With decreased BP, the SNS is stimulated and the PNS is inhibited. This results in an increased heart rate and contractility, arterial and venous constriction to preserve blood flow to the brain and heart, and increased BP.

In the RAAS, the kidneys secrete the protease renin in response to decreased BP, a rise in sympathetic output β stimulation, and a fall in sodium concentration. Renin stimulates the conversion of angiotensinogen to angiotensin I. Angiotensin I is then converted to angiotensin II by angiotensin-converting enzyme (ACE) as the blood travels through the lung. Angiotensin II is a potent vasoconstrictor and raises BP by vasoconstriction and the secretion of aldosterone. Vasoconstriction and sodium and water retention increase BP, which then decreases renin secretion. Various drugs (Figure 3-24) block the RAAS to control BP and decrease preload and afterload in HF. Angiotensin-converting enzyme inhibitors prevent the conversion of angiotensin I to angiotensin II, and angiotensin II receptor blockers (ARBs) block the effects of renin.

Stimulation of the vasoconstrictor area, located in the vasomotor center in the medulla, results in an increase in heart rate, cardiac output, and BP. Venoconstriction decreases vascular capacitance, thus increasing venous return to the heart, preload, and BP. The vasodepressor area causes a decrease in the heart rate, cardiac output, and blood pressure. Venodilation increases vascular capacitance, thus decreasing venous return to the heart, preload, and BP.

Control of Peripheral Blood Flow

Several mechanisms control the regulation of peripheral blood flow. Local autoregulation is the ability of the tissues to control their own blood flow through vasodilation and vasoconstriction. Hypoxia, hypercapnia, and acidosis cause vasodilation. Another mechanism is the precapillary sphincters, which precede every capillary bed, allowing increased blood flow when oxygen tension falls. These sphincters constrict and restrict blood flow when oxygen tension rises.

Oxygen Delivery to the Tissues

The delivery of oxygen to the tissue (DO_2) is the product of the cardiac output and arterial oxygen tension (CaO_2). The arterial oxygen tension is a product of the SaO_2 and the hemoglobin level. Therefore, the three determinants of oxygen delivery to

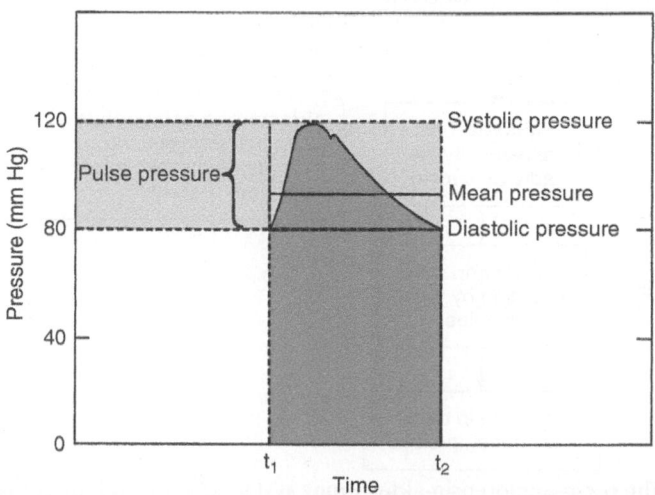

FIGURE 3-23 Blood pressure, pulse pressure (difference between systolic and diastolic pressures), and mean arterial pressure (calculated or measured average pressure). (Modified from Berne, R. M., & Levy, M. N. [1997]. *Cardiovascular physiology* [7th ed.]. St. Louis, MO: Mosby.)

the tissues are Sao_2, hemoglobin, and cardiac output. When using the cardiac index (CI) in place of CO; this calculated parameter is then referred to as the oxygen delivery to the tissues index (Do_2I). While calculating these parameters is not likely in a progressive care unit, the fact that Sao_2, hemoglobin, and cardiac output affects oxygen delivery is an important principle to consider when caring for patients who may have alterations in any of these three parameters. Calculate oxygen consumption by the tissues (Vo_2) using the difference between the Sao_2 and the Svo_2. Situations such as fever, restlessness, and increased work of breathing increase Vo_2. Lactic acidosis results when Do_2 is insufficient to meet Vo_2.

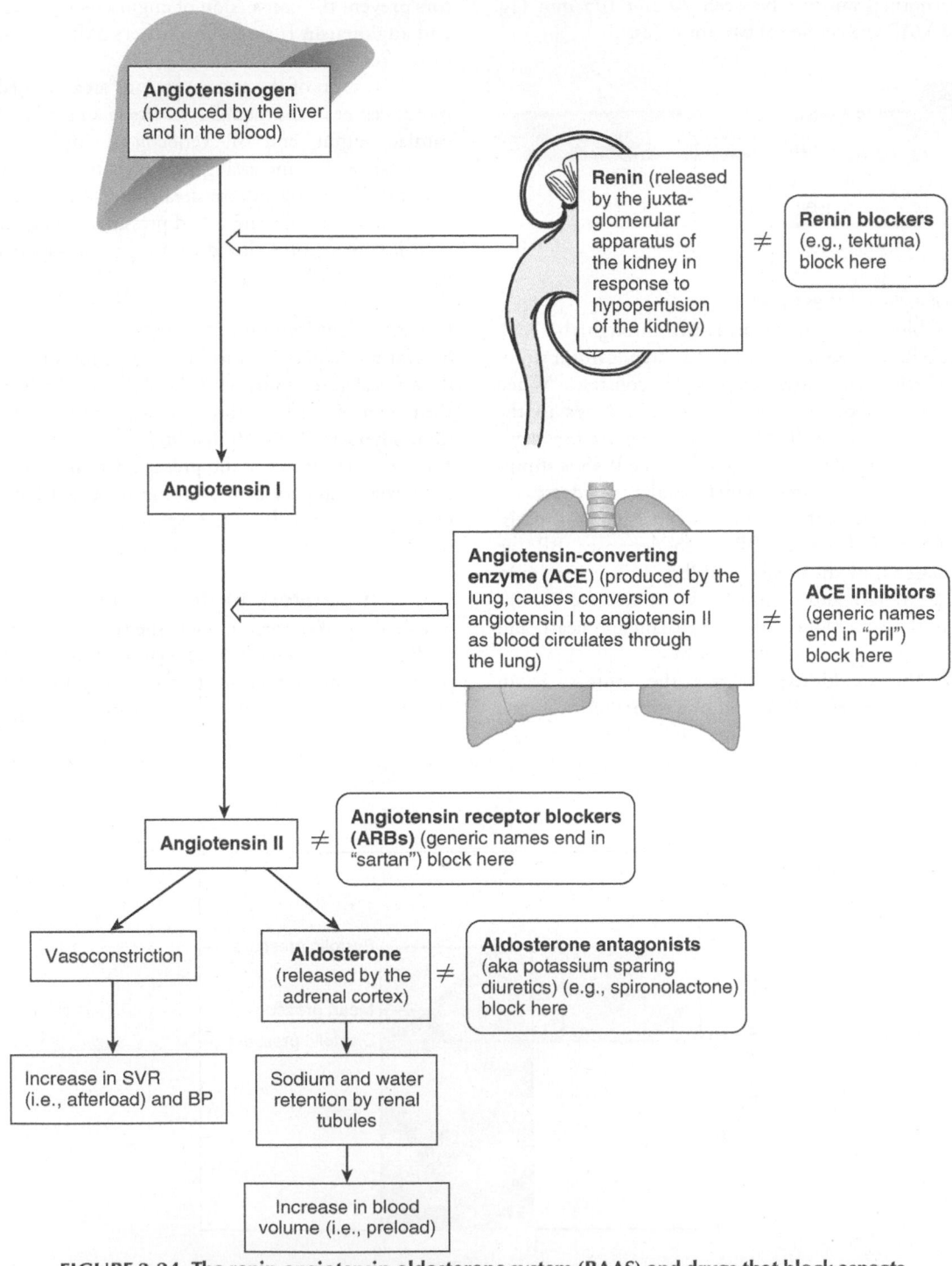

FIGURE 3-24 The renin-angiotensin-aldosterone system (RAAS) and drugs that block aspects of the RAAS. (From Dennison, R. D. [2013]. *Pass CCRN!* [4th ed]. St. Louis, MO: Elsevier.)

3.6 Synthesis Learning Activity: Crossword Puzzle

Complete the following crossword puzzle related to cardiovascular anatomy and physiology.

Answers to this activity can be found in the Answer Key.

ACROSS

6. The term used to describe the effect on contractility

10. These receptors are located in the renal and mesenteric artery bed, and stimulation causes vasodilation of those vascular beds

15. The type of disks that lie between myocardial cells to allow rapid transmission of the cardiac impulse

16. The interatrial pathway is frequently referred to as _____ bundle

17. The calculated parameter used to evaluate left ventricular contractility (abbrev.)

20. This innermost layer of the heart that lines the heart chamber and the heart valves

22. The left bundle branch is divided into left anterior and left posterior _____
23. During this refractory period, the cardiac muscle cell cannot respond no matter how strong the impulse
24. This calculated parameter is used to evaluate left ventricular afterload (abbrev.)
25. The term used to describe the effect on heart rate
26. Rapid depolarization that allows cardiac muscle to contract in concert as if it were one muscle; this is referred to as a functional _____
29. Crossbridging of actin and _____ causes muscle shortening
31. Calcium is necessary for _____, which causes muscle shortening
33. The muscles which contract to close the AV valves
36. The type of pressure that pushes (such as out of the capillary and into the interstitium)
38. This layer of the serous pericardium is synonymous with the epicardium
40. The ability of the cardiac cells to respond to a stimulus
42. Another term for antidiuretic hormone
43. The valve that lies between the right ventricle and the pulmonary artery
45. A mineralocorticoid secreted by the adrenal cortex, which causes sodium and water retention
47. These receptors are located in the right atrium and are sensitive to increased venous pressure
49. This refractory period is frequently referred to as the vulnerable period
51. The relaxation phase of the cardiac cycle
54. A neurotransmitter for the SNS that causes an increase in heart rate and contractility along with vasoconstriction
56. The pressure against which the ventricle must pump in order to open the semilunar valve
57. These fibers penetrate the ventricle to transmit the electrical impulse through to the endocardium

61. Pulse _____ is the difference between systolic and diastolic blood pressure
62. Elevation of this level in the blood is an indication of hypoxia and anaerobic metabolism
64. Occurs when sodium rushes into the cell causing it to become less negative
66. The fluid in the pericardial space acts as a _____
68. This layer of the pericardium acts as a barrier against infection and neoplastic invasion
73. This reflex causes an increase in heart rate with inspiration and a decrease in heart rate with expiration
75. The relationship between filling volume and contractility is frequently referred to as _____'s law of the heart
78. The type of receptors that are located in the carotic and aortic bodies which are sensitive to PaO_2, $PaCO_2$, and pH
79. The basic contractile unit of the myocardium
80. The valve between the left atrium and the aorta
82. DO_2 is a calculated parameter representing the _____ of oxygen to the tissues
86. A precursor of angiotensin
89. An increase in epicardial fat is associated with _____
90. The type of vessel that forms the nutrient bed for the tissues
91. High pressure lower cardiac chambers
92. Vasoconstrictive peptide produced by endothelial cells
93. Phase 1 of the action potential may be referred to as the _____ channel

DOWN

1. The portion of the cardiac wall that includes fibrous and serous layers
2. Fluid accumulation in spaces outside the intracellular and intravascular spaces is referred to as _____ spacing
3. The amount of blood that is ejected by the left ventricle per minute (abbrev.)
4. This peptide is associated with increased intravascular volume and is increased in HF (abbrev.)

5. The atrial contraction is frequently referred to as the atrial _____
7. The valve that lies between the right atrium and the right ventricle
8. The outermost layer of the artery
9. VO_2 is a calculated parameter representing the _____ of oxygen by the tissues
11. The ability of the cardiac cells to initiate electrical impulses regularly and spontaneously
12. Parameter used to evaluate right ventricular preload (abbrev.)
13. Cell layer that lines heart and blood vessels
14. The natural pacemaker of the heart is this node (abbrev.)
18. The function of these structures is to maintain unidirectional blood flow through the heart
19. A rupture of this innermost layer of the artery caused by plaque triggers the intrinsic pathway of clotting in atherosclerosis
21. Parameter used to evaluate right ventricular afterload (abbrev.)
26. The branch of the ANS that is frequently referred to as the "fight or flight" system
27. The contraction phase of the cardiac cycle
28. The type of pressure that pulls (such as into the capillary from the interstitium)
30. The coronary artery that supplies the anterior left ventricle and the anterior two thirds of the septum (abbrev.)
32. Recovery; return to predominance on intracellular potassium and extracellular sodium
34. Vascular resistance dependent on the length and radius of the vessel and the viscosity of the blood is referred to as _____'s formula
35. A cardiac contractile protein used in the diagnosis of myocardial infarction
37. The coronary artery that supplies the right atrium, right ventricle, and inferior wall of the left ventricle
39. A cardiac muscle fiber

41. These receptors are located in the heart and stimulation increases heart rate, contractility, and conductivity
43. The two important factors in coronary artery perfusion are time and _____
44. The coronary artery that supplies blood to the left atrium and the lateral left ventricle (abbrev.)
46. The outmost layer of the cardiac wall
48. Diastolic BP – PAOP (abbrev.)
50. Term for the contractile state of the heart, irrespective of preload
52. Jugular venous distention is an indication of increased preload of the _____ ventricle
53. The _____ fraction is the percentage of blood that was in the ventricle at the end of diastole that was pumped out during systole
55. The substance secreted by the kidney in response to hypoperfusion of the kidney
58. Pressure receptors
59. The valve that lies between the left atrium and the left ventricle
60. This type of cardiac cell has automaticity
61. Phase 3 of the action potential may be referred to as the _____ channel
63. Low pressure upper cardiac chambers
65. The branch of the ANS that maintains a steady state
67. Parasympathetic stimulation is frequently referred to as _____ stimulation
69. The "powerhouse" of the cell that uses nutrients and oxygen to make ATP
70. The effect on conductivity
71. The measured parameter used to evaluate left ventricular preload
72. These receptors are located in the vessels, and stimulation causes vasoconstriction
74. The _____ potential must be met for depolarization to occur
76. The effect of venous return on the heart which stretches the myofibrils and, therefore determines the force of the next contraction

77. During this subphase of diastole and systole, no blood is moving
81. This middle layer of the artery becomes calcified in arteriosclerosis limiting the ability of the artery to dilate
83. The branches of the intraventricular conduction system are referred to as ____
84. Cellular energy (abbrev.)
85. This circulation consists of interarterial vessels that anastomose with each other as the result of gradual coronary artery occlusion
87. Phase 2 of the action potential is referred to as the ____ channel
88. Inflammation or infarction of this layer of the heart is associated with contractility problems

CARDIOVASCULAR ASSESSMENT

Interview

During the interview process, it is very important to identify the chief complaint and history of present illness. Ask first about why the patient is seeking help now and the duration of the problem.

Determine the course of the problem noting the time of the day of the onset, duration, precipitating factors, signs and symptoms, and progression. Differentiation of chest pain (Table 3-5) needs to be ascertained as the patient may identify pain as indigestion, burning, discomfort, tightness, or pressure in the midchest, epigastrium, or left arm. Use the OPQRST format for describing the patient's complaint. O stands for *Onset* (i.e., when did pain begin). P stands for *Provocation* (i.e., What provokes or worsens the pain?) and *Palliation* (What relieves the pain? and What was used but did not relieve pain?). Q stands for *Quality* (i.e., What does the pain feel like?). R stands for *Region* (i.e., Where is the pain?) and *Radiation* (i.e., If the pain radiates, to what area does the pain radiate?). S stands for *Severity* (i.e., How severe is the pain?). T stands for *Timing* (i.e., Is the pain intermittent or continuous?). Attempt to determine what the relationship of the pain is to other events or activities. The most frequently used pain scale in adults is the 1 to 10 scale with 1 being negligible pain and 10 being the worst pain imaginable.

Ascertain if the patient has any complaints of dyspnea. The patient may complain of shortness of breath or breathlessness. The dyspnea may occur at rest or on exertion. In addition, the patient may complain of an inability to lie flat because of dyspnea (orthopnea) and/or a problem with awakening with a feeling of suffocation 1 to 2 hours after going to sleep (paroxysmal nocturnal dyspnea). If wheezing accompanies paroxysmal nocturnal dyspnea, this condition may be called *cardiac asthma.* Patient symptoms may also include a cough. Take into consideration the quality of the cough (e.g., wet or dry), productivity (i.e., appearance of expectorant), frequency, and precipitating factors, including when the cough occurs (e.g., at night or precipitated by supine position, exertion, or by turning to one side). The cough may be a side effect of ACE inhibitors or caused by HF, mitral stenosis, or pulmonary embolism. Hemoptysis may occur with pulmonary edema or pulmonary embolism. Palpitations may also occur, and the patient may describe these as an unpleasant awareness of the heartbeat when at rest or a skipping, pounding, or thumping sensation. Palpitations may be associated with premature beats or other dysrhythmia and may accompany syncope or chest pain.

If the patient reports syncope, the type of syncope should be determined and documented. Effort syncope involves a transient loss of consciousness that occurs shortly after starting a heavy activity. Effort syncope may be associated with aortic or subaortic stenosis. A Stokes-Adams attack might result in dramatic loss of consciousness related to a heart block or dysrhythmia. Pacemaker syncope results from a malfunction or failure of an artificial pacemaker. Hypersensitive carotid sinus syncope may occur caused by pressure applied on a carotid sinus body of a patient with atherosclerotic and hypersensitive carotid arteries.

Other symptoms reported may include a headache, ascites, abdominal pain, edema, weight gain, fatigue, weakness, nocturia, diaphoresis, and leg pain. Associated hypertension may cause headache. Right ventricular failure (RVF) also can cause ascites, which is an accumulation of fluid in the abdominal cavity. Abdominal pain, edema, weight gain, feeling bloated, tightening of clothing, tightening of shoes, and marks left from constricting garments are frequently related to RVF. Fatigue or weakness also stems from RVF. Nocturia results from heart failure (HF) or diuretic use. Patient complaints of diaphoresis may result from SNS stimulation or infection. Intermittent claudication, resulting in hip, thigh, or calf pain that occurs with exercise and ceases with rest, is indicative of peripheral arterial disease. Skin changes, decreases in hair distribution, skin color changes, skin ulcerations that will not heal, or a thin shiny appearance to the skin may also indicate peripheral arterial disease. Elicit how many blocks the patient can walk without symptoms occurring. Complaints of calf tenderness occur with thrombophlebitis, which is accompanied by red, warm skin over the vein or by dilated, sometimes painful varicose veins.

Take a complete past medical history identifying all previous illnesses, injuries, and surgical procedures. Query the patient about general health status for the past several years. Obtain the cardiac history, particularly noting illnesses such as coronary artery disease (e.g., angina, myocardial infarction), cerebrovascular disease (e.g., transient ischemic attacks or stroke), dysrhythmias, and hypertension. Note also if the patient has a history of hyperlipidemia, peripheral vascular disease, rheumatic fever or rheumatic heart disease, heart murmur or known valvular heart disease, pulmonary disease (e.g., asthma, chronic obstructive pulmonary disease [COPD]), pulmonary embolism, connective tissue disorders, endocrine disorders (especially diabetes mellitus), kidney disease, alcoholism, anemia, and/or bleeding disorders. Identify the presence of cardiac risk factors including hypertension, hyperlipidemia, smoking, diabetes, and family history of cardiac disease. Determine the patient's last medical examination, hospitalizations, and prior relevant cardiac diagnostic tests (e.g., echocardiography, stress ECG, cardiac catheterization).

Note if the patient has suffered chest trauma. A history of recent trauma is important to differentiate myocardial infarction from myocardial contusion. A recent chest trauma would also serve as a contraindication for fibrinolytics.

Elicit information on past surgical procedures, especially cardiac surgery. Identify whether the patient has had coronary artery bypass grafting, valve replacement, or other types of cardiac surgery. Determine if the patient has undergone percutaneous coronary intervention (PCI) procedures (e.g., angioplasty, atherectomy, stent placement, or valvuloplasty) or a pacemaker insertion.

Ask about a family history of coronary artery disease (CAD) or cerebrovascular disease, including stroke, congenital heart defects, sudden cardiac death, peripheral vascular disease,

TABLE 3-5	Differentiation of Chest Pain						
Cause	**Provocation**	**Palliation**	**Quality**	**Region/Radiation**	**Severity**	**Timing**	**Associated Signs/ Symptoms**
Angina pectoris	• Exercise • Exertion • Exposure to cold • Emotional stress • Eating • Smoking	• Rest • Oxygen • Nitroglycerin • Calcium channel blocker (e.g., nifedipine)	• Heaviness or pressure • Tightness • Squeezing • Dull ache • Burning • Not always described as pain but as discomfort	• Substernal • May be diffuse and vague • May radiate to arms, neck, jaw, back, upper abdomen	• Mild to severe	• Gradual or sudden onset • Duration: usually 1-4 minutes but may be 5-15 minutes	• Tachycardia, tachypnea • Dyspnea • Nausea, vomiting • Diaphoresis • Weakness • Anxiety • May have ST-T wave changes with pain
Acute myocardial infarction	• No specific precipitator • Lifestyle change and stress • Usually occurs within 3 hours of awakening	• Narcotics • Reperfusion by fibrinolytic or percutaneous coronary intervention (e.g., angioplasty, atherectomy) • No relief with rest and/or nitroglycerin	• As for angina • Heaviness or pressure • May show Levine's sign (clenched fist over sternum)	• As for angina	• No symptoms to severe • Absence of pain is common in patients with diabetes mellitus and in older adults	• Sudden onset • Duration: >30 minutes; usually 1-2 hours	• As for angina • Tachycardia, tachypnea • Dyspnea • Feeling of impending doom • S_4 • ECG changes: T wave inversion, ST segment elevation, eventually Q waves
Dissecting aortic aneurysm	• Peripheral vascular disease • Marfan syndrome • Aortitis • Hypertension and/or hypertensive crisis • Chest trauma	• Narcotics • Surgery • No relief with rest and/or nitroglycerin	• Tearing • Ripping	• Anterior chest • Radiation to shoulders, neck, back, abdomen	• Severe	• Sudden onset • Worse at onset • Duration: hours to days	• Tachycardia, tachypnea • Dysphagia • Confusion • Diaphoresis • Syncope • Dyspnea • Anxiety • Unilateral absence of pulse; BP differences between sides • Motor/sensory changes • Murmur of aortic regurgitation

Condition	Cause	Treatment	Quality	Location/Radiation	Severity	Onset/Duration	Signs and Symptoms
Pericarditis	• Myocardial infarction • Cardiac surgery • Trauma • Infections • Uremia • Lupus Erythematosus	• Nonsteroidal antiinflammatory agents (e.g., ibuprofen; indomethacin) • Sitting up and leaning forward	• Sharp • Stabbing • Knifelike • Worsened by inspiration, coughing, movement, recumbent position	• Precordial • Substernal • Radiation to neck, shoulders, arms, back	• Mild to severe	• Sudden onset • Duration: days	• Tachycardia, tachypnea • Fever • Dyspnea • Pericardial friction rub • Leukocytosis • Diffuse concave ST segment
Pulmonary embolism	• Venous stasis (e.g., immobility, pelvic surgery, atrial fibrillation) • Hypercoagulability (e.g., oral contraceptives, malignancy, polycythemia) • Injury to vessel wall (e.g., IVs, vascular surgery)	• Narcotics • High Fowler's position • Splinting of chest	• Sharp • Knifelike • Shooting • Deep ache • Pressure • Worsened by deep inspiration or coughing	• Substernal or lateral chest • Radiation to shoulder or neck	• Mild to severe	• Sudden onset • Duration: minutes to hours	• Tachycardia, tachypnea • Dyspnea • Pallor or cyanosis • Cough • Anxiety, feeling of impending doom • Sinus tachycardia or atrial dysrhythmias • Accentuated P_2 • Right-sided S_4, possible right-sided S_3 • If RVF: JVD • If pulmonary infarction: pleural friction rub, hemoptysis, fever
Pneumothorax	• Congenital bleb • Emphysematous bullous • Large tidal volumes or PEEP on mechanical ventilator • Chest trauma • Exacerbated by coughing, exertion, or Valsalva maneuver	• Narcotics • Insertion of chest tube	• Tearing • Sharp • Worsened by breathing	• Lateral chest • May radiate to shoulder, back, arms	• Mild to severe	• Sudden onset • Duration: hours to days	• Tachypnea • Tachycardia • Dyspnea • Anxiety • JVD • Hyperresonance to percussion of affected side • Diminished breath sounds on affected side • Subcutaneous emphysema may be seen • Tracheal deviation may be seen, especially with tension pneumothorax

Continued

TABLE 3-5   Differentiation of Chest Pain—cont'd

Cause	Provocation	Palliation	Quality	Region/Radiation	Severity	Timing	Associated Signs/Symptoms
Pleuropulmonary (e.g., pleurisy)	• Respiratory infection • Aspiration	• Narcotics • Relief with sitting up	• Sharp • Worsened by coughing, inspiration, or movement	• Lateral chest • May radiate to shoulder, neck	• Moderate	• Gradual onset • Duration: days to weeks	• Tachypnea • Tachycardia • Dyspnea • Fever • Productive cough • Pleural friction rub
Gastrointestinal chest pain	• Cold liquids • Food intake, especially spicy foods, acidic foods, or foods high in fat • Alcohol • Caffeine • Stress • Smoking • Exercise	• Sitting up • Antacids • Esophageal spasm (may be relieved by nitroglycerin)	• "Heartburn" • Dull, burning • Squeezing • Worsened by eating or supine position	• Retrosternal or lower substernal • Upper abdomen • Midline • May radiate to left arm, neck, jaw, upper abdomen, back, shoulder	• Mild to moderate	• Gradual or sudden onset • Duration: minutes to days	• Dyspnea • Diaphoresis • Anxiety • Dysphagia • Eructation • Vomiting
Musculoskeletal chest pain	• Neck or arm strain • Movement • Coughing • Deep breathing • CPR	• Rest • Heat • Nonsteroidal antiinflammatory agents (e.g., aspirin, ibuprofen)	• Soreness • Stabbing or sticking sensation • Tenderness • Worsened with inspiration and movement	• Localized to one side of chest	• Mild to moderate	• Gradual or sudden onset • Duration: weeks	• Tachypnea • Splinting respirations • Localized tenderness over site of pain
Psychosomatic chest pain	• Stress • Fatigue	• Rest • Anxiolytics	• Dull ache • Sharp • Stabbing • Superficial	• Precordium • Localized; frequently on left side • No radiation	• Mild to moderate	• Gradual or sudden onset • Duration: minutes to days	• Hyperpnea • Dyspnea • Palpitations • Dry mouth • Dizziness • Tingling of hands, mouth • Fatigue • Frequent sighing

TABLE 3-6	Drug and Supplement Effects with the Cardiovascular System
Drugs and Supplements	**Cardiovascular Side Effect**
Ephedrine	Increases BP; prolongs clotting
Tricyclic antidepressants	Dysrhythmias (torsades de pointes)
Phenytoin	Dysrhythmias
Phenothiazines	Dysrhythmias; hypotension
Oral contraceptives	Predisposes to embolism, thrombosis
Doxorubicin	Cardiomyopathy
Lithium	Dysrhythmias
Corticosteroids	Sodium and fluid retention; exacerbation of HF
Theophylline	Tachycardia and dysrhythmias
Cocaine	Tachycardia and dysrhythmias; coronary artery spasm
Alfalfa	Increases risk of bleeding, especially combined with warfarin
Black cohosh	Hypotension
Ephedra	Increases heart rate and BP; fatal drug interactions
Garlic	Increases risk of bleeding of patients taking anticoagulants
Ginger	Potentiates warfarin
Gingko	Increases risk bleeding with warfarin, aspirin, or Cox 2 inhibitors
Ginseng	Hypertension
Goldenseal	Potentiates warfarin: hypertension; hallucinations or delirium
Grapefruit juice	Increases effects of statins and calcium channel blockers
Green tea	Decreases effects of warfarin
Hawthorne	Potentiates the effects of cardiac glycosides and nitrates
Kelp	Increases the effects of antihypertensives and anticoagulants
Licorice root	Hypertension; hypokalemia; digoxin toxicity
Oleander	Heart block; hyperkalemia; dysrhythmias; death
St. John's wort	Increases heart rate and BP; decreases digoxin levels

hypertension, diabetes mellitus, hyperlipidemia, kidney disease, bleeding disorders, or collagen vascular disease.

For the social history, identify present and past work experiences. Determine the current relationship with the spouse or significant other and the family structure. Determine the patient's occupation and education level. Ask whether changes have occurred in the patient's ability to perform job and home responsibilities or activities of daily living. Identify the patient's support system and the presence of any cultural issues or a language barrier. Determine the patient's stress level and usual coping mechanisms. Evaluate the patient for the presence of type A personality, which is associated with a sense of time urgency, hostility, aggression, ambition, competitiveness, impatience, and frustration. Type B personality is the absence of the qualities described as type A. Record the patient's recreational habits, exercise habits, dietary habits, caffeine intake (especially the intake of high-energy drinks), alcohol use, and tobacco use. Record alcohol use as the number of alcoholic beverages consumed per month, week, or day. Record tobacco use as pack-years, which is the number of packs per day times the number of years he or she has been smoking.

Note the presence of allergies and the type of reaction. Determine the patient's exposure to toxins. Ask if there has been recent travel and, if so, the destinations. Inquire about the medication history, including prescribed drugs, dosage, frequency, and time of last dose. List the patient's use of nonprescribed drugs (i.e., over-the-counter drugs, including herbal supplements). Note any substance abuse (e.g., cocaine, amphetamines). It is particularly important to determine the patient's understanding of drug actions, side effects, and if the patient is taking any interacting drugs (Table 3-6) that may be implicated in causing potential problems for patients with cardiovascular disease.

Physical Examination
Landmarks
Anatomical landmarks (Figure 3-25) used in cardiovascular assessment include the clavicle, sternum, ribs, intercostal spaces, angle of Louis, the xiphoid process, the costal margin, and the costal angle. Imaginary lines delineate locations on the thorax. The imaginary lines include the midsternal line (MSL), midclavicular line (MCL), anterior axillary line (AAL), midaxillary line (MAL), posterior axillary line (PAL), scapular line, and the midspinal line. The heart is located between the sternum and spinal column, normally lying between the second ICS and fifth ICS with the apex at the fifth LICS at the MCL.

Inspection and Palpation
Assess vital signs. Take BP while the patient is sitting, lying, and standing. The ideal width of the cuff is 40% of the arm

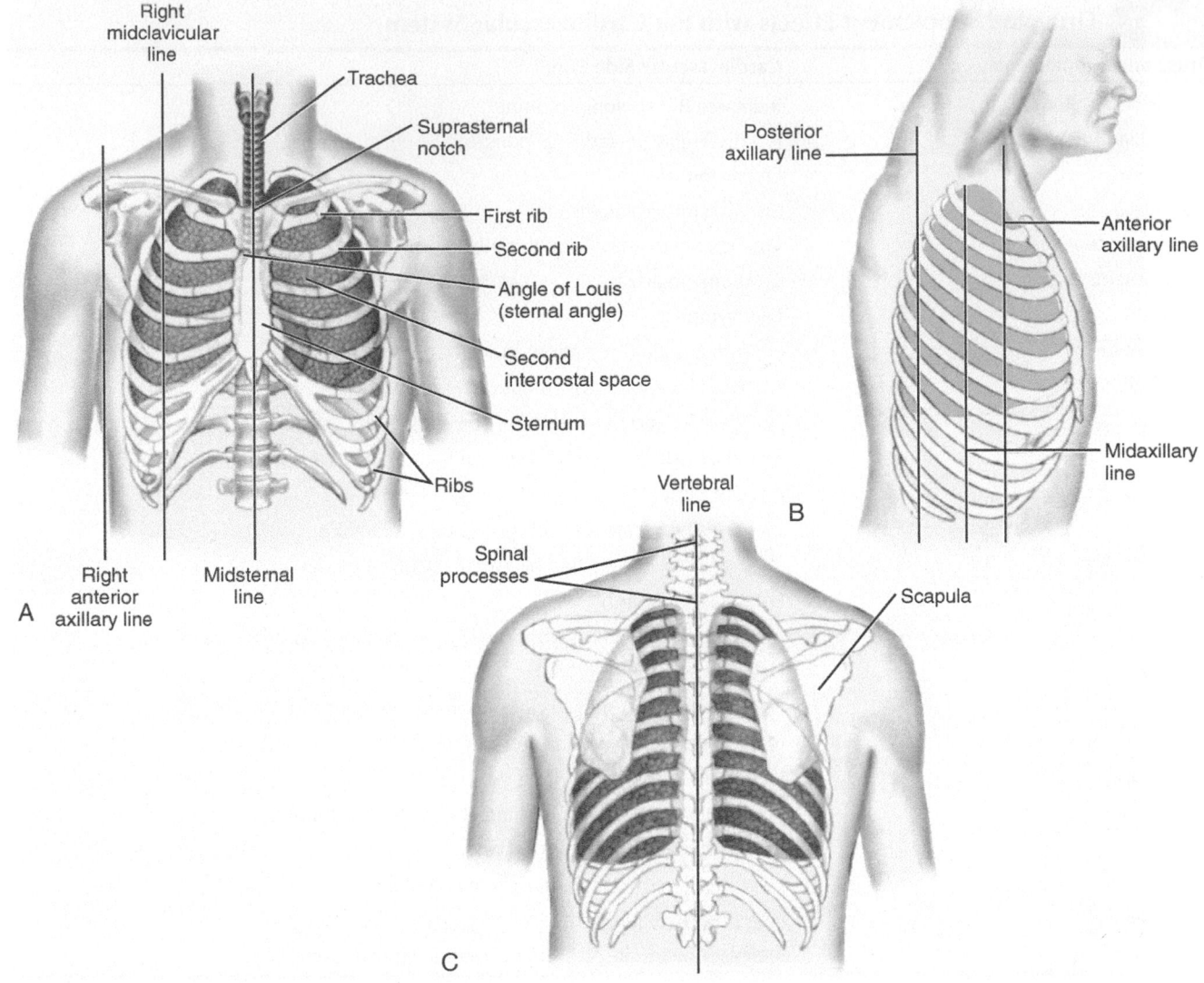

FIGURE 3-25 Landmarks of the thorax. A, Anterior. **B,** Right lateral. **C,** Posterior. (From Urden, L., Stacy, K., & Lough, M. [2014]. *Critical care nursing: Diagnosis and management* [7th ed.]. St. Louis, MO: Mosby.)

circumference; for obese patients, use the large adult or thigh (i.e., 18 cm wide) cuff. The cuff should be positioned no less than 2.5 cm from the antecubital fossa. Take the pressure in both arms. A variation of up to 15 mm Hg between arms is normal. More than 15 mm Hg difference in systolic pressures may indicate diminished arterial flow on the side with the lower reading due to an obstruction or dissection. The BP in the lower extremities is 10 mm Hg higher than it is in the upper extremities. False low measurements occur if the cuff is too large for the arm, the arm is above the heart level, or the listener does not hear the first Korotkoff sound. False high measurements occur if the cuff is too small for the arm, loose, or not centered over the brachial artery, or the arm is below the heart level.

A reduction of up to 15 mm Hg in systolic and 5 mm Hg in diastolic BP upon standing is normal. A greater reduction indicates orthostatic changes. To assess for orthostatic changes, assist the patient to a standing position, wait 2 to 3 minutes, then repeat the measurement of the BP and the heart rate.

A narrowed pulse pressure frequently indicates vasoconstriction, as found with stimulation of the SNS (e.g., hypovolemic shock). A widened pulse pressure frequently indicates excessive vasodilation as found with excessive vasodilatory mediator release (e.g., septic shock).

Pulsus paradoxus is an exaggeration of normal physiologic response to inspiration. A normal decrease in BP during inspiration is 10 mm Hg or less. In pulsus paradoxus, a BP drop of more than 10 mm Hg occurs. Pulsus paradoxus may be an indication of pericardial effusion, constrictive pericarditis, cardiac tamponade, severe lung disease, advanced HF, or hemorrhagic shock.

Determine the patient's heart rate, respiratory rate, and temperature. If an ECG monitor is available, also assess the cardiac rhythm. Tachycardia and tachypnea frequently indicate stimulation of the SNS. Fever may indicate an inflammatory or infectious process (e.g., myocardial infarction, pericarditis, and/or endocarditis).

Determine the patient's height and weight. Body weight is an important indicator of fluid gain or loss. Conduct a general survey including the patient's apparent health status, the consistency of apparent age with the patient's chronologic age, the level of consciousness (LOC), the presence of gross deformities, the nutritional status, and the stature/posture and gait.

Note color of skin and appendages. Pallor may be an indication of anemia, SNS innervation, or sympathomimetic agents (e.g., phenylephrine [Neo-Synephrine], norepinephrine

[Levophed], dopamine [Intropin]). Note any cyanosis and the location. Cyanosis indicates 5 g/dL of deoxygenated hemoglobin. In a dark-skinned patient, cyanosis appears as an ashen color. Peripheral (or cold) cyanosis of the fingertips and toes is associated with peripheral hypoperfusion or vasoconstriction. Central (or warm) cyanosis of the lips, tongue, and mucous membranes is associated with 5 g/dL of deoxygenated hemoglobin. Because patients with chronic bronchitis are frequently polycythemic, they show cyanosis early. Remember that patients with chronic bronchitis are nicknamed *blue bloaters, blue* because of chronic hypoxemia and *bloaters* because of chronic RVF. Central cyanosis may be a late or even an impossible sign of hypoxemia in severely anemic patients who have low hemoglobin levels, because they will not show cyanosis until 5 g/dL of hemoglobin are deoxygenated and they may not even have 5 g/dL desaturated. These conditions explain why it is important to remember that clinical assessment of hypoxemia may be unreliable.

Note any ruddiness, which may indicate polycythemia or hypercapnia. Observe skin moisture; note any diaphoresis or abnormal dryness. Check the temperature of the skin because cold skin indicates hypoperfusion. Evaluate skin turgor. Interstitial dehydration causes tenting, but it may also be related to the normal loss of elasticity of aging. Note the presence and location of edema. Edema indicates an increase in interstitial fluid of 30% above normal levels. Check the face for signs of allergy or profound facial edema in anaphylaxis, exogenous steroid usage (e.g., prednisone), or endogenous conditions (e.g., Cushing syndrome). Renal disease (e.g., nephrotic syndrome) is also associated with dependent edema from RVF. Generalized edema (i.e., anasarca) indicates end-stage HF, end-stage renal failure, or severe hypoproteinemia. Note the degree of any pitting edema. Document the presence of edema according to the following grades:

- Grade 1+ = 0–¼ inch
- Grade 2+ = ¼–½ inch
- Grade 3+ = ½–1 inch
- Grade 4+ = >1 inch

Examine the patient for the presence of lesions. Arterial disease may cause ulcers at the toes or points of trauma. Venous disease may cause ulcers at the sides of the ankles. Check the patient's fingertips and nailbeds for color; a bluish nailbed indicates peripheral cyanosis. Chronic hypoxia is noted by the presence of nail clubbing. Clubbing is an enlargement of the ends of one or more fingers or toes due to proliferation and edema of connective tissue resulting in the loss of the normal angle between the skin and nail plate. Clubbing is present if the angle is greater than 180 degrees. Evaluate the nailbeds for splinter hemorrhages; these are red to black linear streaks under the nailbed that run from the base to the tip of the nail that may indicate bacterial endocarditis. Note Osler nodes on the fingertips; these are painful red subcutaneous nodules that may indicate embolization in infective endocarditis, infected arterial catheter, disseminated gonococcal infection, rheumatoid arthritis, and systemic lupus erythematosus (SLE). Immune complex deposition causes the Osler nodes.

Observe the patient's facial expression and note whether there is facial flushing. Episodic facial flushing may indicate pheochromocytoma, a benign adrenal tumor that causes transient severe hypertension episodes. Head bobbing up and down with each heartbeat is referred to as *de Musset sign.* This indicates the possibility of an aortic aneurysm or regurgitation.

Check the patient's eyes for xanthoma palpebrarum (also called *xanthelasma*). These are benign, fatty, fibrous, yellowish plaques, nodules, or tumors on the eyelids and are

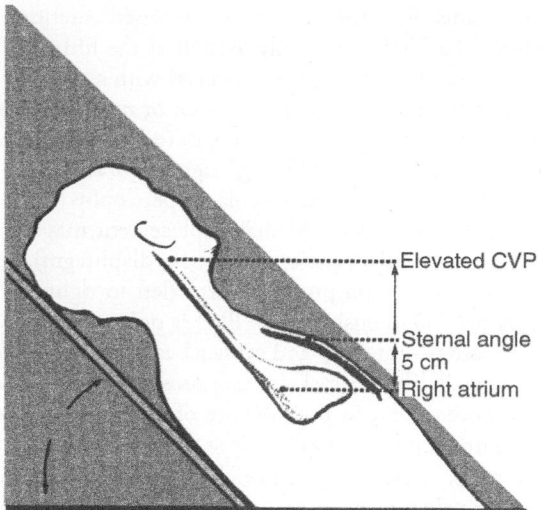

FIGURE 3-26 Jugular venous distention and estimation of central venous pressure (CVP). Assess jugular venous distention with the patient at a 45-degree angle, determine height of jugular venous distention above the sternal angle, and add 5 cm to this measurement to estimate central venous pressure in centimeters of water pressure. (From Guzzetta, C. E., & Dossey, B. M. [1992]. *Cardiovascular nursing: Holistic practice.* St. Louis, MO: Mosby.)

associated with hyperlipidemia. Look for a light-colored ring surrounding the iris; this may be a normal finding in elderly patients (arcus senilis) but is abnormal and associated with hyperlipidemia in younger patients (corneal arcus). Look for bulging of the eyeballs (exophthalmos), which may be seen in patients with advanced HF, pulmonary hypertension, and hyperthyroidism.

Look for diagonal bilateral earlobe creases (referred to as *McCarty sign*), which may indicate CAD if seen in individuals younger than 45 years of age. At the neck, look for JVD. To evaluate JVD (Figure 3-26), place the patient at a 45-degree angle. Identify the sternal angle (also called the *manubriosternal junction* or the *angle of Louis*) located at the raised notch where the manubrium and the body of the sternum join. Measure the height of neck vein distention above the level of the sternal angle. A normal height of neck vein distention is 1 to 3 cm above the sternal angle. A neck vein distention of greater than 3 cm above the sternal angle is indicative of any of the following: right ventricular failure, hypervolemia, tension pneumothorax, or cardiac tamponade. The angle of Louis is assumed to be approximately 5 cm above the right atrium. To estimate the CVP add 5 cm to the height of the neck vein distention above the angle of Louis. A normal CVP is approximately 3 to 8 cm of H_2O pressure.

To evaluate the hepatojugular reflux (also referred to as the *abdominojugular reflux*), have the patient lie at a 45-degree angle and apply pressure over the right upper quadrant for 30 to 60 seconds while evaluating an increase in neck vein distention. A positive result is a sustained increase in neck vein distention of 4 cm or more or a fall of 4 cm or more after release of pressure. A positive result indicates HF.

Examine the shape and contour of the chest, noting the symmetry and breathing pattern. Inspect and palpate the base, apex, and left sternal border of the precordium. Check for pulsations, heaves or lifts, and thrills.

With the patient lying down, palpate the point of maximal impulse (PMI) or the apical impulse. The PMI is frequently visible and usually palpable, but may not be palpable in patients with obesity, a muscular chest wall, or an increased anterior-posterior diameter. The PMI is normally located at the fifth LICS at the MCL. Lateral displacement is associated with any of the following: left ventricular dilation (e.g., aortic or mitral insufficiency), upward displacement of the diaphragm (e.g., pregnancy, ascites), right to left mediastinal shift (e.g., right pleural effusion or tension pneumothorax), left ventricular hypertrophy (LVH), or left ventricular failure (LVF). Medial displacement may occur with COPD (downward displacement of the diaphragm), left pleural effusion, or tension pneumothorax (left to right mediastinal shift). A normal intensity of the PMI is only a light tap. Failure may increase the intensity and cause a heave, which is a lifting of the chest wall. The normal size is approximately 1 to 2 cm, but will be more diffuse in the presence of a ventricular aneurysm. A left ventricular heave can be felt at or near the apex, whereas a right ventricular heave (or lift) is felt at or near the sternum.

As you palpate the thorax, note any thrill. A thrill is a palpable vibration associated with murmur or bruit. The detection of a thrill often occurs where the murmur is loudest or at the location of a bruit. Thrills are associated with murmurs of aortic stenosis, mitral stenosis, patent ductus arteriosus (PDA), and/or ventricular septal defect (VSD) that are at least grade IV.

As you examine the abdomen, note the aortic pulsation, which is normally visible especially during expiration. Palpate the aortic pulsation, which is normally at midline or slightly to the left of midline. It is essential to feel for a pulsatile mass or lateral expansion, which might be indicative of aneurysm.

Examine the extremities for evidence of arterial or venous disease (Table 3-7) using the parameters of pain, pulses, color, temperature, edema, skin changes, and ulcerations. Note the temperature of the extremities; coolness may indicate decreased blood flow due

to hypoperfusion or vasoconstriction. Excessive warmth may indicate hyperthyroidism or fever. Note the capillary refill rate; color should return after blanching within 3 seconds. A delay beyond 3 seconds indicates hypoperfusion. Perform the apical-radial pulse deficit with two nurses using one watch. A deficit (i.e., radial pulse rate less than apical rate) is indicative of dysrhythmia (e.g., atrial fibrillation, ventricular ectopy). Check the rate, rhythm, and amplitude of the peripheral pulses (Figure 3-27): brachial, radial, ulnar, femoral, popliteal, posterior tibialis, and dorsalis pedis. Palpate the lower section of the carotid pulses, but never palpate both carotids simultaneously. Document the amplitude of pulses as follows:

- 0 = not palpable
- 1+(=)weak and thready, easily obliterated
- 2+(=)normal, not easily obliterated
- 3+(=)full and bounding, cannot obliterate

Note the pulse contour (Figure 3-28). Pulsus magnus is a strong, bounding pulse with rapid upstroke and downstroke; this is characteristic of hypertension, thyrotoxicosis, aortic insufficiency, patent ductus arteriosus, or arteriovenous fistula. Pulsus parvus (also tardus [late]) is a small, weak pulse, which is

TABLE 3-7	**Comparison of Clinical Indications of Arterial and Venous Peripheral Vascular Disease**	
	Arterial	**Venous**
Pain	• Excruciating in acute occlusion • Intermittent claudication in chronic occlusion	• Crampy pain • Homan sign in thrombophlebitis
Pulses	• Diminished or absent	• Normal (but may be difficult to palpate due to edema)
Color	• Pale	• Normal or ruddy
Temperature	• Cool or cold	• Warm
Edema	• Absent	• Present; may be severe
Skin changes	• Thin, shiny, atrophic skin • Loss of hair • Thickened toenails	• Brown pigmentation at ankles
Ulcerations	• At toes or points of trauma	• At sides of ankles

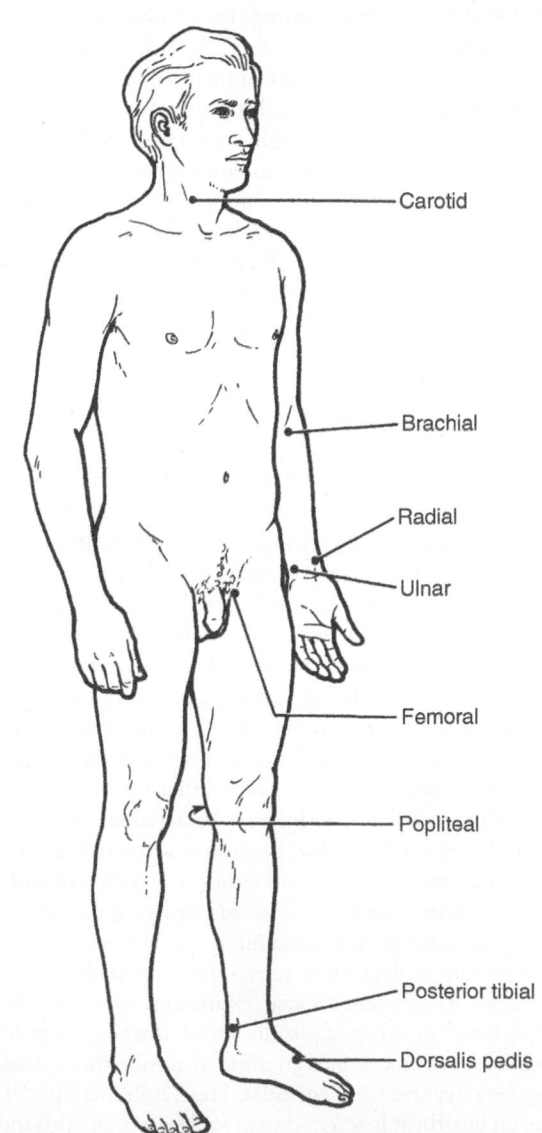

FIGURE 3-27 Locations of peripheral pulses. (From Lewis, S. M., & Collier, I. C. [1992]. *Medical-surgical nursing: Assessment and management of clinical problems* [3rd ed.]. St. Louis, MO: Mosby.)

characteristic of aortic stenosis, mitral stenosis, constrictive pericarditis, or cardiac tamponade. Pulsus alternans occurs in the presence of alternating pulse waves, every other beat being weaker than the preceding one; this is characteristic of left ventricular failure. Pulsus bisferiens is the palpation of two pulses during systole with the second pulse slightly weaker than the first; this may occur with hypertrophic cardiomyopathy, constrictive cardiomyopathy, aortic stenosis, or regurgitation. A water-hammer (or Corrigan's) pulse can be identified by an increased pulse pressure with a rapid upstroke and downstroke and shortened peak; it is characteristic of aortic regurgitation or PDA.

Dorsiflex the patient's foot with the knee slightly bent to elicit Homan sign. Homan sign is present if pain occurs in the patient's calf with this action. Homan sign is suggestive but not definitive evidence of thrombophlebitis or venous thromboembolism (i.e., DVT).

In the presence of petechiae, ecchymosis, or varicose veins, conduct a neurovascular assessment. Also assess the neurovascular status in all of the following situations: after cardiac catheterization, after a PCI procedure (e.g., angioplasty, atherectomy, valvuloplasty), when the patient has an intraaortic balloon pump catheter in place, when the patient has a fracture of an extremity (to monitor for compartment syndrome), and when the patient has a circumferential burn of an extremity. In all of these situations, monitor the patient for clinical indications of acute arterial occlusion (Box 3-1) and the clinical indications of hypoperfusion (see Table 3-2). The state of hypoperfusion is progressive; therefore, the earlier changes are identified, the more appropriate the management and the better the chances for successfully reversing the changes. The six Ps (see Box 3-1) are your format for neurovascular assessment.

Auscultation

Good equipment is imperative to conduct auscultation. A good stethoscope should have snug-fitting earplugs to eliminate extraneous sounds. The tubing should be no longer than 12 to 15 inches. The chest piece should have both a diaphragm and a bell. Hold the diaphragm firmly against the skin. The diaphragm detects high-pitched sounds, such as normal heart sounds (S_1, S_2), splits of S_1 and S_2, pericardial friction rubs, and most murmurs. Hold the bell only tightly enough against the skin to create a seal. The bell detects low-pitched sounds, such as S_3, S_4, or murmurs of AV valve stenosis. Perform cardiac auscultation in a quiet room; turn off the television and radio and ask others to be quiet. The landmarks used to auscultate heart sounds are the right sternal border (RSB), left sternal border (LSB), right intercostal space (RICS), left intercostal space (LICS), and midclavicular line (MCL). The auscultatory areas (Figure 3-29) include the aortic (second RICS at RSB), pulmonic

ARTERIAL PULSE ABNORMALITIES

Type	Description
Pulsus magnus	Pulse is readily palpable, not easily obliterated by fingers, and does not fade Pulse is felt as a brisk impact; can occur with or without increased pulse pressure
Pulsus parvus	Pulse is difficult to feel, easily obliterated by the fingers, and may fade out Pulse is slow to rise, has a sustained summit, and falls slowly If both weak and variable in amplitude, pulse is termed "thready"
Pulsus alterans	Pulses have large amplitude beats followed by pulses of small amplitude Rhythm remains normal
Pulsus paradoxus	Pattern is exaggerated (greater than 10 mm Hg) during inspiration, and amplitude is increased during expiration Heart rate and rhythm are unchanged
Pulsus bisferiens (double-peaked)	Best felt by palpating carotid artery Two systolic peaks occur in disorders that cause rapid left ventricular ejection of large stroke volume with wide pulse pressure
Water-hammer, collapsing	Pulse has greater amplitude than normal pulse Pulse marked by rapid rise to a narrow summit followed by a sudden descent

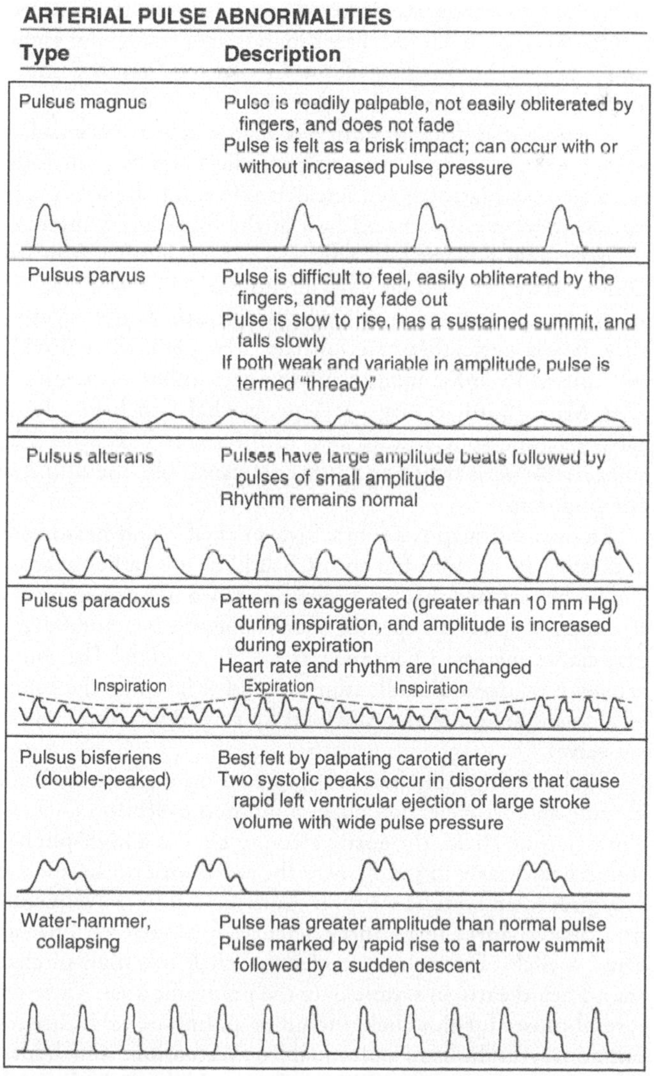

FIGURE 3-28 Pulse contour. (Modified from Cannobio, M. M. [1990]. *Cardiovascular disorders*. St. Louis, MO: Mosby.)

BOX 3-1

Clinical Manifestations of Acute Arterial Occlusion (6 Ps)

- Pain
- Pallor
- Pulselessness
- Paresthesia
- Paralysis
- Polar (cold)

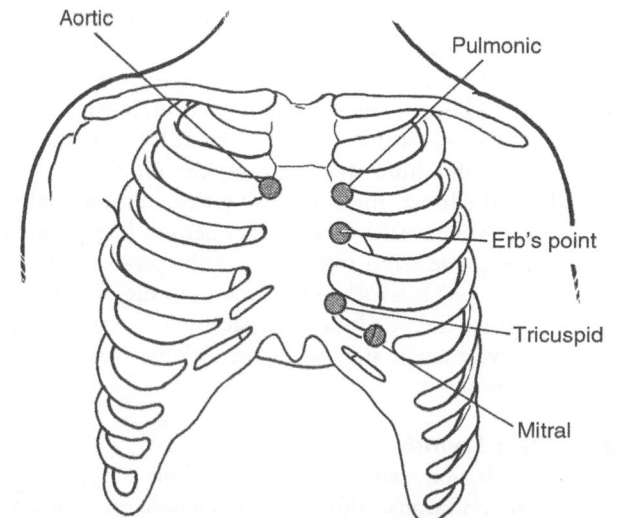

FIGURE 3-29 Cardiac auscultatory areas. (From Price, S., & Wilson, L. [2003]. *Pathophysiology: Clinical concepts of disease processes* [6th ed.]. St. Louis, MO: Mosby.)

(second LICS at LSB), Erb's point (third LICS at LSB), tricuspid (fifth LICS at LSB), and mitral (fifth LICS at MCL). Auscultate all cardiac areas with both the bell and diaphragm. Concentrate on one cardiac event at a time (S_1, S_2, systole, diastole). The usual listening positions include supine, left lateral decubitus position, sitting up, and leaning forward.

An important auscultatory principle is that left-sided heart events precede right-sided heart events. The mitral component (M_1) precedes the tricuspid component (T_1) of the S_1. The aortic component (A_2) precedes the pulmonic component (P_2) of the S_2. The left-sided heart events are normally louder than right-sided heart events. The M_1 is the loudest component of S_1, and the A_2 is the loudest component of S_2. The left-sided heart events are normally loudest during expiration, and the right-sided heart events are normally loudest during inspiration.

S_1 heart sound results from the closure of the AV valves (i.e., the mitral and tricuspid). It marks the end of diastole and the beginning of systole and is loudest at the apex. S_2 is caused by closure of the semilunar valves (i.e., aortic and pulmonic). It marks the end of systole and the beginning of diastole. It is loudest at the base. Therefore, systole is between S_1 and S_2 and diastole is between S_2 and the next S_1. Note if there is a single sound, split sound, or any increase in intensity (i.e., closing snap) of both S_1 and S_2.

A split S_1 occurs when both components (i.e., M_1 and T_1) of S_1 are heard at the tricuspid area. A narrowly split S_1 may be normal; however, a split S_1 is more often abnormal than normal and associated with right bundle branch block (RBBB), left ventricular (i.e., epicardial) pacemaker, and left ventricular ectopy.

A split S_2 occurs when both components (i.e., A_2 and P_2) of S_2 are heard. It is heard best at the pulmonic area. A split of S_2 that occurs only on inspiration is normal and called a physiologic split of S_2. Frequently heard in individuals less than 50 years of age, a physiologic split occurs due to changes in intrathoracic pressure related to ventilation or increased venous return to the right ventricle, and decreased venous return to the left ventricle from a delay in the pulmonic valve closure (P_2) causes the physiologic split of S_2.

An expiratory split of S_2, however, is always abnormal and identified by an increased splitting during inspiration (i.e., split on expiration but split more during inspiration) associated with any of the following: an RBBB, left ventricular ectopy, left ventricular (epicardial) pacemaker, severe mitral regurgitation, pulmonary stenosis, pulmonary hypertension, and a VSD. When splitting does not vary with inspiration, it is a fixed split S_2 usually due to an atrial septal defect (ASD). The ASD creates a left to right shunt that increases the blood flow to the right side of the heart, thereby causing the pulmonic valve to close later than the aortic valve independent of inspiration and expiration. A paradoxical split (i.e., a split on expiration but not on inspiration) is associated with left bundle branch block, right ventricular (i.e., endocardial) pacemaker, right ventricular ectopy, severe aortic stenosis or regurgitation, and a patent ductus arteriosus.

Extra Heart Sounds

During auscultation, extra heart sounds (Table 3-8) heard indicate various conditions. These sounds include atrial and ventricular gallops, rubs, clicks, opening snaps, and crunches.

The S_3 is a left- and right-sided ventricular gallop distinguished by a dull, low-pitched sound occurring early in diastole after S_2. An S_3 sounds like "Ken-tuc-ky" with the "ky" being the S_3. Abnormal in patients over 30 years of age, the sound occurs because of a rapid rush of blood into a dilated ventricle. Use the stethoscope bell with the patient lying on the left side to hear the sound best. The left-sided S_3 is heard best at the apex during expiration. The right-sided S_3 is heard best at the lower left sternum during inspiration. An S_3 is associated primarily with failure. Left ventricular failure causes a left-sided S_3, while right ventricular failure causes a right-sided S_3. An S_3 may also be associated with fluid overload, cardiomyopathy, VSD, PDA, and mitral or tricuspid regurgitation.

The S_4 is a left- and right-sided atrial gallop distinguished by a dull, low-pitched sound occurring late in diastole before S_1. It may sound like "Ten-nes-see" with the "Ten" being the S_4. It occurs from an atrial contraction of blood into a noncompliant ventricle and is abnormal in adults. It is heard best with the bell, with the patient lying on the left side. Left-sided S_4 is heard best at the apex. Right-sided S_4 is heard best at the lower left sternum. The S_4 is associated with myocardial ischemia/infarction and systemic or pulmonary hypertension. Systemic hypertension causes a left-sided S_4, while pulmonary hypertension is a right-sided S_4. Other conditions that cause the S_4 sound are ventricular hypertrophy, AV blocks, and severe aortic or pulmonic stenosis.

All four heart sounds are heard in a quadruple rhythm. In a summation gallop, all four heart sounds are present, but tachycardia causes the merging of the S_3 and the S_4 and causes a louder mid-diastolic sound.

A pericardial friction rub is a high-pitched "to-and-fro" scratchy sound that is usually triphasic because it includes systolic, early diastolic, and late diastolic components. A pericardial friction rub is heard best at the fourth-fifth intercostal space at the lower LSB with the patient leaning forward. Differentiate between pericardial and pleural friction rubs by asking the patient to hold his or her breath; if the rub persists, it is a pericardial friction rub. The pericardial friction rub caused by inflammation of the pericardium is common after MI or cardiac surgery. A pericardial knock is a loud, early-diastolic sound heard best at the lower LSB caused by constrictive pericarditis and it makes a snap like the sound of opening snaps.

An opening snap is a short, high-pitched sound heard early in diastole at the third-fourth LICS at LSB. It is earlier, sharper, and higher pitched than an S_3 and results from the opening of a stenotic AV valve. An opening snap is due to a structural defect that causes increased flow such as a VSD or PDA. The sound usually precedes a diastolic murmur and will mimic the sound of a closing snap (i.e., a really loud S_1, caused by closure of the AV valve).

Clicks are high-pitched sounds heard during systole. These include an aortic ejection click, a pulmonic ejection click, or a midsystolic click. The aortic ejection click is a high-pitched sound heard early in systole over the aortic area to the apex. It may precede a systolic ejection murmur. Aortic valve disease or a dilated aorta (e.g., aortic aneurysm or coarctation) can cause a click. The pulmonic ejection click is a high-pitched sound heard early in systole over the pulmonic area. There are several causes for this click, including pulmonic valve disease, pulmonary embolism, pulmonary hypertension, and hyperthyroidism. The midsystolic click is a high-pitched sound heard best at the apex or LSB. It may occur alone or before

TABLE 3-8   Extra Sounds

Sound	Cause	Timing	Location	Pitch	Position	Respiratory Effect
S3 (also called *ventricular gallop*)	Rapid ventricular filling into dilated ventricle	Early diastole (rapid filling phase of diastole)	Mitral if LV; tricuspid if RV	Low	Heard best in left lateral position	LV S3 increases with expiration; RV S3 increases with inspiration
S4 (also called *atrial with gallop*)	Atrial contraction into noncompliant ventricle	Late diastole (atrial contraction phase of diastole)	Mitral if LV; tricuspid if RV	Low	Heard best in left lateral position	LV S4 increased expiration; RV S4 increased with inspiration
Quadruple rhythm	All four heart sounds are heard	S3 heard in early diastole, and S4 heard in late diastole	Apex	Low	Heard best in left lateral position	As for S3, S4
Summation gallop	S1, S2 heard along with merged S3 and S4; occurs with tachycardia	Mid-diastole	Apex	Low	Heard best in left lateral position	As for S3, S4
Pericardial friction rub	Inflammation of the pericardium	Systolic, early diastolic, and late diastolic components	Lower left sternal border	High	Heard best with patient leaning forward	Heard best if patient holds breath after expiration
Pericardial knock	Constriction of the pericardium	Early diastole	Lower left sternal border	Low	Heard best with patient leaning forward or in left lateral position	Heard best if patient holds breath after expiration
Ejection click	Opening of defective semilunar valve	Early systole	Aortic or pulmonic	High	Heard best with patient leaning forward	Aortic: not affected by respiratory phase Pulmonic: increased with expiration
Midsystolic click	Prolapse of mitral valve leaflet	Midsystole	Mitral	High	Heard best in left lateral position	Increased with expiration
Opening snap	Abrupt recoil of stenotic atrioventricular valve	Early diastole	Mitral	High	Heard best in left lateral position	Mitral: increased with expiration Tricuspid: increased with inspiration
Mediastinal crunch	Pneumomediastinum; heart movements displacing air that is present in the mediastinum	Random	Apex or lower left sternal border	High	Heard best in left lateral position	Increased with inspiration

a late systolic murmur. It usually results from mitral valve prolapse or mitral regurgitation. The prosthetic valve click is a metallic click caused by the opening and closing of the prosthetic valve.

A mediastinal crunch is a crunching sound heard best at the apex or along the LSB in the left lateral position. Air in the mediastinum causes the crunch sound and may be noted in thoracic trauma patients.

Murmurs and Bruits

Murmurs and bruits are the result of turbulence. Causes of turbulence (Figure 3-30) include increased flow across a normal valve (i.e., flow murmur); forward flow through a stenotic valve; backward flow through a regurgitant, also called an *insufficient* or *incompetent* valve; flow through an AV fistula or septal defect; or flow into a dilated chamber or a portion of a vessel. A *murmur* occurs from intracardiac turbulent blood flow. A *bruit* occurs from extracardiac turbulent blood flow. Murmurs may be functional or structural. Functional murmurs are always soft (i.e., not louder than grade II/VI) and systolic, but never holosystolic. Flow murmurs are an example of functional murmurs caused by increased flow across a normal valve. Conditions that cause flow murmurs include hyperthermia, anemia, pregnancy, or hyperthyroidism. A functional murmur is primarily due to physiologic conditions outside the heart, as opposed to structural defects in the heart itself. Disease of the cardiac valves and other cardiac structures results in abnormal turbulent blood flow within the heart, causing structural murmurs.

Differentiate murmurs (Figure 3-31) by timing and location. First, identify if the murmur is systolic or diastolic. A murmur heard between S_1 and S_2 is a systolic murmur. Systolic murmurs are holosystolic, resulting from AV valve regurgitation or a VSD, or midsystolic, resulting from semilunar valve stenosis. A murmur heard between S_2 and the next S_1 is a diastolic murmur. Diastolic murmurs can be early, resulting from semilunar valve regurgitation, or mid- to late diastolic, resulting from AV valve stenosis. Next, identify the location where the murmur is loudest, whether it radiates, and in which direction it radiates. Rate the intensity of the murmur on the Levine scale:

- Grade I/VI: barely audible, difficult to detect
- Grade II/VI: clearly audible but quiet
- Grade III/VI: moderately loud, without a thrill
- Grade IV/VI: loud; with or without a thrill
- Grade V/VI: very loud, thrill present, audible with stethoscope partially off the chest
- Grade VI/VI: loudest possible, thrill present, audible with stethoscope off the chest

Identify the pitch of the murmur by listening with the bell and diaphragm of the stethoscope. A murmur heard best with the bell indicates a low-pitched murmur, while a murmur heard best with the diaphragm indicates a high-pitched murmur. A high-pitched sound might indicate mitral and tricuspid regurgitation, aortic and pulmonic stenosis, or aortic and pulmonic regurgitation. A low-pitched sound indicates mitral and tricuspid stenosis. Describe the quality of the murmur as soft, harsh, blowing, musical, rumbling, or rough. Murmurs may also be described by shape or configuration. Common classifications include the following.

- Crescendo: gets louder
- Decrescendo: gets softer
- Crescendo-decrescendo: louder then softer
- Plateau: same loudness throughout

3.7 Learning Activity

Match the heart sound to its possible cause.

Heart Sound	Possible Cause
_____ 1. S_1	a. Changes in intrathoracic pressure created by ventilation
_____ 2. S_2	b. Atrial septal defect, acute pulmonary hypertension, pulmonic stenosis
_____ 3. Physiologic split of S_2	c. Pericarditis
_____ 4. Paradoxical split of S_2	d. Aortic stenosis, pulmonic stenosis
_____ 5. Fixed, wide split of S_2	e. Mitral stenosis, tricuspid stenosis
_____ 6. S_3	f. LBBB, right ventricular pacemaker or ectopy, severe aortic valve disease, patent ductus arteriosus
_____ 7. S_4	g. Mitral regurgitation, tricuspid stenosis, ventricular septal defect
_____ 8. Pericardial friction rub	h. HF, fluid overload, cardiomyopathy, ventricular septal defect, patent ductus arteriosus
_____ 9. Mid-systolic click	i. Closure of aortic and pulmonic valves
_____ 10. Holosystolic murmur	j. Mitral valve prolapse, mitral regurgitation
_____ 11. Systolic ejection murmur	k. Closure of mitral and tricuspid valves
_____ 12. Early diastolic murmur	l. Aortic regurgitation, pulmonic regurgitation
_____ 13. Mid- to late-diastolic murmur	m. Myocardial ischemia or infarction, hypertension, ventricular hypertrophy, AV block, severe aortic or pulmonic stenosis

Answers to this activity can be found in the Answer Key.

3.8 Learning Activity

Complete the following table describing common murmurs.

Condition	Timing	Location	Pitch
Mitral regurgitation			
Mitral stenosis			
Aortic regurgitation			
Aortic stenosis			
Mitral valve prolapse			
Papillary muscle dysfunction or rupture			
Ventricular septal defect or rupture			

Answers to this activity can be found in the Answer Key.

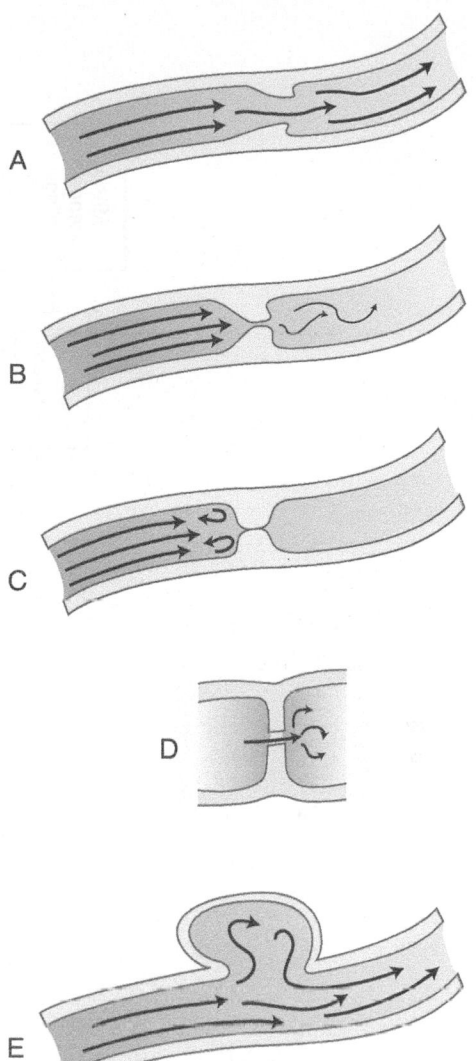

FIGURE 3-30 Causes of turbulence. A, Increased flow across a normal valve. **B,** Forward flow through a stenotic valve. **C,** Backward flow through an incompetent valve. **D,** Flow through a septal defect or an AV fistula. **E,** Flow into a dilated chamber or a portion of a vessel. (From Dennison, R. D. [2013]. *Pass CCRN!* [4th ed]. St. Louis, MO: Elsevier.)

A bruit, Doppler pulse and Doppler pressure are vascular sounds. A bruit is turbulent blood flow that is heard outside of the heart chambers, such as over carotids, aorta, renals, iliacs, and femorals. It is associated with plaque or an aneurysm. If the pulse is difficult to palpate, a Doppler stethoscope is used to confirm that the pulse palpated is the patient's and not the nurse's. A Doppler stethoscope measures the BP distal to vascular lesions or surgery. Apply the sphygmomanometer on the calf or below the graft site and inflate to a pressure above the patient's systolic brachial pressure. Allow the pressure to decrease and note the pressure when the pulse is audible again with the Doppler stethoscope over the posterior tibial artery and then dorsalis pedis artery. Use the best pressure (i.e., posterior tibial or dorsalis pedis) to calculate the ankle-brachial index (ABI). Divide the systolic pressure from the leg by the brachial systolic pressure (ankle/brachial) to calculate the ABI. The toe-brachial index (TBI)—the great toe's systolic pressure divided by the brachial systolic pressure—may also be used; normal and abnormal values are the same as for ABI. The ABI or TBI is an important part of the diagnosis and the evaluation of the extent of arterial disease, and it is classified as follows:

- Unreliable: greater than 1
- Normal: 0.95-1
- Mildly abnormal: 0.95-0.75
- Moderately abnormal: 0.75-0.5
- Ischemia: 0.50-0.25

- Severe ischemia: less than 0.25
- Clinically significant: a decrease of 0.15 or more

Diagnostic Studies

Numerous diagnostic laboratory studies evaluate cardiovascular clinical status. Examine the serum chemistries, hematology, clotting profiles, arterial blood gases, and urinalysis (see Appendix D) in patients with cardiovascular conditions.

Cardiac troponin T and troponin I are a group of compounds that bind to tropomyosin and are involved with the excitation-contraction in muscle. These are the most sensitive markers of cardiac injury or death of myocytes. The levels rise 4 to 6 hours after the onset of ischemic symptoms. The levels peak at 18 to 24 hours after an MI, then fall slowly over a 2-week period. The kidneys clear both compounds, so levels are elevated in chronic renal failure, although troponin I will be more accurate because it is less affected by renal failure. The analysis of troponin facilitates quicker decision making in identification, risk stratification, and treatment of cardiac patients.

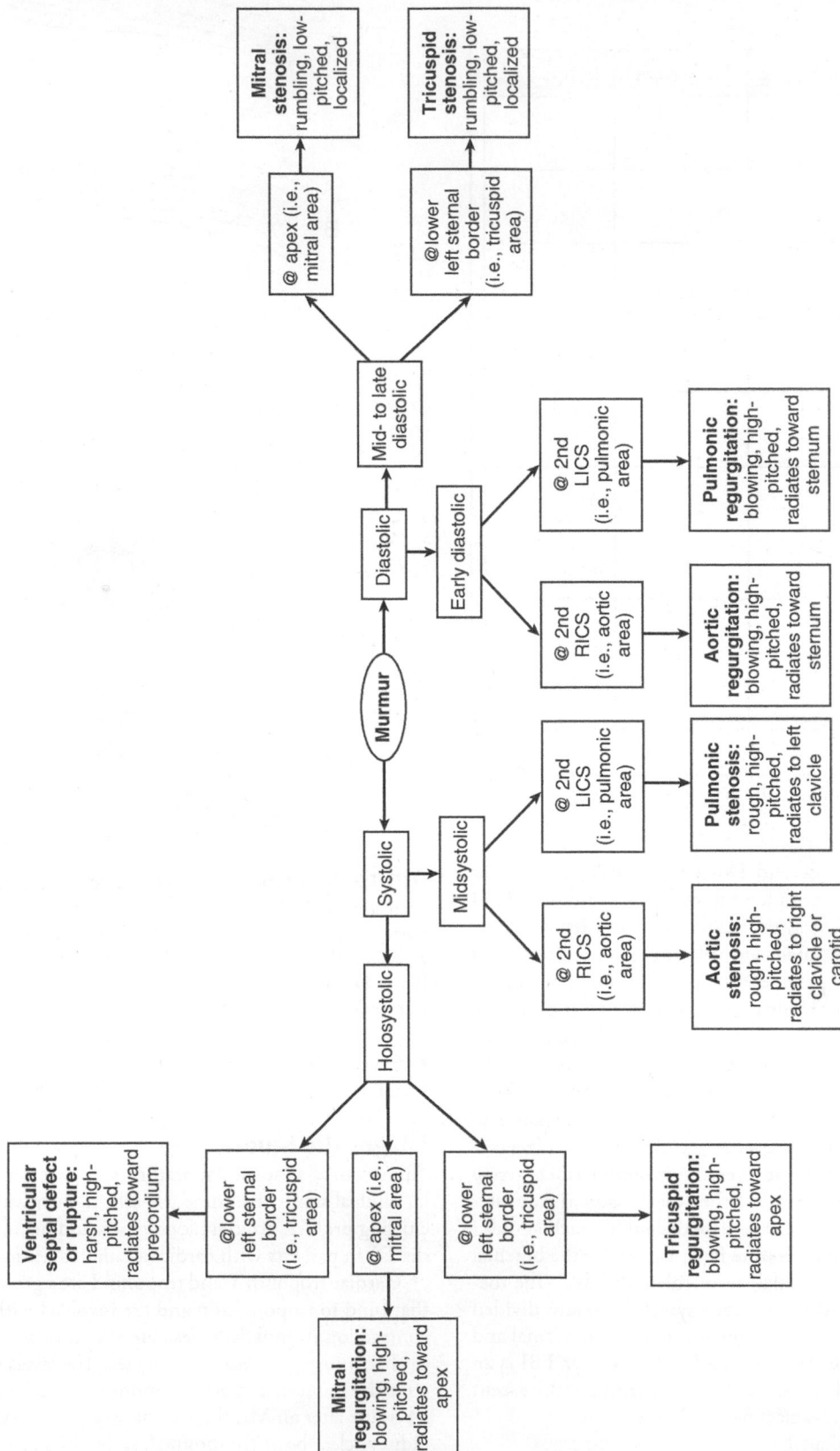

FIGURE 3-31 Murmurs. *LICS,* Left intercostal space; *RICS,* right intercostal space. (From Dennison, R. D. [2013]. *Pass CCRN!* [4th ed]. St. Louis, MO: Elsevier.)

Creatine kinase (CK) and CK-MB isoenzyme are associated with ATP conversion in the contractile muscle tissue. The enzymes are found in heart, brain, and skeletal tissues. MB isoenzyme levels are very sensitive to cardiac tissue. Levels rise 4 to 8 hours after onset, peak in 12 to 24 hours, and return to normal in 24 to 48 hours. A CK-MB concentration of more than 5% of total CK indicates myocardial necrosis.

Myoglobin is a heme-containing protein and a very sensitive marker, but it is not cardiac specific. Myoglobin can elevate with cardiopulmonary resuscitation (CPR), falls, and injections. The level peaks 8 hours after an infarct, then rapidly returns to normal in 18 to 24 hours. This marker is useful in the emergency departments for early MI detection, ruling out of an MI, and reperfusion monitoring. Myocardial stretch releases brain natriuretic peptide (BNP). The level correlates with LV dysfunction. Use the BNP to evaluate HF and the presence of pulmonary emboli. In addition, use the BNP to differentiate cardiac causes from pulmonary causes of pulmonary distress and dyspnea. High BNP levels indicate poor prognosis. False low levels can occur in obese patients because clearance in adipose tissue removes the BNP from the circulation. False high results can occur in the elderly, hypertensive individuals, females, and in patients treated with nesiritide (synthetic BNP).

C-reactive protein is a biomarker of inflammation and can be used as an independent predictor of future cardiovascular risk. An elevation in this protein can indicate an acute infection, inflammatory disease processes, and possible uremia.

In addition to these specific diagnostic labs, a cardiac laboratory's diagnostic profile includes a clotting profile including aPTT, PT/INR, and ACT. The clotting profiles monitor the effectiveness of anticoagulation therapy. Patients with specific disorders such as atrial fibrillation or prosthetic valves have defined recommended therapeutic ranges to maintain with anticoagulants. The therapeutic range for atrial fibrillation is an INR of 2.0 to 3.0. For patients with a prosthetic valve the range is 2.5 to 3.5. The ACT is a bedside test done to measure the time required for blood coagulation. The ACT evaluates heparin's effectiveness to determine whether it is safe to remove a vascular sheath. In addition, complete blood counts, serum electrolyte levels, fasting lipid profile, and homocysteine levels are the routine diagnostic studies completed. The lipid profile examines total cholesterol, high-density lipoproteins, low-density lipoproteins, and triglycerides. Homocysteine levels identify folic acid responsive hyperlipidemia. A normal level is 5 to 15 μmol/L. Elevated levels are considered an independent risk factor for CAD. Other diagnostic studies (Table 3-9) performed to identify specific cardiac conditions and evaluate cardiovascular status include radiologic studies, ultrasounds, cardiopulmonary procedures, nuclear medicine scans, and various ECG testing.

ELECTROCARDIOGRAPHY

General Information

The electrocardiograph measures and records the electrical activity of the heart by measuring electrical potential at the skin surface. The electrocardiogram (ECG) is a recording of that activity. An ECG detects or demonstrates rhythm disturbances, conduction defects, electrolyte imbalances, drug effects and toxicity, chamber enlargement or hypertrophy, and myocardial ischemia, injury, or infarction.

The rule of electrical flow states that impulses traveling toward the positive pole of a lead cause a positive deflection and impulses traveling toward the negative (or away from the positive) pole of a lead cause a negative deflection. On the ECG paper (Figure 3-32), the horizontal axis measures time. Each small box is 1 mm in size and equal to 0.04 second while each large box is 5 mm in size and equal to 0.2 second. The small marks at the top of the paper identify 3-second intervals. The vertical axis measures voltage. This is useful only with standardized measures, such as on multiple-lead ECG. Rhythm strips are not generally standardized because the size (i.e., gain) can be changed. If standardized, each small 1-mm box is equal to 0.1 mV. Each large 5-mm box is equal to 0.5 mV.

Rhythm Strip Analysis
Monitoring Leads

In a five-lead system, the standard electrode placement (Figure 3-33) places the white lead (i.e., right arm) just below the right clavicle and the black lead (i.e., left arm) just below the left clavicle. Place the brown lead for V_1 at the fourth ICS at the RSB or V_6 when placed at the fifth ICS at the left midaxillary line (MAL). Place the green lead (i.e., right leg) on the lower chest, above and to the right of the umbilicus. Place the red lead (i.e., left leg) on the lower chest, above and to the left of the umbilicus. One way to remember lead placement is *White on the right, snow over grass, smoke over fire, brown on the ground* (Barill, 2012).

Other available leads include I, II, III, aVR, aVL, aVF, or V. The V lead you use will depend on the placement of the brown lead. In the typical leads monitored in a three-lead system (Figure 3-34), a lead II places a positive (i.e., red) at the lower left torso, negative (i.e., white) under the right clavicle, and ground (i.e., black) under the left clavicle. The modified chest leads (MCLs) include MCL_1 and MCL_6. For MCL_1, set monitor at lead 1 and place leads as positive (black) at the fourth ICS at RSB, negative (white) under the left clavicle, and ground (red) under the right clavicle. For MCL_6, set the monitor at lead II and place leads as positive (black) at the fifth ICS at the left MAL, negative (white) under the left clavicle, and ground (red) under the right clavicle. The difference between MCLs and true V leads is that V leads are unipolar (and preferred if available) while MCLs are bipolar.

SIDEBAR 3-3	
Lead Placement for Continuous Derived 12-Lead ECG (EASI)	
E (brown)	Lower part of the sternum at the fifth ICS
A (red)	Right midaxillary line at the fifth ICS
S (black)	Upper part of the sternum
I (white)	Left midaxillary line at the fifth ICS
Fifth electrode (green)	Anywhere on the torso; serves as a ground

TABLE 3-9   Cardiovascular Diagnostic Studies

Study	Evaluates	Comments
Aortography	• Aortic valve insufficiency • Aneurysms or dissection of ascending aorta • Coarctation of the aorta • Injuries to the aorta and major branches	• Contrast medium used: check for allergy to iodine, shellfish, dye; ensure hydration following procedure to avoid acute kidney injury (AKI) • Monitor for clinical indications of anaphylaxis (e.g., flushing, urticaria, stridor) • Monitor puncture site
Cardiac biopsy	• Effect of cardiotoxic drugs • Evidence of cardiac transplant rejection • Inflammatory heart disease • Tumors • Cardiomyopathy	• Observe closely for signs of cardiac perforation and/or cardiac tamponade

Cardiac catheterization and coronary angiography	• Severity of coronary artery stenosis
	• Cardiac muscle function
	• Pressures within the heart
	• Cardiac output and ejection fraction
	• Blood gas analysis within chambers
	• Allows angioplasty, atherectomy, intracoronary stents, or lasers to reduce coronary artery obstruction
		• Prior to test:
		  • Check for allergy to iodine, shellfish, dye (contrast medium used)
		• After the test:
		  • Ensure hydration following procedure (contrast medium used) to avoid AKI
		  • Keep extremity in which catheter was placed immobilized in a straight position for 3-6 hours
		  • Monitor arterial puncture point for hemorrhage or hematoma; collagen (e.g., AngioSeal) or stitch device (e.g., Perclose) may be used
		  • Monitor neurovascular status of affected limb
		  • Note complaints of back pain and vital sign changes (may indicate retroperitoneal hemorrhage)

Chest x-ray	• Cardiac size and shape and chamber size • Abnormalities of the lungs, ribs, pleura, pulmonary vasculature • Presence of pleural effusions • Presence of thoracic aneurysm or calcification of the aorta • Presence and location of catheters, pacemaker, and automatic implantable cardiac defibrillator (AICD) leads	• Inquire about possibility of pregnancy
Computed tomography (CT) Electron beam computerized tomography (EBCT): high speed imaging provides improved view of vascular structures including calcification	• Left ventricular wall motion • Cardiac tumors • Myocardial infarction • Pericardial effusion • Aortic aneurysm • Aortic dissection	• May be done with or without contrast medium • If contrast medium used: check for allergy to iodine, shellfish, dye; ensure hydration following procedure to avoid AKI
Digital subtraction angiography	• Vascular disease and degree of occlusion	• Contrast medium used: check for allergy to iodine, shellfish, dye; ensure hydration following procedure to avoid AKI • Monitor for clinical indications of anaphylaxis (e.g., flushing, urticaria, stridor) • Monitor puncture site

Test/Procedure	Uses	Nursing Considerations
Doppler ultrasonography Duplex ultrasonography	• Vascular disease and degree of occlusion	• No preparation required • Wash off conductive paste

Echocardiography
M-mode: single ultrasound beam
2-D: planar ultrasound beam; wider view of heart and structures
Doppler: addition of Doppler to demonstrate flow of blood through the heart
Color flow: Doppler blood flow superimposed on 2-D echocardiogram
Stress echocardiography: images before, during, and after exercise or pharmacologic stress
Transesophageal echocardiography (TEE): transducer placed in esophagus
	• Chamber size and wall thickness
	• Valve functioning
	  • Papillary muscle functioning
	  • Prosthetic valve functioning
	• Ventricular wall motion abnormalities
	• Intracardiac masses
	• Presence of pericardial fluid
	• Intracardiac pressures (Doppler)
	• Ejection fraction and cardiac output (Doppler)
	• Valve gradients (Doppler)
	• Intracardiac shunts (Doppler)
	• Thoracic aneurysm (transesophageal)
		• TEE is better particularly if patient is obese, has COPD, chest wall deformity, chest trauma, or thick chest dressings
		• Monitor for methemoglobinemia if local anesthetic (e.g., Cetacaine) is used
		• If TEE, monitor for clinical indications of esophageal perforation (i.e., sore throat, dysphagia, epigastric or substernal pain)

Electrocardiography (ECG)	• Dysrhythmias • Conduction defects including intraventricular blocks • Electrolyte imbalance • Drug toxicity • Myocardial ischemia, injury, infarction • Chamber hypertrophy	• List what drugs the patient is receiving on ECG request • Be alert to electrical safety hazards
Electrophysiologic studies (EPS)	• Dysrhythmias under controlled circumstances • Best therapy for control of dysrhythmia: drug, required dosage of therapy; pacemaker; catheter ablation	• Patients may have near-death experience during EPS; encourage expression of fears, concerns, anxieties • Monitor puncture site
Holter monitor	• Suspected dysrhythmias over a 24- to 48-hour period • Pacemaker function • Silent ischemia	• Instruct patient regarding importance of diary-keeping
Intravascular ultrasound (IVUS)	• Coronary artery size and patency • Structure of vessel wall • Coronary artery stent position and patency • Aorta and presence of aneurysm; aneurysm dissections	• As for cardiac catheterization

Continued

TABLE 3-9   Cardiovascular Diagnostic Studies—cont'd

Study	Evaluates	Comments
Magnetic resonance imaging (MRI)	• 3-D view of the heart • Anatomy and structure of the heart and great vessels including: cardiomyopathy, congenital defect, masses, aneurysm • Changes in chemistry of tissues before structural changes occur	• Does not involve radiation or dyes • Cannot be used in patients with any implanted metallic device, including pacemakers, implantable defibrillators, metallic heart valves, intracranial aneurysm clips
Multiple-gated acquisition (MUGA) scan (radionuclide angiography)	• Ventricular size and ventricular wall motion • Cardiac output, cardiac index, end-systolic volume, end-diastolic volume, and ejection fraction • Intracardiac shunts	• Assure patient that amount of radioactive material is minimal
Pericardiocentesis and pericardial fluid analysis	• Presence of blood, pus, pathogens, or malignancy • Also used for emergency relief of cardiac tamponade	• Observe closely for signs of cardiac tamponade

Peripheral angiography	*Arterial*
	• Atherosclerotic plaques, occlusion, aneurysms, or traumatic injury
	Venous
	• Patency of peripheral venous system and presence of deep vein thrombosis
		• Prior to test:
		  • Contrast medium used: check for allergy to iodine, shellfish, dye
		• After the test:
		  • Contrast medium used, ensure hydration postprocedure to avoid AKI
		  • Keep extremity in which catheter was placed immobilized in a straight position for 3-6 hours
		  • Monitor arterial puncture point for hemorrhage or hematoma
		  • Monitor neurovascular status of affected limb
		  • Monitor for indications of systemic emboli

Plethysmography: arterial or venous	• Patency of peripheral arteries and presence of occlusive vascular disease	• Requires one normal extremity since one extremity is compared to the other
Positron emission tomography (cardiac PET scan)	• Severity of coronary artery stenosis • Collateral circulation • Patency of bypass grafts • Size and location of infarcted tissue	• Assure patient that amount of radioactive material is minimal
Sestamibi exercise testing and scan Sestamibi-dipyridamole stress test (for patients with physical limitation preventing exercise)	• Myocardial ischemia during exercise (ischemic areas show increased uptake of radioactivity [hot spots])	• Monitor for myocardial ischemia
Signal-averaged ECG	• Presence of late electrical potentials which may be responsible for malignant ventricular dysrhythmias; may be performed before and after ablation	• Patient must lie still for 10 minutes

Test	Findings/Purpose	Nursing Considerations
Stress electrocardiography (also referred to as exercise tolerance test [ETT])	• Persons with high risk for CAD, patients with known CAD, or post-CABG patients for ischemia with exercise or pharmacologic agents (e.g., adenosine, dipyridamole, dobutamine) if patient cannot tolerate exercise • Exercise-induced dysrhythmias	• One millimeter or greater transient ST segment depression 80 msec after the J point is suggestive of CAD • Monitor closely for exercise-induced hypotension or ventricular dysrhythmias • Adenosine is the preferred agent for pharmacologic stress test because it has a short half-life and does not require reversal agent
Technetium-99 pyrophosphate scan	• Size, location of acute MI (infarcted areas show increased uptake of radioactivity ["hot spots"] 1-7 days after MI)	• Assure patient that amount of radioactive material is minimal • Peak accuracy at 12-48 hours after initial symptoms
Thallium stress ECG	• Myocardial ischemia during exercise (ischemic areas show decreased uptake of radioactivity [cold spots])	• Assure patient that amount of radioactive material is minimal
Thallium-201 scan	• Myocardial ischemia (ischemic areas show decreased uptake of radioactivity [cold spots])	• Assure patient that amount of radioactive material is minimal
Vectorcardiography	• Chamber hypertrophy • Bundle branch blocks and hemiblocks • Myocardial ischemia or infarction	
Venography (ascending contrast phlebography)	• Deep leg veins • Presence of deep vein thrombosis (DVT) • Competence of deep vein valves • May be used to locate suitable vein for arterial bypass graft	• Contrast medium used: check for allergy to iodine, shellfish, dye; ensure hydration postprocedure to avoid AKI • Monitor for clinical indications of anaphylaxis (e.g. flushing, urticaria, stridor) • Monitor puncture site
Ventriculography	• Ventricular wall motion • Wall thickness • Ventricular aneurysm • Mitral valve motion • LV end-diastolic volume, end-systolic volume, stroke volume, ejection fraction • Intracardiac shunt	• Contrast medium used: check for allergy to iodine, shellfish, dye; ensure hydration postprocedure to avoid AKI • Monitor for clinical indications of anaphylaxis (e.g., flushing, urticaria, stridor) • Monitor puncture site

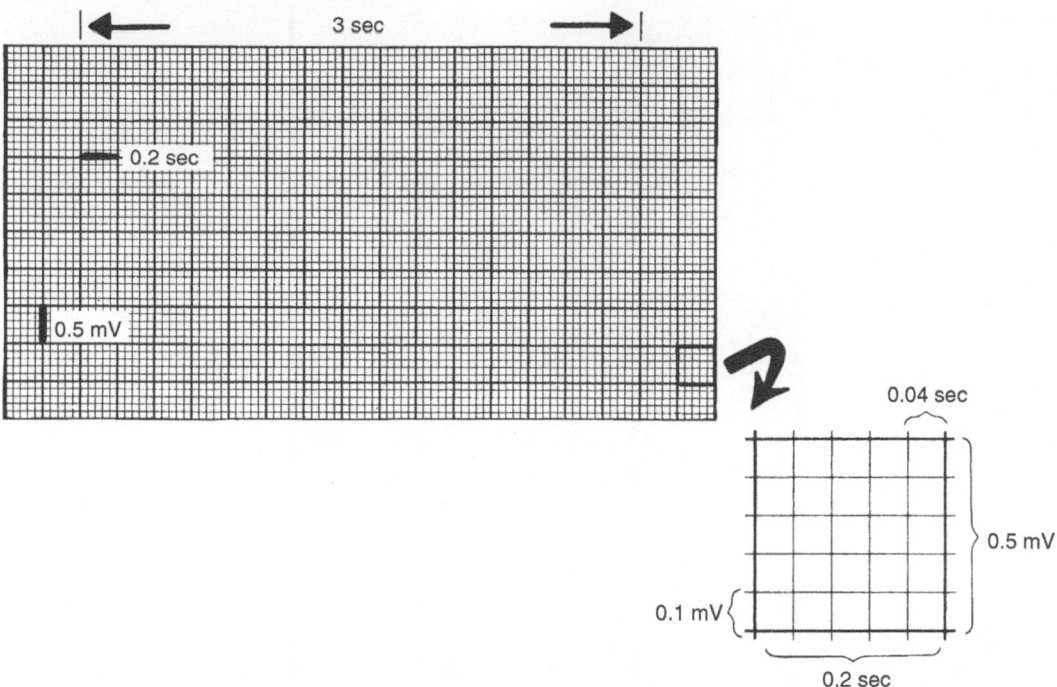

FIGURE 3-32 ECG paper. Horizontal axis represents time with each small block equal to 0.04 second and each large block equal to 0.2 second with 3-second intervals marked off at top of paper; vertical axis represents voltage when standardized with each small block equal to 0.1 mV and each large block equal to 0.5 mV. (From Kinney, M. R., et al. [1998]. *AACN's clinical reference for critical-care nursing* [4th ed.]. St. Louis, MO: Mosby.)

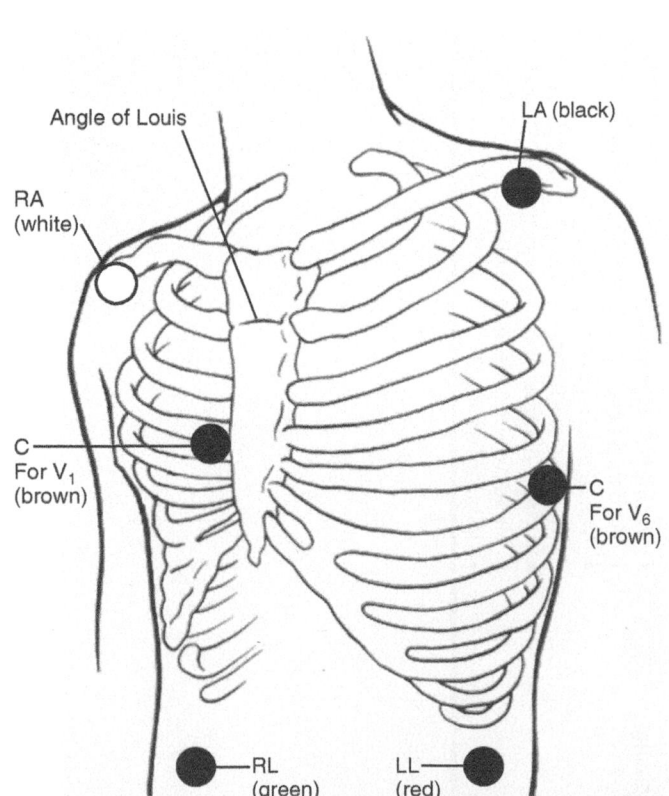

FIGURE 3-33 Standard electrode placement for monitoring with a five-lead system. (From Drew, B. [2002]. *Philips—AACN cardiac monitoring pocket reference*. Philips PN #5990-0487. Aliso Viejo, CA: American Association of Critical-Care Nurses.)

Lead Selection

In lead II, the normal P wave is upright and the normal QRS complex is upright. The primary disadvantage of using lead II is that ectopy and aberrancy look alike. Clinically, lead II is indicated for atrial dysrhythmias. Lead V_1 or MCL_1 provides better differentiation of ectopy from aberrancy, differentiation of left bundle branch block (LBBB) from right bundle branch block (RBBB), and differentiation of LV ectopy from RV ectopy. Disadvantages of V_1 or MCL_1 include the normal biphasic P wave and predominantly negative QRS. V_1 or MCL_1 is indicated for the diagnosis of wide QRS complexes (e.g., differentiation of ventricular ectopy from supraventricular tachycardia with aberrancy, differentiation of RBBB or LBBB). In patients with ischemia, injury, or infarction, two leads are best. The lead with significant ST segment elevation (i.e., patient's ischemic fingerprint) determines the second lead. If the patient's ischemic fingerprint is undetermined, the second lead should be lead III or V_3 until the multiple-lead ECG can be reviewed to determine the lead with the most significant ST segment elevation.

The V_1 is the lead used most often to assess pacemaker function and in cases of HF and/or cardiomyopathy to monitor for the development of bundle branch block. MCL_1 and MCL_6 are substitutes for V_1 and V_6 leads. This may be especially helpful if an incision/dressing prevents placement of the lead at the sternum.

The Cardiac Cycle

Components of a single cardiac cycle (Figure 3-35) are labeled as PQRST. The P wave represents atrial depolarization, the first deflection from the isoelectric line. A normal

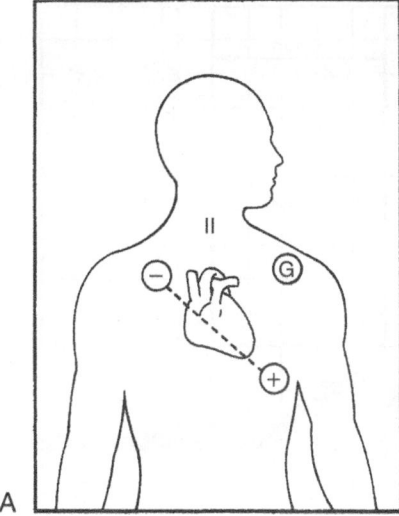

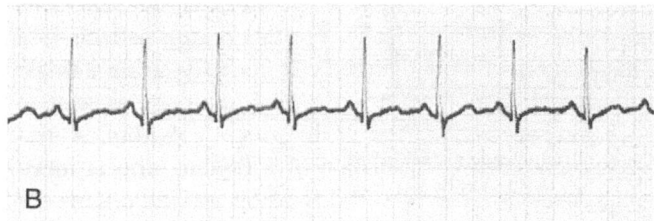

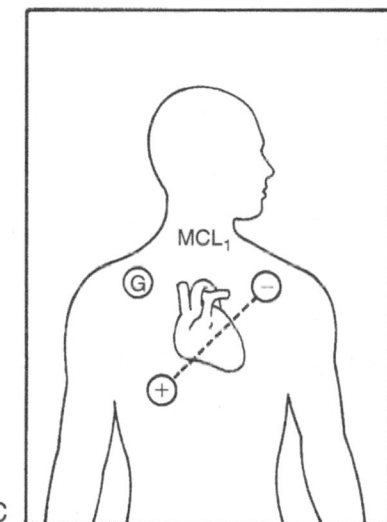

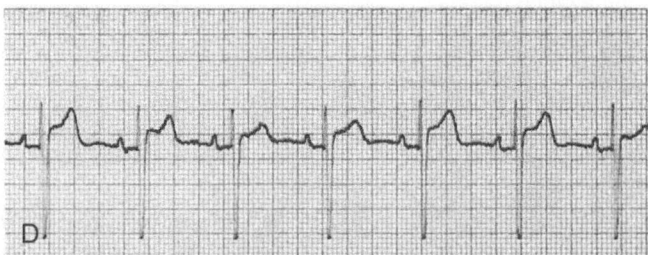

FIGURE 3-34 Monitoring leads. A, Electrode placement for lead II. **B,** Representation of appearance of ECG in lead II. **C,** Electrode placement for MCL₁. **D,** Representation of appearance of ECG in MCL₁. (From Urden L. D., Lough M. E., & Stacy K. M. [1995]. *Priorities in critical care nursing.* St. Louis, MO: Mosby.)

P wave is no more than 2.5 mm tall and no more than 0.11 second wide. The PR segment represents a delay from the AV node, at the isoelectric line between the P wave and the QRS complex. The PR interval represents atrial depolarization as well as the delay in the AV node. The PR interval is measured from the beginning of the P wave to the beginning of the QRS complex. A normal PR interval ranges from 0.12 to 0.2 second. The Q wave is the first negative wave after the P wave but before the R wave. The R wave is the first positive wave after the P wave. An S wave is any negative wave after the R wave.

The QRS complex represents ventricular depolarization and may have one, two, or all three waves: Q, R, and S. The upper or lower case of the letter indicates size (e.g., qRS indicates a small q and large R and S). An apostrophe after an R indicates that it is a second R (i.e., R') as seen in bundle branch blocks. For example, rSR' indicates small R, large S, and a large second R. This QRS configuration is common in bundle branch block. Measure the QRS from the beginning of the first wave of the complex to the end of the last wave of the complex. A normal QRS interval is 0.06 to 0.11, while the normal QRS amplitude is less than 30 mm in chest leads.

The ST segment represents the time beginning from when the ventricles completely depolarized to the beginning of repolarization. It is located between the QRS complex and the beginning of the T wave and is normally isoelectric at baseline.

The J point is the angle at which the QRS complex ends and the ST segment begins. The J point deviates from the isoelectric line if the ST segment is elevated or depressed.

The T wave represents ventricular repolarization. The T wave is after the QRS and may be positive or negative. A normal T wave is less than 5 mm in limb leads and less than 10 mm in the chest lead.

A small wave occurring after the T wave is the U wave, but this is often not seen due to its low voltage. The U wave may represent repolarization of the Purkinje fibers. A normal U wave is less than or equal to 1 mm.

The QT interval represents the time for both ventricular depolarization and repolarization. Measure the QT interval from the first wave of QRS complex to the end of the T wave. A normal QT interval varies based on the heart rate. The slower the heart rate is, the longer the normal QT; the faster the heart rate is, the shorter the normal QT. For heart rates 60 to 100 beats/min, a normal QT interval is less than half of the RR interval. To correct for changes in heart rate, especially for heart rates not 60 to 100 beats/min, calculate the QTc. A normal QTc is 0.32 to 0.44. Many substances interfere with the QT interval (Table 3-10) and clinical indications for monitoring of the QT interval include a congenital long QT syndrome, significant bradycardia (less than 50 beats/min), use of antidysrhythmics that are known to prolong the QT interval, substances that cause electrolyte imbalances, or tricyclic antidepressant and antibiotic use.

SIDEBAR 3-4

QTc Formula

Corrected QT (QT_C) = QT Interval ÷ $\sqrt{}$ RR interval

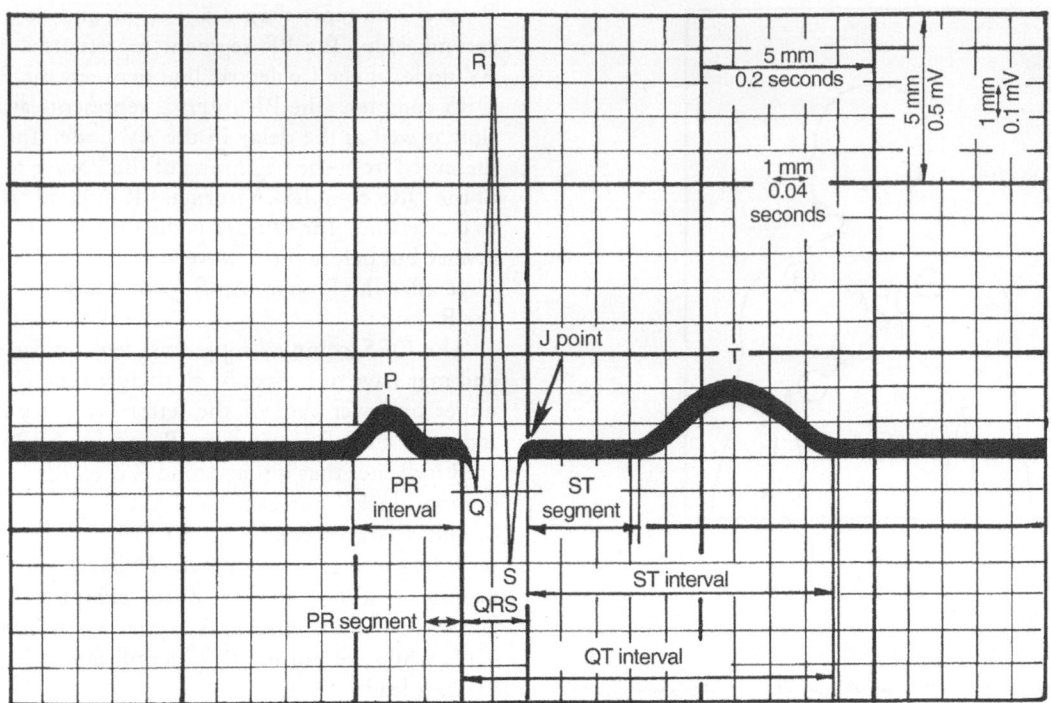

FIGURE 3-35 Components of a single cardiac cycle. (From Seidel, J. C. [1986]. *The Methodist Hospital: Basic electrocardiography: A modular approach.* St. Louis, MO: Mosby.)

TABLE 3-10	Substances and Conditions Interfering with the QT Interval	
Class IA antidysrhythmics	• Quinidine • Procainamide (Pronestyl) • Disopyramide (Norpace)
Class IC antidysrhythmics	• Flecainide (Tambocor) • Propafenone (Rythmol)
Class II/III antidysrhythmics	• Sotalol (Betapace)
Class III antidysrhythmics	• Ibutilide (Corvert) • Dofetilide (Tikosyn)
Tricyclic antidepressants	• Amitriptyline (Elavil) • Nortriptyline (Pamelor)
Antibiotics	• Fluoroquinolones (e.g., gemifloxacin, moxifloxacin) • Macrolides (e.g., azithromycin) • Erythromycin
Electrolyte imbalances	• Hypokalemia • Hypomagnesemia • Hypocalcemia
Pathologic conditions	• Cerebrovascular disease, including intracranial or subarachnoid hemorrhage, stroke, intracranial trauma • Hypothermia • Hypothyroidism • Hypoglycemia • Myocardial ischemia or infarction • HF or cardiomyopathy

Perform rhythm strip analysis (Table 3-11) using a systematic approach. The criteria examined are regularity, rhythm, rate, P waves, PR interval, QRS complex, QT interval, and the patient presentation. Evaluate each criterion in relation to the established norms for sinus rhythm, basic dysrhythmias, and blocks. Evaluate each rhythm based on criteria, significance, and treatment (see Appendix A).

The pacemaker rule is that the fastest rate will control the heart. This is usually the SA node unless an irritable focus (e.g., atrial, junctional, or ventricular) is faster; this is called *irritability*. If an upper pacemaker (e.g., SA node) fails, it is up to lower pacemakers (e.g., junctional or ventricular) to assume control; this is called *escape*.

3.9   Learning Activity

Match the dysrhythmia to the appropriate characteristic.

_____ 1. Normal sinus rhythm
_____ 2. Sinus bradycardia
_____ 3. Sinus tachycardia
_____ 4. Premature atrial contraction
_____ 5. Atrial fibrillation
_____ 6. Atrial flutter
_____ 7. Supraventricular tachycardia
_____ 8. Premature junctional contraction
_____ 9. Junctional escape rhythm
_____ 10. Accelerated junctional rhythm
_____ 11. Junctional tachycardia
_____ 12. Premature ventricular complex
_____ 13. Accelerated idioventricular rhythm
_____ 14. Ventricular tachycardia
_____ 15. Ventricular fibrillation
_____ 16. Asystole
_____ 17. First-degree AV block
_____ 18. Second-degree AV block, type I
_____ 19. Second-degree AV block, type II
_____ 20. Third-degree AV block

a. PR interval >0.20 second
b. Early P wave that looks different from other P waves followed by normal QRS
c. Sawtooth waves on baseline; no clearly identifiable P waves, normal QRS
d. QRS is early, greater than 0.12 second, with T wave in opposite direction of QRS
e. Regular rhythm, normal P waves, normal QRS complexes, rate <60 beats/min
f. Quivering baseline, irregularly irregular occurring QRSs.
g. Normal width QRS complex is early with inverted P wave immediately (<0.12 second) prior to the QRS, in the QRS, or immediately after the QRS
h. Regular rhythm with rate of 40-60 beats/min with normal width QRS with inverted P wave immediately (<0.12 second) prior to the QRS, in the QRS, or immediately after the QRS
i. Flat line, no QRS complexes
j. Regular rhythm, normal P waves, normal QRS complexes, rate >100 beats/min
k. Regular rhythm, normal P waves, normal QRS complexes, rate 60-100 beats/min
l. Progressive PR lengthening until a P wave is not followed by a QRS
m. Regular rhythm with rate of 60-100 beats/min with normal width QRS with inverted P wave immediately (<0.12 second) prior to the QRS, in the QRS, or immediately after the QRS
n. Wide QRS (>0.12 second) rhythm with rate of 40-100 beats/min
o. Regular rhythm with rate of >100 beats/min with normal width QRS with inverted P wave immediately (<0.12 second) prior to the QRS, in the QRS, or immediately after the QRS
p. Regular rhythm with rate with rate 150-250 beats/min without clearly discernible P waves with narrow QRS
q. P wave not followed by QRS without preceding progression of PR interval
r. No relationship between P waves and QRS complexes; escape rhythm established by AV junction or ventricle
s. Irregular baseline, absence of QRS complexes
t. Wide QRS (>0.12 second) rhythm with rate >100 beats/min

Answers to this activity can be found in the Answer Key.

3.10 Learning Activity

Interpret the following 6-second ECG rhythm strips.

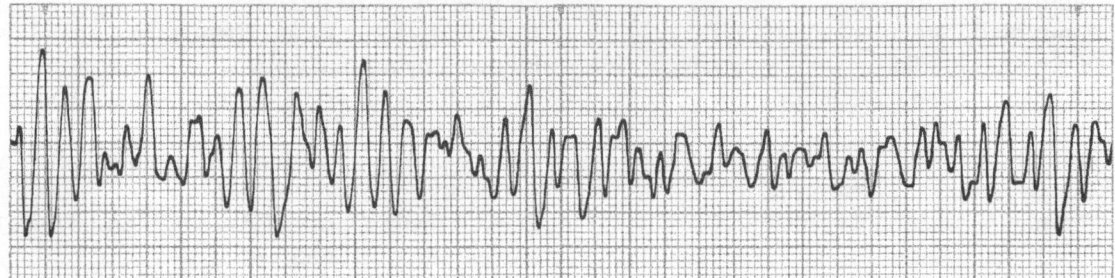

a. Interpretation:

_____

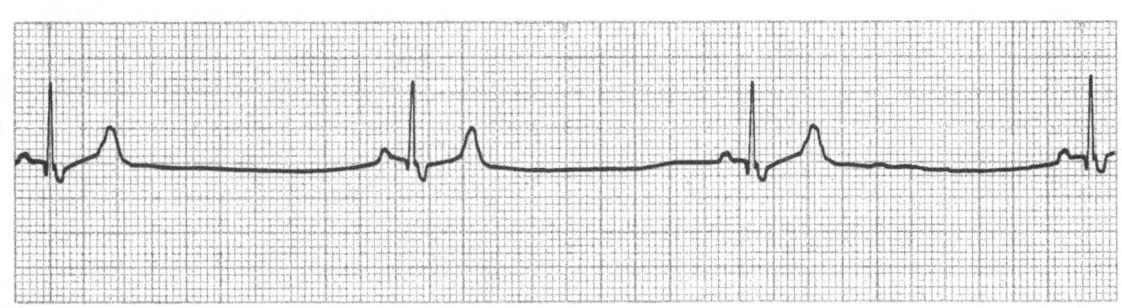

b. Interpretation:

_____

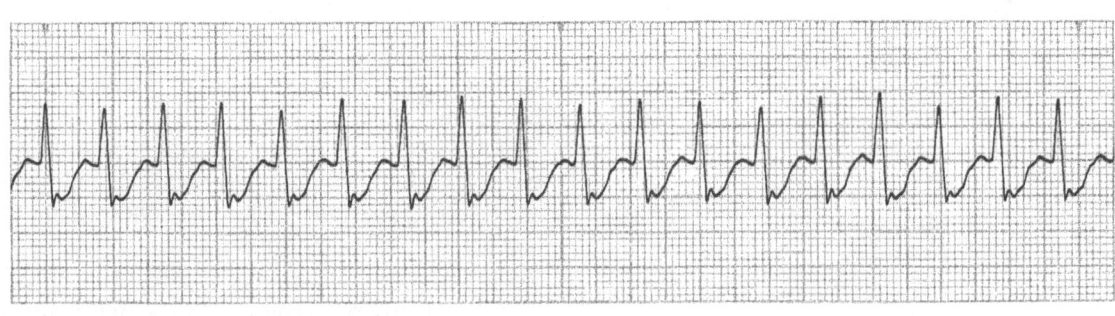

c. Interpretation:

_____

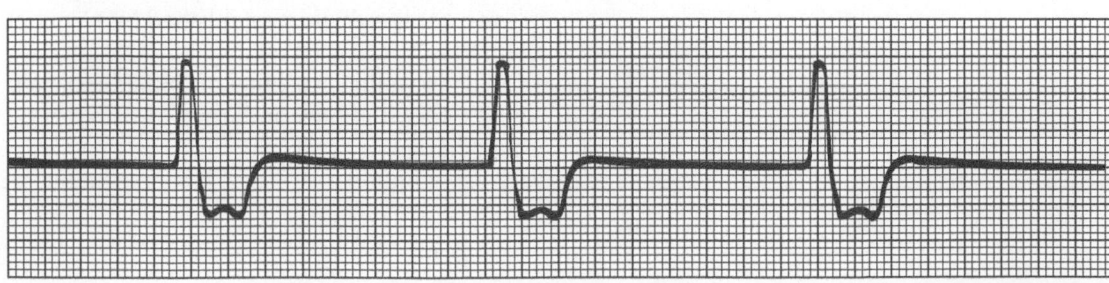

d. Interpretation:

_____

3.10   Learning Activity—cont'd

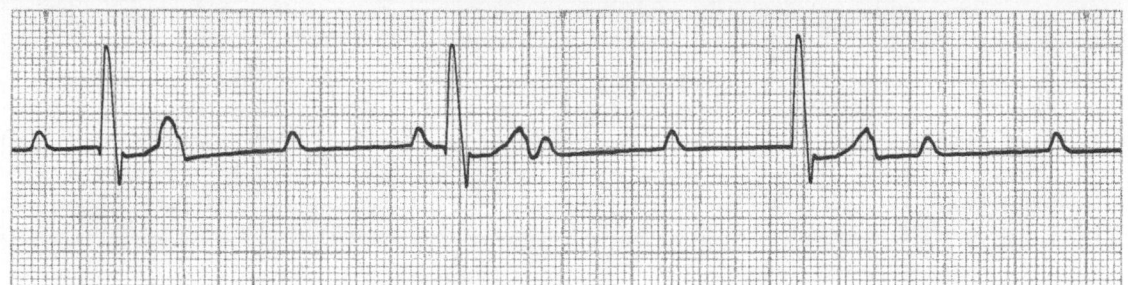

e. Interpretation: _____

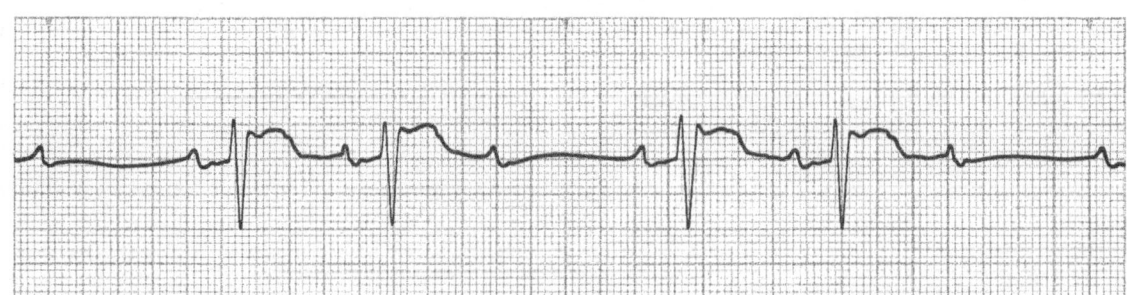

f. Interpretation: _____

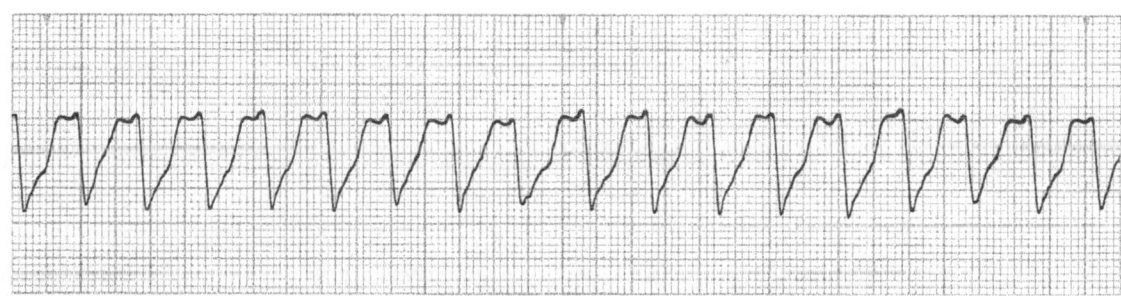

g. Interpretation: _____

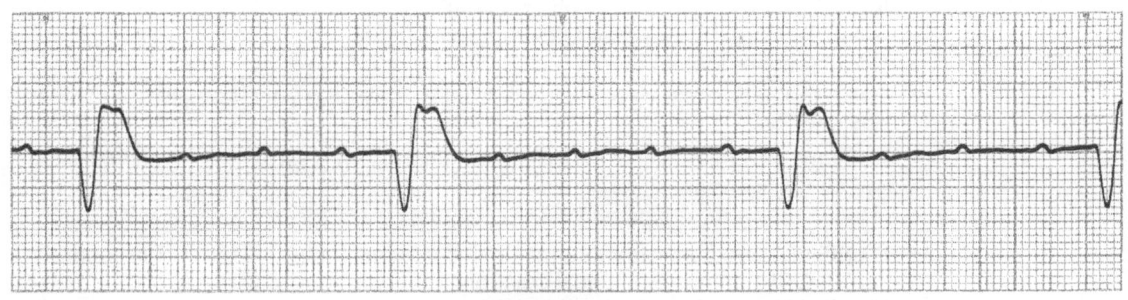

h. Interpretation: _____

Continued

3.10   Learning Activity—cont'd

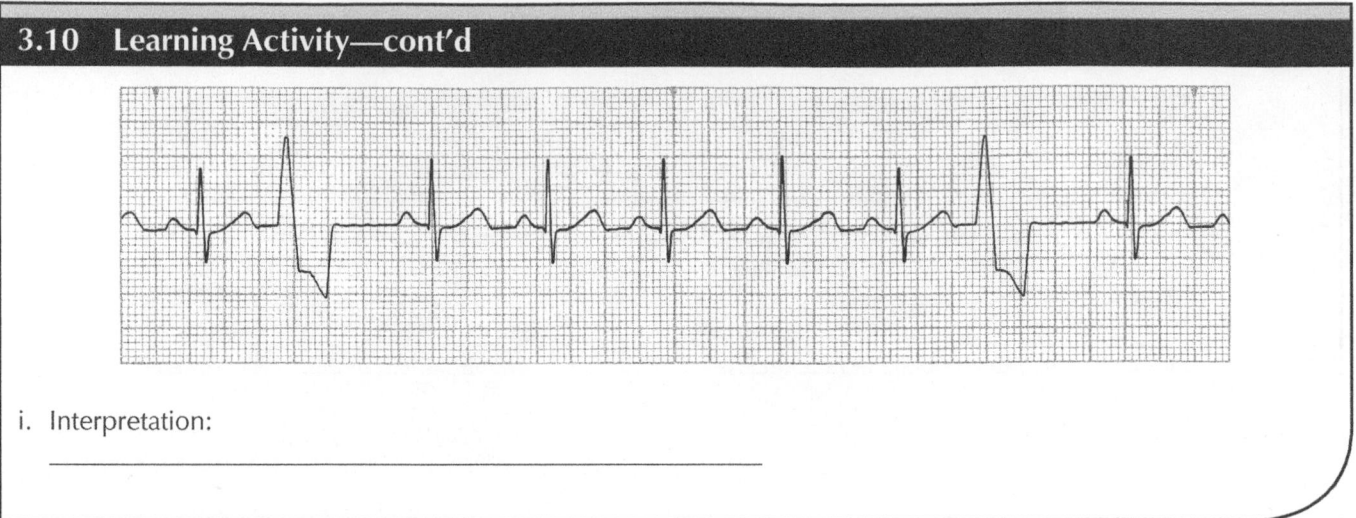

i. Interpretation:

_____

Answers to this activity can be found in the Answer Key.

TABLE 3-11   Rhythm Strip Analysis

Component	Assessment
Regularity (rhythm)	• Is it regular? • Is it irregular? • Are there any patterns to the irregularity? • Are there any ectopic beats; if so, are they early (premature) or are they late (escape)? • Is regularity of P waves and QRS complexes the same? (If there is only one P wave for each QRS, only one regularity needs to be recorded)

Rate	• Methods
	  • Count dark lines between P waves or QRS complexes as 300, 150, 100, 75, 60, 50, 43, 38, 33, 30
	  • Count number of QRS complexes in a 6-second strip and multiply by 10
	  • Use a rate ruler
	• Are atrial and ventricular rates the same? (If there is only one P wave for each QRS, only one rate needs to be recorded)

P waves	• Are the P waves regular? • Is there one P wave for every QRS? • Is there a P wave in front of the QRS or behind it? • Is the P wave normal and upright in lead II? • Are there more P waves than QRS complexes? • Do all P waves look alike? • Are irregular P waves associated with ectopic beats? If so, are they early (premature) or late (escape)?
PR intervals	• Is PRI measurement within normal range? (Normal interval: 0.12-0.20 second) • Are all PRIs constant? • If PRI varies, is there a pattern to the changing measurements?
QRS complexes	• Is QRS measurement within normal limits? (Normal interval: 0.06-0.11 second) • Are all QRS complexes of equal duration? • Do all QRS complexes look alike? • Are unusual QRS complexes associated with ectopic beats? If so, are they early (premature) or late (escape)?
QT interval	• Is the QT measurement within normal limits? (Measured QT less than ½ of previous RR interval or QTc of 0.32-0.44)
Patient presentation	• Is the patient symptomatic? • Are there clinical indications of hypoperfusion such as hypotension, syncope, or chest pain?

Certain drugs and electrolyte imbalances are commonly associated with ECG changes (Table 3-12) and may cause or contribute to cardiac dysrhythmias or hinder resuscitative efforts. Proarrhythmogenesis is the propensity for a drug to cause dysrhythmias. The drugs most likely to cause ECG changes or contribute to dysrhythmia are antidysrhythmics and digitalis. Electrolyte abnormalities are a common cause of cardiac dysrhythmias, and they can cause or complicate attempted resuscitation and post-resuscitation care. In some cases, it may be necessary to initiate treatment for life-threatening electrolyte disorders before laboratory results become available. A high degree of clinical suspicion and aggressive treatment of underlying electrolyte abnormalities can prevent these abnormalities from progressing to cardiac arrest.

Multiple-Lead ECG Analysis

The ECG leads (Figure 3-36) include bipolar limb leads, unipolar augmented limb leads, standard chest, right ventricular, and posterior leads. The bipolar limb leads are leads I, II, and III. The unipolar augmented limb leads are aVR, aVL, and aVF. The standard chest leads are V_1 to V_6. Special leads are used for detecting posterior infarctions and right ventricular infarctions. Right ventricular leads are V_{4R} to V_{6R}. The posterior leads are V_7 to V_9. Accurate placement of the electrodes (Table 3-13) is crucial for diagnostic value of the ECG.

The standard 12 leads plus V_{4R} to V_{6R} and V_7 to V_9 comprise the leads of an 18-lead ECG. The right ventricular leads are assessed on patients with ECG indicators of inferior MI, because 33% to 50% of patients with inferior MI have concurrent right ventricular infarction.

The R wave gets taller across the precordium from V_1 to V_6 (referred to as *normal progression of the R wave across the precordium*); the S wave gets smaller across the precordium (i.e., V_1 to V_6). Conditions associated with poor R wave progression across the precordium include anterior MI, LBBB, and emphysema. Conditions associated with low voltage across the precordium include emphysema, pericardial effusion, myocardial infarction, and obesity.

Bundle Branch Blocks

A bundle branch block (Figure 3-37) is a block of either bundle branch, which causes a delay in the conduction through the ventricles and a prolongation of the QRS interval. Branching (commonly referred to as *rabbit ears*) or slurring at the top of the QRS complex indicates that the two ventricles are asynchronously depolarized. The T wave deflection is in the opposite direction of the QRS. An LBBB is a bifascicular block because there is a loss of both major hemibundles. An LBBB is manifested by a QRS of 0.12 second or more and a QRS that is positive in V_6 and negative in V_1, monophasic QRS, or rsR' complex in V_6, and rS or QS in V_1. An RBBB is a unifascicular block and is manifested by a QRS of 0.12 second or more, a QRS that is positive in V_1 and negative in V_6 (i.e., rSR' in V_1 and a wide terminal S wave in leads I and V_6). Remember *WiLLiaM MaRRoW* (Right bundle branch block, 2010): In LBBB, there is a W in V_1 and an M in V_6; in RBBB, there is an M in lead V_1 and a W in lead V_6.

TABLE 3-12 **ECG Changes Due to Drugs or Electrolyte Imbalance**

Drug or Electrolyte Imbalance	ECG Changes
Class IA, IC, II/III, and III antidysrhythmics	• QT prolongation • T wave flattening
Digitalis	• Scooping of ST-T wave (known as *digitalis effect*) • Shortened QT • Prolonged PR interval possible
Hypokalemia	• If 3 mEq/L or less: flat T with prominent U wave; T wave and U wave have approximately the same amplitude; and there is ST segment flattening and/or depression • If 2 mEq/L or less: U wave will be taller than the T wave, QT interval will be prolonged, ST segment will be depressed • If 1 mEq/L or less, U wave fuses with T wave
Hyperkalemia	• If 6 mEq/L; ST segment disappears; T waves become tall, narrow, and peaked • QRS complex widens; P wave widens and flattens • If 7.5 mEq/L or greater, sinus arrest with disappearance of P waves • If 10-12 mEq/L or greater, wide QRS merged with T wave and ventricular fibrillation or asystole
Hypocalcemia	• Prolonged QT segment • Prolonged ST segment
Hypercalcemia	• Shortened QT segment • Shortened ST segment
Hypomagnesemia	• QT prolonged • Broad, flattened T wave
Hypermagnesemia	• PR, QT prolonged • Prolonged QRS

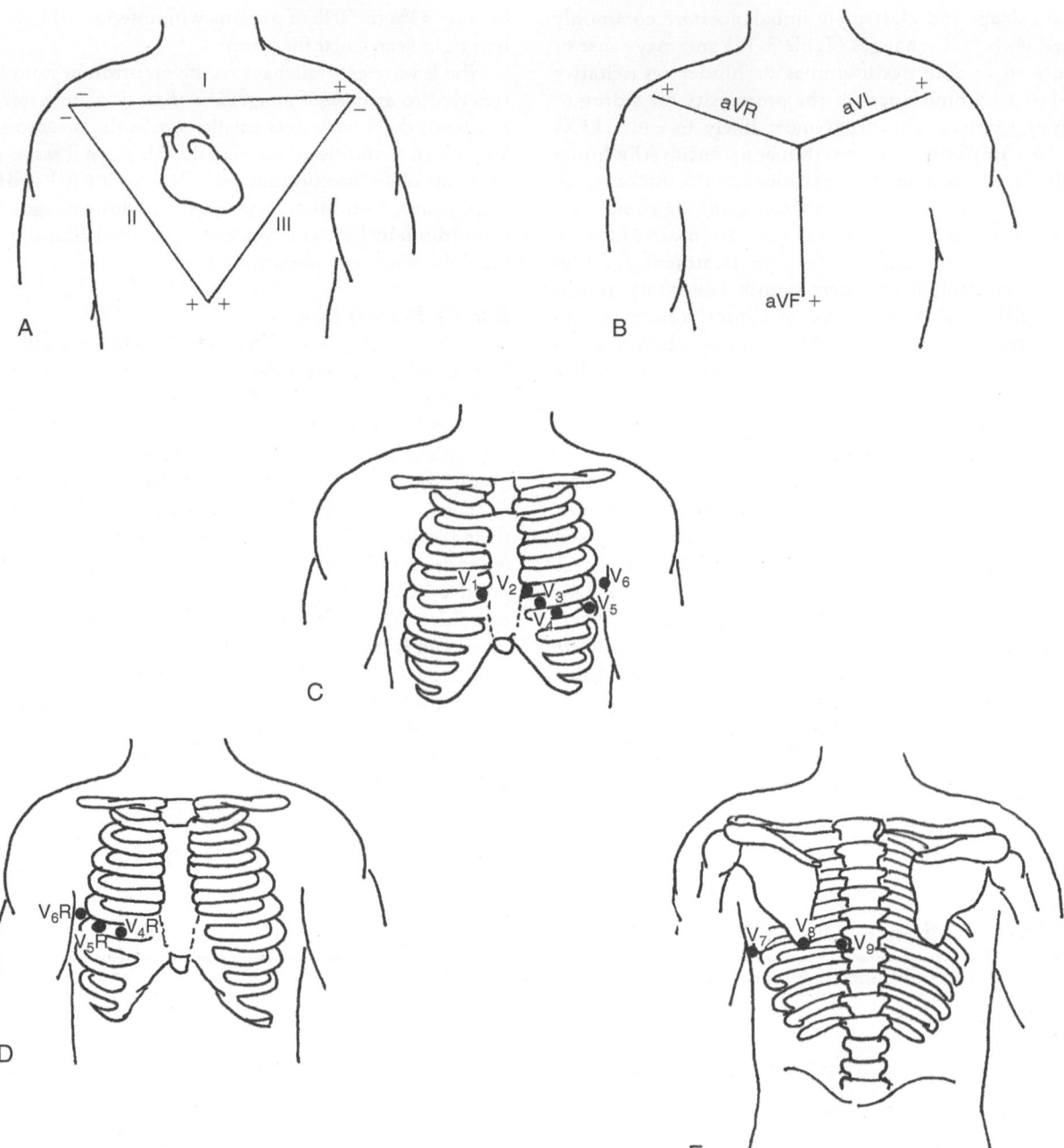

FIGURE 3-36 ECG leads. A, Bipolar limb leads: I, II, III. **B,** Unipolar limb leads: aVR, aVL, aVF. **C,** Standard chest leads: V1-V6. **D,** Right ventricular leads: V4R-V6R. E, Posterior leads: V7-V9. (From Dennison, R. D. [2013]. *Pass CCRN!* [4th ed.]. St. Louis, MO: Elsevier.)

Chamber Enlargement and Hypertrophy

The multiple-lead ECG detects chamber enlargement and hypertrophy. While the atria enlarge, they do not have an increase in muscle mass, hence the term *atrial enlargement*. The ventricles do increase their muscle mass in response to an increase in workload, hence the term ventricular hypertrophy.

The ECG manifests atrial enlargement (Figure 3-38) by changes in the P wave. The two best P wave leads are lead II and lead V_1. Observe for tall or wide P waves in lead II. In lead V_1 or MCL_1, the first half of the normally biphasic P wave represents the right atrium, and the second half of the normally biphasic P wave represents the left atrium. Look for a more dominant initial or terminal phase of the biphasic P wave in V_1 or MCL_1. The ECG manifests right atrial enlargement (RAE) by the following ECG changes: Tall (i.e., greater than 2.5 mm), peaked P wave in II (sometimes referred to as *P-pulmonale*) and a larger initial phase of the biphasic P wave normally seen in V_1. The ECG manifests left atrial enlargement (LAE) by the following ECG changes: wide P (i.e., greater than or equal to 0.12 second), notched P wave in II (sometimes referred to as *P-mitrale*) and a larger terminal phase of the biphasic P wave normally seen in V_1.

TABLE 3-13	Limb and Chest Leads	
Standard limb: Frontal plane	• Lead I: + at LA (left arm); − at RA (right arm) • Lead II: + at F (foot); − at RA • Lead III: + at F (foot); − at LA • Lead aVR: unipolar RA • Lead aVL: unipolar LA • Lead aVF: unipolar F	
Standard chest leads: Horizontal plane	• Lead V_1: 4ICS at right sternal border (RSB) • Lead V_2: 4ICS at left sternal border (LSB) • Lead V_3: halfway between V_2 and V_4 • Lead V_4: 5ICS at left midclavicular line (LMCL) • Lead V_5: 5ICS at left anterior axillary line (LAAL) • Lead V_6: 5ICS at left midaxillary line (LMAL)	
Posterior leads	• Lead V_7: 5ICS at left posterior axillary line (LPAL) • Lead V_8: halfway between V_7 and V_8 • Lead V_9: 5ICS next to vertebral column	
Right ventricular leads	• Lead V_{4R}: 5ICS at RMCL • Lead V_{5R}: 5ICS at RAAL • Lead V_{6R}: 5ICS at RMAL	

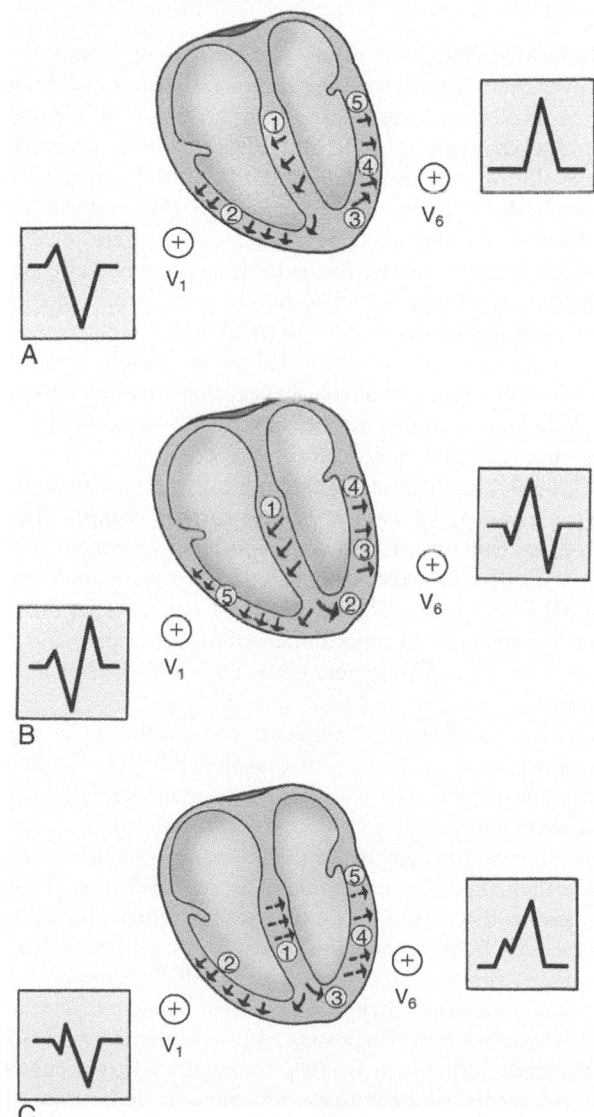

FIGURE 3-37 A, Normal ventricular depolarization. **B,** Right bundle branch block. **C,** Left bundle branch block. (From Urden, L., Stacy, K., & Lough, M. [2014]. *Critical care nursing: Diagnosis and management* [7th ed.]. St. Louis, MO: Mosby.)

The ECG manifests ventricular hypertrophy by changes in the QRS, particularly in the precordial (i.e., V) leads. Right ventricular hypertrophy (RVH) (Figure 3-39) causes a change in the usual left ventricular dominance across the precordial leads. Changes in the QRS amplitude indicative of RVH include the R wave being larger than the S wave in V_1 and V_2 leads or the S wave being larger than the R wave in V_5, V_6. These are changes indicative of a change from the normal dominance of the left ventricle to dominance of the right ventricle. Right axis deviation, manifested by a predominantly negative QRS in I and a predominantly positive QRS in aVF, is seen in RVH. RAE commonly coexists with RVH. Also commonly seen in RVH are ST-T wave changes in V_1, V_2, which indicates a right ventricular strain.

Left ventricular hypertrophy (LVH) (Figure 3-40) causes an exaggeration of the usual left ventricular dominance across the precordial leads. The sum of the height of the tallest R in V_5 or V_6 and the depth of the deepest S in V_1 or V_2 is greater than or equal to 35 mm, or the R in aVL is greater than or equal to 12 mm establishes the voltage criteria for LVH. Left axis deviation is manifested by a positive QRS in I and a negative QRS aVF. LAE commonly coexists in LVH. Also commonly seen in LVH are ST-T wave changes in V_5 and V_6, which indicates a left ventricular strain.

ECG Myocardial Ischemia, Injury, Infarction

Specific ECG indicators (Figure 3-41) are present with myocardial ischemia, injury, and infarction. Indicative changes are seen in the leads over the ischemia, injury, or infarction while reciprocal changes are seen in leads opposite the ischemia, injury, or infarction.

Ischemia is the earliest change in evolution of myocardial infarction. T wave changes manifest ischemia. The indicative change of ischemia is symmetrically inverted T waves in leads over the ischemic area. The reciprocal change of ischemia is tall T waves in leads opposite the ischemic area. ST segment changes manifest injury; these are intermediate changes in the evolution of myocardial infarction.

Condition	P Wave Appearance		Mnemonic Features
	Lead II	Lead V$_1$	
Normal sinus rhythm (NSR)	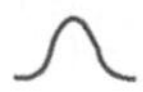	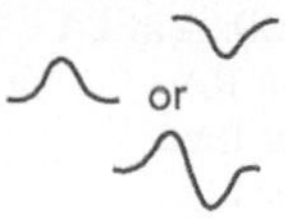 or	• The P should be upright in lead II if there is sinus rhythm • The P may be upright, negative, or biphasic in lead V$_1$ with sinus rhythm
RAE (=P Pulmonale)	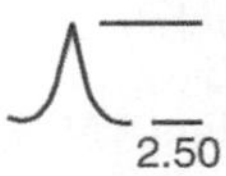 2.50		• Prominent (greater than or equal to 2.5 mm tall) peaked P waves in the pulmonary leads (II, III, and aVF)
LAE (=P Mitrale)	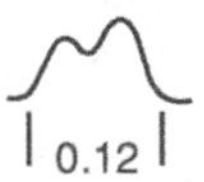 0.12	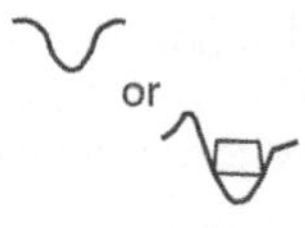 or	• M-shaped, widened (greater than or equal to 0.12 second) P waves in one or more of the mitral leads (I, II, or aVL) • Deep, negative component to the P wave in lead V$_1$

FIGURE 3-38 Atrial enlargement. *RAE*, Right atrial enlargement; *LAE*, left atrial enlargement. (From Grauer, K. [1998]. *A practical guide to ECG interpretation* [2nd ed.]. St. Louis, MO: Mosby.)

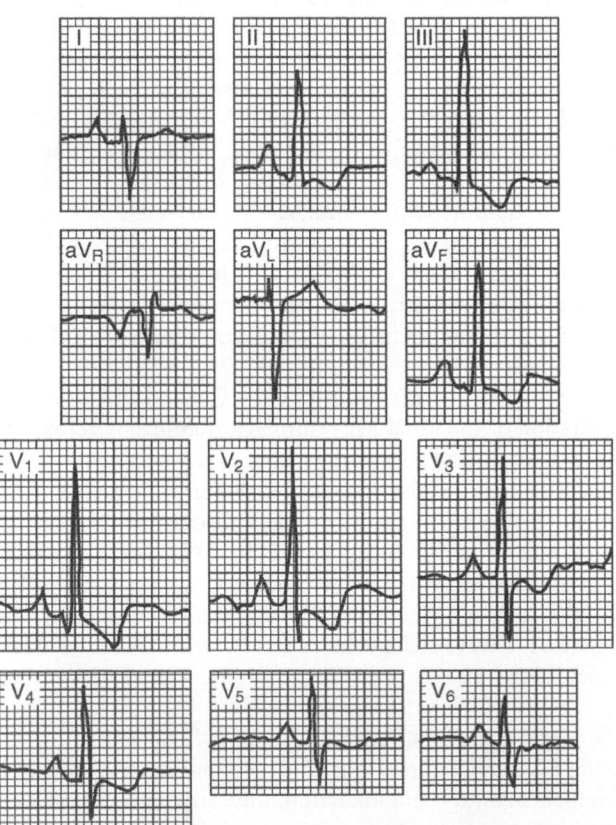

FIGURE 3-39 Right ventricular hypertrophy with right atrial enlargement. Note tall, peaked P waves in lead II with dominant initial component of the P wave in V$_1$ as evidence of right atrial enlargement. Note dominant R wave in V$_1$ and reverse progression of the R wave across the precordium along with right axis deviation and right ventricular strain (ST segment depression and asymmetrical T wave inversion in V$_1$, V$_2$) as evidence of right ventricular hypertrophy. (From Conover, M. B. [2003]. *Understanding electrocardiography* [8th ed.]. St. Louis, MO: Mosby.)

The indicative change of injury is ST segment elevation in leads over the injured area. The reciprocal change is ST segment depression in leads opposite the injured area. Changes in the Q wave manifest infarction; these are the latest changes in the evolution of myocardial infarction. Q waves are normal in many leads. To be considered pathologic (i.e., indicative of infarction), the waves must be 0.4 second wide and/or 25% of the height of the R wave in the leads over the necrotic area. The reciprocal change is tall R waves in leads opposite the necrotic area. Q waves can take up to 24 hours to develop and related to the mass loss of myocardial tissue. Therefore, non-Q wave MIs indicate a loss of less myocardium than do Q wave MIs. Pathologic Q waves can be prevented by successful early reperfusion therapies (e.g., fibrinolytics, PCI).

ECGs are also helpful in determining the age of an MI and discriminating between acute and chronic changes (Table 3-14). Chest pain with T wave inversion and ST segment elevation is indicative of acute ischemia and Q waves may develop as the MI evolves, especially if reperfusion attempts are unsuccessful. A pathologic Q wave alone without chest pain and no T wave inversion or ST segment elevation is indicative of an old Q wave MI.

ECG leads (Table 3-15) correlate to the walls of the heart and coronary arteries that deliver oxygenated blood. The ECG aids in identification of the occluded coronary artery and the compromised wall.

Some conditions may make ECG diagnosis of MI difficult because they affect the morphology of the QRS, the ST segment, and/or the T waves. Conditions that impede ECG diagnosis include Wellens syndrome, atrial fibrillation, ventricular pacemakers, ventricular hypertrophy, Wolff-Parkinson-White syndrome, pericarditis, hypothermia, hemorrhagic stroke, and electrolyte imbalance. Diagnosis of MI in patients with LBBB is particularly difficult; it is likely that acute MI is occurring when symptoms are new onset, ST segment depression is 1 mm in leads V$_1$, V$_2$, or ST segment elevation is more than 5 mm.

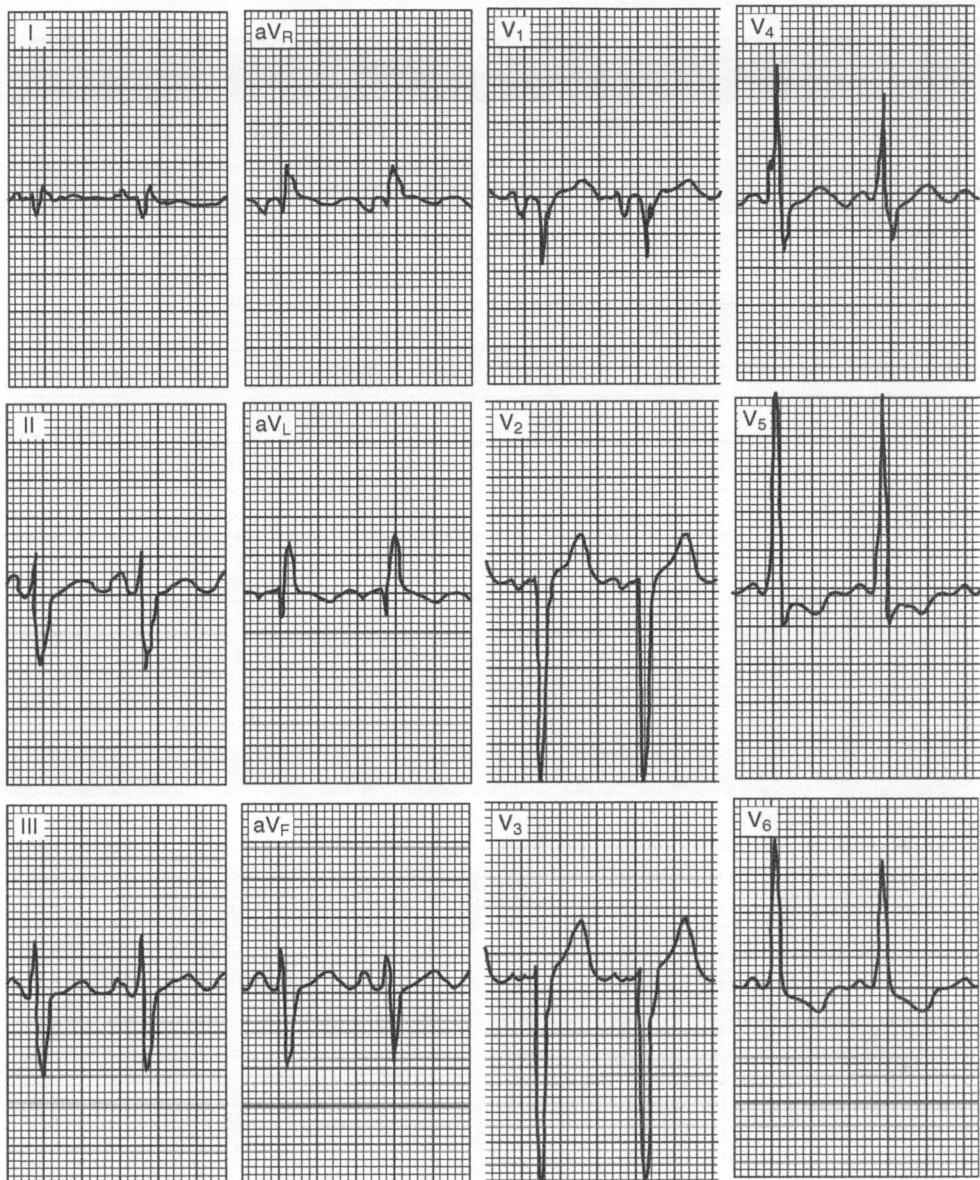

FIGURE 3-40 Left ventricular hypertrophy with left atrial enlargement. Note wide, notched P waves in lead II with dominant terminal component of the P wave in V_1 as evidence of left atrial enlargement. Note deep S wave in V_2 and tall R wave in V_5 with left axis deviation and left ventricular strain (ST segment depression and asymmetrical T wave inversion in V_5, V_6) as evidence of left ventricular hypertrophy. (From Conover, M. B. [2003]. *Understanding electrocardiography* [8th ed.]. St. Louis, MO: Mosby.)

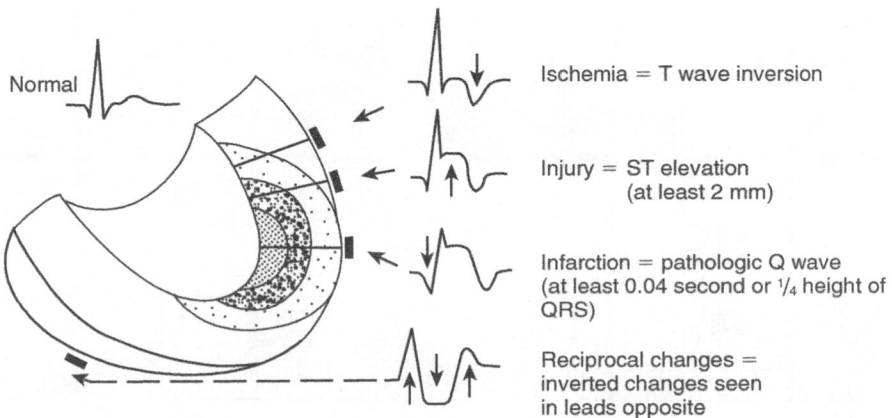

Normal

Ischemia = T wave inversion

Injury = ST elevation
(at least 2 mm)

Infarction = pathologic Q wave
(at least 0.04 second or ¼ height of QRS)

Reciprocal changes = inverted changes seen in leads opposite

FIGURE 3-41 Indicative and reciprocal changes of myocardial ischemia, injury, and infarction. (From Harvey, M. [2000]. *Study guide to core curriculum for critical care nursing* [3rd ed.]. Philadelphia, PA: Saunders.)

3.11   Learning Activity

Match the cardiac wall to the lead grouping that is used to evaluate that wall.

Lead Groupings	Cardiac Wall
_____ 1. II, III, aVF	a. Anterior
_____ 2. V_{4R}	b. Lateral (high)
_____ 3. I, aVL	c. Lateral (low)
_____ 4. V_1, V_2	d. Posterior
_____ 5. V_3, V_4	e. Right ventricular
_____ 6. V_5, V_6	f. Septal
_____ 7. V_8, V_9	g. Inferior

Answers to this activity can be found in the Answer Key.

3.12   Learning Activity

Analyze the following 12-lead ECGs for bundle branch block. Identify if it is a left or right bundle branch block.

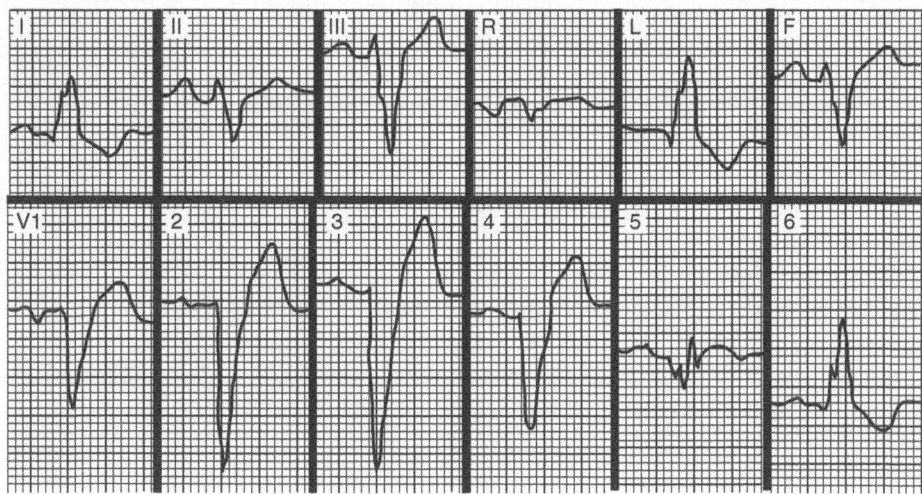

a. Interpretation: _____

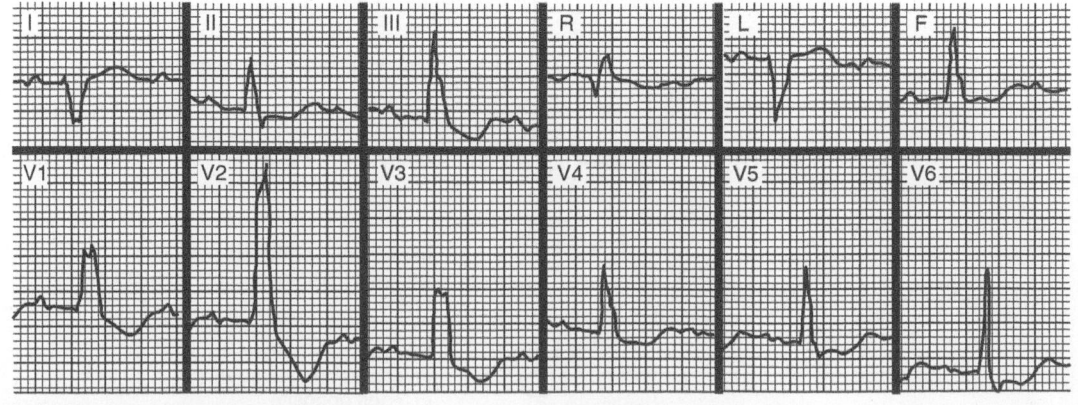

b. Interpretation: _____

Answers to this activity can be found in the Answer Key.

3.13   Learning Activity

Analyze the following 12-lead ECGs for atrial enlargement or ventricular hypertrophy.

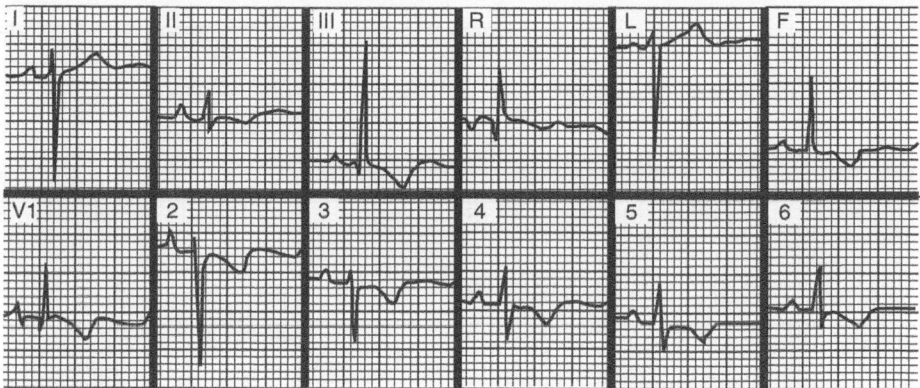

a. Interpretation: _____

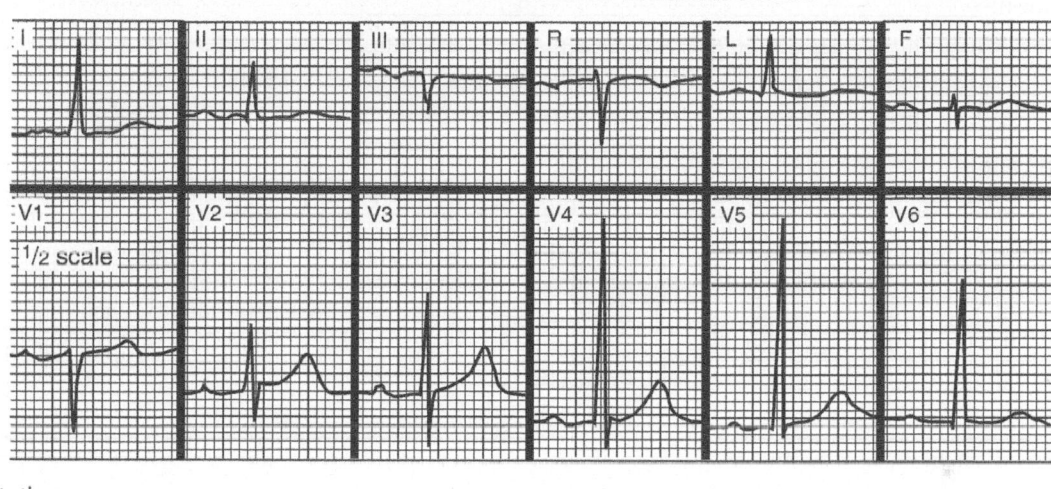

b. Interpretation: _____

Answers to this activity can be found in the Answer Key.

TABLE 3-14	Determination of Age of Myocardial Infarction	
Description	**ECG Characteristics**	**Time from Onset of Pain**
Hyperacute	• ST segment elevation • Tombstone-shaped T waves • T wave inversion	Minutes to hours
Acute	• ST segment elevation • T wave inversion • Pathologic Q waves	Hours to days
Recent	• T wave inversion • Pathologic Q waves	Weeks to months
Old	• Pathologic Q waves	After several months

TABLE 3-15	ECG Lead Correlation with Myocardial Infarction Locations		
Location	**Coronary Artery**	**Indicative Leads**	**Reciprocal Leads**
Anterior	LAD	V_2, V_3, V_4	V_7, V_8, V_9
Septal	LAD	V_1, V_2	V_5, V_6
Anteroseptal	LAD	$V_1, V_2, V_3, (V_4)$	I, aVL
Lateral	LCA	I, aVL (high lateral), V_5, V_6 (low lateral)	II, III, aVF
Anterolateral	LCA	V_3, V_4, V_5, V_6, (I, aVL)	II, III, aVF
Inferior	RCA	II, III, aVF	I, aVL
RV	RCA	V_{4R}, V_{5R}, V_{6R} may be transient	I, aVL
Posterior	RCA and/or LCA	V_7, V_8, V_9 or reciprocal in V_1, V_2, V_3	V_1, V_2, V_3

NOTE: Changes may also be seen in leads in parentheses.

3.14 Learning Activity

Analyze the following 12-lead ECGs from patients with acute chest pain for indications of MI. Identify location and age of MI if present.

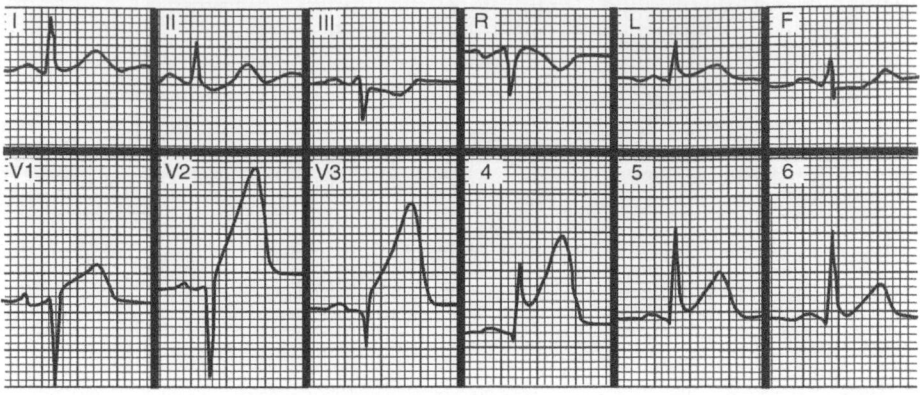

a. Interpretation: _____

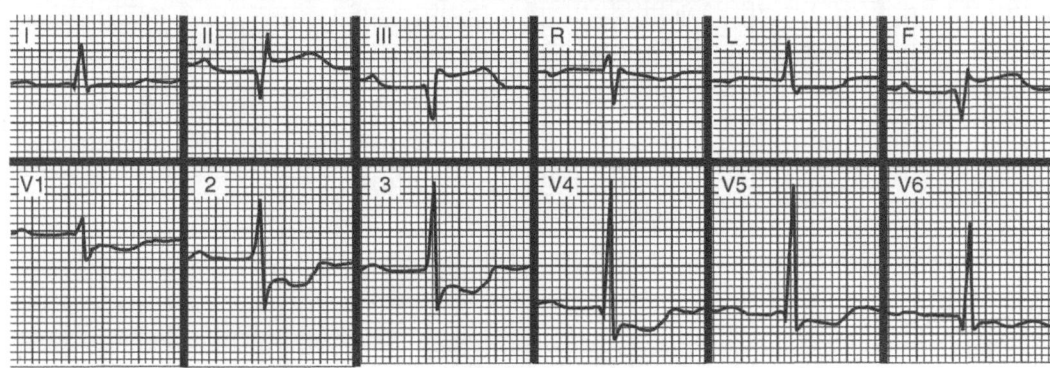

b. Interpretation: _____

Answers to this activity can be found in the Answer Key.

ECG Changes in Angina

A resting ECG is often normal in patients with stable angina pectoris in the absence of a previous MI or a cause for LVH. During pain, the ECG may show transient ST-segment depression, T wave inversion, and/or ventricular dysrhythmia. Abnormal ECG changes are more common with unstable angina pectoris. ST-segment elevation rather than depression occurs during an attack of variant angina. Variant angina, also referred to as *Prinzmetal* or *vasospastic angina*, occurs at rest. Coronary artery spasm causes variant angina and it is manifested by ST segment elevation with pain. Wellens syndrome (Figure 3-42) occurs in a subset of patients with unstable angina who have specific precordial T wave changes. Characterized by a group of signs that are associated with occlusion of the proximal left anterior descending artery, Wellens syndrome has a high risk of sudden cardiac death in a patient with unstable angina; the ECG shows symmetrical, deeply inverted T waves in V_2, V_3 that persist even when the patient is pain free. There is little or no ST segment elevation, little or no enzyme elevation, and no development of Q waves or loss of precordial R waves. The treatment indicated includes cardiac catheterization with PCI.

ECG Changes of Other Conditions

Various conditions may cause ECG changes. In pericarditis, the ST segment is normal in V_1 and aVR, but all other leads show ST segment elevation and T wave changes. If there is a decrease in QRS voltage, suspect a pericardial effusion.

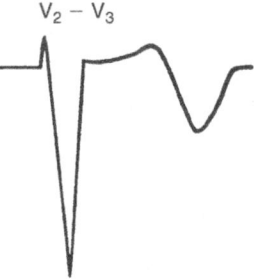

FIGURE 3-42 Wellens syndrome. (From Conover, M. [2003]. *Understanding electrocardiography* [8th ed.]. St. Louis, MO: Mosby.)

In myocardial trauma, nonspecific ST and T wave changes occur with myocardial contusion. There is also a high risk of dysrhythmias and AV nodal blocks. If MI occurs from a myocardial contusion, Q waves will be evident.

Specific ECG changes are evident with severe hypothermia. When core temperatures are less than 30° C, a J wave (also referred to as an *Osborne wave*) occurs. These are rounded waves above the isoelectric line between the QRS complex and the early part of the ST segment. These waves are usually seen best in leads II and V. ST segment elevation and prolonged PR and QT intervals can also occur in hypothermia.

Patients with hypothyroidism may also have ST segment depression and prominent T waves with T wave inversion. Patients with hyperthyroidism may have clinical indications of LVH.

3.15 Learning Activity

Match the following cardiovascular conditions to their major ECG diagnostic features.

Condition	ECG Diagnostic Features
_____ 1. Acute myocardial infarction	a. Symmetrically, deeply inverted T waves in V_2, V_3 with little or no ST segment elevation
_____ 2. Hypercalcemia	b. Prolonged QT, prolonged ST segment
_____ 3. Hyperkalemia	c. R wave larger than S wave in V_1, V_2, S wave larger than R wave in V_5, V_6, right axis deviation, ST-T wave changes in V_1, V_2
_____ 4. Hypocalcemia	d. Diffuse ST segment elevation across the precordium
_____ 5. Hypokalemia	e. Wide (>0.11 second), notched P wave in lead II, dominant terminal component of P wave in V_1
_____ 6. Left atrial enlargement	f. Wide (0.12 second or more) QRS below the baseline in V_1
_____ 7. Left bundle branch block	g. Q waves at least 0.04 second wide and/or ¼ height of R wave along with ST segment elevation and symmetrically inverted T waves
_____ 8. Left ventricular hypertrophy	h. Increased QRS amplitude, left axis deviation, ST-T wave changes in V_5, V_6
_____ 9. Pericarditis	i. Wide (0.12 second or more) QRS above the baseline in V_1
_____ 10. Variant angina	j. Tall (>2.5 mm) peaked P wave in lead II, dominant initial component of P wave in V_1
_____ 11. Right atrial enlargement	k. Shortened QT, shortened ST segment
_____ 12. Right bundle branch block	l. Flat T waves, prominent U wave, ST segment depression
_____ 13. Right ventricular hypertrophy	m. ST segment elevation with pain
_____ 14. Wellens syndrome	n. Tall peaked T waves, widening of QRS complex, atrial asystole

Answers to this activity can be found in the Answer Key.

ST Segment Monitoring

Continuous monitoring of the ST segment is required to detect changes associated with ischemia because ischemia may not cause chest pain (referred to as *silent* ischemia). Indications for continuous ST segment monitoring include acute coronary syndrome, myocardial infarction, post-PCI (depending on clinical indications, such as chest pain and dysrhythmias), during and following cardiac surgery, and during and following noncardiac surgery in patients at risk of myocardial ischemia.

Choose a lead that best demonstrates ST changes during ischemia, evolving MI, or at the time of balloon occlusion at the time of PCI (referred to as the patient's *ischemic fingerprint*). If information regarding the ischemic fingerprint is not available, use leads III and V_3. Significant ST segment changes include either ST segment elevation or depression of at least 1 mm for at least 60 seconds. ST segment elevation represents more severe, usually transmural ischemia. ST segment depression represents less severe, usually subendocardial, ischemia or reciprocal changes of ischemia. Other causes of ST segment deviation include electrolyte imbalances, pericarditis, hypothermia, ventricular aneurysm, hypothyroidism, hyperventilation, pulmonary infarction, and drugs such as digoxin.

CARDIOPULMONARY ARREST

Cardiopulmonary arrest is a sudden cessation of cardiac output and effective circulation. Ventilatory cessation follows cardiac arrest. Causes of cardiopulmonary arrest are most likely dysrhythmias, electrical shock, drowning, asphyxiation, trauma, hypothermia, or the terminal phases of a chronic illness.

Cardiac arrest ceases the delivery of oxygen and the removal of carbon dioxide, causing tissue hypoxia and metabolic (i.e., lactic) acidosis. Ventilatory arrest causes hypercapnia, respiratory acidosis, and hypoxemia. These events cause irreversible damage to the cerebral cortex within 4 to 6 minutes at normal body temperature, during which severe neurologic deficit or biologic death occurs.

A patient in cardiac arrest will experience loss of consciousness and absence of breathing or agonal breathing, which may be a precursor to cardiopulmonary arrest. A cardiopulmonary arrest results in the absence of central pulses, absence of auscultated or palpated BP, loss of consciousness, anoxic seizures, and urinary and bowel incontinence. The ECG will most commonly reveal ventricular fibrillation, less commonly ventricular tachycardia, but rarely asystole. Cardiopulmonary arrest may also occur with a stable electrical rhythm but no effective cardiac output (referred to as *pulseless electrical activity* [PEA]).

The American Heart Association (AHA) has identified factors that are crucial in survival, known as the *chain of survival* (Hazinski et al., 2010). Of utmost importance is the immediate recognition of cardiac arrest, activation of the emergency response system (EMS), and early CPR with emphasis on chest compressions. Recently, CPR guidelines have changed from the airway, breathing, circulation (ABC) sequence to a compression, airway, breathing (CAB) sequence (Field et al., 2010). Because most cardiac arrests occur as a result of ventricular fibrillation or pulseless ventricular tachycardia in adults, chest compressions and defibrillation are most crucial to survival. The former ABC sequence delayed chest compressions due to the time required to look, listen, feel for airflow, open the airway, and start mouth-to-mouth ventilation or retrieve a barrier or other ventilation equipment. In the new sequence, initiate ventilation after a cycle of 30 compressions. Because laypersons are reluctant to give mouth-to-mouth ventilation to a stranger, compressions are more promptly initiated with the new "Hands-Only" CPR. The key is to provide rapid defibrillation, effective advanced life support, and integrated post-cardiac arrest care.

Emergent care includes the recognition of cardiac arrest, activation of the EMS, and completion of a patient assessment. Determine if the person is unresponsive and either not breathing or only gasping. Call for help by initiating a 911 call for out-of-hospital cardiac arrest, or follow the specific hospital protocol (e.g., Code Blue) for an in-hospital cardiac arrest and retrieve the defibrillator. Provide basic life support (BLS) as recommended by current AHA guidelines. Assess the carotid pulse for no more than 10 seconds, and then deliver compressions, placing the heel of one hand over the lower half of the sternum and the other hand over the first hand. Compress the sternum to a depth of at least 2 inches at a rate of at least 100 compressions/min. The new guidelines emphasize that the providers push hard and fast, allowing the chest to completely recoil after each compression. The compression/ventilation ratio is 30:2 for CPR to adults, regardless of whether there are one or two rescuers. Perform all rescue efforts, including defibrillation, insertion of advanced airways, intravenous access, and administration of medications, with minimal interruption of compressions. Maintain compressions without pauses for ventilation.

After the initial 30 compressions, open the airway using the head tilt–chin lift maneuver. The jaw thrust maneuver is no longer recommended in initial establishment of airway. If the patient is breathing adequately, position him or her on the left side in recovery position. If the patient is not breathing or breathing inadequately, deliver two breaths using any of the following methods: mouth to mask ventilation, manual resuscitation with a bag-valve mask secured over nose and mouth, or manual resuscitation with a bag secured to an endotracheal (ET) tube or tracheostomy tube if either tube is already in place. Note that each rescue breath does make the chest rise. After successful intubation, continue rescue breathing every 6 to 8 seconds (8 to 10 breaths/min) to avoid hyperventilation because hyperventilation is associated with poor survival rates.

To coordinate compressions and ventilation, maintain a ratio of 30 compressions to 2 ventilations for one or two rescuers. CPR performed expertly provides only 25% to 30% of normal cardiac output, but most of this goes to the upper body, including the heart and brain. Mortality rates increase despite prompt CPR if advanced cardiac life support (ACLS) is delayed beyond 12 minutes. Resistance of ventricular dysrhythmias to defibrillation occurs over time; therefore, prompt defibrillation is critical to survival.

Initiate rapid defibrillation by delivering a shock of sufficient strength to a critical mass of myocardium. This defibrillation results in a simultaneous depolarization allowing an emergence of a dominant normal rhythm. Use defibrillation in the event of pulseless ventricular tachycardia and ventricular fibrillation (VF) and unstable or refractory ventricular tachycardia with a pulse. It is also used in asystole when the rhythm is unclear and could be fine for ventricular fibrillation. Perform defibrillation as soon as a defibrillator is available and ideally within 3

minutes. Minimize the delay between the cessation of CPR and defibrillation and defibrillation and resumption of CPR.

Manual defibrillation requires checking the patient's pulse. Make sure that the ventricular fibrillation pattern is not merely an artifact caused by a loose ECG electrode. Remove any foil-lined patches from the patient's chest because they may cause arcing and patient burns. The patient must be dry and not in contact with any metallic objects. Turn the defibrillator on and make sure that the synchronizer switch is off so that charge delivers as soon as buttons are pushed. Most defibrillators automatically reset to a nonsynchronized mode so you can immediately defibrillate if ventricular fibrillation occurs after cardioversion.

Monophasic defibrillation requires 360 joules. Apply the paddles to the defibrillation pads or the jellied paddles to the chest using firm (~25 lb) pressure. Say the word *clear* and ensure that no one is touching the patient or the bed. Press both discharge buttons simultaneously. Resume CPR, beginning with chest compressions. Current guidelines recommend only one shock before resuming CPR. Recheck the rhythm after five cycles (~2 minutes) of CPR. Administer antidysrhythmic drug therapy if the rhythm and pulse are restored, otherwise continue with the appropriate algorithm.

Apply defibrillation pads to the chest for paddle placement or apply conductive jelly to the paddles for a "hands-off" defibrillator using biphasic defibrillation. Four pad/paddle positions are equally effective (Link et al., 2010): anterolateral (the default position), anteroposterior (recommended for obese patients, patients with hyperinflated lungs [e.g., COPD], and for patients with an implantable cardioverter-defibrillator [ICD]), anterior-left infrascapular, and anterior-right infrascapular (for patients with pacemakers). For patients with permanent pacemakers, the paddles should not be placed within 8 cm of the pulse generator (Link et al., 2010). If present, turn a temporary pacemaker pulse generator off during defibrillation. Charge the defibrillator to the appropriate voltage. Approximately 150 to 200 joules are required for a biphasic truncated exponential waveform or 120 joules for a rectilinear biphasic waveform. If unknown, use the maximum voltage available. The advantages of biphasic defibrillation are that it offers equal or better efficacy at lower energies than traditional monophasic waveform defibrillators ($\leq$200 joules is safe and offers equal or greater efficiency for terminating VF when compared with higher energy monophasic shock) and there is less risk of myocardial injury and skin burns. In the first phase, the current moves from one paddle to the other (as in monophasic defibrillation) and in the second phase, the current reverses direction.

When using an automatic external defibrillator (AED), attach the device to the patient. Put one pad to the right of the sternum below the right clavicle and the other pad lateral to the apex in the left midaxillary line. Turn the device on. Ensure that the patient is completely still and no one is touching the patient. Press the analyze button. The device signals a "stand clear" and performs a 3-second analysis. If ventricular tachycardia or ventricular fibrillation is detected, the AED will charge to 200 joules (biphasic) and display a "shock indicated" message. Call "clear" and ensure that no one is touching the patient. Press the shock button to deliver the shock. Administer antidysrhythmic drug therapy if the rhythm and pulse are restored; otherwise, continue CPR and apply the appropriate algorithm.

Successful defibrillation is less likely if any of the following are present: hypoxia, severe acidosis, alkalosis, local ionic

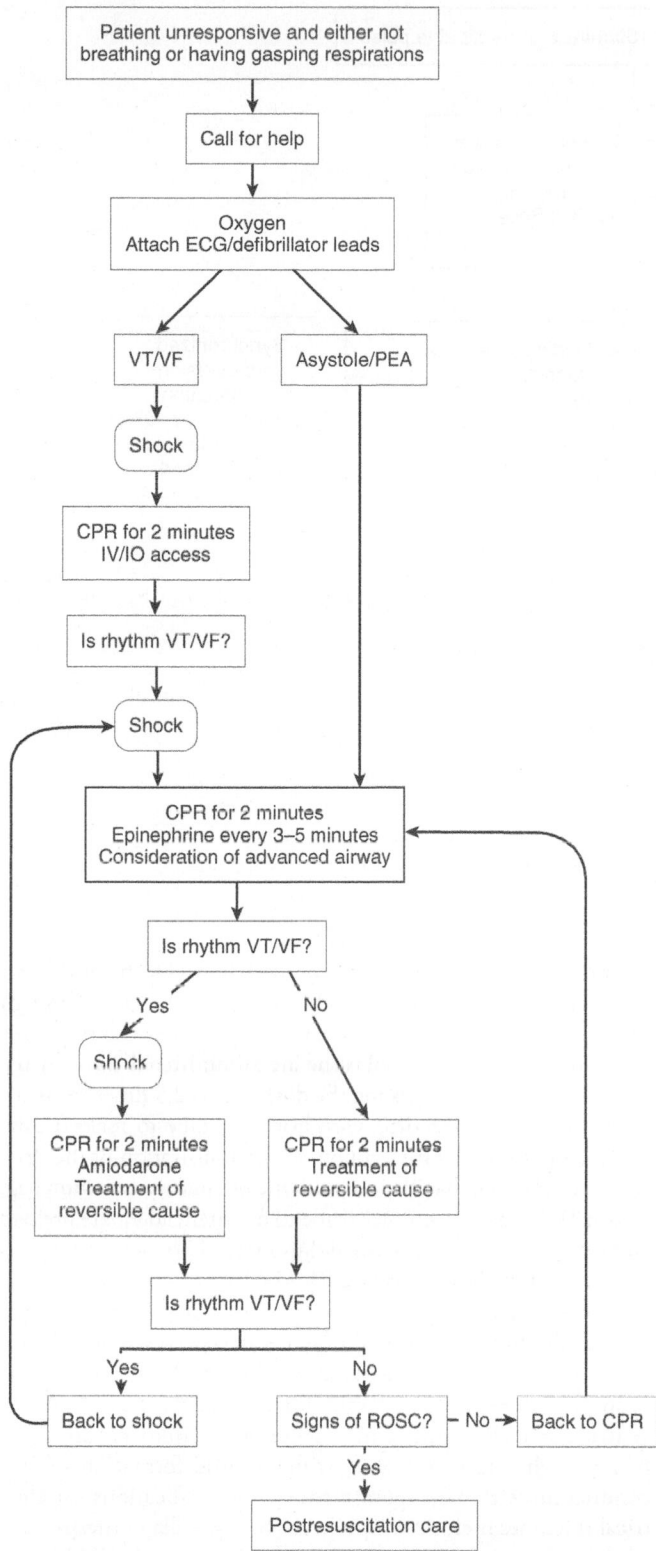

FIGURE 3-43 Advanced cardiac life support cardiac arrest algorithm. *CPR*, Cardiopulmonary resuscitation; *ECG*, electrocardiogram; *PEA*, pulseless electrical activity; *ROSC*, return of spontaneous circulation; *VF*, ventricular fibrillation; *VT*, ventricular tachycardia. (Data from Neumar, R. W., et al. [2010]. Part 8: Adult advanced cardiovascular life support: 2010 American Heart Association guidelines for cardiopulmonary resuscitation and emergency cardiovascular care. *Circulation, 122*[18 Suppl 3], S729-S767.)

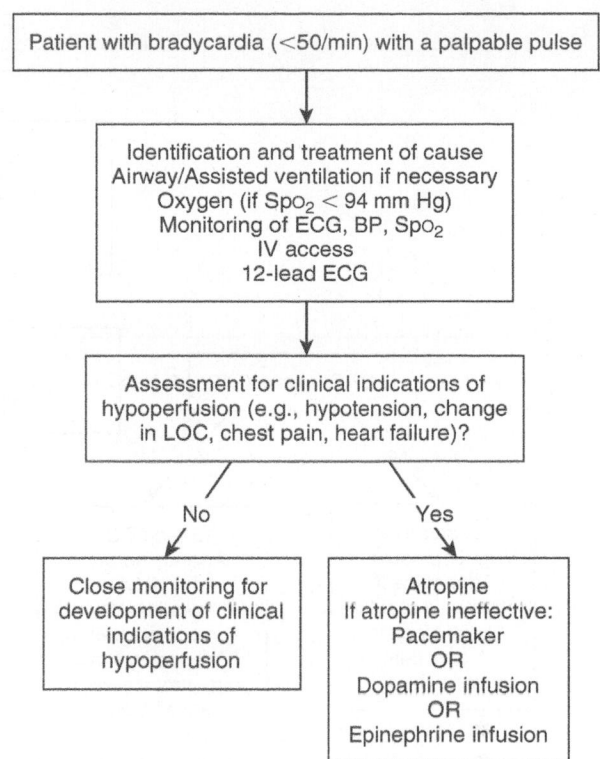

FIGURE 3-44 Bradycardia algorithm. *BP,* Blood pressure; *ECG,* electrocardiogram; *LOC,* level of consciousness; *SpO₂,* oxygen saturation by pulse oximetry. (Data from Neumar R. W., et al. [2010]. Part 8: Adult advanced cardiovascular life support: 2010 American Heart Association guidelines for cardiopulmonary resuscitation and emergency cardiovascular care. *Circulation, 122*[18 Suppl 3], S729-S767.)

imbalance, ischemia, or long VF duration. Complications of defibrillation include dysrhythmias, including asystole, bradycardia, AV blocks; and ventricular fibrillation; hypotension; myocardial damage; pulmonary edema; emboli; muscle pain; and skin burns. Provide effective ACLS as recommended by current AHA guidelines. Use the ACLS algorithms to provide assistance with decision making in a cardiopulmonary arrest (Figures 3-43, 3-44, and 3-45).

Identify and treat the cause of cardiac arrest. This is especially important in the treatment of PEA. Assess for the presence of the 5 Hs (i.e., hypovolemia, hypoxia, hydrogen ion [acidosis], hyper/hypokalemia, and hypothermia) along with the 5 Ts (i.e., tension pneumothorax, tamponade [cardiac], toxins, thrombosis [coronary], and thrombosis [pulmonary]).

Administer 100% oxygen during cardiopulmonary arrest with a bag-valve mask. A reservoir bag or tubing attached to the bag-valve mask is required to achieve as high a concentration of oxygen as possible. Remember that there is no contraindication to 100% oxygen during cardiopulmonary arrest. Determine the patency of existing central or peripheral IV or heparin lock. If a central vein catheter is in place when the arrest occurs, use it to administer drugs during the resuscitation. Antecubital or external jugular veins are preferred if a venous catheter or additional venous catheters must be established. Peak drug concentrations are lower and circulation times are longer when administering drugs via peripheral sites compared with central sites. Administer bolus drugs rapidly, follow with a 20-mL saline, and elevate the extremity for 10 to 20 seconds if peripheral venous access is used for resuscitation drugs.

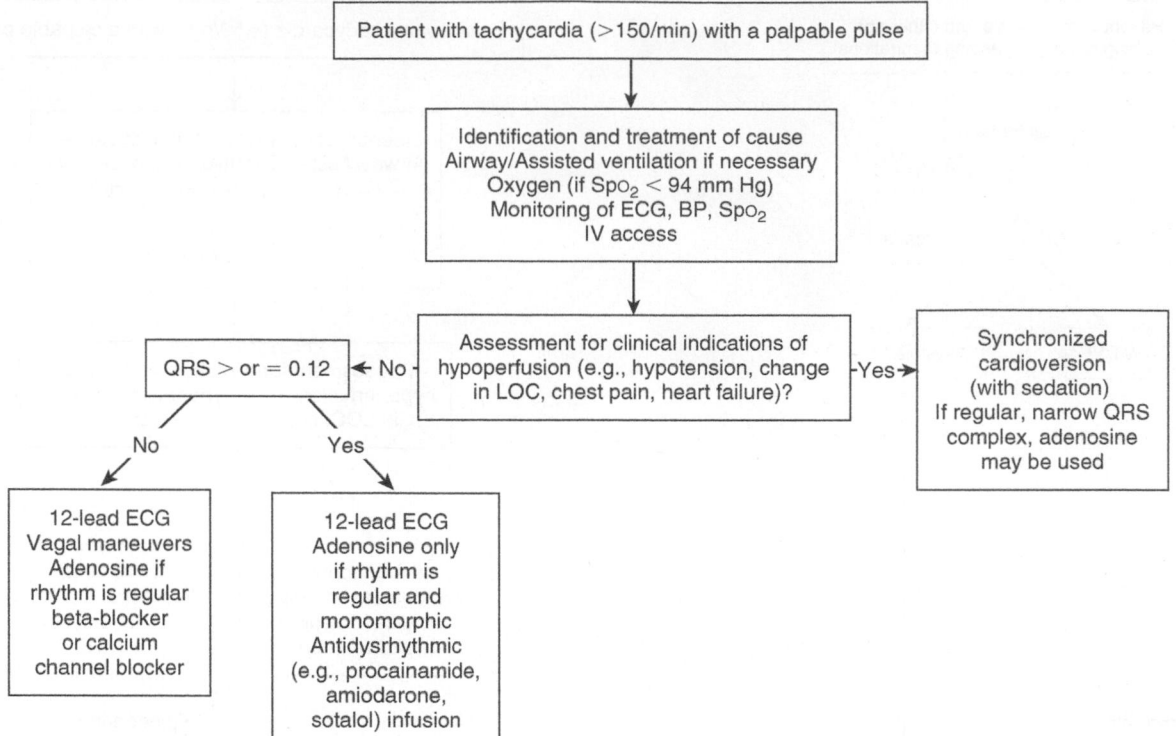

FIGURE 3-45 Tachycardia algorithm. *BP,* Blood pressure; *ECG,* electrocardiogram; *IV,* intravenous; *LOC,* level of consciousness; *SpO₂,* oxygen saturation by pulse oximetry. (Data from Neumar R. W., et al. [2010]. Part 8: Adult advanced cardiovascular life support: 2010 American Heart Association guidelines for cardiopulmonary resuscitation and emergency cardiovascular care. *Circulation, 122*[18 Suppl 3], S729-S767.)

Central vein cannulation is appropriate if needed, but recognize that the major disadvantage of a central vein cannulation during cardiopulmonary arrest is the need to stop CPR. Internal jugular and subclavian sites require cessation of CPR, whereas femoral vein cannulation does not require cessation of CPR. Another consideration is that unsuccessful central vein cannulation may contraindicate the use of fibrinolytics and increase the risk of bleeding with the use of glycoprotein IIb/IIIa agents (e.g., abciximab [ReoPro], eptifibatide [Integrilin], tirofiban HCl [Aggrastat]) and anticoagulants. Distal wrist and hand veins and distal saphenous veins in the legs are the least favorable sites for drug administration during CPR. Use intraosseous (IO) access if IV access is not available, but keep in mind that drugs administered by the IO route take approximately 2 minutes to reach the heart.

Attempt endotracheal intubation as soon as feasible, but defibrillation and administration of epinephrine are the first and second priorities. Hyperventilation with 100% oxygen should precede any intubation attempt. Confirm ET tube placement by listening for equal bilateral breath sounds along with use of an esophageal detector device, end-tidal carbon dioxide indicator, or capnography. Obtain a chest x-ray after stabilizing the patient. Capnography is recommended for confirmation and monitoring of ET tube placement and the quality of CPR (Hazinski, 2010). Advantages of ET intubation include reduction of the risk of vomiting and aspiration and provision of a relative airway seal. Two alternative airway techniques may be placed orally and are inserted past the hypopharynx, but not into the trachea: laryngeal mask airway (LMA) and esophageal-tracheal Combitube (ETC).

If the IV route cannot be established, but ET tube placement has been achieved, some emergency drugs can be given through the ET tube; however, the IV route is preferred. Epinephrine, lidocaine, atropine, and naloxone are administered through the ET tube but require adjusting the dose to 2 to 2.5 times the usual dose and diluting the drug with isotonic saline to make a total volume of at least 10 mL. Follow the administration of the drug with several quick insufflations with the manual resuscitation bag.

For IV fluids, use normal saline to maintain adequate preload and to mix IV drug infusions. Administer pharmacologic agents as indicated in algorithms (see Figures 3-43, 3-44, and 3-45).

If needed, use electrical therapies to change an abnormal cardiac rhythm to a normal one. Treat ventricular fibrillation or pulseless ventricular tachycardia with defibrillation as previously described. Treat unstable supraventricular tachycardia or ventricular tachycardia with a pulse with cardioversion. Treat patients who have problems with impulse formation and/or conduction with a temporary pacemaker. Indications for electrical therapies include symptomatic bradycardia nonresponsive to drug therapy (e.g., atropine) and symptomatic AV blocks. Note that pacing is no longer recommended for patients with asystolic cardiac arrest, as this has not been shown to be effective and delays or interrupts chest compressions (Link et al., 2010).

Apply a transcutaneous pacemaker to the anterior and posterior thorax with large surface skin electrodes. In the posterior position, apply a positive electrode between the spine and left scapula at the level of the heart. In the anterior position, apply a negative electrode at the left fourth LICS at the MCL. Transcutaneous pacing may be painful for patients and should be replaced by a transvenous lead as soon as possible. Use a transvenous pacemaker for patients who do not respond to drugs or transcutaneous pacing. The physician threads the lead into the apex of the right ventricle through the subclavian or internal jugular vein.

Recognize that care after return of spontaneous circulation (ROSC) significantly influences patient survival with optimal quality of life. Provide quality postcardiac arrest care (Peberdy et al., 2010) and facilitate transfer of the patient to a higher acuity level of care. During any wait time for the transfer process to be completed, attempt to identify and treat the reversible causes of cardiac arrest. Optimize ventilation and oxygenation of the patient using the following interventions:

- Avoid hyperventilation and keep $Paco_2$ between 40 and 45 mm Hg.
- Provide oxygen to maintain Sao_2 at 95% or greater.
- Monitor ABGs closely and decrease oxygen when possible to prevent oxygen toxicity.
- Use hyperoxygenation with 100% oxygen during suctioning to avoid hypoxemia.
- Provide advanced airways as required. Limit tidal volume to 6 mL/kg to prevent acute lung injury.
- Use waveform capnography as available and indicated.

Maintain adequate circulation. Treat hypotension (i.e., systolic BP less than 90 mm Hg) and potential causes of hypotension. Provide IV or IO boluses, inotropic or vasopressor agents as indicated, and antidysrhythmics as indicated.

Utilize therapeutic hypothermia if the patient is unresponsive but with an adequate BP following resuscitation. Studies have demonstrated that postresuscitation hypothermia treatment improves neurologic recovery and reduces the mortality rate. This treatment, indicated for in-hospital cardiac arrest patients with persistent changes in neurologic function after ROSC and in patients able to maintain BP with or without vasopressors after ROSC is also indicated for patients suffering a cardiac arrest as the result of ventricular fibrillation or pulseless ventricular tachycardia in the outpatient community setting. It is contraindicated (Seupard & Wilbur, 2011) in patients younger than 18 years of age, patients in a coma of other etiology prior to cardiac arrest, pregnancy, terminal illness (e.g., late-stage cancer), intracerebral hemorrhage, surgery within 14 days, systemic infection or sepsis, and known bleeding or coagulopathy.

Facilitate coronary reperfusion as indicated for ST segment elevation myocardial infarction (STEMI) or high suspicion of STEMI. The patient may go directly to the cardiac catheterization laboratory for a PCI (e.g., angioplasty, atherectomy, stent placement). Provide patient care management as required, including prevention, close monitoring, and/or correction of electrolyte imbalance, hypoglycemia, or hyperglycemia. The patient may require prevention, close monitoring, and/or correction of myocardial stunning with inotropic agents, fluid management, ventilator support, and intraaortic balloon pump (IABP).

In addition, correction of acute renal injury with fluid management and renal replacement therapy and specialized treatment for acute brain injury may be required. Avoid calcium administration, which has been shown to cause cerebral vessel spasm and is associated with poor brain outcomes. Avoid dextrose in water and use isotonic normal saline rather than D_5W for fluid resuscitation and for drug infusions. The dextrose in D_5W quickly metabolizes, leaving only hypotonic water, and this contributes to hypoosmolality, potentially leading to

cerebral edema and poor neurologic outcome. Elevate the head of the bed 30 degrees, avoid neck flexion or rotation, and avoid hip flexion to decrease intracranial pressure (ICP) and increase cerebral perfusion pressure (CPP) as indicated.

Initiate pharmacologic treatment as prescribed according to unit protocol. The administration of multiple common agents occurs in the progressive care unit while waiting on a patient's transfer to higher acuity care. These agents include analgesics to reduce pain, sedatives to reduce anxiety, anticonvulsants (e.g., phenytoin [Dilantin]) to prevent seizures, isotonic or hypertonic solutions to decrease cerebral oxygen requirements, osmotic agents (e.g., mannitol [Osmitrol]) to increase cortical circulation and reduce cerebral edema, calcium channel blockers (e.g., nimodipine [Nimotop]) to prevent cerebral vasospasm, and steroids (e.g., methylprednisolone [Solu-Medrol]) to reduce cerebral edema.

Some circumstances need special attention, such as cardiac arrest with hypothermia when the body temperature is less than 95°F (35°C). Initial treatment requires performance of CPR, defibrillation for ventricular fibrillation or pulseless ventricular tachycardia, and intubation of the patient and ventilation with warm, humidified oxygen. It is also important to obtain IV access and administer warmed IV saline. If the patient's core temperature is less than 86°F (30°C), continue CPR but withhold IV medications until the core temperature reaches 86°F (30°C). Do not attempt repeated defibrillation until after the core temperature reaches 86°F (30°C). Also, continue with warm inspired oxygen and warm IV fluids. Peritoneal lavage with warm saline, extracorporeal rewarming, and esophageal rewarming tubes may be used. If the patient's core temperature is greater than 86°F (30°C), continue CPR and administer IV medications but increase the usual ACLS intervals between doses, and repeat defibrillation for pulseless ventricular tachycardia (VT) or VF as the core temperature rises above 95°F.

Screen the resuscitated patient away from other patients. Make sure other patients are cared for during the resuscitation efforts. During the resuscitation efforts, touch the patient's hand and talk to him or her. Maintain the patient's modesty and dignity with drapes, curtains, and doors and ensure that all team members are respectful of the patient. After the resuscitation, encourage the patient to talk. Patients frequently (~40%) have a near-death experience during cardiac arrest, but are often reluctant to discuss it. As the patient regains consciousness, provide assurance that he or she is not alone and reorient the patient to person, place, and time. Consider asking the patient if he or she remembers anything that occurred during the resuscitation period. If resuscitation efforts are unsuccessful, provide respectful and culturally sensitive care of the body.

The family has a need for information. If the patient's condition has been worsening, inform the family. If the cardiopulmonary arrest was sudden, inform them about what has happened, what has been done, and give an estimate of how long it may be before more information will be available. If information must be conveyed by telephone, the family should be told that the situation is serious, but should not be informed of a death by telephone. If they do ask if the patient is dead, however, you should be truthful.

If the family is present, ensure privacy and escort them to a family conference room where they can grieve apart from other visitors, but do not leave them alone. Ask if they need someone, such as a family member, friend, or religious leader, to be contacted.

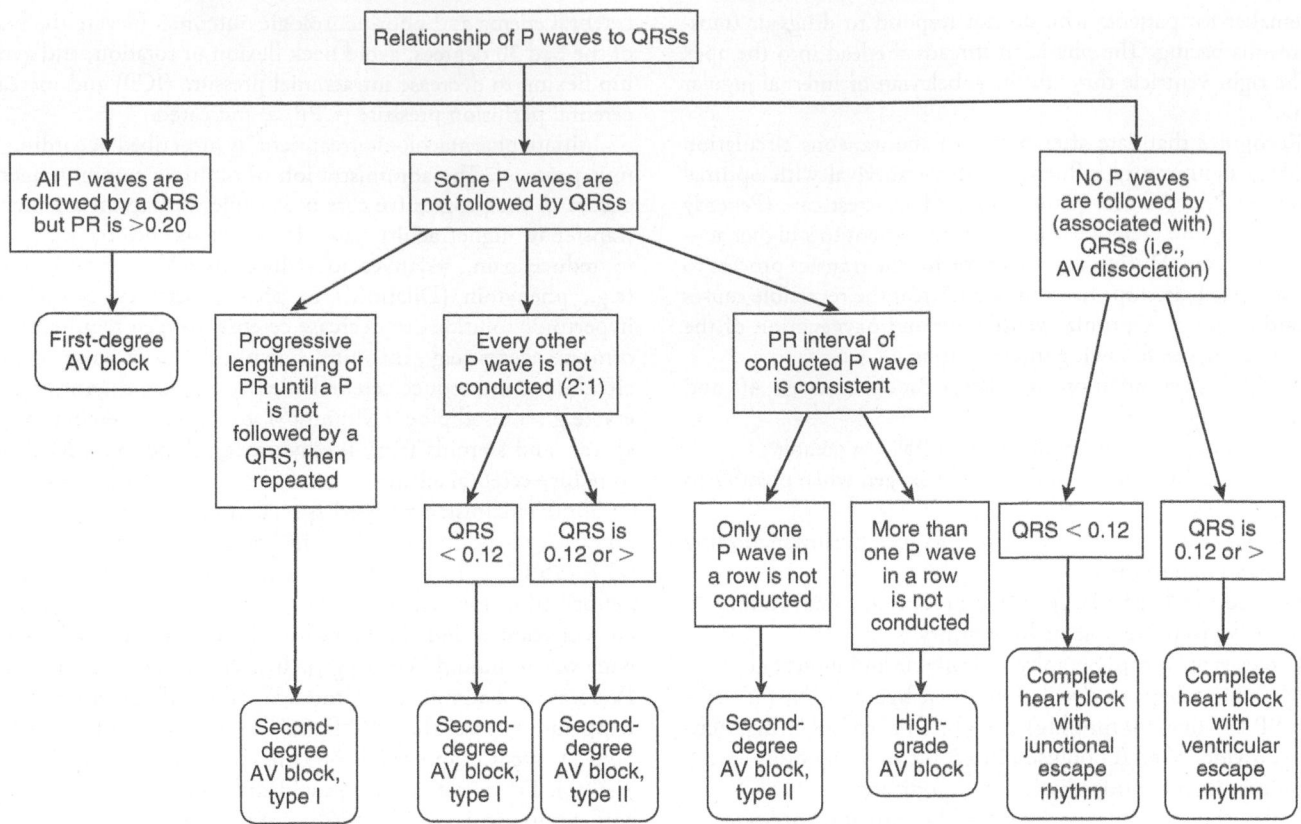

FIGURE 3-46 Differentiation of degrees and types of AV block. (From Dennison, R. D. [2013]. *Pass CCRN!* [4th ed.]. St. Louis, MO: Elsevier.)

Offer to call someone from pastoral services or have a social worker or a volunteer be there with them. Listen and allow the family to tell their story. Be honest, hopeful, warm, and caring, but do not give inappropriate reassurance.

Family presence during cardiopulmonary arrest is being advocated today as part of holistic care. Adhere to the family's wishes if they do not conflict with the wishes of the patient. Give consideration to the family members' coping abilities. If a family member (generally limited to one member) desires to be present during resuscitation efforts, prepare that person for what to expect. Drape the patient appropriately. Set limits prior to the family member entering the room. Explain where he or she may stand and if he or she may touch the patient, such as hold the patient's hand. If the patient is not responding to resuscitation efforts and death is imminent, allow the family member time to talk to the patient. If the code team asks the family member to leave, escort him or her out, and make sure that someone stays with the family member.

If resuscitation efforts are successful, allow family visitation as soon as possible. Consider staff debriefing because constructive multidisciplinary debriefing of resuscitation efforts aids in quality improvement, team building, and stress reduction. The team should continue to perform as a team. Critique of poor performance of an individual member should not occur in a group setting. Counseling services should be available for staff. Also, ensure that supplies and equipment are adequate and restocked for future needs.

Monitor the patient for complications of CPR, including fracture of the sternum or ribs; hemothorax; pneumothorax; laceration of abdominal viscera, especially the liver; myocardial contusion; or cardiac rupture. Successful resuscitation includes continual

evaluation of the patient. Ensure that the patient has adequate oxygenation (i.e., normal PaO_2, SpO_2, and SaO_2) and ventilation (i.e., normal $PaCO_2$) and that there are no signs or clinical indications of respiratory distress. Be sure the patient's cardiac rate and rhythm and hemodynamic status are stable. Check to see if the patient is alert and oriented with no neurologic deficit. Ensure to minimize or eliminate chest pain, discomfort, and dyspnea.

If the resuscitation efforts are unsuccessful, the physician usually informs the family of the patient's death. Express your sympathy and answer whatever questions the family asks. Ask the family members if they desire to see their loved one and prepare them for what they will see. Prepare the body for visitation by discarding trash and removing clutter from the room. Remove the ET tube if legally acceptable (i.e., not a coroner's case) and remove any blood from the face and hands. Place a couple of chairs close to the body and escort the family to the bedside, and stay with them. Contact the organ transplant coordinator if appropriate.

DYSRHYTHMIAS AND BLOCKS

A cardiac dysrhythmia (also referred to as *arrhythmia*) is any cardiac rhythm other than normal sinus rhythm. Dysrhythmias may originate from the sinus node, atria, AV junction, or ventricles. A block is the failure of an intrinsic impulse to be conducted through the conduction system. Differentiation of degrees and types of blocks (Figure 3-46) include first-degree, second-degree type I (previously referred to as Wenckebach or Mobitz I), second-degree type II (previously referred to as Mobitz II), and third-degree blocks along with LBBB and RBBB. A hemiblock is the block of the left anterior or left posterior branch of the LBB.

Many causes of dysrhythmias and blocks exist, including congenital causes (long QT syndrome, Brugada syndrome, and accessory pathways), myocardial ischemia or infarction, hypoxemia and/or hypoxia, electrolyte imbalance, acid-base imbalance, SNS stimulation caused by either endogenous or exogenous catecholamines, PNS (i.e., vagal) stimulation, drug effects, or drug toxicity. One example of drug toxicity is *holiday heart* syndrome caused by excessive alcohol consumption; this may cause dysrhythmias, usually supraventricular tachycardia.

Long QT syndrome is a congenital cause of potentially fatal dysrhythmias. The manifestations include prolonged QT interval and potentially nonsustained or sustained torsades de points with loss of consciousness, seizures, and cardiac arrest. Brugada syndrome is a congenital condition that is more common in Southeast Asian and Japanese populations. It is associated with ST segment elevation and negative T waves in leads V_1 and V_2, RBBB, and a prolonged PR interval. Sudden cardiac arrest may occur from ventricular tachycardia or ventricular fibrillation. Antidysrhythmics (class IA, IC, or III) that prolong the QT interval, antimalarials, antidepressants (e.g., tricyclics, such as amitriptyline [Elavil]), fever, hyperglycemia, cocaine, or lithium may trigger dysrhythmias. Another congenital cause of dysrhythmias is the presence of accessory pathways, such as those associated with Wolff-Parkinson-White (WPW) syndrome.

Arrhythmogenic mechanisms are divided into problems with impulse formation and problems with impulse conduction. Problems with impulse formation include altered automaticity and triggered activity. Altered automaticity may be either enhanced or depressed automaticity. Enhanced automaticity is caused by the resting membrane potential being less negative than normal or the threshold potential being lower than normal; this means that less change in charge is required for the cell to depolarize. Therefore, the cells increase their firing rate, which takes control away from the SA node, causing most atrial, junctional, and ventricular ectopic beats, accelerated junctional rhythm, accelerated idioventricular, and ventricular tachycardia. Causes of enhanced automaticity include hypoxia, hypercapnia, ischemia or infarction, hypokalemia, hypocalcemia, SNS stimulation, hyperthermia, digitalis toxicity, and stretching of atrial muscle such as HF.

Depressed automaticity is caused by the resting membrane potential being more negative than normal or the threshold potential being higher than normal; this means that more change in charge is required for the cell to depolarize. Therefore, the cells decrease their firing rate and responsiveness causing bradycardias and blocks. Causes of depressed automaticity include vagal stimulation, hyperkalemia, hypercalcemia, hypothermia, and beta-blockers.

An afterdepolarization is an abnormal electrical impulse that occurs during or after repolarization of an action potential. If a strong afterdepolarization reaches threshold, a triggered beat or rhythm occurs. This activity is not self-generating but is dependent on the preceding beat. They may be early or late. Early beats occur when the QT is prolonged, resulting from the prolongation of repolarization and effective refractory period; torsades de pointes may result. A delayed response may result from elevated intracellular calcium caused by electrolyte imbalances and/or catecholamine; this is a cause of the dysrhythmias seen in digitalis toxicity.

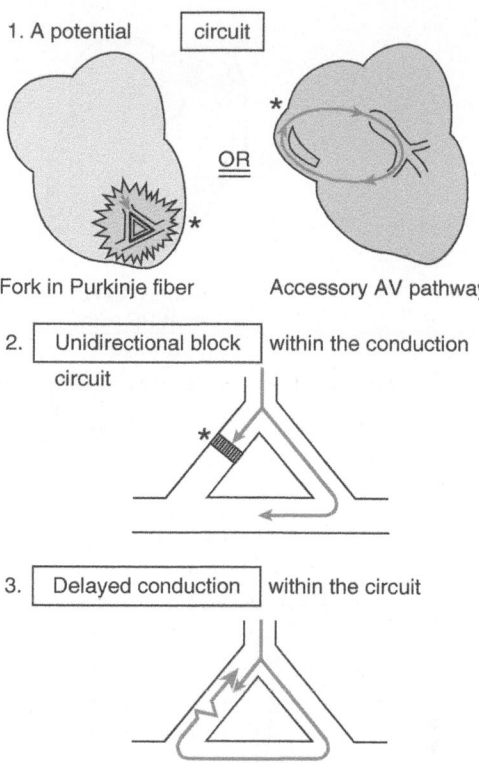

FIGURE 3-47　Reentry. Requirements for reentry include (1) a potential conduction circuit or circular conduction pathway, (2) a block or delay within part of the circuit, and (3) delayed conduction within the remainder of the circuit. *AV,* Atrioventricular. (From Aehlert, B. [2011]. *ECGs made easy* [4th ed.]. St. Louis, MO: Mosby.)

Problems with impulse conduction include reentry, accessory pathways, and aberrant conduction. Reentry (Figure 3-47) is the most common mechanism for tachydysrhythmias. An impulse travels through an area of the myocardium and depolarizes it, but then reenters the same area to depolarize it again. This mechanism requires an available circuit so reentry can occur in areas of the heart where conduction velocity is abnormally slow, where two segments of the circuit have unequal responsiveness (i.e., delay in one limb of the circuit), and where there is an area of slowed conduction or a unidirectional block. Conduction must be slow enough to allow time for the previously stimulated area to recover the ability to conduct. The area of unidirectional block provides a return pathway for the original stimulus to reenter a previously stimulated area and time to repolarize. Impulse reentry occurs with myocardial ischemia or infarction, electrolyte imbalance, or antidysrhythmic drugs. Reentry is the cause of some ectopy, including some ventricular tachycardia and most supraventricular tachycardias, and the tachycardias associated with accessory pathways.

Accessory pathway conduction issues (Figure 3-48) include Lown-Ganong-Levine (LGL) syndrome, WPW syndrome, and Mahaim fiber tachycardia. LGL syndrome is caused by an AV nodal bypass tract, a smaller than normal AV node, and fibers running through the AV node that do not have the built-in delay feature that nodal fibers have. Patients with LGL syndrome have a short PR with a normal QRS and are likely to have a history of palpitations and tachydysrhythmias.

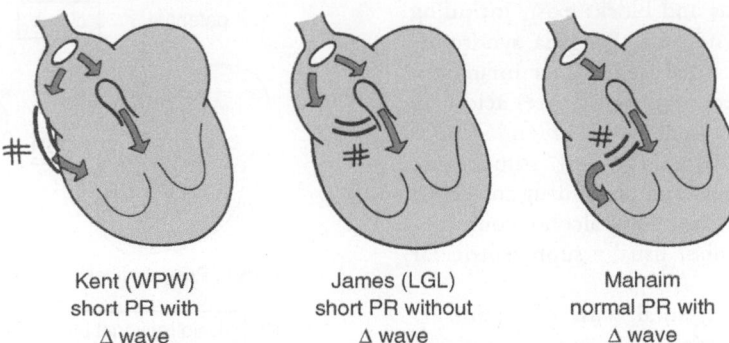

Kent (WPW)
short PR with
Δ wave

James (LGL)
short PR without
Δ wave

Mahaim
normal PR with
Δ wave

FIGURE 3-48 Accessory pathways. Location of accessory pathways and corresponding ECG characteristics. *LGL,* Lown-Ganong-Levine; *WPW,* Wolff-Parkinson-White. (From Aehlert, B. [2009]. *ECGs made easy* [3rd ed.]. St. Louis, MO: Mosby.)

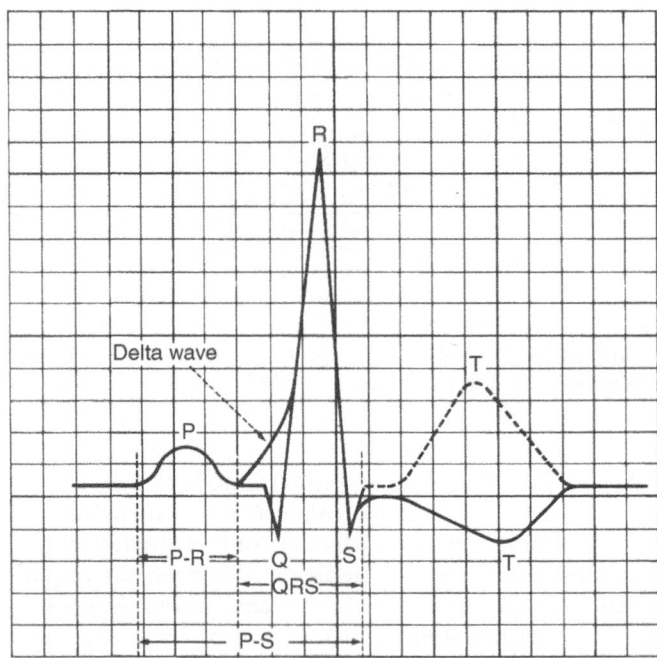

FIGURE 3-49 Wolff-Parkinson-White syndrome. Note the short PR interval, the delta wave, widened QRS complex, and T wave inversion characteristic of preexcitation. (From Kinney, M. R., et al. [1998]. *AACN's clinical reference for critical-care nursing,* [4th ed.]. St. Louis, MO: Mosby.)

WPW syndrome results from a Kent bundle that bypasses the AV node. Type A WPW syndrome occurs with the Kent bundle on the left and causes the ECG appearance of an R wave in V_1 with an inverted T wave and depressed ST segment. Type B WPW syndrome occurs with the Kent bundle on the right and causes the ECG appearance of QS in V_1 with an upright T wave and an elevated ST segment. Patients with WPW have a short PR and a wide QRS with slurring of the first portion of the QRS (Figure 3-49), which is referred to as a delta wave. Patients with WPW are likely to have a history of tachydysrhythmias and palpitations. If the sinus impulse goes through the AV block and then reenters by way of the accessory path, the QRS will be normal. However, if the sinus impulse takes the accessory pathway and then reenters by way of the AV node, the QRS will be wide and many times difficult to differentiate from ventricular tachycardia. Treatment of supraventricular tachycardia in WPW is with

antidysrhythmics, such as amiodarone, flecainide, procainamide, propafenone, or sotalol. Avoid adenosine, calcium channel blockers, and digoxin in patients with tachydysrhythmias with known WPW. If antidysrhythmics are ineffective, cardioversion is used. Definitive treatment of the condition is catheter or surgical ablation.

Mahaim fiber tachycardias results from nodoventricular or fasciculoventricular fibers. The ECG shows a normal PR and a narrow QRS with rS in lead III when in sinus rhythm and has a normal PR interval with an LBBB pattern with tachydysrhythmias and palpitations.

Aberrant conduction occurs when a supraventricular impulse travels through the ventricles outside the normal conduction system. This type of conduction occurs most likely with very rapid rates, premature atrial contractions (PACs), or changes in cycle length. Changes in cycle length are characteristic of atrial fibrillation. The QRS that ends a short cycle length after a previous long cycle length conducted aberrantly because it interrupts the long refractory length of the previous long cycle length; referred to as Ashman's phenomenon. Because one of the bundle branches (usually the right) is still refractory when a supraventricular impulse reaches it, the impulse must travel down the nonrefractory bundle and across to the other ventricle. This causes a wide QRS, which is frequently mistaken for a premature ventricular contraction (PVC) if there is a single complex or for ventricular tachycardia if there are several complexes in a row. Unlike ectopy, aberrancy is no more serious than the supraventricular mechanism that caused it (e.g., atrial fibrillation with aberrancy is no more clinically significant than atrial fibrillation). QRS morphology is the most important criterion in the differentiation between ectopy and aberrancy, but other criteria may also be helpful (Table 3-16). A multiple-lead ECG is often helpful to identify P waves and in looking at the morphology of the QRS. Ectopy is more common than aberrancy. If in doubt, always assume that you are dealing with ectopy and treat it accordingly.

Patients with tachycardia may manifest symptoms of anxiety and restlessness. The patient may have episodes of vertigo and/or syncope and complain of weakness, fatigue, activity intolerance, palpitations, and chest pain. On physical assessment, the patient may exhibit clinical indications of LVF such as dyspnea, S_3, or crackles, and clinical indications of hypoperfusion (see Table 3-2). Diagnostic studies include multiple-lead ECGs, serum electrolyte levels, and drug levels.

3.16 Learning Activity

Match the dysrhythmia with the most appropriate treatment summary. You may choose an answer more than once.

_____ 1. Ventricular fibrillation
_____ 2. Stable monomorphic ventricular tachycardia
_____ 3. Asystole
_____ 4. Symptomatic bradycardia
_____ 5. Pulseless electrical activity
_____ 6. Stable SVT
_____ 7. Acute onset atrial fibrillation
_____ 8. Pulseless ventricular tachycardia
_____ 9. Junctional tachycardia
_____ 10. Complete AV block with ventricular escape rhythm
_____ 11. Sinus tachycardia
_____ 12. Torsades de pointes

a. BLS, epinephrine
b. Treatment of cause; possibly beta-blocker or sedative
c. Cardioversion, or amiodarone or ibutilide
d. Vagal maneuvers and adenosine, calcium channel blocker, beta-blocker
e. Magnesium, overdrive pacing, isoproterenol
f. BLS, defibrillation, epinephrine, amiodarone
g. Procainamide, amiodarone, or lidocaine
h. Transcutaneous pacing or atropine
i. BLS, assess for possible causes, epinephrine
j. Vagal maneuvers, withhold digoxin, administration of adenosine, calcium channel blocker, or beta-blocker

Answers to this activity can be found in the Answer Key.

TABLE 3-16   Differentiation between Ventricular Ectopy and Aberrancy

Features	Favoring Ventricular Ectopy	Favoring Supraventricular Origin with Aberrancy
Rate	• 130-150 beats/min	• >150 beats/min
Regularity	• Regular	• Irregular (because most likely to be atrial fibrillation)
P wave	• None or dissociated (AV dissociation) • Inverted P wave after QRS (retrograde conduction to atria)	• Premature
QRS width	• Greater than 0.14 second	• 0.12-0.14 second
QRS morphology	• Initial vector opposite normal beats • Precordial concordance (all QRSs V_1-V_6 positive or all QRSs V_1-V_6 negative) • QRS morphology similar to previously seen PVCs	• Initial vector same as normal beats
QRS morphology in V_1 NOTE: Upper case letters indicate large waves, lower case letters indicate small waves	• Monophasic R • Rr' with left peak taller • Biphasic qR • Biphasic Rs or rS	• Monophasic QS • Biphasic rS • Triphasic rSR' or rR'
QRS morphology in V_6 NOTE: Upper case letters indicate large waves, lower case letters indicate small waves	• Monophasic QS • Biphasic qR • Biphasic rS	• Monophasic R • Triphasic qRs
Fusion beats	• Yes	• No
Compensatory pause after single beat or at end of run	• Yes	• No
Axis	• Indeterminate or LAD of −30 or greater	• Normal or RAD
Patient history	• History of PVCs • History of heart disease	• History of PACs, atrial fibrillation • History of preexisting bundle branch block
Response to carotid massage	• No effect on ventricular rate	• Often causes at least temporary slowing of ventricular rate
BP	• Usually very low or absent (but may be normal)	• Moderately low or normal
Consciousness	• Frequently unconscious (but may be conscious)	• May complain of lightheadedness
Seizures	• Frequently present (but may be absent)	• Absent

Follow the ACLS algorithms for lethal dysrhythmias. Treat the etiology of the dysrhythmia, for example:

- Decrease psychological and physical stress with therapeutic communication and anxiolytic agents.
- Correct ischemia if possible with coronary artery vasodilators and/or antispasmodics (e.g., nitrates or calcium channel blockers), fibrinolytics, or PCI.
- Correct hypoxemia/hypoxia:
  - Improve the patient's SaO_2 with the administration of oxygen, ET intubation, mechanical ventilation, and positive end-expiratory pressure (PEEP).
  - Augment the patient's cardiac output with inotropes, vasodilators, and/or intraaortic balloon pump treatments.
  - Correct the patient's hemoglobin to improve oxygenated blood flow to the heart.
- Correct electrolyte imbalance with electrolyte restriction, diuretics, ion exchange resins, and dialysis.
- Correct acid-base imbalance by treating the cause:
  - Improve oxygen delivery to the tissues for lactic acidosis.
  - Administer insulin and fluid administration for diabetic ketoacidosis.
  - Initiate dialysis for renal failure with metabolic acidosis.
  - Improve ventilation to correct respiratory acidosis.
- Correct drug toxicity by withholding the suspected drug and administer antidote (e.g., Digibind) or dialysis if appropriate.
- Administer beta-blockers for hyperthyroidism.

It is also important to eliminate the cause of catecholamine release or to block the effects of catecholamine release. Treat the patient's pain with analgesics and decrease anxiety with relaxation techniques and anxiolytics. Administer beta-blockers for cardioprotection as prescribed.

Initiate standing orders, such as IV medications, oxygen, and multiple-lead ECG. Antidysrhythmics are categorized according to the Vaughan-Williams classification (Table 3-17) system. Drugs of the same class have similar electrophysiologic effects and side effects. Administer antidysrhythmics (Table 3-18) as prescribed and monitor closely for adverse effects.

Utilize electrical therapies, such as cardioversion, as indicated. Prepare for urgent cardioversion with tachydysrhythmias, other than sinus tachycardia, that are rapid enough to cause hemodynamic compromise or that have not responded to antidysrhythmic drug therapy. The physician performs elective cardioversion for tachydysrhythmias that are reasonably well tolerated hemodynamically but have not responded to antidysrhythmic drug therapy. Cardioversion is contraindicated in patients with tachydysrhythmias that result from digitalis toxicity, nonsustained tachydysrhythmias, long-standing atrial fibrillation, atrial fibrillation with normal or slow ventricular rate in the absence of AV nodal blocking drugs, and multifocal atrial tachycardia.

The method for cardioversion is the same as for defibrillation except that conscious patients receive sedation with diazepam (Valium), lorazepam (Ativan), or midazolam (Versed). Elective procedures should be preceded by at least a 6-hour fast. Anterior-posterior electrode placement is preferable for cardioversion of atrial fibrillation. When conducting cardioversion, have emergency equipment and drugs available. Turn on the synchronizer switch so that the charge is delivered only during the QRS, avoiding the potential for the shock hitting during the descending limb of the T wave and potentially causing ventricular tachycardia or ventricular fibrillation (R-on-T phenomenon). Voltage should be from 50 to 200 joules (Neumar et al., 2010) according to the following recommendations:

- Narrow and regular: 50-100 J
- Narrow and irregular: 120-200 J biphasic or 200 J monophasic
- Wide and regular: 100 J
- Wide and irregular: defibrillate with 120-200 J biphasic or 360 J monophasic rather than synchronized cardioversion

Provide antidysrhythmic drug therapy to maintain rhythm after sinus rhythm is restored.

Utilize pacemaker therapies for patients who have problems with impulse formation and/or conduction. A pacemaker is

3.17   Learning Activity

Complete the following table by identifying the Vaughn-Williams antidysrhythmic classification of the following drugs. Some drugs are in more than one class.

Drugs	Classification
Adenosine (Adenocard)	
Amiodarone (Cordarone)	
Atropine	
Digoxin	
Diltiazem (Cardizem)	
Dofetilide (Tikosyn)	
Esmolol (Brevibloc)	

Drugs	Classification
Flecainide (Tambocor)	
Ibutilide (Corvert)	
Lidocaine (Xylocaine)	
Metoprolol (Lopressor)	
Procainamide (Pronestyl)	
Propranolol (Inderal)	
Quinidine	
Sotalol (Betapace)	
Verapamil (Calan)	

Answers to this activity can be found in the Answer Key.

TABLE 3-17	Vaughan-Williams Antidysrhythmic Classification System	
Class	**Effect**	**Examples**
IA	• Blocks sodium influx which depresses the rate of depolarization • Delays repolarization and prolongs action potential duration • Decreases contractility (negative inotrope) • Prolongs QT (torsades de pointes potential) and QRS duration	• Quinidine • Procainamide (Pronestyl) • Disopyramide (Norpace)
IB	• Blocks sodium influx during phase 0 which depresses the rate of depolarization • Accelerates repolarization and shortens action potential duration • Suppresses ventricular automaticity in ischemic tissue	• Lidocaine (Xylocaine) • Mexiletine (Mexitil) • Phenytoin (Dilantin)
IC	• Blocks sodium influx which depresses the rate of depolarization • Small delay in repolarization and small increase in effective refractory period • Has pronounced proarrhythmogenic potential	• Flecainide (Tambocor) • Propafenone (Rythmol)

II	• Depresses SA node automaticity
	• Increases refractory period of atrial and AV junctional tissue to slow conduction velocity
	• Shortens action potential duration
	• Inhibits sympathetic activity (i.e., blocks beta receptors)
	• Reduces atrial and ventricular contractility
		• Beta-blockers
		  • Propranolol (Inderal)
		  • Esmolol (Brevibloc)
		  • Acebutolol (Sectral)
		  • Sotalol (Betapace) (both II and III)

III	• Blocks potassium movement during phase III • Delays repolarization • Increases action potential duration • Prolongs effective refractory period	• Amiodarone (Cordarone) • Sotalol (Betapace) (both II and III) • Ibutilide (Corvert) • Dofetilide (Tikosyn)

IV	• Blocks calcium movement during phase II
	• Depresses automaticity in the SA and AV nodes
	• Prolongs the conduction time in the AV junction and increases the refractory period at the AV junction
	• Decreases contractility
		• Calcium channel blockers
		  • Verapamil (Calan)
		  • Diltiazem (Cardizem)

Misc.	• Blocks reentry mechanism • Shortens action potential of atrial tissue with little or no effect on action potential of ventricle • Prolongs AV nodal refractory period • Decreases SA node automaticity and slows sinus rate	• Adenosine (Adenocard)
Misc.	• Blocks parasympathetic nervous system effects to increase SA node firing rate and improve AV nodal conduction	• Atropine
Misc.	• Slows conduction through AV node • Prolongs AV nodal refractory period • Decreases SA node automaticity and slows sinus rate	• Digoxin

an electronic device that delivers an electrical stimulus to the heart to cause depolarization of the myocardium and increase or decrease the heart rate. Specific pacemaker terminology (Table 3-19) is used when discussing pacemakers. The indications for a pacemaker include:

• Sick sinus syndrome with syncope, such as symptomatic bradydysrhythmias, sinus block, or sinus arrest with ventricular asystole, or alternating tachycardia and bradycardia syndrome (also referred to as *tachy-brady syndrome*)
• Hypersensitive carotid sinus syndrome
• AV blocks, including second-degree AV block type I with symptomatic bradycardia, second-degree AV block type II,

or third-degree AV block; bundle branch block with AV block; bifascicular block (i.e., LBBB or RBBB with coexisting hemiblock) with acute MI; trifascicular block (e.g., bilateral bundle branch block)
• Refractory tachydysrhythmias unresponsive to drug therapy or cardioversion; the pacemaker action here is referred to as tachycardia overdrive and is an important treatment modality for torsades de pointes
• Hypertrophic cardiomyopathy or HF, indications for biventricular pacing
• Cardiac surgery in patients with acute coronary syndrome or cardiac dysrhythmias

TABLE 3-18   Selected Antidysrhythmic Agents

Drug	Classification/Actions	Indications	Administration	Adverse Effects	Nursing Implications
Procainamide hydrochloride (Pronestyl)	**Class IA antidysrhythmic** • Increases atrial refractoriness • Decreases automaticity, conductivity, contractility • Causes peripheral vasodilation	• Supraventricular dysrhythmias • Ventricular dysrhythmias	• PO 0.5-1 g every 4-6 hours • IM 250-500 mg every 4-6 hours • IV injection: 50-100 mg every 5 minutes • Stop injections and start maintenance infusion when suppression of dysrhythmia; widening of QRS by 50%; hypotension; or a total of 17 mg/kg occur • IV infusion: mix 2 g in 500 mL (4 mg/mL) and infuse at 1-4 mg/min • Therapeutic blood level 3-10 mcg/mL	• Bradycardia • Hypotension with IV administration • AV block • Dysrhythmias including torsades de pointes • Anorexia, nausea, vomiting, abdominal pain, diarrhea • Hepatic dysfunction • Bitter taste • Rash, urticaria • Fever • Mental depression • Hallucinations • Seizures • Bone marrow depression, thrombocytopenia • Worsening HF • Lupus-like syndrome	• Monitor BP, HR, ECG • ECG effects include increased PR interval, QRS width, and QT interval • Note contraindications: known hypersensitivity, myasthenia gravis, AV block • Use cautiously in renal disease, liver disease, HF, respiratory depression, patient receiving digitalis • Administer PO drug with food • Instruct patient to report fever, rash, muscle pain, bruising or bleeding, diarrhea, chest pain
Lidocaine hydrochloride (Xylocaine)	**Class IB antidysrhythmic** • Decreases ventricular automaticity and excitability • Increases ventricular fibrillation threshold	• Ventricular dysrhythmias	• IV injection: • VF: 1.5 mg/kg repeated every 3-5 minutes • VT: 1 mg/kg repeated every 5-10 minutes • Maximum: 3 mg/kg • IV infusion: mix 2 g in 500 mL (4 mg/mL) and infuse at 1-4 mg/min • Therapeutic blood level: 2-5 mcg/mL	• Hypotension • SA arrest • AV block • Nausea, vomiting • Tremors • Restlessness • Lightheadedness • Anaphylaxis *Clinical indications of toxicity (in relative order of occurrence)* • Perioral paresthesias • Feelings of dissociation • Dizziness • Drowsiness • Euphoria • Mild agitation • Dysarthria • Hearing impairment • Disorientation • Confusion • Muscle twitching • Seizures • Respiratory arrest	• Monitor BP, HR, ECG • Note contraindications: known hypersensitivity, AV block, supraventricular dysrhythmias, sick sinus syndrome • Use cautiously in liver disease, HF, respiratory depression, malignant hyperthermia, and in older adults • Note that toxicity incidence is increased if patient has HF or liver disease, has low lean body mass or is elderly, or is concurrently taking cimetidine (Tagamet) or beta-blocker • Note that the administration of prophylactic lidocaine after MI is no longer recommended; while the incidence of ventricular fibrillation is decreased, the incidence of asystole is increased

| Mexiletine (Mexitil) | **Class IB antidysrhythmic**
• Decreases ventricular automaticity and excitability
• Increases ventricular fibrillation threshold | • Life-threatening ventricular dysrhythmias | • PO: initial dose of 200-400 mg followed by 200-400 bid, tid, or qid; maximum 1200 mg/day | • Proarrhythmia including PVCs, ventricular tachycardia, torsades de pointes, PACs, supraventricular tachycardia, bradycardia, AV block, bundle branch block
• Hypotension
• Nausea, vomiting
• Diarrhea or constipation
• Elevated liver enzymes
• Palpitations
• Chest pain
• Dyspnea
• Headache
• Paresthesia, tremors, nystagmus, ataxia, dysarthria
• Tinnitus
• Blurred vision
• Dizziness
• Drowsiness, insomnia
• Confusion
• Seizures | • Monitor HR, BP, ECG
• Note contraindications: second- or third-degree block or sick sinus syndrome without pacemaker, cardiogenic shock
• Administer with meals to decrease GI adverse effects
• Note that risk of toxicity is greater if patient is concurrently receiving cimetidine (Tagamet) or beta-blocker; dosage is adjusted in HF and liver disease
• Monitor closely for clinical indications of toxicity: tremor, dizziness, ataxia, nystagmus |
| Flecainide (Tambocor) | **Class IC antidysrhythmic**
• Blocks sodium influx during phase 0 which depresses the rate of depolarization
• Does not change repolarization and action potential duration | • Life-threatening or refractory ventricular dysrhythmias
• Atrial or ventricular dysrhythmias that do not respond to other drugs | • PO: 50-200 mg twice daily; maximum dose 400 mg/day | • Proarrhythmia including PVCs, ventricular tachycardia, torsades de pointes, PACs, supraventricular tachycardia, bradycardia, SA block or arrest, AV block, bundle branch block
• Nausea, vomiting, abdominal pain, constipation
• Dyspnea
• Chest pain
• Headache
• Drowsiness
• Dizziness
• Blurred vision
• Tremor
• Dry mouth | • Monitor HR, BP, ECG
• Report widening of QRS of greater than 25%
• Monitor closely for HF
• Note contraindications: known hypersensitivity, second- or third-degree AV block, cardiogenic shock
• Use cautiously in HF, SA or bifascicular blocks or sick sinus syndrome without a pacemaker, renal disease, liver disease, myasthenia gravis
• Use cautiously in patients also receiving another negative inotropic agent (e.g., Verapamil, procainamide, beta-blocker)
• Correct electrolyte imbalance prior to therapy if possible |

Continued

TABLE 3-18   Selected Antidysrhythmic Agents—cont'd

Drug	Classification/Actions	Indications	Administration	Adverse Effects	Nursing Implications
Propafenone (Rythmol)	**Class IC antidysrhythmic** • Blocks sodium influx during phase 0 which depresses the rate of depolarization • Does not change repolarization and action potential duration	• Life-threatening or refractory ventricular dysrhythmias • Atrial fibrillation	• PO: 150-300 mg tid; maximum 900 mg/day	• Proarrhythmia including PVCs, ventricular tachycardia, torsades de pointes, PACs, supraventricular tachycardia, bradycardia, SA block or arrest, AV block, bundle branch block • AV block • Nausea, vomiting, constipation • HF • Dyspnea, bronchospasm • Dizziness • Diplopia • Paresthesia • Headache • Bitter or metallic taste • Leukopenia, agranulocytosis, thrombocytopenia, anemia • Bruising	• Monitor HR, BP, ECG • Report widening of QRS of greater than 25% • Monitor closely for clinical indications of HF • Note contraindications: HF; cardiogenic shock; SA, AV, bifascicular blocks or sick sinus syndrome without a pacemaker; myasthenia gravis; COPD; hypotension • Use cautiously in patients with renal or liver disease; dosage may be adjusted • Use cautiously if the patient is also receiving another negative inotropic agent (e.g., Verapamil, procainamide, beta-blocker) • Use cautiously in patients receiving digitalis as this drug can increase plasma concentration • Use cautiously in patients receiving oral anticoagulants as propafenone can increase plasma concentration • Administer with food to diminish GI adverse effects • Correct electrolytes prior to therapy • Instruct patient to report recurrent or persistent infection

Drug	Action	Use	Dosage	Adverse Effects	Nursing Considerations
Propranolol (Inderal)	**Noncardioselective beta-blocker class II antidysrhythmic** • Decreases HR, contractility, automaticity, excitability, conductivity • Depresses sinus node automaticity • Increases AV nodal refractoriness and decreases conduction velocity • Decreases myocardial oxygen consumption	• Supraventricular and ventricular dysrhythmias • Hypertension • Angina • Pheochromocytoma • Hyperthyroid crisis • Myocardial infarction (primary prevention and secondary prevention of extension and reinfarction) • Hypertrophic cardiomyopathy	• PO: 10-80 mg tid or qid • IV injection: 0.1 mg/kg in 3 divided doses at a rate not to exceed 1 mg/min • IV infusion: mix 20 mg in 250 mL (0.08 mg/mL); usual dose 3-8 mg/hr • Therapeutic blood level 0.04-0.90 mcg/mL	• Bradycardia • AV block • Hypotension • Nausea, vomiting, diarrhea • Fatigue, lethargy • Rash • Syncope • HF • Bronchospasm, especially in patients with asthma • Mental depression • Hyperglycemia in type 2 DM • Asymptomatic hypoglycemia in type 1 DM • Impotence • Emotional lability • Insomnia • Agranulocytosis, thrombocytopenia	• Monitor HR, BP, ECG • Monitor for clinical indications of HF • Note contraindications: known hypersensitivity, sinus bradycardia, AV block greater than first degree, HF, shock, asthma, Raynaud's syndrome • Use cautiously in DM, renal disease, hyperthyroidism, COPD, liver disease, myasthenia gravis, peripheral vascular disease, hypotension • May potentiate the hypoglycemic effects of insulin and prevents sympathetic symptoms of hypoglycemia • Note that this drug limits cardiac reserve and exercise capacity since HR cannot increase • Note that this drug masks sympathetic clinical indications of shock since receptors are blocked
Esmolol (Brevibloc)	**Cardioselective beta-blocker class II antidysrhythmic** • Decreases HR, contractility, automaticity, excitability, conductivity • Depresses sinus node automaticity • Increases AV nodal refractoriness and decreases conduction velocity • Decreases myocardial oxygen consumption	• Supraventricular tachycardia • Intraoperative or postoperative tachycardia and/or hypertension	• IV injection: loading dose of 500 mcg/kg over 1 minute followed by maintenance dose of 50 mcg/kg/min for 4 minutes • If desired effect does not occur, repeat the loading dose of 500 mcg/kg over 1 minute and follow with a dose increased by 50 mcg/kg/min for 4 minutes (e.g., 500 + 100, 500 + 150, 500 + 200) • IV infusion: when desired effect is achieved, no additional loading doses are needed and the maintenance dose is increased by 50 mcg/kg/min and maintained	• Bradycardia • Hypotension • AV block • Nausea, vomiting • Fatigue, lethargy • HF • Bronchospasm, especially in patients with asthma • Urinary retention • Inflammation and induration at injection site	• Monitor HR, BP, ECG • Monitor for clinical indications of HF • Note contraindications: known hypersensitivity, bradycardia, AV block greater than first degree, HF, shock, asthma • Use cautiously in DM, renal disease, hyperthyroidism, COPD, liver disease, myasthenia gravis, peripheral vascular disease, hypotension • May potentiate the hypoglycemic effects of insulin and prevents sympathetic symptoms of hypoglycemia; masks sympathetic clinical indications of shock because receptors are blocked

Continued

TABLE 3-18   Selected Antidysrhythmic Agents—cont'd

Drug	Classification/Actions	Indications	Administration	Adverse Effects	Nursing Implications
Metoprolol (Lopressor)	**Cardioselective beta-blocker class II antidysrhythmic** • Decreases HR, contractility, automaticity, excitability, conductivity • Depresses sinus node automaticity • Increases AV nodal refractoriness and decreases conduction velocity • Decreases myocardial oxygen consumption	• Hypertension • Angina • Myocardial infarction (primary prevention and secondary prevention of extension and reinfarction)	• PO: 100-450 mg daily in one or two doses • IV injection: 5 mg IV slowly at 5-minute intervals to a total of 15 mg	• Bradycardia • AV block • Hypotension • Nausea, vomiting, diarrhea, constipation • Fatigue, lethargy • Rash • Syncope • HF • Dyspnea, wheezing • Mental depression • Hyperglycemia in type 2 DM • Asymptomatic hypoglycemia in type 1 DM • Impotence • Emotional lability • Agranulocytosis, thrombocytopenia	• Monitor HR, BP, ECG • Monitor for clinical indications of HF • Note contraindications: known hypersensitivity, sinus bradycardia, AV block greater than first degree, HF, shock, asthma, Raynaud's syndrome • Use cautiously in DM, renal disease, hyperthyroidism, COPD, liver disease, myasthenia gravis, peripheral vascular disease, hypotension • May potentiate the hypoglycemic effects of insulin and prevents sympathetic symptoms of hypoglycemia • Note that this drug limits cardiac reserve and exercise capacity because heart rate cannot increase • Note that this drug masks sympathetic clinical indications of shock because receptors are blocked
Sotalol (Betapace) NOTE: class II and III	**Class II and III antidysrhythmic** • Depresses SA node automaticity • Increases refractory period of atrial and AV junctional tissue to slow conduction • Shortens action potential duration • Inhibits sympathetic activity • Blocks potassium movement during phase III • Increases action potential duration • Prolongs effective refractory period	• Life-threatening or refractory ventricular dysrhythmias	• PO: initial 80 mg bid followed by 160-320 mg/daily divided into two to three doses • IV injection: 100 mg (1.5 mg/kg) over 5 minutes	• Proarrhythmia including torsades de pointes, sinus bradycardia; second- or third-degree AV block • HF • Hypotension • Dyspnea • Bronchospasm (especially in patients with history of asthma) • Headache	• Monitor HR, BP, ECG • Report prolongation of QT interval to more than half of RR interval or hypotension • Monitor serum glucose in patients with DM • Monitor closely for clinical indications of HF • Note contraindications: second- or third-degree AV block, SA block without pacemaker, QT prolongation • Do not administer concurrently or within 4 hours of class IA antidysrhythmics or other class III antidysrhythmics; do not administer with other drugs that prolong the QT interval such as phenothiazines, tricyclic antidepressants • Correct electrolytes prior to therapy • Warn patient not to discontinue abruptly

| Amiodarone hydrochloride (Cordarone) | **Class III antidysrhythmic**
 • Prolongs the action potential and effective refractory period | • Life-threatening or refractory ventricular dysrhythmias
 • Refractory supraventricular dysrhythmias especially those caused by WPW | • PO: loading dose of 800-1600 mg/day for 1-3 weeks; then 600-800 mg/day for 1 month; then 200-800 mg daily
 • IV injection (loading dose): 150 mg over 10 minutes followed by IV infusion: mix 900 mg in 500 mL (1.8 mg/mL); usual dose is 1 mg/min for the next 6 hours followed by 0.5 mg/min
 • Use central venous catheter if more concentrated solution is used
 • Use solutions diluted in PVC containers within 2 hours; solutions diluted in glass or polyolefin containers within 24 hours
 • Administer through PVC tubing since dosing has taken into account adsorption to tubing
 • Therapeutic blood level 1.5-2.5 mcg/mL | • Hypotension
 • Proarrhythmia including PVCs, ventricular tachycardia, torsades de pointes, PACs, supraventricular tachycardia, bradycardia, SA block or arrest, AV block, bundle branch block
 • HF
 • Nausea, vomiting
 • Dizziness
 • Headache
 • Fatigue, malaise, muscle weakness
 • Corneal microdeposits
 • Rash, photosensitivity
 • Altered liver enzymes, hepatotoxicity
 • Hyperthyroidism, hypothyroidism
 • Blue-gray skin discoloration
 • Tremors, peripheral neuropathies, extrapyramidal symptoms
 • Cough, progressive dyspnea, pulmonary fibrosis | • Monitor HR, BP, ECG, and depth, breath sounds, electrolytes, liver function studies, thyroid function studies, pulmonary function studies, chest x-ray, neurologic symptoms
 • Monitor for clinical indications of HF, pulmonary fibrosis
 • Note contraindications: known hypersensitivity, marked sinus bradycardia, second- or third-degree AV block unless functioning pacemaker, cardiogenic shock
 • Use cautiously in patients with sinus node disease, conduction disturbances, severely depressed ventricular function, and marked cardiomegaly
 • Do not confuse amiodarone (an antidysrhythmic agent) with amrinone (an inotropic agent)
 • Advise methylcellulose ophthalmic solution and annual eye examinations for patients on long-term therapy
 • Advise use of SPF 15 sunscreen and sunglasses for patients on long-term therapy
 • Monitor for drug interactions: interacts with digitalis, anticoagulants, beta-blockers, calcium channel blockers, phenytoin, and class I antidysrhythmics
 • If used concurrently with digitalis, monitor closely for indications of digitalis toxicity
 • Administer PO drug with food to decrease GI adverse effects |

Continued

TABLE 3-18   Selected Antidysrhythmic Agents—cont'd

Drug	Classification/Actions	Indications	Administration	Adverse Effects	Nursing Implications
Ibutilide (Corvert)	**Class III antidysrhythmic** • Blocks potassium movement during phase III • Increases action potential duration • Prolongs effective refractory period	• Recent onset atrial fibrillation or atrial flutter	• IV infusion: mix 1 mg in 50 mL and infuse over 10 minutes for patients weighing over 60 kg (0.01 mg/kg in patients weighing less than 60 kg); may be repeated after 10 minutes if needed • Discontinue if atrial fibrillation or flutter terminates, a new dysrhythmia occurs, or if prolongation of the QT occurs	• Proarrhythmia including PVCs, ventricular tachycardia, torsades de pointes, PACs, supraventricular tachycardia, bradycardia, AV block, bundle branch block • Hypotension	• Monitor HR, BP, ECG • Report widening of QRS by greater than 25% or prolongation of QT interval to more than half of RR interval or hypotension • Correct electrolyte imbalances (especially hypokalemia) before initiating ibutilide • Administer anticoagulants for 2-3 weeks as prescribed for patients with atrial fibrillation of more than 2 to 3 days duration • Note contraindications: patients with second- or third-degree AV block, SA block without pacemaker, hypersensitivity to ibutilide, congenital or acquired long QT syndrome, in patients receiving verapamil or drugs that prolong the QT interval • Use cautiously in patients receiving digitalis as this drug may mask the cardiotoxicity associated with excessive digoxin levels • Do not administer concurrently or within 4 hours of class IA antidysrhythmics or other class III antidysrhythmics; do not administer with other drugs that prolong the QT interval such as phenothiazines, tricyclic antidepressants

Drug	Action	Use	Dosage	Adverse Effects	Nursing Considerations

Dofetilide (Tikosyn)	**Class III antidysrhythmic**
	• Blocks potassium movement during phase III
	• Increases action potential duration
	• Prolongs effective refractory period
		• Recent onset atrial fibrillation or atrial flutter
		• Maintenance of sinus rhythm in patients with highly symptomatic atrial flutter or atrial fibrillation of greater than 1 week duration
			• PO: 500 mcg twice daily
			   • Initiation of this oral therapy requires hospitalization for monitoring of QT interval while dosage is adjusted
			   • Dosage is also adjusted according to creatinine clearance
				• Proarrhythmia including PVCs, ventricular tachycardia, torsades de pointes, PACs, supraventricular tachycardia, bradycardia, AV block, bundle branch block
				• Hypotension
				• Nausea
				• Syncope
				• Chest pain
					• Monitor HR, BP, ECG
					   • Report widening of QRS by greater than 25% or prolongation of QT interval to more than half of RR interval or hypotension
					• Correct electrolyte imbalances (especially hypokalemia or hypomagnesemia) before initiating dofetilide
					• Note contraindications: patients with second- or third-degree AV block, SA block without pacemaker, hypersensitivity to dofetilide, in patients receiving verapamil or drugs that prolong the QT interval
					• Do not administer concurrently or within 4 hours of class IA antidysrhythmics or other class III antidysrhythmics; do not administer with other drugs that prolong the QT interval such as phenothiazines, tricyclic antidepressants

Verapamil (Calan)	**Calcium channel blocker class IV antidysrhythmic** • Depresses rate of SA node • Increases refractoriness of AV node • Relaxes vascular smooth muscle decreasing SVR, BP	• Supraventricular dysrhythmias • Angina • Hypertension • Hypertrophic cardiomyopathy	• PO: 40-120 mg every 6 hours • IV injection: 0.075-0.15 mg/kg (5-10 mg); may be repeated in 15-30 minutes at 5-10 mg • Maximum: 20 mg • IV infusion: mix 50 mg in 250 mL (200 mcg/mL); usual dose is 1-5 mcg/kg/min • Therapeutic blood level 0.1-0.15 mcg/mL	• Bradycardia • AV block • Hypotension • Nausea • Constipation or diarrhea • Elevated liver enzymes • Headache • Dizziness • HF	• Monitor HR, BP, ECG, liver function studies, breath sounds, heart sounds • Note contraindications: known hypersensitivity, AV block, sick sinus syndrome, WPW, advanced HF, cardiogenic shock • Use cautiously in HF, hypotension, liver disease, renal disease, patients receiving digitalis or beta-blockers • Do not give concurrently with IV beta-blockers • Administer calcium (500 mg-1 g IV over 10 minutes) as prescribed prior to IV verapamil to prevent hypotension

Continued

TABLE 3-18	Selected Antidysrhythmic Agents—cont'd				
Drug	**Classification/Actions**	**Indications**	**Administration**	**Adverse Effects**	**Nursing Implications**
Diltiazem (Cardizem)	**Calcium channel blocker** • Relaxes vascular smooth muscle decreasing preload and afterload • Relieves coronary artery spasm • Slows SA and AV nodal conduction times	• Angina • Coronary artery spasm • Mild HF • Hypertension • Hypertrophic cardiomyopathy • Supraventricular tachycardia	• PO: 30-60 mg every 6 hours • IV injection: 0.15-0.25 mg/kg (20 mg average) over 2 minutes, may be repeated in 15 minutes at 0.35 mg/kg (25 mg average) over 2 minutes • IV infusion: mix 125 mg in 100 mL for a total volume of 125 mL (1 mg/mL) and infuse at 5-15 mg/hr	• Bradycardia • Dysrhythmias • AV block • Hypotension • Nausea • Headache • Flushing • Fatigue • Drowsiness • Edema • Rash • Renal failure • Transient elevation in liver enzymes	• Monitor HR, BP, ECG • Note contraindications: known hypersensitivity, severe hypotension, second- or third-degree AV block, SSS, WPW, acute MI, pulmonary edema • Use cautiously in HF, hypotension, liver disease, renal disease, older adults
Digitalis (Digoxin, Lanoxin, Digitoxin)	**Cardiac glycoside** • Increases cardiac contractility to increase CO • Increases the refractory period of the AV node • Decreases sinus node firing rate • Decreases atrial automaticity • Increases ventricular automaticity increases GFR and urine output	• HF • Supraventricular tachycardias, especially in patients with HF	• IV, PO: digitalizing dose: 0.75-1.5 mg dose over 24 hours, usually in 4 doses of 0.25 mg • Administer IV dose over 5 minutes • Maintenance dose: 0.125-0.5 mg daily • Therapeutic blood level 0.5-2.0 ng/mL	*Toxic effects* • Anorexia, nausea, vomiting, diarrhea • Fatigue, muscle weakness • Agitation • Hallucinations • Visual disturbances • SA and AV blocks • Junctional and ventricular dysrhythmias *Treatment of toxicity* • Discontinue drug • Correct hypoxemia, ischemia, acid-base or electrolyte imbalance • Treat tachydysrhythmias as prescribed: usually lidocaine • Treat bradydysrhythmias as prescribed: usually atropine or pacemaker • Administer Digibind as prescribed for life-threatening dysrhythmias or blocks • Correction of hypokalemia is recommended before Digibind • Average dose is 400-800 mg over 30 minutes or IV bolus if cardiac arrest • Administered through inline filter • Reversal of digitalis toxicity occurs within 30-60 minutes but digoxin levels remain elevated	• Monitor apical HR, ECG, serum electrolytes, especially potassium, calcium, magnesium • Note contraindications: known hypersensitivity, sick sinus syndrome, SA or AV block, ventricular tachycardia, hypertrophic cardiomyopathy, WPW • Use cautiously in patients with acute MI, hypothyroidism, liver disease, renal disease, hypothyroidism, older adults • Assess patient for clinical indications of digitalis toxicity • Withhold for 1-2 days before elective electrical cardioversion

| Adenosine (Adenocard) | **Endogenous nucleoside unclassified antidysrhythmic**
• Slows conduction through the AV node
• Interrupts the reentry pathways through the AV node to restore normal sinus rhythm | • Supraventricular tachycardias including those associated with WPW
• Not effective in atrial fibrillation or atrial flutter but may slow rate so that fibrillatory or flutter waves can be identified | • IV injection: 6 mg IV; must be given within 6 seconds; repeat at 12 mg IV if conversion is not achieved within 1-2 minutes; 12 mg dose may be repeated once
  • Must be administered as quickly as possible (referred to as IV "slam") due to very short half-life (10 seconds); administer as quickly as possible into NS flush or insert a Y connector into line to push NS flush as quickly as possible while pushing adenosine as quickly as possible | • Transient dysrhythmias at the time of conversion (including short asystolic pause)
  • Pause may be prolonged especially in patients with sick sinus syndrome
• Hypotension if large doses are used
• Nausea
• Facial flushing
• Headache
• Dyspnea
• Bronchospasm
• Chest pressure
• Recurrence of dysrhythmias | • Monitor HR, BP, ECG, BP, depth of breathing, and breath sounds
• Note contraindications: known hypersensitivity, second- or third-degree AV block, sick sinus syndrome, ventricular dysrhythmias
• Use cautiously in patients with asthma or older adults
• Decrease initial dosage as prescribed in patients receiving dipyridamole (persantine), diazepam (valium), phenobarbital, or carbamazepine (tegretol); initial dose may be prescribed as 3 mg
• Increase initial dosage as prescribed if patient receiving aminophylline or another xanthine; initial dose may be prescribed as 12 mg
• Store at room temperature; solution must be clear at time of use |

Continued

TABLE 3-18   Selected Antidysrhythmic Agents—cont'd

Drug	Classification/Actions	Indications	Administration	Adverse Effects	Nursing Implications
Atropine sulfate	**Anticholinergic (also called parasympatholytic)** • Decreases vagal tone • Increases sinus rate • Slightly increases conduction through the AV node • Relaxes smooth muscle; prevents bronchospasm • Decreases GI, tracheobronchial secretions	• Symptomatic sinus bradycardia • Asystole • Preoperative preparation for surgery • Anticholinesterase insecticide (organophosphate) poisoning	• IV injection: 0.5-2 mg (0.5 mg given as initial dose in sinus bradycardia, 1 mg given as initial dose in asystole, 2 mg given as initial dose in organophosphate poisoning); repeated as needed at 3-5 minute intervals • Maximum: 0.04 mg/kg (usually approximately 3.0 mg)	• Tachycardia, palpitations • Bradycardia if given slowly or in dose of <0.5 mg • Hypotension • Dry mouth • Blurred vision, dilated pupils • Urinary retention • Constipation, paralytic ileus • Headache • Dizziness • Restlessness • Increased myocardial oxygen consumption and chest pain in patients with CAD	• Monitor HR, BP, ECG, urine output, bowel sounds • Note contraindications: known hypersensitivity to belladonna, glaucoma, GI obstruction, myasthenia gravis, thyrotoxicosis, ulcerative colitis, prostatic hypertrophy, tachydysrhythmias • Use cautiously in renal disease, HF, hyperthyroidism, hepatic disease, hypertension • Use cautiously in acute MI: do not administer atropine for bradycardia unless the patient is symptomatic; increasing HR increases myocardial oxygen consumption and can increase infarction size • Do not use pupils as a reflection of brain status after atropine: pupils will be dilated and nonreactive • Use hard candy to help alleviate side effect of dry mouth unless contraindicated
Isoproterenol (Isuprel)	**Unclassified antidysrhythmic; beta-selective adrenergic agent** • Increases HR, contractility, conductivity • Shortens repolarization and QT interval • Causes bronchodilation	• Bradycardia refractory to other drugs • Torsades de pointes	• Mix 1 mg in 250 mL (4 mcg/mL); infuse at 2-20 mcg/min	• Tachycardia, palpitations • Hypotension • Ventricular dysrhythmias • Chest pain • Flushing • Headache • Nausea, vomiting • Anxiety, tremor • Hyperglycemia	• Monitor BP, HR, ECG • Note contraindications: tachydysrhythmias, digitalis toxicity, angina, narrow angle glaucoma • Use cautiously in older adults and those with hyperthyroidism, chest pain, hypertension, psychoneurosis, DM

TABLE 3-19	Pacemaker Terminology
Artifact	The spike recorded on the ECG depicting the electrical energy discharge from the pulse generator
AV interval	In a dual-chamber pacemaker, the period of time between an atrial event (sensed or paced) and a paced ventricular event
Blanking period	The interval of time during which the pacemaker cannot sense any events
Burst pacing	The delivery of rapid, multiple electrical stimuli; typically used to interrupt a fast heart rate
Capture	Depolarization of the atria and/or ventricles by an electrical stimulus delivered by an artificial pacemaker; one-to-one capture occurs when each electrical stimulus causes a corresponding depolarization
Committed (DVI) operation	A characteristic of some DVI pacemakers whereby a ventricular stimulus always follows an atrial stimulus regardless of intrinsic ventricular activity
Cross talk	The phenomenon that can occur in dual-chamber pacemakers in which a stimulus from the atrial lead is sensed by the ventricular lead, or vice versa, resulting in an inappropriate pacemaker response such as inhibiting or resetting of the refractory period
Demand pacemaker	A pacemaker that only discharges when the patient's HR drops below the pacemaker's preset rate
Dual-chamber pacing (i.e., AV sequential)	The pacing in both the atria and the ventricles to artificially restore the natural contraction sequence of the heart; also called *physiologic pacing*
Electrode	The uninsulated conductive portion of a pacing lead that makes electrical contact with tissue
Electromagnetic interference (EMI)	Radiated or conducted energy—either electrical or magnetic—that can interfere with or disrupt the function of a pulse generator
End-of-life	The point at which a pacemaker signals that it should be replaced because its battery is nearing depletion
Escape interval	The time between a paced or sensed cardiac event and the subsequent pacing stimulus of a pulse generator
Fusion beat	A spontaneous cardiac depolarization that occurs coincidentally with a paced depolarization; the paced and natural depolarization waveforms fuse
Hysteresis	A pacing parameter that allows a longer escape interval after a sensed event, allowing perpetuation of the patient's intrinsic rhythm
Inhibited	A common type of pacemaker that does not pace when its output is suppressed by sensed spontaneous cardiac events occurring at a rate more rapid than the pacing rate
Intrinsic	Inherent; belonging to or originating from the heart itself
Lead	The insulated wire or wires that carry electrical signals to and from the heart, a connector pin, and stimulating, sensing electrode(s)
Milliamperage (mA)	The unit of measurement used for electrical stimulus (i.e., output) generated by a pacemaker
Multisite pacing	The ability of a pacemaker to stimulate more than one site, such as biventricular pacing
Myopotentials	Electrical signals that originate in body muscles; these signals may be sensed by the pacemaker and falsely interpreted as depolarization
Output	An electrical stimulus delivered by the pulse generator; measured in milliamperage (mA)
Pacemaker syndrome	A collection of signs and symptoms related to the adverse hemodynamic effects of ventricular pacing, usually attributed to the absence of synchrony between the atrial and ventricular contractions
Pacing mode	The manner in which a pacemaker provides artificial rate and rhythm support in the presence of dysrhythmia; identified by a three- or five-letter code
Programmable	A pulse generator with a pacing mode and/or parameters that can be changed noninvasively at any time by means of an external programmer

Continued

TABLE 3-19   **Pacemaker Terminology—cont'd**

Pulse generator	The portion of the pacing system that produces electrical pulses and contains the power supply and electronic circuit
Pulse width	The duration of the pacing pulse expressed in milliseconds; also called *pulse duration*
Rate responsive or rate modulated pacing	The ability of a pacemaker to increase or decrease its rate in response to the heart's intrinsic rate or detected changes in the body (i.e., body activity, atrial activity, respiratory rate)
Refractory period	The time during which the pacemaker's sensing mechanism becomes nonresponsive to cardiac activity
Safety pacing	In some DVI and DDD pacemakers, following atrial pacing, the pacemaker is designed to trigger a ventricular pacing output if ventricular sensing occurs during the first portion of the programmed AV interval; this ensures a ventricular depolarization if the event sensed was electrical interference
Sensing	The ability of the pacemaker to detect the patient's intrinsic activity and respond appropriately by either triggering or inhibiting output
Sensing threshold	The minimum atrial or ventricular intracardiac signal amplitude required to inhibit or trigger a demand pacemaker
Sensitivity	The degree to which a pacemaker is responsive to levels of electrical activity in the heart
Stimulation threshold	The minimum electrical stimulus needed to obtain consistent capture
Telemetry	The ability of the pacemaker to send information (i.e., programmed status, measurements, signals to the programmer)
Tracking	When ventricular pacing is synchronized to sensed atrial activity
Triggered	To deliver an electrical stimulus upon detecting a spontaneous depolarization
VA interval	With dual-chamber pacemakers, the period of time elapsing from a ventricular event (sensed or paced) to the next scheduled atrial pace

From Medtronic. (2005). *Pacing glossary*. Retrieved September 8, 2012, from https://wwwp.medtronic.com/medtronicconnect/resources/presentationtools//1332879501392/MedtronicPacingGlossary2007.pdf

3.18   Synthesis Learning Activity: Crossword Puzzle

Complete the following puzzle on pacemaker terminology.

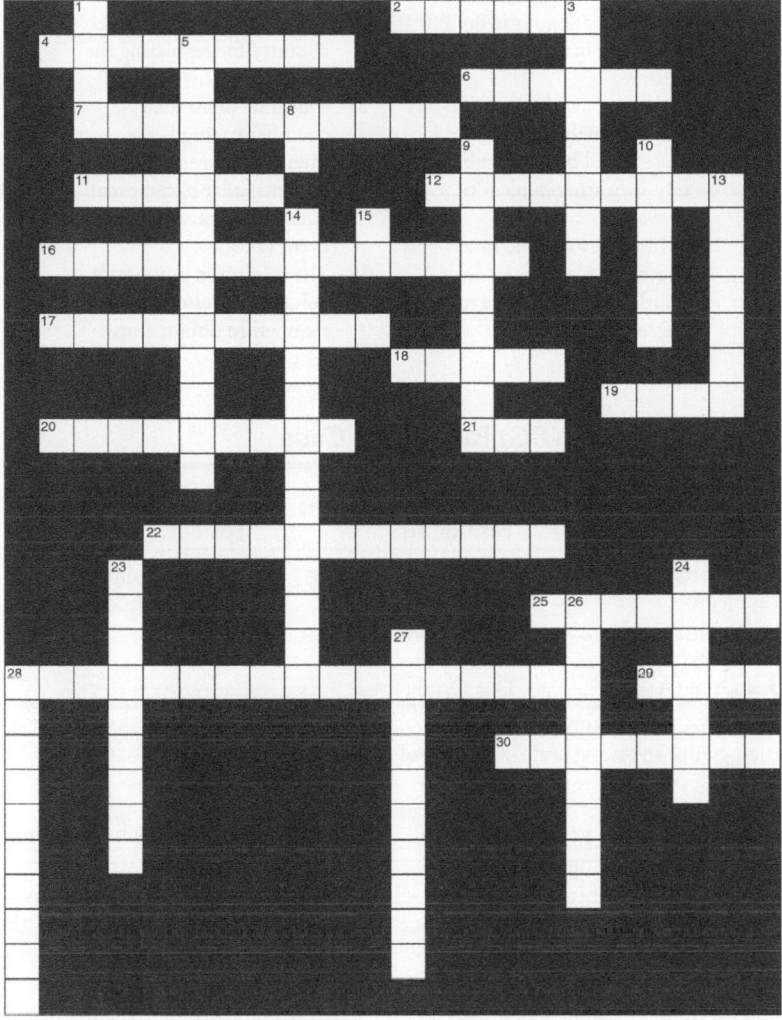

Answers to this activity can be found in the Answer Key.

ACROSS

2. The electrical stimulus delivered by a pacemaker's pulse generator

4. The ability of the pacemaker to send information (i.e., programmed status, measurements, signals) to the programmer

6. This type of pacemaker only discharges when the patient's heart rate drops below the preset rate for the pacemaker

7. This type of pacemaker is capable of stimulating the atria and ventricles (2 words)

11. This type of beat results when an intrinsic depolarization and a paced depolarization occur simultaneously so both contribute to the depolarization

12. Inherent; belonging to or originating from the heart itself

16. The ability of a pacemaker to increase the pacing rate in response to physical activity and physiologic demand (2 words)

17. A pacing parameter that allows a longer escape interval after a sensed event, allowing perpetuation of the patient's intrinsic rhythm

18. Another term for pacemaker artifact

19. This rate is the rate at which the pulse generator discharges when no intrinsic activity is detected

20. To deliver an electrical stimulus upon detecting a spontaneous depolarization

21. Radiated or conducted energy, either electrical or magnetic, which can interfere with or disrupt the function of a pulse generator (abbrev.)

22. A pulse generator with a pacing mode and/or parameters that can be changed noninvasively at any time by means of an external programmer

25. The ability of the pacemaker to detect the patient's intrinsic activity and respond appropriately by either triggering or inhibiting output

28. A collection of signs and symptoms related to the adverse hemodynamic effects of ventricular pacing, usually attributed to the absence of synchrony between the atrial and ventricular contractions (2 words)

29. The manner in which a pacemaker provides artificial rate and rhythm support in the presence of dysrhythmia; identified by a three- or five-letter code

30. The spike recorded on the ECG depicting the electrical energy discharge from the pulse generator

DOWN

1. The wire or wires that carry electrical signals to and from the heart, a connector pin, and stimulating, sensing electrode(s)
3. When ventricular pacing is synchronized to sensed atrial activity

5. The unit of measurement used for an electrical stimulus (i.e., output) generated by a pacemaker
8. This interval in dual-chamber pacing is analogous to the PR interval in intrinsic activity (abbrev.)
9. The point at which a pacemaker signals that it should be replaced because its battery is nearing depletion (3 words)
10. This interval is the time between a sensed intrinsic cardiac event and the next pacemaker output

13. Successful depolarization of the atria and/or ventricles by an artificial pacemaker
14. This portion of the pacemaker system houses the power source and the circuitry for regulating the pacemaker (2 words)
15. This interval in dual-chamber pacing is the interval between a sensed or ventricular paced event and the next atrial paced event (abbrev.)
23. The minimum amount of voltage, expressed in mA, required to obtain consistent capture

24. The lead has both positive and negative electrodes
26. The uninsulated conductive portion of a pacing lead that makes electrical contact with tissue
27. This mode of response to sensing indicates that the pacemaker output is suppressed when an intrinsic event is sensed
28. The duration of the pacing pulse expressed in milliseconds; also called pulse duration (2 words)

TABLE 3-20	The NASPE/BPEG Generic (NBG) Pacemaker Code			
Antibradycardia Function				
Position I	**Position II**	**Position III**	**Position IV**	**Position V**
Chamber(s) paced	Chamber(s) sensed	Response to sensing	Rate modulation	Multisite pacing
0 = None	0 = None	0 = None	R = Rate modulation	0 = None
A= Atrium	A= Atrium	T = Triggered		A= Atrium
V = Ventricle	V = Ventricle	I = Inhibited		V = Ventricle
D = Dual (A + V)	D = Dual (A + V)	D = Dual (T + I)		D = Dual (A + V)

From Bernstein, A. D., et al. (2002). The revised NASPE/BPEG generic code for antibradycardia, adaptive-rate, and multisite pacing. North American Society of Pacing and Electrophysiology/British Pacing and Electrophysiology Group. *PACE, 25*(2), 260-264.

Components of a pacemaker include a pulse generator, a battery, and a microprocessor that controls pacing (i.e., voltage) and sensing. Permanent pacemakers use a lithium-iodide battery that lasts approximately 7 to 10 years. There are several types of pacemakers, including single chamber atrial, single chamber ventricular, dual chamber atrioventricular, and dual chamber biventricular. Pacemakers may have an atrial lead, a ventricular lead, or both. The lead may either have one electrode (i.e., unipolar) or two electrodes (i.e., bipolar). Unipolar electrodes are negative only. The metal of the pulse generator acts as the positive. Bipolar pacemakers have both positive and negative electrodes. The positive electrode placement is proximal and senses. The negative electrode placement is distal and paces. Pacemakers can be temporary or permanent.

Temporary pacemakers have an external pulse generator/battery connected to the pacing wires and may be used for hours to weeks. There are three kinds of temporary pacemakers: transthoracic epicardial, transvenous endocardial, and transcutaneous. The transthoracic epicardial pacemaker is attached to the epicardium of the atrium and/or ventricle during cardiac surgery, then brought through the chest wall. The transvenous endocardial pacemaker is inserted percutaneously, threaded through the internal jugular or subclavian vein, and advanced into the right atrium and/or the right ventricle. The transcutaneous pacemaker electrodes are applied to the chest and back. This type of pacemaker is used during cardiac arrests until a transvenous pacer can be inserted.

A permanent pacemaker has an internal pulse generator and battery, which lasts for 5 to 10 years before requiring replacement, A transvenous endocardial pacemaker has a lead that is inserted into the cephalic vein and advanced into the right atrium or the right ventricle; the pulse generator is implanted in subcutaneous fat under the clavicle. An epicardial pacemaker requires a thoracotomy because the electrodes are sewn onto the epicardium; the pulse generator is then implanted into the subcutaneous fat of the abdomen. These are uncommon today.

An asynchronous pacemaker is also called a *fixed rate pacemaker.* The pacemaker delivers a pacing stimulus at a fixed rate regardless of the heart's intrinsic activity. This type of pacemaker will cause competition with the heart's intrinsic activity and the pacing stimulus may land during the descending limb of the T wave, potentially causing ventricular tachycardia or fibrillation. It is rarely used today.

A synchronous pacemaker is also called a *demand pacemaker.* The pacemaker delivers a pacing stimulus only when the heart's intrinsic pacemaker fails to function at a predetermined rate. The pacing stimulus will be either inhibited or triggered when intrinsic activity occurs.

The generic code (Table 3-20) adopted by the North American Society of Pacing and Electrophysiology (NASPE) describes the pacemaker modes, identifying the chamber paced, sensed, and response to sensing. In atrial modes (i.e., AOO, AAI), the pacing stimulus occurs before the P wave and requires an intact AV nodal conduction. In ventricular modes (i.e., VOO, VAT, VVI, VVT, VDD), the pacing stimulus occurs before the QRS complex. In atrioventricular (AV) sequential modes (i.e., DOO, DVI, DDD), AV synchrony and the hemodynamic benefit of the atrial kick are maintained. The pacing stimulus occurs before the P wave, QRS complex, or both. Sufficient AV delay is set to allow atrial depolarization and contraction to complete ventricular filling.

PACED HEART ACTIVITY

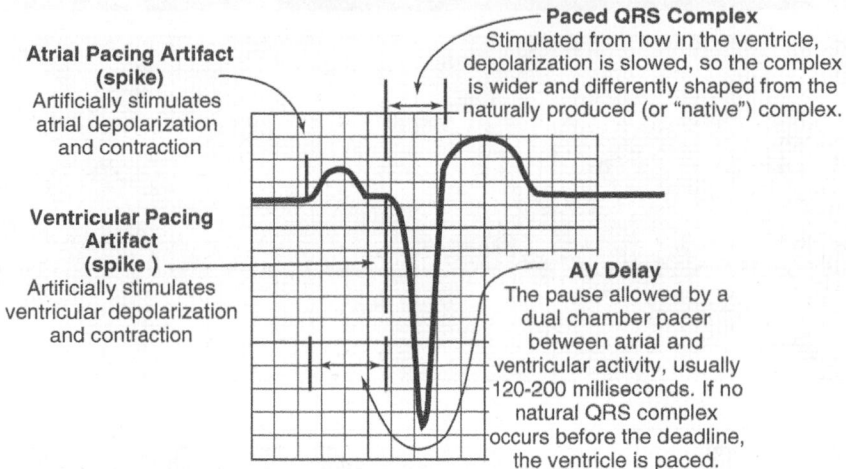

Atrial Pacing Artifact (spike)
Artificially stimulates atrial depolarization and contraction

Ventricular Pacing Artifact (spike)
Artificially stimulates ventricular depolarization and contraction

Paced QRS Complex
Stimulated from low in the ventricle, depolarization is slowed, so the complex is wider and differently shaped from the naturally produced (or "native") complex.

AV Delay
The pause allowed by a dual chamber pacer between atrial and ventricular activity, usually 120-200 milliseconds. If no natural QRS complex occurs before the deadline, the ventricle is paced.

FIGURE 3-50 ECG evidence of pacing. (From Witherall, C. [1990]. Questions nurses ask about pacemakers. *Am J Nurs, 90*[12], 20.)

Multisite atriobiventricular mode, also referred to as *cardiac resynchronization therapy*, is used in severe HF in patients with ventricular depolarization asynchrony. Normally, pacing leads are in the right atria and right ventricle. In this type of pacing, leads are in the right atria, right ventricle, and the left ventricle. A left ventricular lead is placed either directly on the left ventricle (i.e., epicardial) by thoracotomy approach or endocardially through the coronary sinus as well as the right ventricular and right atrial leads. The atrioventricular delay should be adequate enough to allow atrial contraction to contribute optimally to ventricular filling. Optimal timing of stimulation of both ventricles should occur. This may involve one ventricle being stimulated slightly before the other rather than simultaneous stimulation and may or may not include an ICD. The heart rate is adjusted according to demands for cardiac output (i.e., rate responsive). Heart rate changes are stimulated by changes in muscle activity, minute ventilation, or blood changes in temperature or pH. Rate-responsive modes include AAIR, VVIR, and DDDR.

Collaborative management of a patient with a pacemaker focuses on ensuring proper functioning of the pacemaker and detection of any complications. Evaluate ECG evidence of pacing (Figure 3-50), including a spike before a paced event, wide QRS if a ventricular pacer is used, and the presence of T waves to confirm ventricular depolarization. Fusion beats, a merging of the intrinsic impulse, and the paced impulse are common in paced rhythms. The rate is usually set at 60 to 90 beats/min, but will be set higher than the intrinsic rate for tachycardia overdrive. The atria, the ventricles, or both may be paced (Figure 3-51).

Three capital letters delineate the pacemaker modes (Table 3-21). The letters describe the chamber paced, chamber sensed, and the response to sensing. Specific indications, and advantages and disadvantages guide the type of pacemaker mode selected. Assist with establishing a pacing threshold and set the pacing mA two times the pacing threshold, which is the threshold that is determined by decreasing the milliamperes until capture is lost and then increased until regaining capture. A typical pacing threshold is 1 to 1.5 mA. The pacemaker is usually initially set at between 3 and 5 mA, depending on the pacing threshold. Sensitivity is usually set at approximately 2 to 5 mV. The AV interval is similar to the PR interval for AV sequential pacemakers.

3.19   Learning Activity

Analyze the following ECG rhythm strips. Identify the type of pacemaker and if there is a pacemaker malfunction.

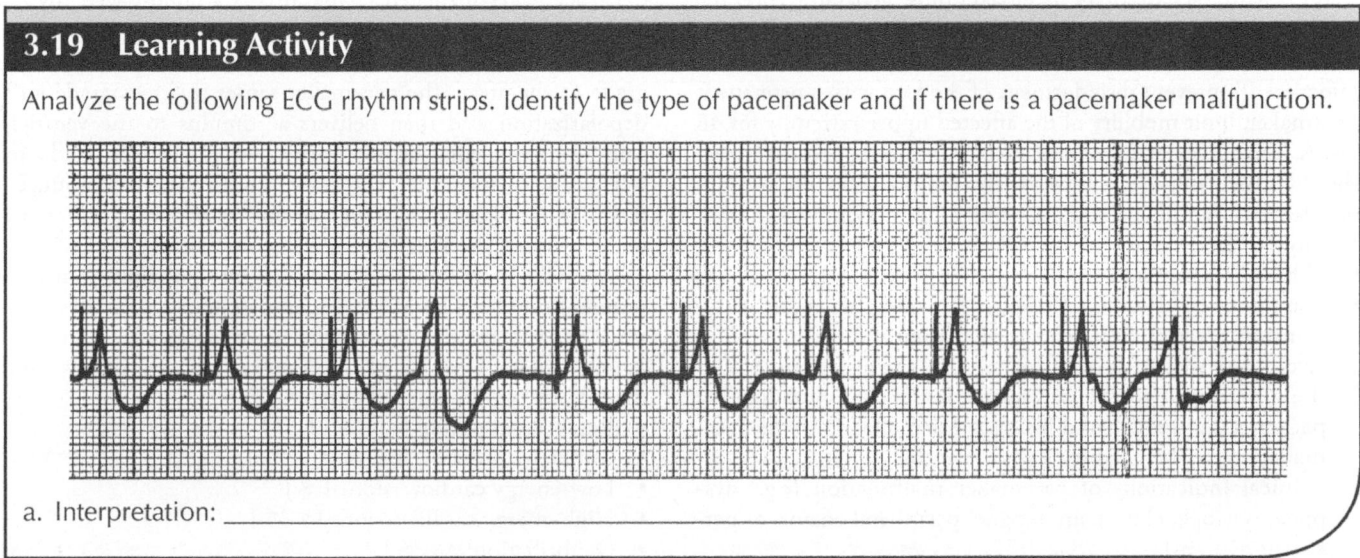

a. Interpretation: _____

Continued

3.19   Learning Activity—cont'd

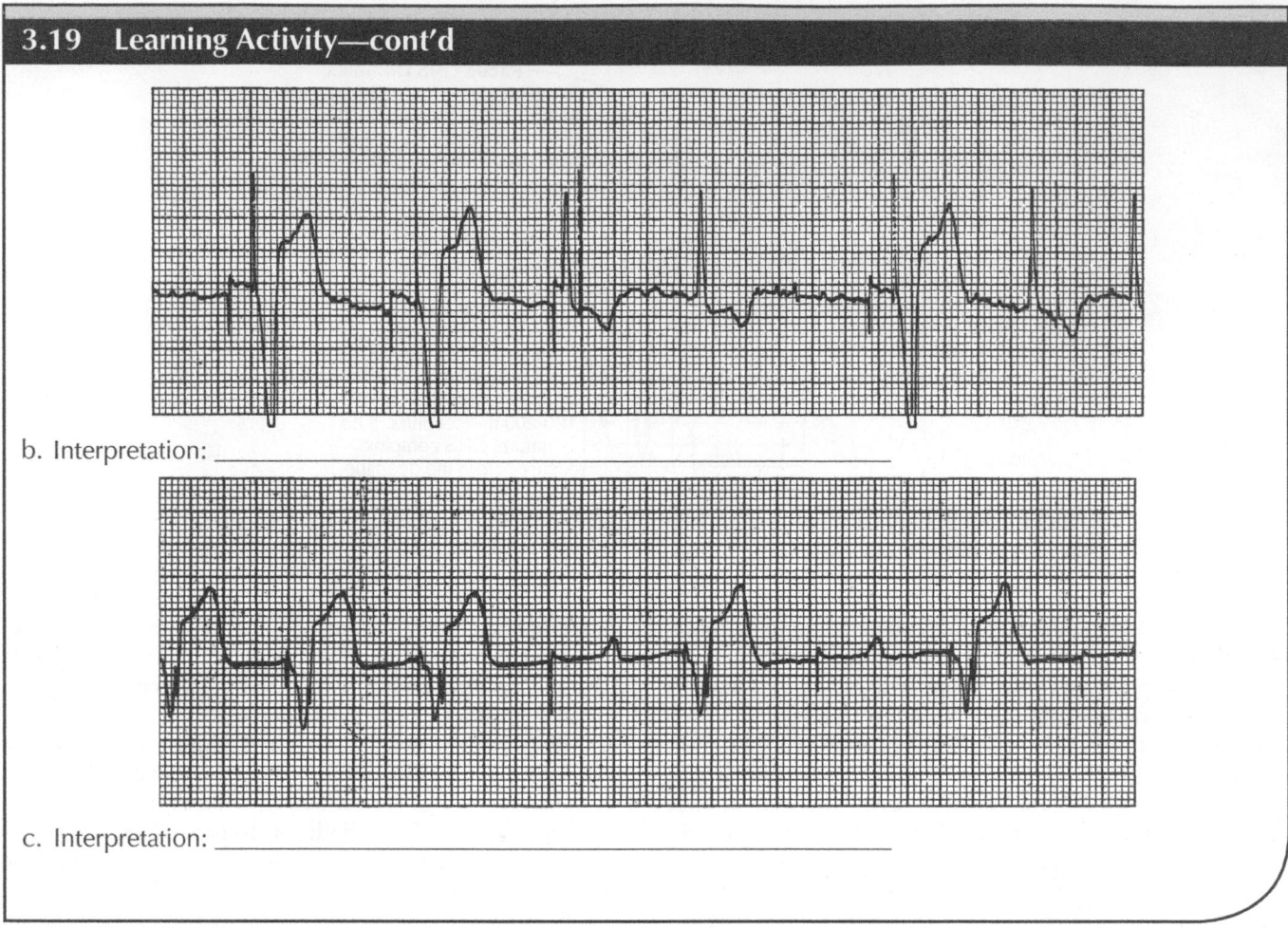

b. Interpretation: _____

c. Interpretation: _____

Answers to this activity can be found in the Answer Key.

For temporary pacemakers, it is important to maintain electrical safety by ensuring proper grounding of equipment. Always touch the side rails before touching the patient to discharge static electricity. Wear rubber gloves when making adjustments. Keep the patient and linens dry at all times. Avoid sources of electromagnetic interference (EMI) (e.g., electrocautery, defibrillation, MRI, transcutaneous electrical nerve stimulation [TENS] units, radiation therapy, lithotripsy). To prevent inadvertent setting changes with the temporary pacemaker pulse generator, cover the dial. Limit mobility of the affected extremity to prevent accidental catheter dislodgement. Observe the catheter site for signs of infection. To prevent dislodgement of the lead with a permanent pacemaker, limit mobility of the affected upper extremity for 48 hours. Encourage arm exercise after 48 hours to prevent frozen shoulder (i.e., ankylosis). Observe the patient's incision for signs of infection. Provide patient and family instruction, including:

- How to take a pulse
- Which symptoms to report
- Sources of EMI to avoid (e.g., MRI, metal detectors, radio transmitters, electrical generating plants)
- Avoid activities such as lifting anything over 5 pounds with the arm closest to the pacemaker for 1 to 2 months. The patient should also avoid lifting the arm closest to the pacemaker above the head for 1 to 2 months.
- Clinical indications of pacemaker malfunction (e.g., dyspnea, syncope, chest pain, fatigue, peripheral edema, or persistent hiccups)

- How to care for the wound, which is usually to just keep it clean and dry until it is healed
- Importance of carrying a pacemaker identification card and informing health care providers of the presence of the pacemaker

Monitor patients for frozen shoulder, infection, pneumothorax, myocardial perforation, catheter or lead displacement, hematoma, dysrhythmias, and pacemaker-mediated tachycardia. Pacemaker-mediated tachycardia is a rapid-paced rhythm that can occur with atrial tracking pacemakers. It begins with and is sustained by ventricular events that are conducted retrograde to the atria. The pacemaker senses this retrograde atrial depolarization and then delivers a stimulus to the ventricle, causing a ventricular depolarization, which again is conducted retrograde to the atria. The cycle repeats itself to produce a tachycardia. Closely monitor patients with temporary or permanent pacemakers for electrical malfunctions (Table 3-22).

An ICD is an implantable device that provides immediate termination of VT or VF in patients in whom these dysrhythmias cannot be pharmacologically or surgically controlled. Tiered therapy (also called *third-generation*) devices have all of the following (Morton & Fontaine, 2012):

- Bradycardia pacing (e.g., VVI, DDD, VDD)
- Antitachycardia pacing: burst
- Low-energy cardioversion: 1-8 J
- High-energy cardioversion: 15-36 J
- Defibrillation: 30-36 J

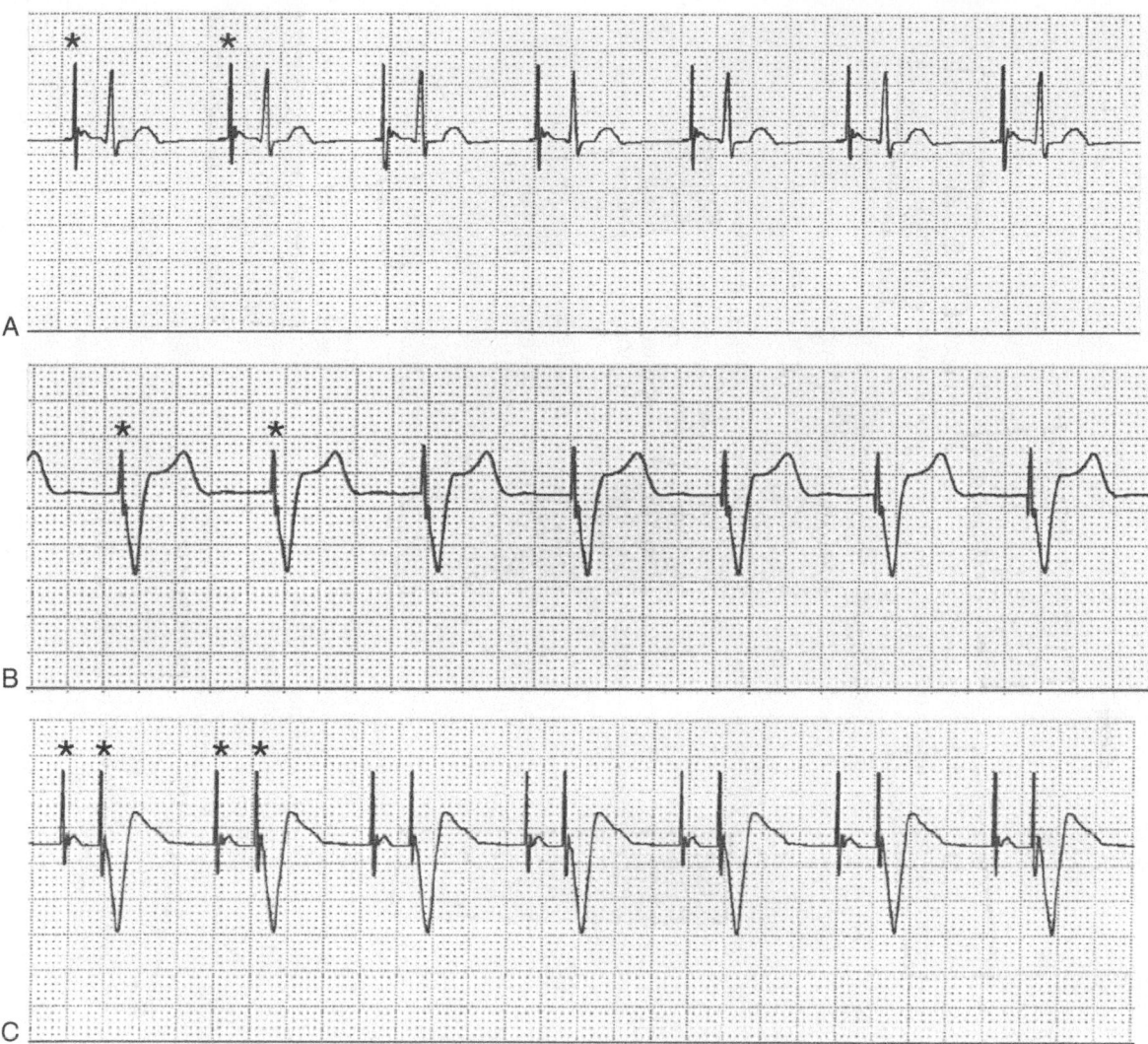

FIGURE 3-51 Pacing examples. A, Atrial pacing. **B,** Ventricular pacing. **C,** Dual-chamber pacing. Each asterisk represents a pacemaker artifact (i.e., spike). (From Urden, L., Stacy, K., & Lough, M. [2014]. *Critical care nursing: Diagnosis and management* [7th ed.]. St. Louis, MO: Mosby.)

ICDs are indicated when there have been one or more episodes of spontaneous VT or VF in a patient in whom electrophysiology studies (EPS) and/or spontaneous ventricular dysrhythmias cannot be used to accurately predict the efficacy of other treatment. Additional criteria for the use of ICD include:

- Recurrent episodes of sustained VT or VF in a patient in whom antidysrhythmic therapy is suboptimal due to intolerance or noncompliance
- Persistent inducibility of sustained VT or VF during EPS despite antidysrhythmic therapy and/or ablation
- VF in a patient with no evidence of structural heart disease and no detectable suppressing triggering factors

ICDs are contraindicated in the presence of frequent episodes of VT or VF (i.e., greater than 2 events/month), uncontrolled HF, when there is less than 6 to 12 months of productive life expectancy, in patients with a history of noncompliance, and when there are extreme psychologic barriers to use of the device.

The generator and the leads are the main components of the defibrillator. The generator processes information from the lead system, delivers the electrical impulses, and stores information about the patient's heart rhythm and therapy delivered. The generator is placed in the left upper quadrant of the abdomen or under the clavicle and usually lasts about 3 to 5 years before replacement is required. The leads record heart rhythm and carry pulses and shocks from the generator to the heart. There are two leads: the atrial lead and the ventricular lead.

The system evaluates heart rate and the probability density function (PDF). PDF diagnoses the amount of time the QRS spends away from the isoelectric baseline. The system is turned on and off by using a donut-shaped magnet. The device is set to off during the early postoperative period due to the frequent occurrence of sinus tachycardia during this period. When the ICD senses VT, the ICD will first initiate antitachycardia pacing. If the VT is not successfully pace-terminated, the ICD will cardiovert the rhythm with low-energy synchronized shocks. If the rhythm deteriorates to VF or if VF is the initial rhythm, the ICD will defibrillate at a higher energy level. After delivering a shock, the device senses the rhythm. If sinus rhythm is not restored, up to five shocks of 25 to 35 joules are delivered. If the electrical rhythm deteriorates to bradycardia or asystole, the bradycardia back-up pacing function is activated.

TABLE 3-21   Pacemaker Modes

Code	Description	Indications	Advantages	Disadvantages
AOO	Fixed rate atrial pacer	• Consistently slow sinus rate with intact AV nodal conduction	• Single lead • Maintains AV synchrony	• Atrial competition • No protection in case of AV nodal block
AAI	Demand atrial pacer	• Sick sinus syndrome • Sinus arrest • Sinus bradycardia • Must have intact AV nodal conduction	• Single lead • Maintains AV synchrony	• No protection in case of AV nodal block
VOO	Fixed rate ventricular pacer	• Complete heart block with slow idioventricular rhythm • Rarely used today	• Single lead • Protection from ventricular asystole	• Ventricular competition with possible stimulation of ventricular dysrhythmias
VAT	Atrial triggered ventricular pacer	• Complete heart block with intact sinus node	• Synchronized AV conduction with atrial "kick" optimizes cardiac output • Ventricular rate increases with atrial rate so more exercise responsive	• Two leads • May cause pacemaker-mediated tachycardia: rapid ventricular response in sinus or atrial dysrhythmias • May cause pacemaker-mediated tachycardia
VVI	Demand ventricular pacer	• Sick sinus syndrome • Sinus bradycardia • Sinus arrest • Complete heart block	• Single lead • Simple and reliable • Inexpensive • Protection from ventricular asystole • Little chance of competitive rhythms	• Loss of synchronized AV conduction and atrial "kick" may reduce cardiac output • Not rate responsive • (Note: VVIR is a VVI with rate-responsiveness)
VVT	Pacing stimulus delivered if needed or not; stimulus depolarizes ventricle if no intrinsic depolarization; stimulus lands harmlessly in QRS if intrinsic depolarization	• Sick sinus syndrome • Sinus bradycardia • Sinus arrest • Complete heart block	• Single lead • Can evaluate pacer function even if intrinsic activity is faster than pacer rate	• Loss of synchronized AV conduction and atrial "kick" may reduce cardiac output • Not rate responsive • Difficult to evaluate QRS morphology
VDD	Ventricular pacer that can be atrial triggered or inhibited by intrinsic ventricular depolarization	• Sick sinus syndrome • Sinus bradycardia • Sinus arrest • Complete heart block	• Maintains AV synchrony • If atrial activity is present as pacer functions in atrial triggered mode; if no atrial activity, paces the ventricle in demand mode with inhibition to intrinsic ventricular depolarization	• Two leads • May cause pacemaker-mediated tachycardia • Does not pace the atria, so loss of atrial contraction if no intrinsic atrial activity
DOO	Fixed rate AV sequential pacer	• Consistently slow atrial and ventricular rate	• Synchronized AV conduction with atrial "kick" optimizes cardiac output	• Two leads • Not rate responsive • Atrial and ventricular competition
DVI	Fixed rate atrial pacer with demand ventricular pacer	• Sick sinus syndrome • Sinus bradycardia • Sinus arrest • Complete heart block	• Synchronized AV conduction with atrial "kick" optimizes cardiac output	• Two leads • Not rate responsive • Blind to intrinsic atrial activity so atrial competition and even atrial fibrillation may occur
DDD	Demand atrial and ventricular pacer; ventricular pacing may be atrial triggered or ventricular inhibited	• Sick sinus syndrome • Sinus bradycardia • Sinus arrest • Complete heart block	• Synchronized AV conduction with atrial "kick" optimizes cardiac output • Near normal physiologic function	• Two leads • Most expensive • May cause pacemaker-mediated tachycardia • Difficult troubleshooting • Is not used in atrial fibrillation

TABLE 3-22	Pacemaker Electrical Malfunctions	
Malfunction	**Causes**	**Interventions**
Failure to fire (pace): pacemaker does not fire when it is physiologically indicated for it to fire • Recognized by pauses longer than the automatic interval and absence of pacer spike at end of escape interval	• Loose connections • Battery depletion • Lead displacement • Lead fracture • Sensing malfunction (e.g., electromagnetic interference [EMI])	• Tighten connections if temporary • Replace battery or pulse generator • Lead repositioning or replacement may be needed • Evaluate patient's own rhythm and patient's response; if inadequate, administer atropine and/or apply external transcutaneous pacemaker; CPR may be required • May be caused by sensing malfunction; to identify a sensing malfunction, convert pacemaker to asynchronous by placing a magnet over an implanted pacemaker or switching to asynchronous on an external pacemaker; if pacer spikes seen in asynchronous mode, sensing malfunction exists • Remove source of EMI
Failure to capture: pacemaker fires but depolarization does not occur • Recognized by spike not followed by depolarization (e.g., P wave if atrial pacer or QRS if ventricular pacer)	• Displacement of lead • Lead fracture • Increased pacing thresholds (e.g., electrolyte imbalance, drug toxicity, acid-base imbalance, ischemia) • Fibrosis or scar tissue at the lead tip • Battery failure • Chamber perforation • Complexes not visible	• Position patient on left side or to the position patient was in when capture was last seen • Increase milliamperes • May require lead repositioning, lead replacement • Replace battery or pulse generator • Check chest x-ray for lead fracture and lead placement • Correct metabolic or electrolyte imbalance • Consider drug levels and toxicity • Check for diaphragmatic pacing and monitor for cardiac tamponade if catheter perforation is suspected • May require external transcutaneous pacing or CPR
Undersensing or failure to sense: pacemaker fails to recognize intrinsic activity (e.g., P wave, QRS) • Recognized by pacer spikes falling closer to the intrinsic beats than the escape interval; spikes land indiscriminately throughout the cardiac cycle including potentially on the descending limb of the T wave	• Displacement of lead • Lead fracture • Sensitivity set too low or set on asynchronous • Disconnection of sensing circuit • Inadequate signal (e.g., low P or QRS voltage) • Battery failure • Increased sensing threshold (e.g., edema or fibrosis at lead tip) • Chamber perforation	• Position patient on left side or to the position sensing was last seen • Lead repositioning or replacement may be necessary • Make sure that pacer is not set on asynchronous • Increase sensitivity (i.e., turn down the millivolts) • Check connections on temporary pacemaker • Administer lidocaine if nonsensed QRSs are PVCs • Check chest x-ray for lead placement or lead fracture • Replace battery or pulse generator • If patient's own rhythm adequate, turn pacer off or heart rate down to minimum • If patient's own rhythm inadequate, increase pacer rate to override patient's own rhythm
Oversensing: pacemaker recognizes extraneous electrical activity or the wrong intrinsic electrical activity as the inhibiting event • Recognized by absence of pacer spikes and failure to fire	• Sensitivity set too high • Electromagnetic interference (EMI) • Oversensing of P waves or T waves • Myopotentials • Crosstalk (no ventricular pacing)	• Decrease sensitivity (i.e., turn up the millivolts) • Remove from EMI; ensure that all equipment is properly grounded • Decrease atrial output, decrease ventricular sensitivity, increase ventricular blanking period • May require external transcutaneous pacing or CPR

Collaborative management is similar to that of insertion of a pacemaker. Monitor for dysrhythmias and evaluate effectiveness of the ICD if firing occurs and administer antidysrhythmic agents as prescribed. If cardiopulmonary arrest occurs, do the following:

1. Obtain emergency equipment and prepare to cardiovert or defibrillate.
2. Treat this patient as you would any patient in cardiopulmonary arrest; do not wait for the device.
3. Do not place defibrillator paddles within 8 cm of the generator.
4. Reposition the paddle or pad placement: anterior-posterior paddle or pad placement may be more effective. Deactivate the ICD using a magnet as requested by the physician.

To monitor further for complications, observe the incision for signs of infection and observe for clinical indications of cardiac tamponade. Encourage the patient to express fears and concerns about being shocked. Consider referring a patient to a support group as warranted. Also, monitor for atelectasis, pneumonia, pneumothorax, lead migration, and lead fracture.

Ablation therapy eradicated dysrhythmias in patients who experience frequent, disabling, or life-threatening dysrhythmias unresponsive to pharmacologic therapy or poorly tolerated. There are two types of ablation therapy: radiofrequency and surgical. In radiofrequency catheter ablation, the physician inserts a catheter in the heart. Radiofrequency energy is then applied to the area in which the dysrhythmia originates or an accessory pathway (e.g., WPW). During this maneuver, controlled localized necrosis occurs. Postprocedure care is the same as it is for cardiac catheterization or angioplasty; monitor the patient closely for dysrhythmias. In a surgical ablation, the surgeon excises the area in which the dysrhythmia originates or eliminates it by cryosurgery or laser.

The maze procedure consists of carefully planned sutures or laser-created cuts to create an electrical conduction route through the atrial myocardium, corralling and herding chaotic atrial impulses from the SA node to the AV node. The procedure is performed by cardiothoracic surgery or PCI and the postoperative management mimics that which is done for cardiothoracic surgery or PCI, depending on procedure performed.

ACUTE CORONARY SYNDROMES

Arteriosclerosis (Figure 3-52) is a group of progressive diseases characterized by the thickening and loss of elasticity of the arterial walls caused by calcification. Atherosclerosis is the most common form of arteriosclerosis. It is a chronic disease process characterized by the buildup of fatty plaque along the subintimal layer of arteries leading to a decrease in arterial lumen.

Coronary artery disease (CAD) is a progressive disease of the coronary arteries that results in the narrowing and obstruction of the vessels and eventually myocardial ischemia. CAD is also referred to as *ischemic heart disease, coronary heart disease,* or *atherosclerotic heart disease.*

Acute coronary syndrome (ACS) describes a group of clinical symptoms compatible with myocardial ischemia and differentiated by ECG findings. ACS includes unstable angina (Figure 3-53), in which patients present with chest pain, no ST segment elevation, and normal cardiac biomarkers. Other types of angina include:

- De novo: new onset effort angina

- Crescendo: angina that has increased in frequency, intensity, or duration
- Preinfarction: angina of prolonged duration that occurs even at rest; may be a precursor of MI
- Wellens syndrome: angina with deep T wave inversion in V_2 and V_3 indicative of critical proximal LAD stenosis
- Prinzmetal or vasospastic: angina with ST segment elevation related to coronary artery spasm

In addition to angina, myocardial infarction (MI) (Figure 3-54) is another form of acute coronary syndrome. The ACS due to an MI involves electrical and mechanical death of a portion of the myocardium. A MI can be either ST segment elevation (STEMI) or non-ST segment elevation. In the former, patients present with chest pain, elevated cardiac biomarkers, and ST segment elevation. In the latter presentation, patients have chest pain and elevated cardiac biomarkers, but without ST segment elevation.

The ECG leads showing indicative changes (Table 3-23) signifies the ventricular wall affected. An MI may occur in the left ventricular myocardial wall (LVMI) or the right ventricular myocardial wall (RVMI). Most MIs are LVMIs; of those, 42% are anterior, 10% are septal, 10% are lateral, 33% are inferior, and 5% are posterior. RVMI (Figure 3-55) may frequently occur with inferior wall MIs. One third of all inferior MIs have concurrent RV infarction. RVMI is rarely isolated. Isolated RVMI is more common in patients with right ventricular hypertrophy (sometimes seen with COPD). RVMI is usually transmural but results in a smaller infarct due to decreased oxygen requirements of the right ventricle.

Arteriosclerosis/atherosclerosis results from a variety of factors, both nonmodifiable and modifiable. Heredity is a nonmodifiable risk factor and is manifested in siblings of parents who developed CAD before 55 years of age. A maternal history of CAD usually occurs in siblings of parents before 65 years of age and conveys a greater risk than a paternal history in women. Genetics plays a role in several diseases that are risk factors. These include hypertension, hyperlipidemia, and diabetes mellitus. Advancing age is a nonmodifiable risk factor, predisposing men older than 45 years and women older than 55 years to heart disease. Males have twice the risk of premenopausal females; however, the risk increases in women after menopause.

Modifiable risk factors include a diagnosis of hypertension or hyperlipidemia. BP greater than 140/90 mm Hg or requiring antihypertensive agents to achieve BP less than 140/90 mm Hg and elevated levels of cholesterol, triglycerides, or low-density lipoproteins (LDL), and/or decreased levels of high-density lipoproteins (HDL) increase cardiovascular risk.

SIDEBAR 3-5

Desirable Lipid Levels

- Cholesterol level less than 200 mg/dL
- LDL level less than 100 mg/dL for patients with heart disease or diabetes mellitus
  - Less than 130 mg/dL for patients with two or more risk factors
  - Less than 160 mg/dL for patients with only one risk factor
- HDL level greater than 40 mg/dL
- Triglyceride level less than 150 mg/dL

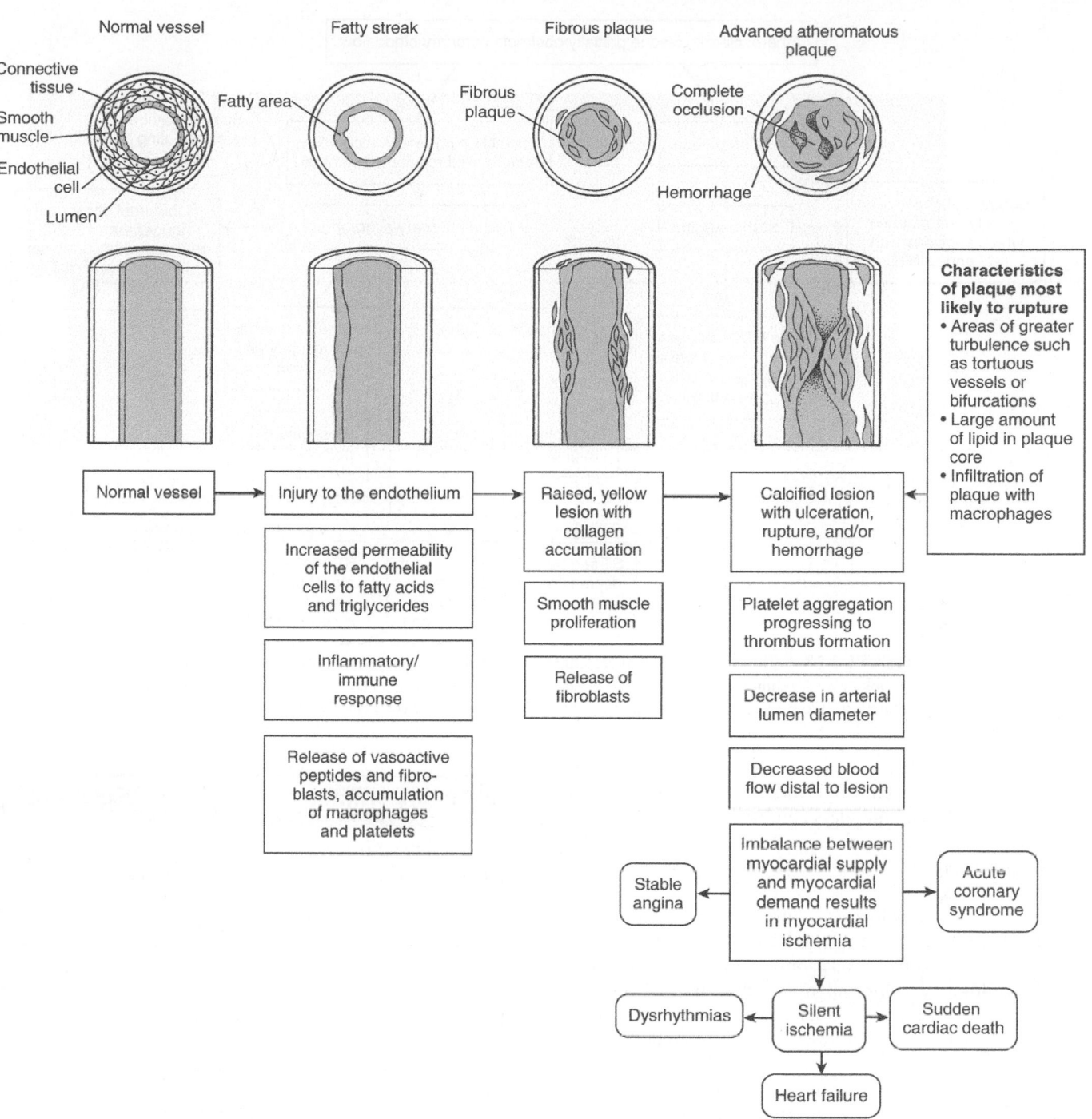

FIGURE 3-52 Progression of atherosclerosis. (Modified from Thelan, L. A., Urden, L. D., Lough, M. E., & Stacy, K. M. [1998]. *Critical care nursing: Diagnosis and management,* [3rd ed.]. St. Louis, MO: Mosby.)

Smoking, another modifiable risk factor, increases LDL level, platelet aggregation, and fibrinogen level and may cause vasospasm. Elevated carbon monoxide levels decrease the oxygen-carrying capacity of hemoglobin. Complete smoking cessation is desirable.

Diabetes mellitus or glucose intolerance also predisposes people to arteriosclerosis and/or atherosclerosis. Control blood glucose in patients with diabetes mellitus to decrease the risk of diabetic complications including CAD. Current recommendations for diabetes control are fasting blood glucose levels and

post prandial glucose close to the upper limits of the normal range (i.e., 110 mg/dL and 140 mg/dL). The recommended 3-month glycosylated hemoglobin (HbA1c) level is less than 7%, which equates to an average blood sugar of 150 mg/dL; therefore, a desirable average glucose level is less than 150 mg/dL. Diabetes is also associated with increased levels of LDL, triglycerides, and obesity.

Homocysteine is an essential sulfur-containing amino acid formed during the processing of dietary protein. Elevated levels are toxic to the vascular endothelium and increase coagulability.

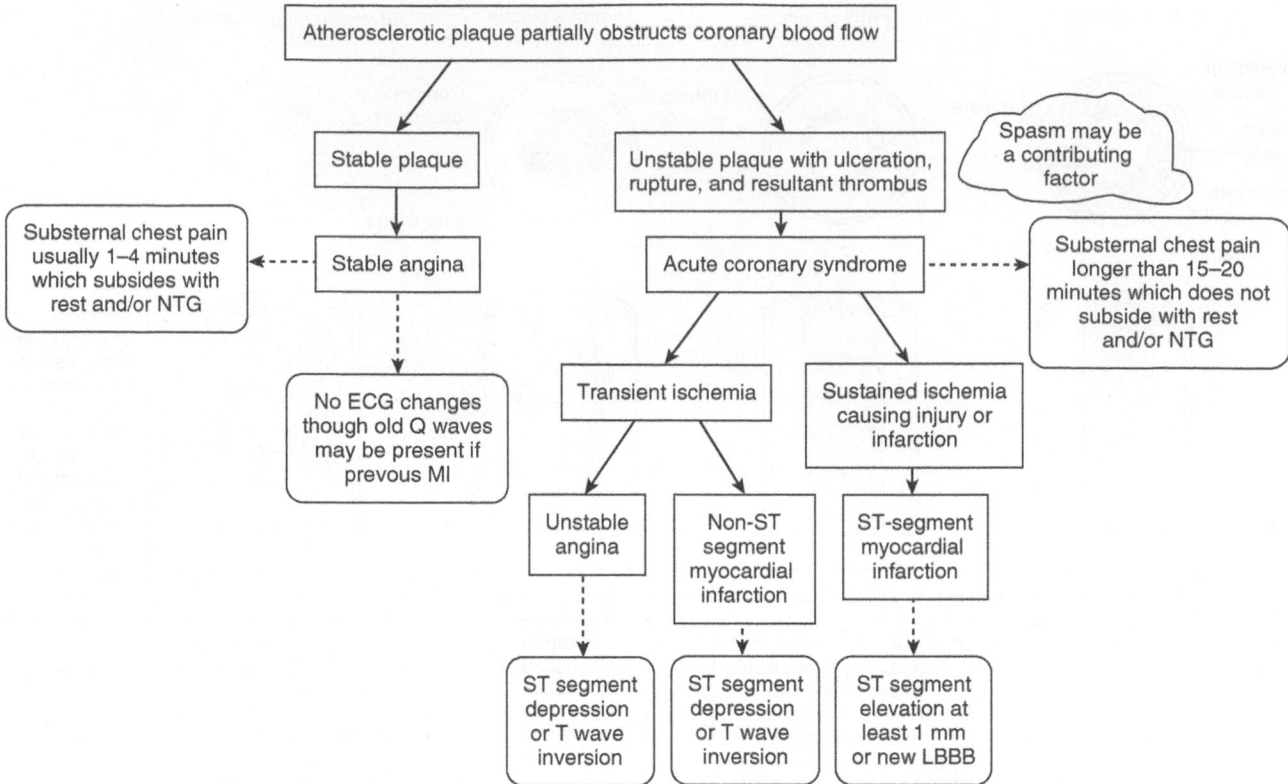

FIGURE 3-53 Differentiation of stable angina from acute coronary syndrome. Dotted lines connect pathology to the clinical presentation. *LBBB,* Left bundle branch block; *NTG,* nitroglycerin; *MI,* myocardial infarction. (From Dennison, R. D. [2013]. *Pass CCRN!* [4th ed.]. St. Louis, MO: Elsevier.)

Folate deficiency, vitamin B_{12}, and vitamin B_6 affect homocysteine levels. Reduce homocysteine levels with folate, vitamin B_{12}, and/or pyridoxine therapy. Patients with homocysteine levels greater than 14 µmol/L are predisposed to developing atherosclerosis.

Health care providers recommend that patients implement changes in an attempt to alter several modifiable CAD risk factors. An inverse relationship exists between exercise and cardiovascular mortality. In addition, sedentary people are more likely to be obese, hypertensive, and diabetic; therefore, changing a sedentary lifestyle to an active lifestyle modifies a health risk and promotes a healthier cardiovascular system. Chronic stress promotes the long-term development of CAD. Acute stress increases catecholamine levels, myocardial oxygen consumption, and dysrhythmia potential. Gaining control and managing a type A personality along with aggression decreases stress. Having an ideal body weight is desirable. Obesity predisposes people to heart disease. Obesity increases risk and is defined as a body mass index (BMI) greater than 30. Obesity also contributes to the other risk factors: hypertension, hyperlipidemia, glucose intolerance, and sedentary lifestyle. Midline fat is a greater risk than hip and thigh fat (i.e., apple vs. pear body shapes). The combination of BMI >30 kg/m², elevated triglycerides, reduced HDL, hypertension, and fasting serum glucose >110 mg/dL or type 2 diabetes (known as *metabolic syndrome*) significantly increases the risk of CAD. Finally, use of oral contraceptives increases the risk of MI, especially in smokers. Using oral contraceptives also increases BP. Thus, smoking cessation is desirable for all people, but especially for women who use oral contraceptives.

3.20 Learning Activity

Complete the following table differentiating cardiac risk factors as nonmodifiable or modifiable.

Nonmodifiable	Modifiable

Answers to this activity can be found in the Answer Key.

Exercise elevates HDL, decreases BP and resting HR, decreases body fat, and increases endogenous tissue plasminogen activator (tPA) levels. To be effective, the exercise must be sufficient enough to increase the heart rate 50% to 80% of the predicted maximal heart rate. Advise patients to exercise for at

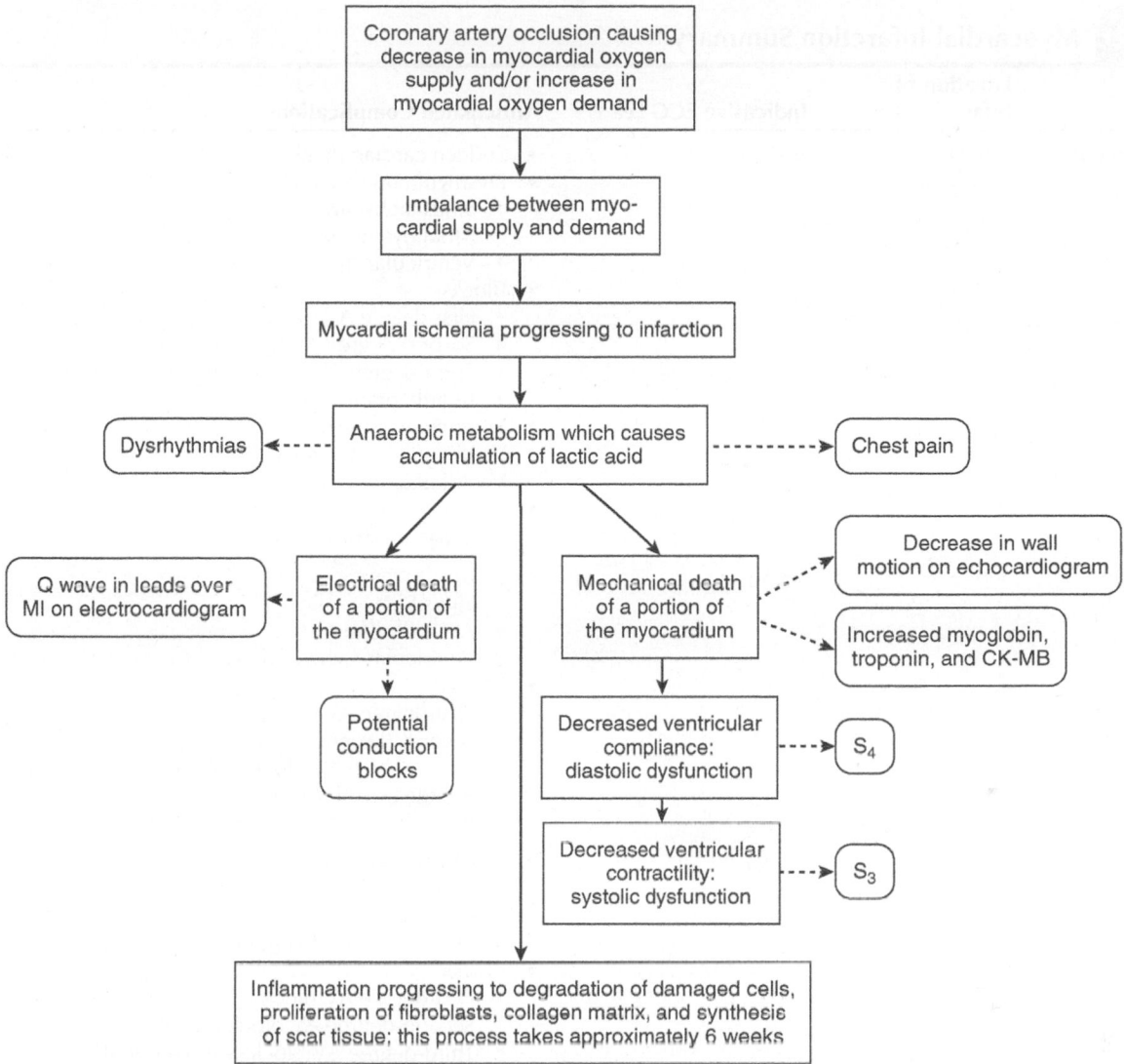

FIGURE 3-54 Pathophysiology of myocardial infarction. Dotted lines connect pathology to the clinical presentation. (From Dennison, R. D. [2013]. *Pass CCRN!* [4th ed.]. St. Louis, MO: Elsevier.)

least 20 to 30 minutes at least three times per week. Patients can vary the type of exercise to prevent boredom, but walking and swimming are excellent forms of exercise for almost all patients.

Stress management can reduce catecholamine levels, decrease BP, and reduce muscle tension. Methods include daily stretching, breathing exercises, meditation, prayer, and yoga. Diets high in fiber and low in fat reduce total cholesterol levels. One to two alcoholic drinks per day increase HDL and may decrease platelet aggregation; however, the overall health benefit diminishes after one to two alcoholic drinks per day.

Enteric-coated aspirin (ECASA) 81 to 325 mg taken daily prevents platelet aggregation and decreases inflammation, which is one postulated contributor to CAD. Omega-3 fatty acids decrease platelet aggregation, increase HDL levels, and decrease triglyceride levels. Alpha linolenic acid found in canola oil, walnuts, flaxseeds and eicosapentaenoic acid (EPA), and docosahexaenoic acid (DHA) found in salmon, trout, and sardines are important adjunctive agents used to prevent CAD. Flavonoids , which are found in tea and cocoa, offer an antioxidant effect, induce nitric oxide formation, and may inhibit platelet aggregation.

Finally, loving relationships decrease the overall incidence of CAD, although the mechanisms are unclear. Loneliness and depression have been identified as contributing factors to

CAD. Pets also have a beneficial effect by decreasing stress and depression.

Atherosclerosis and thrombosis are the primary causes of MIs. A coronary artery spasm can result from Prinzmetal angina and cocaine usage may also result in an MI. A cocaine-induced MI results from excessive sympathetic stimulation that causes tachycardia, hypertension, arterial vasoconstriction, and spasm. Coronary artery spasm and any combination of these factors can result in an MI. Other less commonly seen causes of an MI include severe prolonged hypotension; sudden, severe anemia; chest trauma (e.g., myocardial contusion); trauma to coronary arteries; aortic stenosis or insufficiency; thyrotoxicosis; blood dyscrasias; aortic dissection; arteritis; and carbon monoxide poisoning.

Chest pain is the most common symptom of MI; 75% to 85% of all patients with an MI have chest pain. Emotional or physical stress may provoke an MI, but it may also occur at rest. The pain is usually not relieved by oxygen, rest, and/or nitrates. Narcotics and/or reperfusion (e.g., fibrinolytics or PCI) may provide pain relief. The patient frequently describes the pain as pressure on the chest, but may also describe it as knifelike, stabbing, burning, or like indigestion. The patient may describe the pain of an MI as like their usual anginal pain, only more severe. Consider a dissecting thoracic aneurysm if the pain described is

TABLE 3-23   Myocardial Infarction Summary

Coronary Artery	Location of Infarct	Indicative ECG Leads	Anticipated Complications

Left main coronary artery	Extensive anterior	V_1-V_6	• Sudden cardiac death
			• Dysrhythmias especially:
			  • Sinus tachycardia
			  • Atrial dysrhythmias
			  • Ventricular dysrhythmias
			• Blocks
			  • First-degree AV block
			  • Second-degree AV block type II
			  • Third-degree AV block with ventricular escape
			  • Bundle branch block
			• Ventricular rupture
			• Ventricular septal defect
			• Ventricular aneurysm
			• HF
			• Cardiogenic shock

Left anterior descending artery	Septal	V_1, V_2	• Dysrhythmias especially:
			  • Sinus tachycardia
			  • Atrial fibrillation
			  • Ventricular dysrhythmias
			• Blocks
			  • First-degree AV block
			  • Second-degree AV block type II
			  • Third-degree AV block with ventricular escape
			  • Bundle branch block
			• Ventricular septal rupture

	Anterior	V_3, V_4	• Dysrhythmias especially:
			  • Sinus tachycardia
			  • Atrial fibrillation
			  • Ventricular dysrhythmias
			• Blocks
			  • First-degree AV block
			  • Second-degree AV block type II
			  • Third-degree AV block with ventricular escape
			  • Bundle branch block
			• Ventricular aneurysm
			• HF
			• Cardiogenic shock

Left circumflex artery	Lateral	High: I, aVL Low: V_5, V_6	• Dysrhythmias • HF

Right coronary artery	Inferior	II, III, aVF	• Dysrhythmias especially:
			  • Sinus bradycardia
			  • Sinus arrest
			  • Junctional rhythms
			  • Ventricular dysrhythmias
			• Blocks
			  • SA blocks
			  • First-degree AV block
			  • Second-degree AV block type I
			  • Third-degree AV block usually with AV junctional escape
			  • Bundle branch block
			• Papillary muscle rupture
			• HF

TABLE 3-23	Myocardial Infarction Summary—cont'd		
Coronary Artery	**Location of Infarct**	**Indicative ECG Leads**	**Anticipated Complications**

	Posterior	Reciprocal changes in V_1, V_2
		Indicative changes in V_7-V_9 (especially V_8, V_9)
			• Dysrhythmias especially:
			  • Sinus bradycardia
			  • Sinus arrest
			  • Junctional rhythms
			  • Ventricular dysrhythmias
			• Blocks
			  • First-degree AV block
			  • Second-degree AV block type I
			  • Third-degree AV block usually with AV junctional escape
			• Papillary muscle rupture with acute mitral regurgitation

	Right ventricular	V_{4R}-V_{6R} (especially V_{4R})	• Dysrhythmias especially:
			  • Sinus bradycardia
			  • Sinus arrest
			  • Junctional rhythms
			  • Ventricular dysrhythmias
			• Blocks
			  • First-degree AV block
			  • Second-degree AV block type I
			  • Third-degree AV block usually with AV junctional escape
			  • Bundle branch block
			• Papillary muscle rupture with acute tricuspid regurgitation
			• Right ventricular failure

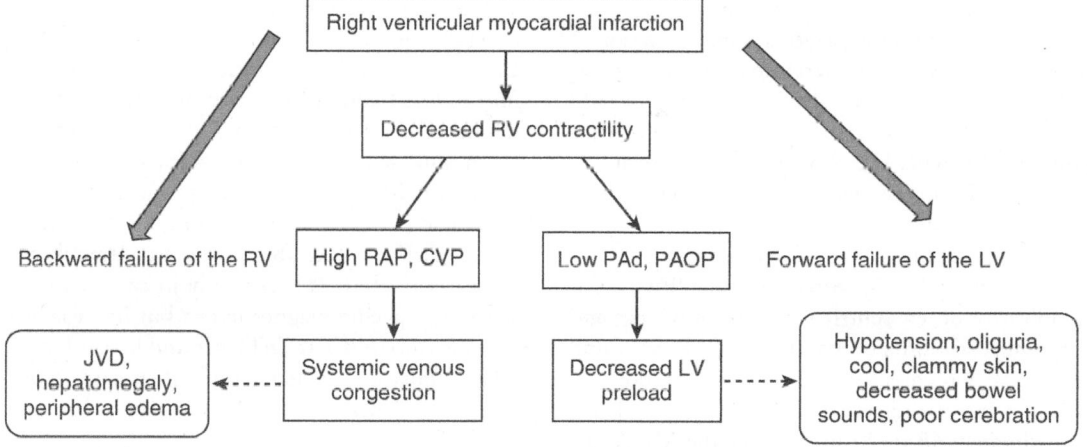

FIGURE 3-55 Pathophysiology of right ventricular MI. Dotted lines connect pathology to the clinical presentation. *CVP,* Central venous pressure; *JVD,* jugular venous distention; *LV,* left ventricular; PAd, pulmonary artery diastolic pressure; *PAOP,* pulmonary artery occlusive pressure; *RAP,* right atrial pressure; *RV,* right ventricular. (From Dennison, R. D. [2013]. *Pass CCRN!* [4th ed.]. St. Louis, MO: Elsevier.)

ripping or tearing. The primary location of the pain is usually the chest, but it may be epigastric especially with an inferior MI. Women often complain of jaw, upper back, or shoulder pain. Pain radiation is usually to the left arm, left elbow, left shoulder, both arms, and/or the jaw. If the pain radiates to the back, consider the possibility of a dissecting aortic aneurysm. The severity of pain ranges widely, from vague, slight discomfort to severe pain. The Levine sign, which is a clenched fist held over the sternum, often accompanies complaints of chest pain. Most MIs occur within 3 hours of awakening. The pain is continuous from onset with duration of 20 minutes or more. A stuttering

MI pattern is pain that comes and goes for as long as several days before the actual MI. Intermittent pain before continuous pain is *preinfarction angina*. A silent (i.e., painless) MI occurs in as many as 25% of all patients with an MI. A silent MI is more likely in an elderly or diabetic patient. Clues suggesting possible silent MI include new onset of HF, acute change in mental status, or unexplained abdominal pain, dyspnea, or fatigue.

Patients with acute MI may also complain of nausea and vomiting; this occurs more often in an inferior or posterior MI. Symptoms of dyspnea, orthopnea, diaphoresis, and palpitations occur more often in an anterior MI. Women frequently

TABLE 3-24   Cardiac Biomarkers for Acute MI

Test	Normal Values	Abnormal Values Consistent with MI	Time to Rise (After Injury)	Peak (After Injury)	Return to Normal (After Injury)
CK-MB	0% of total CK	Greater than 3%	6-10 hours	12-24 hours	2-3 days
LDH_1	17%-25% of total LDH	Greater than 40%	8-24 hours	72 hours	8-14 days
Myoglobin	Men: 20-90 ng/mL Women: 10-75 ng/mL	Men: greater than 90 ng/mL Women: greater than 75 ng/mL	1-4 hours	6-12 hours	1-2 days
Cardiac troponin I (cTnI)	Less than 1.5 ng/mL	Greater than 4 ng/mL	4-6 hours	18 hours	1-2 weeks
Cardiac troponin T (cTnT)	Less than 0.1 ng/mL	Greater than 0.2 ng/mL	3-4 hours	24 hours	2-3 weeks

complain of unusual fatigue, dyspnea, indigestion, sleep disturbances, and anxiety.

Objective findings present during an MI include an alteration in the heart rate and rhythm. Tachycardia occurs more often in patients with anterior MI, while bradycardia occurs more often in patients with inferior MI. Hypertension occurs more often in patients with an anterior MI, while hypotension occurs more often in patients with an inferior MI. BP is normally similar in both arms and inequality between arms indicates possible dissecting thoracic aortic aneurysm.

Tachypnea is a common finding, as either a manifestation of SNS innervation or HF. Elevated temperature frequently occurs 48 to 72 hours after the onset of the MI. The presence of JVD is indicative of RVF, commonly seen in an inferior wall MI with an RV infarction. Patients with MI who have LVF may have an abnormal point of maximum intensity (PMI); it may be displaced downward and laterally.

Heart sound changes are likely. The patient may have diminished heart sounds caused by decreased contractility. An S_4 heart sound is indicative of left ventricular noncompliance and is common in the first 24 hours of an MI. An S_3 heart sound is an early sign of LVF, which is most likely with anterior MI. A pericardial friction rub is indicative of pericarditis, which is most likely approximately 48 to 72 hours after the MI. A systolic murmur associated with mitral regurgitation may indicate LVF or papillary muscle dysfunction or rupture, caused most often by ischemia or infarction of the posterior valve leaflet of the mitral valve in patients with inferior MI. The murmur of mitral regurgitation is a high-pitched, blowing, holosystolic murmur heard loudest at the apex and radiates to the axilla.

A ventricular septal rupture results in a high-pitched, harsh, holosystolic murmur heard loudest at lower left sternal border. Though rare today with successful reperfusion, ventricular septal rupture is more likely with septal infarctions. Carotid, aortic, or femoral bruits may also be present because most patients with MI have more generalized vascular disease. Clinical indications of hypoperfusion (see Table 3-2) may be present. In addition, clinical indications of LVF (e.g., S_3, crackles, dyspnea) in left ventricular infarction or clinical indications of RVF (e.g., JVD, hepatomegaly, and peripheral edema) in right ventricular infarction may be present.

The leukocyte count may be increased (usually 12,000 to 15,000/mm^3) in acute MI at 48 to 72 hours after onset of pain. Erythrocyte sedimentation rate (ESR) may also increase at 48 to 72 hours in acute MI. C-reactive protein increases along with increased interleukin-6 (a marker of increased mortality) in acute MI.

Evaluate the patient's cardiac biomarkers (Table 3-24) indicative of an MI. Note the specific test, normal and abnormal values, along with the peak and duration timing aspects. A positive CK-MB (i.e., greater than 3%) and altered levels of lactate dehydrogenase (LDH_1 and LDH_2) is indicative of MI. This is a highly specific test for MI. Normally, LDH_2 is greater than LDH_1. When LDH_1 is greater than LDH_2, it is referred to as *flipped LDH* and is indicative of MI. This flipped LDH does not occur until 48 to 72 hours after the onset of pain. Increased serum muscle proteins, myoglobin, and troponin are indicative of an MI. Myoglobin is a muscle protein with high sensitivity but low specificity, but it still has an excellent early negative predictive value. Troponin is a contractile protein. Cardiac troponin I (cTnI) is found only in cardiac muscle. Troponin I is a more specific diagnostic test but has a later rise and peak. Cardiac troponin T (cTnT) is found in cardiac muscle as well as skeletal muscle. It is less specific than cardiac troponin I, especially in patients with renal failure, but it has an earlier rise and peak.

An ECG displays ST segment depression in unstable angina and ST segment elevation in variant angina. As a diagnostic tool for acute MI, it is most helpful when clearly abnormal. Repeat ECGs every 30 minutes until pain cessation if the initial ECG is nondiagnostic or the ECG is clearly diagnostic and definitive therapy initiated. Initiate prompt reperfusion therapies (e.g., PCI, fibrinolytics) in an acute MI that meet the criteria of ST segment elevation of greater than or equal to 1 mm in at least 2 continuous leads or a new LBBB.

There are multiple problems with ECG diagnosis of MI, such as the lag time of hours or even days before diagnostic ECG changes become evident. The first ECG is diagnostic only 50% of the time and changes may be subtle. Compare the ECG with a previous ECG if available. Recognize that a competitive condition, such as LBBB or ventricular pacemaker, obscures an anterior MI. Other conditions that obscure ECG diagnostic value are WPW, which can obscure an anterior MI;

left anterior hemiblock, which can obscure an inferior MI; left posterior hemiblock, which can obscure a lateral MI; and ventricular hypertrophy, which can obscure anterior or lateral MI.

To prevent missing an infarction in a traditionally electrically silent area of the heart, perform a 15-lead or 18-lead ECG, which increases sensitivity and inclusion for reperfusion therapy because of the use of right ventricular and posterior leads. An 18-lead ECG includes 12 standard leads, 3 right ventricular leads, and 3 posterior leads. A 15-lead ECG includes 12 standard + V_{4R} + V_8 + V_9 leads. Look for indicative and reciprocal indicators of ischemia, injury, and infarction (see Figure 3-41).

Evaluate ventricular wall motion with an echocardiogram. Normal wall motion is a strong predictor of nonischemic pain. Reduced wall motion is a strong predictor of ischemia/infarction. An echocardiogram may also show mechanical complications (e.g., ventricular septal defect, papillary muscle rupture). A chest x-ray may reveal cardiomegaly, indicating possible HF. Cardiac catheterization will confirm coronary artery occlusion(s) and permit immediate PCI. Radionuclide studies include a technetium-99 pyrophosphate scan, which reveals infarcted areas as "hot spots." A thallium-201 scan will show ischemic or infarcted areas as "cold spots."

Factors affecting mortality in MI include the age of the patient, left ventricular ejection fraction, the number of occluded vessels, whether there is a previous history of MI, and the presence of cardiogenic shock, which is associated with a loss of 40% of LV muscle mass, possibly from one MI or several cumulative MIs. Females have twice the mortality of males; this is probably related to the fact that they tend to be older and have more significant risk factors (e.g., diabetes mellitus, hypertension) when they have an MI.

Collaborative management includes prehospitalized care through emergency treatment and inpatient admission with ACS guidelines (Figure 3-56). Manage cardiopulmonary arrest if required. If ventricular fibrillation occurs, it is frequently within the first hour. Identify early clinical indications of MI and transition the patient to a higher acuity level of care. Perform BLS and ACLS as indicated, and manage airway, oxygenation, and circulation. Also, monitor the ECG, vital signs, physical examination, and hemodynamic parameters for changes.

After any required life-saving measures, the priority of collaborative management is to reduce the size of myocardial infarction using myocardial salvaging techniques. Treat pain promptly and adequately to decrease catecholamine release and, therefore, myocardial oxygen demand. Provide morphine sulfate 2 to 4 mg IV every 5 minutes for pain relief. This intervention causes vasodilation, which decreases preload and relieves pain and decreases anxiety, which decreases catecholamines. Because the SNS increases heart rate and afterload, preventing release of catecholamines and/or blocking the catecholamines with beta-blockers decreases the heart rate and afterload to decrease myocardial oxygen consumption. Give nitroglycerin as prescribed; administration is usually sublingual initially but it may also be given prophylactically at 25 to 100 mcg/min IV for 24 to 48 hours. Nitrates decrease preload, resulting in less myocardial oxygen demand, dilate epicardial coronary vessels to increase myocardial oxygen supply, and augment the analgesic effect of morphine. Use caution with nitrates especially if the patient has changes in the right ventricular ECG leads, such as V_4. In addition, nitrates cause reflex tachycardia, for which beta-blockers may be needed. Titrate carefully if the patient has hypotension.

Administer calcium channel blockers (e.g., nifedipine [Procardia]) for pain, especially for variant angina. Facilitate the patient transfer to a higher level of care for reperfusion therapies (e.g., fibrinolytics, PCI) to relieve pain by reestablishing blood flow and aerobic metabolism, hemodynamic monitoring as required, or IABP for intractable pain to increase CAPP.

In addition to decreasing myocardial oxygen demand, it is also important to increase myocardial oxygen supply. Administer oxygen at 2 to 6 L/min per nasal cannula for 24 to 48 hours, aiming for a SpO_2 of 95% or greater. This probably has little effect on the myocardial arterial oxygen content of otherwise normal individuals, but may significantly improve oxygenation of an ischemic myocardium, especially in patients with hypoxemia from pulmonary edema. Even in the absence of pulmonary edema or other complications, it seems that some patients develop modest hypoxemia early during the course of acute MI.

Reduce STEMI door to balloon time (DTBT). Establish protocols to define the process and facilitate crucial assessment studies (e.g., ECG, troponin) and interventions (Hammond, 2010; Farwell, 2010). These protocols should empower EMS and/or ED physicians to activate the STEMI team. If a hospitalized patient develops clinical indications of MI, contact the attending physician, facilitate transfer to a higher acuity level of care, and activate the STEMI team. Protocols should eliminate unnecessary consults and provide sharing of information through medical record computerization. Administer drugs that affect clotting (Table 3-25), such as platelet aggregation inhibitors and/or anticoagulants, prior to either primary PCI or fibrinolytics. If fibrinolytics are determined to be the appropriate method of reperfusion, administer the prescribed fibrinolytic within a door-to-needle time of 60 minutes. Participate in quality improvement efforts focused on prompt and appropriate interventions and provide feedback to participants so that quality improvements can continue.

Administer platelet aggregation inhibitors, such as ASA (i.e., 160 to 325 mg initially and daily) or another antiplatelet drug (e.g., clopidogrel [Plavix], prasugrel [Effient]) to decrease platelet aggregation and clot extension. Provide glycoprotein IIb/IIIa platelet receptor blockers (e.g., abciximab [ReoPro], eptifibatide [Integrilin], tirofiban HCl [Aggrastat]) as prescribed. Maintain the patient's aPTT of 45 to 60 seconds with anticoagulant therapy, such as unfractionated heparin. Heparin is an indirect thrombin inhibitor prescribed for 24 to 48 hours. Provide initial weight-based dose, followed by an infusion adjusted by aPTT results. The usual dose of unfractionated heparin is a bolus of 60 units/kg, followed by an infusion of 12 units/kg/hr. Low-molecular-weight heparins (LMWH) subcutaneous, another indirect thrombin inhibitor, offers a lower incidence of heparin-induced thrombocytopenia (HIT) than unfractionated heparin. Bivalirudin (Angiomax) is a direct thrombin inhibitor most frequently used after PCI. Warfarin is prescribed for at least 3 months in patients with any of the following: an anterior Q wave MI, HF, severe left ventricular dysfunction, atrial fibrillation, and a previous embolic event.

Provide either emergent PCI or fibrinolytics to reestablish patency of the infarct-related artery (IRA) within the benchmark timeframe. Assist with decision making regarding reperfusion therapies. When PCI facilities are available, PCI is preferred over fibrinolytics for the majority of patients (O'Connor et al., 2010). When PCI facilities are not available, prompt transport

Text continued on p. 141

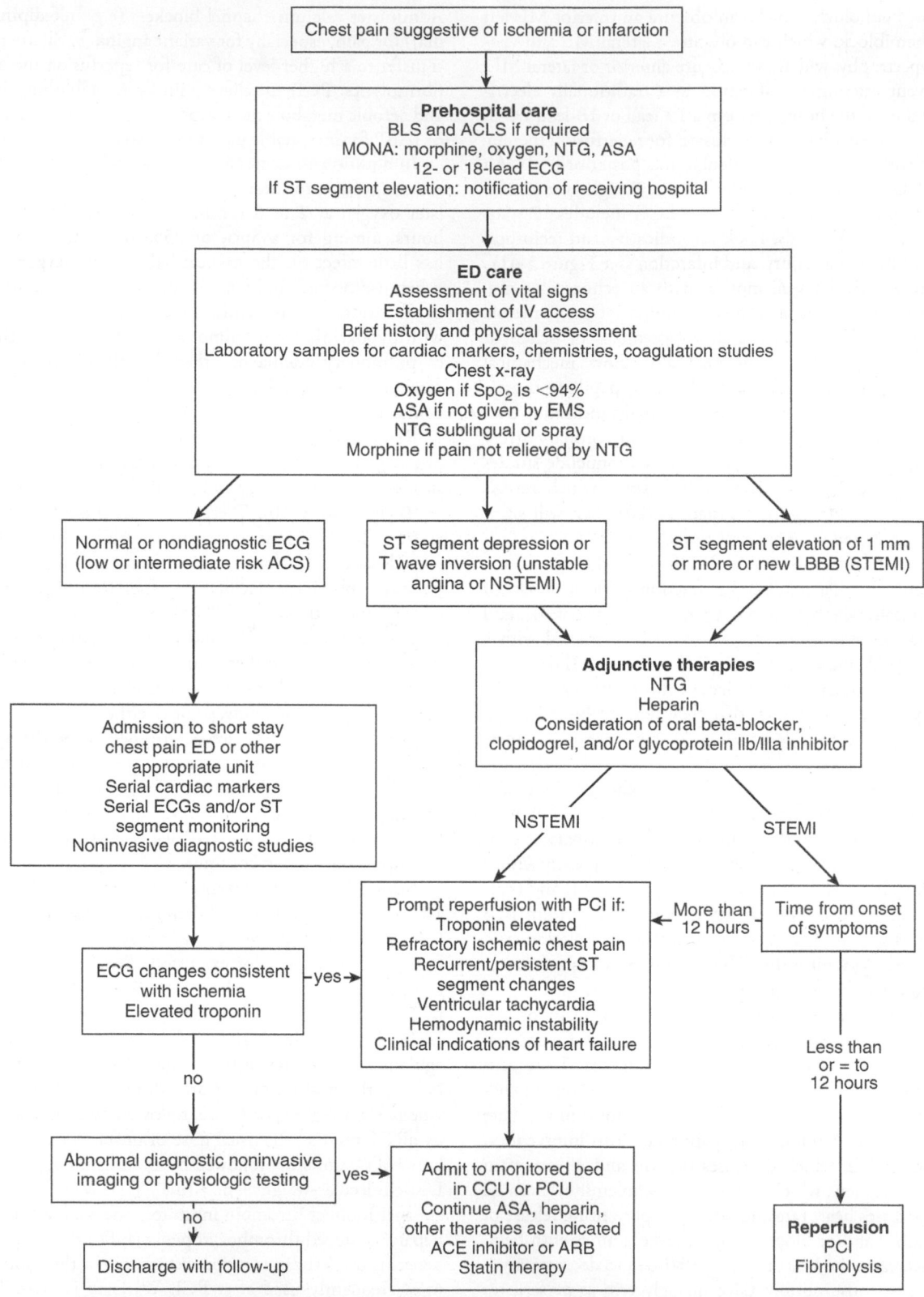

FIGURE 3-56 ACS management algorithm. *ACLS,* Advanced cardiac life support; *ACS,* acute coronary syndrome; *ARB,* angiotensin receptor blocker; *ASA,* aspirin; *BLS,* basic life support; *CCU,* critical care unit; *ECG,* electrocardiogram; *EMS,* emergency medical services; *IV,* intravenous; *LBBB,* left bundle branch block; *MONA,* morphine, oxygen, nitroglycerin, aspirin; *NSTEMI,* non-ST segment elevation myocardial infarction; *NTG,* nitroglycerin; *PCI,* percutaneous coronary intervention; *PCU,* progressive care unit; *SpO₂,* oxygen saturation by pulse oximetry; *STEMI,* ST segment elevation myocardial infarction. (Data from O'Connor, R. E., et al. [2010]. Part 10: Acute coronary syndromes: 2010 American Heart Association guidelines for cardiopulmonary resuscitation and emergency cardiovascular care. *Circulation, 122*[18 Suppl 3], S787-S817.)

TABLE 3-25 Drugs that Affect Clotting Used for Patients with Myocardial Infarction

Drug	Classification/Actions	Indications	Administration	Adverse Effects	Nursing Implications

Abciximab (ReoPro)	**Platelet aggregation inhibitor** (GP IIb/IIIa platelet receptor blocker)
	• Inhibits platelet aggregation and platelet-mediated thrombosis
		• ACS with or without percutaneous coronary intervention (PCI)
		• PCI when risk for thrombosis is high
			• IV injection: 0.25 mg/kg administered between 10 minutes and 1 hour before the start of the PTCA or atherectomy followed by infusion
			• IV infusion: 0.125 mcg/kg/min (10 mcg/min maximum) for 12 hours
				• Bleeding
				  • Intracranial hemorrhage
				  • Hematuria
				  • Hematemesis
				  • Bleeding at sheath site or other puncture point
				• Thrombocytopenia
				• Hypotension
				• Bradycardia
				• Nausea, vomiting, abdominal pain
				• Chest pain
				• Back pain
				• Headache
				• Pain at injection site
				• Allergic reaction, anaphylaxis (especially with repeat administration)
					• Monitor PT, aPTT, or ACT, platelet count
					• Administer with aspirin and heparin therapy as prescribed
					• Note contraindications: patients with active internal bleeding; clinically significant bleeding in the GI or GU tract within the past 6 weeks; bleeding diathesis; history of CVA within the past 2 years or CVA with significant residual neurologic deficit; intracranial neoplasm, aneurysm, or AV malformation; severe uncontrolled hypertension; oral anticoagulants within 7 days unless prothrombin time is less than 1.2 × control; thrombocytopenia; presumed or documented history of vasculitis; major surgery or trauma within the past 6 weeks; pericarditis; known hypersensitivity to abciximab or murine proteins
					• Use cautiously in patients who weigh less than 75 kg, patients older than 65 years of age, patients with a history of GI disease, and patients receiving thrombolytics
					• Do not administer with dextran
					• Monitor oral secretions, sputum, vomitus, NG aspirate, stool, urine for blood
					• Limit venipuncture and urinary catheterization as possible; use IV catheter with saline lock for blood sampling; avoid noncompressible IV sites
					• Avoid nasotracheal and nasogastric tubes if possible
					• Avoid automatic BP cuffs
					• Administer platelets as prescribed for thrombocytopenia
					• Store refrigerated, do not shake (should be clear), administer through filter

Continued

TABLE 3-25   Drugs that Affect Clotting Used for Patients with Myocardial Infarction—cont'd

Drug	Classification/Actions	Indications	Administration	Adverse Effects	Nursing Implications

Eptifibatide (Integrilin)	**Platelet aggregation inhibitor** (GP IIb/IIIa platelet receptor blocker)
	• Inhibits platelet aggregation and platelet-mediated thrombosis
		• ACS with or without percutaneous coronary intervention (PCI)
		• PCI when risk for thrombosis is high
			For acute coronary syndrome:
			• IV injection: 180 mcg/kg over 1-2 minutes followed by IV infusion: 2 mcg/kg/minute for up to 72 hours; decreased to 0.5 mcg/kg/minute during PCI and continued for 24 hours after PCI
			For PCI without acute coronary syndrome:
			• IV injection: 135 mcg/kg over 1-2 minutes before procedure followed by:
			• IV infusion: 0.5 mcg/kg/minute for 24 hours
				• Bleeding
				  • Intracranial hemorrhage
				  • Hematuria
				  • Hematemesis
				  • Bleeding at sheath site
				• Hypotension
					• Monitor PT, aPTT, or ACT, platelet count
					• Note contraindications: active internal bleeding; clinically significant bleeding in the GI or GU tract within the past 6 weeks; bleeding diathesis; history of CVA within the past 2 years or CVA with significant residual neurologic deficit; intracranial neoplasm, aneurysm, or AV malformation; severe uncontrolled hypertension; oral anticoagulants within 7 days unless prothrombin time is less than 1.2 x control; thrombocytopenia; presumed or documented history of vasculitis; major surgery or trauma within the past 6 weeks; pericarditis; known hypersensitivity to eptifibatide; renal failure; thrombocytopenia
					• Administer with aspirin and heparin therapy as prescribed
					• Monitor oral secretions, sputum, vomitus, NG aspirate, stool, urine for blood
					• Limit venipuncture and urinary catheterization if possible; use IV catheter with saline lock for blood sampling; avoid noncompressible IV sites
					• Avoid nasotracheal and nasogastric tubes if possible
					• Avoid automatic BP cuffs
					• Administer platelets as prescribed for thrombocytopenia
					• Store refrigerated

Tirofiban HCl (Aggrastat)	**Platelet aggregation inhibitor** (GP IIb/IIIa platelet receptor blocker)
	• Inhibits platelet aggregation and platelet-mediated thrombosis
		• ACS with or without PCI	• IV infusion: premixed as 25 mg in 500 mL; usual dose is 0.4 mcg/kg/min for 30 minutes and then continued at 0.1 mcg/kg/min (dosage is decreased in renal failure)	• Bleeding
				  • Intracranial hemorrhage
				  • Hematuria
				  • Hematemesis
				  • Bleeding at sheath site
				• Hypotension
				• Bradycardia
				• Pelvic pain
					• Monitor PT, aPTT, or ACT, platelet count
					• Note contraindications: active internal bleeding; clinically significant bleeding in the GI or GU tract within the past 6 weeks; bleeding diathesis; history of CVA within the past 2 years or CVA with significant residual neurologic deficit; intracranial neoplasm, aneurysm, or AV malformation; severe uncontrolled hypertension; oral anticoagulants within 7 days unless prothrombin time is less than 1.2 x control; thrombocytopenia; presumed or documented history of vasculitis; major surgery or trauma within the past month; pericarditis; known hypersensitivity to tirofiban
					• Use cautiously in patients who weigh less than 75 kg, patients older than 65 years of age, patients with a history of GI disease, patients receiving thrombolytics, and patients with thrombocytopenia
					• Administer with aspirin and heparin therapy as prescribed
					• Limit venipuncture and urinary catheterization if possible; use IV catheter with saline lock for blood sampling; avoid noncompressible IV sites
					• Monitor oral secretions, sputum, vomitus, NG aspirate, stool, urine for blood

Drug	Action	Uses	Dosage/Route	Adverse Effects	Nursing Implications

Recombinant tissue plasminogen activator (rt-PA) alteplase (Activase)	**Fibrinolytic**
	• Converts plasminogen to plasmin at fibrin surface
	• Causes clot-specific lysis
		• Acute MI (chest pain strongly suggestive of acute MI; ST segment of at least 1 mm in at least 2 leads)
		• Massive pulmonary embolism (with RVF or refractory hypoxemia)
		• Ischemic stroke
			For acute MI:
			• IV injection: 15 mg followed by IV infusion: 0.75 mg/kg (not to exceed 50 mg) over next 30 minutes, followed by 0.5 mg/kg (not to exceed 35 mg) over the next 60 minutes
			• Heparin started within 1 hour of initial dose
			For ischemic stroke:
			• Total dose: 0.9 mg/kg with maximum dose of ≤90 mg
			• IV injection: 10% of this total dose over 1 minute followed by:
			• IV infusion: remaining 90% of this total dose administered over 60 minutes
			• Anticoagulants and platelet aggregation inhibitors are not used for at least 24 hours
			For acute pulmonary embolism:
			• IV infusion: 100 mg at 50 mg/hr for 2 hours
			For acute arterial occlusion:
			• 0.05 to 0.1 mg/kg/hour by local intra-arterial infusion
			• Reconstitution in sterile water only
				• Severe, spontaneous bleeding including potential cerebral, retroperitoneal, GU, GI bleeding, surface bleeding
				• Reperfusion dysrhythmias
					• Monitor aPTT, PT, thrombin time, fibrinogen, neurologic status, and for signs of hemorrhage
					• Note contraindications: active bleeding; history of cerebral hemorrhage, intracranial neoplasm, AV malformation or aneurysm; recent (within 2 months) intracranial or intraspinal surgery or trauma; known bleeding disorder; severe uncontrolled hypertension; prolonged CPR
					• Use cautiously in recent (within 10 days) major surgery; GI, GU bleeding or trauma; hypertension with SBP >180 mm Hg or DBP >110 mm Hg; high likelihood of left heart thrombus; acute pericarditis; significant liver dysfunction; pregnancy; retinopathy; septic thrombophlebitis; advanced age (>70 to 75 years); patients receiving oral anticoagulants; any condition in which bleeding constitutes a significant hazard or would be particularly difficult to manage because of its location
					• Monitor for indications of reperfusion in MI:
					  • Cessation of pain
					  • ST segments descending back to baseline
					  • Reperfusion dysrhythmias (ventricular ectopy including PVCs, VT or VF, accelerated idioventricular rhythm, junctional escape rhythms, bradycardia)
					  • Early CK peak
					• Note that signs of reperfusion are much more subtle in PE and thrombotic stroke
					• Limit venipuncture and urinary catheterization if possible; use IV catheter with saline lock for blood sampling; avoid noncompressible IV sites
					• Administer all drugs through existing IVs started before initiation of thrombolytic therapy or by mouth
					• Avoid nasotracheal and nasogastric tubes if possible
					• Avoid automatic BP cuffs
					• Monitor oral secretions, sputum, vomitus, NG aspirate, stool, urine for blood
					• Bleeding precautions are maintained for 12 to 24 hours

Continued

TABLE 3-25   **Drugs that Affect Clotting Used for Patients with Myocardial Infarction—cont'd**

Drug	Classification/Actions	Indications	Administration	Adverse Effects	Nursing Implications

Recombinant tissue plasminogen activator (rt-PA) tenecteplase (TNKase)	**Fibrinolytic**
	• Converts plasminogen to plasmin at fibrin surface
	• Causes clot-specific lysis
		• Acute MI (chest pain strongly suggestive of acute MI; ST segment of at least 1 mm in at least 2 leads)	• IV injection over 5 seconds
			  • <60 kg: 30 mg
			  • ≥60-<70 kg: 35 mg
			  • ≥70-<80 kg: 40 mg
			  • ≥80-<90 kg: 45 mg
			  • ≥90 kg: 50 mg
			• Heparin administered concurrently
				• Severe, spontaneous bleeding including potential cerebral, retroperitoneal, GU, GI bleeding, surface bleeding
				• Reperfusion dysrhythmias
					• Monitor aPTT, PT, thrombin time, neurologic status, and for signs of hemorrhage
					• Note contraindications: active bleeding: history of cerebral hemorrhage, intracranial neoplasm, AV malformation or aneurysm; recent (within 2 months) intracranial or intraspinal surgery or trauma; known bleeding disorder; severe uncontrolled hypertension; prolonged CPR
					• Use cautiously in recent (within 10 days) major surgery; GI, GU bleeding, or trauma; hypertension with SBP >180 mm Hg or DBP >110 mm Hg; high likelihood of left heart thrombus; acute pericarditis; significant liver dysfunction; pregnancy; retinopathy; septic thrombophlebitis; advanced age (>70 to 75 years); patients receiving oral anticoagulants; any condition in which bleeding constitutes a significant hazard or would be particularly difficult to manage because of its location
					• Identify indications of reperfusion in MI
					  • Cessation of pain
					  • ST segments descending back to baseline
					  • Reperfusion dysrhythmias (ventricular ectopy including PVCs, VT or VF, accelerated idioventricular rhythm, junctional escape rhythms, bradycardia)
					  • Early CK peak
					• Limit venipuncture and urinary catheterization if possible; use IV catheter with saline lock for blood sampling; avoid noncompressible IV sites
					• Avoid nasotracheal and nasogastric tubes if possible
					• Avoid automatic BP cuffs
					• Administer all drugs through existing IVs started before initiation of thrombolytic therapy or by mouth
					• Monitor oral secretions, sputum, vomitus, NG aspirate, stool, urine for blood
					• Bleeding precautions are maintained for 12 to 24 hours

| Recombinant plasminogen activator (r-PA) reteplase (Retavase) | **Fibrinolytic**
• Converts plasminogen to plasmin at fibrin surface
• Causes clot-specific lysis | • IV injection of 10 units over 2 minutes initially followed by 10 units over 2 minutes after 30 minutes
• Heparin administered concurrently | • Acute MI (chest pain strongly suggestive of acute MI; ST segment of at least 1 mm in at least 2 leads) | • Severe, spontaneous bleeding including potential cerebral, retroperitoneal, GU, GI bleeding, surface bleeding
• Reperfusion dysrhythmias | • Monitor aPTT, PT, thrombin time, neurologic status, and for signs of hemorrhage
• Note contraindications: active bleeding; history of cerebral hemorrhage, intracranial neoplasm, AV malformation or aneurysm; recent (within 2 months) intracranial or intraspinal surgery or trauma; known bleeding disorder; severe uncontrolled hypertension; prolonged CPR
• Use cautiously in recent (within 10 days) major surgery; GI, GU bleeding, or trauma; hypertension with SBP >180 mm Hg or DBP >110 mm Hg; high likelihood of left heart thrombus; acute pericarditis; significant liver dysfunction; pregnancy; retinopathy; septic thrombophlebitis; advanced age (>70 to 75 years); patients receiving oral anticoagulants; any condition in which bleeding constitutes a significant hazard or would be particularly difficult to manage because of its location
• Identify indications of reperfusion in MI
  • Cessation of pain
  • ST segments descending back to baseline
  • Reperfusion dysrhythmias (ventricular ectopy including PVCs, VT or VF, accelerated idioventricular rhythm, junctional escape rhythms, bradycardia)
  • Early CK peak
• Limit venipuncture and urinary catheterization as possible; use IV catheter with saline lock for blood sampling; avoid noncompressible IV sites
• Avoid nasotracheal and nasogastric tubes if possible
• Avoid automatic BP cuffs
• Administer all drugs through existing IVs started before initiation of thrombolytic therapy or by mouth
• Monitor oral secretions, sputum, vomitus, NG aspirate, stool, urine for blood
• Bleeding precautions are maintained for 12 to 24 hours |

Continued

TABLE 3-25   Drugs that Affect Clotting Used for Patients with Myocardial Infarction—cont'd

Drug	Classification/Actions	Indications	Administration	Adverse Effects	Nursing Implications
Heparin sodium	**Anticoagulant; indirect thrombin inhibitor** • Prevents conversion of prothrombin to thrombin • Prevents conversion of fibrinogen to fibrin • Prevents extension of existing clots • Decreases platelet aggregation	• Unstable angina or myocardial infarction • Maintenance of arterial patency after PCI or thrombolytic therapy • Prevention of thrombus formation during periods of inactivity • Deep vein thrombosis • Pulmonary emboli • Peripheral arterial emboli • Transient ischemic attacks or reversible ischemic neurologic deficit • Disseminated intravascular coagulation (controversial) • Maintenance of arterial line patency	• Subcutaneous: usually prophylactic, dose is 5000 units every 12 hours (also called mini-heparin) • IV injection: usually 80 units/kg (maximum 10,000 units) followed by infusion (only 60 units/kg recommended if patient is receiving fibrinolytics or GP IIb/IIIa inhibitors) • IV infusion: mix 25,000 units in 500 mL (50 units/mL) and infuse at 18 units/kg/hour (maximum 1000 units/hour) (only 12 units/kg recommended if patient is receiving fibrinolytics or GP IIb/IIIa inhibitors); dose is adjusted to achieve aPTT of 1½ to 2½ times the laboratory control • Note: the trend in IV weight-dosed heparin is to decrease the amount of heparin (60 units/kg for injection followed by 12 units/kg/hour for infusion) and desirable aPTT (45 to 60 seconds) • Maximum: 40,000 units/day	• Hemorrhage with excessive aPTT • Hypertension or hypotension • Hypersensitivity reaction including bronchospasm • Fever • Hepatitis • Hyperkalemia especially in patients with renal failure • Thrombocytopenia (caused by immune response referred to as heparin-induced thrombocytopenia [HIT])	• Monitor aPTT and platelet count and for signs of hemorrhage • Note petechiae and request platelet count if petechiae noted; heparin usually discontinued if platelet count is <100,000/mm³ • Administer lepirudin (Refludan) or argatroban as prescribed for HIT • Note contraindications: known hypersensitivity, active bleeding, blood dyscrasias (except DIC), suspected intracranial hemorrhage, severe hypertension, peptic ulcer disease, open wounds, recent surgery, endocarditis, shock, threatened abortion • Use cautiously in alcoholism, liver disease, renal disease, older adults • Monitor oral secretions, sputum, vomitus, NG aspirate, stool, urine for blood • Ensure that protamine sulfate (antidote) is available • Avoid IM, arterial, or venous punctures if at all possible • Hold pressure for longer than usual if punctures necessary • Do not discontinue suddenly: warfarin will usually have already been started and the PT within therapeutic range before heparin is discontinued • Do not aspirate before subcutaneous administration and do not massage after administration • Note that NTG interacts with heparin causing more heparin to be required to achieve therapeutic aPTT; monitor aPTT closely with significant NTG dosage changes or discontinuance

Drug	Classification/Action	Indications	Dosages	Adverse Effects	Nursing Considerations
Heparin: low-molecular-weight enoxaparin (Lovenox) dalteparin sodium (Fragmin)	**Anticoagulant; indirect thrombin inhibitor** • Inhibits thrombin activity • Prevents DVT • Does not prevent platelet aggregation	• High risk for DVT • Acute coronary syndrome	Enoxaparin (Lovenox) • SC: 30 mg bid Dalteparin sodium (Fragmin) • SC: 2,500 IU daily starting 1-2 hours before surgery and repeated daily for 5 to 10 days postoperatively Ardeparin (Normiflo) • SC: 50 antifactor Xa international units/kg every 12 hours beginning the evening before surgery and continued until the patient is ambulatory Tinzaparin sodium (Innohep) • SC: 175 anti-Xa international units/kg daily for approximately 6 days or until adequate anticoagulation with warfarin	• Bleeding • Epidural or spinal hematoma (especially when used with patients with epidural or spinal anesthesia) • Fever • Elevation of liver enzymes • Thrombocytopenia • Chest pain	• Note that LMWH does not require routine laboratory monitoring because it does not usually alter PT or aPTT • Note that contraindications and cautions are as for heparin • Obtain baseline platelet count; monitor for petechiae • Monitor oral secretions, sputum, vomitus, NG aspirate, stool, urine for blood • Ensure that protamine sulfate (antidote) is available • Avoid IM, arterial, or venous punctures if at all possible • Hold pressure for longer than usual if punctures necessary • Administer deep subcutaneously but avoid IM injection
Bivalirudin (Angiomax)	**Anticoagulant: direct thrombin inhibitor** • Prevents conversion of prothrombin to thrombin including both free and clot-bound thrombin	• Unstable angina in patients undergoing PCI	• IV injection: 0.75 to 1 mg/kg followed by IV infusion • IV infusion: mix 250 mg in 250 mL of normal saline (1 mg/mL) and infuse at 1.75 to 2.5 mg/kg/hour for 4 hours then decrease infusion to 0.2 mg/kg/hour for an additional 14 to 20 hours if needed	• Bleeding • Back pain • Generalized pain • Headache • Nausea • Hypotension	• Monitor PT, aPTT, CBC, and for signs of bleeding • Note that contraindications and cautions are as for heparin • Obtain baseline platelet count and aPTT; monitor aPTT every 4 hours; ACT may also be used • Anticoagulant effects are increased in patients receiving platelet aggregation inhibitors, fibrinolytics, or other anticoagulants • Monitor oral secretions, sputum, vomitus, NG aspirate, stool, urine for blood • Avoid IM, arterial, or venous punctures if at all possible • Hold pressure for longer than usual if punctures necessary • Protect infusion from direct sunlight

Continued

TABLE 3-25 **Drugs that Affect Clotting Used for Patients with Myocardial Infarction—cont'd**

Drug	Classification/Actions	Indications	Administration	Adverse Effects	Nursing Implications

Warfarin (Coumadin, Panwarfin)	**Anticoagulant**
	• Depresses synthesis of prothrombin by the liver
	• Prevents extension of clot and secondary thromboembolic complications
		• Deep vein thrombosis
		• Valvular heart disease
		• Atrial dysrhythmias
		• Postvalve replacement
			• PO: 2 to 10 mg daily depending on PT and international normalized ratio (INR)
			• INR 2.0 to 3.0
			  — MI
			  — DVT prophylaxis or treatment
			  — Pulmonary embolus
			  — Valvular heart disease
			  — Atrial fibrillation
			  — Tissue heart valve
			• INR 2.5 to 3.5
			  — Mechanical heart valve
				• Hemorrhage with excessive PT
				• Agranulocytosis, leukopenia
				• Hepatitis
				• Diarrhea
				• Fever
				• Rash
				• Skin necrosis: occurs during the first several days of warfarin therapy; lesions occur on extremities, breasts, trunk, penis
				• Cholesterol microemboli causing purple toe syndrome
					• Monitor PT and for signs of hemorrhage
					• Note contraindications: known hypersensitivity, bleeding disorders, leukemia, peptic ulcer disease, liver disease, severe hypertension, endocarditis, acute nephritis, blood dyscrasias, eclampsia, suspected intracranial hemorrhage, open wounds, recent surgery, threatened abortion
					• Use cautiously in alcoholism, pregnancy, lactation, during menses, during use of any drainage tube, older adults, or in any patient in whom slight bleeding is dangerous
					• Ensure that vitamin K (AquaMephyton) is available
					• Avoid IM, arterial, or venous punctures if at all possible
					• Hold pressure for longer than usual if punctures necessary
					• Monitor oral secretions, sputum, vomitus, NG aspirate, stool, urine for blood
					• Do not discontinue suddenly
					• Teach patient to avoid trauma and increased amounts of vitamin K (e.g., green leafy vegetables), and how to monitor for bleeding
					• Teach the patient to report fever or rash; usually necessitates discontinuance

to a facility with PCI capability is preferred over fibrinolytics if transfer to PCI time is less than 120 minutes (O'Connor et al., 2010). Assist in prompt preparation of the patient for emergent PCI if PCI is determined to be the appropriate method of reperfusion. The goal is to achieve a DTBT of 90 minutes or less.

Percutaneous Coronary Intervention

Percutaneous coronary intervention (PCI) opens occluded coronary arteries caused by CAD and restores arterial blood flow to the heart tissue without cardiac surgery. PCI procedures consist of several different techniques. The physician inserts a special catheter into the coronary artery and past the occlusion. The catheter has a small balloon that is inflated once the catheter is in place. The balloon inflation compresses the atherosclerotic plaque in the artery and enlarges the lumen of the artery to improve blood flow. An AngioJet, a high-speed saline jet, may be used to remove the thrombus. In addition, microsurgical blades facilitate maximal dilatation of the lesions. Stents, brachytherapy, and atherectomy procedures maintain long-term patency. PCI collaborative care and management (Table 3-26) focuses on recognizing the indications and contraindications, conducting the postprocedure assessments, providing appropriate care including prevention of and monitoring for complications, and postprocedure education.

Coronary Artery Bypass Graft

Prepare the patient for coronary artery bypass graft surgery (Table 3-27) as indicated. A coronary artery bypass graft procedure provides arterial or venous conduits to redirect coronary blood flow around occluded coronary arteries. Treat anemia if the patient's hemoglobin is less than 12 g/dL. Continually monitor the patient's hemodynamic status and provide preoperative education. The patient is recovered in the critical care unit for a day and then transferred back to the progressive care unit if hemodynamically stable, weaned from inotropic and vasoactive medications, and has had no immediate complications.

After initial myocardial salvaging and reperfusion therapies, the focus of management is on improving myocardial oxygen supply and decreasing myocardial oxygen demand, along with preventing, monitoring for, and treating complications. In addition, before discharge, patient and family education is a priority.

Continue to administer oxygen if required to maintain SpO_2 of 95%. Administer beta-blockers as prescribed to decrease heart rate and contractility and to decrease myocardial oxygen consumption. Beta-blockers decrease the incidence of dysrhythmias and increase the ventricular fibrillation threshold, block the effects of catecholamines offering cardioprotection, and reduce the infarct size and the severity of HF. Metoprolol (Lopressor) is usually administered at 5 mg IV every 2 minutes × 3, but atenolol (Tenormin) or esmolol (Brevibloc) may be substituted. These drugs are contraindicated when the heart rate is less than 50 beats/min, in the presence of second- or third-degree AV block, when the systolic BP is less than 100 mm Hg, or when there is HF or bronchospasm. Avoid beta-blockers in a patient with active bronchospasm. Cardioselective beta-blockers (e.g., metoprolol or esmolol) may be given to a patient with a history of bronchospastic lung disease (e.g., asthma), but avoid noncardioselective beta-blockers (e.g., propranolol).

For cocaine-induced MI, blocking beta-receptors allows unopposed alpha-receptors to increase vasoconstriction and vasospasm. Instead of alpha- and beta-blockers, administer

nitroglycerin and/or a calcium channel blocker (e.g., diltiazem [Cardizem]). In addition, administer benzodiazepine (e.g., diazepam [Valium]) to reduce agitation and seizure potential.

Administer ACE inhibitors (e.g., captopril [Capoten], enalapril [Vasotec]) or angiotensin-receptor blockers (ARBs) (e.g., losartan [Cozaar], valsartan [Diovan]) as prescribed to attenuate ventricular remodeling. This will block the vasoconstriction and sodium and water retention associated with activation of the renin-angiotensin-aldosterone system. Either an ACE or an ARB is indicated for cases of anterior or large inferior MI or where there is evidence of HF with MI. ACE inhibitors block the conversion of angiotensin I to angiotensin II; ARBs block angiotensin II and do not block the breakdown of bradykinin, so they are less likely to cause cough. Either group of drugs can cause hypotension.

Administer vasodilators as prescribed. Venous vasodilators, usually nitroglycerin, decrease preload. Arterial vasodilators, usually nitroprusside, decrease afterload. Take caution as these agents can cause hypotension. If these continuous IV agents are required, transfer the patient to a higher acuity level of care. Careful titration is necessary to decrease myocardial oxygen consumption while preventing hypoperfusion.

Monitor and control dysrhythmias to maintain optimal cardiac output. Tachydysrhythmias decrease the time for coronary artery filling and may decrease cardiac output. Bradydysrhythmias increase the time for coronary artery filling but may decrease cardiac output. Administer calcium channel blockers or nitroglycerin (NTG) for coronary artery spasm; this is especially important in cocaine-induced MI.

Monitor serum glucose and administer insulin as required to maintain serum glucose below 150 mg/dL. Provide physical and emotional rest. Maintain bed rest for 24 hours, and then gradually increase activity as long as the patient is hemodynamically stable. Allow rest after meals, personal hygiene, toileting, and physical therapy. To prevent the patient from initiating the Valsalva maneuver, teach the process of exhaling when turning in bed. Administer stool softeners as prescribed and provide a bedside commode for elimination.

Explain the unit routine and any procedures thoroughly and the reasons for the procedures. Discuss the monitor alarms, equipment, and visiting hours. Keep the family informed of the patient's progress and status.

Provide for the patient's comfort. This includes prompt pain control using prescribed analgesics, oral care, and antiemetics for control of nausea. Also, provide for basic physical comfort by adequately controlling the environmental temperature and lighting and keeping the noise down. Instruct the patient on relaxation techniques and encourage utilization of these techniques. Use calming music, white noise, or nature sounds to aid in relaxation.

Provide appropriate nutrition. A clear liquid to soft diet, usually low in sodium, is best. The patient may have up to four to five caffeinated beverages every 24 hours as long as dysrhythmias do not occur. There is no recommendation on limiting the use of ice water.

If needed, administer anxiolytics as prescribed, usually diazepam (Valium), lorazepam (Ativan), or alprazolam (Xanax). Recognize and treat common emotional responses (Table 3-28) seen in acute MI.

Initiate interventions to prevent complications of MI (Table 3-29) but also monitor closely for indications of complications

TABLE 3-26   **Percutaneous Coronary Interventions**

Procedures	• Percutaneous transluminal coronary angioplasty (PTCA): inflation of a balloon-tipped catheter in an area of coronary artery stenosis from plaque; plaque is pushed back against the wall of the vessel and fractured (controlled trauma)
	   • Cutting balloon microsurgical dilation catheter system: microsurgical blades mounted longitudinally on an angioplasty balloon to open narrowed artery; as the balloon expands radially, the blades are exposed and incise plaque in the arteries; claimed to facilitate maximum dilatation of the target lesion with more precision and less trauma than conventional angioplasty
	• Coronary artery stent: use of a metal mesh tube that acts as a scaffolding device to support a coronary artery and maintain patency after PTCA; previously used only in cases of acute closure, most PTCA procedures include planned stent placements
	   • Stents are usually stainless steel but may be nitinol, tantalum, or another metal
	   • Stents have usually been thought of as a coil but they may be a mesh, slotted tube, ring, or other design
	   • Stents are either deployed by balloon expansion or they may be self-expanding
	   • Stents may be drug-eluting (i.e., drug-eluting stent [DES]) to reduce the risk of neointimal hyperplasia and restenosis rates
	    — Sirolimus, an immunosuppressive agent, prevents proliferation of normal tissue and inflammation
	    — Paclitaxel, an antineoplastic agent, inhibits cell proliferation and migration
	• Brachytherapy: use of intracoronary irradiation to reduce risk of restenosis; combined with PTCA or stent placement
	• Coronary atherectomy: removal of plaque from coronary artery by a high-speed diamond-tipped (rotational) or shaving (directional) device
	   • Directional coronary atherectomy (DCA): a directional device shaves pieces of the atheroma into the catheter tip
	   • Coronary rotational ablation (Rotablator): a diamond-coated burr drills through the atheroma and pulverizes the plaque
	   • Transluminal extraction catheter (TEC): a motorized cutting head shaves the atheroma from the arterial wall and suctions out the pieces
	   • Excimer laser coronary atherectomy (ELCA): use of a laser to vaporize the atheroma
	• AngioJet: high-speed saline jet; most effective for thrombus

Indications	• Unstable or chronic angina • Acute or postacute MI • Postcoronary artery bypass graft with postoperative angina • Patient must be surgical candidate (in case of coronary artery dissection)
Contraindications	• Left main CAD (unless there is a patent bypass around it, referred to as *protected*) • Stenosis of coronary artery at orifice • Variant angina • Critical valvular disease
Action	• The goal of percutaneous coronary interventions is to reduce the degree of coronary artery stenosis; the intervention is considered successful if the degree of stenosis is reduced to 20% to 30% stenosis without serious complications.
Assessment	• Vital signs: BP, HR, RR, T • ECG: monitor closely for ST segment elevation • Sheath insertion site: usually femoral but may be radial • Neurovascular status of affected limb • Any complaints of chest pain • Any complaints of back pain

Brief summary of specific nursing management	• Monitor for myocardial ischemia: note any new chest pain, ST segment elevation (especially if PCI performed for acute ischemia or infarction)
	• Assess puncture site frequently to detect bleeding and/or hematoma formation
	   • Control systolic BP to <150 mm Hg and diastolic BP <90 mm Hg with antihypertensives as prescribed
	   • Monitor platelet count and aPTT (patient will receive platelet aggregation inhibitors and either unfractionated or low-molecular-weight heparin to prevent reocclusion)
	   • Immobilize groin by restraining with sheet stretched over knee on affected side and tucked on each side of bed rather than restraining ankle
	   • Perform neurovascular checks to detect peripheral ischemia related to femoral artery thrombosis

TABLE 3-26 **Percutaneous Coronary Interventions—cont'd**

Brief summary of specific nursing management—cont'd	• Monitor for clinical indications of retroperitoneal hemorrhage: postural tachycardia and/or hypotension; back and/or flank pain; Grey-Turner's sign; decrease in hemoglobin and hematocrit (unfortunately there are no early indications)
	• Keep affected limb straight and immobile; head of bed should be elevated no more than 30 degrees as long as the sheath is in place and for 4 to 8 hours after removal
	• Assist with removal or remove sheath (depending on hospital protocol) if not completed in the cardiac catheterization laboratory; Perclose, VasoSeal, or Angio-Seal may be used when the sheath was removed in the cardiac catheterization laboratory
	  • If IV heparin has been infusing, it will be discontinued and the ACT needs to be less than 150 seconds; if unfractionated heparin is to be restarted, it will be restarted several hours after sheath removal; low-molecular-weight heparin subcutaneously may be used
	  • Pain control and sedation (e.g., local infiltration with lidocaine or IV morphine and/or midazolam [Versed] or lorazepam [Ativan])
	  • Apply pressure to where the sheath entered the artery which is about 1 inch above the skin entry site
	  • Manual pressure or mechanical pressure devices (e.g., C-clamp, FemoStop) may be used
	  • Pressure is held for at least 30 minutes or until hemostasis achieved
	  • Control of bleeding must be maintained while peripheral pulses are still palpated

Complications: prevention and treatment	• Acute reocclusion or closure due to:
	  • Trauma to intima initiating clotting cascade
	    — ASA and heparin are used to prevent thrombosis
	    — GP IIb/IIIa platelet receptor blockers (e.g., abciximab [ReoPro], eptifibatide [Integrilin], or tirofiban HCl [Aggrastat]) are used for PCI in ACS patients who have not been receiving clopidogrel
	    — ASA and clopidogrel (Plavix) are maintained after the procedure
	      — Prasugrel (Effient) is another platelet receptor blocker that may be used but should not be used for ACS patients with stroke or transient ischemic attack
	    — Monitor aPTT; usually maintained at 50 to 70 seconds
	    — Proton pump inhibitor is recommended with dual antiplatelet therapy
	  • Coronary artery spasm
	    — Nitroglycerin infusion and/or calcium channel blockers are frequently used
	    — Note: new onset chest pain or ST segment changes should be reported immediately
	• Coronary artery dissection: due to catheter trauma; necessitates placement of stent or, in severe cases, emergent coronary artery bypass graft
	• Cardiac tamponade: due to cardiac perforation
	• Dysrhythmias: due to ischemia or reperfusion
	• Pseudoaneurysm: due to catheter dissection of artery
	• Hemorrhage or hematoma: due to anticoagulated state
	  • Retroperitoneal hemorrhage or hematoma
	  • Femoral artery puncture site hemorrhage or hematoma
	• Embolic complications (e.g., myocardial infarction, cerebral infarction, peripheral emboli)
	• Chronic restenosis: due to intimal hyperplasia
	• Hypotension, bradycardia (vagal reaction): due to increased parasympathetic nervous system during sheath removal; atropine is effective

Postprocedure education	• Information about devices placed: give the patient a stent identification card with date, facility, type, and site of implant • Care of site used for catheter insertion (femoral or radial) • Need for drugs to maintain stent patency: usually aspirin and clopidogrel • To avoid magnetic resonance imaging (MRI) scans within 8 weeks of stent placement • Symptoms to report: site pain, chest pain, bleeding

TABLE 3-27 **Coronary Artery Bypass Grafting (CABG)**

Procedures	• Types of bypasses
	  • Arterial bypass (preferred because of better long-term patency rates)
	    — Internal thoracic (also called internal mammary) arteries
	    — Gastroepiploic artery
	    — Inferior epigastric arteries
	    — Radial arteries
	  • Vein grafts
	    — Saphenous veins
	    — Brachial veins
	• Surgical approaches
	  • Median sternotomy with cardiopulmonary bypass (CPB)
	    — CPB provides a motionless heart and a bloodless field
	    — Complications of CPB include systemic inflammatory response syndrome (SIRS), coagulopathy, atelectasis, acute respiratory distress syndrome, cerebral microemboli, thrombotic stroke, post-CPB encephalopathy, renal insufficiency, dysrhythmias
	  • Off-pump coronary artery bypass (OPCAB)
	    — May be performed through small median sternotomy or anterior thoracotomy
	    — Bypass is performed on a beating heart
	    — Avoids complications related to cardiopulmonary bypass
	  • Minimally invasive direct (MIDCAB)
	    — Performed through anterior thoracotomy
	    — May be used for proximal LAD and select lesions of RCA or circumflex
	    — Bypass is performed on a beating heart
	    — Avoids complications related to cardiopulmonary bypass
	    — Thoracoscopy may be used

Indications	• Left main artery disease or three-vessel disease • Double-vessel disease if one of the vessels is the proximal LAD • Single- or double-vessel disease with angina unresponsive to medical therapy • CAD with ejection fraction less than 35% • Emergent conditions such as unstable angina, acute MI with persistent pain or shock, or coronary artery dissection during interventional cardiology procedures
Action	• The goal of coronary artery bypass graft is to provide arterial or venous conduits to redirect coronary blood flow around occluded coronary arteries
Assessment	• Vital signs: HR, BP, RR, T • Hemodynamic parameters: RAP, PAP, PAOP, CO, CI, SVR, PVR, LVSWI, RVSWI • Oxygenation parameters: SpO_2, SvO_2; ABGs • Serum electrolytes • Mediastinal and pleural tube drainage • Complaints of incisional pain, chest pain, dyspnea • Incision for bleeding, separation, or redness and induration

Brief summary of specific nursing management	• Relieve pain
	  • Administer narcotics and sedatives for relief of incisional pain
	  • Provide instruction regarding splinting during coughing and turning
	  • Report ischemic pain; titrate NTG for relief of ischemic pain
	• Monitor closely for hemodynamic changes: titrate drug therapy to optimize cardiac output and minimize myocardial oxygen consumption
	  • Pharmacologic support of this patient may include dobutamine, dopamine, nitroglycerin, nitroprusside
	  • Vasopressors may be used to increase coronary artery perfusion pressure and maintain patency of grafts; monitor for excessive afterload and myocardial oxygen consumption as well as excessive vasoconstriction and peripheral hypoperfusion
	  • Nitroglycerin at low dose is frequently used to reduce spasm
	• Monitor closely for hemorrhage: mediastinal tube, pleural tubes, incision
	  • Administer IV fluids, blood and/or blood products, and albumin as prescribed
	  • Maintain patency of mediastinal and pleural tubes
	  • Be alert for sudden reduction of drainage by mediastinal tube since occlusion may cause cardiac tamponade
	• Monitor closely for changes in perfusion
	  • Note any complaints of chest pain, ST segment elevation, dysrhythmias
	  • Note any changes in appearance or volume of urine
	  • Note any changes in level of consciousness or neurologic function
	  • Note any changes in SpO_2, PAP, PVR
	  • Note any changes in bowel sounds, abdominal distention, abdominal pain

TABLE 3-27 Coronary Artery Bypass Grafting (CABG)—cont'd

Brief summary of specific nursing management—cont'd	• Monitor the ECG for dysrhythmias or blocks
	  • Replace electrolytes as prescribed; potassium and magnesium imbalances predispose the patient to dysrhythmias
	  • Administer antidysrhythmics as prescribed; prophylactic antidysrhythmics (e.g., amiodarone) may be given to prevent atrial fibrillation
	  • Utilize epicardial pacing wires for symptomatic bradycardias or blocks
	• Prevent/monitor for complications

Complications: prevention and treatment	• Potential complications during surgery
	  • Cerebral or myocardial infarction
	  • Hemorrhage: greater risk with internal thoracic artery implant
	  • Inability to wean from cardiopulmonary bypass: IABP and/or VAD used
	• Potential complications during postoperative period
	  • Immediate
	    — HF with hypotension and/or pulmonary edema
	    — Hemorrhage
	    — Cardiac tamponade
	    — Dysrhythmias
	    — MI
	    — Hypertension
	    — Cerebral embolism
	    — Acute respiratory failure (e.g., atelectasis, ARDS)
	    — Renal failure
	    — Electrolyte imbalance (e.g., hypokalemia, hypocalcemia, hypomagnesemia)
	    — Graft closure
	    — Coagulopathy
	  • Intermediate
	    — Donor site infection
	    — Sternal wound infection: especially if patient is diabetic and/or internal thoracic (i.e., mammary) artery used for bypass

TABLE 3-28 Emotional Responses Seen in Acute Myocardial Infarction

Response	Indications	Collaborative Management
Anxiety	• Increased verbalization • Inability to concentrate • Restlessness, apprehension • Sleep disturbances • Tremors • Tachycardia • Mild hypertension	• Maintain consistency with patient assignment if possible • Provide orientation to unit, procedures, equipment, etc. • Assess usual coping mechanisms • Invite patient to ask questions • Keep family informed about patient condition • Encourage participation in rehabilitation program
Denial	• Avoidance of discussion of heart attack • Discussions kept on a social, humorous level • Minimization of severity (e.g., "little heart attack") • Noncompliance with activity and diet restrictions; smoking • Overly cheerful demeanor • Repetition of same questions to different staff members	• Listen but do not reinforce denial • Assess consequences of denial: denial decreases inhospital mortality but increases incidence of sudden cardiac death after discharge • Assess the threat causing the need for denial • Provide counseling if patient still in denial at time of discharge • Encourage participation in rehabilitation program
Depression	• Listlessness, disinterest • Expressions of hopelessness, pessimism • Abbreviated verbal responses (e.g., monosyllable answers) • Slowness in movement and speech • Withdrawn behavior • Anorexia • Sad look, crying	• Voice your observations (e.g., "You look sad") • Let patient know that it is normal to feel this way • Encourage verbalization of feelings • Allow and encourage crying • Encourage participation in rehabilitation program

Continued

TABLE 3-28   Emotional Responses Seen in Acute Myocardial Infarction—cont'd

Response	Indications	Collaborative Management
Anger	• Open opposition to treatment regimen • Expressions of disappointment or frustration • Passive-aggressive behavior • Sarcasm • Voices anger, screaming, cursing	• Acknowledge angry or hostile feelings • Explore cause of anger • Let patient know that these feelings are normal • Let spouse and family know that anger is normal • Be matter-of-fact about expressions of anger • Encourage participation in rehabilitation program
Aggressive sexual behavior	• Frequent seductive comments • Frequent initiation of sexually related conversion • Frequent boasts about past sexual interests and prowess • Flirtatious compliments • Attempts to hold, fondle, or kiss parts of nurse's body • Deliberate exposure of genitals	• Be honest and simply tell the patient that his or her behavior makes you uncomfortable if it does • Accept compliments with simple "thank you" • Arrange sexual counseling for patient and spouse • Encourage participation in rehabilitation program

TABLE 3-29   Complications of Myocardial Infarction

Complication	Clinical Indications	Prevention/Treatment
Dysrhythmias and conduction system defects	• Change in rhythm or conduction on rhythm strip or multiple lead ECG • Indications of hypoperfusion may be evident	• Close monitoring for changes in rhythm or conduction • Beta-blocker as a cardioprotective agent as prescribed • Magnesium, potassium, or calcium to correct electrolyte imbalance as prescribed • Antidysrhythmic agents as indicated and prescribed • Application of external pacemaker or insertion of transvenous pacemaker as indicated • Cardioversion or defibrillation as indicated

HF	• Tachycardia, tachypnea
	• Clinical indications of LVF
	  • Dyspnea, orthopnea, cough
	  • S_3
	  • Crackles in lung bases
	• Clinical indications of RVF
	  • Jugular venous distention
	  • Hepatomegaly, splenomegaly
	  • Peripheral edema
	• Chest x-ray shows pulmonary venous congestion, cardiomegaly
	• Increased RAP, PAP, PAOP (PAOP usually >20 mm Hg)
		• Oxygen
		• Sodium and fluid restriction
		• ACE inhibitors (e.g., captopril, enalapril)
		• Beta-blockers (e.g., metoprolol, carvedilol)
		• Diuretics (e.g., furosemide, bumetanide)
		• Vasodilators (e.g., nitroglycerin)
		• Inotropic agents (e.g., dobutamine, milrinone, digoxin)

Cardiogenic shock	• Tachycardia, tachypnea, hypotension
	• Clinical indications of LVF
	• Clinical indications of RVF
	• Clinical indications of hypoperfusion (see Table 3-2)
	• Urine output <0.5 mL/kg/hour
	• Cool to cold skin
	• Diminished to absent bowel sounds
	• Lethargy to confusion to coma
	• Chest x-ray shows pulmonary venous congestion, cardiomegaly
	• Decreased CO/CI (usually <2 L/min/m²)
	• Increased PAOP (usually >18 mm Hg)
	• Increased SVR (usually >2000 dynes/sec/cm⁻⁵)
		• Oxygen
		• Sodium and fluid restrictions
		• ACE inhibitors (e.g., captopril, enalapril)
		• Diuretics (e.g., furosemide, bumetanide)
		• Transfer to higher acuity level of care for:
		  • Inotropic agents (e.g., digoxin, dobutamine, amrinone, or milrinone)
		  • Vasodilators (e.g., nitroglycerin, nitroprusside)
		  • IABP
		  • Ventricular assist devices
		  • Emergent revascularization: fibrinolytics; PCI; CABG

TABLE 3-29 Complications of Myocardial Infarction—cont'd

Complication	Clinical Indications	Prevention/Treatment

Papillary muscle dysfunction/rupture	• New holosystolic murmur loudest at apex
	• Clinical indications of LVF
	• Clinical indications of hypoperfusion
	• Increased PAP, PAOP
	• Large V waves on PAOP waveform
	• ECG shows mitral regurgitation
		• Transfer to higher acuity level of care for:
		  • Vasodilators (e.g., nitroglycerin, nitroprusside)
		  • IABP
		  • Surgical replacement of mitral valve with concurrent CABG

Ventricular septal rupture	• New holosystolic murmur loudest at lower left sternal border (LLSB)
	• Chest pain, dyspnea
	• Syncope
	• Increased PAP, PAOP
	• Increased Svo_2
	• Increased CO/CI by thermodilution method of measurement (inaccurate)
	• Clinical evidence of hypoperfusion
	• Hypotension
		• Transfer to higher acuity level of care for:
		  • Vasodilators (e.g., nitroglycerin, nitroprusside)
		  • IABP
		  • Surgical correction of ventricular septal defect with concurrent CABG unless rupture is small

Cardiac wall rupture	• Clinical indications of hypoperfusion
	• Clinical indications of cardiac tamponade
	  • Jugular venous distention
	  • Muffled heart sounds
	  • Hypotension
	  • Increased RAP, PAP, PAOP with equalization within 5 mm Hg
	• Sinus tachycardia or PEA
	• Eventual cardiopulmonary arrest with PEA
		• Pericardiocentesis
		• CPR; internal cardiac massage may be necessary
		• Surgical repair may be attempted (survival is rare)

Ventricular aneurysm	• Diffuse PMI, left ventricular heave • Atrial fibrillation or ventricular dysrhythmias • Persistent ST segment elevation • Chest x-ray shows left ventricular dilation • Echocardiography shows dyskinesis, left ventricular dilation • Clinical indications of LVF may be present • Clinical indications of systemic emboli may be present: cerebral emboli; peripheral emboli with acute arterial occlusion	• Antidysrhythmics (e.g., amiodarone) • Anticoagulants (e.g., heparin followed by warfarin) • Treatment of HF: ACE inhibitors; beta-blockers; diuretics; vasodilators; inotropes • Surgical resection may be performed • Ablative procedures may be necessary for recurrent ventricular dysrhythmias
Pericarditis	• Fever • Chest pain that worsens with deep breaths and lessens with sitting up and leaning forward • Pericardial friction rub • Elevated WBC, sedimentation rate • Diffuse ST segment elevation across the precordial leads • Chest x-ray may show pericardial effusion	• Aspirin or NSAIDs (e.g., ibuprofen, naproxen); colchicine may also be used • Discontinuance of anticoagulants • Pericardiocentesis may be required for pericardial effusion • Close monitoring for clinical indications of cardiac tamponade
Dressler syndrome (also referred to as *postmyocardial infarction syndrome*); late pericarditis, which is thought to be autoimmune	• Fever • Chest pain that worsens with deep breaths and lessens with sitting up and leaning forward • Pericardial friction rub • Elevated WBC, sedimentation rate • Diffuse ST segment elevation across the precordial leads • Chest x-ray may show pericardial effusion	• Aspirin or colchicine • Corticosteroids (e.g., prednisone) may be prescribed • Pericardiocentesis may be required for pericardial effusion • Close monitoring for clinical indications of cardiac tamponade

Sudden cardiac death	• Cardiopulmonary arrest	• Preventive measures include:
		  • Risk factor modification
		  • Antiplatelet aggregation therapy (e.g., ASA)
		  • Beta-blockers
		  • Encouragement of family members to learn CPR
		• Treatment: BLS and ACLS

and initiate appropriate management as soon as possible. Some complications are more common with specific types of MIs (see Table 3-23).

Patient and family instruction is crucially important after MI to prevent complications including reinfarction. Provide instruction and counseling regarding lifestyle modification and the need for pharmacologic therapy. Discuss cardiac risk factors including which modifiable risk factors the patient has and how to modify them. Emphasize nonpharmacologic therapies including a well-balanced diet to help the patient maintain normal weight. The diet should be low in saturated fat and trans-fatty acids, but should include monounsaturated fats (e.g., olive oil, canola oil). The diet needs to be high in fiber and contain fresh fruit, vegetables, whole grains, and adequate low-fat proteins. Recommend sodium restriction to 2 to 3 g/day. For patients with diabetes mellitus, provide instructions regarding an American Diabetes Association (ADA) diet for control of blood glucose. Counsel patients to abstain from tobacco products and limit alcohol consumption to one to two alcoholic beverages daily. Encourage patients to engage in regular aerobic exercise in moderation and to get adequate rest and relaxation. Include the use of relaxation, imagery, or biofeedback in the patient teaching. Provide instructions regarding sexual modifications to decrease the risk for angina. Teach the patient and the family how to differentiate between symptoms of angina and MI.

Pharmacologic agents should include prescribed medication regimens for the secondary prevention of MI. If indicated, these include aspirin, a beta-blocker, or an ACE inhibitor. To aid in modification of cardiac risk factors, the provider prescribes antihypertensives for hypertension; lipid-reducing agents (e.g., statins) for hyperlipidemia; oral hypoglycemics and/or insulin for diabetes mellitus; and thyroid hormone replacement or suppressive agents for thyroid disorders. Inform the patient of the prescribed drug names along with what the drugs are used for and what adverse effects to be aware of each time the drugs are taken.

Right Ventricular Myocardial Infarction

Clinical presentation and collaborative management of patients with right ventricular myocardial infarction (RVMI) varies from that of an LVMI. Assess for any clinical indications of RVMI, especially in the patient with an acute inferior or posterior MI. Look for ECG changes in V_{4R}, V_{5R}, and V_{6R} and listen for a right-sided S_4 and S_3. In addition, look for other clinical indications of RVF, such as JVD, hepatojugular reflux, and a murmur indicating tricuspid insufficiency (i.e., holosystolic murmur at lower left sternal border). If a central line is present, CVP may be increased. Because the right ventricle cannot propel adequate volumes of blood into the pulmonary circulation and to the left side, there will be minimal or no pulmonary congestion and the patient may have clinical indications of hypoperfusion (see Table 3-2).

Although patients with right ventricular MI will have backward failure of the right ventricle, they will also have forward failure (i.e., poor diastolic filling) of the left ventricle. Maintain adequate filling volumes by administering fluids as prescribed. Fluids may be normal saline or colloids (e.g., dextran, plasma protein fraction, and albumin). Avoid diuretics and/or venous vasodilators. Use selective arterial vasodilators (e.g., hydralazine [Apresoline]) to decrease afterload so that preload is not decreased. Administer inotropic agents (e.g., dobutamine [Dobutrex]) as prescribed to increase contractility of the right ventricle to improve filling of the left ventricle. Transfer patients with significant right ventricular infarction to a higher acuity care unit because these patients usually require hemodynamic monitoring to regulate fluid volume.

3.21 Learning Activity

Match the following treatments for acute MI with rationales for use. More than one may apply.

_____ 1. Fibrinolytics
_____ 2. PCI
_____ 3. ACE inhibitors
_____ 4. Nitroglycerin
_____ 5. Calcium channel blockers
_____ 6. Beta-blockers
_____ 7. ASA
_____ 8. Heparin
_____ 9. Glycoprotein IIb/IIIa inhibitors
_____10. Intra-aortic balloon pump (IABP)

a. Increases myocardial oxygen supply by reestablishing patency of the infarct-related artery
b. Decreases myocardial oxygen demand by blocking the effects of catecholamines
c. Increases myocardial oxygen supply by reducing spasm
d. Decreases myocardial oxygen demand by reducing preload
e. Prevents extension of a clot by decreasing platelet aggregation
f. Prevents extension of a clot by preventing the conversion of prothrombin to thrombin
g. Prevents ventricular dilation and adverse remodeling of the myocardium
h. Used for secondary prevention after MI
i. Decreases myocardial oxygen consumption by decreasing afterload
j. Increases myocardial oxygen supply by increasing coronary artery perfusion pressure.

Answers to this activity can be found in the Answer Key.

3.22 Synthesis Learning Activity: Crossword Puzzle

Complete the following crossword puzzle dealing with coronary artery disease and acute myocardial infarction.

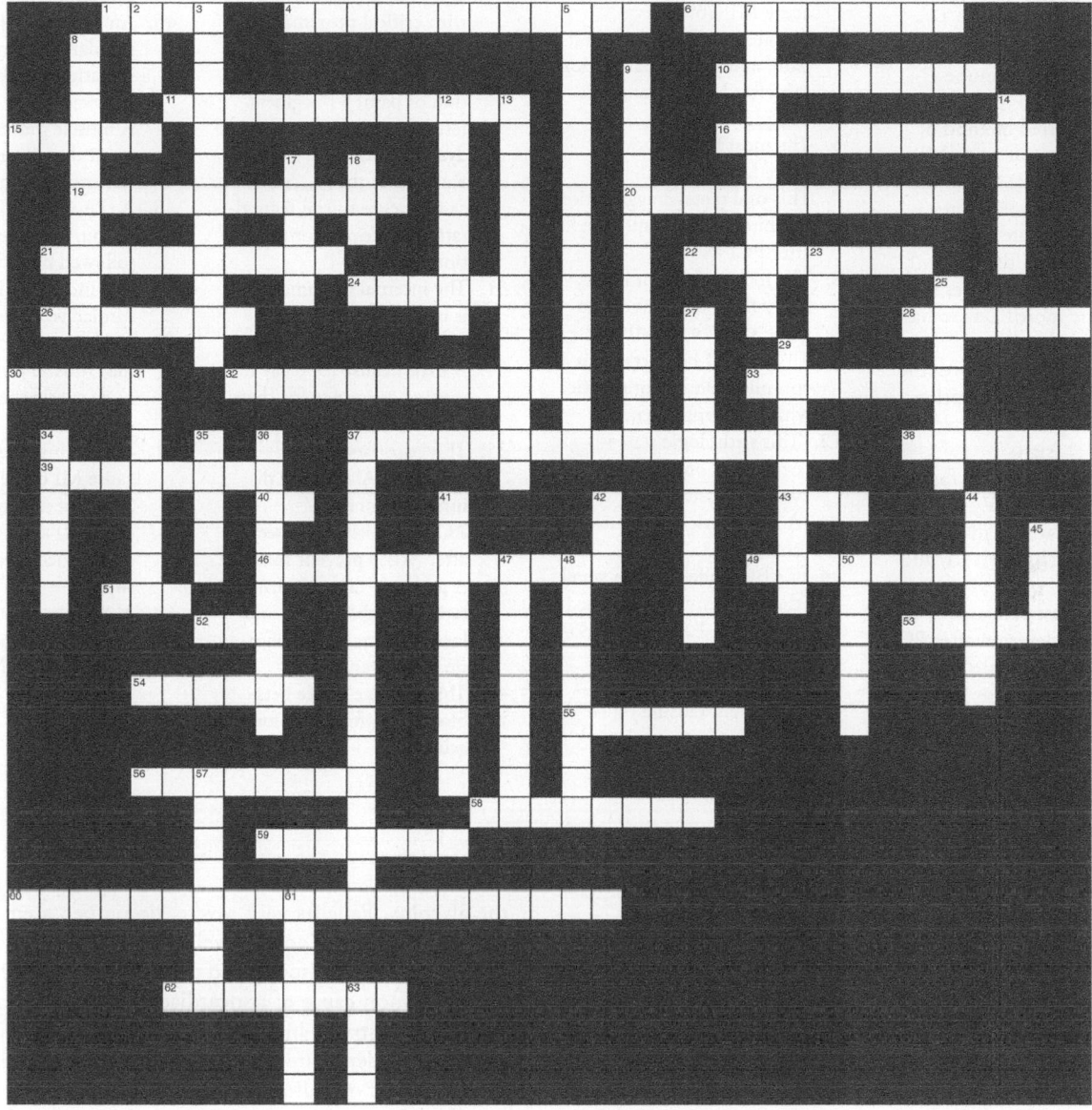

Answers to this activity can be found in the Answer Key.

ACROSS

1. This device is used to decrease afterload and increase myocardial perfusion in cardiogenic shock (abbrev.)

4. This tPA has a longer half-life than others and is administered as a single bolus

6. A glycoprotein IIb/IIIa inhibitor frequently used after PCI (generic)

10. The indicative leads for this cardiac wall are V_8 and V_9

11. The dysrhythmia most likely to cause death in an MI patient is ventricular _____

15. This is the initial therapy for hemodynamic consequences of right ventricular MI

16. This drug is a direct thrombin inhibitor used as an alternative to heparin

19. This PCI procedure opens an occluded artery using a shaving device

20. This PCI procedure opens an occluded artery using balloon dilation

21. This calcium channel blocker is used for coronary artery spasm

22. The analgesic of choice for acute MI

24. The artery sometimes used for CABG that has a high spasm potential

26. An indirect thrombin inhibitor used to prevent extension of a clot or reocclusion

28. A new holosystolic murmur at the lower sternum, increased Svo_2, and shock indicate rupture of the ___

30. A commonly used format for chest pain description

32. These drugs are used to prevent ventricular dysrhythmias post-MI and also for secondary prevention

33. The indicative leads for this cardiac wall are I and aVL and/or V_5 and V_6

37. A group of diseases characterized by thickening and loss of elasticity (calcification) of arterial walls

38. This pathologic state is evidenced on ECG by ST segment elevation

39. An activity that is likely to decrease body weight, BP, lipids, and stress

40. Death of myocardial tissue (abbrev.)

43. S$_3$, dyspnea, and crackles indicate this complication of acute MI (abbrev.)
46. The most common complication of MI
49. _____ syndrome is a late pericarditis that is thought to be an autoimmune response
51. The preferred method of reperfusion for acute MI (abbrev.)
52. Bad cholesterol (abbrev.)
53. These drugs are used to treat pericarditis (abbrev.)
54. Patients with diabetes mellitus are more likely to have this type of MI
55. Clenched fist held over the sternum with description of chest pain is referred to as _____ sign
56. The indicative leads for this cardiac wall are V$_3$ and V$_4$
58. The indicative leads for this cardiac wall are II, III, and aVF
59. Acute chest pain and/or ST segment elevation after PCI may indicate acute ___
60. This risk factor for CAD is treated with folic acid
62. New onset, crescendo, and variant are all categorized as this type of angina

DOWN

2. This platelet aggregation inhibitor is an important aspect of initial treatment of acute MI (abbrev.)
3. Elevated temperature, chest pain, and pericardial friction rub after MI indicates this complication
5. The most likely cause of acute MI
7. This oral platelet aggregation inhibitor is frequently used after PCI
8. The inotropic agent most likely to be used for cardiogenic shock with MI
9. This type of hemorrhage is a complication of fibrinolytics with dire consequences
12. This pathologic state is evidenced on ECG by T wave inversion
13. A nitrate used for acute chest pain
14. CABG done through small thoracotomy incision used for LIMA-LAD anastomosis (abbrev.)
17. A device used during PCI to prevent closure
18. A value of greater than 30 is considered obese (abbrev.)

23. Good cholesterol (abbrev.)
25. This syndrome is characterized by chest pain with deep T wave inversion in V$_2$, V$_3$ and is associated with critical proximal LAD stenosis
27. This is evidenced by cessation of pain, ST segment return to baseline, and dysrhythmias
29. Rupture of the ___ muscle causes acute mitral regurgitation; a serious complication of acute MI
31. The internal mammary is now referred to as the internal ___
34. A major cause for delay in seeking assistance for chest pain
35. This coronary artery supplies RA, RV, and the inferior wall of LV
36. ACE inhibitors are used after MI to prevent this
37. A group of diseases characterized by thickening and loss of elasticity (calcification) of arterial walls
41. This cardioselective beta-blocker is often used for acute MI

42. The general term used for undifferentiated acute ischemic chest pain (abbrev.)
44. This type of angina is caused by spasm
45. An isolated right ventricular MI may be seen in patients with _____ (abbrev.)
47. A muscle protein measurement that is sensitive but not specific for MI
48. A tPA with short half-life so must be given as bolus followed by infusion
50. The indicative leads for this cardiac wall are V$_1$ and V$_2$
57. Measurement of this cardiac muscle protein is the most specific test for acute MI
61. Use of this drug may cause MI by stimulating SNS (increasing oxygen demand) and causing spasm (decreasing oxygen supply)
63. New onset occurrence of this type of block may indicate acute MI (abbrev.)

HEART FAILURE

Heart failure (HF) is a clinical syndrome characterized by dyspnea, activity intolerance, and fluid overload, which adversely affects the patient's functional status and quality of life (Yancy, Jessup, Bozkurt, et al., 2013). Dyspnea, crackles, and edema are clinical indications of intravascular and interstitial volume overload. Fatigue and exercise intolerance are clinical indications of tissue hypoperfusion.

Acute decompensated HF is the sudden or gradual onset of the clinical indications of HF, which necessitate unplanned office visits, emergency department visits, and/or hospitalization. Decompensation is a sustained deterioration in function of at least one New York Heart Association (NYHA) class. A nearly universal finding is pulmonary and systemic congestion due to increased left and right heart filling pressures (Gheorghiade, Vaduganathan, Fonorow et al., 2013).

Pulmonary edema is fluid in the alveolus, which impairs the gas exchange and causes hypoxemia by impairing diffusion between alveolus and capillary. Pulmonary edema may be classified as cardiac versus noncardiac pulmonary edema. Cardiac pulmonary edema stems from acute left ventricular failure and is manifested by an elevated PAP with an elevated PAOP; the difference between PA diastolic and PAOP will be less than 5 mm Hg. The PAOP is an indicator of pulmonary capillary hydrostatic pressure; the elevated PAOP pushes fluid from the pulmonary capillary into the interstitium and finally into the alveolus. Patients with severe, decompensated HF require transfer to a higher acuity level of care. These patients require hemodynamic monitoring and titrated inotropic infusions. The most common cause of noncardiac pulmonary edema is acute respiratory distress syndrome (ARDS). Noncardiac and cardiac pulmonary edema are frequently differentiated using invasive hemodynamic monitoring. Noncardiac pulmonary edema is manifested by an elevated PAP but with a normal PAOP. The difference between PA diastolic and PAOP will be greater than 5 mm Hg, which indicates pulmonary hypertension. In noncardiac pulmonary edema, fluid *leaks* from the pulmonary capillary into the interstitium and alveolus due to the increased permeability of the damaged alveolocapillary membrane. ARDS patients also require a higher acuity level of care; therefore, early identification and the rapid facilitation of transfer are required. There will be more discussion about ARDS in the pulmonary chapter and the remainder of the discussion here will focus on HF and/or cardiac pulmonary edema.

HF can result from many causes (Box 3-2). CAD is the primary risk factor for HF, especially in patients with a history of MI. Congenital heart disease and valvular heart disease are contributory factors in the development of HF. Other conditions such as hypertension, diabetes, obesity, alcoholism, smoking, high or low hematocrit, sedentary lifestyle, obstructive sleep apnea, and consumption of a high-fat/high-salt diet all increase the risk for HF.

BOX 3-2

Etiologic Factors of Heart Failure

Left Ventricular Failure
- CAD/LV infarction
- Cardiomyopathy
- Hypertension
- Dysrhythmias
- Volume overload
- Valvular disease: mitral or aortic
- Ventricular septal defect
- Coarctation of aorta
- Myocarditis
- Cardiac tamponade

Right Ventricular Failure
- LVF
- CAD/RV infarction
- Pulmonary hypertension
- Passive: mitral valve disease
- Active: hypoxemia; pulmonary embolism
- Dysrhythmias
- Volume overload
- Valvular disease: mitral or pulmonic
- Ventricular septal defect
- Cardiomyopathy
- Myocardial contusion

Biventricular Failure
- Increased demand
- Thyrotoxicosis
- Anemia
- Pregnancy
- Systemic infection
- Beriberi
- Paget's disease
- Electrolyte imbalance
- Hyponatremia
- Hypokalemia
- Hypocalcemia
- Hypomagnesemia
- Hypophosphatemia

Patients with HF frequently have comorbidities, especially those conditions that are risk factors for CAD. Common comorbid conditions in a patient with HF include CAD, MI, hypertension (systolic BP greater than 140 mm Hg), renal insufficiency, hyperlipidemia, diabetes mellitus, atrial fibrillation, and COPD and/or asthma.

Decompensation in a patient with HF results from the following:
- Progression of left ventricular dysfunction
- New or worsening ischemia
- Hypoxemia
- Worsening of anemia
- Drugs such as nonsteroidal antiinflammatory drugs (NSAIDs) or the initiation of beta-blocker dosage at too high a dose

Hypertension, new onset of dysrhythmias, particularly atrial fibrillation, missed or suboptimal medication, and dietary indiscretion, such as high-salt foods and alcohol, are additional risk factors for decompensation.

The pathophysiology of HF (Figure 3-57) is characterized by adaptive compensatory processes progressing to maladaptive processes. In the short term, mechanisms compensate for the failing heart, but in the long term, the mechanisms trigger a process of pathologic growth and remodeling. There is also a LVF and RVF interrelationship (Figure 3-58) because most failure begins as a left ventricle problem and due to retrograde pressure and backup, it ultimately results in RVF. Primary

therapies for HF are directed toward blocking dysfunctional compensatory mechanisms with signal-modulating inhibitors, such as beta-blockers, alpha- and beta-blockers, RAAS inhibitors or blockers (e.g., ACE inhibitors and ARBs), and aldosterone antagonists.

HF is classified as left or right, but the most common cause of RVF is LVF. The onset of failure may be acute or chronic. The output state is either low (e.g., myocardial infarction, cardiomyopathy) or high (e.g., thyrotoxicosis, anemia). The pumping defect may either be backward due to high volume and engorgement behind the failing ventricle or forward due to low filling volume for the ventricle in front of the failing ventricle. Finally, HF can be either systolic or diastolic.

Approximately 60% to 70% of HF is due to systolic dysfunction while approximately 30% to 40% is due to diastolic dysfunction. With systolic dysfunction, there is an inability of the ventricle to shorten against a load. The left ventricle loses its ability to contract normally against progressive increases in afterload. Because systolic dysfunction is, in essence, a pump problem, possible causes include MI, myocardial contusion, myocarditis, dilated cardiomyopathy, hypertension, valvular heart disease, electrolyte imbalance, and dysrhythmias. Hemodynamically there will be decreased contractility, increased volumes and pressures, and the EF will be less than 40%. Clinical indications include a displaced PMI, JVD, S_3, crackles, dyspnea, peripheral edema, and cardiomegaly. Direct drug therapy at treating the cause. Provide diuretics in the presence of congestive symptoms. Administer other agents as prescribed, which will likely include an ACE inhibitor or ARB, a beta-blocker or alpha- and beta-blocker, an inotropic agent for diuretic-resistant congestion, antidysrhythmic, and/or anticoagulants. Avoid giving a pure alpha-blocker.

Diastolic dysfunction is a filling problem. There is impairment in left ventricular filling at near normal or mildly elevated left atrial and ventricular pressures. This is due to a decrease in ventricular compliance, so small changes in volume cause a disproportionate increase in pressure. Possible causes of diastolic dysfunction include myocardial ischemia, hypertrophic cardiomyopathy, ventricular hypertrophy, constrictive pericarditis or cardiac tamponade, valvular heart disease, and aging. There will be increased contractility, a normal EF, and increased cardiac pressures with normal or slightly increased cardiac volumes. Clinical indications include S_4, crackles, dyspnea, peripheral edema, precordial heave, and a normal heart sound. Direct drug therapy at treating the cause. Provide diuretics if there are congestive symptoms. Administer other agents as prescribed, which will likely include an ACE inhibitor or ARB, beta-blocker or alpha- and beta-blocker, a calcium channel blocker, and/or an antidysrhythmic.

HF is also classified by functional status. The NYHA Functional Classification system is most typically used and includes the following classifications:
- Class I: patients with cardiac disease but without resulting limitation of physical activity. Ordinary physical activity does not cause these patients undue fatigue, palpitation, dyspnea, or angina.
- Class II: patients with cardiac disease resulting in slight limitation of physical activity. These patients are comfortable at rest but ordinary physical activity results in fatigue, palpitation, dyspnea, or angina.

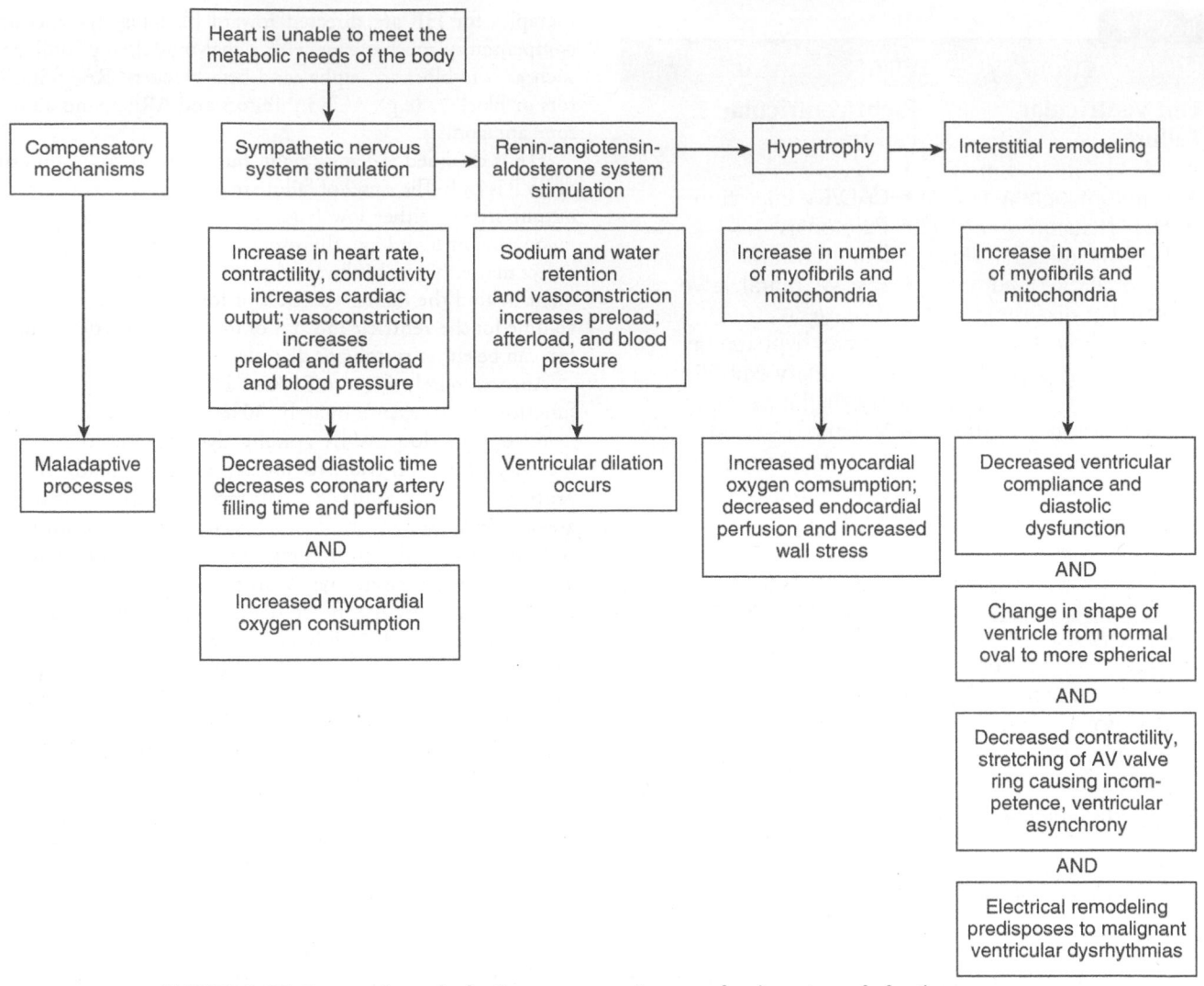

FIGURE 3-57 Progression of adaptive compensatory mechanisms to maladaptive processes seen in heart failure. (From Dennison, R. D. [2013]. *Pass CCRN!* [4th ed.]. St. Louis, MO: Elsevier.)

- Class III: patients with cardiac disease resulting in marked limitation of physical activity. These patients are comfortable at rest but less than ordinary activity causes fatigue, palpitation, dyspnea, or angina.
- Class IV: patients with cardiac disease resulting in an inability to carry on any physical activity without discomfort. These patients may experience fatigue, palpitation, dyspnea, or angina even at rest. If any physical activity is attempted, discomfort is increased.

The American College of Cardiology/American Heart Association (ACCF/AHA) classify HF with the following staging system (Yancy, Jessup, Bozkurt, et al., 2013):

- Class A: These patients are at high risk for developing heart failure and often have hypertension, CAD, diabetes mellitus, and a family history of cardiomyopathy.
- Class B: These patients have asymptomatic heart failure, but have a history of previous MI, left ventricular systolic dysfunction, and/or asymptomatic valvular disease.
- Class C: These patients with symptomatic heart failure have known structural heart disease, shortness of breath and fatigue, and reduced exercise tolerance.
- Class D: These patients with refractory end-stage heart failure have marked symptoms at rest despite maximal medical therapy.

The clinical presentation of a patient with HF stems from multifaceted and complex interrelationships with the pulmonary, hematologic, endocrine, renal, and vascular systems. The first symptoms of HF are usually cough, exertional dyspnea, edema, or fatigue but many clinical findings (Box 3-3) may indicate LVF or RVF. The health care provider uses patient symptoms, diagnostic laboratory findings, ABGs, and radiologic examinations to diagnose HF.

A noninvasive method to evaluate cardiac index is the proportional pulse pressure parameter. Calculate the proportional pulse pressure as the (systolic BP – diastolic BP) / systolic BP. A proportional pulse pressure of less than 25% is associated with a cardiac index of less than 2.2 L/min/m^2 and HF.

Serum electrolyte levels may reveal and/or confirm imbalances, especially hypokalemia, hypocalcemia, and/or hypomagnesemia. Serum albumin levels may show hypoproteinemia, which can contribute to edema. ABGs may show hypoxemia, especially in the presence of pulmonary edema and acid-base imbalances, including lactic acidosis in severe hypoperfusion states. Drug levels may reveal abnormal levels of digoxin and antidysrhythmic agents. The thyroid profile may reveal an abnormal thyroid function, a potential cause

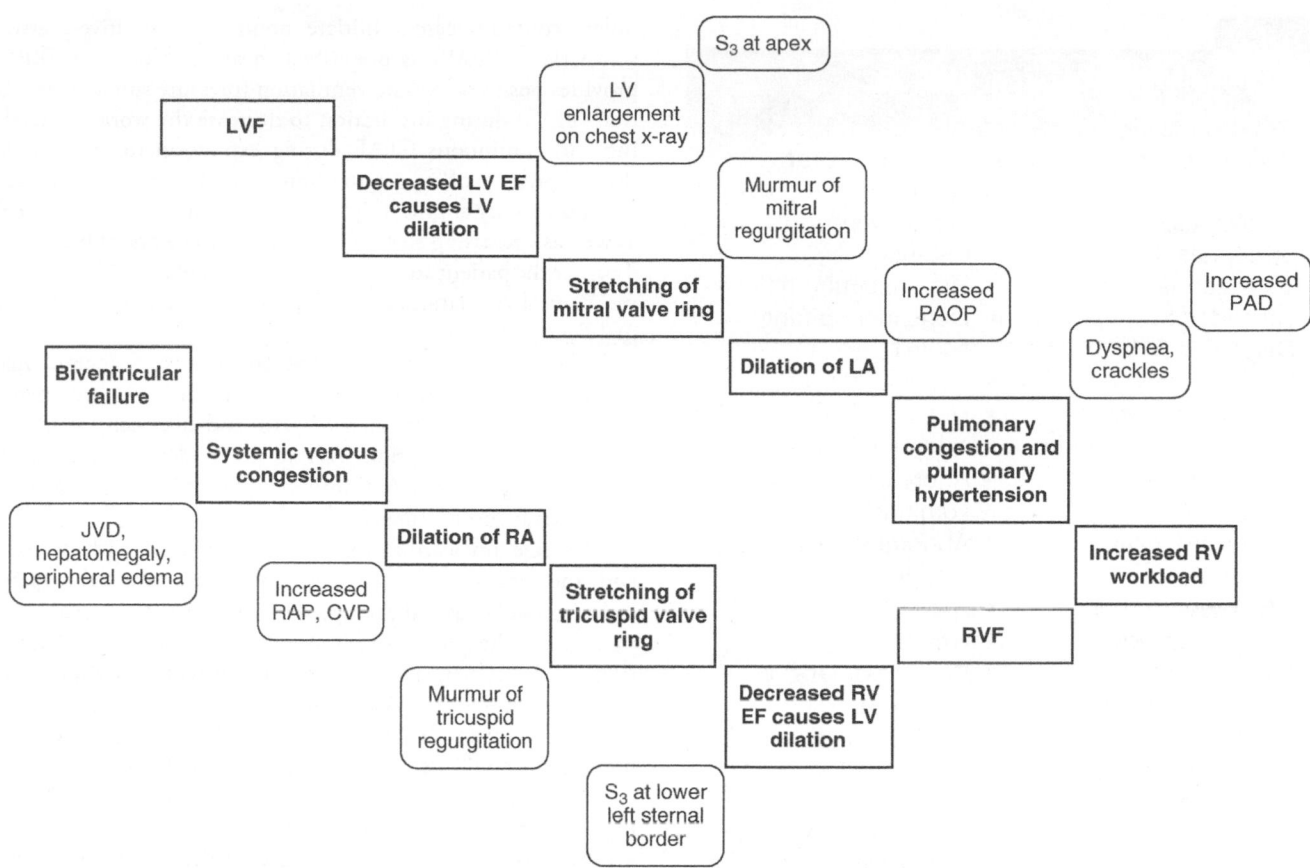

FIGURE 3-58 Left ventricular failure progressing to biventricular failure. Bold square blocks indicate pathophysiologic sequence, while rounded boxes indicate clinical indications associated with the pathophysiologic events. *CVP,* Central venous pressure; *EF,* ejection fraction; *JVD,* jugular venous distention; *LA,* left atrium; *LV,* left ventricular; *LVF,* left ventricular failure; *PAD,* pulmonary artery diastolic pressure; *PAOP,* pulmonary artery occlusive pressure; *RA,* right atrium; *RAP,* right atrial pressure; *RV,* right ventricle; *RVF,* right ventricular failure. (From Dennison, R. D. [2013]. *Pass CCRN!* [4th ed.]. St. Louis, MO: Elsevier.)

of HF. The CBC may show anemia or leukocytosis. BUN and creatinine levels may be elevated, indicating renal impairment. Urine may show proteinuria and/or presence of RBCs or casts.

An elevated BNP level correlates with increased left ventricular end-diastolic pressure and volume. Normal levels are less than 100 g/mL while levels greater than 100 g/mL indicate HF. Other conditions associated with increased BNP levels include cardiac inflammation, primary pulmonary hypertension, renal failure, cirrhosis, and endocrine disorders, such as primary hyperaldosteronism and Cushing's syndrome. BNP may be elevated in elderly patients.

Diagnostic tests are useful in confirming HF and may be helpful in identifying the cause of HF. Chest x-ray will likely show cardiac enlargement, dilation, and possible pulmonary congestion. Cardiac catheterization and coronary angiography may show CAD, valve abnormalities, increased cardiac pressures, decreased ejection fraction in systolic dysfunction, and increased ejection fraction in diastolic dysfunction. Computed tomography (CT) evaluates left ventricular wall motion and detects cardiac tumors, MI, and/or aortic aneurysm. Echocardiography confirms changes in chamber size, wall thickness, and valve motion. Electrocardiography (ECG) indicates myocardial ischemia/infarction, as well as atrial enlargement and/or ventricular hypertrophy. A multiple-gated acquisition (MUGA)

scan evaluates cardiac function, determines ejection fraction, and detects wall motion abnormalities.

Collaborative management of HF begins with treatment of the cause and/or contributing factors of HF. Examples of treating the cause includes the following:

- Reperfusion in acute MI along neurohormonal antagonism with a beta-blocker (e.g., metoprolol [Lopressor]) or an alpha- and beta-blocker (e.g., carvedilol) and ACE inhibitor or ARB
- Revascularization of patients with CAD
- Valve replacement if required, especially for acute valvular disorders such as ruptured papillary muscle with acute mitral regurgitation
- Treatment of symptomatic or life-threatening dysrhythmias with antidysrhythmic agents, electrical therapies (e.g., cardioversion, defibrillation, pacemaker, automatic implantable cardiac defibrillator), or surgical procedures (e.g., ablation)
- Continuous positive airway pressure (CPAP) for obstructive sleep apnea
- Avoidance of certain pharmacologic agents, such as antidysrhythmic agents which decrease contractility, most calcium channel blockers, and NSAIDs, which increase resistance to diuretics

Instruct the patient on recommended medical treatment by ACC/AHA HF stage (Yancy, Jessup, Bozkurt et al., 2013). For patients at stage A, this includes treatment of hypertension and

BOX 3-3

Clinical Indications of Left or Right Ventricular Failure

Left Ventricular Failure
- Tachypnea, dyspnea, orthopnea, PND
- Tachycardia
- Left-sided S_3
- Displaced PMI, heave at apex
- Crackles, wheezes
- Cough, frothy sputum, hemoptysis
- Diaphoresis
- Pulsus alternans
- Oliguria
- Weakness, fatigue
- Mental confusion
- Murmur of MR
- ABGs: decreased Pao_2, Sao_2
- Hemodynamics
  - Elevated PA, PAOP
  - Decreased CO/CI
- Abnormal chest X-ray
  - Cardiomegaly
  - Engorged pulmonary vasculature
  - Kerley B lines
  - Pleural effusion
- ECG
  - Left atrial enlargement
  - Left ventricular hypertrophy
  - Atrial dysrhythmias

Right Ventricular Failure
- Jugular venous distention
- Hepatojugular reflux
- Dependent pitting edema
- Heave at sternum
- Hepatomegaly/ splenomegaly
- Anorexia, nausea, vomiting
- Abdominal pain and bloating
- Ascites
- Nocturia
- Weakness, fatigue
- Weight gain
- Murmur of TR
- Right-sided S_3
- Hemodynamics
  - Elevated CVP, RAP
- Abnormal liver function studies
  - ALT
  - AST
  - LDH
- ECG
  - Right atrial enlargement
  - Right ventricular hypertrophy
  - Atrial dysrhythmias

diabetes, control of metabolic syndrome, avoidance of alcohol and illicit drugs, smoking cessation, regular exercise, and lipid control. For patients at stage B, this includes all recommendations for stage A along with an ACE inhibitor and an ARB as warranted, a beta-blocker or alpha- and beta-blocker as warranted, along with consideration of an ICD. For patients at stage C, this includes all recommendations for stages A and B, along with an ACE inhibitor and an ARB, a beta-blocker or alpha- and beta-blocker, and a diuretic. Selected patients at stage C should also receive an aldosterone antagonist (e.g., spironolactone), digoxin, and/or hydralazine/nitrates. Patients at stage D should receive all the interventions for groups A, B, and C plus a discussion of end-of-life care and consideration of extraordinary measures, such as chronic inotropes, permanent mechanical support, cardiac transplantation, and experimental surgeries or drugs.

For patients with HF with pulmonary edema, provide oxygen by nasal cannula at 2 to 6 L/min to maintain Sao_2 of 95%

unless contraindicated. Initiate noninvasive positive-pressure ventilation (BiPAP) as prescribed to avert intubation. BiPAP provides positive-pressure ventilation (pressure support ventilation [PSV]) during inspiration to decrease the work of breathing and continuous CPAP during expiration to increase the driving pressure of oxygen to improve oxygenation and decrease intrapulmonary shunt. This works by opening collapsed alveoli as well as decreasing surface tension and the work of breathing. Transfer the patient to a higher acuity level of care if intubation, mechanical ventilation, and PEEP are required to maintain normal $Paco_2$ and Pao_2.

To optimize oxygen delivery, treatment of anemia may be required. More than half of patients with HF are anemic with a hemoglobin less than 12 g/dL and treatment of anemia improves cardiac function. Administer packed RBCs if acute anemia is significant. Administer erythropoietin (Epogen) or iron to treat chronic anemia.

Decrease myocardial oxygen consumption with physical and emotional rest. Promote rest after meals, personal hygiene, toileting, and physical therapy. Prevent the Valsalva maneuver by teaching the patient to exhale when turning in bed. Administer stool softeners as prescribed and provide a bedside commode for elimination. Also thoroughly explain procedures and the reasons for procedures, such as visiting hours, and explain monitoring equipment, including monitor alarms. Provide for the patient's physical comfort by control of temperature, lighting, and noise. Provide appropriate nutrition, usually given in a soft, low-sodium (i.e., 2 to 3 g/day) diet. Administer anxiolytics as prescribed (usually diazepam [Valium], lorazepam [Ativan], or alprazolam [Xanax]). Instruct the patient regarding relaxation techniques and encourage their utilization. Keep the patient's family informed regarding the patient's progress and status.

Decrease preload by positioning the patient in the low Fowler's position with legs dependent. Follow sodium and fluid restrictions accurately. Restrict fluids to less than 2000 mL/24 hr and sodium to less than 2 to 3 g/day. Record the patient's weight daily to detect early fluid retention. Administer venous vasodilators (e.g., nitroglycerin [Tridil], morphine) to decrease preload in systolic dysfunction, but they are not recommended in diastolic dysfunction because they would result in decreased ventricular filling volumes. Initiate dialysis if necessary for a patient in renal failure. Manage the overhydration in HF refractory with traditional therapies such as fluid restriction and diuretics with continuous renal replacement therapy (CRRT).

Decrease afterload by the administration of arterial vasodilators. Administer for hypertensive patients. Avoid the use of calcium channel blockers in the treatment of HF, but an exception is the use of amlodipine (Norvasc) and felodipine (Plendil) to treat diastolic dysfunction. Prevent activation of angiotensin II with the resultant vasoconstriction and increase in afterload with ACE inhibitors or ARBs. Transfer the patient to a higher acuity level of care when IABP is required to treat HF and hypotension. Pharmacologic therapies are crucial for patients with HF. Administer beta-blockers or an alpha-blocker plus a beta-blocker (e.g., carvedilol [Coreg]) as prescribed for class II and III HF resulting from systolic and diastolic dysfunction classes. These blockers protect the heart from excessive catecholamines by decreasing left ventricular mass and volume, changing the shape of the ventricle from spherical to elliptical and increasing

TABLE 3-30   Vasodilators

Drug	Arteries	Veins
Clevidipine (Cleviprex)	Yes	No
Fenoldopam mesylate (Corlopam)	Yes	No
Hydralazine (Apresoline)	Yes	No
Milrinone (Primacor)	Yes	Yes
Minoxidil (Loniten)	Yes	No
Morphine sulfate	No	Yes
Nesiritide (Natrecor)	Yes	Yes
Nicardipine (Cardene)	Yes	Yes
Nifedipine (Procardia)	Yes	Yes
Nitroglycerin (Tridil)	Only if greater than 1 mcg/kg/min	Yes
Nitroprusside (Nipride)	Yes	Yes
Phentolamine (Regitine)	Yes	Yes
Prazosin (Minipress)	Yes	Yes

the patient's exercise capacity. Start dosages low and gradually increase while monitoring closely for decompensation. Contraindications for the use of beta-blockers in HF include decompensated HF, cardiogenic shock, acute pulmonary edema, hemodynamic instability requiring IV inotropic support, second- or third-degree AV block, sick sinus syndrome, and severe hepatic impairment. Only cardioselective beta-blockers are used cautiously in asthma.

Administer diuretics for HF with evidence of or a predisposition to fluid retention to eliminate symptoms as well as physical signs of fluid retention, such as JVD and/or edema. Provide loop diuretics (e.g., furosemide [Lasix], bumetanide [Bumex]) as prescribed, but note that continuous infusion may be superior to intermittent boluses. Combine aldosterone-antagonists (e.g., aldosterone [Aldactone], eplerenone [Inspra]) with loop diuretics or administer as a single agent as prescribed. These aldosterone-antagonists have a relatively weak diuretic effect for patients with normal renin but are much more effective in patients who have edema associated with either increased production or decreased elimination of renin. Administer two or more diuretics together; diuretics also act synergistically with ACE inhibitors. Closely monitor potassium levels when the patient is receiving diuretics, ACE inhibitors, or ARBs. Avoid aldosterone-antagonists in patients with renal insufficiency. Increase renal blood flow with a short-term use of a drug such as fenoldopam (Corlopam); however, overuse may decrease blood volume, decrease CO, and lead to organ hypoperfusion and prerenal azotemia. Observe for drug interactions because diuretics may alter the efficacy and toxicity of other drugs used to treat HF (e.g., ACE inhibitors, beta-blockers).

Administer ACE inhibitors and ARBs for HF resulting from systolic and diastolic dysfunction. ACE inhibitors block conversion of angiotensin I to angiotensin II and the resultant vasoconstriction and aldosterone release. ARBs block angiotensin II and the resultant vasoconstriction and aldosterone release. ARBs are frequently used if a patient has angioedema or cough due to ACE inhibitors. They are also preferred for the affected African American population.

ACE inhibitors include captopril (Capoten), enalapril (Vasotec), lisinopril (Zestril, Prinivil), ramipril (Altace), benazepril HCl (Lotensin), quinapril HCl (Accupril), fosinopril (Monopril), moexipril HCl (Univasc), trandolapril (Mavik), and perindopril (Aceon). ARBs include losartan (Cozaar), valsartan (Diovan), telmisartan (Micardis), irbesartan (Avapro), candesartan (Atacand), eprosartan (Teveten), and olmesartan (Benicar). If the patient does not tolerate ACE inhibitors or ARBs, the provider may prescribe a combination of nitrates and hydralazine (Apresoline). Be aware that hypotension and angioedema, especially with ACE inhibitors, may occur. Hyperkalemia may also occur, especially when provided in combination with an aldosterone antagonist, such as spironolactone (Aldactone). Proteinuria and renal failure are also associated with ACE inhibitors and ARBs.

Vasodilators (Table 3-30) prescribed for HF include venodilators to decrease preload and arterial vasodilators to decrease afterload. Mixed vasodilators dilate both the veins and arteries. Many vasodilator drugs require administration by continuous IV infusion, which requires a transfer to a higher acuity level of care.

Nesiritide (Natrecor) is a recombinant form of BNP used for decompensated HF with dyspnea at rest or with minimal activities and clinical evidence of fluid overload as well as for systolic and diastolic dysfunction. The drug binds to the alpha-type natriuretic peptide receptors on the surface of vascular smooth muscle and endothelial cells, which results in:

- Dilation of arteries and reduction of SVR
- Dilation of veins and reduction of intracardiac pressure and volume
- Decreased aldosterone and norepinephrine levels
- Inhibition of the RAAS and endothelin pathways prompting fluid and sodium release

Nesiritide (Natrecor) improves symptoms of decompensated HF more than NTG with less proarrhythmogenesis and tachycardia than dobutamine. It is contraindicated in patients with hypovolemia, profound hypotension (e.g., cardiogenic shock), aortic stenosis, hypertrophic or restrictive cardiomyopathy, and constrictive pericarditis or cardiac tamponade. Recent studies indicate that nesiritide worsens renal function. Consequently, its use has decreased significantly. An endothelin receptor antagonist (tezosentan [Veletri]) acts as a vasodilator. It does not increase heart rate, but higher doses have been associated with hypotension. Recent study has shown mixed results in terms of benefit.

Administer inotropic agents for the temporary treatment of diuretic-refractory decompensation and stage D HF to increase contractility and improve the patient's quality of life. While inotropic agents have hemodynamic effects, they increase myocardial oxygen consumption. Inotropics have not been shown to improve HF survival; therefore, they are generally not recommended. However, cardiac glycosides (e.g., digoxin) along with diuretics, ACE inhibitors, and beta-blockers may improve symptoms in patients with HF due to left ventricular systolic dysfunction with a dilated ventricle. Cardiac glycosides are used to improve cardiac contractility, which increases ejection fraction and exercise tolerance, inhibit the SNS which reduces norepinephrine and renin activity, and slow the heart rate, especially in atrial fibrillation. A major drawback of cardiac glycosides is the narrow therapeutic/toxic ratio.

Administer sympathetic stimulants (e.g., dobutamine) as prescribed; these agents are particularly helpful if HF occurs in the presence of acute MI. They increase contractility by stimulating beta-receptors and thus may increase the potential for ectopy. Dobutamine is preferred unless the patient is hypotensive because it causes less tachycardia and decreases afterload rather than increasing it as with dopamine. Administer parenteral phosphodiesterase (PDE) inhibitors (e.g., milrinone [Primacor], inamrinone [Inocor]) if there is no response to digitalis, diuretics, or vasodilators. PDE inhibitors increase contractility by inhibiting phosphodiesterase and cause vasodilation to decrease preload and afterload.

Atrial dysrhythmias frequently resolve with the treatment of HF because of the decrease in the atrial stretch and irritability. Provide digoxin to decrease the ventricular response rate by increasing the refractoriness of the AV node. Administer anticoagulants to prevent mural thrombi and embolic events. Avoid ventricular antidysrhythmics except for immediately life-threatening ventricular dysrhythmia. Class III antidysrhythmics, such as amiodarone, are preferred over class I agents (e.g., procainamide, lidocaine). Correct electrolyte deficiencies that may cause dysrhythmias and alter the efficacy and safety of antidysrhythmic agents.

Prepare and educate the patient for a dual-chamber pacemaker with rate modulation, if planned. Patients with severe HF and poor activity tolerance often benefit from a pacemaker because it will increase the heart rate in response to physical activity. Provide cardiac resynchronization therapy (CRT) with atriobiventricular pacing in HF patients with an ejection fraction of 35% or less, a QRS of at least 130 milliseconds (0.13 second), and for patients in NYHA classes III to IV. Approximately 30% to 50% of patients with HF have ventricular asynchrony and 80% of patients with advanced HF have LBBB with resultant ventricular asynchrony. Atriobiventricular pacing restores synchronous ventricular contraction to optimize left ventricular filling and improve cardiac output, resulting in improved exercise tolerance, improved quality of life, and a reduction in mortality.

In patients with new pacemakers, monitor for 100% ventricular capture as well as any lengthening of the QRS that might indicate loss of capture of one of the ventricles (usually the left ventricle). Restrict movement of the arm to prevent lead dislodgement or bleeding in the pacemaker pocket. Instruct patients to avoid pushing, pulling, or lifting anything heavier than 5 pounds for 1 to 2 weeks after surgery, what symptoms to report, and other instructions for an implanted pacemaker. Monitor patients for complications such as infection.

Patients with renal artery stenosis are likely to develop hypertension and/or HF. Prepare the patient for renal artery angioplasty and stents for patient with renal artery stenosis, as requested.

Surgical approaches to treat HF include dynamic cardiomyoplasty, partial left ventriculectomy, Dor procedure, left ventricular splints and wraps, and cardiac transplantation. Dynamic cardiomyoplasty involves stimulating the latissimus dorsi muscle (LDM), which is wrapped around the heart, with electrical impulses to contract with each heartbeat. Partial left ventriculectomy (also referred to as the *Batista heart failure procedure*) is most suited for dilated cardiomyopathy. It involves resection of a wedge of the left ventricular wall to restore the volume-mass-diameter relationship of the left ventricle. The mitral and/or tricuspid valve may be replaced concurrently. The Dor procedure (also referred to as *endoventricular circular patch plasty*) involves cutting out areas of hypofunctioning myocardium, then repairing the opening in the wall with a synthetic or autologous tissue circular patch. Current clinical trials are using left-ventricular splints and wraps to arrest and reverse remodeling of the failing heart. Devices in this category include Myocor Myosplint, involving two epicardial pads and a transventricular tension member. The two pads are placed on the surface of the heart with the load-bearing tension member passing through the ventricle, connecting the pads and drawing the ventricular walls toward one another. Another such device is the Acorn Cardiac Support Device, which wraps the heart in a mesh bag to prevent further dilation and failure. A Dacron wrap is pulled over the base of the heart and attached with sutures. All of these procedures are of questionable value and are either not recommended or not addressed by the current ACC/AHA guidelines.

Class II or IV HF patients with a life expectancy of less than 24 hours meet the criteria for cardiac transplantation. Candidates must be younger than 65 years of age at the time of placement listing. If retransplantation or a heart-kidney or heart-liver is required, candidates must be 55 years of age or younger; however, consideration of physiologic age is gaining interest. Candidates must have acute HF or cardiogenic shock from an acute MI that is refractory to medical therapy and requires mechanical support, or the patient must not be able to be weaned from cardiopulmonary bypass.

As the supply of acceptable donor hearts remains insufficient for the number of patients who require them, mechanical devices offer a temporary alternative. Devices continue to be developed and tested as a permanent alternative to cardiac transplantation. The goal is to stabilize and improve the hemodynamic condition of the patient with loss of ventricular function. Complications include infection and thromboembolism, bleeding, and hypertension. The ventricular assist device (VAD) is used in severe cases especially if the patient is a candidate for cardiac transplantation.

Patients with pulmonary disease have primary right ventricular failure due to pulmonary hypertension. Because the most likely cause of pulmonary hypertension is hypoxemia, oxygen is the primary treatment in patients with hypoxemia and pulmonary hypertension; provide oxygen to maintain Sao_2 of at least 90%. Administer pulmonary vasodilators as prescribed; these are especially useful in primary pulmonary hypertension. Administer anticoagulants and fibrinolytics if RVF and/or refractory hypoxemia are due to pulmonary embolism. Administer inotropic agents as required, especially when there is poor right ventricular contractility (e.g., RVMI).

Monitor patients for complications, such as deep vein thrombosis/pulmonary embolism, dysrhythmias, complications of therapy, fluid and electrolyte imbalances (i.e., hypokalemia, hypocalcemia, hypomagnesemia due to diuretic therapy), digitalis toxicity, and progressive deterioration. Manage depression, anxiety, and sleep disturbances. Provide instruction and counseling regarding lifestyle modification and the need for pharmacologic therapy.

Instruct the patient and family about nonpharmacologic therapies. Dietary recommendations include modifications for weight normalization, limitation of saturated fats and sodium, and an ADA diet for control of blood glucose for patients with DM.

Provide recommendations and/or referrals for tobacco cessation. Recommend limiting alcohol consumption to one to two alcoholic beverages daily because moderate alcohol intake has been shown to have a beneficial effect. Larger amounts, however, increase risks. Encourage regular aerobic exercise in moderation. Advocate complementary therapies, such as relaxation, imagery, and biofeedback as stress reduction techniques. Encourage the patient to get vaccinations including pneumococcal yearly influenza vaccines. To detect decompensation, provide instructions regarding recognition of the symptoms of HF and when the patient needs to call the physician. Encourage patients to weigh themselves daily and educate them about self-care guidelines regarding diuretic titration. Teach the patient to notify the physician if he or she gains 2 lb/day for more than 2 days or a total of 5 lb in 1 week. Reinforce that pharmacologic agents should be taken as prescribed for HF, control of hypertension, hyperlipidemia, DM, and thyroid disorders. Warn patients to avoid drugs that may worsen HF, such as over-the-counter NSAIDs.

3.23 Learning Activity

Identify whether the following causes or clinical findings are associated with left or right ventricular failure. Some may be associated with biventricular failure.

Causes	Left	Right
Aortic stenosis		
Cardiac tamponade		
Cardiomyopathy		
Mitral stenosis		
Myocardial infarction (left)		
Myocardial infarction (right)		
Pulmonary embolism		
Pulmonary hypertension		
Systemic hypertension		

Sign/Symptom	Left	Right
Abnormal liver function studies		
Ascites		
Atrial dysrhythmias		
Crackles audible over lungs		
Dyspnea		
Elevated CVP		
Hepatomegaly		

Sign/Symptom	Left	Right
Jugular venous distention		
Mental confusion		
Murmur of mitral regurgitation		
Murmur of tricuspid regurgitation		
Orthopnea		
Peripheral edema		
S_3, S_4 at apex		
S_3, S_4 at sternum		
Weight gain		

Answers to this activity can be found in the Answer Key.

3.24   Synthesis Learning Activity: Clinical Vignette

Patient A is a 75-year-old woman admitted with complaints of increasing dyspnea and fatigue. She has a past medical history of DM, stable angina, and a CABG approximately 10 years ago. Her BP is 136/82 mm Hg and her heart rate is 92 beats/min. The monitor shows atrial fibrillation. An S_3 is heard at the apex, peripheral edema is present to the midcalf, and JVD is visible to 10 cm above the angle of Louis. Current medications include captopril, carvedilol, torsemide, metformin, and warfarin. The patient's last measured ejection fraction was 25%.

a. Does she meet criteria for HF?

_____

_____

b. Is this systolic or diastolic dysfunction?

_____

_____

_____

c. What other medications might be beneficial and why?

_____

_____

_____

d. What other treatments might be helpful?

_____

_____

_____

e. What ACC stage is she in?

_____

_____

_____

Answers to this activity can be found in the Answer Key.

3.25   Learning Activity

Identify whether the following vasoactive agents are arterial or venous dilators; some may be both.

Drug	Arterial Dilator	Venous Dilator
Clevidipine (Cleviprex)		
Dobutamine (Dobutrex)		
Fenoldopam (Corlopam)		

3.25 Learning Activity—cont'd

Drug	Arterial Dilator	Venous Dilator
Hydralazine (Apresoline)		
Milrinone (Primacor)		
Minoxidil (Loniten)		
Morphine sulfate		
Nifedipine (Procardia)		
Nitroglycerin (<1 mcg/kg/min)		
Nitroglycerin (>1 mcg/kg/min)		
Nitroprusside (Nipride)		
Phentolamine (Regitine)		
Prazosin (Minipress)		

Answers to this activity can be found in the Answer Key.

CARDIOMYOPATHY

Cardiomyopathy is a disorder causing destruction of cardiac muscle fibers (i.e., myofibrils) leading to impaired contractility and cardiac output. The main types of cardiomyopathy (Figure 3-59) are dilated cardiomyopathy, hypertrophic cardiomyopathy, and restrictive cardiomyopathy.

Dilated Cardiomyopathy

Dilated cardiomyopathy is the most common type of cardiomyopathy. Dilated cardiomyopathy is idiopathic and may result from a variety of etiologies. Common causes are infection, especially viral (e.g., coxsackievirus B, arbovirus); toxins (e.g., doxorubicin [Adriamycin], daunorubicin [Cerubidine], alcohol, lead, arsenic, cobalt); an electrolyte, vitamin, or nutrient deficiency (e.g., hypokalemia, hypocalcemia, hypophosphatemia, or a thiamine deficiency); pregnancy; neuromuscular disorders (e.g., myasthenia gravis, muscular dystrophy); connective tissue disorders (e.g., lupus, scleroderma, rheumatoid disease); infiltrative disorders (e.g., sarcoidosis, amyloidosis); or hyperthyroidism. The basic pathophysiology of dilated cardiomyopathy (Figure 3-60) is the heart muscle beginning to stretch and becomes thinner (i.e., dilate). This causes the inside of the chamber to enlarge. When the heart chambers dilate, the heart muscle does not contract normally or pump blood very well.

The clinical presentation of dilated cardiomyopathy includes fatigue, weakness, decreased exercise tolerance, chest pain, palpitations, syncope, and symptoms of HF, such as dyspnea and edema. Objective findings include orthostatic BP changes, possible murmurs of tricuspid and/or mitral regurgitation, and signs of biventricular failure, including LVF (i.e., S_3, crackles, or PMI displaced laterally) and RVF (i.e., JVD, peripheral edema, or hepatomegaly).

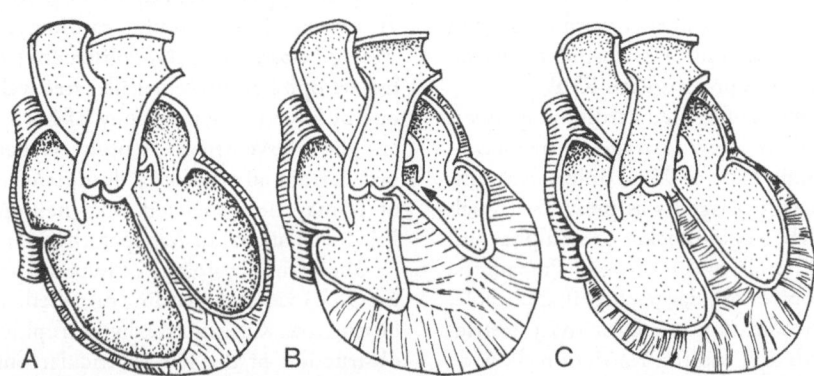

FIGURE 3-59 Cardiomyopathies. A, Dilated. **B,** Hypertrophic. **C,** Restrictive. (From Kinney, M. R., Packa, D. R., & Dunbar, S. B. [1993]. *AACN's clinical reference for critical-care nursing* [3rd ed.]. St. Louis, MO: Mosby.)

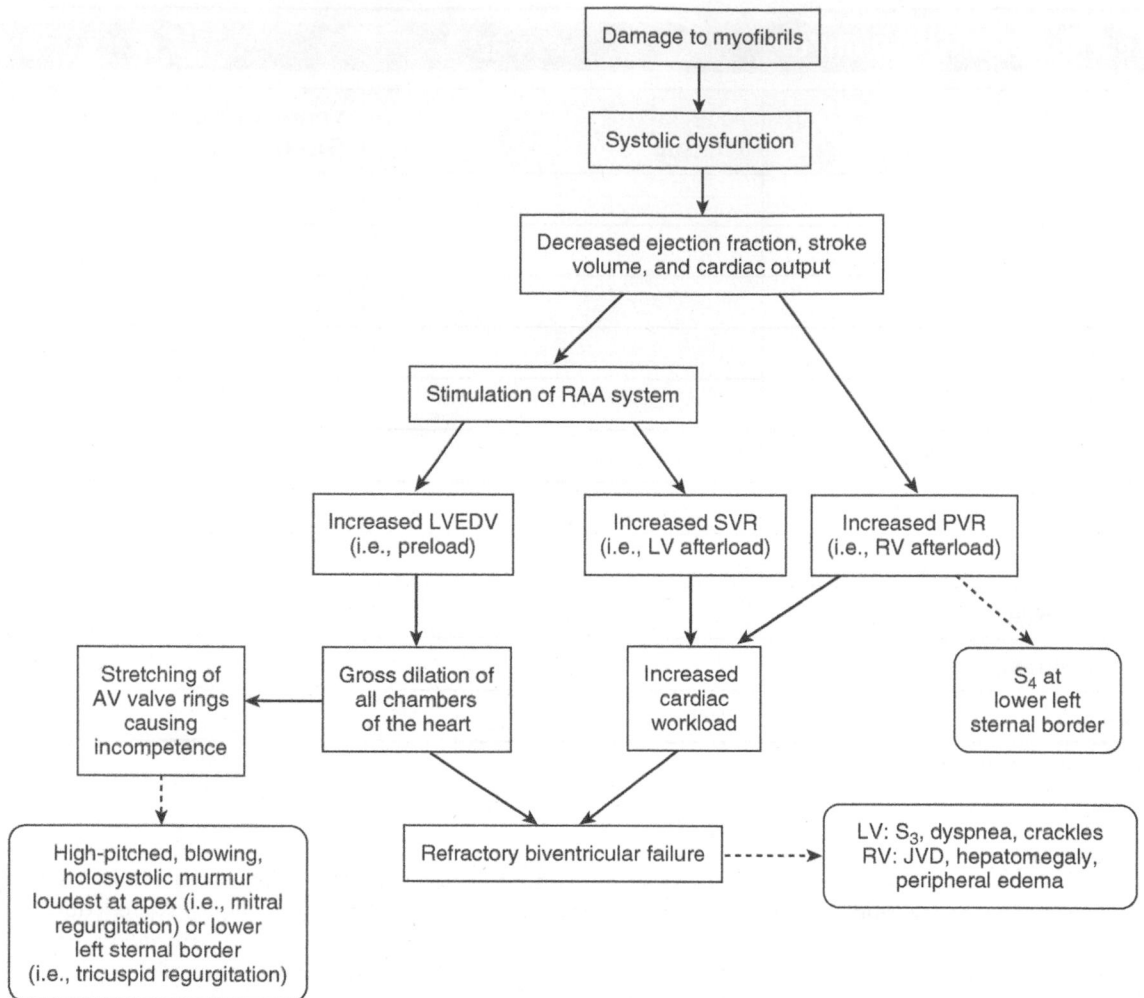

FIGURE 3-60 Pathophysiology of dilated cardiomyopathy. Dotted lines connect pathology to the clinical presentation. *AV,* Atrioventricular; *JVD,* jugular venous distention; *LV,* left ventricular; *LVEDV,* left ventricular end-diastolic volume; *PVR,* pulmonary vascular resistance; *RAA,* renin-angiotensin-aldosterone; *RV,* right ventricular; *SVR,* systemic vascular resistance. (From Dennison, R. D. [2013]. *Pass CCRN!* [4th ed.]. St. Louis, MO: Elsevier.)

Chest x-ray results include cardiomegaly, pulmonary congestion, and pleural effusion. Electrocardiography indicates biventricular hypertrophy and/or biatrial enlargement, dysrhythmias, especially atrial fibrillation, and blocks, especially BBB. Echocardiography confirms decreased ventricular wall motion, decreased ejection fraction, enlarged chamber size, and abnormal wall motion. Cardiac catheterization confirms an elevated PAP, LAP, and LVEDP; decreased cardiac output; decreased ejection fraction; mitral and/or tricuspid regurgitation; and RAP. Elevated RVEDP is present with RVF.

The collaborative management of dilated cardiomyopathy is very similar to management of HF. Provide oxygen by nasal cannula at 2 to 6 L/min to maintain Sao$_2$ of 95%, unless contraindicated. Administer pharmaceutical agents as prescribed, such as an ACE inhibitor or an ARB, a beta-blocker or an alpha- and beta-blocker, vasodilators, diuretics, and inotropes. Prepare the patient for CRT, such as atriobiventricular pacing, if applicable. Decrease myocardial oxygen consumption by activity restrictions and frequent rest periods and sodium restriction. Provide comfort measures by controlling environmental temperature, lighting, and noise control. Administer anxiolytics as prescribed and indicated. Monitor and treat patients for complications, which may include dysrhythmias such as atrial fibrillation and ventricular tachycardia/fibrillation. Monitor patients for prevention and/or treatment of systemic emboli. Provide anticoagulation as prescribed, especially for patients with an ejection fraction of less than 30%. Prepare the patient for mitral valve replacement or cardiac transplantation as requested.

Hypertrophic Cardiomyopathy

Two types of hypertrophic cardiomyopathy exist: nonobstructive and obstructive. Nonobstructive cardiomyopathy involves hypertrophy of the ventricular free wall. Obstructive cardiomyopathy involves hypertrophy of both the ventricular free wall and the interventricular septum. Hypertrophic cardiomyopathy occurs from an autosomal dominant trait, it may be idiopathic, or it may be associated with neuromuscular disorders (e.g., Friedreich ataxia) or hypoparathyroidism.

The pathophysiology of hypertrophic cardiomyopathy (Figure 3-61) varies depending on whether it is obstructive or nonobstructive. Obstructive hypertrophic cardiomyopathy causes obstruction of the left ventricular outflow tract (i.e., subaortic stenosis), resulting in decreased blood flow to both cerebral and coronary arteries. Both obstructive and nonobstructive hypertrophic cardiomyopathy results in diastolic and systolic dysfunction and HF.

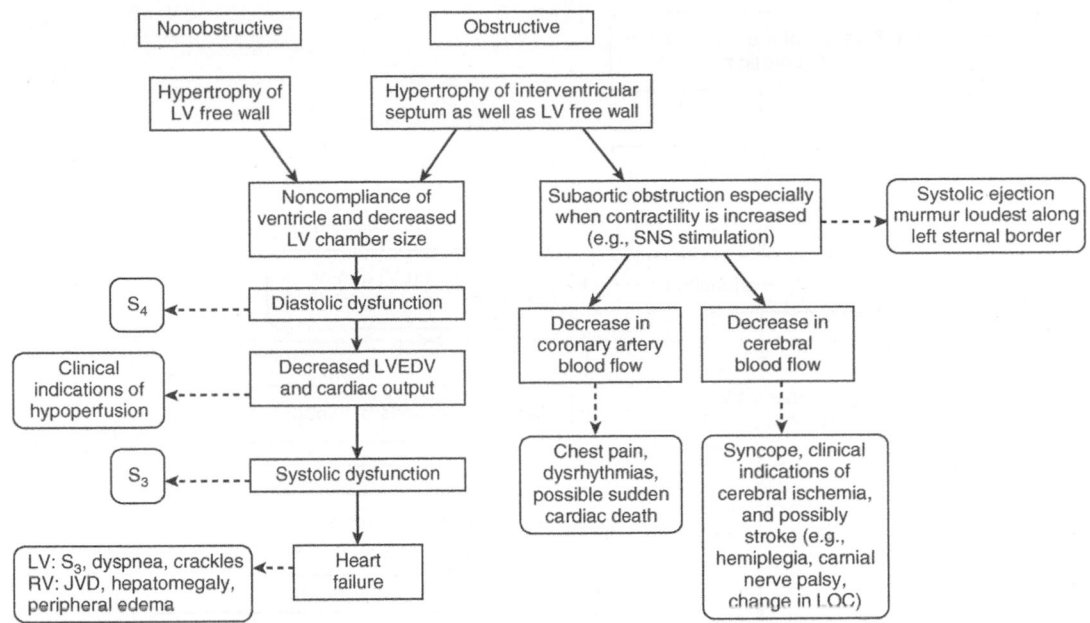

FIGURE 3-61 Pathophysiology of hypertrophic cardiomyopathy. Dotted lines connect pathology to the clinical presentation. *AV,* Atrioventricular; *JVD,* jugular venous distention; *LV,* left ventricular; *LVEDV,* left ventricular end-diastolic volume; *PVR,* pulmonary vascular resistance; *RAA,* renin-angiotensin-aldosterone; *RV,* right ventricular; *SNS,* sympathetic nervous system; *SVR,* systemic vascular resistance. (From Dennison, R. D. [2013]. *Pass CCRN!* [4th ed.]. St. Louis, MO: Elsevier.)

Patients with hypertrophic cardiomyopathy complain of dyspnea, orthopnea, paroxysmal nocturnal dyspnea (PND), and palpitations. If the hypertrophic cardiomyopathy is of the obstructive type, chest pain and syncope are likely. Objective findings include a laterally displaced PMI, S_3, S_4, and crackles. Patients with obstructive hypertrophic cardiomyopathy will have a murmur caused by the subaortic stenosis. This is a systolic ejection murmur heard loudest along the left sternal border. This murmur increases with a Valsalva maneuver and decreases when the patient assumes a squatting position. The patient may also have a murmur of mitral regurgitation, which is holosystolic, blowing, heard loudest at the apex, and radiates to the axilla.

Diagnostic tests used to confirm hypertrophic cardiomyopathy include chest x-ray, ECG, echocardiography, and cardiac catheterization. The chest x-ray shows left atrial dilation, cardiomegaly, and pulmonary congestion. ECG indicates left atrial enlargement and left ventricular hypertrophy, ST and T wave abnormalities, and dysrhythmias. Atrial fibrillation and ventricular dysrhythmias occur with a left anterior hemiblock. Echocardiography confirms left atrial enlargement, increased thickness of the left ventricular free wall and interventricular septum, which causes narrowing of the left ventricular outflow tract; abnormal wall motion especially of the septum; and possible mitral regurgitation. Cardiac catheterization confirms elevated LVEDP, mitral regurgitation, and the left ventricular outflow pressure gradient.

The collaborative management for patients with hypertrophic cardiomyopathy begins with the associated treatment of HF. With patients with obstructive hypertrophic cardiomyopathy, take measures to prevent obstruction of the left ventricular outflow tract. Administer beta-blockers and/or calcium channel blockers as prescribed to decrease contractility to keep the outflow tract open and decrease myocardial oxygen consumption. These agents decrease the heart rate to improve ventricular filling. Avoid inotropic agents that would increase the outflow

tract obstruction. Prepare patients for percutaneous or surgical procedures as requested.

In patients with obstructive hypertrophic cardiomyopathy, a focus of care is to decrease the obstruction of the left ventricular outflow tract. Prepare the patient for the percutaneous transluminal septal myocardial ablation (PTSMA) for left ventricular outflow obstruction if symptoms continue despite optimal medical therapy and if the patient is either a suboptimal surgical candidate or the patient prefers it after a discussion of options. PCI may be necessary to isolate the septal perforator branch of the left anterior descending coronary artery. Injecting 98% ethanol causes selective infarction of a portion of the septum to prevent movement of the septum toward the left ventricular free walls to keep the outflow tract open. In the presence of inadequate septal thickness, RBBB, mitral valve disease, or greater than 50% occlusion of the RCA, a PCI is contraindicated. Monitor the CK-MB and troponin levels, which should peak in 7 hours after ablation. Assist with the insertion and monitor the function of a temporary pacemaker left in place for 24 to 48 hours. Administer any IV or oral analgesics prescribed. Provide nursing care as for any other PCI along with monitoring for dysrhythmias, heart blocks, stroke, cardiac tamponade, and hypotension.

Prepare the patient for a ventricular septal myectomy for left ventricular outflow obstruction if symptoms continue despite optimal medical therapy. This procedure is the surgical removal of a portion of the hypertrophied septum; thoracotomy and cardiopulmonary bypass are required. A mitral valve repair may accompany the septal myectomy if the patient also has primary valvular disease; however, the mitral regurgitation associated with obstructive hypertrophic cardiomyopathy is often relieved with the septal myectomy. Complications include septal perforation, blocks, and dysrhythmias along with the complications of cardiopulmonary bypass.

Maintain adequate filling volumes by administering IV fluids as prescribed. Administer beta-blockers and calcium channel

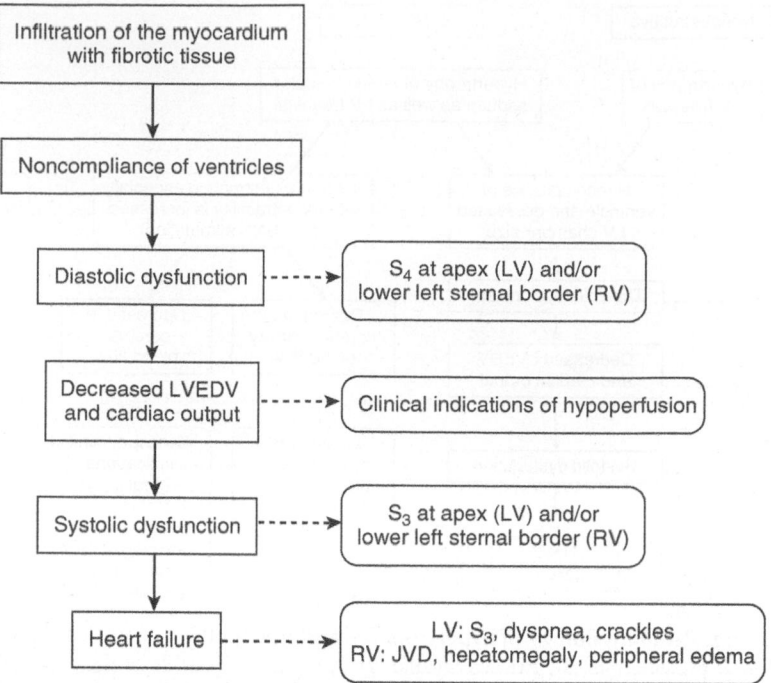

FIGURE 3-62 Pathophysiology of restrictive cardiomyopathy. Dotted lines connect pathology to the clinical presentation. *JVD*, Jugular venous distention; *LV*, left ventricular; *LVEDV*, left ventricular end-diastolic volume; *RV*, right ventricular. (From Dennison, R. D. [2013]. *Pass CCRN!* [4th ed.]. St. Louis, MO: Elsevier.)

blockers, as prescribed, to decrease the heart rate, allowing more time for filling. Employ caution or avoid drugs that decrease preload, such as venous vasodilators and diuretics. Monitor patients for complications such as atrial dysrhythmias. Although digoxin is used to treat atrial fibrillation, its inotropic effect may increase outflow tract obstruction; therefore, do not use in the presence of hypertrophic cardiomyopathy. Manage hypertension and heart rate control with calcium channel blockers, such as diltiazem or verapamil. Administer antidysrhythmics (e.g., amiodarone) for ventricular dysrhythmia as required. Administer anticoagulants as prescribed for systemic emboli, especially for patients with ejection fractions of less than 30%. Monitor the function and settings of the dual-chamber temporary pacemaker while in place the first 24 to 48 hours. The shortening of the AV interval minimizes contraction of the septum and decreases the outflow tract obstruction. Also, prepare the patient for cardiac transplantation as requested.

Restrictive Cardiomyopathy

The least common type of cardiomyopathy is restrictive. This type may be idiopathic or related to infiltrative disorders (e.g., sarcoidosis, amyloidosis), endomyocardial fibrosis, glycogen deposition, hemochromatosis, radiation, lymphoma, and/or connective tissue disorders (e.g., scleroderma). In restrictive cardiomyopathy (Figure 3-62), the ventricles become stiff and rigid because abnormal tissue, such as scar tissue, replaces the normal heart muscle.

The clinical presentation of restrictive cardiomyopathy includes chest pain, fatigue, weakness, dyspnea, orthopnea, and PND. Clinical findings include signs of RVF (e.g., JVD, hepatomegaly, peripheral edema, and right-sided S_3) and LVF (e.g., left-sided S_3, crackles).

A chest x-ray, ECG, echocardiography, and cardiac catheterization are diagnostic tests used to support the diagnosis.

The chest x-ray shows signs of cardiomegaly, pulmonary congestion, and pleural effusion. ECG indicates low QRS voltage and AV blocks, which are common. Echocardiography confirms atrial enlargement, enlarged ventricular outside dimension but small ventricular chamber, and possible pericardial effusion. Cardiac catheterization confirms an elevated RAP, RVEDP, PAP, LAP, and/or LVEDP.

Collaborative management of restrictive cardiomyopathy focuses on the treatment of the cause, which may include steroids. Also, provide care as for HF and assist in preparation of the patient for cardiac transplantation. Provide oxygen by nasal cannula at 2 to 6 L/min to maintain an SaO_2 of 95% unless contraindicated. Administer one or more of the following drugs as prescribed: an ACE inhibitor (e.g., captopril), a beta-blocker (e.g., metoprolol), a vasodilator (e.g., nitrates), a diuretic (e.g., furosemide), and an inotropic agent (e.g., digoxin). Monitor the patient for complications such as dysrhythmias. Digoxin is frequently prescribed for atrial fibrillation. Provide antidysrhythmic agents (e.g., amiodarone) to patients with ventricular dysrhythmias as prescribed. Prepare the patient for a pacemaker insertion to treat AV block if required. Administer prescribed anticoagulants to prevent and/or treat systemic emboli, especially for patients with an ejection fraction of less than 30%.

Indications for Cardiac Transplantation

A cardiac transplant is a treatment choice in the presence of heart disease with severe functional limitations, a poor prognosis, the patient is unresponsive to medical therapy, or when surgery cannot correct problems. In addition, transplantation is indicated for patients with normal pulmonary vascular resistance (PVR) or a high PVR that is reversible with therapy. If pulmonary hypertension is severe and irreversible, the patient may be a candidate for a heart-lung transplant. Patients should be 70 years or

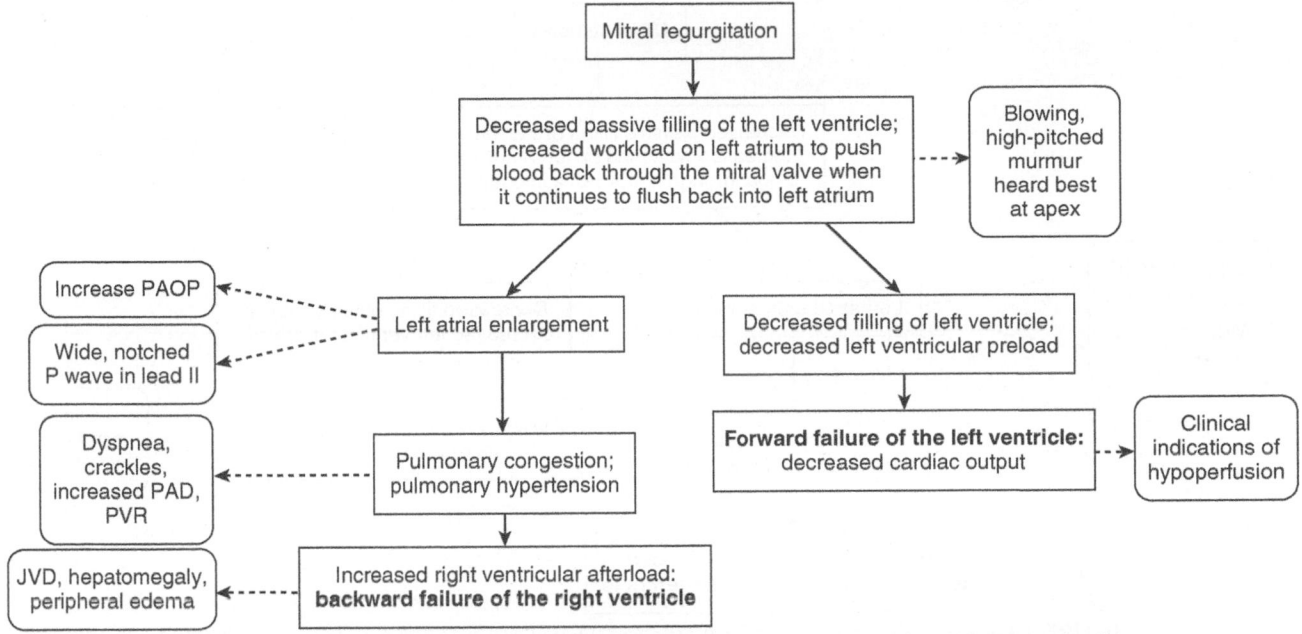

FIGURE 3-63 Pathophysiology of mitral regurgitation. Dotted lines connect pathology to the clinical presentation. *JVD,* Jugular venous distention; *PAD,* pulmonary artery diastolic pressure; *PAOP,* pulmonary artery occlusive pressure; *PVR,* pulmonary vascular resistance. (From Dennison, R. D. [2013]. *Pass CCRN!* [4th ed.]. St. Louis, MO: Elsevier.)

younger and lack intrinsic disease in other organ systems that would limit long-term survival or be worsened by immunosuppressive therapy. In addition, the candidate should have a favorable psychosocial profile and be negative for HIV and HBV.

CONGENITAL HEART DEFECTS

Congenital heart defects are cardiac structural abnormalities present at birth. These defects can involve the interior walls of the heart, the valves inside the heart, and the arteries and veins that carry blood to the heart or the body. Congenital heart defects change the normal flow of blood through the heart. Congenital defects range from simple defects with no symptoms to complex defects with severe, life-threatening symptoms. Although many patients with congenital heart defects do not require treatment, some do. Most patients usually have surgical repair during infancy or childhood, but some patients do require treatment in adulthood. Catheter procedures or surgery is used to repair congenital heart defects. Prepare the patient for the applicable procedure ordered.

Coarctation of the aorta (CoA) is a narrowing of the aorta. This narrowing affects blood flow where the arteries branch out to carry blood along separate vessels to the upper and lower parts of the body. CoA can cause high blood pressure or heart damage.

Atrial septal defect (ASD) is a defect (a "hole") in the septum between the heart's two upper chambers (atria). This defect allows oxygen-rich blood to leak into the oxygen-poor blood chambers in the heart (i.e., shunt). This shunt allows less oxygen to circulate to the rest of the body.

Patent ductus arteriosus (PDA) is an unclosed connection between the aorta and the pulmonary artery. Before birth, the fetus's blood does not need to go to the lungs to get oxygenated. The ductus arteriosus allows the blood to skip the circulation to the lungs. However, after birth, the blood must receive oxygen in the lungs and this connection is supposed to close. If the ductus

arteriosus is still open (patent), the blood may skip this necessary step of circulation; this abnormality is termed a patent ductus arteriosus. It results in oxygenated blood from the aorta mixing with unoxygenated blood from the pulmonary artery, which can result in decreased oxygen circulating to the rest of the body.

Ventral septal defect (VSD) is a hole in the ventricular septal wall. In normal development, the septum closes before the fetus is born so that by birth, oxygen-rich blood is kept from mixing with the oxygen-poor blood. Even if present at birth, most VSDs close on their own. When the hole does not close, it may cause pulmonary hypertension due to the shunting of blood into the right ventricle, and reduced oxygen to the body due to the mixing of oxygen-poor blood into the left ventricle.

VALVULAR HEART DISEASE

Valvular heart disease is an acquired or congenital disorder of a cardiac valve. Valve disorders include those of stenosis, causing obstruction of forward flow, or regurgitation, allowing backward flow of blood.

Mitral Regurgitation (Insufficiency, Incompetence)

Mitral regurgitation (MR) may result from various conditions, including trauma; rheumatic heart disease (RHD) or other forms of infective endocarditis; papillary muscle dysfunction or rupture, including rupture of chordae tendineae; congenital malformation of the mitral valve; left ventricular dilation from hypertrophic cardiomyopathy; Marfan syndrome; calcification of mitral valve leaflets; scleroderma; and prosthetic valve dysfunction. Mitral regurgitation may also be associated with mitral valve prolapse (MVP), also referred to as *Barlow's syndrome* or *floppy mitral valve syndrome.*

The pathophysiology (Figure 3-63) of mitral regurgitation is that backflow occurs due to the incompetence of the heart valve.

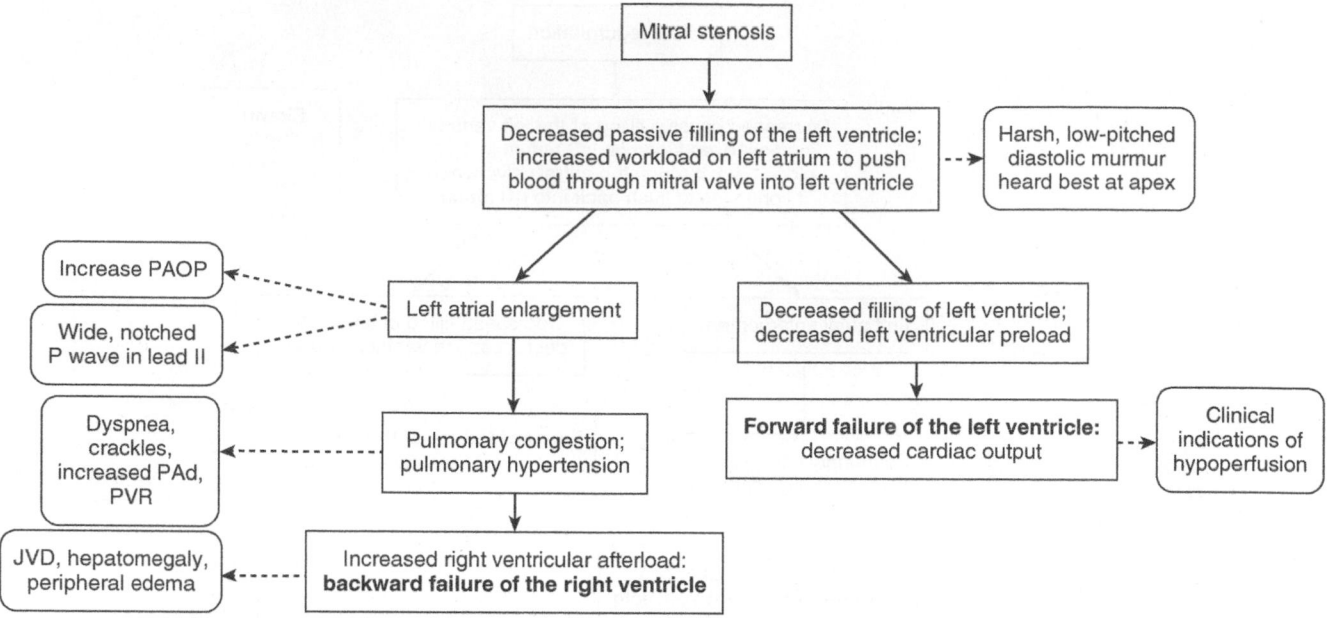

FIGURE 3-64 Pathophysiology of mitral stenosis. Dotted lines connect pathology to the clinical presentation. *JVD*, Jugular venous distention; *PAd*, pulmonary artery diastolic pressure; *PAOP*, pulmonary artery occlusive pressure; *PVR*, pulmonary vascular resistance. (From Dennison, R. D. [2013]. *Pass CCRN!* [4th ed.]. St. Louis, MO: Elsevier.)

The backflow of blood flow creates turbulence, causing a murmur and increased volume and pressure resulting in pulmonary congestion. Ultimately, hypoperfusion results from inadequate forward flow because the ventricle does not adequately fill.

Patients with mitral regurgitation complain of dyspnea, orthopnea, PND palpitations, weakness, fatigue, and anxiety. Some patients complain of cough and chest pain, but this is not common. Physical assessment reveals tachycardia, diaphoresis, confusion, crackles, and a laterally displaced PMI. Heart sound changes include a widely split S_2, right-sided S_3 and S_4, and a murmur. The murmur of mitral regurgitation is a high-pitched, blowing holosystolic murmur that is loudest at the apex and radiates to the axilla. As the condition worsens, signs of RVF, such as JVD, hepatomegaly, and peripheral edema, appear.

A chest x-ray may reveal cardiomegaly, left atrial enlargement, left ventricular hypertrophy, and pulmonary congestion. ECG may reveal left atrial enlargement, left and/or right ventricular hypertrophy, and dysrhythmias. The most frequently occurring dysrhythmia is atrial fibrillation. Echocardiography may show thickening, prolapse, and calcification of the mitral valve along with right ventricular, left atrial, and left ventricular enlargement. Cardiac catheterization may reveal increased left atrial and ventricular pressures and regurgitation of blood from the left ventricle to the left atrium. Cardiac catheterizations or hemodynamic monitoring reveals large v waves on the PAOP and left atrial waveform.

Mitral Stenosis

Mitral stenosis (MS) may be a congenital disorder or stem from RHD, endocarditis, tumors of the left atrium (e.g., atrial myxoma), or calcification of the mitral annulus. The basic pathophysiology of MS (Figure 3-64) is an impediment to the flow of blood into the left ventricle, RVF, and hypoperfusion caused by poor filling of the left ventricle and decreased cardiac output.

Patients with mitral stenosis frequently complain of dyspnea, orthopnea, PND, crackles, cough, hemoptysis, fatigue or weakness, palpitations, syncope, dysphagia, and hoarseness. Chest pain may occur but is uncommon. Clinical presentation may include a ruddy face (i.e., mitral facies). A right ventricular heave is often palpable at the sternum. Heart sound changes include a loud S_1, which is referred to as *closing snap;* a loud P; right-sided S_3 and S_4; and an opening snap. The murmur of mitral regurgitation is a harsh, rumbling mid-diastolic murmur that is loudest at the apex and has an associated thrill. Clinical indications of RVF, such as JVD, hepatomegaly, and peripheral edema, are likely.

Findings on a chest x-ray include left atrial enlargement, pulmonary congestion, right ventricular hypertrophy, and mitral valve calcification. ECG indicates left atrial enlargement, referred to as *P-mitrale;* right ventricular hypertrophy; and dysrhythmias. The most frequent dysrhythmia in patients with mitral regurgitation is atrial fibrillation. Echocardiography would confirm abnormal movement and thickening of valve leaflets and narrowing of mitral valve orifices, left atrial enlargement, and right ventricular hypertrophy. Cardiac catheterization would confirm an elevated pressure gradient across the mitral valve and an elevated RAP, PAP, and LAP.

Aortic Regurgitation (Insufficiency, Incompetence)

The causes of aortic regurgitation (AR) include rheumatic heart disease (RHD), calcification, congenital malformation (e.g., bicuspid aortic valve), endocarditis, syphilis, or Marfan syndrome. Other causes include hypertension, connective tissue disease (e.g., lupus erythematosus), aortic dissection, and trauma. Aortic regurgitation (Figure 3-65) results from the incomplete closure of the aortic valve, resulting in poor left ventricular filling and ejection fraction, which results in hypoperfusion.

Patients with aortic regurgitation report fatigue, cough, symptoms of LVF (e.g., dyspnea, orthopnea, and PND), exertional chest pain, syncope, and palpitations. *Musset sign,* the nodding of the head with each systole, may occur. A widened

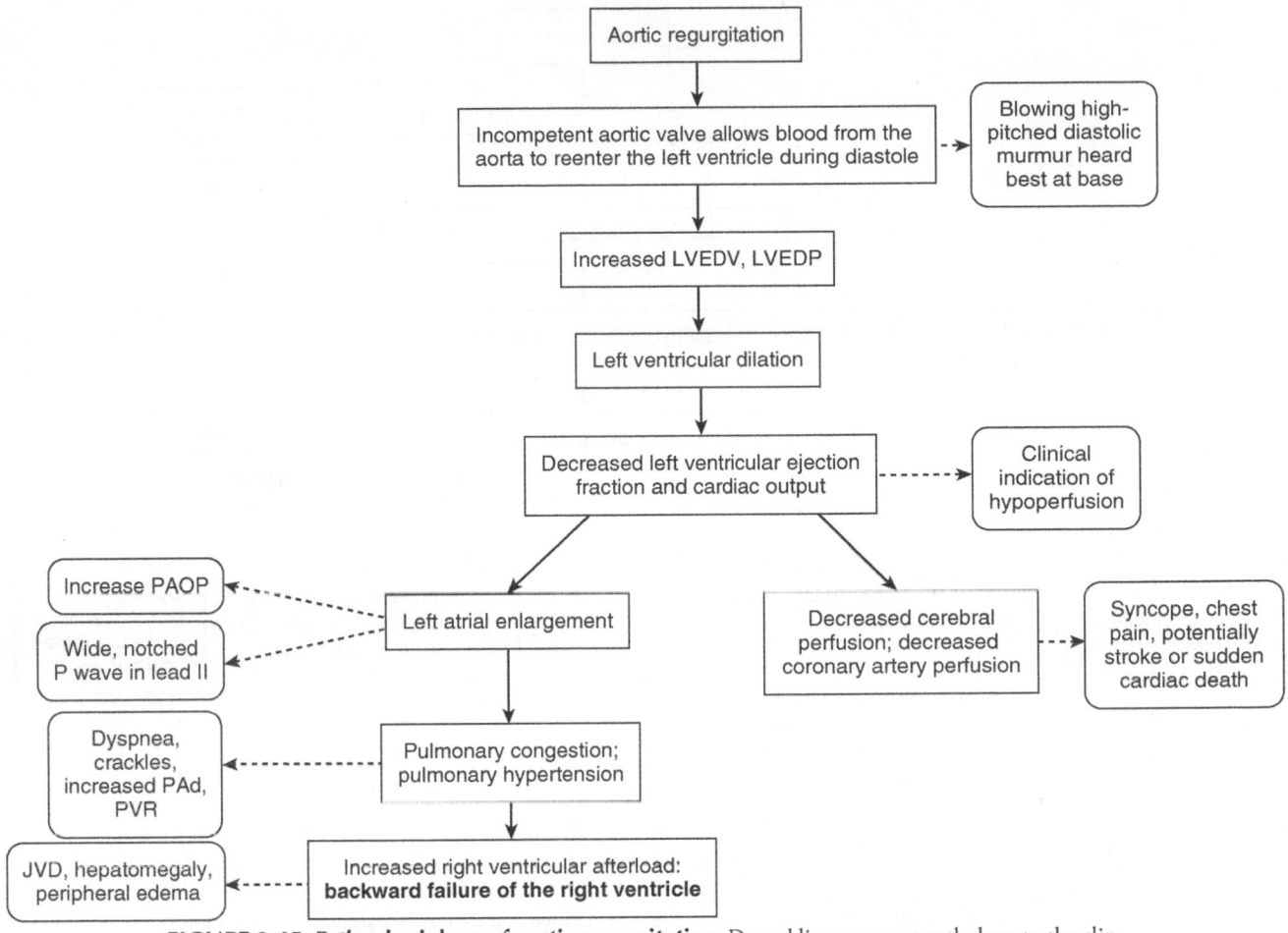

FIGURE 3-65 Pathophysiology of aortic regurgitation. Dotted lines connect pathology to the clinical presentation. *JVD,* Jugular venous distention; *LVEDP,* left ventricular end-diastolic pressure; *LVEDV,* left ventricular end-diastolic volume; *PAd,* pulmonary artery diastolic pressure; *PAOP,* pulmonary artery occlusive pressure; *PVR,* pulmonary vascular resistance. (From Dennison, R. D. [2013]. *Pass CCRN!* [4th ed.]. St. Louis, MO: Elsevier.)

pulse pressure and a downward and laterally displaced PMI are present. Other signs that may be present include Corrigan pulse, Hill sign, and Quincke sign. *Corrigan's pulse,* also called a water-hammer pulse, has a rapid rise that collapses. The Hill sign is present when the popliteal pressure is greater than the brachial pressure by 40 mm Hg or more. The Quincke sign is a visible capillary pulsation of the nailbeds with fingertip pressure. Signs of HF, including S_3, crackles, JVD, hepatomegaly, and peripheral edema, are evident. The murmur of aortic regurgitation is a high-pitched, blowing, diastolic murmur that is loudest at the base, radiates to the apex, and is likely to have an associated thrill. An aortic ejection click may be audible and there may be a systolic ejection murmur.

Findings on a chest x-ray include left atrial enlargement, left ventricular hypertrophy, or pulmonary congestion. The ECG indicates sinus tachycardia, left ventricular hypertrophy, and left atrial enlargement. The echocardiography detects poor aortic valve motion, thickening of the aortic valve, left ventricular hypertrophy, and left atrial enlargement. A cardiac catheterization detects elevated pressures (LAP and LVEDP) along with visualization of regurgitation from the aorta to the left ventricle.

Aortic Stenosis

Aortic stenosis (AS) occurs from RHD, calcification, congenital bicuspid valve, and/or aortic coarctation. The pathophysiology

of aortic stenosis (Figure 3-66) stems from the narrowing of the aortic valve, obstructing blood flow from the left ventricle to the ascending aorta during systole. This results in LVH and LVF along with hypoperfusion.

Patients with aortic stenosis complain of exertional chest pain and syncope, fatigue, weakness, and palpitations. Clinical assessment will likely reveal a narrow pulse pressure, a PMI displaced laterally and/or downward, and clinical indications of LVF (e.g., dyspnea, S_3, crackles). Heart sound changes may include a split S_1, a paradoxical split of S_2, and aortic ejection click. The murmur of aortic stenosis is a harsh, systolic ejection murmur that is loudest at the aortic area radiating to the neck.

The findings on chest x-ray include calcification of the aortic valve, cardiomegaly, left atrial enlargement, left ventricular hypertrophy, pulmonary congestion, and right ventricular hypertrophy. An ECG indicates left atrial enlargement (i.e., *P-mitrale*), left ventricular hypertrophy, and dysrhythmias. The most frequently occurring dysrhythmia is atrial fibrillation, but AV blocks and an LBBB may also occur. Echocardiography reveals a thickened aortic valve leaflet and decreased movement of the leaflets, calcification of the aortic valve, high-pressure gradient between the left ventricle and the aorta, left ventricular hypertrophy, and possible right ventricular hypertrophy. Cardiac catheterization reveals a significant pressure gradient and elevated LAP and LVEDP.

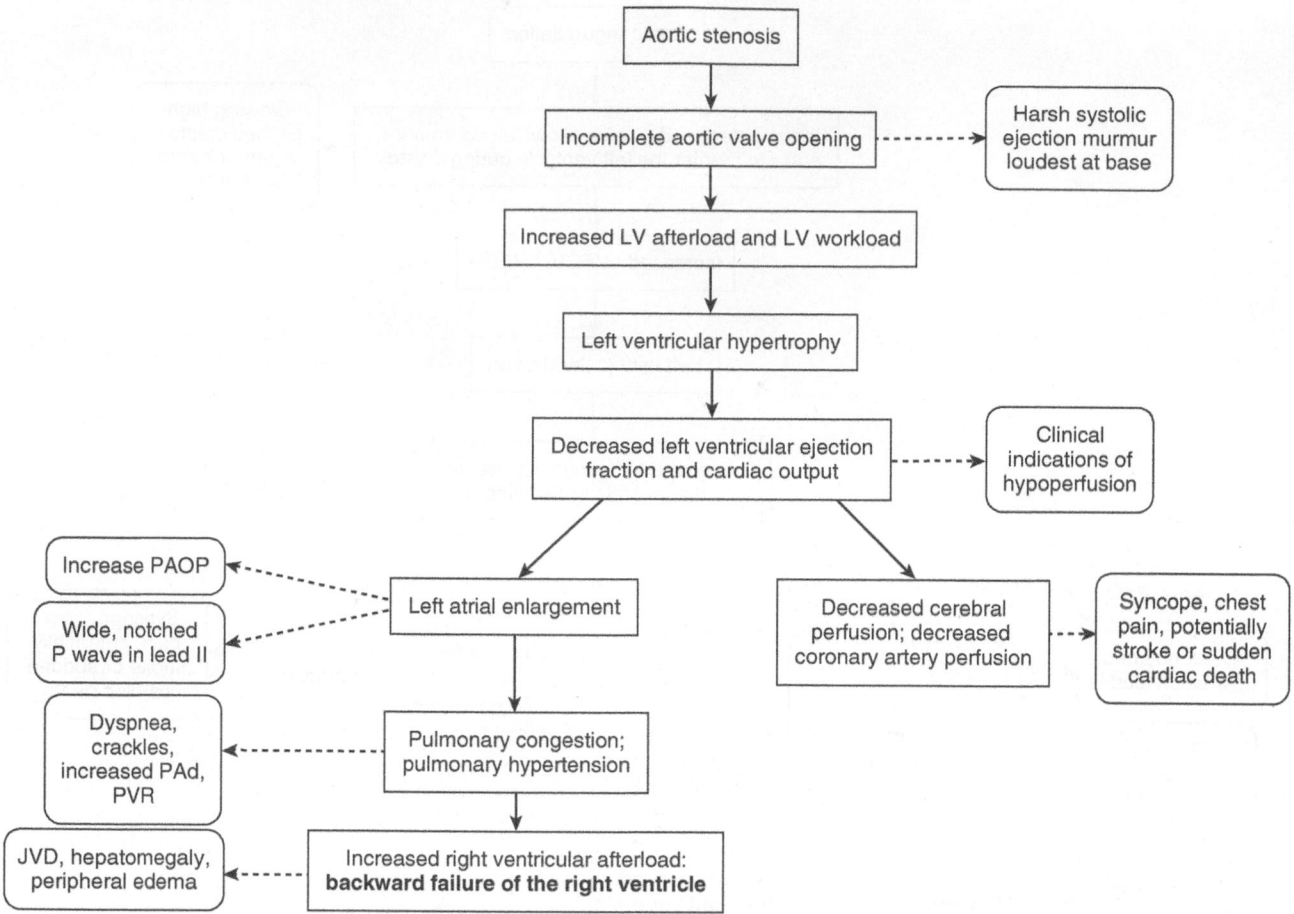

FIGURE 3-66 Pathophysiology of aortic stenosis. Dotted lines connect pathology to the clinical presentation. *JVD,* Jugular venous distention; *LV,* left ventricular; *LVEDP,* left ventricular end-diastolic pressure; *LVEDV,* left ventricular end-diastolic volume; *PAd,* pulmonary artery diastolic pressure; *PAOP,* pulmonary artery occlusive pressure; *PVR,* pulmonary vascular resistance. (From Dennison, R. D. [2013]. *Pass CCRN!* [4th ed.]. St. Louis, MO: Elsevier.)

Collaborative management for patients with AR focuses on improving oxygen delivery to the tissues and decreasing oxygen consumption. Provide oxygen by nasal cannula at 2 to 6 L/min to maintain SaO₂ of 95% unless contraindicated. Restrict sodium in the patient's diet because HF is a commonality in valvular heart disease. Attempt to control temperature, lighting, and noise for the patient's comfort.

Administer anxiolytics as prescribed; diazepam (Valium), lorazepam (Ativan), or alprazolam (Xanax) are most frequently used. Administer drug therapy for HF, such as an ACE inhibitor (e.g., captopril) or an angiotensin receptor blocker (e.g., candesartan), a beta-blocker (e.g., metoprolol), and a vasodilator (e.g., nitrates); however, these drugs are avoided in severe AS. Use caution if administering diuretics (e.g., furosemide) in severe AS. Administer inotropic agents, such as digoxin, as prescribed; digoxin may be especially helpful if supraventricular tachydysrhythmias are present.

Monitor patients for complications, including dysrhythmias (usually atrial fibrillation) and blocks, for which a permanent pacemaker may be necessary. Observe for signs and symptoms of emboli (i.e., mural thrombi), as there is the potential for pulmonary, cerebral, renal, splenic, and mesenteric embolisms. Initiate antiembolic measures including anticoagulation. Monitor patients for endocarditis and provide prophylactic antibiotics before any invasive procedures, such as dental procedures, for prevention.

Prepare patients for surgical repair or replacement of the affected valve as requested. Procedures performed include valvuloplasty, commissurotomy, valve replacement, or valve repair. Valvuloplasty is a PCI to repair a valve. It involves the use of a balloon-tipped intracardiac catheter. This procedure is palliative because the restenosis rate is high. Commissurotomy is the surgical separation of the thickened adherent leaves of a stenosed valve, usually the mitral valve. Valve repair includes an open commissurotomy, during which fused commissures are incised to reestablish mobility. In valve leaflet reconstruction, the fibrous pericardium forms tissue patch material. In an annuloplasty procedure, an inserted ring corrects the dilation of the valve annulus, and suture within or to the side of a papillary muscle repairs the elongated chordae tendineae.

Valve replacement involves replacement of the native valve with a mechanical or biologic prosthetic valve. Postoperative management is the same as for CABG, with close monitoring for AV nodal blocks. Bioprosthetic valves last approximately 5 to 10 years. Homografts involve human cadaver valves specially treated for surgical use. Heterografts use valves from an animal, usually a pig or cow, which have been prepared for surgical use. Administer anticoagulation as prescribed; for homografts and heterografts, anticoagulants are usually only administered for approximately 3 months. A goal of an INR between 2 and 3 is recommended. In cases of atrial fibrillation or left atrial thrombus, the recommendation is long-term anticoagulation therapy. Mechanical valves last approximately 10 to 15 years. Several materials are currently in use, including stainless steel, carbon, or other durable material. Administer long-term anticoagulation to maintain an INR of 2.5 to 3.5 depending on the type of valve. A pulmonary autograft, also referred to as *Ross procedure,* involves the use of the patient's own pulmonic valve to replace a diseased aortic valve with placement of a homograft or heterograft implanted into the pulmonic position.

INFLAMMATORY HEART DISEASE

Inflammatory heart disease pertains to inflammation of layers of the heart. The condition is classified as myocarditis, pericarditis, or endocarditis.

Myocarditis

Myocarditis describes any inflammation that occurs within the heart muscle. Various infections that include viruses like sarcoidosis and distinct immune diseases cause the condition. The most prevalent form of infection is a viral infection that assaults the heart muscle, resulting in local inflammation. Once the infection subsides, the immune response will still endure. Because of this, myocarditis will continue to plague the heart muscle long after the infection has ceased.

Often, the disease is completely asymptomatic. Pain in the chest is the predominant manifestation. In some instances, the disease may progress into degeneration of the heart muscle, at which point HF with its associated findings become apparent. Patients complain of dyspnea, edema of the feet and ankles, and fatigue.

There is much uncertainty about the likelihood of recovery in the early phases of the disease. Some individuals achieve total recovery while others will develop chronic HF due to excessive damage to the myocardium. Infrequently, a person may develop fulminant HF that necessitates a heart transplant.

Pericarditis

Pericarditis is inflammation of the pericardium. The cause of pericarditis may be unexplained; however the following are identified risk factors:
- Some tumors and cancers
- Specific metabolic disorders—such as hypothyroidism and uremia (kidney failure)
- Infection with a virus or bacteria
- Prior impairment to the heart, for example, heart attack, trauma, or heart surgery
- An underlying connective tissue disease such as sarcoidosis or rheumatoid arthritis
- An unexpected reaction to a particular type of medication

Patients with pericarditis usually describe the chest pain as a cutting, intense pain that migrates from the chest area to the shoulder blades, back, and neck. Some patients experience pain near the diaphragm that extends to the back. When inhaling deeply, the chest pain becomes significantly worse. The pain is typically unbearable when lying flat but is eased and better tolerated by leaning forward. Pain on swallowing occurs if the inflammation is close to the esophagus. If the inflammation is due an infection, a slight fever may be present. A pericardial friction rub is an obvious sign of inflammation; however, the rub may be inconsistent. Diagnostic tests include an ECG, chest x-ray, and ultrasound of the heart.

Treat pericarditis with rest and antiinflammatory medications. Administer narcotic analgesics as prescribed. Assist with pericardiocentesis if severe inflammation occurs with restrictive pericarditis. This procedure removes excessive fluid from the pericardial space as well as detects the pathogen of origin causing the condition.

Dressler syndrome is a type of pericarditis associated with an immune system response following damage to heart tissue or the pericardium, such as an MI, surgery, or traumatic injury. Dressler syndrome symptoms include chest pain, much like that experienced during MI, and fever. With recent improvements in MI management, Dressler syndrome is less common than in the past; however, once it occurs it does increase the risk for repeated bouts of the condition. Dressler syndrome is also referred to as postpericardiotomy, postmyocardial infarction syndrome, and postcardiac injury syndrome. Management goals for Dressler syndrome are to manage the pain and reduce the inflammation. Administer NSAIDs, such as aspirin, ibuprofen (e.g., Advil, Motrin IB), and naproxen (Aleve) or indomethacin (Indocin). If these drugs are ineffective, administer colchicine and/or corticosteroids as prescribed to treat persistent or recurring episodes of Dressler syndrome. Because of potential side effects of diarrhea and abdominal pain from colchicine, this treatment is not an option for some people. Administer corticosteroids only when other treatments are not effective because of the risk of serious side effects and because corticosteroids may interfere with the healing of damaged heart tissues after an MI or surgery. Sometimes the complications of Dressler syndrome require more invasive treatments. If the patient develops cardiac tamponade, assist with pericardiocentesis. If thickening or scarring of the pericardium causes a constrictive pericarditis, a portion or the entire pericardium is removed (i.e., pericardial window, pericardiectomy).

Endocarditis

Endocarditis is an infection of the endocardium. Endocarditis results in pronounced inflammation and the development of valve vegetation, caused when pathogens from other regions of the body infect the bloodstream and affix to defective areas of the heart. If not treated promptly, damage to the heart valve occurs. Vegetative emboli can break off and enter the circulation causing ischemia or necrosis in various locations. Patients with valvular damage and patients with an artificial heart valve are at particular risk. In these high-risk patients, administer prophylactic antibiotics for any invasive procedure, including dental procedures. Endocarditis may develop over a long period or may manifest quite suddenly. Its progression will depend on the corresponding heart defect or extent of infection. Administer antibiotics for endocarditis. Assist in preparation of the patient for surgery for correction of valve damage in severe cases.

HYPERTENSIVE CRISES

Hypertension (HTN) is an elevation in BP above 140/90 mm Hg on at least three separate occasions. Hypertensive urgency is an acute or chronic BP elevation not associated with any observable acute organ damage. These conditions do not usually require critical care unit admission and are safely treated with oral antihypertensive agents to reduce BP to baseline over 24 to 48 hours.

Hypertensive emergencies involve an acute elevation of BP that is associated with acute and ongoing organ damage to the kidneys, brain, heart, eyes, or the vascular system. There is no absolute BP level, but the BP is usually greater than 240/140 mm Hg. The BP needs lowering within minutes to a few hours to reduce potential complications of new or progressive end-organ damage. Early recognition of the condition and a transfer to higher acuity level of care for titrated IV antihypertensive therapy (Table 3-31) is required.

A hypertensive crisis (or HTN crisis) involves a rapid rise in BP and occurs when BP elevation is severe enough to cause the threat of immediate vascular necrosis and end-organ damage. The patient's BP is usually greater than 180/120 mm Hg or MAP greater than 150 mm Hg.

A hypertensive crisis is a primary or secondary disorder. A primary crisis arises from untreated or inadequately treated essential (i.e., idiopathic) hypertension. Risk factors include family history, African American race, obesity, hyperlipidemia, diabetes or glucose intolerance, tobacco use, excessive alcohol intake, high-fat and/or high-sodium diet, stress, a sedentary lifestyle, aging, and oral contraceptive use. The HTN crisis is frequently associated with poor compliance. Factors closely related to poor compliance include lack of symptoms (i.e., the silent killer), side effects of pharmacologic agents, and cost of pharmacologic agents.

A secondary HTN crisis arises from cerebrovascular conditions (e.g., thrombotic or hemorrhagic stroke), or CNS injuries, including head injury and spinal cord injury. Spinal cord injury may result in autonomic dysreflexia, which is manifested as hypertension with bradycardia in patients with spinal cord injury T6 or above in response to noxious stimuli. Other secondary causes include aortic dissection or coarctation and renal disease. Increased renin-angiotensin levels may result from a renin-secreting tumor, renovascular disease, acute glomerulonephritis, chronic pyelonephritis, and postrenal transplant. Other secondary causes include preeclampsia, eclampsia, and HELLP (hemolysis, elevated liver enzyme levels, and low platelet count) syndrome. Burn injury and drug side effects from oral contraceptives, steroids, cocaine, amphetamines, methamphetamine, and decongestants may also factor into a secondary hypertension crisis. Drug interactions, especially with MAO inhibitors and tyramine, disulfiram (Antabuse), and alcohol may trigger a HTN crisis. Drug withdrawal from clonidine, beta-blockers, ACE inhibitors, and alcohol can cause secondary hypertensive crisis. Endocrine disorders (e.g., pheochromocytoma, Cushing's syndrome, primary hyperaldosteronism), vasculitis, scleroderma or other connective tissue disease, and perioperative/postoperative hypertension, especially in cardiac or vascular surgery, have also been implicated in the hypertensive crisis.

The pathophysiology of hypertensive crisis (Figure 3-67) starts with either a primary or secondary etiology and ends with significant impact to the target organs of hypertension. The target organs of hypertension are the heart, brain, kidneys, and retinas.

The clinical presentation of a patient with hypertensive crisis includes a significant elevation in BP above normal. BP levels (Table 3-32) have been defined according to the Eight Report of the Joint National Committee (JNC 8) on prevention, detection, evaluation, and treatment of high BP (James et al., 2014).

In addition to elevated BP, epistaxis may occur with a hypertensive crisis. Cardiovascular involvement may be evident by chest pain and clinical indications of LVH and LVF. Indicators for LVH are a PMI displaced to the left, left ventricular heave, presence of a left-sided S_4, and ECG indicators of left ventricular hypertrophy (i.e., deep S in V_1, V_2 and tall R in V_5, V_6). Clinical indications of LFV are dyspnea, orthopnea, S_3, and crackles. Renal involvement presents with nocturia and pressure-related diuresis, which progresses to hematuria and elevated BUN and creatinine levels.

Retinal involvement may occur and manifests as visual disturbances (e.g., blurred vision, reduced visual acuity, photophobia, temporary loss of vision). Funduscopic changes by the Keith-Wagener-Barker classification occur in stages:
- Grade I: arteriolar narrowing
- Grade II: focal arteriolar spasm
- Grade III: hemorrhages and exudates
- Grade IV: papilledema

Neurologic involvement may be present. Patients report severe occipital or anterior headache, especially in the morning. Hypertensive encephalopathy is manifested by altered mental status (e.g., irritability, confusion, agitation progressing to lethargy and coma), and focal neurologic signs (e.g., cranial nerve palsy, sensory or motor deficits, aphasia, positive Babinski reflex) may occur. Seizures may also occur.

Baseline laboratory evaluations include serum potassium levels, BUN and creatinine levels, a lipid profile to evaluate additional cardiac risk, and aldosterone levels. A captopril challenge test, during which plasma renin level is measured before and 1 hour after 25 mg of captopril (Capoten) is administered, is used to confirm or rule out renovascular hypertension. Urinalysis may show hematuria or proteinuria. Cardiomegaly, pulmonary edema, and widening of the mediastinum on chest x-ray suggest dissecting thoracic aortic aneurysm. ECG findings include indications of left atrial enlargement and left ventricular hypertrophy. A CT of the brain provides evidence of any cerebral edema and/or hemorrhage.

Collaborative management in patients with hypertensive crisis begins with maintaining airway, ventilation, and oxygenation. Administer oxygen by nasal cannula to achieve a SaO_2 of 95%. In patients with altered level of consciousness, maintain the airway with an oropharyngeal or nasopharyngeal airway. Endotracheal intubation may be required.

Decrease myocardial oxygen consumption by restricting activity, restricting sodium intake to less than 2 g/24 hr, and restricting smoking. Maintain patient comfort with measures to maintain room temperature, lighting, and noise control. Administer anxiolytics, such as diazepam (Valium), lorazepam (Ativan), or alprazolam (Xanax) as prescribed for some patients.

Decrease a patient's BP gradually. Reduce the MAP by no more than 20% to 25% within the first hour. Aggressive BP reduction may cause neurologic damage by significantly decreasing CPP. If aortic dissection has occurred, BP reduction is more aggressive, but reduction should take place over 5 to 10 minutes. Continue to monitor BP closely. Hypertensive emergency management requires an invasive arterial catheter. If neurologic changes occur, slow or temporarily stop BP reduction.

Antihypertensive agents include predominantly arterial vasodilators (e.g., nitroprusside [Nipride]), but also include mixed arterial and venous vasodilators. Consider vasodilators the first-line agent for hypertensive emergencies. Hydralazine (Apresoline) and clevidipine (Cleviprex) are selective arterial vasodilators as is fenoldopam mesylate (Corlopam) but it has the

TABLE 3-31 Selected Drugs Used for Hypertensive Emergency

Drug	Classification/Actions	Indications	Administration	Adverse Effects	Nursing Implications
Vasodilators					
Clevidipine (Cleviprex)	• Dihydropyridine L-type calcium channel blocker • Decreases SVR	• Reduction of BP when oral therapy is not feasible or not desirable	• IV infusion: 1-2 mg/hr; may be doubled every 90 seconds until BP approaches target; then increased by less than double every 5-10 minutes • Maximum: 21 mg/hr for 24 hours	• Nausea and vomiting • Headache • Insomnia • Tachycardia	• Monitor HR, BP, blood lipids • Metabolized by blood ester hydrolysis to form inactive metabolites; advantage in renal or hepatic insufficiency • Note contraindications: allergy to soybeans, soy products, eggs or egg products; defective lipid metabolism; pancreatitis; hyperlipidemia • Consider lipid calories in daily nutritional plan • Infusion must be changed every 4 hours • Use cautiously in the elderly
Enalaprilat (IV), enalapril (PO) (Vasotec)	**ACE (angiotensin converting enzyme) inhibitor** • Inhibits conversion of angiotensin I to angiotensin II • Prevents vasoconstriction and aldosterone secretion to decrease preload and afterload	• HF • Hypertension	• PO: 5-40 mg daily • IV injection: 1.25 mg over 5 minutes every 6 hours	• Tachycardia • Hypotension, especially after first dose • Anorexia • Fatigue • Headache • Loss of taste • Diarrhea • Rash, angioedema • Dizziness • Photosensitivity • Proteinuria, nephrotic syndrome, renal failure • Pancytopenia • Hyperkalemia • Bronchospasm • Cough	• Monitor HR, BP, urine output, protein in urine, serum potassium, WBC • Monitor WBC and differential before treatment and periodically during treatment • Note contraindications: known hypersensitivity, AV block, hypotension • Use cautiously in renal disease, lupus, scleroderma, hypovolemia, leukemia, DM, thyroid disease, COPD, asthma, hyperkalemia and in patients on drugs that may affect WBC counts or immune response • Monitor for allergic reaction: rash, fever, pruritus, urticaria; antihistamines may be used; discontinuance may be necessary • Administer thiazide diuretics as prescribed; frequently given concurrently • Angiotensin II blocker (e.g., losartan [Cozaar], valsartan [Diovan]) may be prescribed if cough develops • Indicated for hypertension with HF
Fenoldopam mesylate (Corlopam)	**Vasodilator antihypertensive** • Relaxes vascular smooth muscle decreasing preload (PAOP) and afterload (SVR) • Stimulates dopaminergic receptors causing diuresis	• Severe hypertension (short-term treatment) • Need to improve renal flow, such as after use of potentially nephrotoxic dyes and contrast media	• IV infusion: mix 10 mg in 250 mL (40 mcg/mL); usual dose is 0.1-0.3 mcg/kg/min; may be increased in increments of 0.05-0.1 mcg/kg/min every 15 minutes until target BP is reached • Maximum: 1.7 mcg/kg/min	• Tachycardia, hypotension • Ventricular dysrhythmias • Dizziness • Anxiety • Headache • Flushing • Nausea, vomiting, abdominal pain • Hypokalemia • Increased intraocular pressure • Increased intracranial pressure	• Monitor HR, BP, urine output, serum potassium, neurologic status • Note contraindications: known hypersensitivity to fenoldopam or sulfite, intracranial hypertension • Use caution in patients with glaucoma or ocular hypertension and in patients on other drugs that may cause hypotension (e.g., beta-blockers) • Indicated especially for postoperative hypertension or hypertension with renal insufficiency

Continued

TABLE 3-31 Selected Drugs Used for Hypertensive Emergency—cont'd

Drug	Classification/Actions	Indications	Administration	Adverse Effects	Nursing Implications
Hydralazine (Apresoline)	**Vasodilator antihypertensive** • Relaxes arteriolar smooth muscle decreasing SVR, afterload, and BP	• Hypertension • Afterload reduction	• PO: 10-50 mg every 6-8 hours • IV injection: 5-20 mg over 3-5 minutes every 4-6 hours • Maximum: 400 mg/day	• Tachycardia • Orthostatic hypotension • Anorexia, nausea, vomiting, diarrhea • Sodium retention • Weight gain • Palpitations • Flushing • Headache • Tremors • Dizziness • Lupus-like syndrome • Exacerbation of HF or chest pain • Leukopenia, agranulocytosis	• Monitor HR, BP, ECG • Note contraindications: known hypersensitivity to hydralazine, coronary artery disease, mitral valve disease, severe aortic stenosis • Use cautiously in renal disease, cerebrovascular disease • Administer beta-blockers as prescribed for reflex tachycardia as it may cause myocardial ischemia • Indicated for pregnancy-related hypertension (i.e., eclampsia)
Nicardipine (Cardene)	**Calcium channel blocker** • Relaxes vascular smooth muscle, decreasing preload and afterload	• Hypertension • Angina pectoris	• PO: 20 mg tid initially; may be increased to 20-40 mg tid after 3 days if tolerated well • IV infusion: mix 25 mg in 240 mL (0.1 mg/mL) and infuse at 5 mg/hr (50 mL/hour); may be increased by 2.5 mg/hour (25 mL/hr) every 5 minutes until desired BP reduction is achieved • Do not mix in lactated Ringer's solution • Maximum: 15 mg/hr	• Tachycardia • Hypotension • Nausea, vomiting, heartburn • Flushing • Headache • Chest pain • HF • Hepatitis • Renal failure • Local irritation at injection site	• Monitor HR, BP • Note contraindications: known hypersensitivity, sick sinus syndrome, second- or third-degree AV block, severe aortic stenosis systolic BP <90 mm Hg, • Use caution in HF, hypotension, liver disease, renal insufficiency or failure, and in the elderly • Indicated for postoperative hypertension

| Nitroglycerin (Tridil) | **Nitrates**
• Relaxes smooth muscle to reduce preload (PAOP) (and afterload [SVR] if >1 mcg/kg/min)
• Dilates coronary collateral circulation
• Relieves coronary artery spasm | • Acute angina
• Prophylactic use before activities that may cause angina
• HF (preload reduction) | • Sublingual: 0.3-0.4 mg at 5-minute intervals to a maximum of three tablets or metered-dose sprays
• PO (isosorbide): 5-40 mg every 6 hours
• Transdermal: 1-4 inches every 8 hours
• IV infusion: mix 50 mg in 250 mL (200 mcg/mL); initial dose 5-10 mcg/min, increase by 5-10 mcg/min every 5 minutes until desired results are achieved (e.g., control of chest pain, preload reduction)
• Maximum: 400 mcg/min
• Administer in glass bottle and with non-PVC tubing | • Tachycardia or bradycardia
• Hypotension or hypertension
• Palpitations
• Weakness
• Apprehension
• Flushing
• Dizziness
• Syncope
• Headache
• Methemoglobinemia with resultant reduction in SaO_2, SpO_2, and tissue oxygen delivery | • Monitor HR, BP, urine output
• Monitor RAP, PAP, PAOP, SVR, CI if hemodynamic monitoring, if nitroglycerin is being administered through IV, and a pulmonary artery catheter has been inserted
• Note contraindications: known hypersensitivity, anemia, intracranial hypertension, cerebral hemorrhage, hypertrophic cardiomyopathy, right ventricular infarction, sildenafil (Viagra) or vardenafil (Levitra) within the past 24 hours
• Use cautiously in hypotension; IV nitroglycerin is titratable and preferred in acute situations
• Decrease nitrate tolerance by scheduling oral nitrates with nitrate-free period at night and by removing transdermal nitrates at night
• Administer ASA or acetaminophen for headache; usually dose-related
• Teach patient to protect tablets from light and moisture and replace every 3 months
• Teach patient to limit NTG to 3 tablets every 5 minutes and if no relief is obtained, to go to the ED
• Teach patient to apply NTG paste to any relatively hairless area between the knees and shoulders and to rotate sites to prevent maceration
• Note that patients receiving IV NTG and heparin IV concurrently require more heparin to achieve therapeutic aPTT; monitor aPTT closely with NTG dosage changes or discontinuance
• Indicated especially for hypertension with chest pain |

Continued

TABLE 3-31   Selected Drugs Used for Hypertensive Emergency—cont'd

Drug	Classification/Actions	Indications	Administration	Adverse Effects	Nursing Implications

Nitroprusside (Nipride)	**Vasodilator antihypertensive**
	• Relaxes vascular smooth muscle decreasing preload (PAOP) and afterload (SVR)
		• Hypertensive crisis
		• HF (preload and afterload reduction)
		• Cardiogenic shock
		• BP control during and after vascular surgery
			• IV infusion: mix 50 mg in 250 mL (200 mcg/mL) and infuse at 0.25-10 mcg/kg/min
			• Maximum: 10 mcg/kg/min for 10 minutes only
			• Protect from light by wrapping aluminum foil around bag or bottle; it is not necessary to foil tubing but avoid exposure of tubing to direct sunlight
				• Nausea, vomiting, abdominal pain
				• Headache
				• Tinnitus
				• Dizziness
				• Diaphoresis
				• Apprehension
				• Hypotension
				• Tachycardia
				• Palpitations
				• Coronary artery steal causing myocardial ischemia and chest pain
				• Intrapulmonary shunt causing hypoxemia (referred to as nitroprusside-induced intrapulmonary shunt)
				• Methemoglobinemia with resultant reduction in SaO_2, SpO_2, and tissue oxygen delivery
				• Thiocyanate toxicity
					• Monitor HR, BP, urine output, neurologic status
					• Note contraindications: known hypersensitivity; use cautiously in liver disease, renal disease, anemia, hypovolemia, hypothyroidism; older adults, CAD; neurologic injury
					• Discard solution after 24 hours
					• Foil bottle to protect from light
					• Discard solution if dark brown, blue, green, or red
					• Monitor for thiocyanate toxicity
					  • Thiocyanate levels should be determined daily if drugs are used longer than 72 hours
					  • Signs of thiocyanate toxicity: metabolic acidosis; confusion; hyperreflexia; seizures
					  • Treatment includes amyl nitrate, sodium nitrate, and/or sodium thiosulfate
					  • Simultaneous infusion with thiosulfate with nitroprusside may prevent thiocyanate toxicity

Adrenergic Blocking Agents

Esmolol (Brevibloc)	Beta adrenergic blocker	• Ventricular rate control in SVT, atrial fibrillation, atrial flutter and noncompensatory sinus tachycardia
		• Control of perioperative tachycardia and hypertension
			• Administer intravenously
			• Titrate using ventricular rate or BP at 4-minute intervals
			• Optional loading dose: 500 mcg/kg infused over 1 minute
			• Then 50 mcg/kg/min for the next 4 minutes
			• Adjust dose as needed to a maximum of 200 mcg/kg/min
			• Additional loading doses may be administered
			• Perioperative tachycardia and hypertension
			• Loading dose: 500 mcg/kg over 1 minute for gradual control (1 mg/kg over 30 seconds for immediate control)
			• Then 50 mcg/kg/min for gradual control (150 mcg/kg/min for immediate control) adjusted to a maximum of 200 (tachycardia) or 300 (hypertension) mcg/kg/min
				Adverse effects:
				• Bradycardia,
				• Chest pain, HA, pain at injection site, bronchospasm (rare), seizures (rare)
					• Monitor BP, ECG, HR, respiratory rate, IV site
					• Check for drug interactions with:
					  • Digitalis glycosides: Risk of bradycardia
					  • Anticholinesterases: Prolongs neuromuscular blockade
					  • Antihypertensive agents: Risk of rebound hypertension
					  • Sympathomimetic drugs: Dose adjustment needed
					  • Vasoconstrictive and positive inotropic effect substances: Avoid concomitant use

Continued

TABLE 3-31   **Selected Drugs Used for Hypertensive Emergency—cont'd**

Drug	Classification/Actions	Indications	Administration	Adverse Effects	Nursing Implications
Labetalol hydrochloride (Normodyne, Trandate)	**Alpha- and beta-adrenergic blocker** • Blocks response to alpha and beta stimulation • Causes decrease in BP without reflex tachycardia • Causes decrease in HR	• Hypertension • Hypertensive crisis	• PO: 100-400 mg/12 hr • IV injection: 20 mg over 2 minutes, may repeat 40 mg every 10 minutes • IV infusion: mix 300 mg in 250 mL for a total volume of 300 mg in 300 mL (1 mg/mL); usual dose if 1-2 mg/min until satisfactory response is achieved • Maximum: 300 mg	• Bradycardia • Orthostatic hypotension • Ventricular dysrhythmias • AV blocks • HF • Nausea, vomiting, diarrhea • Dizziness • Lethargy • Hypoglycemia without symptoms in type 1 DM • Hyperglycemia in type 2 DM • Agranulocytosis, thrombocytopenia • Bronchospasm in patients with COPD, asthma	• Monitor HR, BP, ECG, breath sounds, daily weight • Note contraindications: known hypersensitivity, shock, second- or third-degree AV block, sinus bradycardia, sick sinus syndrome, New York Heart Association (NYHA), class IV HF, asthma • Use cautiously in DM, renal disease, hepatic disease, thyroid disease, COPD, CAD, bronchospasm, peripheral vascular disease • Keep patient supine for 3 hours after IV administration (labetalol) • Do not discontinue suddenly • Indicated for hypertension postoperatively or aortic dissection
Phentolamine (Regitine)	**Alpha adrenergic blocker** • Blocks response to alpha stimulation • Causes decrease in BP without reflex tachycardia	• Hypertension, especially autonomic dysreflexia; pheochromocytoma; monoamine oxidase inhibitor-tyramine interaction • Infiltration of vasopressor agents	• IV injection: 5-15 mg; may be repeated every 5-15 minutes • Maximum: 15 mg	• Tachycardia • Flushing • Headache	• Monitor HR, BP • Use cautiously in CAD • Beta-blocker may be given concurrently to control tachycardia

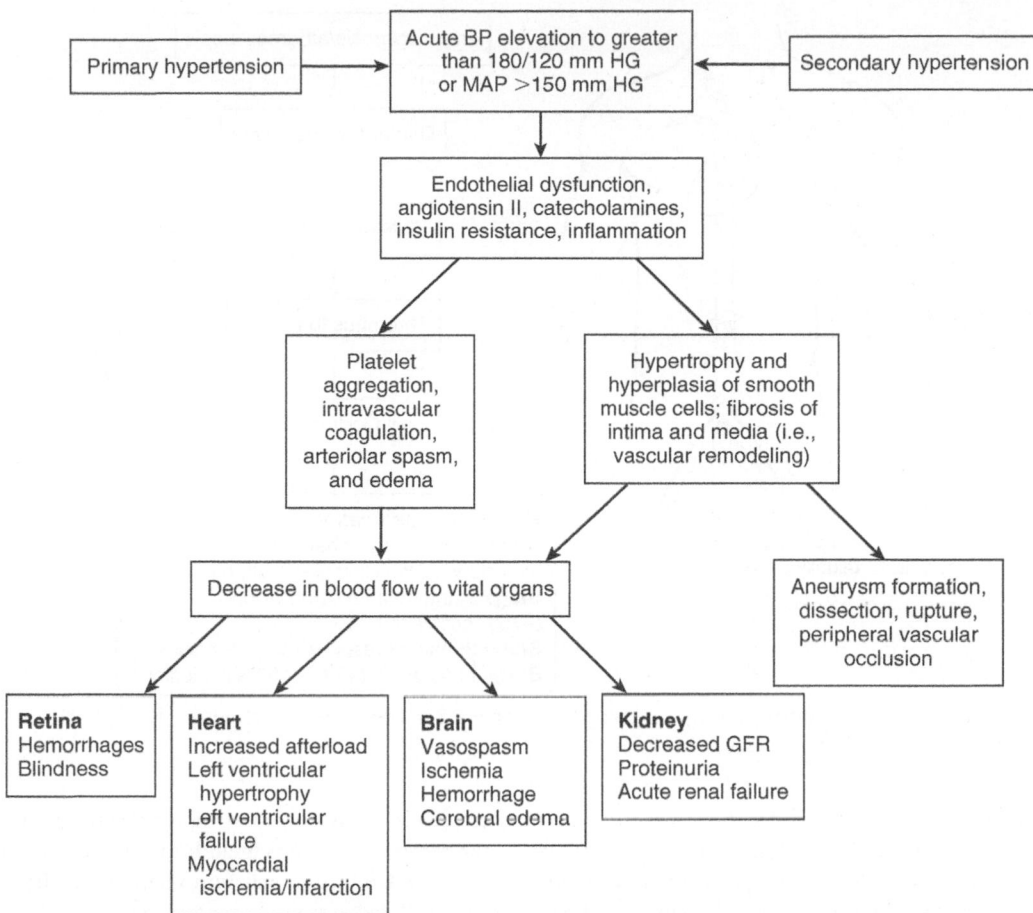

FIGURE 3-67 Pathophysiology of hypertensive crisis. *BP,* Blood pressure; *GFR,* glomerular filtration rate; *MAP,* mean arterial pressure. (From Dennison, R. D. [2013]. *Pass CCRN!* [4th ed.]. St. Louis, MO: Elsevier.)

| TABLE 3-32 | Joint National Committee (JNC 8) on Prevention, Detection, Evaluation, and Treatment of High Blood Pressure |

BP Category	Systolic (mm Hg)	and/or	Diastolic (mm Hg)
Prehypertension	120 to 130		80 to 89
Normal	<130	and	<85
Hypertensive			
Stage 1	140 to 159	or	90 to 99
Stage 2	160 or greater	or	100 or greater

James, P.A., Oparil, S., Carter, B.L., et al. (2014). Evidence-based guideline for the management of high blood pressure in adults. Report From the Panel Members Appointed to the Eighth Joint National Committee (JNC 8). *JAMA, 311*(5): 507-520.

addition of a dopaminergic stimulation effect. Nitroglycerin is dose-dependent; a dose of less than 1 mcg/kg/min causes venous vasodilation while a dose greater than 1 mcg/kg/min causes arterial and venous vasodilation. Arterial and venous vasodilators include nicardipine (Cardene) and nifedipine (Procardia).

Sympathetic blockers include alpha-blockers, which block vasoconstriction. Phentolamine (Regitine) can be especially helpful if the hypertension is a result of autonomic dysreflexia,

because bradycardia contraindicates the use of a beta-blocker. Phentolamine may also be particularly helpful in pheochromocytoma. Beta-blockers block the reflex tachycardia associated with vasodilators. Esmolol (Brevibloc) is a rapid acting, cardioselective beta-blocker contraindicated in HF and heart block. Alpha- and beta-blockers block both vasoconstriction and tachycardia. Labetalol (Normodyne) is an alpha- and noncardioselective beta-blocker. It is particularly helpful in patients with intracranial hypertension because direct vasodilators would increase intracranial volume and pressure.

ACE inhibitors block angiotensin and aldosterone, which decreases BP. Enalaprilat (Vasotec) is the only IV ACE inhibitor. Loop diuretics (e.g., furosemide [Lasix], bumetanide [Bumex]) may be prescribed, but using diuretics remains controversial in these patients because they may have significant diuresis related to an excessive glomerular filtration rate. Preferred pharmacologic agents are condition specific (Vadera, 2011). Conditions and useful drugs include:

- Hypertensive encephalopathy: labetalol, nicardipine, nitroprusside
- HF: nitroglycerin, nitroprusside
- Myocardial ischemia: nitroglycerin
- Aortic dissection: labetalol or nitroprusside and esmolol
- Adrenergic crisis: phentolamine or nitroprusside and esmolol
- Preeclampsia/eclampsia: hydralazine
- Perioperative/postoperative: clevidipine, nicardipine, esmolol, nitroprusside, nitroglycerin, or fenoldopam

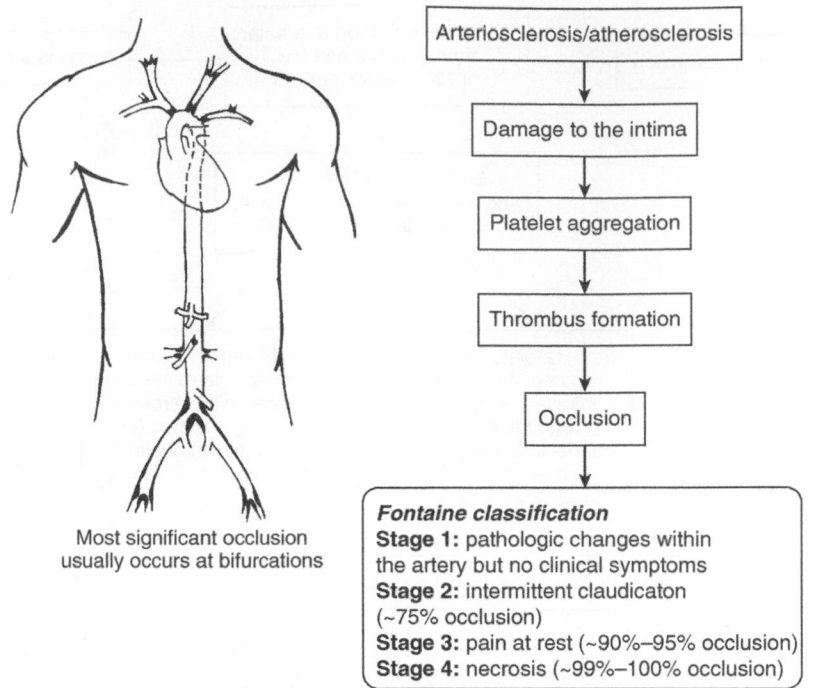

Most significant occlusion
usually occurs at bifurcations

Fontaine classification
Stage 1: pathologic changes within the artery but no clinical symptoms
Stage 2: intermittent claudicaton (~75% occlusion)
Stage 3: pain at rest (~90%–95% occlusion)
Stage 4: necrosis (~99%–100% occlusion)

FIGURE 3-68 Pathophysiology of peripheral arterial disease. (From Dennison, R. D. [2013]. *Pass CCRN!* [4th ed.]. St. Louis, MO: Elsevier.)

Assist in preparation of the patient for surgical procedures to treat the cause of hypertension. Angioplasty may be performed for renovascular disease. Adrenalectomy is performed for pheochromocytoma after tachycardia and hypertension have been adequately controlled.

Monitor the patient for complications. Serious complications of hypertensive crisis include stroke, MI, HF/pulmonary edema, aortic dissection, and renal failure.

Provide instruction and counseling regarding lifestyle modification and need for pharmacologic therapy. Nonpharmacologic management includes weight normalization, smoking cessation, and dietary modifications. Patients are encouraged to follow a low-fat, no-added-salt (i.e., 2 to 3 g/day) diet that includes fresh fruits, vegetables, and fish, especially fatty fish such as salmon or trout. The diet recommends the inclusion of nuts, low-fat dairy, and monounsaturated fatty acids (e.g., extra-virgin olive oil). Encourage an increase intake of potassium, magnesium, and calcium. Recommend a moderate intake of alcohol (i.e., one glass of wine or equivalent/day) as long as they do not have a history of substance abuse. Aerobic exercise should be encouraged along with complementary therapies, such as relaxation, biofeedback, and acupuncture. Caring for pets can also be relaxing and lower BP.

Initiate pharmacologic management in the presence of mild hypertension with end-organ damage or DM, moderate hypertension that has not responded to conservative treatment, and severe hypertension. Choice of drug and/or combination is guided by need and preexisting condition. Diuretics and beta-blockers are usually first line. For patients with HF, recommendations include thiazide diuretics and an ACE inhibitor or ARB and/or beta-blocker (e.g., carvedilol [Coreg]) and/or aldosterone antagonist (i.e., potassium-sparing diuretics)(e.g., spironolactone [Aldactone], eplerenone [Inspra]). For post-MI patients, a beta-blocker and an ACE inhibitor or ARB and/ or aldosterone antagonist (e.g., spironolactone [Aldactone],

eplerenone [Inspra]) may be required. For patients with DM, the recommendations include an ACE inhibitor, ARB, diuretic, beta-blocker and/or calcium channel blocker. Elderly patients with isolated systolic hypertension generally require a diuretic or calcium channel blocker. Hypertensive and hypercholesteremic patients require a statin (e.g., pravastatin). Patients with renal insufficiency require an ACE inhibitor or an ARB.

VASCULAR DISEASE

Peripheral Arterial Disease

Peripheral arterial disease results in partial or total occlusion of an artery. The occlusion is primarily due to atherosclerosis/arteriosclerosis obliterans. The risk factors for arteriosclerosis/atherosclerosis are the same as those discussed for CAD. Atherosclerosis is the most common cause, but arteriosclerosis is a significant cause in older patients. Also implicated are the conditions of hypertension and arteritis.

The pathophysiology of peripheral arterial disease (Figure 3-68) stems from the arteriosclerosis and atherosclerosis processes. Fatty material (i.e., plaque) builds up on the walls of the arteries outside of the heart and makes them narrower. The walls of the arteries become stiffer and cannot dilate to allow greater blood flow when needed.

Occlusive disease of the terminal aorta and iliac arteries may manifest as intermittent claudication in the thigh and hip. Pain increases with exercise and decreases with rest. Impotence may also occur. Objective findings include coolness and hair loss over the lower extremities, decreased or absent iliac or femoral pulses, and the presence of a bruit or thrill over the iliac area. Occlusive disease of the femoral and popliteal arteries may manifest itself as intermittent claudication in the lower leg progressing to pain at rest and decreased sensation or paresthesia of the lower extremities. Objective findings include coolness and hair loss over the lower extremities, pallor and mottling of the

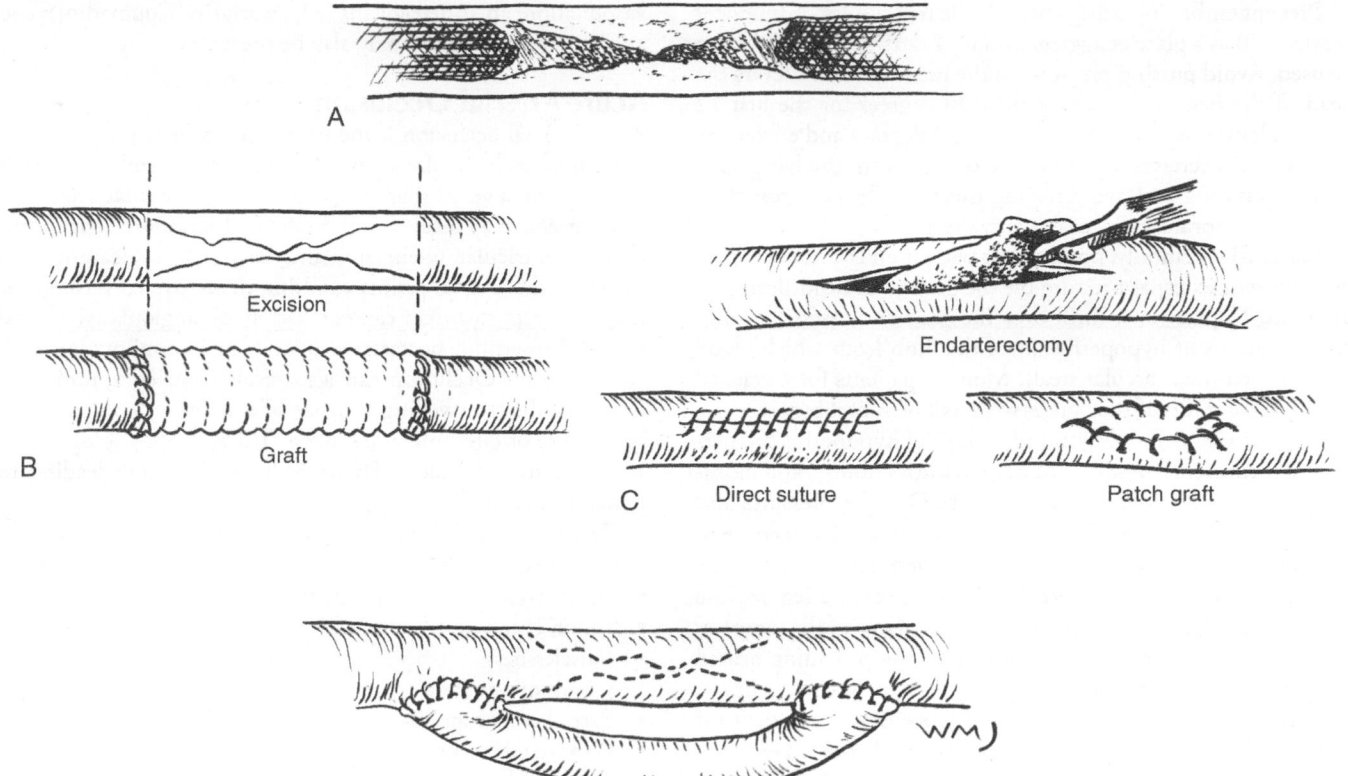

FIGURE 3-69 Surgical procedures for peripheral vascular disease. A, Occluded vessel. **B,** Excision and circumferential graft. **C,** Endarterectomy with direct suture or patch graft. **D,** Bypass graft. (Drawing by Wendy M. Johnson.)

lower extremities, nonhealing ulcers on toes or points of trauma, decreased motor strength in the lower extremities, decreased or absent femoral and popliteal pulses, or the presence of a bruit or thrill over the femoral or popliteal area. Diagnostic studies include arteriography and Doppler and duplex ultrasonography, which will indicate partial to complete vascular occlusion.

Collaborative management focuses on reduction of peripheral oxygen requirements. Instruct the patient to stop activities when pain occurs, maintain bed rest during acute occlusion, maintain normothermia and hydration, and to prevent trauma. Administer appropriate pharmacologic agents to reestablish blood flow. Fibrinolytics (e.g., urokinase, streptokinase, rt-PA) may be administered intravenously or locally by an intraarterial infusion and then followed by an anticoagulant such as heparin.

Assist in preparing the patient for percutaneous procedures (e.g., percutaneous balloon angioplasty, laser angioplasty, and atherectomy) aimed at removing the occlusion. The insertion of a flexible coil stent may accompany these procedures. Provide postprocedure care as for PCI. Monitor the catheter insertion site closely for bleeding and/or hematoma formation. Monitor peripheral perfusion closely. Report any indications of arterial occlusion (i.e., the six Ps) immediately. Provide anticoagulants and/or platelet aggregation inhibitors as prescribed. Assist in preparation of the patient for surgery aimed at improving flow and provide postoperative management.

Surgical procedures (Figure 3-69) include an arterial embolectomy to remove an occlusive clot from an artery. Clot removal occurs with a balloon-tipped catheter. Thromboendarterectomy (aortofemoral, aortoiliac, or femoral-popliteal) may also

be indicated, involving excision of a thickened layer of artery. Bypass surgery involves anastomosing a graft proximal and distal to the occlusion. The graft used may be an autologous vein, usually the saphenous, human umbilical vein, or an artificial graft (i.e., Dacron or polytetrafluoroethylene [PTFE]). Commonly performed bypasses include aortobifemoral, femoral to femoral, femoral-popliteal, and femoral-tibial.

Extra-anatomical bypass (EAB) involves the use of prosthetic material tunneled subcutaneously from the femoral to femoral or axillary to femoral arteries. It is frequently used for patients who are at high risk for an open abdominal procedure or who have numerous previous surgical procedures or peritonitis (sometimes referred to as a *hostile abdomen*). A sympathectomy requires interruption of the sympathetic tract to decrease local vascular resistance to improve local blood flow. When attempts to revascularize the limb have failed, an amputation is performed.

Postoperative management includes focus on maintaining airway, oxygenation, and ventilation. Assess the patient's ventilatory status frequently. Assess respiratory rate, rhythm, excursion, effort, and the use of accessory muscles. Note the presence of stridor or other adventitious sounds. Monitor oxygen saturation with pulse oximetry. Administer oxygen at 2 to 5 L/min as necessary to achieve SpO_2 of at least 90%. Encourage deep breathing and incentive spirometry.

Maintain adequate flow and pressure at the graft site. Maintain and control systolic BP at less than 120 mm Hg. Administer antihypertensives, such as nitroprusside (NTP), nicardipine (Cardene), or clevidipine (Cleviprex), as prescribed. Also, administer analgesics as indicated.

Prevent emboli by using antiembolic techniques. Administer Dextran 40 as a platelet aggregation inhibitor. Heparin may also be used. Avoid putting pressure on the incision sites. Elevate the head of the bed to no greater than 30 degrees for the first 72 hours. Elevate the patient's legs 20 to 30 degrees and encourage foot and leg exercises. Mobilize the patient from the lying position to standing and avoid having them sit, flex, or cross their legs after femoral artery revascularization.

For EAB specifically, position the patient on the nonoperative side. Prevent external pressure on the graft and avoid flexion of the graft. Palpate for a thrill over the graft and assess for clinical indications of hypoperfusion of the limb from which blood was diverted (i.e., vascular steal). Monitor patients for a brachial plexus nerve injury if they underwent axillofemoral bypass.

Assess patients for clinical indications of hypoperfusion, perform neurovascular assessment of extremities hourly, and monitor for the six Ps. Measure the patient's Doppler pressures and calculate the ankle-brachial index (ABI). Report any decrease in ABI of 0.15 or more. Do not measure Doppler pressure if the bypass location was the most distal arteries of the leg because this is painful for the patient and may cause graft compression. Maintain normal body temperature by providing heated blankets or an automatic warming blanket or warming lights. Administer analgesics to treat pain and position the patient for comfort. Inspect skin, bony prominences, and affected extremities frequently. Prevent skin breakdown related to ischemia and immobility by frequent position changes. Utilize an alternating air mattress or a special bed, depending on other risk factors. Keep the patient's heels elevated and off the bed. Also, maintain adequate hydration, administering IV fluids as indicated. Monitor the patient's urine output closely and report urine output of less than 0.5 mL/kg/hr.

Monitor the patient for postoperative complications, such as hemorrhage and infection. Assess incision and wounds for indications of infection and provide aseptic wound care. Monitor WBC and body temperature. Assess patients for arterial thrombosis, cerebral embolus, peripheral ischemia, infarction, loss of limb, and graft infection. Monitor the patient for fever, malaise, back pain, anorexia, paralytic ileus, and leukocytosis, which indicate graft infection and administer antibiotics as prescribed. If the patient requires a removal and replacement of a graft, prepare the patient for surgery.

Provide instructions and counseling regarding lifestyle modification and the importance of pharmacologic therapy. Patients should be encouraged to lose weight, if applicable. Recommended diet modifications include low saturated fat intake and adherence to an ADA diet for control of a diabetic patient's blood glucose. Smoking cessation is a major component of treatment; so offer smoking cessation resources. Recommend regular aerobic exercise in moderation, but not to the point of pain.

Provide special attention to any lesions of the foot, because healing may be impaired due to ischemia. Instruct the patient to avoid wearing constrictive clothing. Also, encourage complementary therapies of relaxation techniques, imagery, and biofeedback to decrease stress and cortisol response.

Teach the patient about the pharmacologic agents prescribed. These are usually platelet aggregation inhibitors (e.g., ASA, clopidogrel [Plavix]), agents that increase the flexibility of the red blood cells (e.g., pentoxifylline [Trental]), and peripheral vasodilators. A phosphodiesterase III inhibitor (e.g., cilostazol [Pletal]), which inhibits platelet aggregation and causes

vasodilation; an anticoagulant (e.g., warfarin [Coumadin]); and antihypertensive agents may also be prescribed.

Acute Arterial Occlusion

Acute arterial occlusion is the complete occlusion of an artery. A thrombosis in an already narrowed artery, an embolism, and/or trauma to a vessel that most likely causes the total occlusion. These events may result from arterial embolization, atrial fibrillation, ventricular aneurysm, and bacterial endocarditis. An injury to the arterial intima resulting in an arterial thrombosis may occur postcardiac catheterization or angioplasty, related to IABP insertion, postarterial bypass, or in conjunction with an aneurysm. Occlusion can also result from compression of an artery due to swelling because of a fracture (compartment syndrome) or circumferential burn. The pathophysiology of an acute arterial occlusion (Figure 3-70) is occlusion leading to ischemia and necrosis.

The clinical presentation of acute arterial occlusion can be remembered as the six Ps:
- Pain: severe and sudden
- Pallor, cyanosis
- Pulselessness
- Paresis or paralysis
- Paresthesia or anesthesia
- Polar (cold) or poikylothermia

A Doppler stethoscope is used to determine the presence or absence of a pulse when it cannot be palpated. Angiography is useful for confirming arterial occlusion.

Initiate emergency measures immediately for suspected acute arterial occlusion. Provide oxygen at 2 to 5 L/min to maintain Sao_2 at 95%, unless contraindicated. Position the limb properly, keeping the extremity straight, warm, and dependent. Initiate an IV infusion of NS at KVO rate in an unaffected limb. Notify the physician immediately and assist in preparation for diagnostic studies, such as an arteriogram and/or emergent surgery or procedure. Administer narcotics (e.g., morphine) for pain, which will be severe. To reestablish patency of the artery, assist with initiation of an intraarterial fibrinolytic (e.g., urokinase, rt-PA) followed by an anticoagulant. If a surgical procedure is indicated, assist in preparation of the patient and instruction of the patient and family. Explain the procedures thoroughly to the patient to minimize stress. Surgical procedures include a surgical embolectomy, balloon embolectomy, thromboendarterectomy, and bypass grafting. Provide postoperative care as for other vascular surgery. Monitor the patient closely for complications, including reocclusion, loss of limb, and/or infection. Before discharge, provide patient teaching as for peripheral arterial disease.

Aortic Aneurysm

An aortic aneurysm is a permanent localized dilation of the aorta with an increase to at least 1.5 times its normal diameter. The aneurysm is caused by degenerative changes associated with aging and familial predisposition, congenital weakness of the aorta, hypertension, pregnancy (especially in the third trimester), coarctation of the aorta, syphilis, severe systemic infection (e.g., bacterial aneurysm, mycotic aneurysm), Marfan syndrome, trauma (especially blunt trauma with acceleration-deceleration injury), or arterial cannulation (e.g., PCI, IABP).

The pathophysiology of an aortic aneurysm (Figure 3-71) stems from the atherosclerotic process. Five types of aneurysms exist. The *false* type does not involve all layers of the

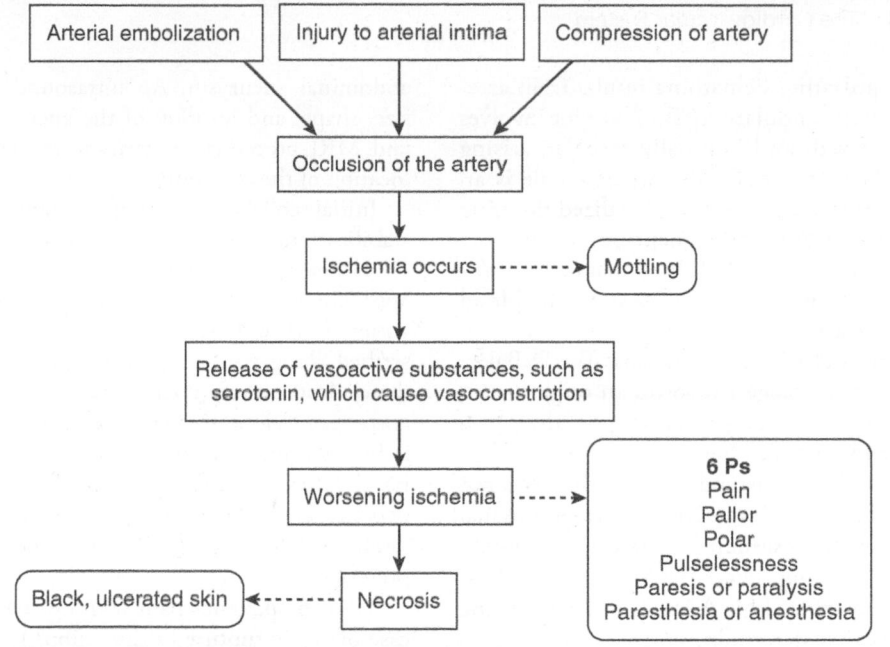

Arterial embolization | Injury to arterial intima | Compression of artery

↓

Occlusion of the artery

↓

Ischemia occurs ----> Mottling

↓

Release of vasoactive substances, such as serotonin, which cause vasoconstriction

↓

Worsening ischemia ---->

6 Ps
Pain
Pallor
Polar
Pulselessness
Paresis or paralysis
Paresthesia or anesthesia

↓

Black, ulcerated skin <---- Necrosis

FIGURE 3-70 Pathophysiology of acute arterial occlusion. Dotted lines connect pathology to the clinical presentation. (From Dennison, R. D. [2013]. *Pass CCRN!* [4th ed.]. St. Louis, MO: Elsevier.)

Atherosclerotic plaque erodes the vessel wall

↓

Elastin fragmentation allows formation of the aneurysm

↓

Collagen deposition and degradation allows enlargement and rupture of the aneurysm

Torn intimal
Blood flow
Dissection

Ruptured area
Blood flow
Rupture

Aortic dissection results from a tear in the intimal layer of the aorta

↓

Blood flows into the medial layer creating a false channel (lumen)

↓

Pressure change in the aorta caused by left ventricular ejection is a factor in progressive dissection ----> "Ripping" or "tearing" pain; BP differences comparing left and right

↓

Perfusion to major arteries arising from the section of the aorta is reduced as blood flows into the false lumen ----> Clinical indications of diminished perfusion to areas supplied by affected branches

Aortic rupture is more likely as the aneurysm increases in size

↓

Rupture results in leakage of blood into the peritoneal cavity or the mediastinum ----> Sudden severe pain in chest or back

↓

Hypovolemic shock ----> Clinical indications of hypoperfusion

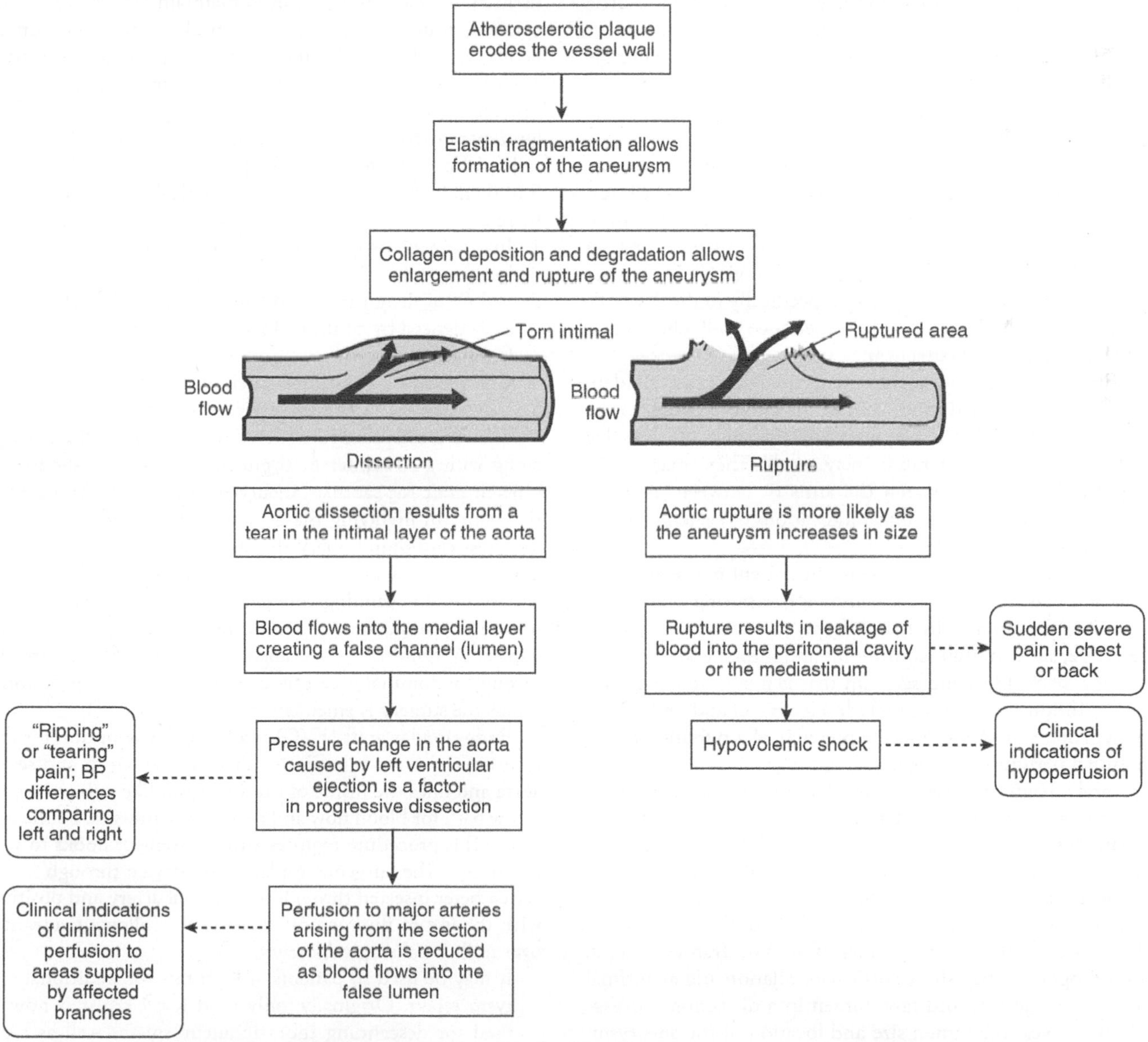

FIGURE 3-71 Pathophysiology of aneurysm dissection. Dotted lines connect pathology to the clinical presentation. (From Dennison, R. D. [2013]. *Pass CCRN!* [4th ed.]. St. Louis, MO: Elsevier.)

artery. The associated pulsating hematoma results from arterial trauma, such as arterial cannulation. The *true* type involves all layers of the arterial wall and is usually saccular, arising from a distinct portion of the wall. The *saccular* type is an outpouching from an artery resulting from localized thinning and stretching of the media. A *fusiform* aneurysm involves the total circumference of the artery with diffuse dilatation. A *dissecting* aneurysm results from a cavity formed by the blood between the layers of the arterial wall.

Aneurysms have several classification systems. The DeBakey system describes three stages. Stage I involves an original intimal tear that begins in the ascending aorta with the dissection extending to the descending aorta. Stage II involves an original intimal tear beginning in the ascending aorta that does not extend to the descending aorta. Stage III involves an original intimal tear beginning in the descending aorta with the dissection confined in the descending aorta. The Stanford classification system describes two types. Type A involves the ascending aorta and type B involves the descending aorta.

Rupture of the aortic wall results in leaking of arterial blood into the mediastinum (if a thoracic aortic aneurysm) or into the abdominal cavity (if an abdominal aortic aneurysm). Aortic aneurysms are usually asymptomatic until dissection or rupture occurs. Clinical findings include normal to high BP, a pulsatile mass, increased aortic diameter on palpation, and a bruit over the aorta. The sudden occurrence of hypotension suggests cardiac tamponade or an aortic rupture.

Although thoracic aortic aneurysms may be asymptomatic, the patient may also experience dyspnea, chest pain, or clinical indications of aortic regurgitation, such as diastolic murmur, LVF, and/or widened pulse pressure. Aneurysms occurring on the aortic arch result in dyspnea, stridor, cough, JVD, hoarseness, or a weak voice. For aneurysms specifically in the descending thoracic arch, patients may experience dull chest pain, upper back pain, and hoarseness.

A dissecting thoracic aortic aneurysm may cause sudden, sharp, tearing, and/or ripping pain in the chest radiating to the shoulders, neck, or back. Hypotension, dyspnea, syncope, leg weakness, or transient paralysis may result. There may be BP and pulse differences between the arms or between the arms and the legs, and possible clinical indications of ischemic stroke and/or cardiac tamponade.

For abdominal aortic aneurysms, the patient may experience dull abdominal and back pain, nausea and vomiting, abdominal bloating, and pulsation in the abdomen. Patients may experience severe, sudden, dull, continuous abdominal pain radiating to the low back, hips, and scrotum that is unaffected by movement. Additional symptoms include a feeling of abdominal fullness, syncope and shock, and the presence of a pulsation in the abdominal periumbilical area.

Several diagnostic tests may determine the differential diagnosis of an aneurysm. If there is a dissection or rupture, the patient's hemoglobin and hematocrit decreases. The chest x-ray will reveal mediastinal widening in a thoracic aneurysm and the presence of aortic calcification; ECG may show left ventricular hypertrophy, nonspecific ST and T wave changes, and an absence of ECG indicators of an MI. Transesophageal echocardiography may show aortic root dilation and an intimal flap dividing the true and false lumen in a dissection. Aortography will reveal the lumen size and location of the aneurysm. A flat plate of abdomen (i.e., KUB) provides an outline of the abdominal aneurysm. An ultrasound confirms the presence, size, shape, and location of the aneurysm. The diagnostic CT and MRI procedures determine the exact presence, size, and location of the aneurysm.

Initial collaborative management focuses on circulatory stabilization. Obtain IV access with two large-bore, short IV catheters. Maintain and control mean arterial pressure at approximately 60 to 75 mm Hg if dissection occurs. If the patient is hypertensive, administer nitroprusside (NTP) as prescribed along with propranolol (Inderal). Labetalol (Normodyne) decreases contractility and the pulsatile pressure on the aorta. Send blood for typing and crossmatching. If the patient is hypotensive, provide normal saline or lactated Ringer's by rapid infusion until replacement blood and/or blood products are available. Administer colloids (e.g., albumin, hetastarch, and dextran) along with blood and blood products, as prescribed.

Treat the patient's pain with opiates (i.e., morphine) in the case of aortic rupture or dissection. Use extreme caution with these drugs if the patient is hypotensive. Restrict patient activity to decrease tissue oxygenation requirements. Provide oxygen by nasal cannula at 2 to 6 L/min to maintain SaO_2 of 95%, unless contraindicated. Intubation and mechanical ventilation may be necessary. Provide for the patient's physical comfort, paying attention to temperature control, lighting, and noise control. Provide anxiolytics as prescribed, usually diazepam (Valium), lorazepam (Ativan), or alprazolam (Xanax). Assist in the preparation of patients for surgical repair for aneurysmal dilation of 5 to 6 cm in diameter. Immediate surgical repair is indicated if there is:

1. Involvement of the ascending aorta and subsequent aortic insufficiency
2. Failure of drug therapy to control progression of dissection as evidenced by continued pain and progressive symptoms
3. Cardiac tamponade
4. Compromise of a major branch of the aorta
5. Indications of cerebral or cardiac ischemia

The surgical procedure includes resection of the aneurysm along with a circumferential graft for a fusiform aneurysm or a patch graft for saccular aneurysm. Repair of a thoracic aortic aneurysm involving the ascending aorta and/or aortic arch requires cardiopulmonary bypass. Concurrent aortic valve repair or replacement may be needed for ascending thoracic aneurysms. Descending thoracic aortic aneurysms are usually repaired by thoracotomy and do not require cardiopulmonary bypass. Abdominal aortic aneurysm (AAA) repairs are done through abdominal incisions; a bowel preparation is performed unless the surgery is emergent.

Endovascular graft (EVG) is a less invasive option for aneurysm repair. A modular device that expands to fit and seal the aorta and lines the inside of the aneurysm like a sleeve provides a new path for blood flow and reduces the pressure on the aneurysm. This procedure requires either a stent or hooks to secure the sleeve. The surgeon implants the device through a delivery catheter inserted through the femoral artery and positioned with the use of fluoroscopy. It offers the following advantages over traditional surgical aneurysm repair:

- It may be used in patients at high risk for traditional aneurysm repair. Originally, only used for AAA, it is now also used for descending thoracic aneurysms as well as type B dissections.

- Intubation is not required and patients may not require critical care unit stay.
- This process offers fewer complications, including less blood loss than with an open repair, less hypothermia than with laparotomy, a shorter hospital stay, and lower early mortality.

Long-term mortality is comparable for EVG and open repair of aortic aneurysm. Disadvantages of the EVG option compared with traditional surgical repair include the fact that not all patients are candidates because of the location of the aneurysm and the size of the patient's arteries above and below the aneurysm may preclude the implant. Finally, it may be more costly in both the short and long term because lifelong surveillance is required.

Postoperative management after aneurysm repair focuses first on maintaining airway, oxygenation, and ventilation. Assess the patient's ventilatory status frequently. Assess respiratory rate, rhythm, excursion, effort, and the use of accessory muscles. Note the presence of stridor or other adventitious sounds. Monitor oxygen saturation with pulse oximetry. Administer oxygen at 2 to 5 L/min as necessary to achieve SpO_2 of at least 95%. Encourage deep breathing and incentive spirometry.

Maintain adequate flow and pressure at the graft site. Maintain and control systolic BP less than 120 mm Hg, using prescribed nitroprusside (NTP), nicardipine (Cardene), and analgesics as indicated. Prevent emboli by using antiembolic techniques. Administer Dextran 40 as a platelet aggregation inhibitor. Heparin may also be used. Avoid pressure on the incision sites. Elevate the patient's head of bed to no greater than 30 degrees for the first 72 hours. Elevate the patient's legs 20 to 30 degrees and encourage foot and leg exercises. Mobilize the patient from lying to a standing position; avoid the sitting position and flexing or crossing of the legs.

Assess patients for clinical indications of hypoperfusion. Perform a neurovascular assessment of the extremities hourly, monitoring for the six Ps. Use heated blankets, an automatic warming blankets, or warming lights to maintain a normal body temperature. Treat pain, administering analgesics as indicated, and position the patient for comfort. Prevent skin breakdown related to ischemia and immobility. Inspect skin, bony prominences, and affected extremities frequently and reposition patients often. Utilize an egg crate mattress, an alternating air mattress, or a special bed, depending on the patient's other risk factors. Keep the patient's heels elevated and off the bed. Maintain adequate hydration by administering IV fluids as indicated; monitor the patient's urine output closely and report urine output of less than 0.5 mL/kg/hr.

Monitor patients for postoperative complications. Dyspnea, hypoxemia, tachypnea, tachycardia, and/or fever may indicate acute respiratory failure. Note hypotension, tachycardia, clinical manifestations of hypoperfusion, and decreased CVP, which could indicate hemorrhage, hypovolemia, or hematoma. Monitor the patient for myocardial ischemia and infarction by assessing the patient for chest pain, dyspnea, dysrhythmias, ST segment changes, and clinical indications of hypoperfusion. Monitor for cerebral ischemia and infarction by assessing the patient for alterations in LOC, pupillary changes, aphasia, and motor or sensory changes. Monitor the patient for dyspnea, chest pain, pleural friction rub, and hypoxemia, which may indicate pulmonary ischemia and/or infarction. For renal ischemia and infarction, monitor the patient for flank pain, decreased urine output, changes in BUN or creatinine, and hematuria. For mesenteric ischemia and infarction,

monitor the patient for watery, bloody diarrhea; abdominal pain; and changes in bowel sounds. For splenic ischemia and infarction, monitor the patient for left upper quadrant pain radiating to the left shoulder and abdominal rigidity. For spinal cord ischemia and infarction, monitor the patient for paralysis of the lower extremities and bowel/bladder paralysis. Drainage of cerebral spinal fluid (CSF), naloxone, osmotic diuretics, steroids, and/or calcium channel blockers are treatments used to prevent and/or treat spinal cord hyperemia and edema.

To monitor for arterial thrombosis, look for sudden, painful ischemia of the feet (sometimes referred to as *trash foot*) and/or lower leg and diminished or absent peripheral pulses with a decreased ABI. For complications specific to endovascular aneurysm repair, monitor for an endoleak. An endoleak is the persistence of blood flow outside the lumen of the endoluminal graft but within the aneurysmal sac. Manage endoleaks by observation, further endovascular procedures, or an open repair. An endoleak increases the risk for continued aneurysm expansion and rupture.

Monitor the patient for postimplant syndrome manifested as back pain and fever without leukocytosis or other signs of infection that last up to 7 days. The cause of this syndrome is unknown. Graft limb thrombosis may occur, requiring thrombectomy or embolectomy.

Provide instruction and counseling regarding required lifestyle modification as for peripheral arterial disease. Also, provide instruction regarding prescribed pharmacologic therapy.

Carotid Arterial Stenosis

Carotid arterial stenosis, referred to as *extracranial cerebrovascular disease,* is a form of vascular disease that shares the same risk factors as for CAD and peripheral vascular disease (i.e., atherosclerosis/arteriosclerosis). During a vascular workup, all cardiovascular conditions are assessed. The carotid disease is repaired first before the other cardiovascular conditions are surgically repaired (i.e., stent the carotids prior to aneurysm repair). Stenosis also occurs from trauma, fibromuscular dysplasia, cervical irradiation, and/or arteritis. The process involves the accumulation of atherosclerotic plaque at the bifurcation of the internal and external carotid arteries. Fragments of this plaque or associated thrombi break away causing cerebral emboli. Eventually, ischemia or infarction of the brain occurs. A transient ischemic attack (TIA) is a focal neurologic deficit lasting less than 24 hours caused by ischemia. An infarction is a completed ischemic stroke, resulting in permanent neurologic deficit, although there is some reversible ischemic neurologic deficit (RIND) that shows full improvement over time.

Carotid stenosis is usually asymptomatic unless it results in a TIA, RIND, or a completed stroke. There will be a bruit or thrill over one or both carotid arteries. Signs of a TIA or stroke may include slurred speech or aphasia, ataxia, paresis or paralysis, and temporary loss of consciousness. Duplex ultrasonography of the carotid arteries is the initial diagnostic test for patients with known or suspected carotid stenosis. Magnetic resonance angiography or CT angiography is used if sonography cannot be obtained or yields nondiagnostic results. Cerebral arteriography is a diagnostic examination used in some cases.

Collaborative management requires administering pharmacologic agents as prescribed. These include platelet aggregation inhibitors (e.g., ASA, clopidogrel [Plavix] or ASA plus dipyridamole [Aggrenox]). Avoid concomitant administration of ASA and clopidogrel. Another agent used is pentoxifylline (Trental) because it increases the flexibility of the red blood cells. Administer anticoagulants (e.g., warfarin [Coumadin]) as prescribed for patients with atrial fibrillation or a mechanical prosthetic cardiac valve to maintain an INR of 2.5. To control BP, administer prescribed antihypertensive agents. Prepare the patient for percutaneous or surgical procedure as requested. Indications for a surgical procedure include an occlusion of 70% or greater of the internal carotid artery, a mild stroke within the previous 6 months, and no surgical contraindications. Procedures include a carotid endarterectomy (CEA), involving removal of an atheroma at the carotic artery bifurcation, and carotid artery stenting, especially for patients who are a high surgical risk. CEA is a standard intervention for carotid artery stenosis, while angioplasty/stenting (CAS) is gaining acceptance. Stenting may require balloon dilation of the stenotic area and placement of a crush-resistant stent. A stent is especially useful in patients with recurrent carotid stenosis, lesions distal in the internal carotid artery or high in the neck, or a history of cervical irradiation. It is important to optimize cerebral blood flow and minimize myocardial stress during these procedures. MI, cranial nerve injury, wound infection, and venous thromboembolism are unlikely with the CAS procedure. There is no risk of injury to the cranial nerves with carotid artery stenting.

After either procedure, it is essential to maintain the patient's airway, oxygenation, and ventilation. Assess ventilatory status frequently and monitor the patient's rate, rhythm, excursion, effort, use of accessory muscles, presence of stridor or other adventitious sounds, and pulse oximetry. Encourage patients to breathe deeply and use incentive spirometry. Assess patients frequently for edema, hematoma, tracheal deviation, and dysphagia. Elevate the patient's head of bed to 30 degrees. Keep emergency equipment on hand for cricothyroidotomy, tracheostomy, and suctioning. Until the gag reflex returns, patients need to avoid taken anything by mouth (NPO). To prevent aspiration, have the patient assume the high Fowler's position while eating. Administer oxygen at 2 to 5 L/min as prescribed to maintain a Sao_2 of 95%. Monitor patients to prevent alterations in cerebral perfusion related to cerebral embolism, ischemia, and infarction, especially after procedures. Assess BP and HR frequently. Maintain the BP within 20 mm Hg of preoperative values. Assess the patient's neurologic and cranial nerve function, including loss of consciousness, pupillary response, motor function, sensory function, and cranial nerves. Report changes in the LOC, pupillary changes, paresis or plegia, visual changes, dysphasia or aphasia, seizures, or complaints of headache immediately.

SIDEBAR 3-6

Cranial Nerve Assessment Post Carotid Endarterectomy

To detect injury to cranial nerves and spinal nerves after carotid endarterectomy, assess the following:

- Cranial nerve (CN) VII: Ask the patient to smile.
- CN IX, X: Check swallowing, speech, and gag reflex.
- CN XI: Ask the patient to shrug against your hands.
- CN XII: Ask the patient to stick the tongue out and check for the midline position.
- Spinal recurrent laryngeal nerve: Check speech.
- Spinal great auricular nerve: Note perception of sensation on face and ear.

Administer antiplatelet aggregation drugs (e.g., ASA, clopidogrel [Plavix], Dextran 40) as prescribed. Administer the antiplatelet aggregation therapy before surgery and for at least 30 days after carotid artery stenting. Continue to monitor patients for hemorrhage, hematoma, or tracheal deviation. Assess the BP and HR frequently. Assess the neck dressing for hematoma or hemorrhage, making sure to observe the patient's posterior neck. Observe for the presence of any drainage from the drain. Monitor the patient's hemoglobin and hematocrit. Administer antihypertensives (e.g., nitroprusside [Nipride], labetalol [Normodyne]) as prescribed to maintain systolic BP between 100 and 160 mm Hg and diastolic BP less than 100 mm Hg.

Monitor for complications, such as MI, cerebral hemorrhage/embolism/infarction, carotid hemorrhage, hematoma, cranial nerve injury, and seizures. Provide instruction and counseling to the patient regarding lifestyle modification and the need for pharmacologic therapy as for peripheral arterial disease.

BLUNT CARDIAC INJURY

Blunt cardiac injury (i.e., myocardial contusion) may result in transient or permanent myocardial dysfunction and may include myocardial necrosis without coronary artery disease. This type of injury is common in acceleration/deceleration injuries sustained in motor vehicle collisions (MVC). In a MVC, a cardiac injury occurs when the sternum hits the steering wheel or the dashboard. The shoulder strap of the seat belt can also cause injury. This same type of injury occurs with other vehicular collisions such as motorcycle collisions and auto-pedestrian collisions. Other etiologies of blunt chest trauma include large animal kicks in the chest, assault with a blunt instrument, industrial crush injury, explosions, vigorous CPR, and projectile objects (e.g., baseball, hockey puck).

The pathophysiology of cardiac trauma (Figure 3-72) stems from a resultant injury due to compression of the cardiac structures between the sternum and spine. Because the right ventricle is anterior, injury occurs there more often than the left ventricle. Right ventricular MI may occur.

The patient will report a history of events and mechanism of injury, precordial angina-like chest pain that frequently increases with inspiration, cough, and movement that is unresponsive to nitroglycerin. The chest pain is frequently responsive to oxygen, antiinflammatory agents, or narcotics. The patient may also complain of dyspnea and palpitations. Objective findings include persistent tachycardia despite adequate fluid replacement, tachypnea, hypotension, ecchymosis on the anterior chest, chest wall tenderness with palpation, clinical indications of RVF (i.e., JVD, peripheral edema, and hepatomegaly), clinical indications of left ventricular noncompliance (left-sided S_4), and clinical indications of hypoperfusion (see Table 3-2). Cardiac arrest because of fatal ventricular dysrhythmias may occur.

Diagnosis requires serum analysis of cardiac markers. The CK-MB and cardiac troponin will be positive depending on the severity of the injury. An ECG including the right ventricular leads will show ST segment changes, T wave inversion in V_1-V_4, and Q waves indicating a severe injury and/or a lacerated or thrombosed coronary artery. A blunt cardiac injury often results in a prolonged QT interval and dysrhythmias including atrial dysrhythmias (e.g., PACs, atrial fibrillation, atrial flutter); ventricular dysrhythmias (e.g., PVCs, ventricular tachycardia, ventricular fibrillation); and blocks (e.g., AV blocks, RBBB).

Echocardiography is useful in detecting decreased regional wall motion, increased end-diastolic wall thickness, and decreased RV ejection fraction. The echocardiogram reveals complications such as an apical thrombi, pericardial effusion, and cardiac tamponade. Radionuclide studies indicate decreased RV ejection fraction.

Collaborative management of blunt cardiac injury requires treating pain. Administer opiates (e.g., morphine) and anti-inflammatory agents. Ensure that the patient has adequate right ventricular contractility, left ventricular filling, and cardiac output. Administer isotonic fluids as prescribed to ensure adequate left ventricular filling. Avoid venous vasodilators and diuretics because they decrease left ventricular filling volumes. Administer inotropes (e.g., dobutamine) as prescribed to improve right ventricular contractility. Decrease myocardial oxygen demand by imposing bed rest. Provide oxygen by nasal cannula at 2 to 6 L/min to maintain the SaO_2 at 95% unless contraindicated. Administer anxiolytics as prescribed and indicated.

Treat dysrhythmias as indicated:
- Atrial dysrhythmias are usually treated with digoxin and/or cardioversion.
- Ventricular dysrhythmias usually respond to amiodarone.
- Blocks may require a temporary pacemaker and/or permanent pacemaker

Assist in the assessment for other thoracic injuries (e.g., fractured ribs, sternum, or clavicle, and pulmonary contusion). Monitor the patient for complications, including ventricular rupture, cardiac tamponade, coronary artery thrombosis, intracardiac thrombus, valve rupture, conduction defects, HF, ventricular aneurysm, and cardiogenic shock. Also, monitor the patient for clinical manifestations of hypoperfusion (see Table 3-2) and systemic emboli. Use sequential compression devices to prevent deep vein thrombosis (DVT) until the patient resumes normal activity level; avoid anticoagulation therapy unless there are intramural thrombi present.

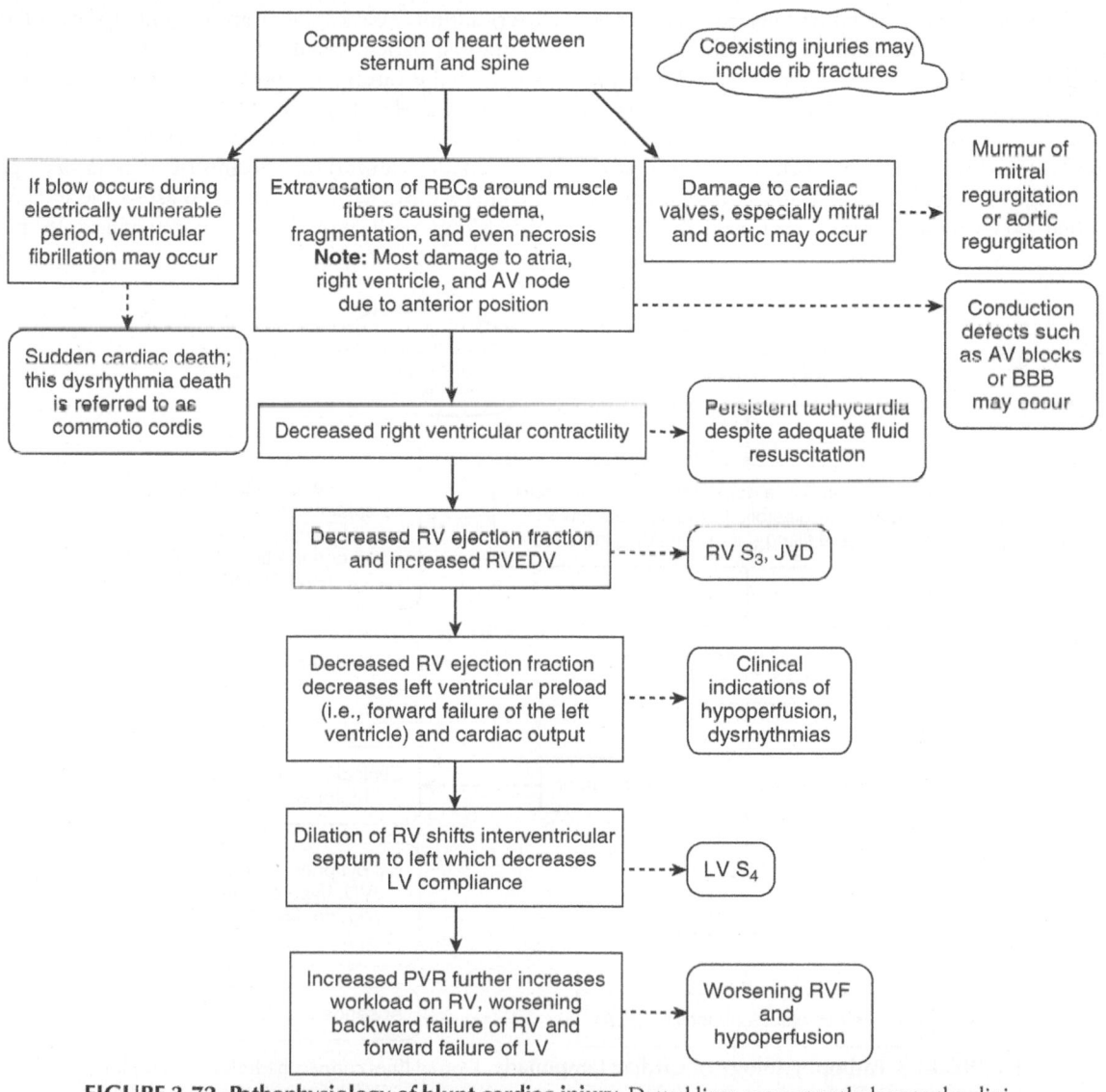

FIGURE 3-72 **Pathophysiology of blunt cardiac injury.** Dotted lines connect pathology to the clinical presentation. *BBB,* Bundle branch block; *JVD,* jugular venous distention; *LV,* left ventricular; *PVR,* pulmonary vascular resistance; *RV,* right ventricular; *RVEDV,* right ventricular end-diastolic volume; *RVF,* right ventricular failure. (From Dennison, R. D. [2013]. *Pass CCRN!* [4th ed.]. St. Louis, MO: Elsevier.)

CARDIAC TAMPONADE

Cardiac tamponade occurs when fluid (i.e., blood, effusion fluid, pus) in the pericardial space compromises cardiac filling and cardiac output. Tamponade is not dependent on the amount of fluid in the pericardial space but on the presence of hemodynamic consequences of the pericardial fluid.

Cardiac tamponade may occur for a variety of reasons. Common etiologies include blunt or penetrating injury to the heart, occlusion of a postcardiotomy mediastinal tube, or after removal of a mediastinal tube and/or epicardial pacing wires. Cardiac tamponade may also occur post-MI, manifesting as pericarditis especially in the anticoagulated patient, and/or cardiac rupture. Iatrogenic causes include perforation of the myocardium by transvenous pacemaker wires, invasive catheters, intracardiac injection, or cardiac needle biopsy. Other causes of tamponade include several different treatments, injury or disease processes and drug treatments. Treatments that may cause cardiac tamponade include transmyocardial revascularization, CPR, and electrical cardioversion. The injury or disease processes that may cause cardiac tamponade include the: rupture of great vessels, dissecting aortic aneurysms, malignancy and/or radiation therapy, connective tissue disease, metabolic disease, and inflammation or infection. Connective tissue diseases include rheumatoid arthritis (RA), systemic lupus erythematosus (SLE), and scleroderma. Metabolic diseases include renal failure, hepatic failure, or myxedema. Inflammatory conditions such as pericarditis or viral, bacterial (e.g., tuberculosis), or fungal infections may result in cardiac tamponade. Drugs implicated in cardiac tamponade include fibrinolytic or anticoagulant therapy, procainamide (Pronestyl), hydralazine (Apresoline), minoxidil (Loniten), phenytoin (Dilantin), daunorubicin (Cerubidine), methyldopa (Aldomet), sulfasalazine (Azulfidine), isoniazid (INH), methysergide (Sansert), sargramostim (Leukine), and tetracycline derivatives.

The underlying pathophysiology process for cardiac tamponade (Figure 3-73) is compression with a decrease in diastolic filling. This results in decreased cardiac output.

A patient with cardiac tamponade will complain of precordial fullness or pain, dyspnea with improvement when sitting upright, anxiety, or a feeling of impending doom. Tachycardia is usually an early objective sign. Hypotension and a narrowed pulse pressure may occur, as well as pulsus paradoxus. An increased JVD may result, but it may not be visible if the patient is hypotensive. There will be an absence of the PMI, dullness to percussion below the left scapula (i.e., Ewart's sign), and heart sound changes. If the tamponade is associated with pericarditis, a pericardial friction rub is heard. There may be distant, muffled, or absent heart sounds. Hypotension, distended neck veins, and muffled heart sounds (Beck's triad) are present. In a cardiac surgery or trauma patient, mediastinal tube drainage may suddenly stop. As the cardiac tamponade progresses, the patient may become pulseless (i.e., PEA).

In a patient at risk for or suspected of having a cardiac tamponade, important diagnostic laboratory parameters include a CBC with differential to assess the patient for anemia along with typing and crossmatching in preparation

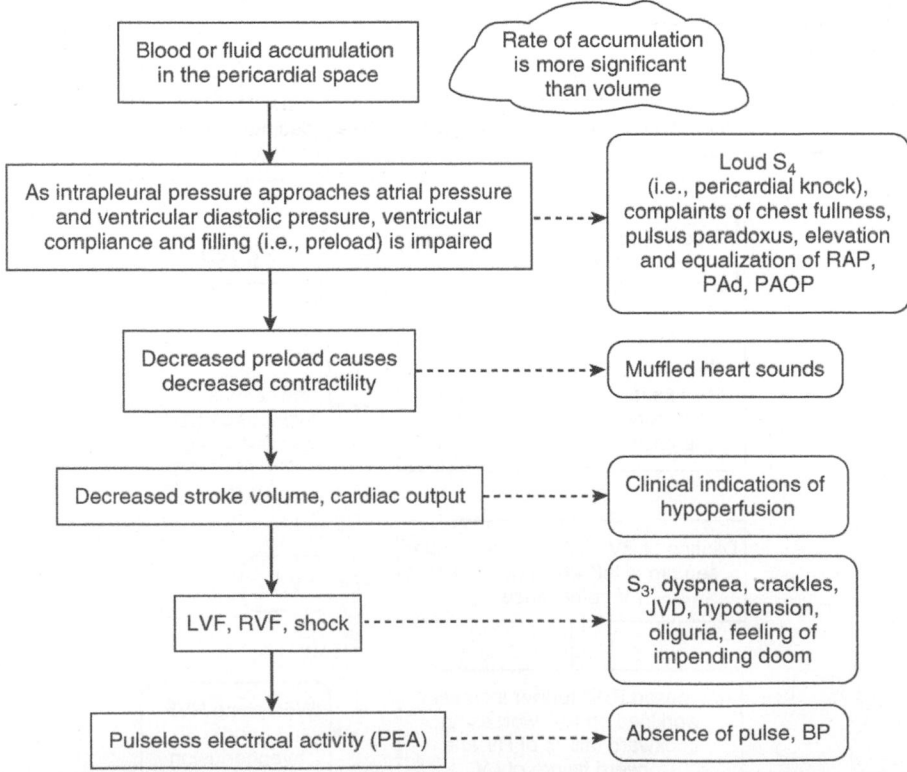

FIGURE 3-73 Pathophysiology of cardiac tamponade. Dotted lines connect pathology to the clinical presentation. *BP,* Blood pressure; *JVD,* jugular venous distention; *LVF,* left ventricular failure; *PAd,* pulmonary artery diastolic pressure; *PAOP,* pulmonary artery occlusive pressure; *PEA,* pulseless electrical activity; *RAP,* right atrial pressure; *RVF,* right ventricular failure. (From Dennison, R. D. [2013]. *Pass CCRN!* [4th ed.]. St. Louis, MO: Elsevier.)

for possible blood administration. A chest x-ray may reveal a widened mediastinum, dilated superior vena cava, and an enlarged heart (i.e., water-bottle silhouette). ECG is useful in revealing diffuse ST segment elevation across the precordial leads, a decrease in the amplitude of the QRS or electrical alternans (i.e., alternating tall and small QRSs) across the precordial leads, bradycardia possibly indicating impending PEA, and ventricular dysrhythmias. A 2-D or transesophageal echocardiogram will reveal any evidence of an echo-free space between the pericardium and epicardium, right atrial and ventricular collapse, respiratory variation in cardiac chamber dimension, and transvalvular flow velocities. Other diagnostic modalities include focused assessment with sonography (FAST), a CT of the chest, and fluoroscopy of the chest during pericardiocentesis.

The priority of collaborative management is providing airway, oxygenation, and circulation support, using BLS and ACLS, if needed. Oxygen (100%) should be provided by face mask during resuscitation efforts. Intubate and mechanically ventilate the patient as indicated.

Prepare to replace circulating volume by initiating two large-bore IVs. Replace the vascular volume as necessary. Provide normal saline, usually 200 to 500 mL over 10 to 15 minutes. Administer fresh frozen plasma (FFP), Dextran, albumin, and blood replacement as prescribed. Administer inotropic agents (e.g., dobutamine) as prescribed. Administer atropine or initiate transcutaneous pacing for bradydysrhythmias if indicated.

Prepare to assist with a pericardiocentesis for an emergency cardiac tamponade. Place the patient in a semi-Fowler's position. The subxiphoid and left parasternal approaches are the most commonly used sites. Apply the ECG machine and electrodes. Apply the limb leads and attach the chest lead wire to the exploring needle with an alligator clamp if requested. This technique assesses needle position because when the needle touches the epicardium, it triggers ST segment elevation and PVCs may occur. Have fluoroscopy at bedside and the echocardiography technician available to assist with 2-D echo guidance. Ensure that the emergency equipment including a transcutaneous pacemaker is at the bedside. Assist with administration of the local anesthetic and administer sedation if the patient is anxious. Assist with the slow aspiration of the fluid, label appropriately, and send it to the laboratory department for analysis. Assist with the placement of a pericardial catheter, if the plan of care includes the injection of sclerosing agents, corticosteroids, fibrinolytics, or chemotherapeutic agents.

Monitor the patient for complications, including laceration of the coronary artery or conduction system, myocardial perforation, pneumothorax, dysrhythmias, and hypotension (usually reflexogenic). Administer drugs or therapies related to the cause. Discontinue any drug that contributed to the tamponade. Initiate dialysis for patients with renal failure. Provide other pharmacologic agents as needed.

- Administer protamine sulfate or vitamin as prescribed if the patient is receiving anticoagulants.
  - Administer antibiotics as prescribed in the presence of a purulent effusion.
  - Administer thyroid hormone replacement as prescribed for myxedema.
  - Administer corticosteroids as prescribed for drug-related pericardial effusions, uremia, and pericarditis.

Assist in preparing the patient for surgical intervention if the pericardiocentesis does not resolve the tamponade. This failure to resolve the tamponade is common in the case of a posterior effusion or in the presence of purulent or hemorrhagic effusion. A subxiphoid pericardiotomy or a thorascopic procedure is often required.

Monitor/assist with the treatment of recurrent pericardial effusion or tamponade. Monitor the patient for recurring clinical indications of tamponade. Prepare the patient for the selected surgical procedure: percutaneous balloon pericardiotomy, intrapericardial instillation of a sclerosing agent, or pleuropericardial or peritoneal-pericardial window.

3.26   Learning Activity

Identify the physical findings from the following list observed in these pathologic conditions. More than one physical finding may be listed for each pathologic condition.

_____ 1. Right ventricular failure
_____ 2. Left ventricular failure
_____ 3. Left ventricular MI
_____ 4. Right ventricular MI
_____ 5. Cardiac tamponade
_____ 6. Valvular dysfunction
_____ 7. Chronic arterial insufficiency

a. Jugular venous distention
b. Displaced PMI
c. S_3 at apex
d. S_3 at sternum
e. S_4 at apex
f. S_4 at sternum
g. Murmur
h. Muffled heart sounds
i. Intermittent claudication
j. Peripheral edema
k. Peripheral pallor
l. Crackles in lung bases
m. Hepatomegaly
n. Pulsus paradoxus

Answers to this activity can be found in the Answer Key.

3.27   Synthesis Learning Activity: Clinical Vignette

Patient B is a 65-year-old man with a 10-year history of essential hypertension who came to the emergency department with complaints of headache. He rubs the back of his head and says that it has been hurting for the last several days even though he has been taking acetaminophen. He says that he had a "heart attack" 5 years ago and was prescribed metoprolol (Lopressor) and enalaprilat (Vasotec). Patient states he has "gout" and has been on allopurinol (Zyloprim) for a number of years. The patient recently started taking indomethacin (Indocin) for an acute exacerbation of gout. The only other change in his health status reported is a weight gain of about 20 pounds over the past 2 months. Current weight is 80 kg. The patient denies chest pain, but he is significantly dyspneic. BP is 220/140 mm Hg supine and 200/136 mm Hg when sitting upright. The heart rate is 62 beats/min; respiratory rate is 32 breaths/min and labored. The PMI is palpable at the sixth left intercostal space, anterior axillary line. Cardiac auscultation reveals S_1, S_2, and an S_3. Bibasilar crackles are audible. Pulse oximeter reads 88%. Oxygen therapy is initiated with 5 L by nasal cannula. An IV catheter is inserted and blood specimen is collected for CBC, electrolytes, BUN, and creatinine. A urinalysis is sent to the lab for analysis from a voided 50 mL of concentrated urine specimen. The chest x-ray reveals cardiomegaly and pulmonary edema. Multiple lead ECG shows a left ventricular strain pattern in V_5, V_6 and R waves in V_6 that measure 30 mm. Abnormal laboratory results include a creatinine of 3.0 mg/dL and BUN of 35 mg/dL.

a. Identify the findings that indicate hypertensive emergency.

_____

b. What is the most likely cause of this abrupt increase in BP?

_____

c. Hypertension and hypertensive crisis affect what organs?

_____

d. Does patient meet admission criteria? If yes, which unit? Progressive care unit or critical care unit?

_____

e. What is the therapeutic goal for BP reduction within the next 2 hours?

_____

f. List a parenteral drug in each of the following categories.
   Vasodilator:_____
   ACE inhibitor:_____
   Alpha-blocker:_____
   Beta-blocker:_____
   Alpha- and beta-blocker:_____

g. The physician prescribes nitroprusside (Nipride) to be started at 1 mcg/kg/min. Patient B weighs 80 kg. You reconstitute 50 mg of nitroprusside with 3 mL of sterile water and put it in 250 mL of normal saline. At what rate should infusion be started for the 1 mcg/kg/min prescription?

_____

h. List adverse effects of nitroprusside and how to monitor for them.

_____

i. Could sublingual nifedipine be used instead of the nitroprusside in this patient?

_____

j. Which drug would have been most appropriate if the CT had shown cerebral hemorrhage?

_____

k. What signs and/or symptoms could indicate that Patient B is experiencing thoracic aortic dissection?

_____

Answers to this activity can be found in the Answer Key.

3.28   Synthesis Learning Activity: Crossword Puzzle

Complete the following crossword puzzle dealing with cardiovascular pharmacology. Use only generic names.

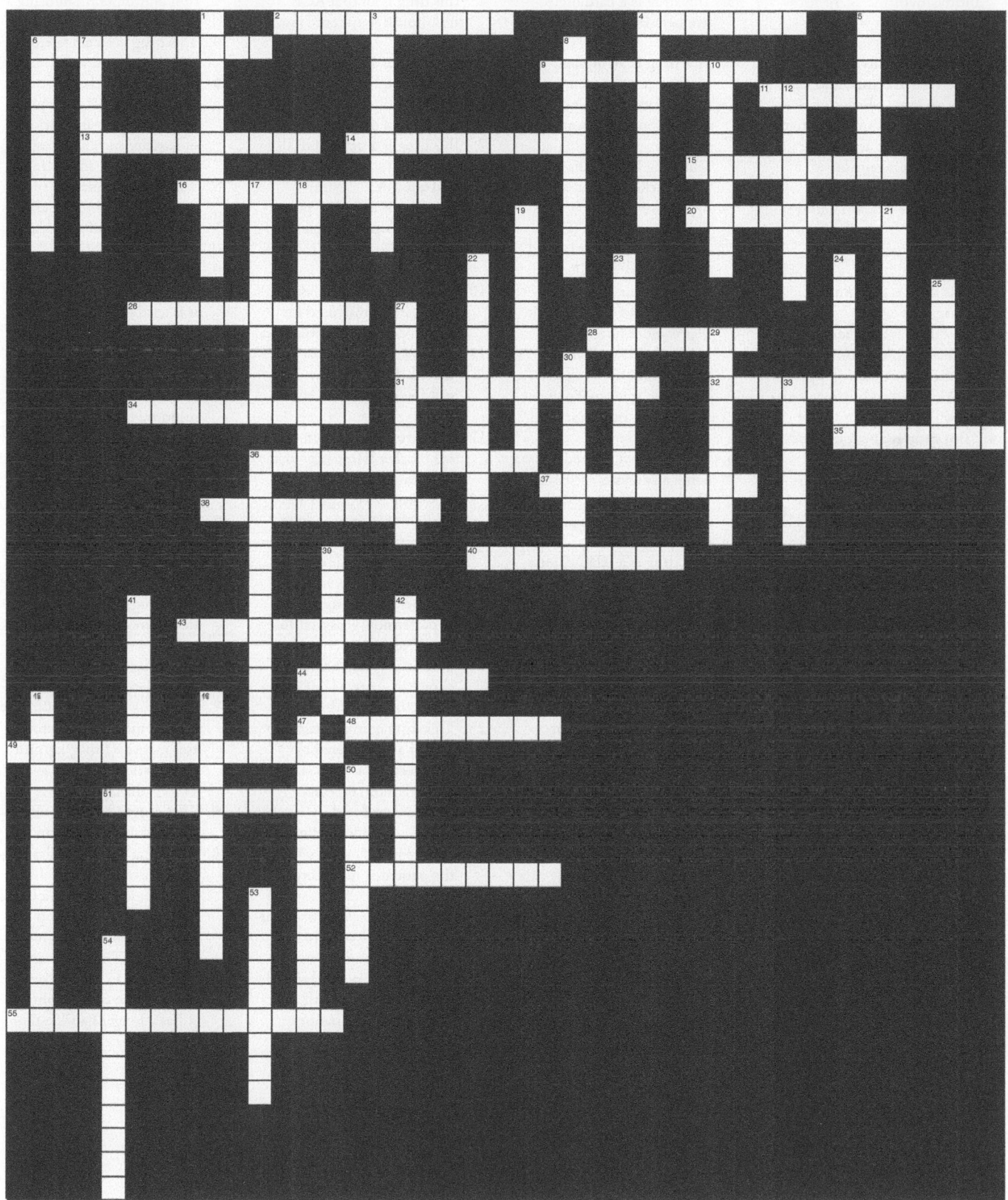

Answers to this activity can be found in the Answer Key.

ACROSS

2. This drug is a class III antidysrhythmic; it is the first-line antidysrhythmic agent for pulseless VT or VF

4. This electrolyte is used in hyperkalemia, hypermagnesemia, hypocalcemia, and calcium channel blocker toxicity

6. This drug is a cardioselective beta-blocker; it is used for secondary prevention of acute MI

9. This drug is a class IV antidysrhythmic; it is frequently used in supraventricular tachycardia

11. This drug is a vitamin K antagonist

13. This drug is an arterial dilator with dopaminergic stimulation used in hypertension and to improve renal flow

14. This drug is an alpha- and beta-blocker used in HF

15. This drug is a phosphodiesterase inhibitor used for short-term treatment of HF

16. This drug is an adrenergic agent used in pulseless VT, VF, asystole, and PEA

20. This drug is a class IV antidysrhythmic agent that decreases contractility less than verapamil

26. This drug is a beta-type natriuretic hormone used in HF

28. This drug is a low-molecular-weight form used as a platelet aggregation inhibitor especially after vascular surgery

31. This drug is an intravenous ACE inhibitor that may be used for hypertension or HF

32. This drug is an adrenergic agent with dose-dependent effects; it may be used as an inotropic agent or vasopressor

34. This drug is a loop diuretic; rapid administration of this drug may cause temporary deafness

35. This drug is a cardioselective beta-blocker with short half-life

36. This drug is an alpha-blocker; it is frequently used for vasopressor drug infiltration to prevent tissue necrosis

37. This drug is an alpha- and beta-blocker; it is used for hypertension

38. This drug is a class IC antidysrhythmic; it is used for refractory ventricular dysrhythmias

40. This drug is a loop diuretic that is more potent and longer duration than furosemide

43. This drug is an oral platelet aggregation inhibitor used after MI or stroke

44. This drug is a benzodiazepine anxiolytic

48. This electrolyte is usually included in postoperative fluid replacement

49. This drug is a RBC colony-stimulating factor used for anemia

51. This drug is a pure beta stimulant; it may be used in torsades de pointes to shorten repolarization

52. This drug is a nucleoside used to break reentrant mechanism in paroxysmal supraventricular tachycardia (PSVT)

55. This drug is used in peripheral arterial disease to increase the flexibility of the RBCs

DOWN

1. This drug is an arterial selective IV calcium channel blocker used as an antihypertensive especially postoperatively

3. This drug is an adrenergic-type inotropic agent; it is most frequently used in cardiogenic shock

4. This drug is an oral ACE inhibitor; it may cause rash or cough

5. This drug is an indirect thrombin inhibitor

6. This electrolyte is indicated for torsades de pointes

7. This drug is a newer GP IIb/IIIa inhibitor; it is frequently used after PCI

8. This drug is an antihypertensive with dopaminergic qualities; it is also used to improve renal perfusion

10. This drug is an IV class III antidysrhythmic used for acute onset atrial fibrillation

12. This drug was the first IV GP IIb/IIIa inhibitor; it is still frequently used after PCI

17. This drug is a calcium channel blocker frequently used in variant angina

18. This drug is a class IA antidysrhythmic; it may cause prolongation of the QT interval and torsades de pointes

19. This drug is a calcium channel blocker used for hypertension; it is available for IV use

21. This drug is an analgesic of choice in acute MI; it is also a venous vasodilator

22. This drug is an arterial dilator administered by IV injection; it is used in hypertension, especially if pregnancy-related

23. This drug is a loop diuretic; it is frequently used when the patient is refractory to furosemide

24. This drug is used in bradycardia but is no longer recommended for asystole or PEA

25. This drug is an antidysrhythmic agent; it has both class II and class III qualities

27. This drug is an oral class III antidysrhythmic agent used for new onset atrial fibrillation; it requires hospitalization and ECG monitoring during initiation of therapy

29. This drug is an aldosterone antagonist used in HF

30. This drug is a class IB antidysrhythmic; it requires monitoring for indications of toxicity such as paresthesia, confusion, and seizures

33. This drug is a platelet aggregation inhibitor used for primary and secondary prevention of MI

36. This drug is an alpha selective adrenergic agent; it is used as a vasopressor especially when tachycardia is very undesirable

39. This drug is a cardiac glycoside; it decreases ventricular response rate in atrial fibrillation and flutter

41. This drug is a predominantly arterial nitrate-type vasodilator

42. This drug is a tissue plasminogen activator with a longer half-life; it is given as a single bolus

45. This drug is an alpha dominant adrenergic agent; it is used as a vasopressor

46. This drug is a noncardioselective beta-blocker

47. This drug is a predominantly venous nitrate-type vasodilator; a dose >1 mcg/kg/min causes arterial as well as venous dilation

50. This drug is an ACE inhibitor available in IV form

53. This drug is a tissue plasminogen activator with a short half-life; it is given as a bolus followed by an infusion

54. This hormone is used in pulseless VT or VF as an alternative to the first or second dose of epinephrine; it has a longer half-life than epinephrine

The Pulmonary System

ANATOMY AND PHYSIOLOGY

The pulmonary system consists of lungs, conducting air passages, muscles of ventilation, central nervous system control, thoracic cage, and alveoli. The functions of the pulmonary system include the following:

- Allows interchange of gases between the atmosphere and the bloodstream
- Assists in maintenance of acid-base balance
- Contributes to phonation (i.e., process to produce sounds)
- Acts as a reservoir for blood for the left atrium and ventricle
- Assists in clearing metabolic wastes

Upper Airway

The conducting pathways of the upper airway conduct airflow from the nose to the terminal bronchioles (Figure 4-1). No gas exchange occurs in these airways as the air is conducted toward gas exchange units. The air in these branching tubes accounts for approximately one third of the inspired tidal volume and is referred to as *anatomic dead space.*

The upper airway is from the nose or mouth to the external opening of the vocal cords and serves as a passageway for food and inspired gases. The functions of the upper airway are to warm, humidify, and filter the inspired air. While air is in the upper airway, the relative humidity is approximately 80% to 100% at body temperature; this accounts for insensible water loss of 400 mL/24 hours.

The nose has a large surface area due to the presence of the turbinates and ciliated epithelium to trap particulate matter and bacteria from the inspired air. Four sinuses (frontal, maxillary, ethmoid, and sphenoid) drain into the nasal cavity. The septum divides two nasal fossae, and skeletal rigidity keeps the nasal passages open during inspiration. The mucous membrane of the nose contains cilia and mucus-producing cells to protect the lower airway from foreign material, filtering inspired air of particles 5 microns or larger. The nose has a rich supply of blood vessels beneath the mucous membranes, which warms inspired gases to body temperature. The smaller inlet and larger outlet allows air to have maximal contact with the nasal mucosa to enhance this warming effect. However, because there is two to three times more resistance in the nose than in the mouth, dyspneic patients are more likely to breathe through their mouth.

The nose provides the sense of olfaction; the olfactory area is located in the superior turbinate and sniffing directs air toward this area. The nose is also involved in production of sound in phonation.

The next portion of the upper airway is the pharynx, which is from the posterior nasal cavity to the opening of the esophagus. The pharynx divides into three distinct areas: the nasopharynx, oropharynx, and laryngopharynx. The primary functions of the pharynx are swallowing and protection of the lower area. During swallowing, the uvula and soft palate move posteriorly and superiorly to keep food and liquid from entering the nasopharynx. The pharynx is rich in lymphatic tissues that contribute to protection of the lower airway from microorganisms.

The nasopharynx is between the posterior nasal cavity and the soft palate and contains the pharyngeal tonsils and the eustachian tubes. The pharyngeal tonsils, also referred as adenoids, are a dense concentration of lymphatic tissue that guards the entryway to the respiratory and gastrointestinal tracts. The eustachian tubes connect the nasopharynx to each middle ear; they open during swallowing to equalize pressure in the middle ear. If the eustachian tube closes, middle ear pain or infection may develop.

The oropharynx is between the soft palate and the base of the tongue. The palatine and lingual tonsils are located in this area. The gag reflex defends the lower airway against aspiration and is located in this area. Cranial nerves IX (glossopharyngeal) and X (vagus) control the gag reflex.

The laryngopharynx, also referred to as the hypopharynx, is where both food and air pass. It is located from the base of the tongue to the epiglottis between the hyoid bone, larynx, and esophagus.

The larynx divides the upper airway from the lower airway. It is the upper portion of the trachea and connects the laryngopharynx with the trachea. The functions of the larynx are to allow speech, to prevent aspiration through the valve action of the epiglottis, and to allow for cough reflex and Valsalva maneuver. The larynx consists of the thyroid cartilage, the vocal cords, and the cricoid cartilage. The epiglottis, a flexible cartilage attached to the thyroid cartilage, overhangs the thyroid cartilage like a lid to prevent food from entering the larynx and trachea during swallowing. The thyroid cartilage, frequently referred to as the *Adam's apple*, is the largest laryngeal cartilage and contains the vocal cords. This is the narrowest part of the conducting airways in the adult. The vocal folds are two pairs of membranes that protrude into the lumen of the larynx. The upper pair of membranes are the false vocal cords, which play no part in vocalization. The true vocal cords, the lower pair, form the triangular glottis that leads to the trachea. The true vocal cords change shape and vibrate in response to contraction of muscles

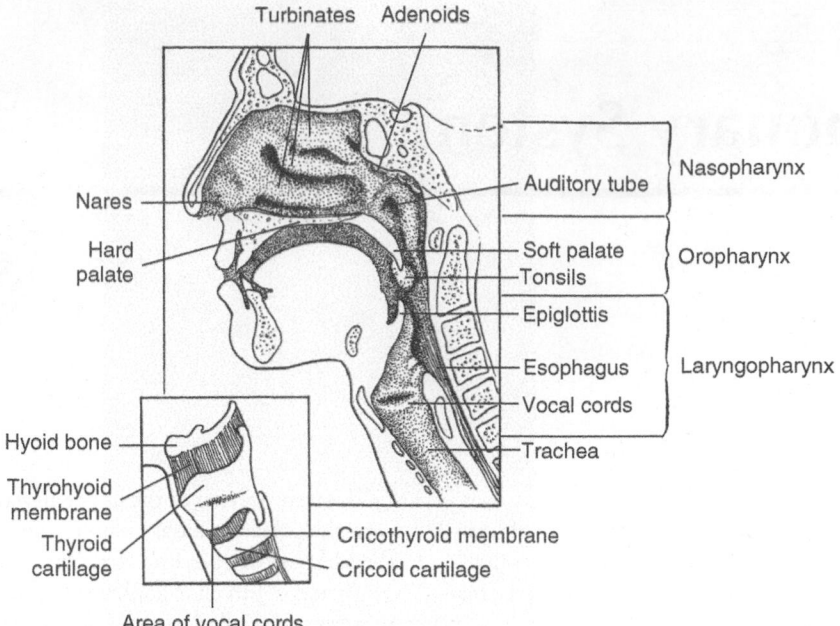

FIGURE 4-1 The upper airway (lateral view). (From Luce, J. M., & Pierson, D. J. [1998]. *Critical care medicine.* Philadelphia: W. B. Saunders.)

in the larynx to result in phonation. Speech is a joint function of the vocal cords, lips, tongue, soft palate, and respiration, with control by temporal and parietal lobes of the cerebral cortex. The cricothyroid membrane is an avascular structure that connects the thyroid and cricoid cartilages. This membrane may be punctured (i.e., cricothyrotomy) to establish an open airway in an emergency. The cricoid cartilage is the only complete rigid ring; the inner diameter also sets the limit for the size of an endotracheal tube (ETT).

Lower Airway

The lower airway (Figure 4-2) is below the larynx and conducts air to the gas exchange surfaces of the lung. The first portion of the lower airway and the tracheobronchial tree is the trachea, which consists of 16 to 20 C-shaped rings that stabilize the airway and prevent collapse with coughing. It is 10 to 12 cm long. The trachea warms and humidifies the air, has mucosal cells that trap foreign material, and has cilia that propel mucus upward through the airway. The trachea and the esophagus share a common wall. Erosion through this wall creates a tracheoesophageal fistula. An overinflated tracheostomy tube cuff may cause such a fistula. A cough reflex is present, especially at the carina. The carina is the point of bifurcation of the trachea into the left and right mainstem bronchi. This area is rich in parasympathetic fibers.

4.1   Learning Activity

Because the carina is rich in parasympathetic fibers, what may occur if a suction catheter stimulates this area?

Answers to this activity can be found in the Answer Key.

There are two mainstem bronchi, one going to each lung. The right mainstem bronchus is almost straight (25 degrees) off the trachea and larger in diameter than the left (40-60 degrees);

therefore, aspiration of liquid or food, foreign bodies, a suction catheter, and endotracheal (ET) tube go to the right preferentially. The conducting airways continue to branch. These branches are called *generations* or *levels* (Figure 4-3): mainstem (first level), lobar (second level), segmental (third level), subsegmental (fourth through ninth levels), and bronchioles (tenth through fifteenth levels).

4.2   Learning Activity

Which lung is most likely to be affected by aspiration? Why does this occur?

Answers to this activity can be found in the Answer Key.

The bronchi continue the function of the upper airway in warming, humidifying, and filtering inspired air. Cartilage and smooth muscle support the bronchi and are responsible for most of total airway resistance in a healthy person. Mast cells lie just beneath the bronchial epithelium near the smooth muscle and blood vessels. These mast cells secrete histamine and other mediators of the inflammatory process when stimulated by the antigen-antibody response.

The sixteenth and final branch of the conducting bronchioles is referred to as the *terminal bronchioles.* They are 1 mm in diameter, consist of fibrous, elastic smooth muscle with no cartilage, and they have no mucus glands or cilia. The terminal bronchiole is the most peripheral bronchiole not to have alveoli in its wall. The terminal bronchioles are particularly sensitive to CO_2 and dilate in response to increased CO_2 levels. Bronchospasm may significantly narrow the lumen and increase airway resistance.

The Lungs

The right lung divides into three lobes and the left lung divides into two lobes. A fissure divides the upper left lung from the

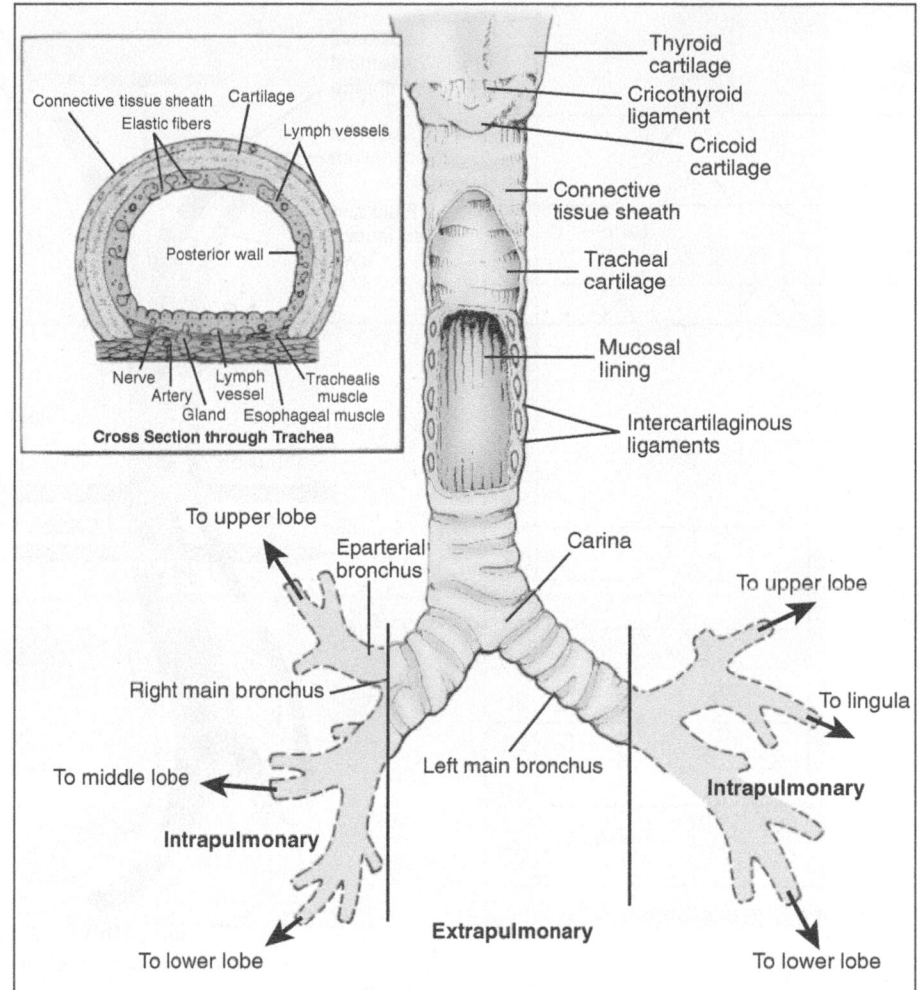

FIGURE 4-2 The lower airway. (From Martin, D. E. [1988]. *Respiratory anatomy and physiology.* St. Louis, MO: Mosby.)

lower left lung. The lower portion of the left upper lobe (lingual) is approximately the same size as the right middle lobe. The right lung divides into 10 segments and the left lung divides into 8 segments. These segments divide into subsegments, and subsegments divide into lobules. The acinus is the primary gas exchange unit; it is distal to each terminal bronchiole and consists of four levels (17th through 19th generations) of respiratory bronchioles leading to three alveolar ducts (20th through 22nd generations). Alveolar ducts lead to alveolar sacs (23rd generation). There are approximately 300 million alveolar sacs, with one-half of the alveoli in the ducts and one-half in the alveolar sacs in grapelike clusters of 15 to 20 alveoli. The surface area of the alveoli is approximately 80 m². The pores of Kohn are openings in the intraalveolar septa between the alveoli thought to contribute to collateral ventilation but may also contribute to the movement of microorganisms between alveoli and the rapid transmission of infection.

Alveolar epithelium lines the entire acinus from respiratory bronchioles through the alveolar sacs, which is the site of diffusion of oxygen and carbon dioxide between the inspired air and the blood. The alveolar-capillary membrane of the adult human lung has a surface area of one square meter per kilogram of ideal body weight and is 0.5 micron in thickness. The diffusion pathway (Figure 4-4) for the diffusion of gases from the alveolus to

the blood for oxygen and from the blood to the alveolus for carbon dioxide consists of the following layers:

- Alveolar epithelium
- Epithelial basement membrane
- Interstitial space
- Capillary basement membrane
- Capillary endothelium

The immense surface area and thinness of the alveolar-capillary membrane allow for rapid transfer of oxygen and carbon dioxide by diffusion. Loss of surface area, such as lobectomy, pneumonectomy, or emphysema, or widening of the diffusion pathway, such as pulmonary edema or pulmonary fibrosis, will cause impaired diffusion and hypoxemia.

There are several types of pulmonary cells, each with specific functions. Pulmonary capillary endothelial cells produce and degrade prostaglandins, metabolize vasoactive amines, convert angiotensin I to angiotensin II, and at least partly produce coagulation factor VIII. Type I pneumocytes cover 90% of total alveolar surface and are responsible for the integumentary air-blood barrier; the cytoplasmic junctions are very tight and impermeable to water under normal circumstances. These flat, large, squamous cells are very susceptible to injury. Type II pneumocytes are small, cuboidal, granular cells that cover only 5% of the total alveolar surface. These cells produce, store, and secrete surfactant, a lipoprotein that

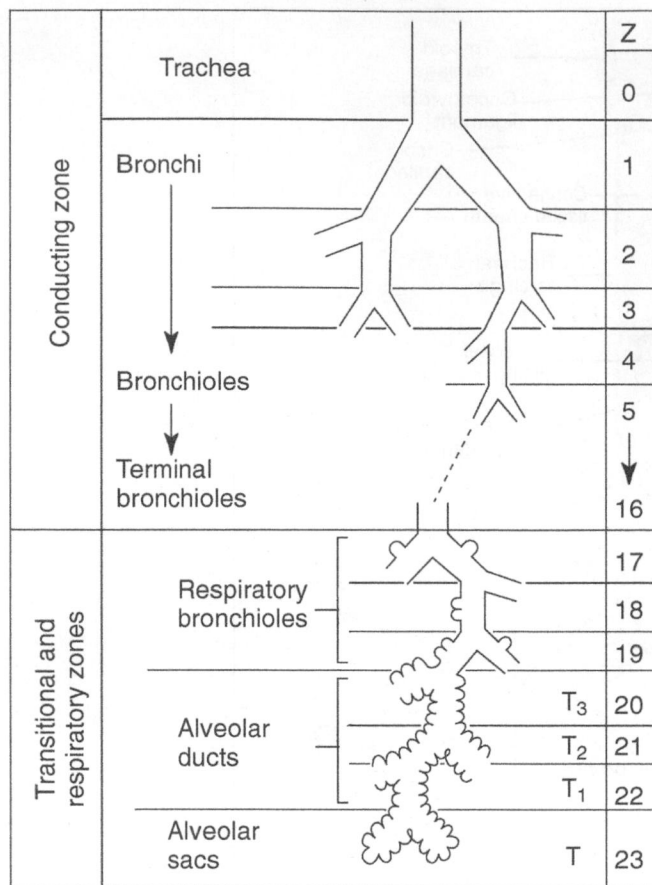

FIGURE 4-3 Airway generations.

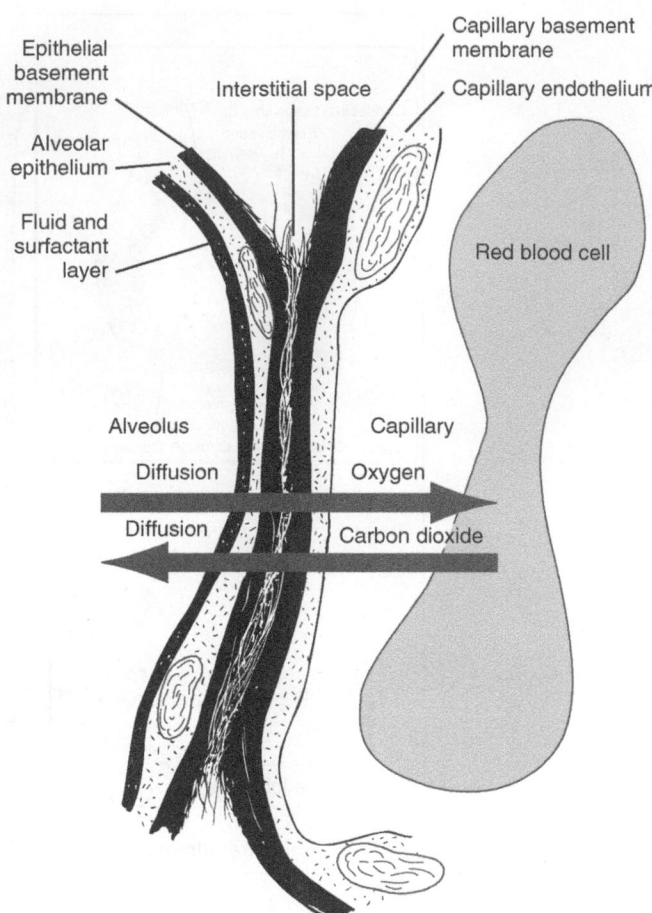

FIGURE 4-4 The diffusion pathway. (From Carlson, K. K. [Ed.]. [2009]. *Advanced critical care nursing* St. Louis, MO: Saunders Elsevier.)

lines the inner aspect of the alveolus. Surfactant decreases surface tension of the fluid lining the alveoli and prevents alveolar collapse at the end of expiration, especially at low volumes. This is especially important in the inferior portions of lung where alveoli are small and distending pressures are low. A deficiency of surfactant causes alveolar collapse, poorly compliant lungs, and alveolar edema. Because the half-life of surfactant is only 14 hours, injury to these cells quickly results in massive atelectasis. If type I pneumocytes are injured, type II pneumocytes increase mitosis to replicate and form a cuboidal cell line and may differentiate to type I.

4.3   Learning Activity

How long after a hypoxic injury, such as shock, do the indications of acute respiratory distress syndrome occur? Why?

Answers to this activity can be found in the Answer Key.

Defense Mechanisms of the Pulmonary System
The following defense mechanisms protect the pulmonary system:
- Nasal cilia to filter particles larger than 5 mm
- Sneeze as a reaction to irritation in the nose
- Cough as a reaction to irritation in the upper airway distal to the nose

- Mucociliary escalator, the combination of mucus and cilia, to filter particles smaller than 5 mm; particles are trapped in mucus and then moved upward by cilia to be expelled by cough or swallow
- Lymphatics to remove interstitial fluid to keep lungs free of excess fluid and remove inhaled particles from distal areas of the lung
- The immune system
- Alveolar macrophages to engulf and remove bacteria and other foreign substances

Loss of normal defense mechanisms may result from disease, injury, anesthesia, corticosteroids, smoking, malnutrition, sedating substances (such as ethanol), uremia, artificial airways, or hypoxia. Any of these conditions may lead to pulmonary infection.

Pulmonary Circulation
The pulmonary circulation (Figure 4-5) is a low pressure, low resistance system. The lungs receive the entire cardiac output of approximately 5 L into the main pulmonary artery from the right ventricle. The main pulmonary artery divides into the right and left pulmonary arteries, which divide into arterioles and then capillaries, which spread over the surface of the alveoli. This network of capillaries is very dense, and the pulmonary capillaries are so small that they barely accommodate erythrocyte passage. Red blood cells (RBCs) move through the capillaries in a single file to allow diffusion of gases and the attachment of oxygen to hemoglobin.

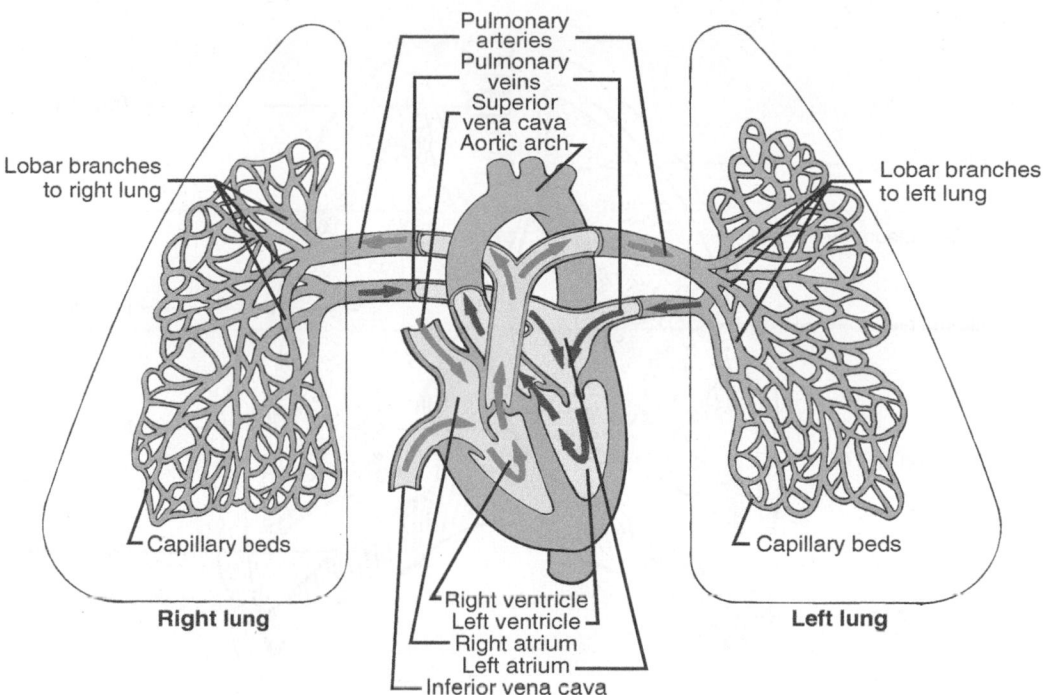

FIGURE 4-5 The pulmonary circulation. (From McCance, K. L., & Huether, S. E. [2014]. *Pathophysiology: The biologic basis for disease in adults and children* [7th ed.]. St. Louis, MO: Elsevier.)

There is a corresponding arteriole and venule for every bronchiole. Veins move out of the lung toward the pleura. Numerous veins gradually form four pulmonary veins that empty into the left atrium. The venous system serves as an immense reservoir of blood for the left atrium and left ventricle.

The normal mean pressure in the pulmonary artery is 10 to 20 mm Hg. Pulmonary hypertension is when the mean pulmonary artery pressure (PAP) is >20 mm Hg. Causes of pulmonary hypertension can be categorized as primary or secondary. Primary pulmonary hypertension is idiopathic. Secondary pulmonary hypertension is either active or passive. Active secondary pulmonary hypertension results from hypoxemia that occurs in COPD, pulmonary embolism, or acute respiratory distress syndrome because pulmonary vasoconstriction occurs in response to hypoxemia. Passive secondary pulmonary hypertension is the result of back pressure as occurs in mitral valve disease or left ventricular failure.

The bronchial circulation consists of the nutrient and oxygen circulation for the tracheobronchial tree down to terminal bronchioles, visceral pleura, interstitial and connective tissue, some arteries and veins, lymph nodes, and nerves within the thoracic cavity. There are two bronchial arteries to the left lung, which originate directly from the aorta. One bronchial artery goes to the right lung; it is a branch of the intercostal artery, which originates from the right subclavian or internal mammary artery. Bronchial venous blood enters the pulmonary veins and causes some desaturation of the oxygenated blood in the pulmonary vein; this venous blood and the blood from the thebesian veins account for the normal physiologic shunt of 3% to 5%. The pulmonary circulation supplies gas exchange units with nutrients and oxygen.

Thoracic Cage
The thoracic cage (Figure 4-6) consists of muscular walls reinforced by bones. The anterior aspect of the thoracic cage is

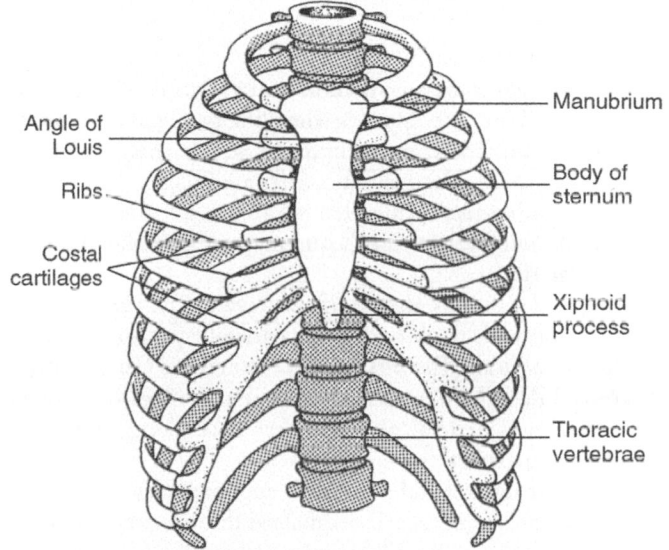

FIGURE 4-6 The thoracic cage. (From Scanlan, C. L., Wilkins, R. L., & Stoller, J. K. (Eds.). [1999]. *Egan's fundamentals of respiratory care* [7th ed.]. St. Louis, MO: Mosby.)

comprised of the sternum, which consists of three connected flat bones: the manubrium, body, and xiphoid. The posterior aspect of the thoracic cage is comprised of the spine, and 12 pairs of ribs attached to the vertebrae. These ribs are anterior, lateral, and posterior. The true ribs are the seven pairs of ribs attached to the sternum. The clavicles are superior to the thoracic cage and the diaphragm forms the inferior border of the thoracic cage.

The thoracic cage is rigid to protect the lungs, but it is resilient to allow expansion and reduction of lung volume that occurs during ventilation. The heart, lungs, esophagus, great vessels, liver, and spleen are within the thoracic cage.

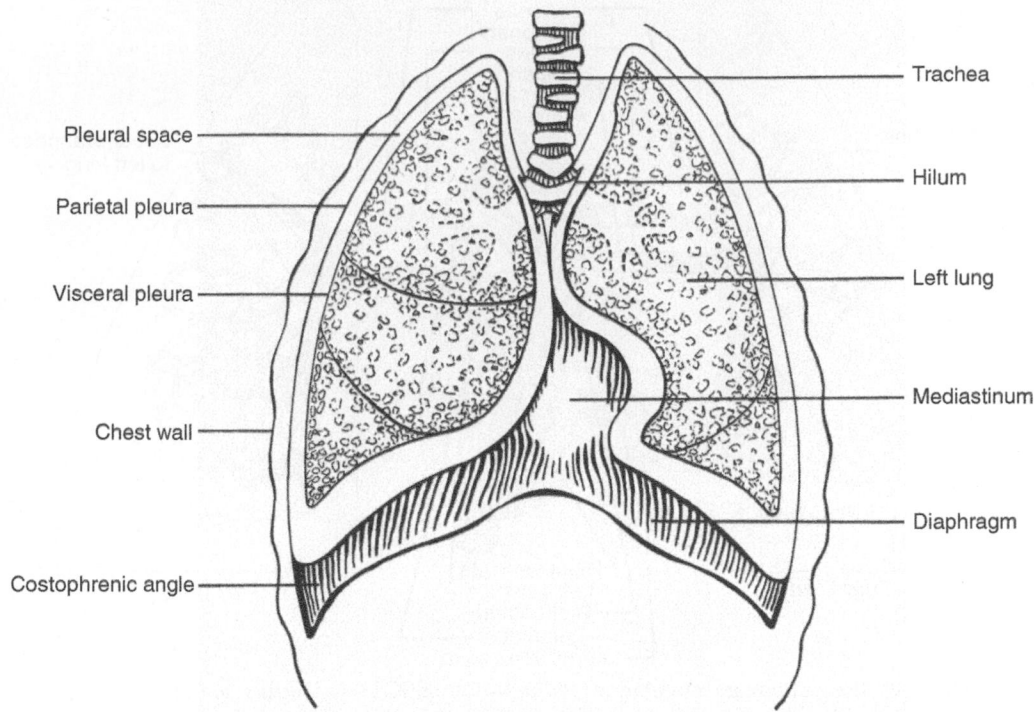

FIGURE 4-7 Internal structures of the thorax, including pleural cavities. (From Dettenmeier, P. A. [1992]. *Pulmonary nursing care.* St. Louis, MO: Mosby.)

Pleural Cavities

Each lung hangs in its own pleural cavity (Figure 4-7) attached only at the hilum. The hilum is where the two mainstem bronchi branch and where the pulmonary vessels enter and leave the thoracic space. The pleural cavities are independent of one another. The borders of the pleural cavities are formed by the chest wall laterally, the mediastinum medially, and the diaphragm inferiorly.

The pleural linings consist of two layers. The visceral layer is contiguous with the lung and the parietal layer is contiguous with the chest wall. The pleural space contains a few milliliters of serous fluid, which acts as a lubricant and adhesive between the visceral and parietal pleura as they slide along each other with each ventilatory cycle.

A negative intrapleural pressure of approximately –5 mm Hg below atmospheric pressure is maintained throughout the respiratory cycle, but this pressure becomes more negative (–10 mm Hg) during inspiration. Loss of this negative intrapleural pressure causes the lung to collapse (e.g., pneumothorax).

Mediastinum

The mediastinum is the center of the thoracic cavity. It contains the following:

• Heart and great vessels
• Trachea and mainstem bronchi
• Esophagus
• Phrenic nerve, vagus nerve, and other nerves
• Lymph nodes and ducts
• Thymus gland

Muscles of Ventilation

The muscles of ventilation (Figure 4-8) include both primary and accessory muscles. The primary muscle of inspiration is

the diaphragm, which accounts for 70% of the tidal volume during quiet breathing. The diaphragm consists of two hemidiaphragms connected by a central membranous tendon; this tendon is contiguous with the fibrous pericardium. The phrenic nerve arises from the spinal cord from C3 to C5 and innervates the diaphragm. When the diaphragm is stimulated, the contraction flattens the diaphragm, which increases the size of the thorax superior-inferior. Relaxation makes the diaphragm dome shaped and decreases the volume of the thoracic cavity. The other muscles used during normal inspiration are the external intercostals, which are innervated at spinal levels T1 to T12. Contraction raises the ribs, increasing the size of thorax anteroposteriorly.

Normal resting ventilation does not use the accessory muscles of inspiration. Patients use the accessory muscles of inspiration during exercise and with compromised inspiration such as upper airway obstruction. Accessory muscles are also innervated during the inspiratory phase of a sneeze or cough. The scalene muscles are located in the neck, stretching from the first cervical vertebrae to the first and second ribs. Contraction of the scalene muscles enlarges the upper rib cage. The sternocleidomastoid muscles are located in the neck, stretching from the manubrium and clavicle to the mastoid process and occipital bone. Contraction of the sternocleidomastoid muscles elevates the sternum to increase the anteroposterior and transverse diameter of the chest.

Expiration is normally passive. It occurs when the diaphragm and external intercostals relax and return to a resting position. The natural tendency of the lungs is to collapse, as they are made of elastic tissue; elastance is the quality of the lungs to recoil after inspiration.

Accessory muscles of expiration include the internal oblique, external oblique, rectus abdominis, internal intercostal, and

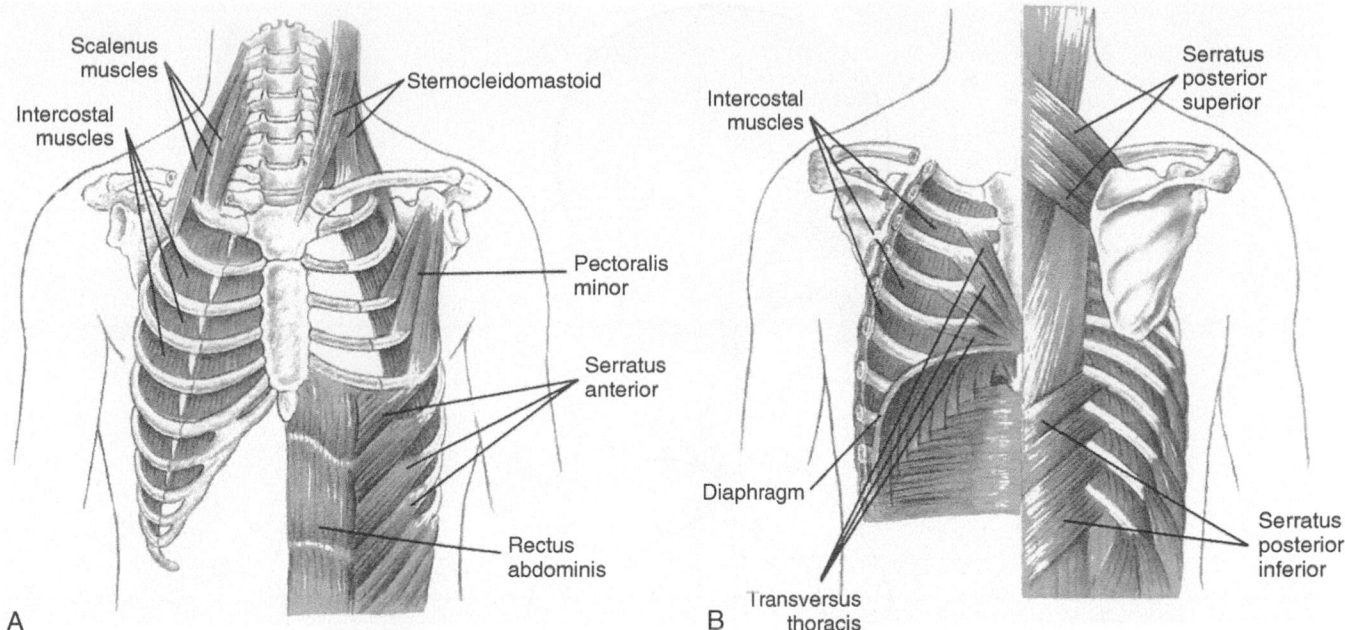

FIGURE 4-8 Muscles of ventilation. A, Anterior. **B,** Posterior. (From Urden, L. D., Stacy, K. M., & Lough, M. E. [2010]. *Critical care nursing: Diagnosis and management* [6th ed.]. St. Louis, MO: Mosby.)

transverse abdominis. Contraction of these muscles depresses the lower ribs and pulls down the anterior portion of the lower chest causing increased pressure in the abdominal cavity and compression of the abdominal viscera up against the diaphragm. The muscles are used when increased levels of ventilation are needed and are important in forceful expiration, coughing, and sneezing.

4.4 Learning Activity

Fill in the primary and accessory muscles of inspiration and expiration.

	Primary	Accessory
Inspiration		
Expiration		

Answers to this activity can be found in the Answer Key.

Neuroanatomy

There are several neural influences on ventilation and the pulmonary system. In addition, drugs, brain trauma, edema, increased intracranial pressure, and chronic hypercapnia may modify these effects.

Central chemoreceptors sensitive to cerebrospinal fluid (CSF) pH ($\uparrow$ $Paco_2 \rightarrow$ acidosis) are located in the medulla. Central chemoreceptors, along with the $Paco_2$ and pH levels, control ventilation. Chemoreceptors respond to minimal changes in $Paco_2$ very quickly by adjusting alveolar ventilation. An increase in $Paco_2$ causes an increase in the rate and depth of ventilation. A decrease in $Paco_2$ causes a decrease in the rate and depths of ventilation.

Arterial chemoreceptors located in the aortic arch and carotid bodies are sensitive to pH and Pao_2. These peripheral chemoreceptors and Pao_2 levels provide secondary control of ventilation. They respond when Pao_2 falls below approximately 60 mm Hg; this is particularly important in patients with chronically elevated levels of $Paco_2$, such as patients with COPD.

The pons controls the rhythmicity of ventilation. The apneustic center in the pons stimulates the inspiratory center and the pneumotaxic center inhibits inspiratory activity.

Stretch receptors in alveoli (i.e., Hering-Breuer reflex) inhibit further inspiration to prevent overdistension of alveoli. They may cause bronchodilation, tachycardia, and vasodilation. Proprioceptors in muscles and tendons increase ventilation in response to body movements. Baroreceptors in the aortic arch and carotid bodies inhibit ventilation in response to an increase in blood pressure (BP). Stimulated by an increase in interstitial fluid volume, the juxtacapillary receptors (also called pulmonary J receptors) may cause laryngeal constriction, hypotension, bradycardia, mucous production, and dyspnea.

The lung parenchyma does not have pain receptors. The parietal pleura pain receptors transmit impulses via intercostal nerves and thoracic ganglia. Pulmonary edema and chemical or mechanical irritation stimulate irritant receptors that cause bronchospasm, cough, and mucus production.

Physiology

The crucial processes in pulmonary physiology (Figure 4-9) include ventilation, distribution of inspired air, diffusion of oxygen and carbon dioxide, transportation of oxygen to the cells and carbon dioxide from the cells, and cellular utilization of oxygen in the production of ATP.

Ventilation

Ventilation (Figure 4-10) is the movement of air between atmosphere and alveoli and distribution of air within the

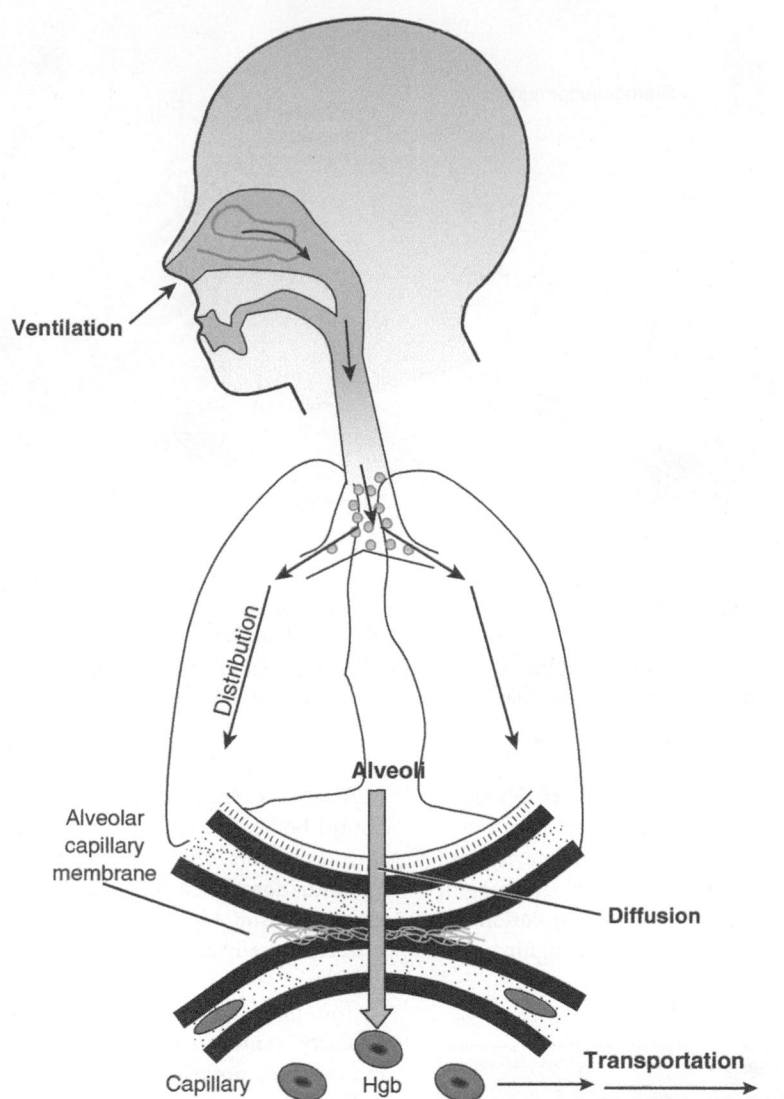

FIGURE 4-9 Respiratory process: ventilation, distribution, diffusion, transportation, cellular utilization. *Hgb,* Hemoglobin.

lungs to maintain appropriate concentrations of oxygen and carbon dioxide in the alveoli. It includes the process of inspiration and expiration. Inspiration, also referred to as inhalation, is the movement of atmospheric air into the alveoli. The process by which this occurs includes the following steps:

- Message from medulla travels down phrenic nerve to diaphragm
- Diaphragm and external intercostals contract
- Size of thorax increases
- Lungs stretch and intrapulmonary pressure decreases to less than atmospheric pressure (–1 cm H_2O)
- Air movement into lungs to equalize the difference between atmospheric and alveolar pressure

Expiration, also referred to as exhalation, is the movement of air from alveoli to the atmosphere. This passive process includes the following steps:

- Diaphragm and external intercostals relax

- Recoil of lungs to their resting size and a concomitant increase in alveolar pressure above atmospheric pressure (+1 cm H_2O)
- Air moves out of the lungs to equalize the pressure difference

The $Paco_2$ evaluates the efficiency of ventilation. When the $Paco_2$ is greater than 45 mm Hg, it indicates hypoventilation. When the $Paco_2$ is less than 35 mm Hg, it indicates hyperventilation.

Pulmonary function studies measure lung volumes (Figure 4-11 and Table 4-1). Tidal volume is the amount of air moved into and out of the lungs in each breath. This volume is normally 7 mL/kg or approximately 500 mL. Of that 7 mL/kg, 2 mL/kg, which is approximately 150 mL, is in the conducting pathways and referred to as *anatomic dead space*; therefore the amount of air that reaches the gas exchange units during each breath is 5 mL/kg or approximately 350 mL per breath. Alveolar ventilation, the volume of air per minute participating in gas exchange, is the most important portion of minute ventilation.

Alveolar ventilation is the minute ventilation minus dead space ventilation.

Dead space ventilation (Figure 4-12) is the volume of air per minute that does not participate in gas exchange. It is the sum of the anatomic dead space and alveolar (i.e., pathologic) dead space, which is the volume of air in contact with nonperfused alveoli.

4.5 Learning Activity

Match the following volumes, capacity, and indices to their description.

_____ 1. Tidal volume (V$_T$)
_____ 2. Total lung capacity (TLC)
_____ 3. Forced vital capacity (FVC)
_____ 4. Residual volume (RV)
_____ 5. Forced expiratory volume (FEV$_1$)
_____ 6. Vital capacity (VC)
_____ 7. Functional residual capacity (FRC)

a. Volume of air exhaled in the first second of forced vital capacity
b. Volume of air inhaled and exhaled with each breath
c. Maximum volume that can be exhaled after a maximal inspiration
d. Maximum volume of air that the lungs can contain
e. Amount of air that can be quickly and forcefully exhaled after a maximum inspiration
f. Volume of air remaining in the lungs after forced expiration
g. Volume of air remaining in the lungs at the end of a normal exhalation

Answers to this activity can be found in the Answer Key.

Work of Breathing
The work of breathing is normally negligible, accounting for only 2% to 3% of the total energy expenditure of the body. The work of breathing is the combination of the work of deforming the elastic system (i.e., compliance) and the work of producing airflow through the airways (i.e., airway resistance) (Figure 4-13).

Compliance is the change in pressure for a given change in volume. Normally the lungs expand to a normal tidal volume

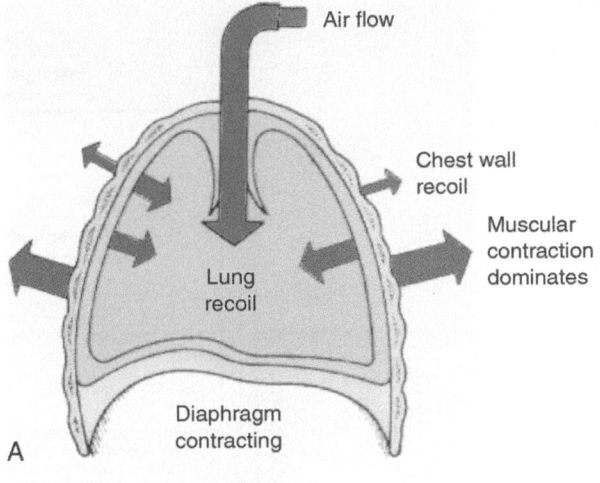
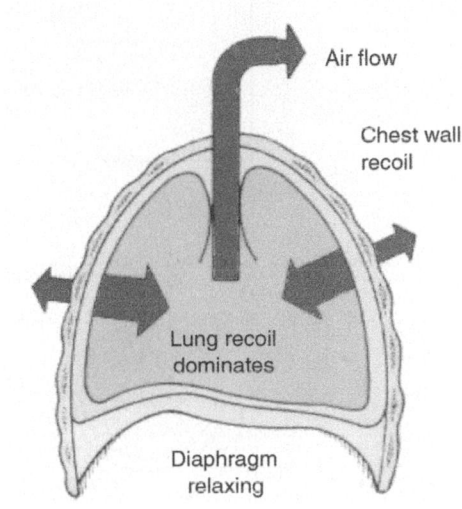

FIGURE 4-10 The process of ventilation. A, Diaphragm contracting during inspiration. **B,** Diaphragm relaxing during expiration. (Modified from McCance, K. L., & Huether, S. E. [2014]. *Pathophysiology: The biologic basis for disease in adults and children* [7th ed.]. St. Louis, MO: Elsevier.)

with only 5 to 10 cm/H$_2$O pressure. Factors that affect compliance include the following:
- Chest wall changes such as kyphoscoliosis, flail chest, thoracic pain with splinting, or obesity
- Lung changes such as atelectasis, pneumonia, pulmonary edema, pulmonary fibrosis, pleural effusion, or pneumothorax

Airway resistance is the pressure required to produce airflow. Airway caliber and length determine airway resistance. Factors affecting airway resistance include bronchospasm, mucus, artificial airways, mucosal edema, and bronchial tumor.

Restrictive disorders affect compliance. Patients with restrictive disorders tend to have a decreased tidal volume and an increased respiratory rate. Obstructive disorders affect airway resistance. These patients tend to have stridor, wheezes, or rhonchi and/or a prolonged expiratory time.

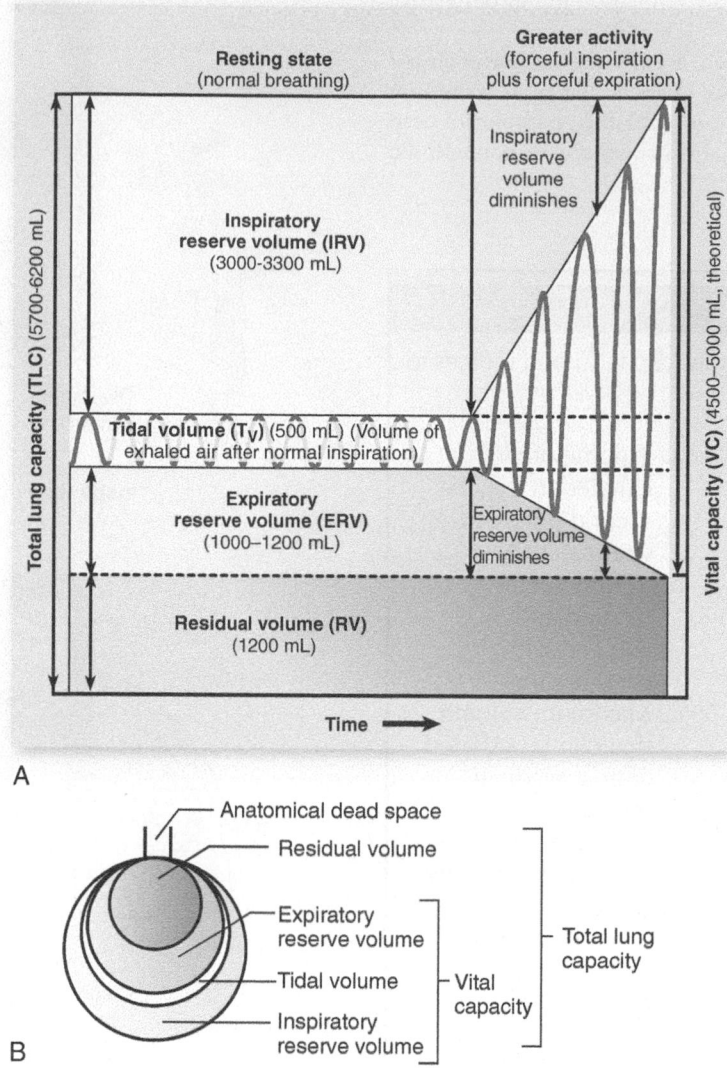

FIGURE 4-11 Lung volumes and capacities. A, Spirometry. Note that upward deflection reflects inspiration and downward deflection reflects expiration. **B,** Capacities. (From Patton, K. T. & Thibodeau, G. A. (2010). *Anatomy & physiology* [7th ed.] St. Louis, MO: Mosby.)

TABLE 4-1   Lung Volumes, Capacities, and Mechanics

Volume	Definition	Normal
Tidal volume (V_T)	The volume of air moved in and out of the lungs with each normal breath	7 mL/kg or approximately 500 mL
Inspiratory reserve volume (IRV)	The volume of air that can be maximally inspired above the normal inspiratory level	3000 mL
Expiratory reserve volume (ERV)	The volume of air that can be maximally exhaled beyond the normal expiratory level	1000 mL
Residual volume (RV)	The volume of air remaining in the lungs at the end of a maximal expiration	1000 mL
Inspiratory capacity (IC)	V_T + IRC; the volume of air that can be maximally inspired from a normal expiratory level	3500 mL
Functional residual capacity (FRC)	RV + ERV; volume of air remaining in the lungs at the end of normal expiration	2000 mL
Vital capacity (VC)	V_T + IRC + ERV; the volume of air that can be maximally expired after a maximal inspiration	4500 mL

Volume	Definition	Normal
Total lung capacity (TLC)	V_T + IRC + ERV + RV; the volume of air that the lungs can hold with maximal inspiration	5500-6000 mL
Respiratory rate or frequency (f)	The number of breaths per minute	12-20
Minute ventilation (M_E)	V_T x f; the volume of air expired per minute	5-10 L
Dead space (V_D)	V_D/V_T = $Paco_2$ − $Peco_2$ /$Paco_2$ $Paco_2$ (arterial); $Peco_2$ (exhaled); the volume or percentage of the V_T that does not participate in gas exchange; includes the volume of air in the conducting pathways (anatomic dead space) plus the volume of alveolar air that is not involved in gas exchange due to pathology (alveolar dead space)	V_D/V_T ratio is normally <0.4; V_D/V_T >0.6 usually indication for mechanical ventilation
Alveolar ventilation (V_A)	V_T - V_D; the volume of tidal air that is involved in alveolar gas exchange	350 mL
Forced vital capacity (FVC)	The volume of air in a forceful maximal expiration	Normally same as VC: 4500 mL
Forced expiratory volume (FEV)	The volume of air exhaled in a given time period; FEV_1: the volume of air exhaled in 1 second; FEV_3: the volume of air exhaled in 3 seconds	FEV_1: >75% of VC FEV_3: >95% of VC

TABLE 4-1 Lung Volumes, Capacities, and Mechanics—cont'd

4.6 Learning Activity

Identify the following conditions as restrictive or obstructive. Remember: If compliance of the lung or chest wall is affected, the condition is restrictive; if airway resistance is affected, the condition is obstructive.

	Restrictive	Obstructive
Obesity hypoventilation syndrome		
Asthma		
Pneumothorax		
Atelectasis		
Pneumonia		
Kyphoscoliosis		
Pulmonary edema		
Mucus plugs		
Lung cancer (bronchial)		
Lung cancer (parenchymal)		
Chronic bronchitis		
Artificial airway		
Bronchospasm		

Answers to this activity can be found in the Answer Key.

Perfusion

Perfusion is the movement of blood through the pulmonary capillaries so that oxygen can move into the blood and carbon dioxide can move out of the blood. The pulmonary vasculature is a low-pressure circuit. Resistance varies to accommodate the blood flow that it receives. Localized pulmonary vasoconstriction occurs as a protective mechanism to decrease blood flow to an area of poor ventilation, which shunts blood to areas of better ventilation. Generalized pulmonary vasoconstriction and resultant pulmonary hypertension occurs when all alveoli have low oxygen levels as occurs with alveolar hypoventilation. Pulmonary hypertension usually occurs when PaO_2 is less than 60 mm Hg or SaO_2 is less than 88% to 90%. When pulmonary vascular resistance and pulmonary artery pressures are elevated, the right ventricular afterload and workload is increased. This contributes to right ventricular hypertrophy and failure (i.e., cor pulmonale). This can occur acutely in conditions such as pulmonary embolism or chronic conditions such as pulmonary fibrosis or emphysema.

Ventilation (V)/Perfusion (Q) Ratio

The ventilation/perfusion ratio or V/Q ratio (Figure 4-14) compares ventilation to perfusion. Normal alveolar minute ventilation is approximately 4 L and the normal cardiac output is approximately 5 L; 100% of the cardiac output goes to lungs so that the normal V/Q ratio is 0.8. There are normal positional mismatches (Figure 4-15) that occur. Ventilation is greater than perfusion in the superior areas and perfusion is greater than ventilation in the inferior areas.

4.7   Learning Activity

How should you position a patient after a lobectomy and why? How should you position a patient after a pneumonectomy and why?

_____

_____

_____

Answers to this activity can be found in the Answer Key.

Pathologic mismatch (Figure 4-16) occurs when pathologic conditions cause a decrease in either ventilation or perfusion. When ventilation is greater than perfusion (i.e., high V/Q ratio), it is referred to as pathologic dead space unit. Examples of this condition include pulmonary embolism and shock. When perfusion is greater than ventilation (i.e., low V/Q ratio), it is referred to as a *shunt unit*. Examples of conditions that cause shunt include atelectasis, pneumonia, and acute respiratory distress syndrome. Silent units are areas with no ventilation or perfusion. An example of a silent unit is emphysema, which is decreased ventilation and perfusion.

Distribution

The process of air distribution is the movement of inspired air into lobes, segments, and lobules. Bronchiolar occlusion adversely affects the distribution of gases. Positional changes such as prone position or continuous lateral rotation beds positively affect the distribution of gases.

Diffusion

Diffusion, movement of gases between the alveoli, plasma, and RBCs, occurs when the inspired gases are in contact with the alveolar-capillary membrane. Gases diffuse from areas of higher concentration to areas of lower concentration so oxygen, which is in higher concentration in the alveolus than the blood, moves from the alveolus to the blood. Carbon dioxide, which is in higher in concentration in the blood than in the alveolus, moves from the blood to the alveolus.

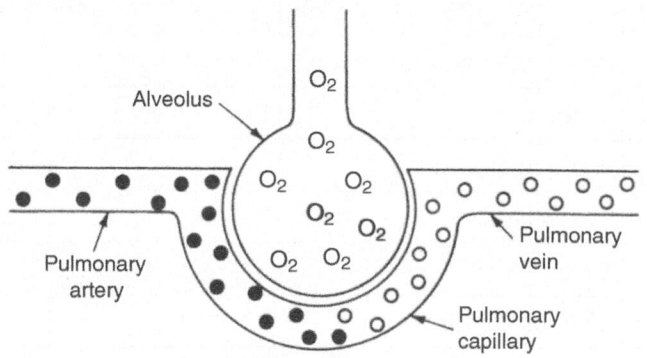

FIGURE 4-14 Normal V/Q ratio. Normal alveolar ventilation is approximately 4 L/min, and normal perfusion (cardiac output) is approximately 5 L/min; normal V/Q ratio is 0.8. (From Kinney, M. R., Packa, D. R., & Dunbar, S. B. [1998]. *AACN's clinical reference for critical-care nursing*. [4th ed.]. St. Louis, MO: Mosby.)

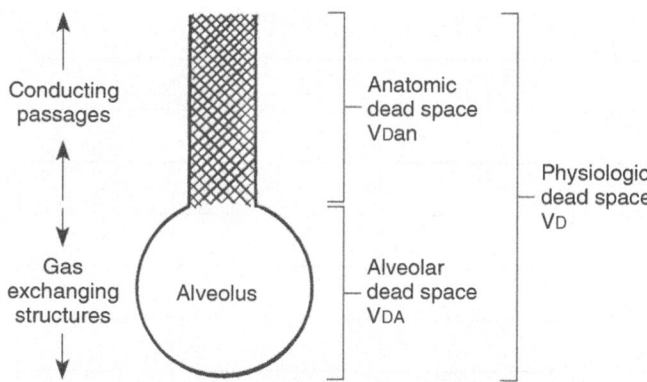

FIGURE 4-12 Physiologic dead space: anatomic dead space and alveolar dead space. (Drawing by Wendy W. Johnson.)

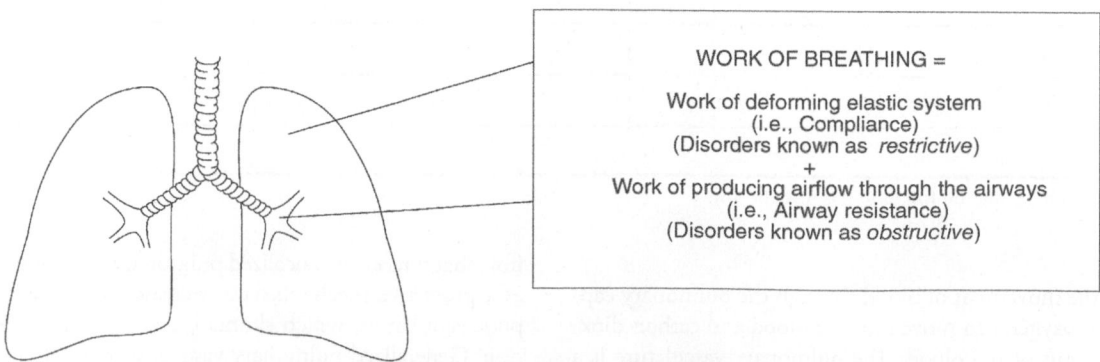

FIGURE 4-13 The work of breathing.

Multiple factors affect the efficiency of diffusion. The surface area available for gas transfer affects diffusion, so lobectomy, pneumonectomy, and emphysema all impair diffusion. Factors that affect the thickness of the diffusion pathway, such as pulmonary edema or pulmonary fibrosis, also impair diffusion. The diffusibility of the specific gas also affects diffusion. Because CO_2 is about 20 times more diffusible than O_2, conditions that affect diffusion cause a decrease in O_2 rather than an increase in CO_2.

The final factor that affects diffusion is the driving pressure of the gas. The driving pressure is calculated as the fraction of the gas times the barometric pressure. Therefore, the driving pressure of oxygen in room air is 0.21 (room air is 21% oxygen) × 760 mm Hg (the barometric pressure at sea level). This calculation adjusts accordingly for low barometric pressure at high altitudes. The partial pressure of oxygen in the alveolus (PAO_2) and resultantly the arterial blood (PaO_2) would be negatively affected by low inspired fraction of oxygen (e.g., smoke inhalation) or low barometric pressure (e.g., high altitudes) and positively affected by higher than normal fraction of inspired oxygen (FiO_2) (e.g., supplemental oxygen) or higher than normal barometric pressure (e.g., hyperbaric oxygen chamber).

Dalton's Law of Partial Pressure indicates that the pressure of a gas mixture is the sum of the partial pressures of the individual components and the partial pressures in the alveolus cannot add up to more than atmospheric pressure. Therefore, when a patient is breathing room air and the $PaCO_2$ increases, the partial pressure of oxygen in the alveolus decreases and the PAO_2 decreases.

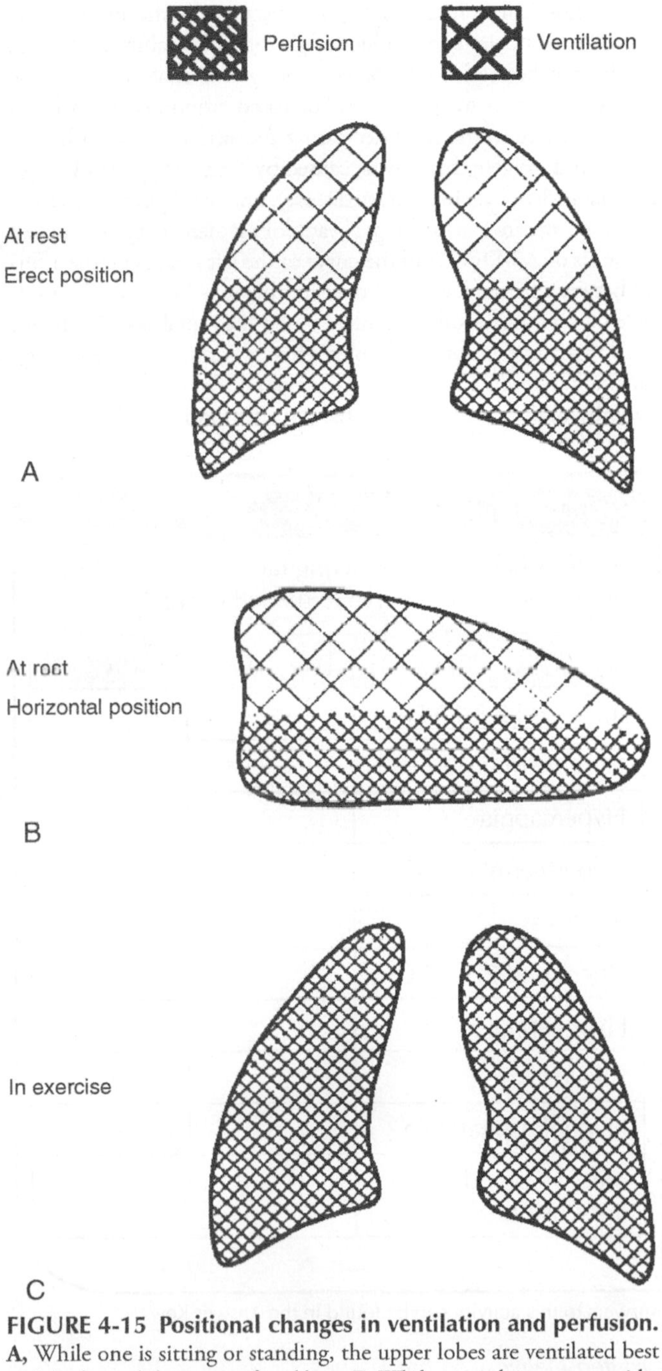

Transport of Gases in Blood

Ninety-seven percent of oxygen is transported combined with hemoglobin; this is represented by SaO_2. The remaining 3% of oxygen is dissolved in the plasma; this oxygen is represented by PaO_2.

One molecule of hemoglobin can carry four molecules of oxygen. The amount of oxygen that the hemoglobin actually carries depends on the affinity of the hemoglobin for oxygen. There is normally more affinity at the lung level and less affinity at the tissue level. The ability of hemoglobin to deliver oxygen to the tissues is negatively affected by anemia and abnormal hemoglobins (e.g., methemoglobinemia, carboxyhemoglobin, or hemoglobin S [sickle cell]).

The oxyhemoglobin dissociation curve (Figure 4-17) shows the relationship between PaO_2 and hemoglobin saturation. When there is a normal midline curve, the correlation between PaO_2 and SaO_2 is predictable (Table 4-2). Crucial levels to

FIGURE 4-15 Positional changes in ventilation and perfusion. A, While one is sitting or standing, the upper lobes are ventilated best and the lower lobes are perfused best. **B,** While one is lying on one side, the superior lung is ventilated best and the inferior lung is perfused best. **C,** In exercise, ventilation and perfusion are increased and optimally matched throughout. (From Wade, J. F. [1982]. *Comprehensive respiratory care.* St. Louis, MO: Mosby.)

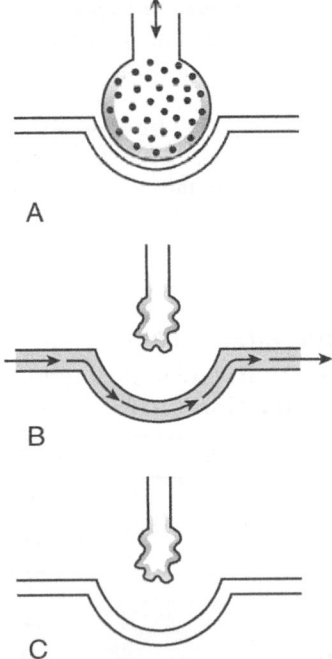

FIGURE 4-16 Abnormal V/Q ratio. A, High V/Q ratio with ventilation exceeding perfusion; also called a dead space unit. **B,** Low V/Q ratio with perfusion exceeding ventilation; also called a shunt unit. **C,** Absent ventilation and perfusion, referred to as a silent unit. (From Kinney, M. R., Packa, D. R., & Dunbar, S. B. [1998]. *AACN's clinical reference for critical-care nursing* [4th ed.]. St. Louis, MO: Mosby.)

remember include Pao_2 of 100 mm Hg correlates to a Sao_2 of close to 100%, a Pao_2 of 80 mm Hg correlates to a Sao_2 of 95%, Pao_2 of 60 mm Hg correlates to a Sao_2 of 90%, and a Pao_2 of 40 mm Hg correlates to a Sao_2 of 75%.

The critical point on the oxyhemoglobin dissociation curve is at a Pao_2 60 mm Hg. If the Pao_2 is above 60 mm Hg, it is on the horizontal limb of the curve and increases in Pao_2 above 60 mm Hg result in minimal increases in oxygen saturation. If the Pao_2 is below 60 mm Hg, it is on the vertical limb of the curve, and decreases in Pao_2 below 60 mm Hg result in dramatic decreases in oxygen saturation. The partial pressure of oxygen at which hemoglobin is 50% saturated with a pH of 7.40 is referred to as the P_{50}: it is usually Pao_2 of 27 mm Hg. The curve shifts left or right due to pathologic conditions or situations. Decreased P_{50} and shifting of the oxyhemoglobin dissociation curve to the left increases the affinity of hemoglobin for oxygen; therefore, hemoglobin is more saturated for a given Pao_2 and less oxygen is unloaded for a given Pao_2. Factors that shift the oxyhemoglobin dissociation curve to the left include alkalemia, hypothermia, hypocapnia, and decreased 2,3-diphosphoglycerate (2,3-DPG). Increased P_{50} and shifting of the oxyhemoglobin dissociation curve to the right decreases affinity of hemoglobin for oxygen; therefore, hemoglobin is less saturated for a given Pao_2 and more oxygen is unloaded for a given Pao_2. This means that it is more difficult to pick up oxygen at the lung level but easier to drop off oxygen at the tissue level.

One of the factors that affect shifting of the oxyhemoglobin dissociation curve is 2,3-DPG, a substance in the erythrocyte. 2,3-DPG is a chief end product of glucose metabolism and a link in the biochemical feedback control system that regulates the release of oxygen to the tissues. Increased amounts of 2,3-DPG shift the curve to the right decreasing the affinity between hemoglobin and oxygen; this may be caused by chronic hypoxemia (e.g., high altitude, congenital heart disease), anemia, hyperthyroidism, and the inherited disorder pyruvate kinase deficiency. Decreased amounts of 2,3-DPG shift the curve to the left increasing the affinity between hemoglobin and oxygen; this may be caused by multiple blood transfusions of banked blood (i.e., total body exchange [~10 units] over minutes to hours), hypophosphatemia (e.g., malnutrition, refeeding syndrome, treatment of diabetic ketoacidosis), hypothyroidism, and the inherited disorder hexokinase deficiency.

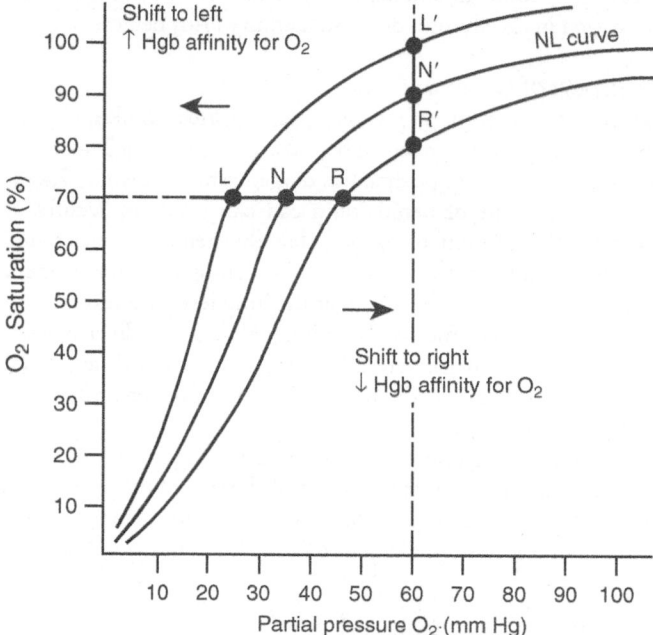

FIGURE 4-17 Oxyhemoglobin dissociation curve. Normal curve (N) optimizes pickup of O_2 at the lung and drop-off of O_2 at the tissue level; left shift (L) increases the affinity between O_2 and Hgb, which optimizes pickup of O_2 at the lung level but impairs drop-off of O_2 at the tissue level; right shift (R) decreases affinity between O_2 and Hgb, which impairs pickup of O_2 at the lung level but optimizes drop-off of O_2 at the tissue level. (From Dettenmeier, P. A. [1992]. *Pulmonary nursing care*. St. Louis, MO: Mosby.)

TABLE 4-2	Correlation between Pao_2 and Sao_2 with Normal Oxyhemoglobin Dissociation Curve

Pao_2 (mm Hg)	Sao_2 (%)
100	98
90	97
80	95
70	93
60	90
50	85
40	75
30	57
27	50

4.8 **Learning Activity**		
Identify whether the following factors cause a shift of the oxyhemoglobin curve to the left or right.		
	Left	**Right**
Increased 2,3-DPG		
Hypothermia		
Hypercapnia		
Hyperthermia		
Acidosis		
Decreased 2,3-DPG		
Hypocapnia		
Alkalosis		
Hypophosphatemia		
Massive blood transfusion		

Answers to this activity can be found in the Answer Key.

Oxygen Delivery to the Tissues
The maximal amount of oxygen the blood can carry, referred to as *oxygen capacity*, is calculated as the hemoglobin × 1.34 because that number represents the amount of oxygen 1 gram of hemoglobin can carry if 100% saturated. The oxygen content

in the arterial blood (CaO_2) is the actual amount of oxygen that arterial blood is carrying and is calculated by multiplying the oxygen capacity × SaO_2 as a decimal (i.e., Hgb [in g/dL] × 1.34 × SaO_2 [as a decimal such as .95 for 95%]). Normal CaO_2 is 18 to 20 mL/dL. Finally, factor the cardiac output into the delivery of oxygen to the tissues (DO_2) by multiply the CaO_2 × CO × 10 (a conversion constant). Normal DO_2 is 1000 mL/min. Remember that anything that decreases hemoglobin, SaO_2, or cardiac output impairs oxygen delivery to the tissues.

CO_2 is mostly transported as bicarbonate when carbonic acid and water in the presence of carbonic anhydrase form bicarbonate in the erythrocyte. The 5% of dissolve CO_2 in plasma ($PaCO_2$) combines with hemoglobin as carbaminohemoglobin. CO_2 attaches to hemoglobin at a different bonding site than oxygen.

Pressure gradients allow diffusion. Oxygen diffusion to peripheral tissues is affected by the following:
- Quantity and rate of blood flow
- Difference in capillary and tissue oxygen pressures
- Capillary surface area
- Capillary permeability
- Intracapillary distance

Cellular respiration is the utilization of oxygen by the cell and estimated by the amount of carbon dioxide produced and the oxygen consumed. The ratio of these two values is referred to as the respiratory quotient (RQ), which is normally 0.8. Changes occur according to the nutritional substrate being utilized. Primary carbohydrate metabolism changes the ratio to 1.0 as carbohydrate metabolism produces more carbon dioxide than does the metabolism of protein or fat.

During the Krebs cycle, food is converted to H_2O and CO_2 and cellular energy (ATP). The mitochondria use oxygen in the production of cellular energy; oxygen deficit may result in lethal cell injury if prolonged. Oxygen deficit may result from either impaired delivery (e.g., decreased hemoglobin, SaO_2, or cardiac output) or increased oxygen consumption. Variables that increase oxygen consumption include the following:
- Increased work of breathing
- Hyperthermia
- Trauma
- Sepsis
- Anxiety
- Hyperthyroidism
- Muscle tremors or seizures
Oxygen consumption may be reduced by the following:
- Hypothermia
- Sedation
- Neuromuscular blockade
- Anesthesia
- Hypothyroidism
- Inactivity

4.9 Learning Activity

List the three determinants of oxygen delivery to the tissues.

1. _____
2. _____
3. _____

Answers to this activity can be found in the Answer Key.

Metabolic Functions of the Lung
In addition to providing oxygen for cellular functions and removal of carbon dioxide, the lung has several metabolic functions, including the synthesis of interferon and tumor inhibiting factor. Many vasoactive substances, including bradykinin, serotonin, heparin, histamine, prostaglandins E and F, and certain polypeptides such as angiotensin I, are produced, converted, or removed in the pulmonary circulation.

PULMONARY ASSESSMENT

Pulmonary assessment uses the methods of interview, inspection, palpation, percussion, and auscultation. This section also includes discussion of diagnostic studies important in diagnosis and monitoring of pulmonary conditions.

Interview
Chief Complaint and History of Present Illness
Recognize possible symptoms related to pulmonary disorders in the chief complaint. These symptoms may include dyspnea, chest pain, coughing, and wheezing. If the patient complains of dyspnea or shortness of breath, ask about onset, duration, and frequency. Ascertain if the time of day, weather or season, physical activity, eating, talking, or deep breathing influences the dyspnea. Ask if it is associated with a certain position, such as lying down (i.e., orthopnea). Grade the severity of dyspnea using the following subjective scale:
- Grade 1: Shortness of breath with mild exertion, such as running a short distance or climbing a flight of stairs
- Grade 2: Shortness of breath while walking a short distance at a normal pace on level grade
- Grade 3: Shortness of breath with mild daily activity such as shaving or bathing
- Grade 4: Shortness of breath while sitting at rest
- Grade 5: Shortness of breath while reclining at rest

Additional characteristics of the dyspnea to ask about include the effect that the dyspnea is having on the patient's ability to do activities of daily living (ADLs). Determine whether anxiety accentuates the problem. Inquire about what the patient has tried to relieve the dyspnea and if anything has been effective. In addition, ask the patient about accompanying symptoms such as cough, chest pain, or wheezing.

If the patient reports a cough, ask about when it started, how long has it been an issue, how often the coughing occurs, and whether it is affected by position, time of day, weather or season, physical activity, eating, talking, position, or deep breathing. Ask if it occurs on a regular basis or only occasionally. Also, ask if there are accompanying symptoms such as chest pain, dyspnea, or wheezing. Note any relationship between medications and the cough as cough is a common side effect of ACE inhibitors (e.g., captopril [Capoten], enalapril [Vasotec]).

If the patient indicates a productive cough, ask for a description of the sputum and if there has been any blood noted in the sputum. Ask about the frequency, color, consistency, and odor of the sputum production. Suggest household measurements (e.g., teaspoons, tablespoons, shot glass, Dixie cup, or iced tea glass) when asking a patient about the amount of sputum. Inquire about treatments used to relieve a cough such as sips of water, cough drops, and an expectorant. Smokers frequently indicate that a cigarette helps to control the cough. Ask specifically about blood in the sputum (i.e., hemoptysis) and the amount of blood. Ask if it is blood-tinged, blood-streaked, or grossly bloody. Hemoptysis may occur with tuberculosis, lung cancer, bronchiectasis, pneumonia, and pulmonary embolism. To differentiate hemoptysis from hematemesis, consider that hemoptysis is typically frothy, alkaline, and accompanied by coughing and sputum and hematemesis is typically nonfrothy, acidic, dark red or brown, and accompanied by food particles.

Chest pain may be associated with pulmonary, cardiac, musculoskeletal, or gastrointestinal problems. Review Table 3-5 in Chapter 3 for information regarding differentiation of chest pain. As with cardiac pain, the OPQRST format is helpful in describing the pain.

- **Onset of the event**: What the patient was doing when it started. Was it sudden, gradual, or part of an ongoing chronic problem?
- **Provocation or palliation**: Pulmonary pain is frequently provoked by trauma, coughing, deep breathing, or movement. Pulmonary pain may be relieved by sitting upright or by narcotics
- **Quality of the pain**: Pulmonary pain is most frequently sharp and increased by coughing, inspiration, and/or movement
- **Region and radiation**: Pulmonary pain is usually located at the lateral chest. Pulmonary pain may radiate to the shoulder or neck
- **Severity**: Pulmonary pain is usually moderate but may be severe
- **Time (history)**: Pulmonary pain onset is usually gradual. Pulmonary pain duration is usually days to weeks

If the patient complains of wheezing, ask about the onset, duration, and timing. Timing questions should include relationship to time of day, weather or season, physical activity, eating, talking, deep breathing, and position. Ask if the wheezes are inspiratory, expiratory, or both. Ask if there are identifiable triggers, such as dust, pollen, or propellants, and if there are effective treatments.

Though nasal or sinus problems, nasal stuffiness, postnasal drip, and sinus pain are not reasons for admission to a progressive care unit, they may be coexisting conditions the patients complains about. Epistaxis may be minor, but it could cause significant blood loss. Chronic hoarseness may be related to cancer of the larynx.

Ascites, abdominal pain, edema and weight gain, and fatigue or weakness may occur in patients with pulmonary hypertension and cor pulmonale. Fever indicates possible pulmonary infection. The symptom of night sweats indicates several disorders such as tuberculosis, cancer, and hormonal imbalances. Anorexia results from cor pulmonale, dyspnea, or drug side effects (e.g., xanthine bronchodilators). Weight loss may occur because of dyspnea, fatigue preventing food preparation, or hypermetabolism. Sleep disturbances may occur due to dyspnea or coughing.

Past Medical History

When asking patients about their past medical history, questions should be included to determine conditions that predispose to pulmonary conditions, such as childhood diseases, frequent respiratory infections, allergies, and asthma. In addition, ask if the patient has had pulmonary conditions such as the following:

- Pneumonia
- Cystic fibrosis
- Asthma
- Emphysema
- Chronic bronchitis

- Tuberculosis
- Lung cancer
- Occupational lung diseases such as pulmonary fibrosis, pneumoconiosis (i.e., coal worker's lung disease), asbestosis, or silicosis
- Fungal disease (e.g., histoplasmosis)
- Pulmonary embolism
- Pneumothorax
- Granulomatous diseases (e.g., sarcoidosis)
- Connective tissue disorders (e.g., lupus, scleroderma)
- Immunosuppression
- Cor pulmonale

Also ask about past chest trauma or surgery, such as a thoracotomy. Determine whether and when the patient has had any diagnostic procedures related to the pulmonary system, such as allergy testing, tuberculin and/or fungal skin tests, chest x-ray, pulmonary function studies, bronchoscopy, or laryngoscopy,

Determine whether there is a family history of genetically predisposed disease, such as asthma; emphysema, particularly alpha$_1$-antitrypsin deficiency–related emphysema; tuberculosis; cystic fibrosis; and cancer. Social history pertinent to the pulmonary system includes questions about work environment and occupation, environmental hazards (i.e., chemicals, vapors, dust, pulmonary irritants, and allergens) and use of protective devices, home environment, type of heating system, allergens (i.e., pets, plants, trees, molds, dust mites), and use of an air conditioner and/or humidifier. Determine whether the patient participates in recreational habits that cause exposure to inhalants and allergens. Ask about usual exercise and activity habits.

Ask about tobacco use, present and past, including type of tobacco products used and duration of use. Cigarette use is recorded as pack-years (i.e., number of packs per day times the number of years he or she has been smoking). Document the usage of chewing or rubbing tobacco as the type and amount per day. Note marijuana usage and record as joints per day. Ask about efforts to quit using tobacco products including previous attempts and current desire to quit. In addition, inquire about secondhand smoke exposure.

Information about eating habits should be determined. Ask about the quality and quantity of meals along with the number of meals per day. Ask about pulmonary symptoms during meals, such as dyspnea, cough, or wheezing.

Medication history should include both prescribed and nonprescribed drugs. Ask about prescribed drugs including dose, frequency, and time of last dose. Determine whether the patient understands drug actions and side effects. Determine the patient's knowledge and skill regarding the maintenance and use of respiratory devices prescribed (i.e., inhaler, CPAP, BiPAP).

Nonprescribed drugs include over-the-counter drugs, street drugs, and herbal preparations. The following herbal preparations may have pulmonary implications:

- *St. John's wort* can worsen asthma symptoms if taken with theophylline or amitriptyline (Elavil)
- *Guarana* can increase the likelihood of side effects if taken with respiratory medications because it contains theophylline
- *Ginseng* reduces the effectiveness of beta blockers
- *Licorice* elimination is reduced if taken with corticosteroids
- *Blue cohosh* and *lobelia* may increase the side effects of nicotine patches
- *Ma hang* can increase toxicity of methylxanthines in asthmatics

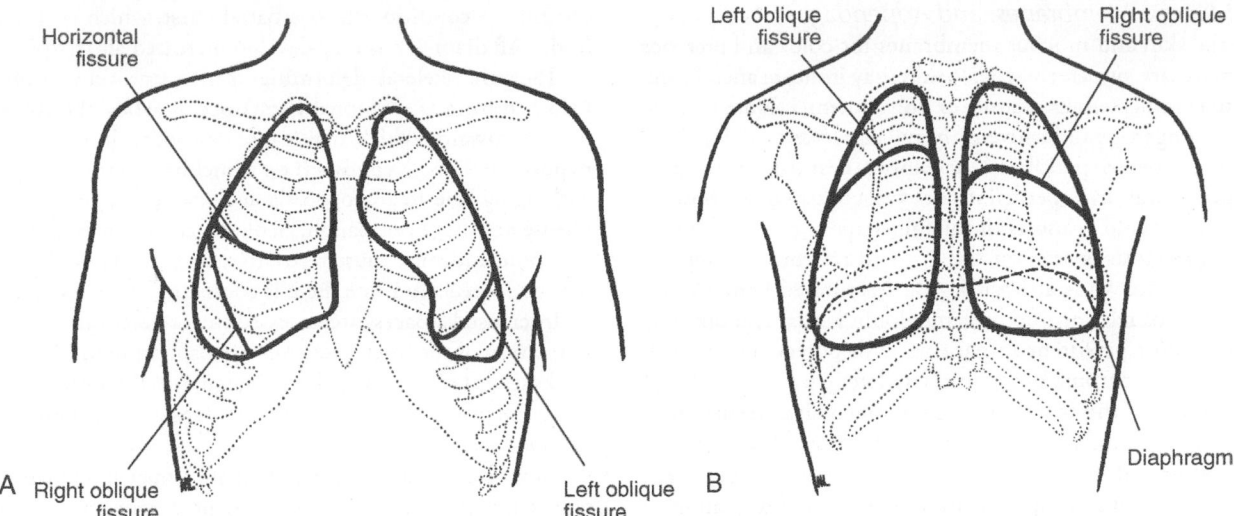

FIGURE 4-18 Location of the lungs. A, Anterior. **B,** Posterior. (From Wilkins, R. L., Sheldon, R. L., & Krider, S. J. [2005]. *Clinical assessment in respiratory care.* [5th ed.]. St. Louis, MO: Mosby Elsevier.)

Physical Assessment

Anatomic landmarks and imaginary lines on the thorax (see Figure 3-25) define the location of changes to the thorax. The lungs are located within the thorax (Figure 4-18). The apex of the lungs extend 2 to 4 cm above the inner third of the clavicle and the inferior border anteriorly is at the 6th rib at the midclavicular line (MCL) and at the 8th rib at the midaxillary line (MAL), posteriorly at T10 on expiration and at T12 with deep inspiration. The fissure dividing the upper and lower lobes is at T3 posteriorly. The upper lobes are primarily anterior and the lower lobes are primarily posterior. The trachea bifurcates at the angle of Louis anteriorly or T4 posteriorly.

Inspection and Palpation

The initial aspect of assessment of the pulmonary system is measurement of height and weight and determination of vital signs including blood pressure, heart rate, respiratory rate, and temperature. A general survey of the patient should note the following:

- Apparent health status: compare apparent age relative to chronologic age
- Level of consciousness: note restlessness and/or confusion, which is frequently the first sign of hypoxia
- Increased work of breathing: note use of accessory muscles
- Speech pattern: note pausing midsentence to take a breath
- Presence of injury, abrasion, deformity
- Nutritional status
- Stature/posture

Respiratory distress in a patient is always of concern. Note clinical indications of respiratory distress (Box 4-1).

The Pao_2 determines hypoxemia (i.e., decreased oxygen in the blood). Hypoxemia occurs when the Pao_2 is less than 80 mm Hg and Sao_2 less than 95% on arterial blood gases (ABGs) or the Spo_2 is less than 95% by pulse oximetry. Note hypoxia (i.e., decreased oxygen in the tissues) by clinical indications of hypoxia (Box 4-2) and increased serum lactate level.

Hypoventilation leads to hypercapnia (i.e., increased Co_2 in the blood), which may be identified as increased $Paco_2$ on ABGs. Clinical indications of hypercapnia are listed in Box 4-3.

Note whether the patient is using pursed-lip breathing. This may be instinctive or the patient received instruction to use this technique during times of dyspnea. Note the presence of an

> **BOX 4-1**
>
> ### Clinical Indications of Respiratory Distress
>
> - Pursed lip breathing
> - Tripod positioning
> - Speaking only one or two words between breaths
> - Cough
> - Use of accessory muscles
> - Intercostal retractions

> **BOX 4-2**
>
> ### Clinical Indications of Hypoxia
>
> - Restlessness ⇒ confusion ⇒ lethargy ⇒ coma
> - Tachycardia ⇒ dysrhythmias
> - Tachypnea
> - Dyspnea
> - Use of accessory muscles
> - Mild hypertension (early) ⇒ hypotension (late)
> - Cyanosis may be present (depending on hemoglobin level)

> **BOX 4-3**
>
> ### Clinical Indications of Hypercapnia
>
> - Headache
> - Irritability
> - Confusion
> - Inability to concentrate ⇒ somnolence ⇒ coma
> - Bradypnea
> - Tachycardia ⇒ dysrhythmias
> - Hypotension
> - Facial rubor (plethora)

artificial airway or oxygen therapy. If the patient is receiving supplemental oxygen, note the administration device and flow rate. If there are nasogastric, nasointestinal, orogastric, or intestinal tubes, note the size, centimeter mark at nose or teeth, condition of the nares or oral mucosa, and the presence of any halitosis. Halitosis suggests poor oral hygiene, poor dental health, or sinus infection.

Skin, Mucous Membranes, and Appendages

Assess the skin and mucous membranes for color and presence of edema, scars, or petechiae. Pale skin may indicate anemia and rubor may indicate hypercapnia or polycythemia. Note tobacco stains on fingertips indicative of heavy cigarette smoking. Differentiate between peripheral or central cyanosis. Associated with peripheral hypoperfusion or vasoconstriction, observe peripheral, or cold cyanosis in the fingertips and toes. Central, or warm, cyanosis is seen on the lips and mucous membranes and is associated with at least 5 g of desaturated hemoglobin. Because of this relationship to hemoglobin levels, cyanosis may be early and/or persistent in patients with polycythemia, such as patients with chronic bronchitis, and late in patients with significant anemia. This is why patients with massive bleeding may not manifest cyanosis despite profound hypoxia. Also, consider that cyanosis is difficult to detect in dark-skinned individuals. Cherry-red skin may indicate carbon monoxide intoxication.

Note any scars, especially on the thorax. Petechiae, if noted, may indicate blood dyscrasias that affect platelets, such as disseminated intravascular coagulation (DIC), platelet aggregation inhibitors (e.g., ASA, nonsteroidal antiinflammatory agents, clopidogrel [Plavix]), liver disease, severe infection, or fat embolism. Peripheral edema may be associated with cor pulmonale, such as occurs with chronic hypoxemia.

Assess the nail bed for cyanosis or clubbing. Early clubbing is flattening of the angle between the nail bed and the nail; late clubbing is an increase in the angle (i.e., >180 degrees) between the nail bed and the nail. Clubbing indicates chronic hypoxia and is frequently seen in restrictive disorders or late obstructive lung disease.

Neck

The trachea should be midline but may be deviated from either local conditions, such as hematoma or goiter, or mediastinal conditions. Mediastinal conditions that can cause tracheal shifts toward the affected side include spontaneous pneumothorax, atelectasis, or pneumonectomy. Mediastinal conditions that can cause tracheal shifts away from the affected side include tension pneumothorax, large pleural effusion, and hemothorax.

When observing the neck veins, consider that they are normally distended 2 cm above the angle of Louis with the patient's head of bed (HOB) elevated at 45 degrees. If the neck veins are distended more than 2 cm, consider right ventricular failure (e.g., cor pulmonale), tension pneumothorax, cardiac tamponade, or superior vena cava syndrome. If the neck veins are flat when the patient is in a flat position, it is indicative of hypovolemia. Superior vena cava syndrome may occur in lung cancer and edema of the neck, eyelids, and hands accompanies the jugular vein distention.

Evaluate the patient for enlargement of lymph nodes (infraclavicular, supraclavicular, and/or axillary nodes), which may be seen in lung cancer. In addition, note the use of accessory muscles indicative of respiratory distress.

Thorax

Note the patient's posture and the contour of the thorax. Patients in respiratory distress will frequently assume a tripod position, which is sitting up and leaning forward, to achieve optimal chest excursion and ventilation. The normal contour of the chest is symmetric with a costal angle of less than 90 degrees and an anterior-posterior (AP) diameter of one half the lateral diameter (i.e., AP to lateral diameter ratio of 1:2). Patients with obstructive conditions have a barrel chest, which is an increase in the AP diameter as they develop increased air trapping.

Thoracic skeletal deformities can affect ventilation. Pectus excavatum (i.e., funnel chest) occurs when the sternum is pushed inward, which may cause restrictive lung disease and hypoventilation. Kyphosis (i.e., hunchback) frequently occurs with aging due to osteoporosis and may cause restrictive lung disease and hypoventilation. Scoliosis causes an S curvature of the spine and may cause restrictive lung disease and hypoventilation, especially when there is coexisting kyphosis of aging.

Intercostal spaces are assessed for retraction or bulging. Retraction of the interspaces during inspiration may occur with tracheal obstruction or asthma. Bulging of the interspaces during expiration may occur in asthma, tension pneumothorax, or pleural effusion.

Note impaired chest movement, unequal expansion, or reduced respiratory excursion. Impaired movement is associated with thoracic pain with splinting or restrictive lung disease. Unequal expansion is associated with unilateral conditions such as massive atelectasis or pleural effusion, pneumonia, pneumothorax, or pulmonary resection. In addition, note unequal expansion with intubation of the right main stem bronchus; the right chest expands, but the left chest does not.

Paradoxical breathing is a type of breathing in which all or part of a lung inflates during inspiration and balloons out during expiration; this usually results from traumatic injury to the thorax (e.g., flail chest). Respiratory excursion is normally 2 to 6 cm during normal breathing, but airway obstruction or restrictive conditions reduce normal excursion. Note the respiratory rate, rhythm (Table 4-3), and quality of respirations.

Normally the inspiration to expiration (I:E) ratio is 1:2 with expiration lasting twice as long as inspiration. In obstructive conditions, prolonged expiration will be noted with I:E ratios 1:3 or greater. Use of abdominal and internal intercostal muscles may also be noted.

Although the point of maximal impulse (PMI) is normally palpated at the 5th left intercostal space (LICS) at MCL, it may be shifted medially in patients with chronic lung disease and pulmonary hypertension due to right ventricular hypertrophy. The PMI may also move in either direction with a mediastinal shift depending on the side and type of condition creating the mediastinal shift. A right ventricular heave may be felt at the sternum or in the epigastric area due to right ventricular hypertrophy and/or failure.

When palpating the thorax, note any chest wall tenderness, which may result from a fracture, tumor, or costochondritis. Evaluate vocal fremitus by asking the patient to say "99" while palpating the thorax with the ball of your hand. Conditions that decrease vocal fremitus include the following:

- Thick chest wall
- Bronchial obstruction
- Pleural effusion
- Pleural thickening
- Pneumothorax
- Emphysema

Vocal fremitus is increased when palpating over large airways or with any of the following conditions:

- Pneumonia
- Tumor
- Pulmonary fibrosis
- Pulmonary infarction

TABLE 4-3	Respiratory Rhythms	
Rhythm	**Description**	**Possible Causes**
Eupnea	Rate 12-20/breath/min and normal depth of ventilation; regular with occasional sigh	• Normal
Bradypnea	Slow (<10/min), regular ventilation	• Depression of respiratory center with opium, alcohol, or tumor • Sleep • Increased intracranial pressure • CO_2 narcosis • Metabolic alkalosis
Tachypnea	Rapid (>30/breath/min) ventilation; depth may be normal or decreased	• Restrictive lung disease • Pneumonia • Pleurisy • Chest pain • Fear • Anxiety • Respiratory insufficiency
Hypopnea	Shallow ventilation, normal rate	• Deep sleep • Heart failure • Shock • Meningitis • Central nervous system depression • Coma
Hyperpnea	Deep ventilation; rate may be normal or increased	• Exercise • Hypoxia • Fever • Hepatic coma • Midbrain or pons lesions • Acid-base imbalance • Salicylate overdosage
Cheyne-Stokes	Increasing and decreasing rate and depth of ventilation followed by apnea lasting 20-60 seconds	• Increased intracranial pressure • Heart failure • Renal failure • Meningitis • Cerebral hemisphere damage • Drug overdose
Kussmaul	Deep, gasping, rapid (usually >35/breath/min) ventilation	• Metabolic acidosis (e.g., diabetic ketoacidosis, renal failure) • Peritonitis
Apneustic	Prolonged gasping inspiration followed by short inefficient expiration	• Lesion of pons
Biot	Periods of apnea alternating with a series of breaths of equal depth; breathing may be slow and deep or rapid and shallow	• Meningitis • Encephalitis • Head trauma • Increased intracranial pressure
Ataxic	Lack of any pattern to ventilation	• Brainstem lesion
Obstructive	I:E ratio of 1:4 or greater	• Asthma • Emphysema • Chronic bronchitis
Apnea	Cessation of ventilation for longer than 15 seconds	• Central nervous system damage • Sleep apnea

Two types of pathologic fremitus associated with pulmonary conditions may be noted during palpation of the thorax; these are pleural friction fremitus and rhonchal fremitus. Pleural friction fremitus is a grating sensation that occurs with pleural inflammation. Rhonchal fremitus is the vibration felt with movement of secretions through the tracheobronchial tree.

Assess for subcutaneous emphysema (i.e., air in subcutaneous tissue around a tracheostomy, chest tube, or stab wound; it feels like bubble wrap. Also, note the presence of a chest tube, central venous catheter, or wounds on the thorax.

Although the liver is not normally palpable below the costal margin, a normal liver may be palpable in patients with hyperinflated lungs because the lungs push the liver downward.

TABLE 4-4	Percussion Tones				
Tone	**Intensity**	**Pitch**	**Duration**	**Quality**	**Normal Location**
Tympanic	Loud	High	Medium	Drumlike	Stomach, bowel
Hyperresonant	Loud	Low	Long	Booming	Hyperinflated lungs
Resonant	Medium	Low	Long	Hollow	Normal lung
Dull	Soft	High	Medium	Thudlike	Liver, spleen, heart
Flat	Soft	High	Short	Extreme dullness	Muscle, bone

An enlarged and tender liver may occur and be palpated in patients with cor pulmonale.

Percussion

Percussion of the thorax is very helpful in identification of pulmonary pathologic states. There are five percussion tones (Table 4-4) and these are normal in specific locations.

Lung tissue normally produces a resonant percussion tone, the heart is normally dull, and the diaphragm is flat. A hyperresonant percussion tone produced is indicative of trapped air such as in asthma, emphysema, or pneumothorax. Dullness over lung tissue indicates atelectasis, pneumonia, or tumor. The flat tone occurs over a pleural effusion.

Percussion also evaluates diaphragmatic excursion. Percuss the flatness of the diaphragm with expiration and then percuss the new position of the diaphragm at full inspiration. Normal diaphragmatic excursion is 3 to 5 cm, but a decreased excursion may exist by the following:

- Conditions that increase intrathoracic volume such as emphysema
- Conditions that increase intraabdominal volume and pressure such as ascites, hepatomegaly, pregnancy, and gaseous abdominal distention
- Conditions that decrease chest excursion and tidal volume such as thoracic or abdominal pain
- Phrenic nerve injury

Percussion also evaluates the size of the liver. Starting in the MCL at about the third ICS, lightly percuss and move down. Percuss inferiorly until dullness denotes the liver's upper border (usually at the fifth intercostal space in MCL). Hyperresonance that continues below these boundaries can be suggestive of hyperinflation (e.g., emphysema). Resume percussion from below the umbilicus on the MCL in an area of tympany. Percuss superiorly until dullness indicates the liver's inferior border. Measure the span in centimeters. The span of dullness in the right midclavicular line that is indicative of normal liver size is 6 to 12 cm. Hepatomegaly (i.e., liver span >12 cm in the right MCL) may occur with cor pulmonale.

Auscultation

Auscultate lungs using the diaphragm because they are high-pitched sounds. Ask the patient to take deep breaths through his or her mouth and listen for at least one full breath at each location while comparing symmetric areas.

Evaluate breath sounds for intensity, quality, and the presence of adventitious sounds. The intensity (i.e., loudness) of breath sounds increase with hyperventilation and anything that decreases the distance between the lung and your stethoscope, such as a thin chest wall. The intensity of breath sounds decrease by hypoventilation, such as occurs in emphysema, thoracic pain, or restrictive lung disease and anything that increases the distance between the lung and your stethoscope, such as a muscular or obese chest, pneumothorax, hemothorax, or pleural effusion. Breath sounds may be absent in severe bronchospasm, massive atelectasis, pneumonectomy, pneumothorax, or hemothorax. A malpositioned endotracheal tube will cause breath sounds to be absent over the left lung.

Breath sound quality varies with location (Figure 4-19 and Table 4-5) or presence of pathologic states. Bronchial breath sounds audible in areas other than the normal location indicates consolidation (e.g., atelectasis, pneumonia, tumor). Bronchovesicular breath sounds audible in areas other than the normal location indicates partial consolidation and partial aeration, such as developing or resolving atelectasis or pneumonia.

4.10 Learning Activity

Identify the primary breath sound change that occurs in the following conditions.

Condition	Breath Sound Change(s)
Emphysema	
Atelectasis	
Pneumonia	
Chronic bronchitis	
Pneumothorax	
Pulmonary fibrosis	
Asthma	
Pulmonary edema	
Pleurisy	
Hemothorax	
Pleural effusion	
Pulmonary embolism	

Answers to this activity can be found in the Answer Key.

Adventitious sounds (Table 4-6) are extra sounds, which may be heard at points in the ventilatory cycle or throughout the ventilatory cycle. These sounds are associated with pulmonary pathology.

Bedside Assessment of Pulmonary Function

Bedside parameters (also referred to as *ventilatory mechanics*) are measured with a Wright respirometer. Tidal volume (V_T), vital capacity (VC), and minute ventilation (V_E or MV) are all measured. A normal V_T, the amount of air moved in and out with each breath, is 7 mL/kg. A V_T less than 5 mL/kg indicates the need for an artificial airway and/or mechanical ventilation. VC is the maximal amount of air exhaled after a maximal inspiration, and is normally 15 mL/kg. A VC less than 10 mL/kg indicates the need for an artificial airway and/or mechanical ventilation. Minute ventilation is the amount of air moved in and out per minute (i.e., f x V_T); a normal rate is 5 to 10 L/min. The maximal voluntary ventilation (MVV) is the volume of air moved into and out of the lungs with maximal effort over a short period (usually 10 to 15 seconds). It is

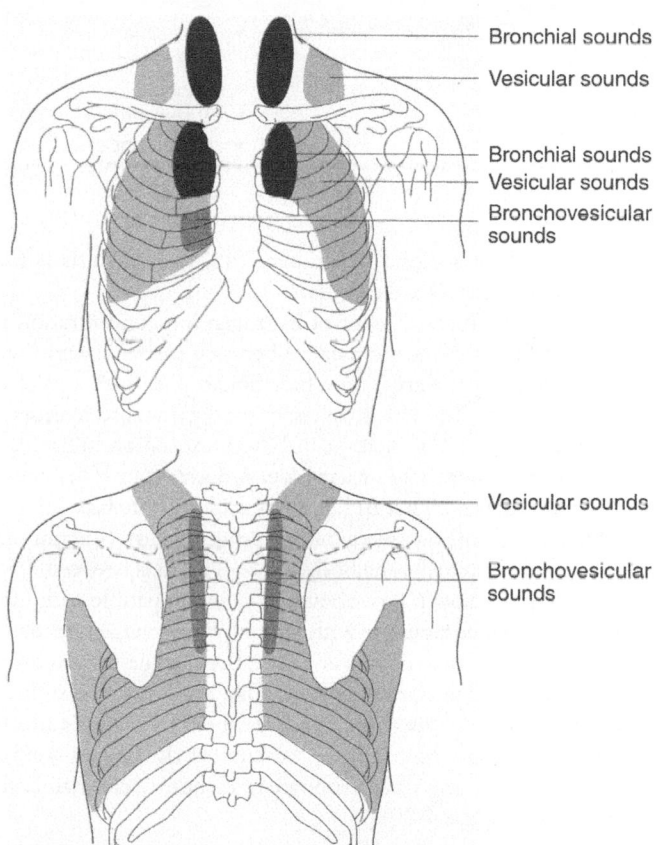

FIGURE 4-19 Breath sounds: normal locations. (From Barkauskas, V. H., et al. [1994]. *Health and physical assessment.* St. Louis, MO: Mosby.)

normally 170 L/min, though only one quarter of this total is actually measured in a 15-second period for patients are not asked to ventilate at this intensity for an entire minute. MVV reflects the status of the ventilatory muscles, compliance of the lung and thorax, and airway resistance. This parameter may provide a quick assessment of the patient's ventilatory reserve before surgery.

Pulse oximetry (SpO_2), the continuous noninvasive method of monitoring arterial oxygen saturation (SaO_2), is very important in assessing patients with oxygenation problems. Pulse oximetry allows the assessment of adequacy of oxygenation; however, it does not adequately evaluate ventilation because $PaCO_2$ increases with hypoventilation but PaO_2 and O_2 saturation do not decrease until much later.

The method of pulse oximetry includes a sensor with a light source, which is placed on the fingertip, toe, bridge of the nose, forehead, or earlobe; care must be taken to use the appropriate sensor for the location (i.e., a finger sensor should not be attached to the earlobe). The beams of light that pass through the tissue determine the amount of arterial hemoglobin saturated with oxygen.

The normal SpO_2 value is greater than 95%. Suspect moderate to severe hypoxemia if it is less than 90%. Causes of decreased SpO_2 include a decrease in SaO_2 and PaO_2 or a decrease in cardiac output. Patients with changes in SpO_2 require prompt assessment and ABGs for analysis.

Although SpO_2 is a valuable parameter, it has many limitations. Factors that result in inadequate pulsations, such as significant hypotension, vasopressors, severe hypothermia, or arterial compression cause an overestimation of SaO_2. Carboxyhemoglobin, a result of carbon monoxide poisoning or heavy tobacco use, results in overestimation of SaO_2. Other variables that may impair accuracy of SpO_2 and the relationship to SaO_2 include the following:

- Intravenous dyes (e.g., methylene blue, indocyanine green) result in inaccurate readings
- Increased bilirubin (>20 mg/dL results in inaccurately low readings
- Ambient light may affect accuracy
- Motion artifact may affect accuracy
- Edema may result in inaccurately low readings
- Sensor on finger with nail polish; blue, green, gold, black, or brown nail polish needs to be removed
- Sensor on pierced earlobe results in inaccurate reading

Laboratory studies used in the diagnosis and management of pulmonary conditions include serum chemistry, hematology and ABGs. Normal values for these studies are included in Appendix D

Obtain sputum for culture and sensitivity, Gram stain, acid-fast stain, and cytology. Sputum for analysis is collected in the morning by cough, but may also be obtained by induced tracheobronchial aspiration or by bronchoscopy.

TABLE 4-5	Breath Sounds: Quality				
Quality	**I:E Ratio**	**Intensity**	**Pitch**	**Description**	**Normal Location**
Bronchial	I < E	Loud	High	Hollow	Trachea
Bronchovesicular	I = E	Medium	Medium	Breezy	Mainstem bronchi
Vesicular	I > E	Soft	Low	Swishy	Peripheral lung

TABLE 4-6	Breath Sounds: Adventitious Sounds			
Sound	**Alternative Terms**	**Phase**	**Description**	**Cause**
Stridor	Croupy	Inspiratory	High pitched whistle audible without a stethoscope	• Upper airway obstruction • Epiglottis • Foreign body • Laryngospasm • Laryngeal edema

Wheezes	Whistles; sibilant rhonchi	Inspiratory or expiratory	High-pitched whistling sound	• Decrease in airway lumen
				  • Bronchospasm
				  • Mucus plug
				  • Tumor

Crackles	Rales	Inspiratory	Discontinuous crackling sound; similar to rubbing hair between fingers	• Pulmonary edema • Atelectasis • Pulmonary fibrosis
Rhonchi	Gurgles, sonorous rhonchi, coarse crackles	Expiratory	Continuous gurgling sound	• Fluid or mucus in airways
Pleural friction rub		Inspiratory and expiratory	Grating or scratching sound	• Pulmonary infarction • Pleurisy • Tuberculosis • Lung cancer

Note the characteristics of the sputum including color, odor, viscosity, and presence of blood. The physician performs a thoracentesis to obtain pleural fluid for analysis. Total protein differentiates between exudative pleural effusion and transudative pleural effusion. A Gram stain, acid-fast stain, and cytology analysis on the pleural fluid is also performed. Skin tests are used to identify type I hypersensitivity tests (i.e., "allergy tests"), type II hypersensitivity tests (e.g., purified protein derivative [PPD] for tuberculosis), and fungal diseases (e.g., *candida*).

Many diagnostic studies (Table 4-7) may be required for diagnosis and monitoring of patients with pulmonary conditions. Many of these require preparation of the patient.

ACID-BASE BALANCE AND ARTERIAL BLOOD GAS INTERPRETATION

Physiology Review

Acids are substances that can give up a H^+ ion; they are produced by the body as a result of cellular metabolism. Volatile (i.e., exhalable) acids result from the aerobic metabolism of glucose. The best example of a volatile acid is carbonic acid, which the lungs eliminate. Nonvolatile (also called fixed) acids are nonexhalable and cannot be converted to a gas. These fixed acids result from the aerobic metabolism of protein and fat and the anaerobic metabolism of glucose. Examples of nonvolatile acids include sulfuric, phosphoric, and uric. The kidney must eliminate these acids or be neutralized by a salt (base). Acidemia is the condition characterized by a blood pH of below 7.35 and acidosis is the process that causes the acidemia.

A base is a substance that can accept a H^+ ion. The primary base in the body is bicarbonate. Alkalemia is the condition characterized by a blood pH above 7.45, and alkalosis is the process that causes the alkalemia.

The indirect measurement of hydrogen ion concentration is the pH, which reflects the balance between carbonic acid (i.e., acid regulated by the lungs) and bicarbonate (i.e., base regulated by the kidneys). The pH is inversely proportional to hydrogen ion concentration. An increase in H^+ concentration indicates a lower pH and more acid or less base. A decrease in H^+ concentration indicates a higher pH and less acid or more base.

Maintain the pH within a narrow range to allow functioning of enzymatic systems in the body. A normal pH is between 7.35 and 7.45; pH below 6.8 or above 7.8 is incompatible with life. Note that the incompatible with life pH values range includes a 0.6 change toward acidosis but only a 0.4 change toward alkalosis (from midline normal of 7.4). This is because the shift of the oxyhemoglobin dissociation curve caused by alkalosis affects tissue oxygenation more adversely than does the shift caused by acidosis. A 20:1 ratio of bicarbonate to carbonic acid maintains normal pH (Figure 4-20).

Acid-Base Regulation

There are three primary mechanisms involved in maintenance of a normal pH. The first, physiologic buffers, consist of weak acids and their salt. These buffering pairs allow an immediate response when a change in acid-base status occurs by the salt combining with excess acid or the acid combining with the base. The most important buffer system is the bicarbonate-carbonic acid buffer system. The kidney generates bicarbonate and aids in the elimination of H^+. The phosphate system aids in the excretion of H^+ by the kidney. The ammonium system allows for greater excretion of H^+ by the kidney; H^+ is added to ammonia (NH_3) in the renal tubule to form ammonium

TABLE 4-7	**Pulmonary Diagnostic Studies**	
Study	**Evaluates**	**Comments**
Bronchography	• Detects obstruction or malformation of the tracheobronchial tree	• Patient inspires radiopaque substance and then x-rays are taken • Inquire about possibility of pregnancy
Chest x-ray	• Detects lung pathology (e.g., Pneumonia, pulmonary edema, atelectasis, tuberculosis, etc.) • Determines size and location of lung lesions and tumors • Verifies placement of endotracheal tube, central venous catheters, chest tubes	• Noninvasive test with minimal radiation exposure • Inquire about possibility of pregnancy • Posteroanterior (PA) and lateral films are done most commonly but in critical care areas anteroposterior (AP) portable films are frequently necessary due to inability to transport patient • Lateral decubitus films aid in identification of pleural effusion
Exercise testing	• Identify early disability • Differentiate between cardiac and pulmonary disease	• Monitor for changes in Spo_2 during exercise • Monitor closely for exercise-induced hypotension or ventricular dysrhythmias
Laryngoscopy, bronchoscopy, mediastinoscopy	• Obtain cytology specimen or biopsy • Identify tumors, obstructions, secretions, foreign bodies in tracheobronchial tree • Locate a bleeding site • May be used therapeutically to remove secretions, foreign bodies, other contaminants	• Patient is sedated before the procedure, usually with a benzodiazepine (e.g., diazepam, midazolam) • Monitor the patient for subcutaneous emphysema after study; indicates tracheal or bronchial tear • Monitor for hemoptysis; some blood in sputum is normal after biopsy but frank hemoptysis requires immediate attention
Lung biopsy Transthoracic needle lung biopsy Open lung biopsy	• Obtain specimen for cytology evaluation	• Transthoracic needle biopsy performed under fluoroscopy; inquire about possibility of pregnancy • Open lung biopsy requires thoracotomy
Magnetic resonance imaging (MRI)	• Distinguishes tumors from other structures (e.g., tumor, pleural thickening, fibrosis)	• Noninvasive test • Contraindicated for patients with pacemakers or implanted metallic devices
Pulmonary angiography	• Detects changes in lung tissue (e.g., masses) • Diagnoses abnormalities in pulmonary vasculature include thrombi and emboli • Identifies congenital abnormalities of the circulation	• Invasive test • Inquire about possibility of pregnancy • Contrast media injected into pulmonary artery: ensure adequate hydration after study • Monitor arterial puncture point for hematoma or hemorrhage
Pulmonary function studies (see Table 4-1 for lung volumes and parameters with normal spirometry: volumes and capacities) RV, FRC, TLC require nitrogen washout technique Ventilatory mechanics Flow-volume loop studies Diffusing capacity	• Measures lung volumes, capacities, and flow rates • Identifies features of restrictive or obstructive lung disease • Evaluates responsiveness to bronchodilator therapy • Aids in evaluation of surgical risk • Documents a disability or cause of dyspnea	• Noninvasive study • Frequently repeated after bronchodilator therapy
Sleep studies	• Diagnose and differentiate between obstructive sleep apnea, central sleep apnea, and cardiac sleep apnea	• Restrict caffeine before testing • Usually done during normal sleep hours
Thoracentesis (may include pleural biopsy)	• Obtain pleural fluid and/or tissue specimen • May be used therapeutically to remove pleural fluid	• Monitor patient for indications of pneumothorax • Monitor for leakage from puncture point

Continued

TABLE 4-7	Pulmonary Diagnostic Studies—cont'd	
Study	**Evaluates**	**Comments**
Thoracic computerized tomography (CT)	• Defines lesions, masses, cavities, or shadows seen on a normal chest x-ray • Evaluates tracheal or bronchial narrowing • Aids in planning radiation therapy	• X-rays taken at different angles
Ultrasonography	• Evaluates pleural disease • Visualizes diaphragm and detects disease around diaphragm (e.g., subphrenic hematoma or abscess)	• Noninvasive test
Ventilation scan Lung perfusion scan Ventilation/perfusion (V/Q) scan	• Diagnoses ventilation and/or perfusion abnormalities including emphysema, pulmonary emboli	• Invasive test: radioisotope inspired and injected intravascularly • Inquire about possibility of pregnancy • Nuclear scan study: assure patient that amount of radioactive material is minimal

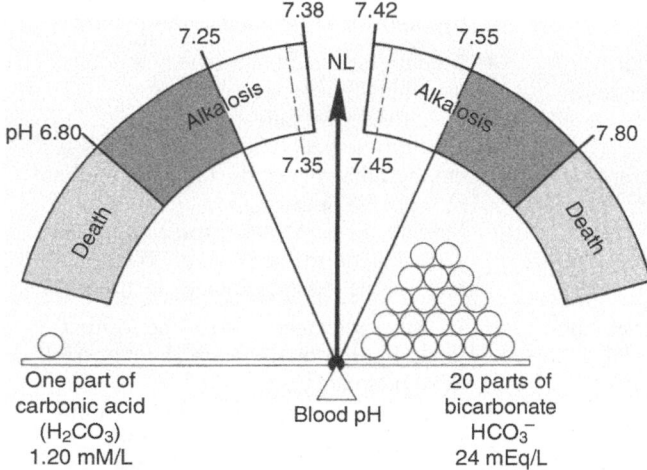

FIGURE 4-20 Acid-base balance. Twenty parts of HCO_3^- are required to buffer one part carbonic acid; pH normally is maintained within the narrow range (NL) of 7.35 to 7.45; pH below 6.8 or above 7.8 is incompatible with life. (From Price, S. A., & Wilson, L. M. [2003]. *Pathophysiology: Clinical concepts of disease processes.* [6th ed.]. St. Louis, MO: Mosby.)

(NH_4). Hemoglobin and other proteins aid in buffering extracellular fluid.

The respiratory system regulates the excretion or retention of carbonic acid. If the pH decreases, the rate and depth of ventilation increases; if the pH increases the rate and depth of ventilation decreases. This response occurs within minutes; however, although this response is fast, it is weak.

The kidneys regulate the excretion or retention of bicarbonate and the excretion of hydrogen and nonvolatile acids. If the pH decreases, the kidneys retain bicarbonate and if the pH increases, the kidney excretes bicarbonate. This response occurs within 48 hours; however, although this response is slow, it is powerful.

Acid-Base Imbalances

Acid-base imbalances (Figure 4-21) associated with respiratory conditions include respiratory acidosis, respiratory alkalosis, and metabolic acidosis. When the pH is below 7.35, acidemia exists. Acidosis, the process causing acidemia, stems from either an acid gain or a base loss. If the acidosis is caused by an acid gain, it is

respiratory acidosis if the acid is carbonic acid, which is reflected by an increase in $Paco_2$, and metabolic acidosis if the acid is a nonvolatile acid, which is reflected by a decrease in HCO_3^-. The anion gap, calculated as ($Na^+ + K^+$) − ($Cl^- + CO_2^-$), is used to differentiate between metabolic acid gain and base loss as the cause of the metabolic acidosis. If the anion gap is normal (i.e., between 5 and 15), the metabolic acidosis is due to a base loss. However, if the anion gap is increased (i.e., >15), the metabolic acidosis is due to acid gain. Remember the causes of metabolic acidosis with an increased anion gap by the MUDPILES mnemonic (Box 4-4). Metabolic acidosis also occurs if the acid is a nonvolatile acid, which an increase in HCO_3^- reflects.

When the pH is above 7.45, alkalemia exists. Alkalosis, the process causing alkalemia, stems from either a base gain or an acid loss. If an acid loss causes alkalosis, it is respiratory alkalosis if the acid is carbonic acid, which a decrease in $Paco_2$ reflects. If a base gain causes alkalosis, it is a metabolic alkalosis, which an increased HCO_3^- reflects.

A mixed ABG disorder (Figure 4-22) occurs when more than one disorder coexists with another. When a respiratory acidosis and a metabolic acidosis occur together, severe acidosis occurs. When a respiratory alkalosis and a metabolic alkalosis occur together, severe alkalosis occurs. However, if one acidosis and one alkalosis (i.e., respiratory acidosis and metabolic alkalosis or respiratory alkalosis and metabolic acidosis) occur, the pH will be normal or only slightly abnormal.

Compensation occurs when the body normalizes the pH by mechanisms aimed at increasing or decreasing acid or base. In respiratory acidosis, the kidneys reabsorb more bicarbonate or excrete more H^+, so the bicarbonate and base excess levels increase. In respiratory alkalosis, the kidneys excrete more bicarbonate, so bicarbonate and base excess levels decrease. Renal compensation for respiratory disorders is slow and may take as long as 2 to 3 days. Because respiratory alkalosis is predominantly a short-term process (e.g., hyperventilation anxiety syndrome), compensation for respiratory alkalosis is rarely seen because it takes too long and the problem would be resolved.

In metabolic acidosis, the lungs increase the rate and depth of ventilation, so the $Paco_2$ level decreases. In metabolic alkalosis, the lungs decrease the rate and depth of ventilation, so the $Paco_2$ level increases. These changes will be rapid, usually within minutes to hours.

In partial compensation, the pH is still abnormal, but the secondary parameter is outside normal range in the direction to move the pH toward normal. In full compensation, the pH is normal and the secondary parameter is outside normal range in the direction to move the pH toward normal. On the other hand, correction occurs when the pH is normal and both indicators ($Paco_2$, HCO_3^-) are normal. Correction may be a physiologic process or the result of appropriate therapeutic measures.

Arterial Blood Gas Analysis

The purposes of ABGs include evaluation of ventilation as evidenced by $Paco_2$, evaluation of acid-base status as evidenced by pH, and evaluation of oxygenation as evidenced by Pao_2 and Sao_2. Be familiar with the parameters of an ABG report, normal values and what abnormal values indicate (Table 4-8).

To analyze ABGs (Figure 4-21), start by looking at the pH; is it normal, acidotic, or alkalotic. To determine the cause of an abnormal pH, determine which parameter is abnormal. If the $Paco_2$ is abnormal, this is a respiratory disorder. If the HCO_3^- is abnormal, this is a metabolic disorder. If the pH is normal, is it leaning toward the acidic or alkalotic range? If so, consider compensation. Now look at the other parameter (either $Paco_2$ or HCO_3^-). If this parameter is abnormal but the pH is not normal yet, this is partial compensation. If this parameter is abnormal and the pH is within normal range, this is full compensation. The last step in ABG analysis is to look at the Pao_2 and Sao_2 to evaluate oxygenation.

Some technical problems may affect accuracy of ABG values. Some examples of situations that may affect accuracy include the following:
- Too much heparin: decrease in $Paco_2$, decrease in HCO_3^-, increase in base excess except with point of care analyzers (e.g., ISTAT)
- Air bubble: increase in pH, decrease in $Paco_2$, increase in Pao_2
- Not chilled immediately: decrease in pH, decrease in Pao_2, increase in $Paco_2$ except with point of care analyzers (e.g., ISTAT)
- Inadequate discard volume when drawing from catheter with flush solution: decreased $Paco_2$

The clinical implications of acid-base imbalances include anticipating or postulating the cause of an acid-base imbalance. This is accomplished by being familiar with etiologic factors, recognizing the signs and symptoms of the typical clinical presentation and being knowledgeable about medical and nursing management of acid-base imbalances (Table 4-9). Remember that close monitoring of laboratory data and clinical status is important in patients who are predisposed to acid-base imbalance. Treatment of acid-base balance always begins with treatment of the cause.

4.11 Learning Activity

Analyze the following arterial blood gases. Identify any acid-base imbalance, any partial or total compensation, and the presence of hypoxemia. Assume all patients are under 60 years of age.

	pH	$Paco_2$	HCO_3^-	Pao_2	Answer
1.	7.30	54	26	64	
2.	7.48	30	24	96	
3.	7.30	40	18	85	
4.	7.50	40	33	92	
5.	7.35	54	30	55	
6.	7.21	60	20	48	
7.	7.54	25	30	95	
8.	7.40	58	33	72	
9.	7.40	30	18	89	
10.	7.40	40	24	98	
11.	7.33	40	21	62	
12.	7.34	60	34	70	
13.	7.29	32	15	98	
14.	7.52	28	22	95	
15.	7.49	48	38	72	

4.12 Learning Activity

Identify the acid-base imbalance likely to occur in each of these situations.

a.	A patient admitted to your unit with epidural analgesia being delivered. Her ventilatory rate is 8/min.	
b.	A patient has had large volumes of NG drainage for the last several shifts.	
c.	A postoperative patient has a history of COPD. He is now having problems with retained secretions.	
d.	A postoperative patient has a history of heart failure (HF). She has been on diuretics before and after surgery.	
e.	A postoperative thoracotomy patient is complaining of chest pain and has a RR of 32/min. She is complaining of tingling around her mouth and fingertips.	
f.	A postoperative patient has large volumes of ileal drainage from the new ileostomy.	

Answers to this activity can be found in the Answer Key.

Answers to this activity can be found in the Answer Key.

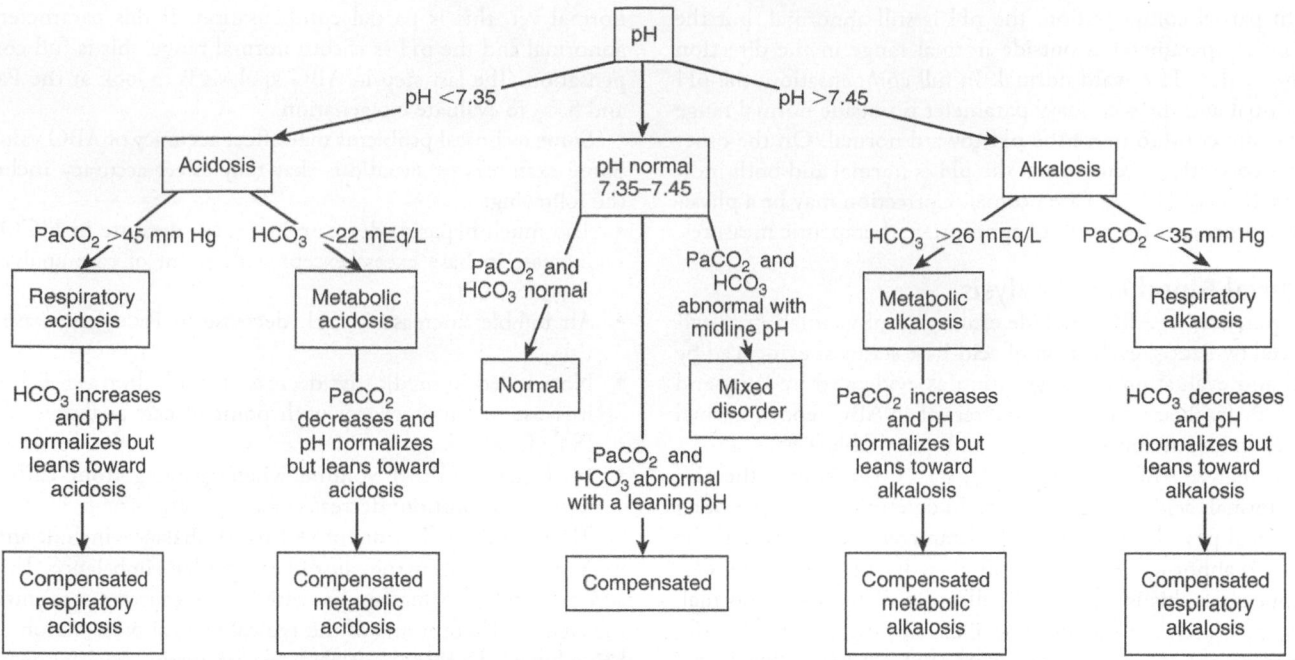

FIGURE 4-21   Determination of acid-base balance or imbalance. (From Dennison, R. D. [2013]. *Pass CCRN!* [4th ed.]. St. Louis, MO: Elsevier.)

BOX 4-4

Causes of Metabolic Acidosis with Increased Anion Gap

M	Methanol or ethanol ingestion
U	Uremia
D	Diabetic ketoacidosis or alcoholic ketoacidosis or starvation
P	Paraldehyde ingestion
I	Iron or isoniazid (INH)
L	Lactic acidosis
E	Ethylene glycol ingestion
S	Salicylate toxicity

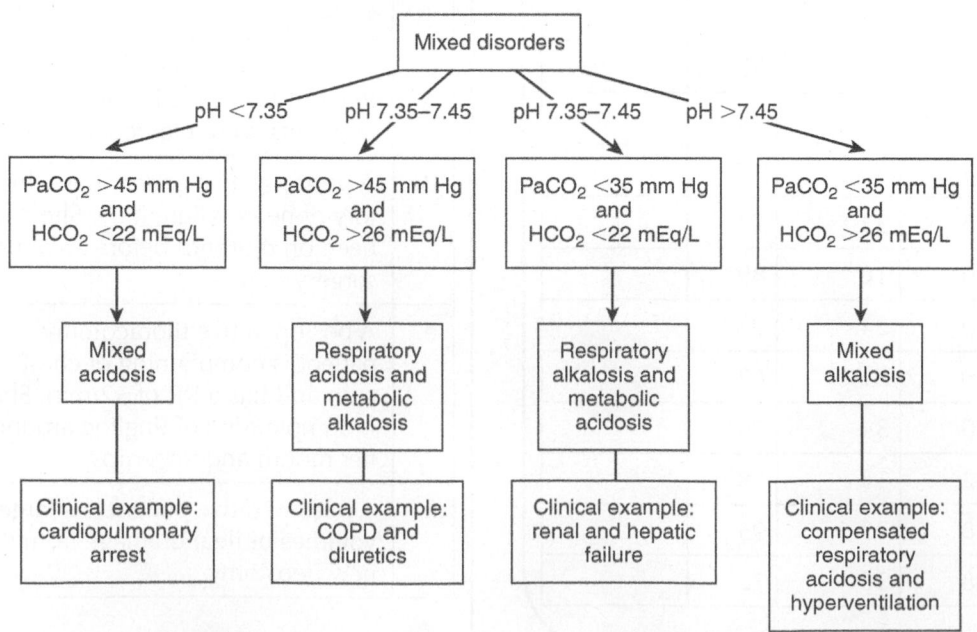

FIGURE 4-22   Mixed disorders and clinical examples. (From Dennison, R. D. [2013]. *Pass CCRN!* [4th ed.]. St. Louis, MO: Elsevier.)

| TABLE 4-8 | Parameters and Normals |

Parameter	Description	Normal	Increased Levels	Decreased Levels
pH	Negative logarithm of hydrogen ion concentration in arterial blood	7.35-7.45	Levels below 7.35 indicate an acidosis	Levels above 7.45 indicate an alkalosis
$Paco_2$	Partial pressure of carbon dioxide in arterial blood	35-45 mm Hg	Levels below 35 indicate a respiratory alkalosis or respiratory compensation for a metabolic acidosis	Levels above 45 indicate a respiratory acidosis or respiratory compensation for a metabolic alkalosis
HCO_3	Bicarbonate ion level in arterial blood	22-26 mEq/L	Levels below 22 indicate a metabolic acidosis or metabolic compensation for respiratory alkalosis	Levels above 26 indicate a metabolic alkalosis or metabolic compensation for respiratory acidosis
Base excess (BE)	Difference between acid and base levels in arterial blood	+2 - −2	Levels below -2 (actually a base deficit) indicate a metabolic acidosis or metabolic compensation for respiratory alkalosis	Levels above +2 indicate a metabolic alkalosis or metabolic compensation for respiratory acidosis
Pao_2	Partial pressure of oxygen in arterial blood	80-100 mm Hg	Levels above 100 indicate hyperoxemia	Levels below 80 indicate mild hypoxemia Levels below 60 indicate moderate hypoxemia Levels below 40 indicate severe hypoxemia Acceptable Pao_2 should be adjusted for age; one method is to subtract 1 mm Hg for each year greater than 60 years from 80 mm Hg; this gives acceptable Pao_2 on room air for a patient of that age
Sao_2	Saturation of hemoglobin by oxygen	95% or greater		Levels below 95% indicate mild desaturation of hemoglobin Levels below 90% indicate moderate desaturation of hemoglobin Levels below 75% indicate severe desaturation of hemoglobin

| TABLE 4-9 | Discussion of Acid-Base Imbalances |

Imbalance	Etiology	Clinical Presentation	Collaborative MGT
Respiratory acidosis pH low; $Paco_2$ high	Hypoventilation • Airway obstruction • CNS depression from drugs, injury, or disease • Chest wall injury (e.g., flail chest) • Obstructive lung disease (e.g., chronic bronchitis, emphysema, late asthma) • Restrictive lung disease (e.g., kyphoscoliosis, obesity hypoventilation syndrome) • Oxygen-induced hypoventilation in patients with chronic hypercapnia • Neuromuscular abnormality (e.g., Guillain-Barré syndrome, myasthenia gravis, multiple sclerosis) • Atelectasis, pneumonia • Pulmonary edema • Respiratory arrest	Initially • Sympathetic nervous system stimulation symptoms (e.g., tachycardia, tachypnea, diaphoresis) Later • Bradypnea • Hypotension • Dysrhythmias • Confusion • Headache • Blurred vision • Flushed face (plethora) • Somnolence leading to coma These late symptoms are also referred to as *CO₂ narcosis.*	Increase ventilation and treat cause • Maintain patent airway • Positioning for optimal ventilation • Implement bronchial hygiene measures • Administer drug therapy (e.g., bronchodilators, mucolytics, antibiotics) • Mechanical ventilation may be necessary • If patient is on mechanical ventilation • Increase rate • Increase tidal volume

Continued

TABLE 4-9 **Discussion of Acid-Base Imbalances—cont'd**

Imbalance	Etiology	Clinical Presentation	Collaborative MGT

Respiratory alkalosis pH high; $Paco_2$ low	Hyperventilation
	• Anxiety or hysteria
	• Thoracic pain
	• Early asthma
	• Pneumothorax
	• Pulmonary embolus
	• Early salicylate intoxication
	• Hyperthyroidism
	• Hepatic failure
	• Fever
	• Gram-negative septicemia
	• CNS infection or injury
	• Excessive mechanical ventilation
		• Tachycardia
		• Palpitations
		• Dry mouth
		• Anxiety
		• Profuse perspiration
		• Paresthesia around mouth and extremities
		• Dizziness, vertigo, syncope
		• Increased muscle irritability, twitching
		• Tetany
		• Inability to concentrate
		• Seizures
		• Coma
			Decrease ventilation and treat cause
			• Provide reassurance and maintain a calm attitude
			• Administer sedatives (frequently given intravenously)
			• Ask patient to breathe into and out of a paper bag or use a rebreathing mask
			• If patient is on mechanical ventilation
			  ○ Decrease rate
			  ○ Decrease tidal volume
			  ○ Change from assist-control to IMV
			  ○ Consider improved sedation

Metabolic acidosis pH low; HCO_3^- low	Acid gain (increased anion gap)
	• Tissue hypoxia (e.g., shock [lactic acidosis])
	• Ketoacidosis (diabetic ketoacidosis or starvation)
	• Renal failure
	• Drugs and toxins (e.g., salicylates; methanol, ethylene glycol)
	Bicarbonate loss (normal anion gap)
	• Bile drainage
	• Pancreatic fistula
	• Diarrhea
	• Acetazolamide (Diamox) therapy
		• Nausea, vomiting, abdominal discomfort
		• Weakness
		• Tremors
		• Malaise
		• Headache
		• Tachypnea progressing to Kussmaul breathing
		• Hypotension
		• Dysrhythmias
		• Confusion
		• Lethargy → coma
			• Treat cause as appropriate
			  ○ Improvement of oxygenation and/or perfusion (lactic acidosis)
			  ○ Insulin for DKA
			  ○ Dialysis for renal failure
			  ○ Antidiarrheals for diarrhea
			• Administer buffer
			  ○ Bicarbonate IV or orally for pH 7.0 or less

Metabolic alkalosis pH high; HCO_3^- high	Acid loss
	• Nasogastric suction or severe vomiting
	• Potassium-wasting diuretic therapy
	• Steroid therapy
	• Cushing's disease
	• Hyperaldosteronism
	• Hepatic disease
	• Hypokalemia, hypochloremia
	Bicarbonate gain
	• Bicarbonate administration
	• Excess infusion of lactated Ringer's solution
	• Lactate administration in dialysis solution
		• Bradypnea
		• Nausea, vomiting, diarrhea
		• Paresthesia around mouth and extremities
		• Confusion
		• Dizziness
		• Increased muscle irritability
		• Tetany
		• Seizures
		• Coma
			• Treat cause
			  ○ Antiemetic
			  ○ Electrolyte replacement: potassium and/or chloride
			  ○ Discontinuance of sodium bicarbonate or lactated Ringer's solution
			• Administer carbonic anhydrase inhibitor
			  ○ Acetazolamide (Diamox)
			• Administer buffer (rare)
			  ○ Arginine monohydrochloride
			  ○ Ammonium chloride
			  ○ Weak HCl acid solution

4.13   Synthesis Learning Activity: Crossword Puzzle

Complete the following crossword puzzle to review pulmonary anatomy, physiology, and assessment.

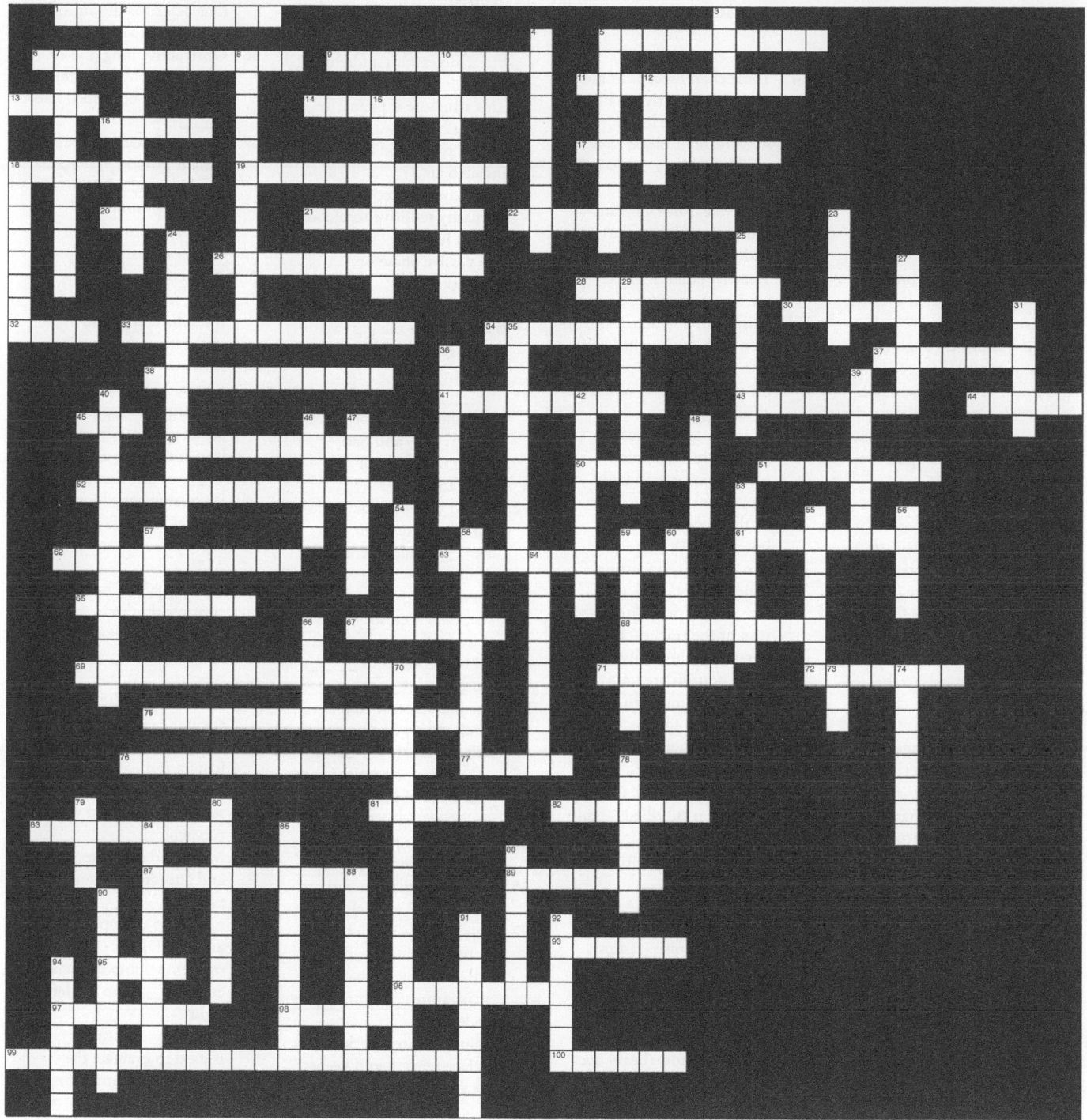

Answers to this activity can be found in the Answer Key.

ACROSS

1. These structures increase the surface area in the nose

5. The flexible cartilage attached to the thyroid cartilage; closes to protect the larynx

6. The avascular membrane that can be punctured or opened with a scalpel to provide an emergency airway

9. The change in pressure for a given change in volume

11. Measurement of lung volumes

13. The type of cell that secretes histamine

14. This acid-base imbalance would cause the oxyhemoglobin dissociation curve to shift to the left

16. When deoxygenated blood comes in contact with nonventilated alveoli; V<Q

17. Rapid breathing

18. A pulmonary embolism would decrease _____ relative to ventilation

19. These cellular organelles use oxygen and nutrients to make ATP

20. A decrease in surfactant would cause a decrease in compliance and an increase in _____ (abbrev.)
21. Alkalosis increases the _____ between hemoglobin and oxygen, which impairs oxygen drop off at the tissue
22. A phagocyte in the alveoli
26. In this type of acid-base imbalance, one system (i.e., respiratory or renal) changes as a result of an abnormality in the other system
28. These are normal breath sounds auscultated over the peripheral lung
30. The passage through the vocal cords
32. A shift of the oxyhemoglobin dissociation curve to the _____ would improve pickup at the lung but impair drop off to the tissues
33. This gas is 20 times more diffusible than oxygen (2 words)
34. The area between the soft palate and the base of the tongue; the center for the gag reflex is located here
37. The area of the left lung that corresponds to the right middle lobe
38. The movement of air into and out of the lungs
41. Airway _____ affects the work of breathing
43. This nail bed change is associated with chronic hypoxia
44. Decreased compliance of the chest wall occurs in _____
45. This adventitious breath sound is associated with pleurisy
49. The eustachian tubes open into the _____
50. A dense concentration of lymphatic tissue that guards entryways into the GI or respiratory tracts
51. Noninvasive method of measuring arterial oxygen saturation
52. The lowest portion of the pharynx
61. The type of dead space that describes the air in the alveoli that are not perfused; V>Q
62. Measurement of expired carbon dioxide tension

63. This type of disorder is when expansion of the alveolus, lung, or chest wall is impaired resulting in decreased compliance
65. An enzyme that breaks down elastic tissue
67. These chemoreceptors are primarily sensitive to blood carbon dioxide levels
68. A decrease in blood oxygen; manifested by a decrease in Pao_2 and Sao_2
69. These are normal breath sounds heard over the mainstem bronchi
71. The first portion of the trachea
72. Shift of this structure is seen with mediastinal shift
75. The cause of hypoxemia in myasthenia gravis would be alveolar _____
76. These receptors cause an increase in ventilation rate in response to body movement
77. In this type of acid-base imbalance, there are two disorders occurring concurrently
81. The area at the bifurcation of the trachea; rich in parasympathetic fibers
82. These sounds are heard when listening with a stethoscope to a patient with pneumonia or chronic bronchitis
83. The nutrient circulation of the lung is supplied by this artery
87. Surfactant is produced by the type II _____
89. A decrease in tissue oxygen; manifested by SNS innervation, cyanosis, restlessness, or confusion
93. A cause for hypoxia even though the patient has a normal Pao_2
95. Percussion tone heard over pleural effusion
96. This acid-base imbalance causes vasodilation resulting in headache, flushed face, and hypotension
97. Shortness of breath
98. The terminal respiratory unit that has an alveolar-capillary membrane for the exchange of oxygen and carbon dioxide
99. This is caused most commonly by hypoxemia (2 words)

100. Respiratory pattern with normal rate and depth

DOWN

2. A procedure to view the bronchioles with a fiberoptic scope
3. This structure is primarily responsible for warming, humidifying, and filtering inspired air
4. These chemoreceptors are primarily sensitive to blood oxygen levels
5. The passive phase of ventilation
7. The first bronchial branch that is part of the gas exchange unit is the _____ bronchiole
8. The _____ dissociation curve shows the relationship between Pao_2 and Sao_2
10. The active phase of ventilation
12. A shift of the oxyhemoglobin dissociation curve to the ___ would decrease the affinity between hemoglobin and oxygen
15. The main accessory muscles of expiration are the internal intercostal and _____ muscles
18. The pleural layer that is contiguous with the chest wall
23. _____'s law is why the Pao_2 goes down if the $Paco_2$ goes up (assuming room air)
24. Percussion tone heard over hyperinflated lung
25. Area of ventilation without perfusion (2 words)
27. This pressure is calculated by multiplying the Fio_2 (as a decimal) by the barometric pressure (760 mm Hg at sea level)
29. A lipoprotein that decreases surface tension and keeps the alveoli open at low distending pressure
31. The type of compliance that reflects the compliance of the lung and the chest wall
35. Air and gas are _____ and appear black on chest x-ray
36. The last branch of the conducting airways is the _____ bronchiole
39. The pleural layer that is contiguous with the lung

40. These receptors are stimulated by an increase in interstitial fluid volume
42. The type of dead space that describes the air in conducting pathways
46. Obstructive lung disease, such as emphysema, causes the chest to be shaped like a _____
47. Bluish skin color associated with at least 5 g of desaturated hemoglobin
48. Hairlike projections that move mucus with entrapped particles upward to be coughed out
53. These sounds are heard when listening with a stethoscope to a patient with atelectasis, pulmonary edema, and ARDS
54. The primary responsibility of the pulmonary system is to ensure the delivery of _____ to the tissues
55. Percussion tone heard over normal lung
56. This cycle converts food to ATP
57. The area of the brain that controls rhythmic ventilation; contains both the apneustic and pneumotaxic centers
58. The center of the thoracic cavity
59. The primary muscle of inspiration
60. Bloody sputum; may be seen in lung cancer or tuberculosis
64. Metal and bone are _____ and appear white on chest x-ray
66. pH, $Paco_2$, temperature, and 2,3-DPG cause the oxyhemoglobin dissociation curve to _____ to the left or right
70. This diagnostic study is used to evaluate the adequacy of ventilation (3 words)
73. This may be caused by pulmonary hypertension (abbrev.)
74. The primary functions of the nose is to filter, warm, and _____ inspired air
78. The type of compliance that reflects both compliance of the lung and airway resistance

79. These openings between the alveoli are called pores of _____

80. This type of chest pain is sharp pain that occurs with deep inspiration

84. Increased $Paco_2$

85. Most carbon dioxide is transported in the blood as _____

86. These sounds are heard when listening with a stethoscope to a patient with asthma (plural)

88. The ability of the lung to return to its original size after inspiration

90. The process by which oxygen and carbon dioxide move across the alveolar-capillary membrane

91. Respiratory pattern with rate less than 10 breaths/min

92. Transfusion of greater than 10 units that causes decreased 2,3-DPG and impaired oxygen release from hemoglobin

94. Central chemoreceptors are located in this area of the brain

AIRWAY MANAGEMENT

Airway Obstruction

Airway obstruction occurs when there is a blockage of airflow preventing air from entering the lungs. The primary cause of upper airway obstruction in an unconscious patient is relaxation of the tongue back against the hypopharynx. The most likely cause of upper airway obstruction in a conscious person is aspiration of food. Vomitus or dentures may also be causes of obstruction. The upper airway may also be obstructed or compromised by tumor, hematoma, laryngeal spasm or edema, vocal cord paralysis, infection (e.g., epiglottitis), trauma (e.g., fractured trachea), or inflammation (e.g., angioedema, ingestion of caustic agents). Foreign bodies, secretions, hemorrhage, pneumonia, space-occupying lesions or tumors, or bronchospasm may obstruct or compromise the lower airway.

The clinical presentation of airway obstruction varies depending on if the obstruction is partial or complete. With partial obstruction, there is air movement but there is evidence of respiratory distress, such as tracheal tug, intercostal retractions, and use of accessory muscles. The patient is restless, agitated, and anxious. Cyanosis may be present. The patient may be coughing and there will be altered speech. Snoring or stridor may be audible. Breath sounds are likely to reveal wheezes and rhonchi. With complete obstruction, there is no air movement. If the patient is conscious, he or she will be very anxious. Cyanosis will be present, and the patient will be unable to speak, cough, or produce any sound. If conscious, the patient will likely be exhibiting the universal sign of choking: clutching of the throat with his or her hand. There will be indications of respiratory distress, including tracheal tug, intercostal retractions, and use of accessory muscles. As oxygen levels to the brain are significantly reduced, the patient will quickly lose consciousness.

Management of respiratory distress and potential airway obstruction begins with the evaluation of the patency of the airway; look, listen, and feel for airflow. Maintain optimal airway and thoracic position. Use head-tilt, chin-lift (also called *sniffing*) position for optimal airway position; avoid true hyperextension. Use a jaw thrust instead of the head-tilt, chin-lift position if a cervical spine fracture is possible. Position the HOB in a semi-Fowler's to high Fowler's position for optimal chest excursion.

Remove any obstruction. Inspect the mouth for blood, teeth, loose dentures, food, or anything else that may cause obstruction. Use your fingers to remove visible foreign bodies. Avoid blind sweeps due to a potential concern of pushing the obstruction deeper into the airway. Use Magill forceps, but take care not to push the obstruction deeper into the airway. If the obstruction persists, use abdominal thrusts to relieve an upper airway obstruction. Alternate five abdominal thrusts with a ventilation attempt in an unconscious patient. Avoid abdominal thrusts (use chest thrusts) if the patient is too obese for you to get your arms around him or her, has had recent abdominal surgery, or is pregnant. After relieving the upper airway obstruction, place the patient in recovery position (i.e., lying on left side).

Deep Breathing and Coughing

Encourage patients to take deep breaths to prevent atelectasis. Deep breathing before coughing increases the effectiveness of coughing. Use incentive spirometry, especially postoperatively, to provide graded incentives for sustained inspiration.

Remove secretions as required. If the patient can effectively cough, it is preferable to encourage the patient to cough rather than suctioning the patient's airway. A cough is a forceful expiration to dislodge and remove secretions from the tracheobronchial tree. Indications to encourage a patient to cough include audible rhonchi and between position changes during postural drainage. Instruct patient to avoid coughing in a head down position. Although coughing should be encouraged in the previously identified situations, routine coughing may increase the incidence of atelectasis so preventive measures (e.g., postoperative patients) should focus on deep breathing with sustained inspiration rather than forced expiration (e.g., coughing). For effective coughing, assist the patient to a comfortable position and instruction the patient to inhale deeply and then cough two to three times with the mouth open. They should expectorate any sputum and then inhale slowly and deeply.

Huff coughing is a special coughing method that may be helpful for patients with COPD to allow the airways to stay open. Instruct the patient to perform forced expiration with the glottis open. Another special method, augmented coughing is used for patients with abdominal muscle weakness or paralysis. This method requires an assistant to deliver a subxiphoid thrust during expiration.

A flutter valve is a small plastic handheld device that consists of a small plastic cone containing a steel ball. Use of a flutter valve promotes airway clearance by causing vibration to loosen secretions, maintaining open airways during exhalation, and creating a series of minicoughs. Instruct the patient to use any prescribed bronchodilator before use of the flutter valve. Instruct the patient to inhale deeply, hold their breath for 2 to 3 seconds, and then exhale into the flutter valve. Use of the flutter valve is usually recommended 3 to 4 times daily with 10 to 15 repetitions each session.

Suctioning

If a cough is ineffective, suctioning of the oropharynx or airway may be necessary to clear the airway of secretions. Suctioning removes secretions from the oropharynx via a suction catheter and negative pressure Perform suctioning before deflation of the endotracheal tube cuff to prevent oropharyngeal secretions from draining into the tracheobronchial tree and after suctioning of the tracheobronchial tree to prevent accumulation of oropharyngeal secretions that can result in a silent aspiration around the endotracheal tube cuff. Use an oral suction device to clear the oropharynx of secretions, but if the suction catheter that was used to suction the tracheobronchial tree is used, suction the oropharynx only **after** suctioning the tracheobronchial tree and rinsing the catheter. Currently, specialized endotracheal tubes allow for continuous aspiration of subglottic secretions (CASS); these CASS tubes reduce the incidence or delay the onset of ventilator-associated pneumonia.

Suctioning the tracheobronchial tree removes secretions from the tracheobronchial tree. Avoid "routine" suctioning of the tracheobronchial tree and perform only when clinically indicated. Clinical indications for the need to suction include the following:

- Sympathetic nervous system stimulation (i.e., tachycardia, tachypnea)
- Change in BP (i.e., hypotension, hypertension)
- Dyspnea
- Noisy or shallow ventilation
- Rhonchi, obvious visible secretions
- Frequent or sustained coughing, especially during the inspiratory cycle of the ventilator
- A high pressure alarm from the ventilator
- Clinical indications of hypoxia (see Box 4-2) or hypercapnia (see Box 4-3).

Use the methods described here for suctioning the tracheobronchial tree to prevent complications. Suction only if indicated and limit the number of passes to the minimum required. Choose a catheter size with the outer diameter of the catheter no more than half the inner diameter of the ET tube or tracheostomy. Use a closed suction system if possible, which allows continued oxygenation and reduction in loss of positive-end expiratory pressure (PEEP) to decreased incidence of hypoxemia. Closed suction systems also decrease cost and nursing time for suctioning and decrease the risk of aerosolization of secretions, which protects the patient's and nurse's eyes. They also decrease the risk of introducing bacteria into the patient's airway.

Use sterile technique if suctioning through ET tube or tracheostomy. Use two gloves and wear goggles to protect the eyes. Explain the procedure to the patient and the family. If not using a closed suction system, also protect the patient's eyes. Hyperoxygenate with 100% oxygen before, during, and after suctioning and ensure that the SpO_2 reflects this increase in oxygen before initiating suctioning. Advance the catheter to no farther than 1 cm past the end of the ET or tracheostomy tube to avoid contact with the trachea and carina. Avoid the previously used technique of advancing the catheter to the point of obstruction, then pulling back slightly before applying suction to prevent contact trauma to the tracheobronchial tree. Shallow suctioning decreases mucosal damage, decreases mucous production, and results in less mucosal inflammation. Limit suctioning to 10 seconds. There is no difference in patient outcomes with intermittent versus continuous suction as long as the duration is limited to 10 seconds. Avoid excessive negative pressure; keep pressure at 100 mm Hg or less unless using a closed suction system, where the recommendation is 120 mm Hg.

Liquefy secretions through humidification and hydration rather than the instillation of saline (also referred to as *saline lavage*). Research has shown instillation of saline is ineffective and potentially harmful because it contributes to hypoxemia and ventilator-associated pneumonia. If increased oral or parenteral fluids cannot be given (e.g., renal failure), saline by inhalation or acetylcysteine (Mucomyst) may be prescribed. Saline by inhalation allows the small particle size to penetrate deeper into tracheobronchial tube and liquefies mucus. Acetylcysteine (Mucomyst) by inhalation breaks down disulfide bonds to liquefy mucus. A concurrent bronchodilator is frequently required.

If performing nasotracheal suctioning in a patient who does not have an endotracheal or tracheostomy tube, use aseptic technique and provide oxygen with a nonrebreathing mask before suctioning. Place the patient in "sniffing" position while sitting up or place a towel roll between the shoulders if the patient is supine. Lubricate the catheter with water-soluble lubricant before insertion. Ask the patient to cough and advance the catheter during that time, as the glottis is open; if the patient cannot follow commands, advance the catheter during inspiration. Indications that the catheter is in the trachea are that the patient becomes anxious and cannot speak. Complete suctioning as for a patient with an endotracheal or tracheostomy tube providing hyperoxygenation after each suctioning pass. After the suctioning is complete, rinse the catheter and appropriately discard a disposable catheter. To prevent injury to the nasal and oral mucosa when frequent suctioning is required, place a nasopharyngeal or oropharyngeal airway; endotracheal intubation or tracheostomy may be required.

Chest Physiotherapy

Chest physiotherapy promotes bronchial hygiene, improves breathing efficiency, and stimulates physical reconditioning. Postural drainage (PD) is the sequential positioning of the patient, which utilizes gravity to drain secretions from peripheral areas into the major bronchi or trachea so that they can be coughed and expectorated or suctioned. Postural drainage prevents and treats respiratory complications, lobar atelectasis, and disorders with significant mucus production (e.g., cystic fibrosis, bronchiectasis, COPD). The respiratory therapist usually implements, but the PCU nurse may assist. Administer any prescribed bronchodilator before PD, and turn off enteral feedings for 30 minutes before PD or avoid PD for at least 1.5 hours after meals. Also, ensure that the cuff of the endotracheal or tracheostomy tube is inflated. Place the patient in the following positions to drain selected areas of the lungs:

- Left side with hips higher than head
- Right side with hips higher than head
- Supine with hips higher than head
- Prone with hips higher than head

Maintain each position for 10 to 30 minutes though prone position will not be used for patients with neurologic injury. Encourage the patient to cough between position changes but never in a head down position. PD is contraindicated in patients with obesity, spinal fracture, rib fracture, flail chest, pulmonary hemorrhage, embolism, malignancy, pneumothorax, empyema, large pleural effusion, tuberculosis, asthma, acute bronchospasm, bleeding disorder, seizures, intracranial hypertension, acute myocardial infarction, heart failure, hemodynamic instability, recent pacemaker insertion, and increased risk of aspiration.

Percussion is the clapping of the chest with cupped hands to mechanically dislodge secretions from the bronchial walls into the major bronchi or trachea so that they can be coughed and expectorated or using a specialty bed with a vibropercussion mode in conjunction with continuous lateral rotation therapy (CLRT). Avoid percussing over the spine, liver, kidneys, spleen, and female patients' breasts. Percussion is contraindicated in patients with known bleeding disorder, lung cancer, and pneumothorax. Use extreme caution in elderly patients with osteoporosis and after thoracotomy.

Vibration is the application of vibration during expiration to areas of the chest with either an open hand or a vibrating device to loosen secretions from the bronchial walls into the major bronchi or trachea so that they can be coughed and expectorated or suctioned. Either hold your hand flat against the patient's chest and vibrate the hand during expiration or use a hand vibrator. The contraindications are the same as with percussion.

Turning

Ensure that all patients either turn themselves or are turned at least every 2 hours, especially immobile patients or patients with pulmonary problems. Consider the "good lung down" principle for patients with unilateral lung conditions with the exception of patients after pneumonectomy when the rule is "no lung down."

Consider the use of a specialty bed for kinetic therapy or CLRT. With kinetic therapy, the patient is continuously turned from side to side with a rotation of 40 degrees or greater. In CLRT, the rotation is less than 40 degrees. The effect of therapeutic rotation is that it promotes redistribution of ventilation, promotes redistribution of perfusion, and optimizes ventilation/perfusion (V/Q) matching. Rotation therapy is indicated for patients with acute respiratory distress syndrome (ARDS) or for patients with high risk for ARDS or pneumonia. It is also indicated for prevention of ventilator-associated pneumonia (VAP) and lobar atelectasis. Start this therapeutic modality as early as possible. Explain the process to the patient before initiating the therapy. Monitor blood pressure and Spo_2 frequently, especially initially until acclimation. This therapy is contraindicated in patients with severe claustrophobia (though most of these patients will be sedated), uncontrolled diarrhea, weight of greater than 300 pounds, unstable spinal cord injury, and skeletal traction.

Artificial Airways

Artificial airways are crucial for airway maintenance and require special attention for patient safety and comfort. Always provide adequate humidification because the airway bypasses natural humidification mechanisms. Use aseptic technique with upper airway artificial airways; use sterile technique with lower airway artificial airways. Suction as indicated; because ET tubes splint the epiglottis open, effective coughing is impaired and suctioning, when indicated, is required. Always provide a method of communication; this is the most significant stressor experienced by intubated patients. Use a picture communication board, alphabet board, or magic slate.

Some patients have weakness that inhibits the ability to apply the needed pressure for writing with pens and pencils so felt-tip pens or markers may work better. Fenestrated or Passy-Muir tracheostomy tubes allow air to flow past the vocal cords; therefore, do not impede speech.

Selection of an appropriate artificial airway (Table 4-10) is determined by many factors. Consider the problem requiring the artificial airway and the anticipated duration of the need for the artificial airway. Many types of artificial airways exist (Table 4-11), each with its own advantages and disadvantages. Upper airway artificial airways maintain patency of the airway when compromised by the relaxation of the tongue against the hypopharynx. Artificial airways that extend down into the lower airway with a cuff are required when a sealed airway is required, such as for mechanical ventilation.

Endotracheal Tubes

Intubation

Indications for intubation with an ET tube are generally a tidal volume of less than 5 mL/kg and/or a vital capacity less than 10 mL/kg, maximal inspiratory pressure less than 20 cm H_2O, inability to adequately cough and clear the airway, loss of protective reflexes, and need for a sealed airway (e.g., mechanical ventilation, risk for aspiration). Before the insertion of the ET tube, prepare the planned oxygen delivery system; usually this is a T-piece with nebulizer, CPAP, BiPAP, or mechanical ventilator. A manual resuscitation bag with reservoir bag with 100% oxygen may be used during cardiac arrest or until a mechanical ventilator is ready. The usual tube size is 7.5 to 8.0 for females and 8.0 to 8.5 for males. Other equipment needed includes laryngoscope with straight (Miller) and curved (MacIntosh) blades with working lights, stylet, Magill forceps, lubricant, syringe, tape or device

TABLE 4-10	Selection of Appropriate Artificial Airway	
Problem	**Preferred Artificial Airway**
Tongue against hypopharynx	Oropharyngeal or nasopharyngeal
Need for frequent nasotracheal suctioning	Nasopharyngeal
Inability to open mouth (e.g., seizure)	Nasopharyngeal
Facial or jaw fracture	Nasopharyngeal or nasotracheal tube
Complete upper airway obstruction when endotracheal intubation is impossible (e.g., laryngeal edema or spasm, tracheal fracture)	Cricothyrotomy or tracheostomy
Need for sealed airway (e.g., mechanical ventilationor potential for aspiration)	Endotracheal tube or tracheostomy
Need for long-term lower airway access and sealed airway	Tracheostomy

TABLE 4-11   Summary of Artificial Airways

Type of Airway	Advantages	Disadvantages	Miscellaneous

Oropharyngeal airway	• Easy to insert
	• Inexpensive
	• Effectively holds tongue away from pharynx
		• Improper insertion technique can push tongue back and occlude airway
		• Easily dislodged
		• Poorly tolerated by conscious patients as it may stimulate gag reflex
		• Causes increased oral secretions
		• Contraindicated in patients with trauma to lower face, recent oral surgery, loose or avulsed teeth
			• Determine appropriate size: with flange at teeth, end of airway should not extend beyond the angle of the jaw
			  • Large adult: usually 100 mm (size 5)
			  • Medium adult: usually 90 mm (size 4)
			  • Small adult: usually 80 mm (size 3)
			• Insert by holding tongue down with tongue blade and sliding into place; alternative method: insert upside down and turn over when into pharynx; take care not to traumatize palate
			• Do not use as a bite block; likely to cause vomiting and potential aspiration in conscious patients
			• Remove, wash, and give oral care every 4 hours; check mucous membranes for ulcerations

Nasopharyngeal airway (also called a *trumpet airway*)	• Easy to insert
	• Inexpensive
	• Effectively holds tongue away from pharynx
	• May be used in conscious or unconscious patients
	• Prevents trauma to nasal mucosa during nasotracheal suctioning
	• May be inserted when mouth cannot be opened (e.g., during seizures, jaw fractures)
		• May cause nosebleeds, pressure necrosis, or sinus infection
		• Kinks and clogs easily
		• Contraindicated in patients predisposed to nosebleeds, nasal obstruction, bleeding disorder, and sepsis and in patients with basal skull fracture
			• Determine appropriate size: 1 inch longer than nose to earlobe; lumen smaller than naris
			  • Large adult: usually 8-9 mm internal diameter
			  • Medium adult: usually 7-8 mm internal diameter
			  • Small adult: usually 6-7 mm internal diameter
			• Insert with bevel against septum
			• Use viscous Xylocaine as a lubricant for insertion to decrease discomfort
			• Do not use in patients receiving anticoagulants
			• Provide humidification of inspired air
			• Confirm placement by visualizing the tip of the airway next to the uvula
			• Rotate naris to naris every 8 hours
			• Limit the duration of use to reduce risk of sinus infection

Esophageal-tracheal Combitube	• Allows ventilation whether the tube is inserted into the trachea or the esophagus • Reduces risk of aspiration over mask ventilation • Permits easier placement over endotracheal tube because visualization of the vocal cords is not necessary • Provides comparable ventilation and oxygenation to that achieved with an endotracheal tube	• Incorrect identification of the position of the distal lumen may result in absence of ventilation • May cause esophageal trauma • Cannot mechanically ventilate the patient with a Combitube	• Use of an end-tidal CO_2 or esophageal detector device is recommended to confirm placement as either being in the trachea or esophagus

TABLE 4-11   **Summary of Artificial Airways—cont'd**

Type of Airway	Advantages	Disadvantages	Miscellaneous
Laryngeal mask airway (LMA)	• Permits easier placement than endotracheal tube because visualization of the vocal cords is not necessary • Provides comparable ventilation and oxygenation to that achieved with an endotracheal tube • Allows placement when there is a possibility of unstable neck injury or when appropriate positioning of the patient for tracheal intubation is impossible • Reduces risk of aspiration over mask ventilation • Permits coughing and speech	• Small proportion of patients cannot be ventilated with an LMA, so an alternative strategy is needed • Cannot prevent aspiration because it does not separate the GI tract from the respiratory tract • May cause laryngospasm or bronchospasm • May be difficult to ventilate patients who require high airway pressures to attain adequate tidal volumes	• If lubrication is required, only the posterior aspect of the airway should be lubricated • If used for mechanical ventilation, an audible air leak may occur

Endotracheal tube (general)	• Provides relatively sealed airway for mechanical ventilation, prevention of aspiration
	• Permits easy suctioning
	• Prevents gastric distention with air during CPR
		• Requires skilled personnel for insertion
		• Splints epiglottis opens and prevents effective cough
		• Causes loss of physiologic PEEP because epiglottis is splinted open; patient should receive 3-5 cm PEEP to reestablish physiologic PEEP
		• May kink and clog
		• Causes aphonia
		• May cause laryngeal or tracheal damage
		• Contraindicated in patients with laryngeal obstruction caused by tumor, infection, or vocal cord paralysis
			• Determine appropriate size
			  • Females: usually 7.5-8.0 mm internal diameter
			  • Males: usually 8.0-8.5 mm internal diameter
			  • Tube may need to be 0.5-1.0 mm smaller if to be inserted nasally
			• Provide humidification of inspired air
			• Mark tube at corner of mouth or at naris to assess any movement
			• Use minimal occlusive volume or minimal leak volume for cuff inflation; ensure that cuff pressure does not exceed 18 mm Hg (if pressure >18 mm Hg required to achieve seal, tube is too small and needs to be replaced with larger tube)
			• Confirm placement by chest x-ray: tip of tube should be 3-5 cm above carina
			• Provide oral care every 4 hours; observe oral or nasal mucosa for signs of ulcerations or necrosis
			• Position to prevent kinking; utilize mechanical ventilator's support arms to support ventilator tubing

Oral (specific) endotracheal tube	• Easier insertion than nasal intubation • Permits larger tube than nasal intubation	• Less stable and comfortable than nasal tube • May stimulate gag reflex • May be bitten or chewed • May cause necrosis at corner of mouth • Increases oral secretions; makes oral care more difficult • Contraindicated in patients with acute unstable cervical spine injury due to need for neck extension (blind nasotracheal intubation may be attempted in these patients)	• Reposition tube from one side of the mouth to the other and retape when indicated; avoid unnecessary manipulation of tube

Continued

TABLE 4-11   **Summary of Artificial Airways—cont'd**

Type of Airway	Advantages	Disadvantages	Miscellaneous
Nasal (specific) endotracheal tube	• More comfortable for patient than oral endotracheal tube • Permits good oral hygiene • Cannot be bitten or chewed	• More difficult insertion than oral intubation • May cause pressure necrosis or sinus infection • Requires smaller size • Contraindicated in patients with nasal obstruction, fractured nose, sinusitis, bleeding disorder, basal skull fracture	• Monitor for clinical indications of sinus infection: fever, increased pharyngeal drainage, halitosis, leukocytosis, sinus pain, or headache
Cricothyrotomy	• Provides immediate airway access, especially helpful if complete upper airway obstruction	• May cause bleeding • Only temporary; very small opening if established with large needle; larger if airway opened with scalpel and small tracheostomy tube used	• Provide humidification of inspired air • Use large bore over-the-needle catheter; adaptor required to attach to manual resuscitation bag • Physician may use scalpel and insert small tracheostomy tube • Monitor for bleeding, subcutaneous emphysema
Tracheostomy	• Provides long-term airway access • Minimizes risk of vocal cord damage from an endotracheal tube during long-term airway maintenance • Decreases dead space and decreases work of breathing • Provides a relative seal to prevent aspiration • Allows the patient to eat, swallow • Allows easier suctioning • Permits Valsalva maneuver and effective cough • Is more comfortable for patient • Is less likely to be dislodged than endotracheal tube • Bypasses upper airway obstruction	• May require surgery but may be performed percutaneously • Causes aphonia • May cause false passage anterior to trachea in patients with thick necks • May cause erosion of innominate artery with tip of tube or low stoma • Causes scar • May cause tracheocutaneous or tracheoesophageal fistula	• Usually considered if artificial airway is required longer than 2-3 weeks • Determine appropriate size: usually 5-6 mm • Requires humidification of inspired air • Preferred if airway obstruction (e.g., tumor or laryngeal edema or spasm) • Provide tracheostomy care that includes cleaning stoma and tube every 8 hours with saline; keep stoma dry (if 4 × 4 used, change often if secretions present) • Keep obturator, extra tracheostomy tube, and tracheal spreader at bedside

for stabilization of tube, and suction equipment including a suction catheter and oral suctioning device. During the intubation procedure, monitor ECG and Spo$_2$. Prior to the intubation, the patient is hyperoxygenated with 100% oxygen for at least 2 minutes. Place the patient in head-tilt, chin-lift position. A trained, qualified and experienced person (usually a physician or nurse anesthetist) performs the Intubation within 30 seconds; if not, attempts should be ceased and the patient should again be hyperoxygenated. To confirm placement of the ET tube:
• Feel air movement through tube
• Assess bilateral chest excursion
• Auscultate bilateral breath sounds; if breath sounds are audible on the right but not on the left, right mainstem intubation has occurred; pull the tube back slightly and then recheck breath sounds

• Use a capnometer to confirm consistent exhalation of CO_2
• Auscultate over epigastrium: air movement should not be audible
• Radiographic confirmation is necessary for positioning: the distal tip of the tube should be 3 to 5 cm above the carina

After confirmation of tube placement, inflate the cuff using either minimal occlusive volume or minimal leak volume. To inflate the cuff to minimal occlusive volume, listen over the trachea with a stethoscope and inflate the cuff until no air leak is audible during the inspiratory cycle of the ventilator. To inflate the cuff using the minimal leak volume technique, listen over the trachea with a stethoscope and inflate the cuff until no air leak is audible when the manual resuscitation bag is squeezed and then remove 0.1 cm of air or until a minimal leak is audible when the manual resuscitation bag is squeezed. Cuffs in current use are high volume, low-pressure cuffs; these cuffs distribute the low pressure over a larger area of the trachea and decrease the incidence of tracheal ischemia and stenosis. Cuffed tubes provide a relative seal for patients receiving mechanical ventilation and aid in prevention of aspiration. Note that cuffs do not establish an absolute seal and silent aspiration of oropharyngeal or gastric secretions is common. Measure and record cuff pressure every 8 hours with a cuff pressure gauge. Recommended pressure is between 20 and 30 cm H_2O.

Secure the tube using tape or a commercial stabilization device. Take care to minimize pressure areas on the face and corners of the mouth if using an oral ET tube. If a commercial stabilization devise is used, monitor the oral mucosa frequently for evidence of excessive pressure. Cut the ET tube so that only 2 to 3 inches of tube extends beyond the mouth or nose to decrease airway resistance and potential for kinking. Attach an oxygen delivery system or mechanical ventilator.

Extubation

Criteria for extubation include the patient being awake and oriented or able to keep his or her airway open. Protective reflexes must be intact (e.g., gag) and the patient should not be paralyzed or excessively narcotized or sedated. Physiologic parameters include the following:

- Vital signs stable; acceptable hemoglobin and hemodynamics
- ABGs within acceptable limits after a trial of 30 minutes on nebulizer (T-piece) at 40% oxygen: PaO_2 60 mm Hg or greater, SaO_2 90% or greater, $PaCO_2$ 35 to 45 mm Hg or consistent with patient's normal values
- Acceptable bedside ventilatory parameters: tidal volume 5 mL/kg or greater, vital capacity 10 mL/kg or greater, and maximal inspiratory pressure (MIP) of -20 cm H_2O or greater

Before extubation, have the planned oxygen delivery system ready. An intubation kit should also be available in case of an emergent reintubation. Suction the trachea and then the pharynx. Deflate the cuff, and remove the tube during expiration. Apply an oxygen delivery system. Encourage the patient to cough, and suction if needed. Repeat ABGs 20 to 30 minutes after extubation and as indicated thereafter.

Monitor the patient's tolerance to extubation by clinical observation, ventilatory measurements, and ABG studies. During the first several hours after extubation, observe the patient for laryngospasm as evidenced by stridor, dyspnea, and tachypnea. Should laryngospasm occur, treatment usually includes high humidity, steroids, racemic epinephrine, or reintubation.

There are many complications of airway intubation. Physiologic alterations created by airway diversion include the following:

- Inadequate humidification of inspired air
- Increased risk of nosocomial pneumonia caused by accumulation of secretions
- Increased mucus caused by the tube because it is a foreign body
- Impaired ciliary movement
- Aphonia, which is the most significant stressor identified by patients
- Ineffective cough: an ET tube splints the epiglottis open preventing effective intrathoracic pressure to achieve an effective cough; patients can cough with a tracheostomy because the epiglottis is not splinted open

- Loss of physiologic PEEP because ET tubes splint the epiglottis open and remove physiologic PEEP; physiologic PEEP is reestablished with 3 to 5 cm H_2O of PEEP for intubated mechanically ventilated patients (Note: may be contraindicated with thoracotomy patients)

Complications that can occur during endotracheal intubation include the following:

- Trauma: damage to teeth, mucous membranes, and perforation or laceration of the pharynx, larynx, trachea
- Aspiration
- Laryngospasm, bronchospasm
- Tube malposition: esophageal or endobronchial intubation
- Hypoxia, anoxia if attempts are prolonged
- Tracheostomy
- Barotrauma: pneumothorax; pneumomediastinum
- Hemorrhage
- Tracheoesophageal fistula
- Laryngeal nerve injury
- Cardiopulmonary arrest

Complications that may occur while an ET tube is in place include the following:

- Tube obstruction or displacement
- Cuff rupture
- Disconnection between tracheal tube and ventilator including self-extubation
- Pressure necrosis
- Pressure sores at corners of mouth if oral endotracheal tube
- Pressure ulcers at superior nasal concha if nasal endotracheal tube
- Local infection; otitis media; sinus infection with nasotracheal tubes
- Bronchospasm
- Leaks due to broken cuff balloon
- Trauma: laryngeal injury; tracheal ischemia, necrosis, or dilation

Complications that may occur postextubation include the following:

- Need for reintubation
- Acute laryngeal edema
- Hoarseness (common)
- Aspiration if swallowing is impaired
- Stenosis of larynx or trachea (late complication)

Complications that may occur with a tracheostomy include the following:

- Difficulties with decannulation of a tracheostomy
- Tracheoesophageal fistula
- Tracheo-innominate artery fistula
- Tracheocutaneous fistula
- Tracheal stenosis

Tracheostomy

Transition from ET tube to tracheostomy usually occurs approximately 2 weeks after intubation. Advantages of tracheostomy over ET intubation include decreased dead space and airway resistance, increased effectiveness of cough, and improved airway clearance. Criteria for weaning patients from a tracheostomy tube are the same as for extubation of an ET tube and several methods are used. One method is to progress to a smaller size uncuffed (or cuff not inflated) tracheostomy tube to allow the patient to use both his upper airway and the tracheostomy tube opening. Another method is to change to a fenestrated tube; the opening at the top of the tube allows air to leak upward so that the patient can use the upper airway. The movement of air over the vocal cords allows the patient to speak. The final method is a trach button to close the opening in the trachea so that the patient uses his upper airway. This method greatly increases airway resistance and the work of breathing so patients must be physiologically able to tolerate this increased work. Possible complications of tracheostomy include difficulties with decannulation of a tracheostomy, tracheoesophageal fistula, tracheo-innominate artery fistula, tracheocutaneous fistula, and tracheal stenosis.

Oral Care

Oral care is an important aspect of airway management because it aids in the prevention of nosocomial pneumonia and enhances patient comfort. Factors contributing to poor oral hygiene include artificial airways, poor nutrition, nothing by mouth status, mouth breathing, tachypnea, oxygen administration, anxiety, and drugs such as antihistamines, antiemetics, and antibiotics. Assess the lips, oral mucosa, tongue, gums, teeth, and soft and hard palate at least twice daily. Provide oral care every 2 to 4 hours if intubated. Use suction foam swabs over the teeth, tongue, and oral mucosa followed by moisturizing swabs and water-soluble lip balm. Avoid lemon glycerin swabs, which are drying to the oral mucosa. Suction the oropharynx with an oropharyngeal suction catheter (i.e., Yankauer) and then rinse after each use. Between uses store the oropharyngeal suction catheter in a nonsealed bag and replace the oropharyngeal suction device, tubing, and suction canister every 24 hours.

Brush teeth twice daily to prevent dental plaque colonization. Brushing the teeth with a toothbrush removes dental plaque and reduces the number of oral microorganisms. Use a soft-bristle

pediatric toothbrush along with toothpaste, preferably with an alkaline pH. Remove dentures and partials and clean thoroughly. Administer chlorhexidine gluconate (Peridex) by spray or rinse as prescribed. Chlorhexidine is a broad-spectrum antibacterial agent that is not absorbed through the skin or mucous membranes; concentration recommendations vary from 0.12% to 0.2%.

OXYGEN THERAPY

Hypoxemia and Hypoxia

Administer oxygen therapy for hypoxemia and hypoxia. Hypoxemia is a decrease in arterial blood oxygen tension; it is diagnosed by ABGs with a PaO_2 of less than 80 mm Hg or SaO_2 of less than 95%. Degrees of hypoxemia are:

- Mild hypoxemia: PaO_2 less than 80 mm Hg (~SaO_2 95%)
- Moderate (significant) hypoxemia: PaO_2 less than 60 mm Hg (~SaO_2 90%)
- Severe hypoxemia: PaO_2 less than 40 mm Hg (~SaO_2 75%)

A decrease in the driving pressure of oxygen or a pulmonary condition may cause hypoxemia. A decrease in the driving pressure of oxygen may occur because of a low concentration of oxygen (e.g., smoke-filled room) or a low barometric pressure (e.g., high altitudes). Pulmonary causes of hypoxemia (Figure 4-23) include hypoventilation (e.g., respiratory depression caused by drugs or head injury), V/Q mismatch, or diffusion abnormalities (e.g., pulmonary edema, pulmonary fibrosis). V/Q mismatch may be either low V/Q mismatch (shunt) (e.g., ARDS) or high V/Q mismatch (dead space) (e.g., pulmonary embolism).

Hypoxia is a decrease in tissue oxygenation affected by PaO_2 and SaO_2, hemoglobin, cardiac output, patent vessels, and

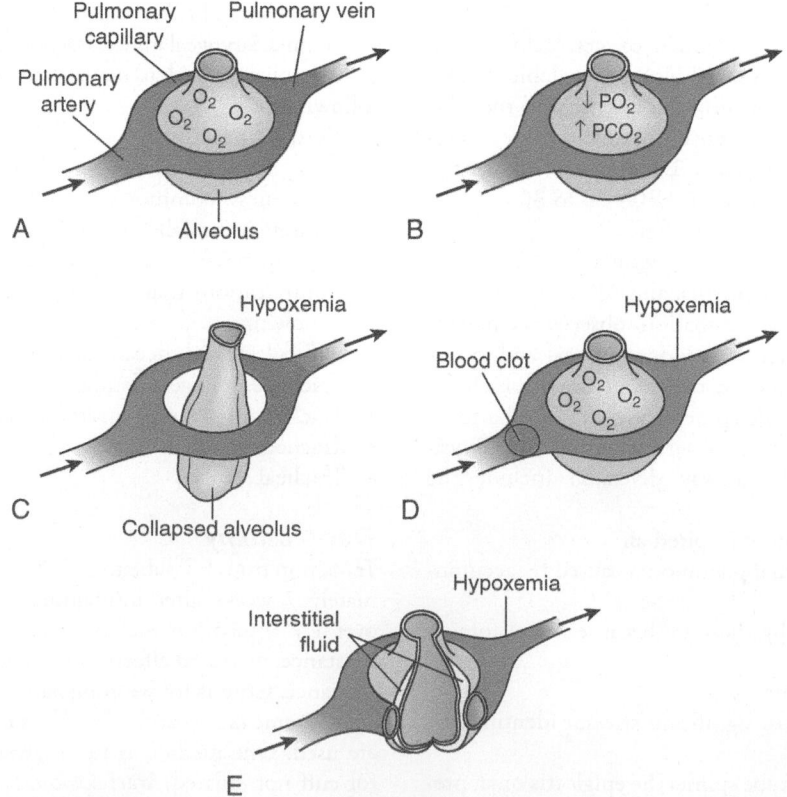

FIGURE 4-23 Pulmonary causes of hypoxemia. A, Normal alveolar-capillary unit. **B,** Hypoventilation. **C,** Low V/Q (i.e., shunt). **D,** High V/Q (i.e., dead space). **E,** Diffusion abnormality. (From Sole, M. L., Klein, D. G., & Moseley, M. J. [2013]. *Introduction to critical care nursing* [6th ed.]. Philadelphia, PA: Elsevier.)

cellular demand. Specific clinical indications (see Box 4-2) and elevated serum lactate levels determine the presence of hypoxia. The following are causes of hypoxia:

- Hypoxemic hypoxia: secondary to a gas exchange problem (e.g., V/Q mismatch, shunt, diffusion abnormalities)
- Anemic hypoxia: secondary to reduced oxygen-carrying capacity of the blood (e.g., anemia, carbon monoxide poisoning, methemoglobinemia)
- Circulatory hypoxia: secondary to a reduced blood flow in the body or a reduction in cardiac output (e.g., shock)
- Histotoxic hypoxia: secondary to the inability of the cells to utilize oxygen (e.g., cyanide poisoning)

A decrease in PaO_2 initially stimulates the sympathetic nervous system (SNS). The tissues increase oxygen extraction, which reduces oxygen reserve. When the PaO_2 becomes critically low, tissue oxygenation becomes inadequate and hypoxia occurs. Nutrient metabolism changes from aerobic to anaerobic, which results in less ATP than aerobic metabolism and lactic acid as a waste product. Acidosis and decreased cellular energy results. Cellular edema results from failure of the sodium-potassium pump.

Hypoxemia does not result in clinical findings; the only indications of hypoxemia are by ABG results (i.e., PaO_2 <80 mm Hg, SaO_2 <95%). The clinical findings of hypoxia are manifestations of SNS stimulation, such as tachycardia and tachypnea. Hypotension occurs as lactic acidosis progresses because acidosis causes vasodilation. Central cyanosis may occur if the patient is not anemic. Evidence of organ dysfunction occurs as the hypoxia progresses such as:

- Cerebral: altered sensorium
- Myocardial: decreased cardiac output; dysrhythmias
- Renal: decreased urine output

4.14 Learning Activity

Answer the following questions.

a. What is the difference between hypoxemia and hypoxia? _____

b. What are the indications of hypoxemia? _____
_____

c. What are the indications of hypoxia? _____
_____

d. Can hypoxemia occur without hypoxia? If so, how? _____

e. Can hypoxia occur without hypoxemia? If so, how? _____

Answers to this activity can be found in the Answer Key.

Indications for Oxygen Therapy

The primary indication for oxygen therapy is significant hypoxemia (i.e., PaO_2 <60 mm Hg or SaO_2 or SpO_2 <90% on room air). Administer oxygen for suspected hypoxemia (e.g., asthma, pulmonary embolism, aspiration, drug overdose, seizure or postictal state, pneumothorax, and/or trauma) or any acute care situation in which hypoxemia is likely such as:

- Increased myocardial workload (e.g., heart failure, hypertensive crisis, MI)
- Decreased cardiac output (e.g., shock, hypotension, cardiopulmonary arrest)
- Increased oxygen demand (e.g., sepsis, increased ventilatory work, trauma)
- Before procedures that may cause hypoxemia (e.g., suctioning, during and after anesthesia, transportation of the unstable patient, bronchoscopy)
- Decreased oxygen carrying capacity (e.g., carbon monoxide or cyanide poisoning, methemoglobinemia, sickle cell disease, anemia)

Principles of Oxygen Therapy

Airway patency is always the first priority because oxygen is useless without an adequate airway. The effectiveness of oxygen therapy is affected by the pathologic state; for example, oxygen therapy is ineffective for shunt because alveoli must be open to get the oxygen to the alveolar-capillary membrane, so PEEP is required in these cases.

The objective is to improve tissue oxygenation so the goal is to maintain PaO_2 at approximately 60 mm Hg and SaO_2 or SpO_2 at approximately 90%. Serial serum lactate levels are also helpful in monitoring progression or improvement of hypoxia and degree of anaerobic metabolism. Administer oxygen as prescribed for it is a potent drug. It may be prescribed as flow rate, oxygen concentration (expressed as a percentage), or fraction of inspired oxygen (FiO_2) (expressed as a decimal). Measure and document the exact concentration of inspired O_2 with an O_2 analyzer.

Ensure safety during oxygen therapy. Keep the oxygen source at least 10 feet from open flame and do not allow smoking in a room with supplemental oxygen. Also, do not use electrical appliances within 5 feet of an oxygen source. Use only water-based lubricants around an oxygen source; avoid any petroleum-based products. Turn the oxygen off when not in use. When using oxygen tanks, secure the tank to prevent accidental dropping and keep it away from heat or direct sunlight.

Oxygen Delivery Systems

Oxygen delivery systems are either low flow or high flow. This categorization is determined by what portion of the inspired air is accounted for by the oxygen delivery system not the flow rate.

Low-flow oxygen delivery systems do not provide the total inspired gas so the remainder of the patient's inspiratory volume is met by the patient breathing varying amounts of room air. The FiO_2 is dependent on the rate and depth of ventilation and the fit of the device. If the minute ventilation increases, the oxygen concentration decreases because the amount of room air (i.e., diluent) increases in relation to the amount of oxygen via the oxygen delivery system. If the minute ventilation decreases, the oxygen concentration increases. For a low-flow oxygen delivery system to be acceptable for use, the patient must have a normal or near-normal tidal volume (i.e., ~7 mL/kg of ideal body weight [IBW]), a respiratory rate that is normal or near normal (i.e., ~15-25/min), have a regular respiratory pattern, and the specific oxygen concentration is not critical to the patient's care. Examples of low-flow oxygen delivery devices include nasal cannula, simple face mask, partial rebreathing mask, and nonrebreathing mask. One method of estimating inspired oxygen concentration with an oxygen delivery system is to count the number of reservoirs; the more reservoirs, the higher the oxygen concentration (Sidebar 4-1).

A high-flow delivery system provides the entire inspired gas by high flow of gas or entrainment of room air. They provide a predictable FiO_2. Criteria requiring the use of a high-flow oxygen delivery system include:

- Tidal volume is significantly less than or more than normal (~7 mL/kg of IBW)
- Respiratory rate less than 15/min or more than 25/min
- Irregular respiratory rhythm
- Specific oxygen concentration is critical to patient's care
- Evidence of alveolar hypoventilation with hypercapnia

Examples of high-flow oxygen delivery devices are a Venturi mask, a T-piece if high-flow rate, a trach collar if high-flow rate, and mechanical ventilator.

SIDEBAR 4-1

Estimating O_2 Concentration by Counting Number of Reservoirs

1. Nose and pharynx only (1) = <40%: e.g., nasal cannula
2. Nose and pharynx + mask (2) = 40% to 60%: e.g., simple face mask
3. Nose and pharynx + mask + reservoir bag (3) = 60% to 80%: e.g., partial rebreathing mask
3+ Nose and pharynx + mask + reservoir bag + one-way valves (3+ decrease in dilution) = 80% to 100%: example nonrebreathing mask

---

There are many oxygen delivery devices (Table 4-12). The desired oxygen concentration and specific patient condition determines the choice of device.

4.15 Learning Activity

Match the type of oxygen delivery with the description.

_____ 1. Nonrebreathing mask
_____ 2. Venturi mask
_____ 3. Nasal cannula
_____ 4. Tracheostomy collar
_____ 5. Partial rebreathing mask

a. Most comfortable method of oxygen administration
b. May cause aspiration of condensed fluid
c. Delivers approximately 40%-60% oxygen concentration
d. Provides the highest oxygen concentration
e. Ensures a reliable oxygen concentration regardless of change in respiratory rate and/or depth

Answers to this activity can be found in the Answer Key.

Hazards of Oxygen Therapy

Oxygen-induced hypoventilation is most likely to occur in patients with an elevated $PaCO_2$, such as patients with COPD, airway obstruction, or respiratory center depression from drugs or a head injury. Use O_2 with caution, but remember low PaO_2, not FiO_2, is the stimulus to breathe; use only enough oxygen to bring PaO_2 up to approximately 60 mm Hg or the SaO_2 or SpO_2 up to approximately 90%.

High concentrations of oxygen (an absorbable gas) that washes out the nitrogen (a nonabsorbable gas) that normally holds the alveoli open at the end of expiration causes absorptive atelectasis. Other contributing factors include the effects of oxygen on pulmonary surfactant and depression of ciliary function. Prevent this complication by administering oxygen only when indicated, and not administering oxygen prophylactically.

A high concentration of oxygen over too long a period of time (i.e., hours to days) is the cause of oxygen toxicity. The high concentrations of oxygen cause the overproduction of oxygen free radicals, which overwhelm the supply of neutralizing enzymes. There is injury to the capillary endothelium and interstitial edema along with injury to type I pneumocytes and intraalveolar edema. Thickening of the alveolar-capillary membrane and pulmonary fibrosis occurs. Early clinical indications of oxygen toxicity include substernal chest pain that increases with deep breathing, dry cough and tracheal irritation, dyspnea, upper airway changes (e.g., nasal stuffiness, sore throat, eye and ear discomfort), anorexia, nausea, vomiting, fatigue, lethargy, malaise, and restlessness. Later, chest x-ray changes occur, indicating atelectasis and patchy pneumonia along with progressive ventilator difficulty with decreased capacity, decreased compliance, and hypercapnia. Intrapulmonary shunt develops and causes an oxygenation deficit manifested by a decreased PaO_2/FiO_2 ratio and refractory hypoxemia.

The most important method to prevent oxygen toxicity is to use the lowest FiO_2 possible to maintain a PaO_2 of at least 60 mm Hg or SaO_2 of 90%. If patients require 100% oxygen (i.e., FiO_2 of 1.0), limit the duration to 24 hours if possible. Concentrations above 60% (i.e., FiO_2 0.6) should be limited to 2 to 3 days if possible. Assess ABGs frequently if FiO_2 is above 0.40 to ensure that high concentration is still required. A FiO_2 of 0.40 or less is relatively safe. One method to reduce the concentration of oxygen required to achieve desirable PaO_2 and SaO_2 levels is the addition of PEEP to increase the driving pressure of oxygen. The use of PEEP achieves the same PaO_2 at a lower FiO_2 or a better PaO_2 at the same FiO_2. Hypoxia requires correction and is far more common than O_2 toxicity. Do not allow actual hypoxemia to persist because of concern regarding potential oxygen toxicity.

NONINVASIVE POSITIVE PRESSURE VENTILATION

Noninvasive positive pressure ventilation (NPPV) is positive pressure ventilation of a nonintubated spontaneous breathing patient. It is delivered primarily with a face or nasal mask attached to a standard ventilator or a machine specifically for noninvasive ventilation (NIV). The purpose of NPPV is to augment alveolar ventilation. There are two possible modes (Table 4-13). In continuous positive airway pressure (CPAP), there is a preset positive airway pressure during spontaneous breaths. In bilevel positive airway pressure (BiPAP), there is a preset positive pressure to be delivered during inspiration and preset pressure to be maintained during expiration; this is a combination of pressure support ventilation (PSV [I-PAP]) and CPAP (E-PAP).

TABLE 4-12 **Summary of Oxygen Delivery Devices**

Device	Advantages	Disadvantages	Miscellaneous
Nasal cannula 1 lpm = ~24% 2 lpm = ~28% 3 lpm = ~32% 4 lpm = ~36% 5 lpm = ~40% 6 lpm = ~44%	• Safe and simple • Comfortable • Effective for low oxygen concentration • Allows eating and talking • Inexpensive	• Contraindicated in nasal obstruction • May cause drying and irritation of nasal mucosa • May cause necrosis at ears • Cannot be used when patient has nasal obstruction • Variable concentrations of oxygen depending on tidal volume, ventilatory rate, flow rate, and nasal patency	• Ensure that flow rates do not exceed 6 L/min • Provide humidification if flow rates exceed 4 L/min • Use gauze pads under cannula at tops of ears to prevent pressure ulceration • Give oral and nasal care every 8 hours; moisten lips, nose with water-soluble lubricant
Reservoir nasal cannula; mustache-style or pendant-style • Delivers ≥50% oxygen	• As for nasal cannula • Captures water vapor with patient exhalation and returns the moisture during inhalation so no need for humidification	• As for nasal cannula • Pendant-style may weigh down the ear loops	• As for nasal cannula • Must be replaced regularly • Used most often in home care • Conserves oxygen use
Simple face mask 5 lpm = ~40% 6 lpm = ~45%-50% 7 lpm = ~50%-55% 8 lpm = ~55%-60%	• Delivers high oxygen concentration • Does not dry mucous membranes of nose and mouth • Can be used in patients with nasal obstruction	• Hot, confining, uncomfortable • Tight seal necessary • Frequently poorly tolerated in dyspneic patient • Interferes with eating and talking • May cause CO_2 retention if flow rate is <6 L/min • Variable concentrations of oxygen depending on tidal volume, ventilatory rate, and flow rate • Cannot deliver <40% • Potential for oxygen toxicity • Impractical for long-term therapy	• Place pads between mask and bony facial parts • Wash and dry face every 4 hours • Clean mask every 8 hours • Ensure flow rate of at least 5 L/min • Check ABGs frequently • Watch for signs of oxygen toxicity
Partial rebreathing mask 6 lpm – ~35%-40% 8 lpm = ~45%-50% 10 lpm = ~60%	• Delivers high oxygen concentrations • Doesn't dry mucous membranes	• As for face mask • May cause CO_2 retention if reservoir bag is allowed to collapse	• Ensure that bag does not totally deflate during inhalation (increase flow rate) • Keep mask snug • Check ABGs frequently • Watch for signs of oxygen toxicity
Nonrebreathing mask 6 lpm = ~60% 7 lpm = ~70% 8 lpm = ~70% 9 lpm = ~90% 10 lpm = close to 100%	• As for other masks • One-way valves prevent rebreathing of CO_2 and increases oxygen concentrations	• As for other masks except does not cause CO_2 retention	• As for partial rebreathing mask • Check ABGs frequently • Watch for signs of oxygen toxicity
Venturi mask 4 lpm = ~24%-28% 8 lpm = ~35%-40% 12 lpm = ~50%	• Delivers accurate oxygen concentration depending on flow rate and diluter jet inserted despite changes in patient's respiratory pattern • Oxygen concentration can be changed • Does not dry mucous membranes	• Fio_2 can be lowered if mask does not fit snugly, if tubing is kinked, if oxygen intake ports are blocked, or if less than recommended liter flow is used • Hot, confining, uncomfortable • Tight seal necessary • Frequently poorly tolerated in dyspneic patient • Interferes with eating and talking	• Check ABGs frequently • Watch for signs of oxygen toxicity • As for other masks

Continued

TABLE 4-12   **Summary of Oxygen Delivery Devices—cont'd**

Device	Advantages	Disadvantages	Miscellaneous
Trach collar • Delivers 21%-70% at 10 lpm or to provide visible mist	• Does not pull on tracheostomy • Elastic ties allow movement of mask away from tracheostomy without removing it	• Oxygen diluted by room air • Increased likelihood of infection and skin irritation around stoma because of high humidity • Condensation can collect in the tubing and drain into patient's airway especially during turning	• Ensure that oxygen be warmed and humidified • Empty condensation from tubing frequently; empty into water trap or container for appropriate discard; do not empty water back into humidifier
T-piece or tube • Delivers 21%-100% with flow rate set at 2.5 times the patient's minute ventilation	• Delivers variable concentrations • Less moisture around tracheostomy than with tracheostomy collar	• May cause CO_2 retention at low flow rates • Weight of T-piece can pull on tracheostomy tube • Condensation can collect in the tubing and drain into patient's airway especially during turning	• Requires heated nebulizer • Use extension on open side to act as a reservoir and increase oxygen concentration as prescribed • Empty condensation from tubing frequently • Check ABGs frequently • Watch for signs of oxygen toxicity
Mechanical ventilation • Delivers 21%-100%	• Delivers predictable, constant concentrations of oxygen • Supports ventilation as well as oxygenation • Addition of positive end-expiratory pressure (PEEP) augments the driving pressure of oxygen; this aids in the achievement of acceptable Po_2 levels at lower oxygen concentrations	• Requires skilled personnel • Requires electricity and backup power generator (plug into red outlet) • Condensation can collect in the tubing and drain into patient's airway especially during turning	• Requires heated humidifier • Empty condensation from tubing frequently • Check ABGs frequently • Watch for signs of oxygen toxicity

TABLE 4-13   **Noninvasive Positive Pressure Ventilation Modes**

Mode	Description	Comments
Continuous positive airway pressure (CPAP)	• Elevates end-expiratory pressure to above atmospheric pressure to increase lung volume and oxygenation. • Depending on machine type, CPAP is delivered via a continuous flow or demand valve system	• All breaths are spontaneous; therefore an intact respiratory drive required. • Can be used in intubated, as well as nonintubated patients via a face or nasal mask. • Prevents lung overdistention while maintaining inflation of newly recruited alveoli. • Maintains lower mean and peak airway pressures. • Less hemodynamic compromise than traditional modes. • Contraindicated in patients with obstructive lung disease.
Bilevel positive airway pressure (BiPAP)	• Noninvasive ventilator assist device that employs a spontaneous breathing mode with the baseline pressure elevated above zero • CPAP with two different levels; CPAP-high and CPAP-low • Allows separate regulation of inspiratory and expiratory functions	• Essentially a combination of PSV with CPAP. • The differences between inspiratory and expiratory positive airway pressure contribute to total ventilation. • Enhances the capabilities of home CPAP for obstructive sleep apnea to provide nocturnal support in a variety of restrictive and obstructive disorders. • Affords a noninvasive means of augmenting alveolar ventilation in hypercapnic respiratory failure.

Possible indications for NPPV include acute respiratory failure, especially in COPD, cardiac pulmonary edema, weaning of a patient from traditional mechanical ventilation and/or PEEP, sleep apnea, and terminal care to avoid intubation, such as a patient with end-stage COPD. There are advantages of NPPV over traditional mechanical ventilation in some situations. NPPV does not require intubation; therefore, it avoids the complications associated with intubation such as VAP. NPPV can be used intermittently and only initiated, discontinued, and reinitiated when required. There is improved patient comfort, though some patients may find the mask uncomfortable, and lower sedation requirements with NPPV.

The disadvantages of NPPV include discomfort caused by a mask tight enough to create a seal, difficulty creating a seal if an orogastric or nasogastric tube is in place, and inability of the patient to eat due to high risk of aspiration. Absolute contraindications of NPPV include hemodynamic instability, problems with airway patency (e.g., copious secretions), risk for aspiration, altered level of consciousness (i.e., patients without airway protective reflexes), and recent upper airway or esophageal surgery. Relative contraindications of NPPV include an uncooperative patient, morbid obesity, unstable angina or acute MI, inability to fit the mask, and agitation.

Monitor the patient closely for complications including facial skin breakdown, nasal congestion, conjunctivitis, gastric distention, aspiration, and pneumothorax. Patients will need to be intubated and mechanically ventilated if there is worsening of $Paco_2$ and respiratory acidosis, worsening Pao_2 and Sao_2, severe tachypnea, hemodynamic instability, altered level of consciousness, inability to clear airway secretions, or inability to tolerate the face mask (Williams, Cox, & Hargett, 2012).

MECHANICAL VENTILATION

Indications and Objectives

Impaired alveolar ventilation results from the inability to maintain spontaneous ventilation. Clinical findings include ineffective breathing patterns, dyspnea, tachypnea or apnea, accessory muscle use, abnormal ABG levels, and the excess work of breathing. The collaborative health team works to restore adequate alveolar ventilation by promoting normal rest and sleep patterns. Plan patient care activities to allow rest periods. Rest allows replenishment of energy reserves and sleep deprivation blunts the patient's respiratory drive. If indicated, implement an appropriate level of mechanical ventilator support. The indications for mechanical ventilation include:

- Acute ventilatory failure with respiratory acidosis not relieved by ordinary methods
- Hypoxemia despite maximum oxygen therapy
- Relief of hypoxemia causes increased CO_2 retention. Hypercapnia alone is not an indication for mechanical ventilation. Acidosis must accompany the hypercapnia to be an indication for mechanical ventilation. For example, a patient with COPD has chronic hypercapnia (not an indication for mechanical ventilation) but develops an even greater $Paco_2$ level and decompensated respiratory acidosis with acute respiratory infection (a potential indication for mechanical ventilation)
- Apnea: consideration needs to be given to the reversibility of the situation (i.e., mechanical ventilation is not indicated to prolong a terminal condition)

The prevention of the development of complications associated with ventilator support along with optimal methods for weaning patients from continuous mechanical ventilation are priority interventions from the onset of support.

The physiologic objectives of mechanical ventilation are to support pulmonary gas exchange, increase lung volume, and reduce the work of breathing. Measure alveolar ventilation by the arterial partial pressure of carbon dioxide ($Paco_2$) and pH. Measure arterial oxygenation by the partial pressure of oxygen (Pao_2), arterial oxygen saturation (Sao_2), and oxygen content (Cao_2). Evaluate changes in lung volume by end-inspiratory lung inflation and the functional residual capacity (FRC).

The clinical objective of mechanical ventilation is to reverse hypoxemia, acute respiratory acidosis, atelectasis, and ventilatory muscle fatigue. In addition, the achievement of these objectives will relieve respiratory distress, prevent further atelectasis, and decrease systemic or myocardial oxygen consumption. Other clinical objectives for the use of mechanical ventilation include sedation and/or neuromuscular blockade, reduce intracranial pressure, and/or stabilize the chest wall.

Ventilator Type and Classification

In positive pressure ventilation, used almost exclusively today, positive pressure is applied to the airways. The clinician determined both the delivery system and ventilation settings in response to the patient's efforts. Positive pressure pushed into the airway creates inspiration. Expiration occurs passively when the positive pressure stops.

The gas delivery is the flow from the ventilator regulated or limited by a set flow or set pressure. A preset volume, time, or flow terminates the cycling of the gas delivery. Insensitive or unresponsive triggering systems can force significant ventilator loads. Oversensitive valves can result in spontaneous ventilatory cycling independent of patient effort.

Cycling Classifications

The pressure-cycled ventilation used in adults delivers inspiratory flow until a preset pressure is met. The pressure is set, and tidal volume varies dependent on compliance of the lung and the integrity of the ventilatory circuit. This type of ventilation requires a sealed airway (e.g., cuffed ET tube or tracheostomy tube). Positive intrathoracic pressure decreases venous return to the right atrium, which may decrease cardiac output, especially in hypovolemic patients. There is also a risk of ventilator-induced lung injury (VILI).

The volume-cycled ventilation delivers inspiratory flow until a preset volume is met. The tidal volume set delivers the volume regardless of changes in lung compliance and the pressure varies. Volume-cycled ventilation may decrease cardiac output especially in hypovolemic patients. There is also a risk of VILI.

Standard Modes of Ventilation

Modes of ventilation (Table 4-14) are classified according to the initiation of the inspiratory cycle. In essence, the mode is how the machine senses or signals the initiation of inspiration. The standard ventilation modes used in a progressive care setting are assist control (AC), synchronized intermittent mandatory ventilation (SIMV), pressure support ventilation (PSV), CPAP, and BiPAP.

Ventilator Settings and Controls

Ventilator controls and settings (Table 4-15) are adjusted according to the patient's underlying disease process and the results

TABLE 4-14	Modes of Ventilation	
Mode	**Description**	**Comments**
Volume Modes		
Assist/control (also called assisted mandatory ventilation)	• Preset tidal volume, minimum rate (control rate), and inspiratory effort required to "trigger" the ventilator to cycle to assist breaths (sensitivity); the ventilator delivers the control breaths of the specified tidal volume and responds by cycling additionally if the patient's inspiratory effort (negative pressure) is adequate	• More comfortable than control mode • Less work of breathing for patient than spontaneous breathing or IMV • Allows ventilatory muscle rest • Risk for hyperventilation because each assisted breath is delivered at same tidal volume as mandatory breaths; sedation may be necessary to decrease number of spontaneously triggered breaths
Synchronized intermittent mandatory ventilation (SIMV)	• Preset tidal volume and minimum rate; the ventilatory circuit is open between the mandatory breaths so that the patient may take additional breaths; because the ventilator does not cycle to assist these breaths, the tidal volume of these breaths varies • Mandatory breaths are synchronized so that they do not occur during the patient's ventilatory efforts	• Allows muscle reconditioning better than control or assist/control • Less potential for hyperventilation because patient-initiated breaths are at the tidal volume determined by the patient • More work of breathing for patient than assist-control because patient-initiated breaths are not assisted • Less need for sedation than assist/control or control modes • Does not decrease cardiac output as much as assist/control or control modes • Frequently used for weaning
Pressure Modes		
Pressure support ventilation (PSV)	• Preset inspiratory support pressure level; when the patient initiates a breath this positive pressure flows to assist the patient's spontaneous breaths; tidal volume and rate is patient controlled	• Low level (5-10 cm H_2O) helps to eliminate the increased work of breathing associated with an endotracheal tube; higher levels help to augment the patient's own intrinsic tidal volume • Lessens work of breathing but also allows use of respiratory muscles to lessen muscular atrophy • Lower mean airway pressures than volume ventilation • May be used with IMV or alone; if used alone, patient must be spontaneously breathing • There is no preset ventilatory rate, and apnea occurs if the patient does not initiate a breath

Note: CPAP and BiPAP are also pressure modes, but they are noninvasive positive pressure modes.

of ABG analysis. The respiratory therapist changes the ventilator controls and settings under the supervision of the clinician. The nurse is an important member of the collaborative team. In caring for patients who are receiving mechanical ventilation, guidelines (Table 4-16) for ventilator adjustment are crucial for understanding.

Assessment of the Mechanically Ventilated Patient

The patient's response to ventilator setting requires constant vigilance. Mechanical ventilation alters the volumes and pressures within in the airways and lungs along with ABG values. The respiratory assessment in conscious and semiconscious patients warrants careful evaluation. Ventilator-induced alterations result in a change of rate (ventilator demand), depth, and timing of respiratory efforts (synchrony between patient and ventilator) through neural reflexes, chemoreceptors, and behavioral responses.

Monitor and clinically observe all patients on mechanical ventilation according to institutional policies. A complete physical nursing assessment should be performed each shift. Assess the ventilator system and its current settings. A manual self-inflating resuscitation bag should be open and ready for use at the bedside. Suction equipment should also be in working order and ready for use. Many of these patients have an arterial line, intravenous line, and urinary catheter in place, so assess all these invasive lines for patency, function, and signs of infection.

General monitoring for a patient on continuous ventilator support may include hemodynamic monitoring (arterial, central, or pulmonary catheter) if indicated. Cardiac monitoring, heart sounds, pulses, and pulse pressure evaluation is part of the standard evaluation. The respiratory therapist conducts pulmonary function studies such as vital capacity, negative inspiratory pressure, minute ventilation, and maximal voluntary ventilation tests as required. Routine chemistry and hematology laboratory tests, intake and output measurements, body weight, focused respiratory assessments, inspection of dressings and drainage from all tubes, catheters, and suction apparatus are part of the routine assessment of a patient requiring mechanical ventilation.

TABLE 4-15	Guidelines for Volume-Cycled Ventilator Adjustments
Control	**Setting**
Minute ventilation	Usually 6-10 L/min but may be higher dependent on patient needs
Tidal volume	Governed by estimated tidal volume. Normally varies from 8-10 mL/kg ideal body weight to prevent lung overinflation and potential stretch injury to lung tissue. Preset tidal volume may be decreased to 6-8 mL/kg. Intentional use of lower tidal volumes may cause an increase in arterial CO_2; therefore this is often referred to as permissive hypercapnia. Low tidal volumes have been shown to lower mortality in some settings. Intermittent sighs during mechanical ventilation is no longer routinely recommended.
Respiratory rate	Varies from 8-12 breaths/min for most clinically stable patients. Rates above 20 breaths/min are sometimes necessary.
Flow rate	Adjusted so that inspiratory volume delivery can be completed in a time frame that allows adequate time for exhalation. Inspiratory flow rate range of about 40-100 L/min is most commonly used. Slow flow rates are preferred for optimal distribution in normal lungs; faster flow rates are beneficial in patients with obstructive lung disease. Altering the flow rate may reduce the work of breathing, improve patient-ventilator synchrony, and increase the comfort of patients who are restless while undergoing mechanical ventilation.
I/E ratio	Normal ratio is 1:2-1:3
Inspiratory flow of gas from ventilator	Depending on model, gas can be delivered using one of several flow patterns: decelerating, square wave, or sine wave.
Oxygen concentration	Initially, the fraction of inspired oxygen (Fio_2) is deliberatively set high (often at 0.1) to ensure adequate oxygenation. An ABG is obtained and the Fio_2 is adjusted according to the patient's Pao_2 and Sao_2. The Fio_2 is adjusted so that the Pao_2 is acceptable for the patient condition. This is usually a Pao_2 higher than 55 mm Hg or a Sao_2 of 88% or higher. Excessively high levels for prolonged periods can cause oxygen toxicity. The lowest Fio_2 that achieves an acceptable Pao_2 and Sao_2 should be used.
Positive end-expiratory pressure (PEEP)	Used as appropriate to reduce the Fio_2 to safe levels.
Humidification	Continuous humidification is mandatory with inspired air warmed to near body temperature. Standard humidifiers using a water feed system must be monitored closely for water condensation in the tubing and emptied routinely. Heat and moisture exchanges (HME) are sometimes used.
Sensitivity	Sensitivity refers to when the patient can trigger the machine for assistance. Sensitivity is adjusted so that minimal patient effort is required. The usual setting is -0.50 to -1.5 cm H_2O. Certain ventilators allow for a flow-triggering mechanism and should be set to their maximum sensitivity (1-3 L/min).
Pressure limit alarms	Should be set at approximately 10-15 cm H_2O above the patient's normal peak inflation pressure (PIP) or airway pressure. The goal is to keep PIP below 35-30 cm H_2O if possible. The peak inspiratory plateau is equal to or less than 35 cm H_2O. Certain ventilators provide a low-airway-pressure alarm feature. Check that all other alarms are operational and on at all times.

TABLE 4-16	Mechanical Ventilator Parameter Changes to Make According to Arterial Blood Gases

If $Paco_2$ is >45 mm Hg (or above the patient's normal if the patient has COPD)	• Increase ventilation
	  • Increase rate
	  • Increase tidal volume (if it does not currently exceed 10 mL/kg)

If $Paco_2$ is <35 mm Hg	• Decrease ventilation
	  • Decrease rate
	  • Decrease tidal volume
	  • If patient on assist/control mode: change mode from AC to IMV
	  • Consider sedation and/or analgesia
	  • Mechanical dead space may be considered (tubing which acts as a rebreathing device)

If Pao_2 is <60 mm Hg	• Increase Fio_2 • Add or increase PEEP (especially if Fio_2 already >0.6 [60%])
If Pao_2 is >100 mm Hg	• Decrease Fio_2 • Decrease PEEP (especially if Fio_2 is <0.4 [40%])

Ventilatory Monitoring

Perform ventilator checks per institutional policy. At a minimum, ventilator checks are performed routinely each shift and when blood gas samples are drawn, and changes are made in settings. Hourly checks are required for any unstable patient. The components recorded on the nursing flow sheet include blood gas values and ventilator settings. Record the following ventilator settings:

- Mode, tidal volume, and Fio_2
- Preset rate, pressure support level, PEEP, minute volume, inspiratory flow rate and time, inspiration/expiration (I:E) ratio
- Temperature of the humidification device, temperature of the inspired gas
- Alarms on

Routinely record ventilator measurements of tidal volume, peak inspiratory pressure, plateau airway pressures, exhaled minute ventilation, respiratory rate, and exhaled tidal volume. Additional measurements that may be used in assessment include PEEP levels, auto PEEP, A-a gradient, static and dynamic compliance curves, dead space, and I:E ratio.

Respiratory monitoring techniques used during mechanical ventilation include pulse oximetry and end-tidal CO_2 ($Petco_2$) monitoring. Pulse oximetry is a noninvasive estimate of arterial oxygen saturation (Spo_2). End-tidal CO_2 ($Petco_2$) monitoring is a noninvasive sampling and measurement of exhaled CO_2.

Patient Discomfort and Anxiety

Communicate with the patient frequently. Orient the patient to place and time, and inform him or her about what is happening. Reinforce the need for the patient to communicate his or her needs using the various communication aides available. Provide distraction (e.g., music, television, radio) along with nonpharmacologic comfort measures (e.g., massage, aromatherapy).

Drug Therapy for Maintenance of Ventilation

Administer narcotics (morphine sulfate, meperidine, and fentanyl) dosed to effect to control pain and discomfort. Narcotics act as a respiratory depressant, and are good euphoric agents and excellent analgesics. Narcotics also provide sedation and good control of ventilation without adverse effects in a well ventilated, well oxygenated, acid-base balanced patient. For a sedative effect, combine a narcotic and benzodiazepine. The administration of these agents reduces the sensation of dyspnea; however, use with caution, especially with large dosages as they may cause increased venous capacitance. Drug tolerance may develop with prolonged use.

Administer sedatives such as benzodiazepines (e.g., diazepam [Valium], lorazepam [Ativan], and midazolam [Versed]) to manage patient anxiety as prescribed. These drugs cause a central nervous system (CNS) depressant effect, which can lead to alveolar hypoventilation and respiratory acidosis, particularly in geriatric patients and those with liver disease. Severe respiratory depression and apnea can result with a combination of sedatives and other CNS depressant drugs. As with any sedative agent, the routine use of validated sedation, agitation, and mobility scales (Tables 4-17, 4-18, and 4-19) for monitoring and assessing the degree of sedation is important.

TABLE 4-17   Ramsay Sedation Scale

Score	Description
1	Anxious, agitated or restless, or both
2	Cooperative, oriented, tranquil
3	Responding to commands only
4	Asleep but with brisk response to light glabellar tap or loud auditory stimulus
5	Asleep with sluggish response to light glabellar tap or loud auditory stimulus
6	Asleep, nonresponsive

From Ramsay, M., Savege, T., Simpson, B., & Goodwin, R. (1974). Controlled sedation with alphaxalone-alphadolone. *British Medical Journal, 2,* 656.

TABLE 4-18   Sedation-Agitation Scale

Score	Definition	Description
7	Dangerous agitation	Pulling at ET tube, trying to remove catheters, climbing over bed rail, striking at staff, thrashing side to side
6	Very agitated	Does not calm despite frequent verbal reminding of limits; requires physical restraints, biting ET tube
5	Agitated	Anxious or mildly agitated, attempting to sit up, calms down to verbal instructions
4	Calm and cooperative	Calm, wakes easily, follows commands
3	Sedated	Difficult to rouse, awakens to verbal stimuli or gently shaking but drifts off again, follows simple commands
2	Very sedated	Arouses to physical stimuli but does not communicate or follow commands; may move spontaneously
1	Unarousable	Minimal or no response to noxious stimuli, does not communicate or follow commands

From Riker, R., Picard, J., & Fraser, G. (1999). Prospective evaluation of the Sedation-Agitation Scale for adult critically ill patients. *Critical Care Medicine, 27,* 1325.

Complications

Complications from mechanical ventilation (Table 4-20) affect several body systems. Preventing and monitoring the patient for the onset of complications is a priority of care.

Weaning

Weaning, also referred to as liberation, is the gradual withdrawal of ventilatory support for patients mechanically ventilated for more than 24 hours. The process of weaning occurs in phases.

TABLE 4-19	Motor Activity Assessment Scale
Score	Definition
0	Unresponsiveness
1	Responsive only to noxious stimuli
2	Responsive to touch
3	Calm and cooperative
4	Restless and cooperative
5	Agitated
6	Dangerously agitated

From Devlin, J. W., Boleski, G., Mlynarek, M. et al. (1999). Motor activity assessment scale: A valid and reliable sedation scale for use with mechanically ventilated patients in an adult surgical intensive care unit. *Critical Care Medicine, 27*(7), 1271-1275.

The preweaning phase is an assessment to determine whether the patient is capable of attempting spontaneous ventilation. The readiness assessment for weaning includes resolution or improvement of the disease process that necessitated mechanical ventilation, respiratory factors, and nonrespiratory factors. The patient's strength, vigor, fluid and electrolyte balances, and nutritional status needs to be adequate. The patient should be conscious, removed from deep sedatives along with being cooperative and psychologically prepared for weaning. Stable oxygenation status, hemodynamic parameters, and hemoglobin level are required. The patient needs to have acceptable values for ABGs, tidal volume, vital capacity, minute ventilation, respiratory rate, and maximal inspiratory pressure. Common factors that impede the weaning process include:

- Underlying illness has not resolved sufficiently
- Malnutrition
- Excessive secretions
- Presence of auto-PEEP
- Impaired muscle function secondary to electrolyte imbalance (e.g., hypokalemia, hypophosphatemia, hypomagnesemia)
- Respiratory muscle fatigue

During the actual weaning phase, several methods may be used. The methods used are the spontaneous breathing trial (SBT) with a T-piece, intermittent mandatory ventilation, pressure support ventilation, and CPAP. SBT with a T-piece for short-term mechanical ventilation (i.e., <72 hours) or spontaneous breathing for 120 minutes through the ventilator with PSV of 0 or CPAP of up to 5 cm H_2O is tried. If trial is successful, extubate the patient. If unsuccessful, allow the patient to rest and try again the next day. A tracheostomy may also be considered. The advantage of this trial method is a quicker weaning process than the intermittent mandatory ventilation (IMV) or PSV methods. A disadvantage is that recurrent wean attempts and failures discourage and frighten the patient.

To wean with IMV, gradually reduce the IMV rate. The advantages of this method is that it provides exercise for ventilatory musculature, more physiologic $Paco_2$ may be achieved, and large ventilator-provided breaths help to prevent atelectasis. It is safer than the trial-and-error method and has a good acceptance by patients. The disadvantage is that the method may take longer than the SBT method.

Using the PSV method, gradually decrease the amount of pressure support assisting the patient. Usually started at 15 to 25 cm H_2O, gradually decrease the pressure by 3 to 6 cm H_2O every 1 to 3 days as long as the patient maintains a satisfactory minute ventilation. When the patient can maintain adequate ventilation with the PSV at 5 cm H_2O, extubation is considered. The advantages of this method is patient comfort is frequently greater with PSV because there is less work of breathing than with IMV or the SBT method.

CPAP may be used for patients whose Pao_2 is PEEP-dependent. The patient is weaned from the ventilator by one of the previously discussed methods but left on CPAP to provide the improved driving pressure needed to maintain an adequate Pao_2.

Position the patient for optimal ventilation. This is usually the semi-Fowler's to high Fowler's position. Avoid depressing the patient's ventilatory drive and muscle strength by avoiding sedatives. Treat the patient's pain but do not overnarcotize. Optimize nutrition status. If indicated, reduce carbohydrates and give equivalent calories in the form of fats. Utilize Pulmocare if being fed enterally. This feeding supplement has high fat and protein but low carbohydrates. Decrease glucose and increase fat (Intralipids) if being fed parenterally. Begin weaning attempts in the early morning, and do not attempt to wean the patient at night.

Complementary therapies such as biofeedback and music may be helpful. Because the mechanical ventilator may provide security for the patient, it may be helpful to leave the ventilator in the room with the patient for 24 hours after weaning. Monitor closely for clinical indicators of fatigue and ventilatory failure and abort weaning if necessary.

The weaning outcomes phase results in a completed weaning process in which the patient is able to maintain a normal respiratory rate and tidal volume while breathing spontaneously. A partial weaning outcome occurs when the patient is able to maintain spontaneous ventilation for short time. Terminal weaning is followed by death.

CHEST TUBES

Chest tubes may be either pleural or mediastinal tubes. Pleural tubes remove free air, drain the intrapleural space, and reestablish negative pressure in pleural space. Mediastinal tubes drain air and blood from the mediastinum after cardiac or other mediastinal surgery.

Pleural chest tubes remove free air, such as in a pneumothorax, and are placed anterior and superior (i.e., second ICS at MCL). A small spontaneous pneumothorax will be resolved without a chest tube, but a pneumothorax greater than 15% or if the patient is being mechanically ventilated requires a pleural chest tube.

Pleural chest tubes to drain the intrapleural space are placed lateral and inferior (i.e., fifth or sixth ICS at midaxillary line). A pleural chest tube is indicated for hemothorax (i.e., blood in the pleural space) if greater than 500 mL. A pleural chest tube is also indicated for pleural effusion (i.e., liquid in the pleural space) especially if the patient is dyspneic. Pleural effusion may be transudate or exudate. A transudate occurs if there is a rise in pulmonary venous pressure (e.g., HF) or hypoproteinemia (e.g., malnutrition, cirrhosis); this fluid tends to accumulate at the base of the lungs. An exudate results from increased capillary permeability or impaired lymphatic absorption (e.g., involvement of the pleura by inflammation or malignancy); this fluid has a higher specific gravity and protein content than a

TABLE 4-20   Complications of Mechanical Ventilation

Complication	Causes	Prevention	Clinical Presentation	Treatment
Decreased cardiac output	• Increased intrathoracic pressures that • Decrease venous return to the right heart • Increase RV afterload • Decrease LV distensibility	• Ensure adequate preload before mechanical ventilation • Avoid excessive tidal volumes • Adjust PEEP carefully	• Tachycardia, hypotension • Cool, clammy skin • Decrease in urine output • Change in level of consciousness	• Administer fluids to increase preload • Administer inotropes as prescribed
Ventilator-induced lung injury (VILI)	• Barotrauma: high inflation pressures may cause pneumothorax, pneumo-mediastinum, subcutaneous emphysema • Volutrauma: high inflation volumes and repeated end-expiratory collapse followed by repeated reopening during inspiration may cause release of inflammatory mediators, injury to the lung ultrastructure, and ARDS • Oxygen toxicity • High end-inspiratory lung volume, such as occurs with high levels of PEEP, auto-PEEP (e.g., IRV), and high functional residual capacity, such as elderly patients (i.e., senile emphysema) or patients with COPD	• Avoid excessive tidal volumes; now recommended to be within 5-10 mL/kg of IBW with even lower tidal volumes for patients with ARDS (~6 mL/kg of IBW) • Keep plateau pressure <30 cm H$_2$O • Keep Fio$_2$ <0.60 (60%) • Adjust PEEP carefully	• Pneumothorax: chest pain, dyspnea, sudden increase in peak inspiratory pressure, decreased breath sounds and chest movement on affected side, tracheal shift, hypotension, JVD if tension pneumothorax, clinical indications of hypoxia, decreased Spo$_2$, chest x-ray changes • ARDS: high peak and plateau pressures, refractory hypoxemia (P/F ratio <300 mm Hg), noncardiac (PAOP <18 mm Hg) pulmonary edema, patchy atelectasis on chest x-ray	• If pneumothorax suspected: take patient off ventilator and manually ventilate with a manual resuscitation bag; assist with insertion of chest tube for pneumothorax • Decrease tidal volume or PEEP if possible to decrease mean airway pressure and prevent alveolar overdistention
Fluid retention	• Decrease in insensible loss via respiratory system • Overhydration by humidification • Decreased urine output due to ADH and aldosterone secretion	• Avoid decrease in cardiac output, which stimulates renin-angiotensin-aldosterone system	• Weight gain • Intake greater than output • Crackles • Decreased compliance	• Utilize therapies above to prevent decrease in cardiac output
Atelectasis	• Airway obstruction • Small tidal volumes or lack of sighing • Infrequent turning of patient	• Use periodic sighing • Turn frequently • Provide adequate humidification • Perform tracheal suctioning as indicated • Provide chest physical therapy (PT) as indicated • Reposition frequently	• Diminished breath sounds • Crackles • Abnormal chest x-ray • Increased A-a gradient • Decreased compliance	• Provide periodic sighing • Provide chest PT

Continued

Complication	Etiology	Signs and Symptoms	Nursing Interventions	
Hypercapnia; hypocapnia	• Inadequate or excessive ventilation • Hypermetabolism may contribute to hypercapnia	• Increased (>45 mm Hg) or decreased (<35 mm Hg) $PaCO_2$	• Initiate ventilation with tidal volume at 10-15 mL/kg and rate of 8-12 breaths/min • Make ventilator changes after initial ABGs	• Hypercapnia: increase tidal volume (or rate) • Hypocapnia: decrease rate (or tidal volume); change to IMV or PSV
Oxygen toxicity	• Too high a concentration of O_2 over too long a time	• Substernal distress • Paresthesias in extremities • Anorexia, nausea, vomiting • Fatigue, lethargy, malaise • Restlessness • Dyspnea, progressive respiratory difficulty • Decreased compliance • Increased A-a gradient	• Maintain FiO_2 as low as possible to maintain a SaO_2 (or SpO_2) of 90% and limit duration of FiO_2 of greater than 0.40 if possible; addition of PEEP allows reduction of FiO_2 while maintaining the same SaO_2 • REMEMBER: hypoxemia is far more common than O_2 toxicity and must be corrected	• Decrease O_2 concentration as soon as possible • Provide supportive management
Aspiration	• Stomach contents • Tube feedings • Oral secretions • Gastric distention • Impaired gastric emptying • Esophageal reflux	• Increased tracheal secretions • Fever • Rhonchi, wheezes • Signs/symptoms of hypoxemia/hypoxia • Infiltrate on chest x-ray	• Maintain cuff inflation using minimal occlusive volume • Keep head of bed elevated 30-45 degrees • Check for gastric retention at least every 4 hours • Check NC tube placement at least every 4 hours	• Provide supportive management • Administer antibiotics as prescribed • Administer steroids as prescribed
GI effects: stress ulcer, ileus, gastric dilation	• Hyperacidity • Endogenous or exogenous steroids • Gastric or mesenteric ischemia • Inadequate nutrition	• NG aspirate, vomitus, or stools positive for blood • Decreased bowel sounds • Gastric distention • Increased gastric retention	• Utilize enteral feedings • Administer antacids (e.g., cimetidine [Tagamet]); H_2 receptor antagonists (e.g., cimetidine [Tagamet]); barrier agents (e.g., sucralfate [Carafate]) as prescribed	• Note effect of hemoglobin loss of tissue oxygenation; blood administration may be necessary • Administer antacids, sucralfate, H_2 receptor antagonists, and/or PP, as prescribed

TABLE 4-20   Complications of Mechanical Ventilation—cont'd

Complication	Causes	Prevention	Clinical Presentation	Treatment
Infection	• Immunosuppression • Artificial airways bypass normal upper airway defense mechanisms • Ventilatory equipment: warm, moist environment is good for bacterial growth • Suctioning procedure • Silent aspiration of GI bacteria when PPIs, H_2 antagonists, or antacids used for ulcer prophylaxis; controversial issue • Cross-contamination may be cause	• Use good handwashing techniques • Use sterile technique for suctioning • Provide aseptic airway management, tubing changes, etc. • Avoid change in usual acidic gastric pH; use enteral feedings for ulcer prophylaxis if gastric mobility adequate • Keep head of bed elevated during tube feedings • Keep ET tube or trach cuff inflated to 18 mm Hg • Drain humidifier condensation into water trap or container and not back into humidifier • Routine change of ventilator circuit is no longer indicated but the circuit should be changed if visibly soiled or malfunctioning • Additional information in Pneumonia section of this chapter	• Tachycardia, tachypnea • Fever • Crackles, rhonchi, or wheezes • Hypoxemia • Change in color or character of sputum • Positive cultures • Infiltrate on chest x-ray	• Administer antibiotic specific to culture
Patient-ventilator asynchrony (patient "fighting" ventilator)	• Incorrect ventilator setup for the patient's needs • Acute change in patient's status • Obstructed airway • Ventilator malfunction • Anxiety	• Ensure proper setup of ventilator equipment; monitor settings every hour • Monitor peak inspiratory pressure • Suction as indicated • Talk to patient, keep him or her informed • Administer anxiolytics as indicated	• Anxiety, agitation • Increase in peak inspiratory pressure • Ventilator alarm sounding • Change in pulse oximetry or ABGs	• Perform rapid check of patient and ventilator • Disconnect patient from ventilator and provide manual ventilation via manual resuscitation bag • Check vital signs, breath sounds, pulse oximetry • Assess ABGs • Suction airway • Check patency of endotracheal or tracheostomy tube

Anxiety	• Loss of autonomy over vital body function (breathing) • Inability to communicate • Sensory overload (e.g., alarms, repeated interruptions for vital signs, noise of ventilator) • Sensory deprivation (e.g., separation from family, work, meaningful activities) • Discomfort (e.g., arterial punctures, endotracheal tube, nasogastric tube, Foley catheter, etc.)	• High-pressure alarm because the patient is breathing out of synch with ventilator • Tachycardia • Tachypnea, excessive triggering of ventilator if on assist/control, potentially causing hypocapnia and respiratory alkalosis • Complaints of being "nervous"
	• Explain to patient why he or she cannot speak; provide method of communication • Explain all procedures thoroughly; keep patient informed regarding progress and plans • Add familiar objects to patient's environment (e.g., family photos, cards) • Have a calendar and clock in the room; have window shades or curtains open to orient patient to light and dark • Allow uninterrupted time for rest and sleep • Put eyeglasses and hearing aide on patient if appropriate • Encourage expression of fears • Be available; answer call bell promptly • Promote as much independence as possible • Provide emotional support to the family • Avoid uncomfortable or painful procedures if possible (e.g., arterial catheter instead of arterial punctures) • Use complementary therapies such as music, aromatherapy	• Stay with patient during times of extreme anxiety • Use therapeutic touch (e.g., hold hand) • Utilize soft restraints only as necessary to prevent self-extubation • Encourage family visitation and participation if appropriate
Inability to wean	• COPD: occurs when $Paco_2$ is corrected instead of pH • Malnutrition: catabolism and muscle breakdown • Neuromuscular blocking agents: disuse syndrome	• Increased $Paco_2$, increased ventilatory rate, tachycardia with weaning efforts
	• Correct pH instead of $Paco_2$ in patients with COPD • Provide adequate calories to prevent catabolism; adequate protein and high calories are given; adequate calories must be given to prevent the protein from being utilized for energy; calories given are predominantly fat because CHO metabolism produces more CO_2 • Avoid neuromuscular blocking agents if possible; limit duration of use	• COPD: allow $Paco_2$ to increase so that the kidney will hold on to bicarbonate to compensate; keep Pao_2 close to patient's normal (e.g., 60-65 mm Hg) • Provide adequate protein and calories; avoid high-carbohydrate feedings during weaning • Discontinue several days before weaning

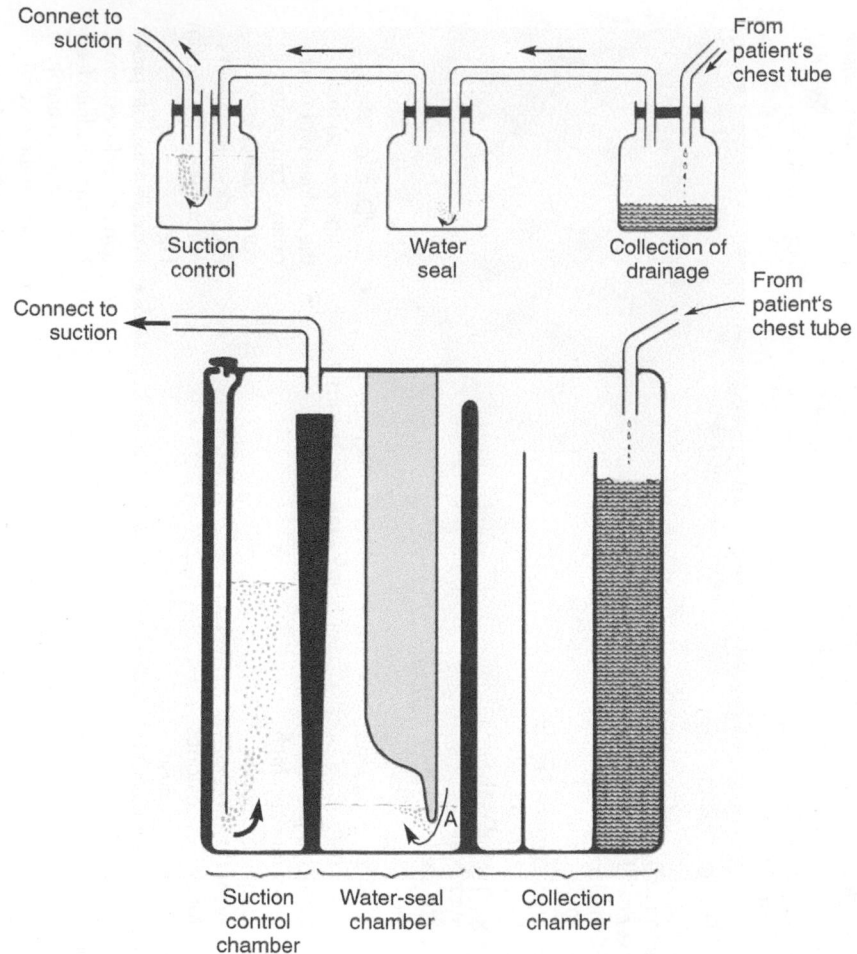

FIGURE 4-24 Comparison of a commercially available chest tube drainage system with a three-bottle system. (From Urden, L. D., Stacy, K. M., & Lough, M. E. [2006]. *Thelan's critical care nursing: Diagnosis and management* [5th ed.]. St. Louis, MO: Mosby.)

transudate. Other fluid accumulations that may require insertion of a chest tube include empyema (also called *pyothorax*) (pus in the pleural space), chylothorax (lymph fluid and triglyceride fat in the pleural space), and hydrothorax (water [e.g., IV fluid] in the pleural space).

Chest tubes are inserted during surgery when the thoracic cavity must be invaded during the procedure, in the interventional radiology department, or at the bedside. Informed consent is required and the procedure starts with an explanation to patient and family given by the physician and reinforced by the nurse. The chest drainage system is set up before insertion of the tube. A local anesthetic is used but the patient feels pressure with insertion of the trocar. The physician sutures the tube in place and then applies an occlusive dressing with the tube taped securely to avoid tugging. Obtain a chest x-ray to confirm placement.

Chest drainage systems (Figure 4-24) are comprised of up to three components. The drainage collection bottle or chamber collects liquid drainage. This is the bottle or chamber closest to the patient and connects to the water-seal bottle or chamber. The water-seal bottle or chamber provides a one-way valve to allow air to escape, but does not allow atmospheric air to go into the pleural space. Fill it until the tube is underwater or the chamber fluid reaches to the 2-cm mark. This means that there must be more than 2 cm of pressure to allow drainage. If that

bottle or chamber is overfilled, it reduces the effectiveness of the chest tube. The water-seal bottle or chamber vents to allow the air from the chest to escape through the drainage system. The suction control bottle or chamber controls the amount of suction. It is connected to the water-seal bottle or chamber as well as the suction source, usually wall suction but it could be a free-standing suction device. Another tube is submerged under water to the prescribed suction amount measured in centimeters (cm) of water (usually 20 cm of H_2O) for a bottle or the chamber is filled to the prescribed level. Adjust the wall suction so that there is a gentle bubbling in this bottle or chamber. Note that vigorous bubbling does not increase the amount of suction but rather just makes the water evaporate more quickly so that you must keep refilling it. The actual amount of suction is determined by the depth that the tube is submersed (or the height that the chamber is filled) minus the water-seal. Suction is not necessary to remove air and free-flowing fluid, but suction may be applied if the liquid does not respond to gravity water-seal drainage.

All-in-one systems are convenient and less cumbersome than the bottle system. Only the water-seal and drainage collection chambers may be used, but if suction is desired, all three chambers are used. In a wet system (e.g., Atrium, Pleur-evac, Thora Seal, Aqua Seal, Medi-Vac), adjust the amount of suction by filling the water level in the suction control chamber and adjust

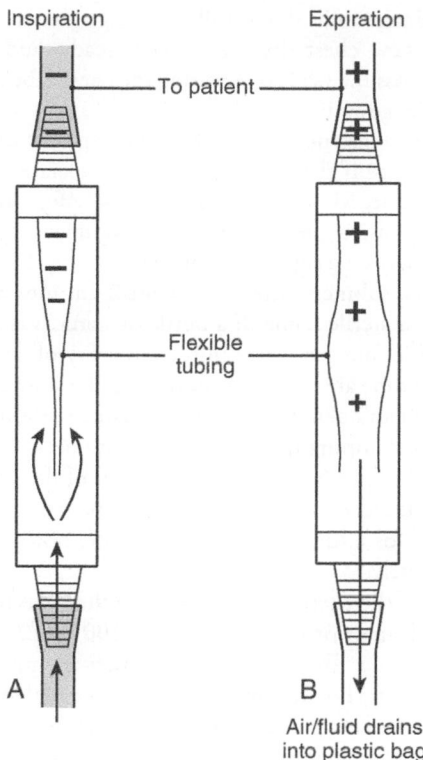

Inspiration   Expiration

To patient

Flexible
tubing

A   B

Air/fluid drains
into plastic bag

FIGURE 4-25 Heimlich one-way valve. A, During inspiration, negative pressure collapses the flexible tubing and prevents outside air from entering the pleural space. **B,** During expiration, positive pressure opens the flexible tubing and allows air and fluid to drain into an attached plastic bag. (From Kersten, L. D. [1989]. *Comprehensive respiratory nursing: A decision-making approach.* Philadelphia, PA: W. B. Saunders.)

TABLE 4-21	Assessment Parameters for the Patient with a Chest Tube	
Parameter	**Note**	
Patient	• Ventilatory effort • Chest discomfort or pain • Anxiety • Level of understanding • Cough • Sputum production	
Breathing	• Rate • Regularity • Depth • Breath sounds (disconnection of suction from suction control chamber is required for accurate assessment of breath sounds)	
Entry site	• Intactness of dressing • Drainage on dressing • Subcutaneous emphysema around insertion site	
Tubing	• Tight, taped connections • Absence of kinks, compressions, or dependent loops	
Drainage collection chamber	• Volume (normal 50-100 mL/hr for first few hours after thoracotomy, then 10-20 mL/hr) • Type: color, consistency, odor • Bottle below chest level	
Water-seal chamber	• Filled to 2 cm or prescribed amount • Fluctuations with respirations (also referred to as *tidaling*) • Any bubbling • If not on suction: air vent open	
Suction control chamber	• Filled to prescribed amount (usually -20 cm H_2O) • Gentle, continuous bubbling	
Suction source	• If no control bottle: suction set at ordered level • If control bottle: suction set so that gentle, continuous bubbling occurs	

the suction so that gentle bubbling occurs in the suction control chamber. Remember that the actual amount of suction is the height of the suction control chamber minus the height of the water-seal chamber. In a dry system (e.g., Sentinel Seal, Thora-Klex, Argyle Altitude, Pleur-evac Sahara, Atrium Oasis), adjust the amount of suction until the indicator appears.

For patient transportation, use a portable chest drainage system (e.g., Atrium Express). These systems have only one chamber to collect chest drainage and a dry seal. The portable drainage system is usually used as a gravity drain only but may be used with suction, which is automatically regulated to –20 cm H_2O when connected to suction. Another possibility for patient transport or for home use is a Heimlich valve (Figure 4-25). This is a one-way flutter valve made of rubber tubing encased in a clear, plastic chamber used for uncomplicated pneumothorax with little or no liquid drainage. The valve may be connected to a small drainage bag, but it is usually not used if there is more than 50 mL of fluid. Note the fluttering of the valve as air escapes from the pleural space. The advantages of a Heimlich valve include that it is small, lightweight, and the patient can move around easily. A patient may be discharged with a chest tube attached to a Heimlich valve in some instances.

Assessment of a patient (Table 4-21) with a chest tube is important for patient comfort, safety, and resolution of the need for the chest tube. Assessment includes the patient, the chest tube, and the chest drainage system.

Management of a patient with a chest tube begins with the consideration of pain. Assess the patient for pain and discomfort

and administer analgesics and/or local anesthetics as prescribed to relieve pain, and encourage deep breathing. Instruct the patient regarding how to splint the chest when coughing and instruct the family how to assist the patient.

Maintain airway patency and adequate oxygenation and ventilation. Position the patient for optimal V/Q matching. Elevate the HOB to 30 to 45 degrees. "Good lung down" optimizes ventilation to encourage reexpansion of the affected lung and optimizes perfusion to the nonaffected "good" lung. Note that the exception to this rule is to position a post pneumonectomy patient on the operative lung side or back. Remember these positioning guidelines as "good lung down, no lung down." An occluded chest tube can cause a tension pneumothorax. Assess the position of the trachea and report immediately any shift from the normal midline. Encourage deep breathing and use of the incentive spirometer. Note that removal of air from the pleural space occurs by the positive pressure of expiration and the negative pressure of suction on the chest tube; deep breathing is *very* important in reexpansion of the lung. To maintain airway clearance, focus on sustained inspiration maneuvers such as deep breathing and incentive spirometry. This frequently stimulates the patient to cough if coughing is needed. Suction only if the patient is unable to clear secretions. Administer oxygen as indicated by ABGs and SpO_2. Assist with weaning from mechanical ventilation and extubation as soon as possible, as positive pressure ventilation increases risk of air leak.

Nursing interventions to ensure patient safety include maintaining the water-seal drainage system and the patency of chest tubes. Assess the chest drainage system hourly. Ensure that connections are taped, and position the tubing to prevent kinks and dependent loops. Maintain the suction level at the prescribed level; water may need to be added to the suction control chamber, as water evaporates in wet chest drainage systems. Assess the water-seal chamber for fluctuation with ventilation (also referred to as *tidaling*); this indicates that the tube is patent. If fluctuation in the water-seal chamber is absent, consider the following:

- The lung is reexpanded; confirm by assessment of chest x-ray
- The tube is kinked; follow the tube from chest to chest drainage system and position the tube to prevent kinking
- The tube is occluded

The dangers of an occluded tube, especially in a patient on mechanical ventilation, are tension pneumothorax, mediastinal shift, and potential tearing of great vessels. Although routine milking or stripping is not recommended, efforts to reestablish patency of an occluded tube (and prevent tension pneumothorax) require the milking or stripping in some instances. Milking is hand over hand squeezing of the chest tube; stripping is to clamp with the thumb and forefinger of the nondominant hand while pulling the tube between the thumb and forefinger of the dominant hand followed by release of the thumb and forefinger of the nondominant hand. Milk the tube first and if unsuccessful in reestablishing fluctuation in the water-seal chamber, strip short sections. Milking and stripping chest tubes create negative pressure within the pleural space; although these processes may help to move a clot along, they may create trauma to the pleura. If milking or stripping short sections are unsuccessful in reestablishing fluctuation in the water-seal chamber, notify the physician; a new tube may be required.

Assess for air leak and differentiate between expected removal of air from the pleural space (i.e., occasional bubble) from a break in the chest tube system. An occasional bubble indicates that the tube is still needed because air is still escaping from the pleural space. Excessive bubbling indicates the need to search for a leak in the system. Brief clamping with hemostats moving from the chest drainage system to the insertion site can be helpful in identifying the location of the leak. Ensure that all connections are connected and taped. Assess the insertion site for displacement of the tube so that the proximal eyelet is outside the skin; notify the physician of displacement and prepare to assist in the repositioning of the tube. Suspect a bronchopleural fistula if no external air leak identified.

Keep the chest drainage system lower than the patient's chest. Also, avoid intentionally occluding (e.g., clamping) the tube. Clamp the tube only if one of the following occurs:

- The chest drainage system must be lifted above the level of the chest (e.g., putting the patient in helicopter for transport) so that chest drainage does not drain back into the pleural space; clamp as briefly as possible.

- If the drainage collection is full (e.g., large pleural effusions), have the new chest drainage system ready, and clamp as briefly as possible while connecting the chest tube to the new chest drainage system.
- If specifically instructed to by the physician before chest tube removal to see if the patient is likely to tolerate not having the chest tube. Monitor the patient closely for clinical indications of tension pneumothorax during this time.

If there has been a significant air leak and the chest drainage system breaks, submerse the tube about 2 cm into a bottle of sterile water or sterile saline. If a bottle of sterile water or saline is not available, put tap water into a clean Styrofoam cup and submerse the tube about 2 cm into the cup. Because a patient is better off with an open pneumothorax than a tension pneumothorax, avoid clamping the tube. If there has been a significant air leak and the tube accidentally comes out of the chest, apply a dressing to the chest with your hand or tape it on 3 sides (i.e., as you would for a sucking chest wound) and notify the physician immediately.

Removal of the chest tube occurs when there has been no air leak from the anterior tube or less than 100 mL/24 hours for the posterior tube. The physician may order the tube clamped for up to 24 hours before removal. Administer analgesics before chest tube removal; music may also be helpful to relax the patient. Recommended analgesics include Ketorolac (Toradol) 30 mg IV 60 minutes before and morphine 4 mg IV 20 minutes before. While the physician cuts the suture, instruct the patient to hold his or her breath while the physician removes the tube. There is no difference in the occurrence rate of a pneumothorax post removal using either end-inspiration or end-expiration timing (Bauman, 2011). Apply an occlusive dressing after tube removal. Monitor the patient for clinical indications of recurrent pneumothorax: dyspnea, chest pain, asymmetric chest excursion, and/or diminished breath sounds. Obtain a chest x-ray for confirmation of reexpansion.

CHEST SURGERY

Procedures

There are many commonly performed surgical chest procedures. A *thoracotomy* is a procedure to create an opening into the thorax or pleural cavity. A *video-assisted thoracotomy* is the use of two or more small incisions in the chest for visualization and instrumentation for exploration, biopsy, or resection. When required for chest trauma, a surgeon performs a thoracotomy to repair penetrating or nonpenetrating trauma, drain the pleural cavity, or control a hemorrhage. A thoracotomy performed to obtain a biopsy or locate a source of bleeding is referred to as an *exploratory thoracotomy*. Thoracotomies are frequently performed for removal of masses. Removal of one or more lobes of the lung is a *lobectomy*. A *segmental resection* is the removal of a segment or segments of a lobe and a *wedge resection* is the removal of a small peripheral section of the lung without regard to segments. A *pneumonectomy* is the removal of an entire lung with or without mediastinal lymph node resection; it is indicated when a tumor is centrally located at the hilus or bronchus. *Bronchoplastic reconstruction* (i.e., sleeve resection) is the removal of a mass that involves or protrudes into the airway; a section of the airway and lung is removed and then reanastomosis of the airway proximal and distal to the resected area is performed. A thoracotomy may also be required to remove a cyst, tumor, or abscess from the mediastinum.

A *thoracostomy* is the creation of an opening into the thorax for the insertion of a chest tube. A *closed thoracostomy* is the insertion of a chest tube through an intercostal space into the pleural space; the chest drainage system connects to the inserted tube. An *open thoracostomy* is insertion of a chest tube during a rib resection; this is usually used in empyema when the pleural space is fixed.

A *bullectomy* is the removal of cysts or bullae in the lung; it may be performed with a laser to avoid a thoracotomy. A *reduction pneumoplasty* (i.e., lung volume reduction surgery) is a resection of hyperinflated areas of lung to allow more normal function of the diaphragm and expansion of more normal areas of the lung; this may be performed for COPD.

For patients with recurrent spontaneous pneumothorax, the surgeon may perform a *decortication,* which is the removal of the fibrinous membrane covering the visceral and parietal pleura to cause adhesion and eliminate the pleural space. A *pleurodesis* is a process of fusing the two layers of the pleura by instilling agents (e.g., doxycycline, minocycline, or sterile talc), which causes a fibrotic reaction to prevent pleural fluid formation. This procedure may be used for recurrent malignant pleural effusion. A *thoracoplasty* is the surgical collapse of a portion of chest wall by multiple rib resections. This is performed to decrease volume in the hemithorax; this procedure may be used after pulmonary resection if the lung cannot reexpand to fill thoracic space or after pneumonectomy to reduce the size of the thoracic cavity on the operative side and decrease the chance of mediastinal shift toward that side.

A *thymectomy* is the removal of the thymus. This procedure requires a median sternotomy. This procedure may be performed for myasthenia gravis because it is considered an autoimmune disorder and the thymus is the site of T-cell distribution. A *tracheal resection* is the removal of a stenotic area of the trachea or tumor. After the resection, an end-to-end anastomosis is performed.

Some thoracotomies are performed for gastrointestinal problems. A *diaphragmatic hernia repair* is repositioning of the abdominal contents back into the abdominal cavity and closure of the diaphragm with suture or patch. An *esophagogastrectomy* is the resection of a part of the esophagus and upper portion of the stomach for cancer of esophagus or corrosive esophagitis. Either an end-to-end anastomosis or a colon interposition using a portion of the large intestine is performed.

Postoperative Management

The priority of care for a patient after thoracotomy is the maintenance of airway patency and adequate oxygenation and ventilation. Administer oxygen as indicated by ABGs and SpO_2. Position the patient for optimal V/Q matching. The head of the bed should be elevated from 30 to 45 degrees.

Turn the patient frequently and ambulate them early. Encourage deep breathing and use of the incentive spirometer. Note that air removal from the pleural space occurs from the positive pressure of expiration and the negative pressure of suction on the chest tube; therefore, deep breathing is *very* important to reexpand the lung. Be sure also to maintain airway clearance. Encourage sustained inspiration through deep breathing and incentive spirometry. Coughing will occur if needed, but avoid routine coughing because the forced expiration increases

the risk of atelectasis. Coughing also causes pain and may cause splinting, decreasing chest excursion and increasing the risk of atelectasis.

Suction the patient only if he or she is unable to clear secretions. Use caution when suctioning the patient because leakage from the bronchial stump may occur, especially with pneumonectomy patients. Assess the position of the trachea, and immediately report any shift from the normal midline. To prevent gastric distention with resultant pressure against the diaphragm, gastric suction may be required.

To control pain, administer analgesics and/or local anesthetics as prescribed to relieve pain and encourage deep breathing. Provide intravenous analgesia by regularly scheduled IV injection or by patient-controlled analgesia (PCA). During the surgical procedure, the patient may have received interpleural analgesia, which involves injecting a local anesthetic (e.g., bupivacaine [Marcaine]) into the pleural space. Epidural analgesia, which involves infusion of an opiate and/or local anesthetic into the epidural space with a basal rate (i.e., continuous infusion) or PCA is used to provide pain management. Administer a nonsteroidal antiinflammatory agent (e.g., ketorolac [Toradol]) to augment the pain relief of the narcotics provided as prescribed. Instructing the patient how to splint the chest when coughing and instructing the family on how to assist the patient may further reduce pain.

Maintain the water-seal drainage system and patency of the chest tubes. Monitor the amount and appearance of the drainage. It should progress from bloody to serosanguineous to serous in 2 to 3 days. Expected drainage is 100 to 300 mL for the first 2 hours and then less than 50 mL/hr for the next several hours with negligible drainage within 2 days. Assess the patient for an air leak. Expect an occasional bubble as air is removed from the pleural space, but note that a continuous bubbling in the water-seal chamber indicates a leak in the chest tube system or a bronchopleural fistula.

Monitor the patient for common complications. Monitor patients for clinical indications of hypoperfusion (see Table 3-2). In the event of hemorrhage/shock, replace blood and fluid volume as prescribed. Thoracic surgery patients generally receive less fluid in the early postoperative period than other surgical patients to prevent ARDS and pulmonary edema.

To prevent infection, utilize sterile technique while dressing the insertion site, setting up the chest drainage system, and replacing the system. Monitor patients for fever, purulent drainage, leukocytosis, and other clinical indications of infection. Assess the incision and the insertion site for redness, induration, and drainage. Culture the drainage if purulent. Monitor sputum and chest drainage for signs of infection, and culture as necessary. Administer antibiotics as prescribed.

Tension pneumothorax may occur if the chest drainage system becomes occluded. For prevention, maintain the patency of the chest tube and functioning of the chest drainage system and avoid clamping the chest tube except for reasons identified earlier. Monitor the patient for clinical indications of tension pneumothorax, including dyspnea, chest pain, tracheal shift away from the affected side, hyperresonance to percussion, and decreased breath sounds on the affected side. Contact the provider immediately if these indications of tension pneumothorax occur; emergency needle decompression and replacement of chest tube may be indicated.

Monitor patients for dysrhythmias, especially atrial dysrhythmias in patients having pneumonectomy. Administer prophylactic antidysrhythmics preoperatively as prescribed. Use caution with fluid administration. Hemodynamic monitoring in these patients may be necessary. Monitor patients for changes in ventilatory effort and SpO_2, which may indicate the development of ARDS. To prevent pulmonary embolism, minimize the risk of deep vein thrombosis. Progress the patient's activity if hemodynamically stable. Have the patient sit on the edge of the bed the evening of surgery. Have them get out of bed and into a chair within 24 to 36 hours of surgery. Ambulate the patient as soon as possible. Bronchopleural fistula causes an air leak and is usually related to empyema. In the event of empyema, treat infection with drainage and antimicrobials. For patients experiencing frozen shoulder (i.e., impairment in shoulder mobility), encourage range-of-motion exercises to the shoulder on the operative side. Administer analgesics to allow movement and encourage the use of the affected arm for self-care activities.

ACUTE RESPIRATORY FAILURE

Acute respiratory failure occurs when there is failure of the respiratory system to provide the exchange of oxygen and carbon dioxide between the environment and tissues in quantities sufficient to sustain life. The characteristics of hypoxemic normocapnic respiratory failure (i.e., type I) include a PaO_2 lower than 60 mm Hg with a normal $PaCO_2$. The characteristics of hypoxemic hypercapnic respiratory failure (i.e., type II) include a low PaO_2 with a $PaCO_2$ greater than 50 mm Hg.

Diffusion defects without hypoventilation cause type I acute respiratory failure. Examples include the following:
- Pneumonia
- Pulmonary edema
- Pulmonary fibrosis
- Pleural effusion
- Pneumothorax
- Asthma
- Atelectasis
- Aspiration pneumonitis
- ARDS (early)
- Smoke inhalation
- Pulmonary embolism
- Kyphoscoliosis
- Fat embolism

Hypoventilation and the resultant hypoxemia cause type II acute respiratory failure. Examples include the following:
- COPD with acute exacerbation (Sidebar 4-2)
- Status asthmaticus
- CNS depressant drugs
- Anesthesia
- Neuromuscular blocking drugs, aminoglycosides, and organophosphate poisoning
- Head trauma
- Poliomyelitis
- Amyotrophic lateral sclerosis
- Spinal cord injury
- Guillain-Barré syndrome
- Myasthenia gravis
- Multiple sclerosis
- Muscular dystrophy
- Morbid obesity
- Chest trauma

- Surgery, especially thoracic, abdominal, and flank incision
- Obstructive sleep apnea (Sidebar 4-3)
- Tracheal obstruction
- Epiglottitis
- Cystic fibrosis
- Near-drowning

SIDEBAR 4-2
Chronic Obstructive Pulmonary Disease

Chronic obstructive pulmonary disease (COPD) with acute exacerbation is an acute process (usually caused by respiratory infection) in a patient with a chronic condition. COPD, also known as *chronic obstructive lung disease* (COLD), is a disease state characterized by the presence of airflow obstruction due to chronic bronchitis or emphysema. The airflow obstruction is progressive and accompanied by airway hyperactivity. Inflammation and cough with excessive mucus secretion clinically defines chronic bronchitis which may be partially reversible. The enlargement of the air spaces distal to the terminal bronchioles with destruction of the alveolar walls defines emphysema, which is not reversible. Many patients with chronic bronchitis or emphysema have some degree of asthma. An acute exacerbation of COPD involves worsening dyspnea, an increase in sputum volume, and an increase in sputum purulence.

SIDEBAR 4-3
Obstructive Sleep Apnea

The relaxation of the throat muscles intermittently with resultant airway obstruction during sleep causes the condition known as obstructive sleep apnea (OSA). OSA occurs more often in men and postmenopausal women; additional risk factors include aging, obesity, smoking, alcohol use, and diabetes and anatomic factors include increased neck circumference, tonsillar hypertrophy, and a small or receding jaw. OSA may cause hypertension, stroke, and mood or hormonal changes. It may be a contributing factor to motor vehicle collisions, reduced productivity, and disrupted relationships. Sleeping partners may report loud snoring with periods of apnea and the patient may report difficulty staying asleep, sudden awakening with dyspnea, morning headaches, daytime sleepiness, and mood changes such as irritability or depression. Diagnosis is based on either an in-laboratory polysomnogram or an at-home sleep study. These studies will show apnea, oxygen desaturations, brief awakenings, and increased heart rate and blood pressure. The primary treatment of OSA is positive airway pressure using CPAP or BiPAP using a well-fitting face mask or nasal pillows. An oral device may be used as an alternative to positive airway pressure in some patients; these devices work by bringing the jaw forward or holding the tongue away from the hypopharynx. Surgery, such as a uvulopalatopharyngoplasty or a maxillomandibular advancement, may be used in some patients. Patient instruction should include discussion of modification of contributing factors. If obesity is a contributing factor, weight reduction should be encouraged. Advocate regular exercise, avoidance of alcohol before bedtime, and smoking cessation. The patient should be encouraged to avoid sleeping on his or her back.

4.16   Learning Activity

List 10 possible causes of acute respiratory failure.

1. _____
2. _____
3. _____
4. _____
5. _____
6. _____
7. _____
8. _____
9. _____
10. _____

Answers to this activity can be found in the Answer Key.

The pathophysiology of acute respiratory failure (Table 4-22) may result from hypoventilation, V/Q mismatching, shunt, and diffusion defects. Clinical presentation and management vary with the mechanism of acute respiratory failure.

The clinical findings of acute respiratory failure vary with the mechanism of the hypoventilation and/or hypoxemia. The history may include an identifiable precipitating factor. Subjective and objective findings of respiratory distress (see Box 4-1), hypoxia (see Box 4-2), and hypercapnia (see Box 4-3) are likely to be present. Acute respiratory failure can be confirmed by ABG changes (i.e., PaO_2 <50-60 mm Hg or a $PaCO_2$ >50 mm Hg with a pH of <7.3). A chest x-ray may identify the cause.

Collaborative management begins with the treatment of the cause of the acute respiratory failure as well as maintenance of a patent airway and optimal ventilation. Position the patient for optimal ventilation, which includes keeping the head of the bed from 30 to 45 degrees, using an overbed table for the patient to lean on, and maintaining the "good lung down" if a unilateral lung condition exists. Use continuous lateral rotation therapy as prescribed, especially if the PaO_2/FiO_2 ratio (i.e., P/F ratio) is less than 250 mm Hg. The P/F ratio is calculated by dividing the PaO_2 by the FiO_2 (remember to use the FiO_2 as a decimal so 50% is 0.5) Normal P/F ratio is 300 mm Hg and <200 mm of Hg is considered ARDS. Utilize prone positioning, especially for patients with ARDS.

Maintain adequate hydration, usually 2 to 3 L/24 hours unless contraindicated by cardiac or renal disease. Provide only noncaffeinated oral fluids along with IV fluids, usually D_5NS. Provide bronchial hygiene and chest physiotherapy as indicated. Inspiratory maneuvers, such as deep breathing, incentive spirometry, and flutter valve, encourage reexpansion of alveoli and generate cough if needed. Provide adequate analgesics doses to allow the patient to breathe deeply and cough as indicated. Suction patients who are unable to clear their airways. Early activity and ambulation is important for these patients. Postural drainage, percussion, and vibration may be necessary. Bronchoscopy may also be necessary, if airway clearance techniques are inadequate. Noninvasive ventilation may be used to avert intubation in either the CPAP or BiPAP mode. If the patient previously required nocturnal CPAP or BiPAP at home, direct the family to bring in the equipment. Intubation and mechanical ventilation may be necessary if $PaCO_2$ continues to rise and acidosis develops. The goal of mechanical ventilation is to normalize the pH, not necessarily the $PaCO_2$. It is not appropriate to normalize the $PaCO_2$ in patients with COPD and chronic hypercapnia because this causes metabolic alkalosis with eventual excretion of sodium bicarbonate and weaning difficulties. Administer appropriate drug therapy. Administer bronchodilators to relax smooth muscle and provide bronchodilation as prescribed. Indications for drug therapy include asthma (i.e., reactive airway disease), acute bronchospasm related to anaphylaxis, and pulmonary hypertension (specifically xanthines).

Bronchodilators (Table 4-23) are commonly used medications in patients with acute respiratory failure. These include sympathomimetics (i.e., beta-adrenergic agents) (e.g., epinephrine, albuterol [Proventil]), isoetharine (Bronkosol), metaproterenol (Alupent), terbutaline sulfate (Brethine), and salmeterol (Serevent). $Beta_2$-adrenergic agonists are preferred over nonrespiratory-selective beta stimulants such as epinephrine and isoproterenol because they cause fewer cardiovascular side effects. These respiratory selective agents include albuterol (Proventil), isoetharine (Bronkosol), metaproterenol (Alupent), terbutaline sulfate (Brethine), salmeterol (Serevent), and levalbuterol (Xopenex). Anticholinergics work by blocking the parasympathetic nervous system so that the sympathetic nervous system is dominant. These anticholinergics, such as ipratropium (Atrovent), are weaker bronchodilators than are the sympathomimetic agents. Combivent is a combination of albuterol and ipratropium and administered by inhalation. Methylxanthines, such as aminophylline (Aminophyllin), oxtriphylline (Choledyl), and theophylline (Theo-Dur), are smooth muscle relaxants, so they vasodilate as well as bronchodilate, therefore, also reducing pulmonary hypertension. Magnesium also has a smooth muscle relaxant effect and may also be used as a bronchodilator.

Corticosteroids (e.g., betamethasone [Vanceril]) may be used in acute respiratory failure, especially with reactive airway disease. Although hydration is most important, expectorants (e.g., guaifenesin [Robitussin], potassium iodide [SSKI]) and mucolytics (e.g., acetylcysteine [Mucomyst]) may be used to decrease the tenacity of the mucus. Avoid using antitussives unless a nonproductive cough is causing the patient fatigue. Avoid sedatives unless the patient is very agitated.

4.17   Learning Activity

List four classifications of bronchodilators and an example of each.

Classification	Example
1.	
2.	
3.	
4.	

Answers to this activity can be found in the Answer Key.

Optimize oxygen delivery and decrease oxygen consumption. Administer oxygen as indicated for hypoxemia, using a nasal cannula or mask. The flow rate or oxygen concentration should maintain SpO_2 at approximately 95%, unless contraindicated.

TABLE 4-22   **Mechanisms of Acute Respiratory Failure**

Mechanism	Pathophysiology	Causes	Clinical Presentation	Management

Hypoventilation	Hypoventilation causes CO_2 retention and hypoxemia	Damage to/depression of the neurologic control of ventilation
		• Head injury
		• Cerebral thrombosis or hemorrhage
		• CNS depressant drugs
		• Oxygen-induced hypoventilation
		Neuromuscular defects in the ventilatory mechanism
		• Myasthenia gravis
		• Multiple sclerosis
		• Muscular dystrophy
		• Guillain-Barré syndrome
		• Poliomyelitis
		• Spinal cord injuries
		• Botulism
		• Tetanus
		• Neuromuscular blocking drugs
		Obstructive lung conditions
		• Asthma
		• Chronic bronchitis
		• Emphysema
		• Airway obstruction
		• Cystic fibrosis
		Restrictive lung conditions
		• Kyphoscoliosis
		• Obesity hypoventilation syndrome
		• Recent thoracic, abdominal, or flank incision
		• Lung cancer
		• Flail chest
		• Pleural effusion
		• Pneumothorax
			• Physical examination
			  • Neurologic status may be altered
			  • Abnormal chest wall motion
			  • Abnormal breath sounds
			  • Clinical indications of hypoxemia, hypercapnia
			• ABG: hypoxemia with increased $Paco_2$ and normal A:a gradient
			• May have abnormal chest x-ray, PFTs
				• Improve oxygenation by increasing alveolar ventilation (e.g., positioning, bronchial hygiene, drug therapy)
				• Specific therapy is dependent on the specific etiology

V/Q mismatching	Low V/Q units, with perfusion in excess of ventilation, result in hypoxemia because the blood traversing these alveolar units is not fully oxygenated
	High V/Q units, with ventilation in excess of perfusion, result in oxygenated alveolar units, which are not perfused
		Regional ventilation abnormalities
		• Asthma
		• Chronic bronchitis
		• Emphysema
		• Atelectasis
		• Pneumonia
		• Bronchospasm
		• Mucus plugs
		• Foreign bodies
		• Tumor
		Regional perfusion abnormalities
		• Pulmonary embolus
		• Decreased cardiac output/index
		• Excessive PEEp
			• Physical examination
			  • Abnormal chest wall motion
			  • Abnormal breath sounds
			  • Clinical indications of hypoxemia
			• ABG: hypoxemia with a widened A:a gradient; $Paco_2$ dependent on ventilation status
			• Abnormal chest x-ray, PFTs, and/or V/Q scan
				• Oxygen
				• Specific therapy dependent on the specific etiology

TABLE 4-22	Mechanisms of Acute Respiratory Failure—cont'd			
Mechanism	**Pathophysiology**	**Causes**	**Clinical Presentation**	**Management**

Shunt	Blood transverses from the right heart to the left heart without being oxygenated: anatomic shunt is when the blood bypasses the alveolar-capillary unit and physiologic shunt is when the blood goes through the alveolar-capillary unit but it is nonfunctional	Anatomic shunts
		• Normal anatomic shunts: bronchial, pleural, thebesian veins
		• Intrapulmonary shunts: pulmonary A-V fistula
		• Intracardiac shunts: tetralogy of Fallot
		• Other pathologic shunts (e.g., shunts associated with neoplasms)
		Physiologic shunts
		• Alveolar collapse
		  • Atelectasis
		  • Pneumothorax
		  • Hemothorax
		  • Pleural effusion
		• Alveoli filled with a fluid or foreign material
		  • Cardiac pulmonary edema
		  • Noncardiac pulmonary edema (e.g., near-drowning, ARDS)
		  • Pneumonias
			• Physical examination
			  • Abnormal breath sounds
			  • Clinical indications of hypoxemia
			• ABG: hypoxemia with a normal or decreased $Paco_2$
			  • Widened A:a gradient
			  • Shunt >6%
			• May have abnormal chest x-ray, PFTs
				• Oxygen administration has little or no effect
				• Specific therapy dependent on the specific etiology
				• Positive end-expiratory pressure is frequently used for physiologic shunt

Diffusion abnormalities	Increased diffusion pathway: diffusion between alveolar oxygen and pulmonary capillary blood is impaired; blood exiting the gas exchange unit is hypoxemic
	Decreased diffusion area: decrease in alveolar-capillary membrane surface area available for diffusion and/or loss of pulmonary capillary bed
		Increased diffusion pathway
		• Accumulation of fluid
		• Pulmonary edema: cardiac or noncardiac
		• Accumulation of collagen in the pulmonary interstitium
		  • Pulmonary fibrosis
		  • Sarcoidosis
		  • Collagen vascular disease
		Decreased diffusion area
		• Pulmonary resection (e.g., lobectomy, pneumonectomy)
		• Destructive lung diseases
		  • Emphysema
		  • Tumor
		  • Obliterative pulmonary vascular diseases
			• History and physical examination findings are compatible with the diagnosis
			• ABG: hypoxemia with normal or low $Paco_2$
			  • Widened A:a gradient
			  • Further decrease in Pao_2 with exercise
			• PFTs: decreased diffusing capacity for CO
			• Chest x-ray may show cause
				• Oxygen
				• Home oxygen therapy is frequently indicated

In patients with chronic hypercapnia, adjust the flow rate or oxygen concentration to keep Spo_2 approximately 90%. Masks are contraindicated in hypercapnic patients because the high concentration of oxygen provided by these delivery systems would likely further elevate $Paco_2$ levels. Ensure rest periods, especially after meals or activities. Provide a quiet, restful environment. Treat fever with antipyretics, such as acetaminophen (Tylenol), but be aware that doing so is controversial because pyrogens can be helpful in mobilizing the immune system. Cooling blankets may be used, but avoid shivering due to its negative effect on oxygen consumption.

To improve oxygen delivery, optimize Sao_2, cardiac functioning, and hemoglobin. Improve Sao_2 with oxygen. Optimize cardiac status by controlling an adequate heart rate and blood pressure. Improve hemoglobin by administering packed RBCs

as required. If a patient requires hemodynamic monitoring, mechanical ventilation, and vasoactive agents to improve oxygen delivery, facilitate a rapid transfer to a higher-acuity level of care.

Investigate the source and type of infection and obtain cultures of sputum. Treat infection by administering the prescribed antimicrobials, either empirically or specific to the cultured microorganism. Utilize bronchial hygiene techniques. Monitor and teach the patient and family how to monitor for clinical indications of infection. Monitor the patient for complications such as dysrhythmias, pulmonary infections, pulmonary edema, pulmonary embolism, barotrauma (e.g., pneumothorax), pulmonary fibrosis, oxygen toxicity, and renal failure. Also, monitor for acid-base imbalances; electrolyte imbalances; GI complications, such as abdominal distention; ileus; ulcer;

TABLE 4-23   **Bronchodilators**

Drug	Administration	Adverse Effects	Nursing Implications
Short-Acting Beta$_2$-Adrenergic Agents*			
Albuterol (Proventil, Ventolin)	• PO: 2-4 mg every 6-8 hours • Handheld inhaler: 1-2 inhalations every 4-6 hours • Nebulizer: 0.5 mL (2.5 mg) in 3-5 mL of normal saline over 10-15 minutes every 6 hours	• Tachycardia • Palpitations • Nausea, vomiting • Anxiety • Tremor • Headache	• Monitor HR, BP, breath sounds • Note contraindications: known hypersensitivity, glaucoma, tachydysrhythmias; do not give with MAO inhibitors • Use cautiously in older adults and patients with diabetes mellitus, hypertension, hyperthyroidism, cardiac disease, seizure disorder, prostatic hypertrophy • Do not administer with beta-blockers (they block effect)
Metaproterenol (Alupent, Metaprel)	• PO: 20 mg every 6-8 hours • Handheld inhaler: 2-3 inhalations every 3-4 hours • Nebulizer: 0.2-0.3 mL of undiluted 5% solution or 2.5 mL of a 6% solution every 6-8 hours	• Tachycardia • Palpitations • Nausea, vomiting • Anxiety • Tremor • Headache	• Monitor HR, BP, breath sounds • Note contraindications: known hypersensitivity, glaucoma, tachydysrhythmias; do not give with MAO inhibitors • Use cautiously in older adults and patients with diabetes mellitus, hypertension, hyperthyroidism, cardiac disease, seizure disorder, prostatic hypertrophy • Do not administer with beta-blockers (they block effect)
Anticholinergic Agents			
Ipratropium (Atrovent)	• PO: 20 mg every 6-8 hours • Handheld inhaler: 2-3 inhalations every 3-4 hours • Nebulizer: 0.2-0.3 mL of undiluted 5% solution or 2.5 mL of a 6% solution every 6-8 hours	• Tachycardia • Palpitations • Anxiety • Restlessness • Dizziness • Headache • Cough • Blurred vision • Gastrointestinal distress • Dry mouth	• Monitor HR, BP, ECG, respiratory rate and rhythm, breath sounds, urine output and fluid status • Note contraindications: known sensitivity, cardiac dysrhythmias • Use cautiously in older adults and patients with acute MI, HF, hypertension
Methylxanthines			
Aminophylline (Theophylline, Elixophyllin, Tedral, Quibron, Choledyl)	• PO: 250-500 mg every 6-8 hours • IV: loading dose of 5-6 mg/kg (250-500 mg) over 20 minutes followed by infusion • IV infusion: mix 500 mg in 250 mL (2 mg/mL) and infuse at 0.1-0.9 mg/kg/hr • HF, liver disease: ~0.1-0.2 mg/kg/hr • COPD: ~0.3 mg/kg/hr • Smokers: ~0.8 mg/kg/hr • Therapeutic blood level 10-20 mcg/mL	• Tachycardia • Hypotension • Palpitations • Anxiety • Restlessness • Insomnia • Dizziness • Tremors • Headache Signs of toxicity • Anorexia, nausea, vomiting • Ventricular dysrhythmias • Agitation, seizures	• Monitor HR, BP, ECG, respiratory rate and rhythm, breath sounds, urine output and fluid status • Note contraindications: known sensitivity, cardiac dysrhythmias • Use cautiously in older adults and patients with acute MI, HF, hypertension, hepatic disease, acute peptic ulcer, hyperthyroidism, diabetes mellitus • Administer PO drug with meals to decrease GI adverse effects

TABLE 4-23	Bronchodilators—cont'd		
Drug	**Administration**	**Adverse Effects**	**Nursing Implications**
Electrolytes			
Magnesium sulfate	• IV infusion: mix 1-2 g in 100 mL and infuse over 1-4 hours • May also be given by inhalation	• Bradycardia • Hypotension • Diaphoresis • Flushing • Hypermagnesemia resulting in respiratory muscle weakness and arrest	• Monitor HR, BP, respiratory rate, ECG, urine output, deep tendon reflexes (DTRs), mental status • Note contraindications: renal disease • Use cautiously in renal insufficiency, patients on digitalis • Monitor closely for clinical indications of hypermagnesemia: hypotension, AV block, CNS depression, depressed or absent DTRs, muscle weakness or paralysis, respiratory arrest • Administer calcium IV as prescribed for hypermagnesemic effects • Have intubation equipment and mechanical ventilator available

Additional short-acting beta$_2$-adrenergic agents include terbutaline (Brethine, Brethaire), levalbuterol (Xopenex), pirbuterol (Maxair), and bitolterol (Tornalate). Long-acting beta$_2$-stimulants include salmeterol (Serevent) and formoterol (Foradil).

hemorrhage; thromboembolism; disseminated intravascular coagulation (DIC); sepsis or septic shock; and psychological responses, such as psychosis or depression. Provide the patient and family with instructions regarding smoking cessation.

4.18   Learning Activity

Match the cause of acute respiratory failure to the primary treatment.

_____ 1. Upper airway obstruction
_____ 2. Airway secretions
_____ 3. Overdosage of narcotics
_____ 4. Bronchospasm
_____ 5. Pneumothorax
_____ 6. Pneumonia
_____ 7. Postoperative pain
_____ 8. ARDS
_____ 9. Myasthenic crisis
_____ 10. Atelectasis

a. Antimicrobials
b. Deep breathing and incentive spirometry
c. Chest tube
d. Positioning and airway placement
e. Cholinergic drugs and mechanical ventilator
f. Encouragement of coughing; suctioning if patient cannot effectively cough
g. Mechanical ventilation with PEEP
h. Bronchodilators
i. Naloxone (Narcan)
j. Analgesics

Answers to this activity can be found in the Answer Key.

POSTSURGICAL PULMONARY PROBLEMS

Pulmonary problems are a major cause of complication and morbidity after surgery, especially following abdominal and thoracic surgery. Changes in pulmonary function occur normally during the immediate postoperative period. There is a reduction in the forced vital capacity (FVC), functional residual capacity (FRC), and reduced lung compliance resulting in reduced tidal volume and increased respiratory rates. Arterial hypoxemia due to V/Q mismatching is common in the postoperative period in normal patients and is exaggerated in patients with pulmonary conditions like COPD. Microatelectasis is the most common cause of hypoxemia, and the increased respiratory rate frequently leads to respiratory alkalosis. Bacterial invasion of lower airways and reduced clearance after surgery predisposes the patients to postoperative respiratory infection. Patients often have a disturbance in consciousness, which puts them at risk for aspiration of gastric and oropharyngeal contents.

Preoperative hypercapnia, a history of COPD, cigarette smoking, and prolonged anesthesia time are serious risk factors for postoperative complications. Obesity results in a decreased vital capacity, which increases risk. The very young and elderly persons are also at an increased risk. Maximal inspirations are voluntarily limited because of pain, which thereby increases the risk of atelectasis.

The postoperative patient may present with a cough with or without sputum production and the patient may demonstrate a fear of or reluctance to cough, deep breathe, and move about after surgery. Tachypnea, or shallow respirations, may be due to splinting with incision pain and may progress to signs of respiratory distress, increased work of breathing, and dyspnea. If atelectasis progresses to pneumonia, clinical signs include those related to fever and infection. Crackles are heard indicating small airway collapse due to shallow breathing; rhonchi are heard indicating secretions in the larger airways; wheezing indicating airway obstruction; and bronchial breath sounds indicating consolidation may be auscultated.

The priority care focus is on prevention with proper patient positioning and pulmonary hygiene measures. Guide the patient to perform intensive deep breathing using incentive spirometry and early ambulation. Delivery of care is dependent on the severity of the patient's signs and symptoms. Assess the patient frequently for evidence of pulmonary complications after surgery. Treatment measures can range from encouraging pulmonary hygiene measures, oxygen, antibiotics, breathing treatments, and facilitating a transfer to a higher-acuity level of care.

ACUTE RESPIRATORY DISTRESS SYNDROME

ARDS is an acute diffuse, inflammatory lung injury, leading to increased pulmonary vascular permeability, increased lung weight, and loss of aerated lung tissue. It is associated with hypoxemia and bilateral radiographic opacities, associated with increased venous admixture, increased physiological dead space, and decreased lung compliance (Phillips, 2013; Ramieri, Rubenfeld, & Thomson et al., 2012)

Causes of ARDS are categorized into direct injuries that affect the lung directly and indirect injuries that affect the lung indirectly. The risk of death increases if more than one of these conditions occurs simultaneously. Direct injuries include the following:

- Chest trauma, especially pulmonary contusion
- Submersion injury
- Hypervolemia or pulmonary edema
- Inhalation of toxic gases and vapors, such as smoke, chemicals, or high concentrations of oxygen (i.e., oxygen toxicity)
- Pneumonia, including viral, bacterial, or fungal pneumonia
- Aspiration pneumonitis
- Radiation pneumonitis
- Pulmonary embolism, especially fat or amniotic fluid embolism
- Radiation injury
- Drugs such as bleomycin, known to be associated with pulmonary toxicity

The most common cause of ARDS is sepsis. Other indirect causes include the following:

- Prolonged hypotension or shock
- Multisystem trauma, especially with multiple fractures
- Blood transfusion (i.e., transfusion-related lung injury)
- Burns
- Cardiopulmonary bypass
- Disseminated intravascular coagulation (DIC)
- Toxemia of pregnancy
- Acute pancreatitis
- Diabetic coma
- Central nervous system (CNS) injury
- Drug overdosage from heroin, methadone, barbiturates, aspirin, or thiazide diuretics
- Abdominal trauma

4.19 Learning Activity

List five pulmonary and five nonpulmonary causes for ARDS.

Pulmonary	Nonpulmonary
1.	1.
2.	2.
3.	3.
4.	4.
5.	5.

Answers to this activity can be found in the Answer Key.

The pathophysiology of ARDS (Figure 4-26) is the result of a direct or indirect injury to the lung, which triggers an immune/inflammatory response, increased capillary pulmonary edema, and noncardiac pulmonary edema. Refractory hypoxemia, decreased lung compliance, and pulmonary hypertension characterize ARDS.

Early identification of the syndrome and rapid initiation of treatment is required to improve outcomes. The progressive care nurse's role is early identification, initiating treatment and facilitating a rapid transfer to a higher-acuity level of care. Knowledge of the risk factors for ARDS along with an awareness of the four phases of ARDS (Table 4-24) provides a basis for early identification, initiation of treatment and rapid transfer. It is important to note the progression from phase I to phase II includes a normal Pao_2 with hyperventilation causing respiratory alkalosis to normal or slightly decreased Pao_2 with continuing hyperventilation and respiratory alkalosis. In phase III, the Pao_2 is significantly decreased causing tissue hypoxia and metabolic (i.e., lactic) acidosis. Ventilation in phase III is more difficult due to the decreased compliance of the lung increasing the work of breathing which may increase $Paco_2$ and cause a respiratory acidosis. In phase IV, profound hypoxemia occurs, causing tissue hypoxia and metabolic acidosis along with hypoventilation and respiratory acidosis. The progressive care nurse needs to carefully monitor patient with identified risk factors and observe for severe oxygen defect despite oxygen administration. Identification of patients in phase I or II is optimum.

The criteria used in ARDS diagnosis include the following:
- Acute, onset over 1 week or less
- Bilateral opacities consistent with pulmonary edema must be present and may be detected on CT or chest radiograph
- P/F ratio less than 300 mm Hg with a minimum of 5 cm H_2O PEEP (or CPAP)
- Findings not be fully explained by cardiac failure or fluid overload (i.e., an echocardiogram should be performed in most cases if there is no clear cause such as trauma or sepsis).

Diagnostic studies support the diagnosis of ARDS and may also provide information regarding possible causes. ABG results (see Table 4-24) show refractory hypoxemia (i.e., hypoxemia despite high concentration of oxygen). Pulmonary function studies may show decreased lung volumes, including tidal volume

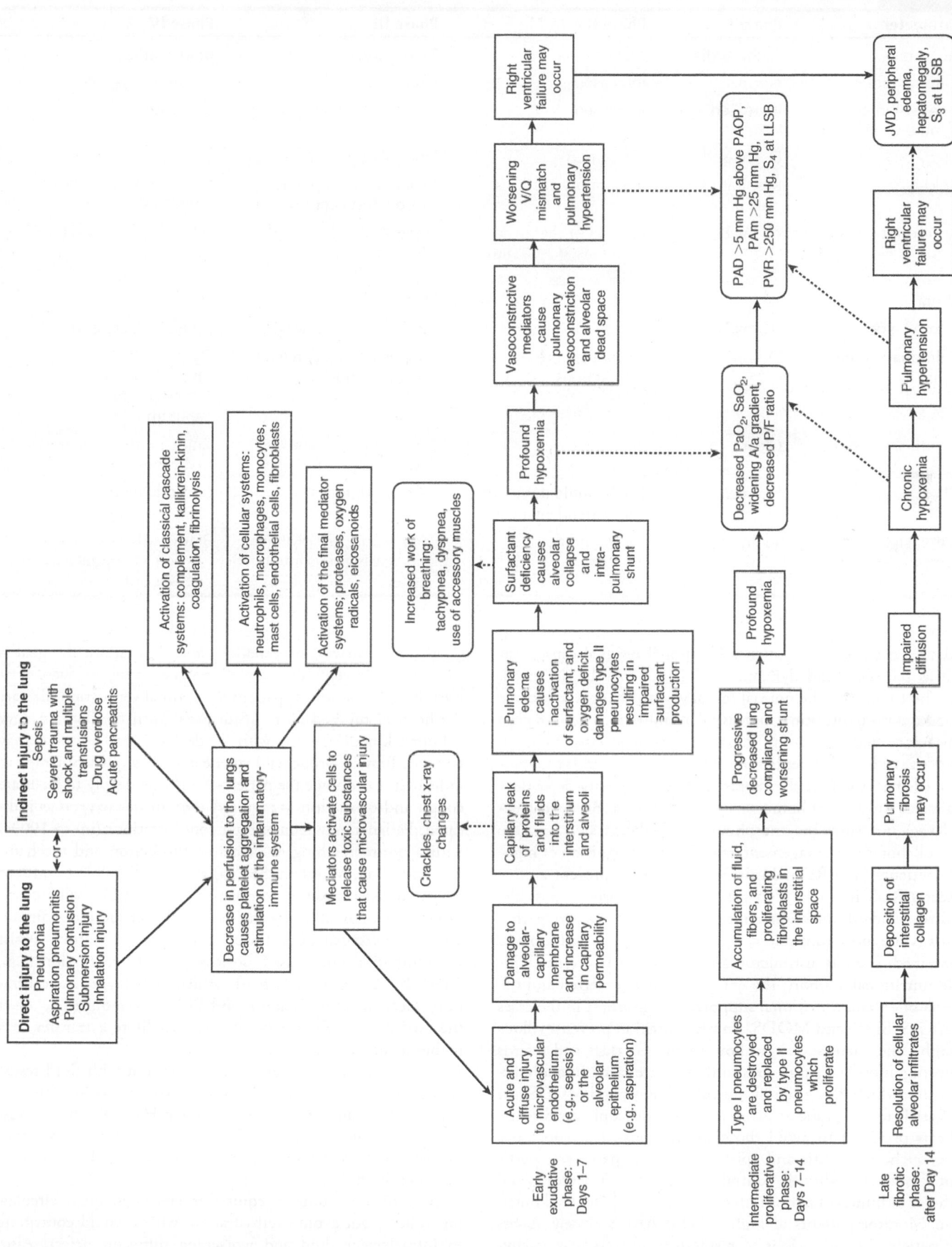

FIGURE 4-26 Pathophysiology of ARDS. Dotted lines connect pathology to the clinical presentation. (From Dennison, R. D. [2013]. *Pass CCRN!* [4th ed.]. St. Louis, MO: Elsevier.)

TABLE 4-24 **Phases of ARDS**

Parameter	Phase I	Phase II	Phase III	Phase IV
Heart rate	Tachycardia	Tachycardia	Tachycardia	Bradycardia
Cardiac index	Normal	Increased	Increased	Decreased
Tidal volume/ Minute ventilation	Increased	Increased	Normal or decreased	Decreased
Paco$_2$	Decreased	Decreased	Normal or increased	Increased
Acid-base	Respiratory alkalosis	Respiratory alkalosis	Metabolic (and possibly respiratory) acidosis	Respiratory and metabolic acidosis
PaO$_2$ on room air	Normal	Normal or slightly decreased (~60 mm Hg)	Significantly decreased (~40 mm Hg)	Severely decreased (~25 mm Hg)
Shunt	<6%	10%	20%	>30%
Compliance	Normal	Slightly decreased	Moderately decreased	Severely decreased
Pulmonary clinical manifestations	Dyspnea	Dyspnea; fatigue; retractions	Dyspnea; fatigue; retractions; cyanosis	Dyspnea; fatigue (may have had respiratory arrest); cyanosis; rusty sputum
Breath sounds	Clear	Fine crackles	Coarse crackles and/or wheezes	Crackles, rhonchi, and/or wheezes
Chest x-ray	Normal	Patchy infiltrates usually in dependent areas	Diffuse infiltrates	Consolidation
Other signs/ symptoms	Tachycardia	Tachycardia	Tachycardia; dysrhythmias; decreasing sensorium	Bradycardia; dysrhythmias; hypotension; decreasing sensorium

and vital capacity. The patient's functional residual capacity as well as the static and dynamic compliance may be decreased. The chest x-ray may be normal initially, with changes to include bilateral diffuse interstitial and alveolar infiltrates, a ground glass appearance, and "white-out" due to massive atelectasis. A normal heart size aids in differentiation of ARDS from cardiac pulmonary edema. A CT of the thorax may reveal gravity-dependent infiltrates and lack of homogeneity of infiltrates. Bronchoalveolar lavage may show polymorphonuclear leukocytes.

Collaborative management begins with recognition of high-risk patients for ARDS. Institute measures to prevent and/or detect ARDS in these high-risk patients as early as possible. Utilize standard infection control measures considering that sepsis is the most common cause. Treat precipitating factors as prescribed, such as antimicrobials if infection is present. Provide nutritional support; the enteral route is preferred and the effects of enteral nutritional support are significant in the cases of ARDS, SIRS, and MODS. Enteral nutrition prevents villous atrophy and increases blood flow to the GI tract and retards transmigration (i.e., translocation) of bacteria or lipopolysaccharides, which play a significant role in sepsis and MODS. An orogastric feeding tube or percutaneous endoscopic gastroscopy tube is preferred to avoid the complications of a nasogastric tube, such as sinusitis and epistaxis. Provide parenteral nutrition if enteral feeding is contraindicated. Use a dedicated IV catheter or lumen of a multilumen catheter for parenteral nutrition. Monitor patients at high risk for ARDS closely. Assess the patient for indications of respiratory distress (e.g., tachypnea, use of accessory muscles) and monitor pulse oximetry for changes in Spo$_2$.

Maintain airway, oxygenation, and ventilation; the goal is to maintain acceptable oxygenation (i.e., Spo$_2$ or Sao$_2$ of at least 90%). Position the patient for optimal ventilation. Elevate the head of the bed 30 to 45 degrees. Turn the patient every 2 hours; kinetic therapy with 60-degree lateral rotation may be used. Provide bronchial hygiene and chest physiotherapy as indicated. Encourage the patient to breathe deeply to facilitate cough and/or suction as required. Administer oxygen as indicated. Patients may require high concentrations (up to 100%) with a nonrebreathing mask before intubation and mechanical ventilation. Maintain the Fio$_2$ as low as possible to prevent oxygen toxicity; positive pressure (CPAP or PEEP) will increase driving pressure, allowing the use of a lower Fio$_2$ to maintain acceptable oxygenation. Ensure adequate ventilation. Assist with initiating noninvasive positive pressure ventilation (e.g., CPAP, BiPAP) with a face mask. When high oxygen concentration, mechanical ventilation, and PEEP are required to meet the goal of a Spo$_2$ or Sao$_2$ of 90%, facilitate a transfer to a higher-acuity level of care.

Avoid overhydration and exercise caution with fluid resuscitation of shock patients. Administer volume as indicated by CVP readings and maintain CVP ~6 cm H$_2$O after fluid resuscitation is achieved (i.e., MAP of at least 60 mm Hg without vasopressors). Administer diuretics as prescribed to decrease intraalveolar fluid.

Administer volume as required to ensure adequate circulating volume but avoid overhydration, which would contribute to intraalveolar fluid and worsening diffusion defect. Also, ensure adequate hemoglobin levels. Provide blood as prescribed for hemoglobin of less than 7 g/dL, but an infusion may be necessary if the hemoglobin is between 8 and 10 g/dL when there is impaired oxygen delivery as evidenced by Svo_2 or $Scvo_2$. (Carson, Carless, & Hébert, 2013). Because there is a known relationship between transfusion and ARDS, try to avoid blood transfusions in patients at risk of ARDS after completion of fluid resuscitation. In this case, erythropoietin (Epogen) may be prescribed (Collins, 2013). Administer inotropes, such as dobutamine (Dobutrex), as prescribed for patients with poor contractility.

In addition to increasing the oxygen delivery to the tissues, it is important to decrease the patient's oxygen consumption. Eliminate unnecessary activity. Provide rest periods after meals and other activities that increase oxygen consumption. Decrease the patient's anxiety by providing anxiolytics or sedatives. Treat fever using antipyretics (e.g., acetaminophen [Tylenol]) and a cooling blanket. The debate continues regarding the benefits of fever reduction because the pyrogens are thought to be essential in mobilizing the immune system. Reducing a patient's fever does reduce their oxygen requirements and may be necessary to reduce the tissue oxygen deficit. Care must be taken while using a cooling blanket to prevent shivering.

Provide treatment for pulmonary hypertension as prescribed. The primary reason for pulmonary hypertension in patients with ARDS is hypoxemia, so utilizing oxygen and CPAP or PEEP to reduce hypoxemia is most important.

Provide nutritional support to prevent respiratory muscle atrophy. Utilize the enteral route if possible. Administer a high-protein and high-calorie diet rich in omega-3 and omega-6 fatty acids (1-2 g/kg of ideal body weight (IBW) of protein). To prevent exogenous protein and muscle tissue from catabolism and to meet nutritional requirements, patients should take in 20 to 25 kcal/kg of IBW of nonprotein calories. Nonprotein carbohydrate calories increase carbon dioxide production. Reduced carbohydrate formulas, such as Pulmocare, may be preferable, especially in patients with hypercapnia. Replace multivitamins and minerals, particularly vitamins A, C, and E; zinc; and selenium.

Monitor for complications, including secondary infections, such as nosocomial pneumonia, sepsis, shock, MODS, airway trauma, dysrhythmias, pulmonary embolism, pulmonary fibrosis, pneumothorax, GI hemorrhage, DIC, heart failure, and renal failure.

PULMONARY ARTERIAL HYPERTENSION (PAH)/PULMONARY HYPERTENSION (PH)

Pulmonary arterial hypertension is the abnormal elevation of the pressure in the blood vessels of the lungs. It may be primary pulmonary arterial hypertension (PAH) or secondary pulmonary hypertension (PH). Primary pulmonary arterial hypertension affects the small to medium-size arteries in the vascular bed of the lung, which causes high pulmonary vascular pressures. Idiopathic PAH is more likely in women, usually between the ages of 20 and 40 years (Gin-Sing, 2010). Other risk factors include oral contraceptive use, elevated catecholamines, hepatic dysfunction, and hereditary factors. Toxins or drugs (e.g., fen-phen) may induce PAH. Other possible causes include pulmonary veno-occlusive disease or pulmonary capillary hemangiomatosis, connective tissue disease, HIV, portal hypertension, congenital heart disease, chronic hemolytic anemia, and

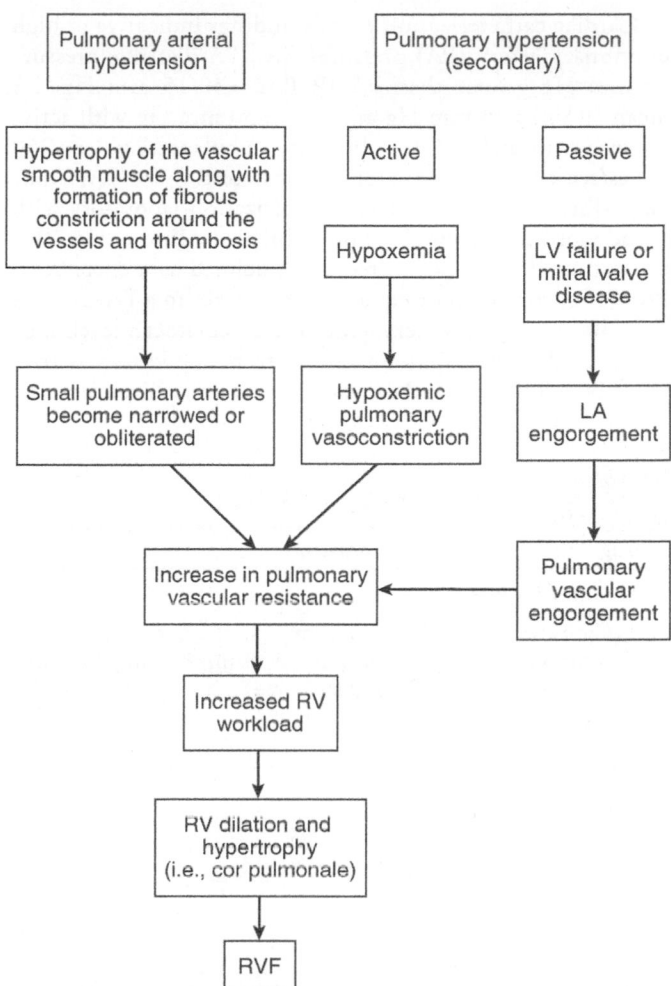

FIGURE 4-27 Pathophysiology of pulmonary arterial hypertension and pulmonary hypertension. (From Dennison, R. D. [2013]. *Pass CCRN!* [4th ed.]. Philadelphia, PA: Elsevier.)

schistosomiasis. Secondary PAH is when high pulmonary vascular pressures are secondary to another pathologic state. Possible causes include left ventricular failure, lung disease and/or hypoxemia, and chronic thromboembolic disease. Thyroid disorders, chronic renal failure, sarcoidosis, and vasculitis may cause PH, but the mechanism is unclear.

The pathophysiology of primary PAH and secondary PHPAH (Figure 4-27) causes an increase in pulmonary vascular resistance (PVR). This increased PVR increases the workload on the right ventricle and right ventricular failure (RVF).

Patients with primary PAH or secondary PH complain primarily of dyspnea, initially exertional dyspnea progressing to dyspnea with mild exertion to dyspnea at rest. They may also report fatigue, lethargy, chest discomfort, palpitations, syncope, and cyanosis. Clinical findings include tachypnea, use of accessory muscles, cough with possible hemoptysis, and an accentuated P_2 (i.e., the second component of S_2). Patients may also have clinical indications of right ventricular hypertrophy (RVH) (i.e., right ventricular heave and/or right-sided S_4). They may also exhibit clinical indications of RVF, including jugular venous distention (JVD), peripheral edema, hepatomegaly, and a murmur of tricuspid regurgitation (i.e., systolic murmur at lower left sternal border).

Cardiac catheterization reveals findings indicative of high pulmonary artery (PA) pressures (i.e., PA diastolic pressure >5 mm Hg greater than PAOP, PAP >30/15 mm Hg, PA mean [PAm] >25 mm Hg at rest or >30 mm Hg with activity with a normal PAOP, pulmonary vascular resistance >250 dynes/sec/cm^{-5}). Vasodilator response testing for PAH may be performed in the cardiac catheterization laboratory with IV adenosine or epoprostenol or inhaled nitric oxide. This test can confirm an acute response, defined as a decrease in PAm of greater than or equal to 10 mm Hg to a PAm of less than 40 mm Hg. The hemoglobin and hematocrit levels may be elevated. Erythropoietin release from the kidney is triggered by hypoxemia and causes polycythemia. Liver function studies may be elevated. ABGs may be normal at rest, but hypoxemia occurs with exertion. Eventually hypoxemia will occur even at rest. The chest x-ray may show cardiomegaly with dilated central pulmonary vessels. The ECG may reveal right atrial enlargement and right ventricular hypertrophy. Echocardiograms evaluate heart size, function, and blood flow. A V/Q scan evaluate for the presence of a pulmonary embolism.

Collaborative management begins with treatment of the cause. Discontinue any causative drug. Provide fibrinolytics, pulmonary embolectomy, and/or anticoagulants as prescribed if pulmonary embolism is the cause. To decrease pulmonary vascular pressures, administer pulmonary vasodilators (Table 4-25)

TABLE 4-25   Pulmonary Vasodilators

Drug	Administration	Adverse Effects	Nursing Implications
Calcium Channel Blockers			
Nifedipine (Procardia)	• PO immediate release: 10-30 mg tid or qid; maximum 180 mg/24 hour • PO sustained release: 30-120 mg daily	• Tachycardia • Dysrhythmias • Hypotension • Nausea, vomiting, heartburn • Diarrhea or constipation • Headache • Flushing • Fatigue • Dizziness • Rash • Pedal edema • Hypokalemia	• Monitor HR, BP, potassium • Note contraindications: known hypersensitivity, severe aortic stenosis • Use caution in HF, sick sinus syndrome, second- or third-degree AV block, systolic BP <90 mm Hg, liver disease, renal insufficiency or failure, and in the elderly
Methylxanthines			
Aminophylline (Theophylline, Elixophyllin, Tedral, Quibron, Choledyl): see Table 4-22			
Direct Vasodilators			
Prostanoids			
Epoprostenol (Flolan)	• IV infusion by central venous catheter: 2-15 ng/kg/min titrated based on symptoms and adverse effects • Inhalation	• Flushing • Hypotension • Headache • Nausea/vomiting • Diarrhea • Anxiety • Skeletal pain • Jaw pain • Flulike symptoms • Thrombocytopenia • Central venous catheter infections	• Monitor HR, BP, and for clinical indications of central venous catheter infection and/or sepsis • Requires refrigeration • Administered by central venous catheter if given IV • Do not stop abruptly; can lead to worsening of PH • Monitor for indications of platelet dysfunction (i.e., petechiae, bleeding)
Iloprost (Ventavis)	• PO: 50-300 mcg bid • IV infusion by central venous catheter: 2-4 ng/kg/min • Inhalation: 2.5-5 mcg 6-9 times/day but not more than every 2 hours	• Flushing • Hypotension • Supraventricular tachycardia • Headache • Insomnia • Nausea/vomiting • Flulike symptoms • Cough (from inhalation) • Infusion site pain	• Monitor HR, BP, and for clinical indications of central venous catheter infection and/or sepsis • Administered by central venous catheter if given IV

TABLE 4-25	Pulmonary Vasodilators—cont'd		
Drug	**Administration**	**Adverse Effects**	**Nursing Implications**
Treprostinil (Remodulin [IV], Tyvaso [inhalation])	• IV or subcutaneous infusion: 1.25 ng/kg/min (or 0.625 ng/kg/min if it is not tolerated or the patient has mild to moderate hepatic insufficiency); dose should be increased based on clinical response in increments of 1.25 ng/kg/min per week for the first 4 weeks of treatment and 2.5 ng/kg/min per week after that • Inhalation: 3 breaths (18 mcg of treprostinil) per treatment session, qid	• Rash • Flushing • Headache • Nausea • Diarrhea • Jaw pain • Thrombocytopenia • Pain at infusion site • Cough, throat irritation with inhalation	• Monitor HR, BP, ECG • Administered IV by central venous catheter; continuous subcutaneous administration is preferred • Monitor for indications of platelet dysfunction (i.e., petechiae, bleeding) • Use cautiously in patients with hepatic insufficiency
Endothelin Receptor Antagonists			
Bosentan (Tracleer)	• PO: started at 62.5 mg bid for 4 weeks and then increased to 125 mg bid	• Elevation of liver enzymes, hepatotoxicity • Anemia • Headache • Flushing • Hypotension • Chest pain • Syncope • Respiratory tract infections • Peripheral edema	• Monitor HR, BP, ECG, liver function studies • Requires liver function studies monthly and hematocrit every 3 months
Ambrisentan (Letairis)	• PO: 5-10 mg daily	• Elevation of liver enzymes • Anemia • Peripheral edema • Headache • Flushing • Hypotension • Syncope	• Monitor HR, BP, ECG, liver function studies • Requires liver function studies monthly and hematocrit every 3 months
Phosphodiesterase Type 5 Inhibitors			
Sildenafil (Viagra, Revatio)	• PO: 20 mg tid	• Headache • Dyspepsia • Flushing • Dyspnea • Epistaxis • Hearing loss	• Monitor HR, BP, ECG • Should not be administered with nitrates
Tadalafil (Adcirca)	• PO: 2.5-40 mg daily	• Headache • Flushing • Hypotension • Myalgias • Nasopharyngitis • Respiratory tract infections • Hearing or vision loss	• Monitor HR, BP, ECG • Should not be administered with nitrates

as prescribed. These drugs are useful for relaxing the smooth muscle of the pulmonary vascular system and are indicated for PAH and are sometimes used for secondary PH. Because the most common cause of secondary PH is hypoxemia, first administer oxygen to maintain SpO_2 and SaO_2 greater than 90%. Secondary PH caused by left ventricular failure requires treatment of the heart failure. Administer diuretics as prescribed

and maintain a sodium-restricted diet (2-3 g/day) for congestive symptoms. Administer inotropic agents, such as digoxin, as prescribed.

Prepare patients for surgery, as requested to treat the cause (e.g., valve repair or replacement). Balloon dilation atrial septostomy for severe primary PH is a palliative treatment for patients with primary PH refractory to vasodilator therapy.

BOX 4-5

Microorganisms Most Commonly Associated with Pneumonia

Bacteria
Bacterial Agents Associated with Community-Acquired Pneumonia (CAP)
- *Streptococcus pneumoniae* (most common)
- *Haemophilus influenzae*
- *Staphylococcus aureus*
- *Enterobacter* species
- *Streptococcus pyogenes*
- *Chlamydia pneumoniae*
- *Legionella pneumophila*
- *Mycoplasma pneumoniae*
- *Moraxella catarrhalis*
- *Bacteroides fragilis*
- *Mycobacterium tuberculosis*

Bacterial Agents Associated with Health Care–Associated Pneumonia (HCAP)
- *Pseudomonas* species
- *Staphylococcus aureus*
- *Enterobacter* species
- *Klebsiella pneumoniae*
- *Escherichia coli*
- *Haemophilus influenzae*
- *Serratia marcescens*
- *Streptococcus* species
- *Proteus mirabilis*
- *Acinetobacter* species
- *Legionella pneumophila*

Bacterial Agents Associated with Ventilator-Associated Pneumonia (VAP)
Early Onset
- *Staphylococcus aureus*
- *Streptococcus pneumoniae*

- *Haemophilus influenzae*
- *Moraxella catarrhalis*
- *Proteus* species
- *Serratia marcescens*
- *Klebsiella pneumoniae*
- *Escherichia coli*

Late Onset (More Likely to Be Antibiotic Resistant)
- Methicillin-resistant *Staphylococcus aureus*
- *Pseudomonas aeruginosa*
- *Klebsiella pneumoniae*
- *Acinetobacter* species
- *Enterobacter* species

Viruses
- Adenovirus
- Hantavirus
- Influenza types A and B
- Respiratory syncytium virus (RSV)

Fungi
- *Histoplasma capsulatum*
- *Coccidioides immitis*
- *Candida* species
- *Aspergillus* species

Parasitic involvement
- *Pneumocystis carinii*

Mycoplasma
- *Mycoplasma pneumonia*

In this procedure, the surgeon creates an atrial septal defect. The resultant right-to-left shunting improves left ventricular filling and cardiac output, offsetting the desaturation of the blood that bypassed the lung. Patients may also require lung or heart-lung transplantation. Patients with primary PH who fail to respond to therapy may meet the criteria for a single or double lung transplant. Patients with left ventricular disease or congenital structural abnormalities may meet the criteria for a heart-lung transplant.

Provide the patient and family with instruction and counseling regarding lifestyle modification and the need for pharmacologic therapy. Inform the patient and family that continuous oxygen therapy is prescribed and teach them safety measures associated with oxygen therapy. Patients should avoid high altitudes, which would decrease the driving pressure of oxygen and worsen hypoxemia. They will require oxygen when flying. Additional recommendations include a low-sodium (2-3 g) diet, smoking cessation, moderate exercise while avoiding overexertion, and energy conservation methods. Instruct the patient to avoid the use of oral anticoagulants, decongestants, aspirin, and NSAIDs. The patient needs to avoid pregnancy, so recommend another method of birth control other than oral contraceptives.

PNEUMONIA

Pneumonia is an infectious, inflammatory process of the lung parenchyma, including the alveolar spaces and interstitial tissue. Community-acquired pneumonia (CAP) is an infection of the lungs in individuals who have not been recently hospitalized. Health care–associated pneumonia (HCAP) involves an acute infection of the lungs that develops after 48 hours of hospitalization. HCAP is also referred to as *nosocomial pneumonia* or *hospital-acquired pneumonia*. HCAP is associated with a more virulent organism than CAP. These organisms are often resistant to multiple antibiotics. Ventilator-associated pneumonia (VAP) is a subtype of HCAP and, as the name implies, is associated with intubation and mechanical ventilation. Early-onset VAP usually develops within 4 days of intubation and mechanical ventilation. Late-onset VAP develops 5 or more days after intubation and mechanical ventilation. The most likely microorganisms of pneumonia vary for CAP, HCAP, and VAP (Box 4-5).

Patient-related risk factors for pneumonia include advanced age; a history of smoking; the presence of periodontal disease; an altered level of consciousness; chronic illness, such as COPD; diabetes mellitus; cardiovascular disease; malignancy; and severe acute illness, such as shock, head

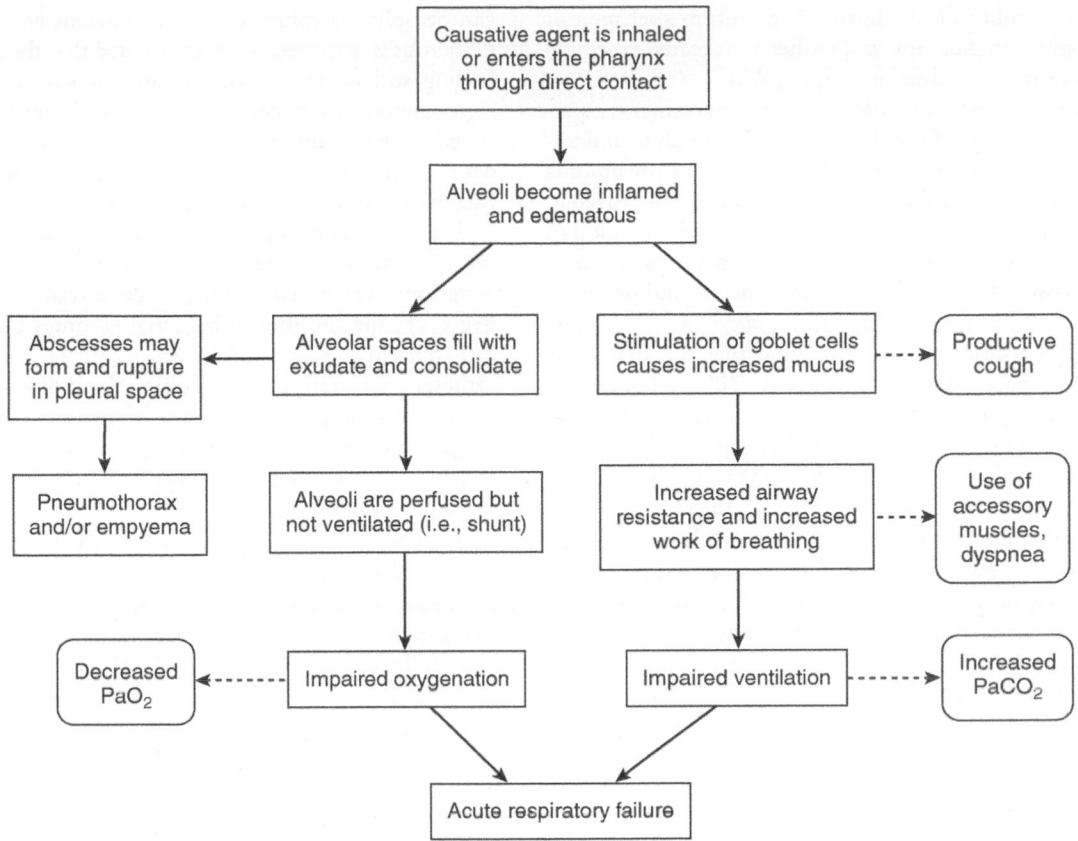

FIGURE 4-28 Pathophysiology of pneumonia. Dotted lines connect pathology to the clinical presentation. (From Dennison, R. D. [2013]. *Pass CCRN!* [4th ed.]. St. Louis, MO: Elsevier.)

injury, or chest trauma. Malnutrition increases the risk of pneumonia. Alcoholism, malignancy, eating disorder, and/or poverty may cause malnutrition. Immunocompromised patients, such as patients with neutropenia resulting from acute leukemia or cytotoxic agents, are particularly susceptible to pneumonia. Chronic immobility also increases risk of pneumonia.

Treatment-related risk factors for pneumonia include surgery, artificial airways, bronchoscopy, nasogastric tubes, and mechanical ventilation. Thoracic, abdominal, or flank incisions, craniotomy, long anesthesia time, and prolonged hospitalization increase the risk of pneumonia. Aspiration of colonized material is also implicated in development of pneumonia; antibiotic therapy allows colonization of the oropharynx. Proton pump inhibitors, H_2-receptor antagonists, and antacids allow bacteria that are normally killed by the extreme acid environment of the stomach to survive and be aspirated into the lungs. Supine position and broad-spectrum antibiotics also increase risk of pneumonia.

Other risk factors for pneumonia are related to poor infection-control practices. These include inadequate hand washing, failure to change gloves between contacts with patients, failure to wear appropriate protective equipment (especially when antibiotic-resistant bacterial strains have been identified), inadequate disinfection/sterilization of devices, contaminated water in a humidification system, and contaminated respiratory therapy or anesthesia equipment.

The pathophysiology of pneumonia (Figure 4-28) includes alveolar consolidation and increased mucus. These result in a shunt, increased airway resistance, and increased work of

breathing, which impairs both oxygenation and ventilation and potentially leads to acute respiratory failure.

A patient with pneumonia frequently complains of cold or flulike symptoms such as chills, fever, malaise, headache, and myalgia. They may also complain of chest pain, which is frequently pleuritic-type pain. Some patients exhibit confusion; this is more common in elderly patients. Tachycardia, tachypnea, diaphoresis, and fever are common, though elderly patients may be hypothermic. Clinical indications of dehydration (i.e., oliguria, poor skin turgor, dry mucous membranes) may be present. A productive cough with mucoid or rusty, bloody, or purulent sputum that may have a foul odor may be present. Splinting of the chest with decreased chest excursion and use of accessory muscles may be evident with breathing. There will be dullness to percussion over areas of consolidation and breath sound changes. The breath sounds may be diminished and bronchial breath sounds may be present over the area of consolidation. Crackles, rhonchi, and/or a rub may be audible.

An elevated WBC count with a shift to the left (i.e., increased in bands) indicates bacterial involvement, but levels may be normal in elderly patients, immunocompromised patients, or in patients with overwhelming infection. The WBC count may be normal or decreased if the pneumonia is of viral origin. ABGs will likely show a decrease in Pao_2 and the $Paco_2$ may increase, decrease, or remain stable depending on ventilation.

A blood culture will be positive for a specific organism in bacteremia. Obtain a Gram stain, acid-fast stain and a culture and sensitivity tests to identify a specific bacterial organism. An acid-fast stain rules out tuberculosis. A PPD skin test also rules out exposure to tuberculosis. Induce the sputum specimen or obtain through bronchoscopy with either a protected specimen brush (PSB) or bronchoalveolar lavage (BAL).

A chest x-ray localizes the infection and determines the pattern of inflammation. Bronchopneumonia involves inflammation of the bronchioles and alveoli. Interstitial pneumonia involves inflammation of the tissue around the alveoli. Alveolar pneumonia, usually caused by a virus, involves inflammation of the alveoli. Necrotizing pneumonia involves necrosis of a portion of lung tissue. Diffuse changes can indicate viral pneumonia. Pleural effusion may indicate empyema.

CURB-65 is a clinical scoring method that can determine mortality in patients with CAP (Lim et al., 2003). The criteria include **C**onfusion, **U**remia (i.e., BUN >20 mg/dL), **R**espiratory rate (i.e., ≥30 breaths/min); low **B**lood pressure (i.e., systolic BP <90 mm Hg or diastolic BP ≤60 mm Hg; and age ≥**65** years. The number of criteria determines the recommended level of care. A patient with one criterion are likely to be treated as an outpatient, a patient with two criteria should be admitted to an inpatient unit, such as a progressive care unit, and a patient with three or more criteria often requires critical care admission.

The first goal for all patients, especially for high-risk patients, is to prevent nosocomial pneumonia (HCAP). In patients with pneumonia, it is important to maintain standard precautions and prevent cross-contamination. Wash your hands with soap and water or a waterless antiseptic agent before and after any contact with the patient and after contact with mucous membranes, respiratory secretions, or objects contaminated with respiratory secretions. Wear gloves for handling respiratory secretions or any object contaminated by respiratory secretions. Avoid wearing jewelry, artificial nails or tips, and nail polish because bacteria can accumulate underneath.

To prevent colonization, which can contribute to pneumonia, avoid unnecessary antibiotics (e.g., prophylactic antibiotics in situations where not warranted). To prevent stress ulcers, use the enteral route for nutrition and use agents such as sucralfate (Carafate) rather than agents that reduce the acidity of gastric secretions. Agents that alter the pH of gastric secretions, such as H_2-receptor antagonists, and proton pump inhibitors increase the risk of HAP and CAP (Fohl & Regal, 2011).

Provide oral care every 2 to 4 hours. Use suction foam swabs to clean teeth and tongue, followed by moisturizing swabs and water-soluble lip balm. Suction the oropharynx twice daily. Rinse the oral catheter with sterile water or saline after each use. Store the oropharyngeal suction catheter in an unsealed bag when not in use. Replace the oropharyngeal suction device, tubing, and suction canister every 24 hours. Brush the patient's teeth to prevent dental plaque colonization with a small soft-bristle toothbrush along with toothpaste, preferably with an alkaline pH. Remove partial dentures and thoroughly cleaned. Use chlorhexidine gluconate (Peridex) 0.12% by spray or rinse as prescribed. Chlorhexidine is a broad-spectrum antibacterial agent that is not absorbed through the skin or mucous membranes. Prophylactic preoperative care may include this oral care to prevent the occurrence of postsurgical infection.

Use aseptic preparation and maintenance of enteral feedings to prevent contamination and gastric colonization. An orogastric tube is preferred over a nasogastric; however, the risk of gastric reflux is still present because it also causes incompetence of the gastroesophageal sphincter. A percutaneous endoscopic gastrostomy tube is preferred if it is anticipated that the need for enteral feeding will be prolonged. To prevent gastric distention and regurgitation, ensure correct placement of a feeding tube. Evaluate gastric retention for patients receiving enteral feedings. Duodenal or jejunal feedings may be beneficial to prevent aspiration. Remove the nasogastric or orogastric tube as soon as possible.

Perform suctioning of the airway only when necessary and avoid saline lavage. Saline lavage is ineffective in liquefying secretions, accentuates oxygen desaturation and dislodges five times the number of bacterial colonies than the suction catheter alone (Zahran & El-Razik, 2011). Rinse the suction catheter after suctioning by pulling the inline suction catheter back to the black line and injecting saline injected into the irrigation port while suction is maintained. Elevate the head of bed to 30 to 45 degrees. Turn and reposition the patient every 2 hours.

To detect HCAP and VAP, obtain a culture for any patient with a new or changing infiltrate on chest x-ray who also exhibits at least two of the following: fever, leukocytosis, or purulent sputum. Assist with the acquisition of high-quality cultures, such as bronchoalveolar lavage (BAL) or protected specimen brush (PSB) cultures if indicated. Nonbronchoscopic collection of endotracheal aspirates from the lower airways or nonbronchoscopic bronchoalveolar lavage may be used, but these produce a lower-quality culture (Baselski & Klutts, 2013).

Administer antimicrobials as prescribed for bacterial infection. Patients with CAP should be started on antibiotics within 4 hours of arrival to the hospital; broad-spectrum antibiotics are generally prescribed initially empirically (i.e., for the most likely organism[s] as determined by experience). The patient response and/or culture results determine whether the antibiotic is changed. Administer other antimicrobials as prescribed for nonbacterial infections.

Provide adequate hydration (2-3 L/24 hr) unless contraindicated by cardiac or renal disease. Oral fluids should be noncaffeinated. Provide IV fluids (usually D_5NS). Maintain patent airways and improve ventilation first by positioning the patient for optimal ventilation. Elevate the head of bed to 30 to 45 degrees. Turn the patient from "good lung down" to supine. To prevent atelectasis and pneumonia, especially in postoperative or immobile patients, encourage the patient to breathe deeply and use incentive spirometry. Provide adequate analgesia so that the patient can breathe deeply.

Maintain bronchial hygiene and provide chest physiotherapy as indicated. Inspiratory maneuvers should include deep breathing and incentive spirometry. Provide humidified air and/or oxygen. Encourage the patient to cough or suction the patient if the patient is unable to clear airways. Provide postural drainage, percussion, and vibration, if necessary. Provide bronchodilators as prescribed. Although expectorants (e.g., guaifenesin [Robitussin], potassium iodide [SSKI]) may be used, hydration is most important. Water is the best expectorant. If necessary, administer mucolytics (e.g., acetylcysteine [Mucomyst]) to decrease the tenacity of the mucus. Sedatives should be generally avoided unless the patient is very agitated or on mechanical ventilation. Avoid the use of antitussives unless the cough is nonproductive and causing fatigue. Prepare the patient for bronchoscopy as requested. Bronchoscopy may be necessary if airway clearance techniques are inadequate.

Ensure intubation and mechanical ventilation as indicated, particularly if the $PaCO_2$ continues to rise and acidosis develops. The goal of mechanical ventilation is to normalize the pH, not necessarily the $PaCO_2$. Optimize oxygen delivery and decrease oxygen consumption. Administer oxygen via nasal cannula or mask. Avoid masks in chronically hypercapnic patients because the high concentration of oxygen provided by these delivery systems would likely further elevate the $PaCO_2$ level. The flow rate or oxygen concentration should be maintained to keep the SpO_2 approximately 95% unless contraindicated. In patients with chronic hypercapnia, adjust the flow rate or oxygen concentration to keep the SpO_2 approximately 90%. Provide rest periods, especially after meals or activities. Treat fever with antipyretics and a cooling blanket.

Monitor patients for complications. The most significant complications include acute respiratory failure, acute respiratory distress syndrome, pleural effusion, empyema, lung abscess, sepsis, and septic shock. If the $PaCO_2$ continues to rise and acidosis develops, the patient will require intubation and mechanical ventilation. Facilitate a transfer to a higher-acuity level of care.

Provide instruction and counseling to the patient and family on the need to modify lifestyle and adhere to pharmacologic therapy. Include the importance of immunizations (e.g., influenza, *Pneumococcus, Haemophilus*), hydration, proper nutrition, smoking cessation, hand washing techniques, disposal of tissues, and prevention of cross-contamination. Emphasize the recognition of symptoms to report to the physician and the importance of taking the entire prescription of prescribed antimicrobials.

ASPIRATION LUNG DISORDER

Aspiration lung disorder describes several clinical syndromes. The disorder generally relates to a lung injury caused by the inhalation of gastric contents, oropharyngeal secretions, food, or other foreign material into the tracheobronchial tree. Another related syndrome is aspiration pneumonitis (also referred to as *Mendelson syndrome*), a chemical injury of the lung caused by aspiration of gastric contents, oropharyngeal secretions, or exogenous liquids. Aspiration pneumonia is a lung infection caused by aspiration of colonized oropharyngeal or gastric contents.

Aspiration-related lung disorders are more common in patients with altered consciousness and/or altered gag reflex. They are associated with increased age; sedation; anesthesia, especially in emergency surgery when the patient has eaten recently; CNS disorders, including cerebral infarction or hemorrhage, seizures, and neuromuscular diseases; and drug or alcohol intoxication. They may also be associated with altered anatomy, resulting from an endotracheal tube, which keeps the epiglottis splinted open. A tracheostomy tube also impairs the swallowing mechanism. A nasogastric or orogastric tube causes incompetence of the gastroesophageal sphincter. Other etiologies include GI tamponade (e.g., Sengstaken-Blakemore tube); facial, neck, or oral trauma; and poor oral hygiene. Associated GI conditions include esophageal abnormalities (e.g., tracheoesophageal fistula or stricture) and gastroesophageal reflux, which is further associated with obesity, hiatal hernia, and pregnancy. Decreased GI motility (e.g., diabetic gastroparesis); GI hemorrhage; vomiting; and intestinal obstruction, both functional (e.g., ileus) and structural (e.g., tumor, volvulus), have also been associated aspiration lung disorder. Patients on enteral nutritional support frequently experience impaired gastric motility especially when complicated by perfusion deficits, sepsis, or drugs (e.g., propofol, opioid). Problems may occur in patients improperly positioned, especially those on enteral feedings. Certain drugs decrease gastroesophageal sphincter tone, including anticholinergics (e.g., atropine), adrenergics (e.g., dopamine), nitrates, caffeine, calcium channel blockers (e.g., nifedipine), and estrogen.

The pathophysiology of aspiration lung disorder (Figure 4-29) varies with the nature of the aspirate. The most significant possible changes are airway obstruction and asphyxia, shunt and hypoxemia, bronchospasm and increased airway resistance, damage to type II pneumocytes and decreased lung compliance, pneumonia, and acute respiratory failure.

The patient's history may include an episode of vomiting followed by coughing and dyspnea. The patient may also report chest pain, usually pleuritic in nature, and anxiety. Note the presence of tachycardia, tachypnea, fever, and increased work of breathing, including use of accessory muscles and intercostal retractions. The patient may have a productive cough, or food or stomach contents may be visible in secretions suctioned from lungs. If enteral feedings are aspirated, the suctioned secretions will positive for glucose. A pink, frothy sputum may occur with acidic aspiration. Breath sounds may include stridor if an obstruction of the upper airway occurs. The breath sounds may be diminished and adventitious sounds, such as crackles, rhonchi, or wheezing, may be audible. Hypoxemia (i.e., decreased SpO_2, SaO_2, PaO_2) and clinical indications of hypoxia (see Box 4-2) may also occur.

Diagnostic findings include increased WBC and changes in ABGs. Hypoxemia (i.e., decreased PaO_2 and SaO_2) will be present. The $PaCO_2$ may be normal, decreased, or increased depending on the ventilation pattern (i.e., may be low due to hyperventilation or high due to hypoventilation). Analysis of sputum may reveal the presence of polymorphonuclear leukocytes. Culture and sensitivity would identify the infecting organism in the presence of pneumonia. The chest x-ray may show bilateral patchy infiltrates or atelectasis, and pulmonary edema may be present.

It is important to examine tracheal aspirate, visually or via analysis, to determine whether aspiration has occurred. Pepsin, a proxy for gastric contents, will likely be the most sensitive indicator of aspiration. Glucose oxidase reagent strips can detect the presence of glucose and the strips are more sensitive than the dye method. Potential problems with the diagnosis of aspiration of enteral feedings can occur when there is blood in tracheal secretions, which may cause a false-positive test result. Low glucose formulas may not cause a positive result. Concerns regarding specificity have arisen because some patients not fed via the enteral route have had positive results. There have also been concerns about the validity of using strips intended for blood or urine for tracheal aspirate. The outdated practice of adding blue dye (i.e., blue food coloring) to enteral feedings to aid in the visual assessment of tracheal aspirate for discoloration is no longer practiced. Blue dye may result in generalized absorption from the GI tract, particularly in patients with multiple organ failure, causing discoloration of body fluids and tissues, possible fatal liver toxicity, and questionable specificity as discoloration of tracheal secretions may have occurred by the systemic route. Dyes may also result in infection due to contamination of the food coloring, interfere with occult blood testing, trigger allergic reactions in some

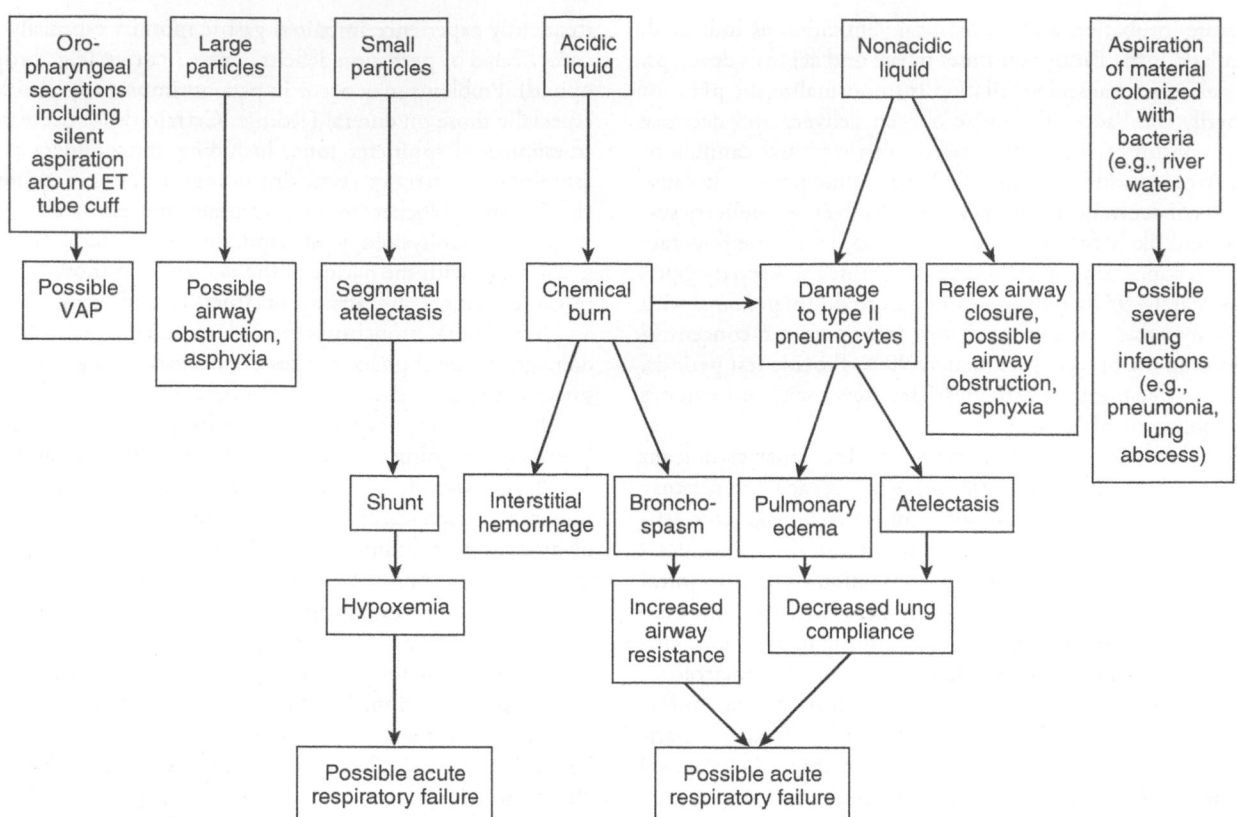

FIGURE 4-29 Pathophysiology of aspiration lung disorder. (From Dennison, R. D. [2013]. *Pass CCRN!* [4th ed.]. St. Louis, MO: Elsevier.)

people due to presence of FD&C yellow No. 5, and provide relatively low sensitivity.

A priority of management for all patients at high risk for aspiration is to institute appropriate preventive measures. Utilize appropriate positioning to reduce the risk of aspiration and reduce the volume aspirated should vomiting occur. Place unconscious patients in a side-lying position. Avoid using the flat position, especially in patients receiving enteral feedings. Keep the HOB elevated to 45 degrees continuously for patients on continuous feedings and for at least 30 minutes after intermittent feedings. Stop continuous enteral feedings at least 30 minutes before any procedure that requires lowering the HOB except for brief lowering of the HOB for repositioning. If the HOB cannot be elevated, position the patient on the right side as much as possible to facilitate movement of gastric contents through the pylorus and allow drainage of emesis out of the mouth to prevent aspiration. Do not restrain patients in such a way that they cannot protect their airway if vomiting occurs.

Select an appropriate tube and site for enteral feeding. Use intragastric feedings when GI motility is normal because they are easier and less expensive to place than small intestinal tubes. However, small lumen feeding tubes cause less gastroesophageal incompetence than do larger lumen nasogastric tubes. Tubes that do not go through the gastroesophageal sphincter (e.g., percutaneous endoscopic gastrostomy [PEG] or needle jejunostomy tubes) are best for long-term enteral feeding. Use small intestinal tubes and feedings when GI motility is impaired. However, because these feedings do increase gastric secretions and duodenal feedings may reflux back into the stomach, aspiration is still possible.

Maintain proper functioning of the nasogastric, orogastric, or intestinal tube utilized for gastric suctioning or enteral feeding. More than one method to verify tube placement should be utilized (Metheny, 2009). During the procedure, note any indications of respiratory distress. Use capnography if available unless the patient is on proton pump inhibitors or other acid-suppressing medications, or continuous tube feedings. Measure the pH of aspirate from the tube. Gastric secretions have a pH of 4 or less unless the patient is receiving acid-suppressing medications or continuous feedings. Intestinal secretions have a pH of greater than 7. Radiographic confirmation is the recommended practice for blindly inserted gastrointestinal tubes. Ensure that a health care provider has read the x-ray. Auscultatory (i.e., air bolus) and water bubbling methods are unreliable. Reassess placement every 4 hours. Be alert to any change in the length of tubing outside of the patient by monitoring the markings on the tube.

Monitor patients receiving gastric enteral feedings for gastric retention (i.e., gastric residual). Though currently controversial, the recommendation remains is still to check for retention before the administration of each intermittent enteral feeding and every 4 to 6 hours for continuous enteral feedings. If more than 200 mL with continuous feedings or greater than 50% of the bolus volume for intermittent feedings is aspirated, consider the following interventions: (1) Change to continuous feedings if feeding method a bolus or intermittent feedings; (2) change the enteral feeding site to the duodenum or jejunum (though this does not completely eliminate the risk); (3) administer metoclopramide (Reglan) or erythromycin as prescribed to increase gastric motility; and (4) continue feedings, but reassessing patients in 1 hour. If more than 500 mL residual is obtained, withhold feeding for 1 hour and then recheck for retention. Holding or discontinuing feedings can result in malnutrition, so notify the physician and consider the changes stated earlier rather than automatically discontinuing feedings. Aspiration of small-lumen feeding tubes is difficult because they may collapse with suction. An increase in abdominal girth, absent bowel sounds, and nausea are indications of retention, which prompts an evaluation for the cause of delayed gastric emptying.

Monitor the secretions suctioned or expectorated. Perform glucose testing to confirm presence of enteral feeding in sputum. Keep appropriate equipment at the patient's bedside, including airway suctioning equipment and wire cutters for patients with wired jaw. Prepare patients for surgery for intractable aspiration (e.g., tracheoesophageal diversion or laryngotracheal separation) as requested.

Prevent aspiration in patients with artificial airways. Keep the cuff of the endotracheal or tracheostomy tube inflated to 20 to 30 cm H_2O. If the patient is not on a mechanical ventilator, inflate the cuff of a tracheostomy tube during meals and suction the mouth and oropharynx before deflating the cuff.

Maintain the patient's airway, ventilation, and oxygenation if aspiration does occur. Position the bed in a slight Trendelenburg position with the patient in a right lateral decubitus position. Suction the airway immediately and provide adequate oxygenation during suctioning. Bronchoscopy may be required for the removal of large particles if indicated. Stop enteral feeding if being administered. Monitor ABGs and pulse oximetry; a decrease in SpO_2, SaO_2, and PaO_2 may indicate the development of acute respiratory distress syndrome. Administer oxygen therapy if hypoxemia is present. Use of a CPAP or PEEP may be necessary to maintain adequate oxygenation. Administer bronchodilators as prescribed. Administer antibiotics as prescribed; avoid prophylactic antibiotics, but administer prescribed antibiotics specific to positive sputum or blood cultures. Prepare the patient for pulmonary resection if abscess develops. Monitor patients continually for complications such as acute respiratory failure, acute respiratory distress syndrome, pneumonia, lung abscess, and empyema. Endotracheal intubation may be necessary. Initiate mechanical ventilation as prescribed if hypercapnia develops and facilitate a transfer to a higher-acuity level of care.

4.20 Learning Activity

List four nursing interventions to prevent aspiration in a patient on enteral feedings.

1. _____
2. _____
3. _____
4. _____

Answers to this activity can be found in the Answer Key.

ASTHMA

Asthma is a recurrent, reversible airway disease characterized by increased airway responsiveness to a variety of stimuli that produces airway narrowing. Status asthmaticus is an exacerbation of acute asthma characterized by severe airflow obstruction that is not relieved after 24 hours of maximal doses of traditional therapy.

Extrinsic factors (haptens and antigens) trigger an allergic response that results in asthma. Common extrinsic haptens and antigens include dust and dust mites, animal dander or feathers, pollen, mold, smoke, propellants, air pollution, and preservatives (e.g., bisulfites). Common food allergens include nuts, legumes (e.g., peanuts), chocolate, eggs, shellfish, food additives, and alcohol. Changes in inspired air such as cold or hot air or very high or very low humidity; and medications, such as aspirin, nonsteroidal noninflammatory drugs (NSAIDs), and beta-blockers can also trigger an allergic response. Intrinsic triggers of asthma attack are seemingly unrelated to a specific allergen. Intrinsic triggers include infection, such as bacterial or viral pneumonia, bronchitis, or sinusitis; stress; exercise; gastroesophageal reflux disease (GERD); aspiration; fear, anger, crying, or laughing; and the menstrual cycle.

The pathophysiology of asthmat (Figure 4-30) is initiated by either an intrinsic or extrinsic trigger. Bronchial muscle contraction, inflammation and mucosal swelling, and an increase in mucus in the airways cause airway narrowing and increased airway resistance, which leads to an increased work of breathing, shunt, and airway trapping.

Patients with a history of asthma may be asymptomatic between episodes. During asthma attacks, the patients complain of dyspnea, chest tightness, and anxiety. They may also indicate fatigue and insomnia. Clinical findings include tachycardia, tachypnea, and an inability to speak in full sentences due to dyspnea. In addition, the patients may have a cough with thick tenacious sputum production; use of accessory muscles; intercostal retractions; prolonged expiration (more than a 1-3 I:E ratio); diaphoresis; and peak expiratory flow rate (PEFR) below 80% of the patient's personal or predicted best and frequently below 50% of the patient's personal best. Clinical indications of dehydration may be present, including poor skin turgor, dry mucous membranes, and increased specific gravity of urine. Clinical indications of hypoxia (Box 4-2), clinical indications of hypercapnia (Box 4-3), and breath sound changes, such as rhonchi and wheezing, are present.

A history of a slow, progressive worsening of airflow obstruction over the course of several days or weeks may be signs of impending status asthmaticus. Indications of potential imminent respiratory arrest include a change in consciousness, such as drowsiness or confusion; paradoxical thoracoabdominal movement; the absence of rhonchi and wheeze, which may occur in critical stages indicating the absence of airflow; bradycardia; and pulsus paradoxus greater than 20 mm Hg.

Diagnostic studies may include an increased WBC count if infection is the cause of the asthma attack or status asthmaticus. An increased eosinophil count is likely if the patient is not receiving steroids. Because dehydration is common, the hematocrit may be increased. Serum potassium and/or magnesium may be low during an acute attack. ABGs (Table 4-26) are crucial in evaluating the severity of the oxygenation and ventilation impairment. Sputum may show increased viscosity and an eosinophil stain may be positive. An increased number of eosinophils indicate an allergic reaction.

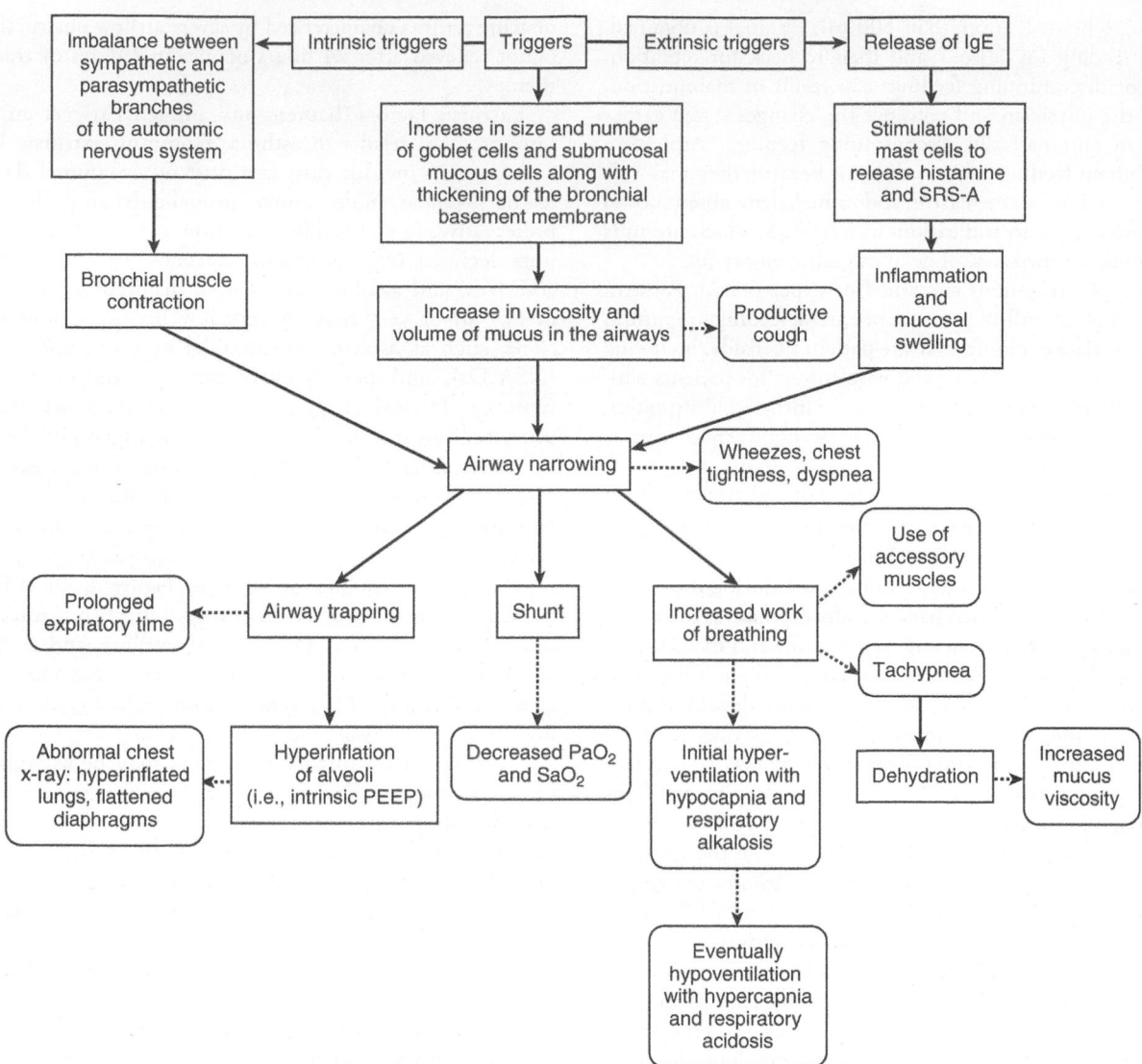

FIGURE 4-30 Pathophysiology of asthma. Dotted lines connect pathology to the clinical presentation. (From Dennison, R. D. [2013]. *Pass CCRN!* [4th ed.]. St. Louis, MO: Elsevier.)

TABLE 4-26	Asthma: ABG Analysis			
Stage	**PaO$_2$**	**PaCO$_2$**	**pH**	**Acid-Base Imbalance**
I	Normal	Decreased	Increased	Respiratory alkalosis
II	Decreased	Decreased	Increased	Respiratory alkalosis Mild to moderate hypoxemia
III	Very low	Normal	Normal	Significant hypoxemia
IV	Extremely low	Elevated	Decreased	Respiratory acidosis Critical hypoxemia

Pulmonary function studies may be impossible to do during an attack because the patient is too dyspneic; however, if performed, patients may have a decreased tidal volume and vital capacity, increased residual volume, and/or a diminished PEF or FEV$_1$ with improvement after bronchodilators. A combination of the patient's best FEV$_1$ and patient report of symptoms is a better predictor of mortality than best peak expiratory flow in patients with asthma. An ECG might reveal sinus tachycardia. A chest x-ray may show normal or hyperinflated lungs with flattened diaphragms. A chest x-ray is also helpful to rule out a foreign body, aspiration, pulmonary edema, pulmonary embolism, pneumonia, or pneumothorax.

4.21 Learning Activity

Complete the following table identifying the stage of asthma.

Pao$_2$ (mm Hg)	Paco$_2$ (mm Hg)	pH	Stage
68	30	7.48	
88	25	7.52	
45	55	7.28	
52	40	7.40	

Answers to this activity can be found in the Answer Key.

Collaborative management initially includes measures to lessen the severity of an asthma attack. Determine the patient's predisposing factors and attempt to eliminate and/or treat the cause. Administer prescribed antibiotics to treat infection. Eliminate exposure to pulmonary irritants and pollutants as well as drugs or foods that may have triggered an attack.

Maintain airway and improve ventilation. Elevate the patient's HOB to between 30 and 45 degrees. The overbed table may be helpful for the patient to lean on. Administer pharmacologic agents as prescribed. Note that cromolyn sodium (Intal) or nedocromil (Tilade) are inhaled mast cell stabilizers that prevent the release of histamine from the mast cells. These agents have no direct bronchodilation or antiinflammatory effect; therefore, will not be helpful during an acute attack.

Bronchodilators can help relax bronchial smooth muscle. Leukotriene inhibitors/leukotriene receptor antagonists are prescribed as preventative agents (e.g., zafirlukast [Accolate], zileuton [Zyflo], montelukast sodium [Singulair]), but they are not helpful for treatment of acute bronchospasm. Beta$_2$-stimulants cause smooth muscle to relax by stimulating beta$_2$ receptors. Administer long-acting agents (e.g., salmeterol [Serevent] by metered-dose inhaler) as prescribed to the patient with a diagnosis of asthma. Short-acting beta$_2$-agonists include metaproterenol (Alupent, Metaprel), albuterol (Proventil, Ventolin), pirbuterol (Maxair), bitolterol (Tornalate), and terbutaline (Brethaire). A metered-dose inhaler is usually used and may be as effective as a nebulizer treatment when used with a spacing device. Administer a nebulizer treatment as prescribed if the PEFR is less than 50% of the patient's personal best. Administer a beta$_2$-agonist by nebulizer every 20 minutes or continuously for 1 hour. Continuous nebulizer treatments are effective with no more side effects than intermittent nebulizer treatments and require less clinician time. Avoid intravenous beta-agonists if inhalation therapy is possible because they do not produce better results but instead increase adverse effects significantly. Monitor patients closely for adverse effects such as significant tachycardia, dysrhythmias, hypertension, headache, tremor, anxiety, or hypokalemia. In severe attacks, an anticholinergic (e.g., ipratropium bromide [Atrovent]) may augment the effects of beta$_2$-agonists. These agents block parasympathetic stimulation, thereby making sympathetic stimulation dominant and causing smooth muscle relaxation. They may be especially helpful for asthma stimulated by an intrinsic trigger. Administer the anticholinergic medication as a metered-dose inhaler or a nebulize treatment. In addition, administer an anticholinergic medications combined with a beta$_2$-agonist (e.g., ipratropium bromide and albuterol sulfate [Combivent]) as prescribed. Administer an intravenous Xanthine (e.g., theophylline, aminophylline) for a refractory attack. Xanthines cause smooth muscle relaxation resulting in bronchodilation; however, they are less effective than nebulized beta$_2$-agonists and have more adverse effects than beta$_2$-agonists. Their immune-modulating effects include inhibition of T lymphocytes and other inflammatory cells and inhibition of cytokine release. Primarily because of a narrow therapeutic window and interactions with other commonly prescribed drugs, Xanthine intravenous therapy is no longer considered a first line agent. Continue Xanthine therapy in patients on oral xanthine therapy at home. Obtain a theophylline level for patients who have been receiving xanthines at home and monitor them closely for indications of theophylline toxicity, including GI upset (e.g., anorexia, nausea, or vomiting), cardiac complications, such as dysrhythmias, and neurologic problems, such as restlessness or seizures. Xanthine, prescribed orally for long-term therapy at home, is usually given by intravenous infusion in acute asthma.

Administer magnesium as prescribed in acutely ill asthmatic patients with severe exacerbation. Magnesium causes muscles to relax, resulting in bronchodilation and improved airflow. Consider it for patients who have not responded to other bronchodilators after 1 hour. Administer magnesium as an intravenous infusion. The usual dose is 1 to 2 g over 20 minutes. Avoid magnesium in patients with hypotension or renal failure. Monitor the patient's blood pressure and deep tendon reflexes (DTRs) during infusion and report significant hypotension or loss of DTRs.

Administer prescribed corticosteroids to reduce inflammation. Corticosteroids work by decreasing mucosal swelling, blocking the release of histamine by the mast cells, and potentiating bronchodilators. It is likely that the patient will have administered steroids (e.g., beclomethasone [Vanceril, Beclovent], flunisolide [Aerobid], triamcinolone [Azmacort], or fluticasone [Flovent]) via metered dose inhaler before hospitalization. Steroids by inhalation diminish, but do not eliminate the systemic effects of steroid administration. Steroids may be initially administered intravenously (e.g., methylprednisolone [Solu-Medrol]) or orally (prednisone and prednisolone) in status asthmaticus. Initial large doses are titrated downward over days to weeks. Alternate-day oral dosing decreases the potential for adrenal suppression. In steroid-resistant asthma, intravenous immunoglobulin may be administered.

Expectorants (e.g., guaifenesin [Robitussin], potassium iodide [SSKI]) may be used, but hydration is most important; water is the best expectorant. Avoid mucolytics (e.g., acetylcysteine [Mucomyst]) because of their adverse effect of bronchospasm. Avoid using antitussives because airway clearance is important and coughing is preferred to suctioning as long as the cough is effective and the patient is not fatigued. Administer prescribed antibiotics only in the presence of infection to avoid antibiotic resistance.

Maintain bronchial hygiene. Encourage patients to use abdominal (i.e., deep) breathing to permit effective coughing. Suction patients only if coughing is ineffective. Chest physical therapy is not generally recommended and may be unnecessarily stressful for a patient with status asthmaticus.

Assist in initiation of noninvasive ventilatory methods (CPAP, BiPAP) as required. These methods use a mask, and they may prevent further deterioration as well as intubation and mechanical ventilation by unloading the respiratory muscles and reducing the work of breathing. In the long-run, noninvasive methods may improve survival rates (Young, 2010). Facilitate intubation and mechanical ventilation as necessary, especially if the $Paco_2$ continues to rise and acidosis develops. The goal of mechanical ventilation is to normalize the pH, not necessarily the $Paco_2$. Patients requiring intubation and mechanical ventilation for status asthmaticus require a higher-acuity level of care. Facilitate a transfer.

Tachypnea increases insensible fluid losses by the respiratory track and the resultant dehydration contributes to thick, tenacious mucus and difficulties with airway clearance. Provide adequate rehydration with noncaffeinated oral fluids or intravenous fluids (i.e., D_5NS or $D_5\frac{1}{2}NS$).

Provide the patient and family with instruction and counseling regarding lifestyle modification and the need for pharmacologic therapy. Discuss triggers and encourage the patient to identify his or her common triggers. Encourage follow-up for allergy testing and desensitization if needed. Discuss methods of monitoring symptoms including measuring the PEFR twice daily. Instruct the patient to call the physician when the PEFR drops by 20% or more below its usual level, when there is an increase in symptoms such as dyspnea, and when there are indications of a respiratory infection. Drug therapy includes inhaled bronchodilators, corticosteroids, cromolyn, and antimicrobials. Teach patients how to use and clean a metered-dose inhaler or nebulizer, to use corticosteroids after the bronchodilator, and to rinse the mouth after inhaled corticosteroids to avoid oral fungal infections (e.g., candidiasis).

Using the teach-back method, instruct the patient how to perform slow deep breathing and pursed-lip breathing. Discuss the need to maintain up-to-date on immunizations (e.g., influenza, *Pneumococcus, Haemophilus)*. Teach the patient how to control GERD with prescribed medications such as H_2 receptor antagonists or proton pump inhibitors (e.g., omeprazole [Prilosec], lansoprazole [Protonix], rabeprazole [Aciphex]). Also, encourage avoiding large meals, avoiding the supine position after eating, and normalizing body weight.

Monitor the patient for complications, such as asphyxia, acute respiratory failure, barotrauma/volutrauma (e.g., pneumothorax), pneumonia, dysrhythmias, and hypovolemia. Monitor for hypotension related to hypovolemia, decreased venous return caused by lung hyperinflation, or tension pneumothorax.

PULMONARY EMBOLISM/INFARCTION

Pulmonary embolism/infarction results in the obstruction of blood flow to one or more arteries of the lung by a thrombus lodged in a pulmonary vessel. The most common type of pulmonary embolism (PE) is a thrombus but other types of emboli include fat, air, amniotic fluid, tumor, and foreign body (e.g., catheter fragment). The embolism may be massive or submassive. A massive embolism involves more than a 50% occlusion of pulmonary blood flow and caused by the occlusion of a lobar artery or larger artery. A submassive embolism involves less than a 50% occlusion of pulmonary blood flow. In patients with preexisting heart or lung disease, hemodynamic deterioration may occur with less than 50% pulmonary vascular obstruction.

The three primary risk factors for thrombus formation are hypercoagulability, alterations in the blood vessel wall, and venous stasis; referred to as the *Virchow triad*. The state of hypercoagulability may be caused by the following:

- Malignancy, especially of the breast, lung, pancreas, or GI or GU tracts
- Estrogen use in the form of oral contraceptives or postmenopausal hormone replacement therapy; this risk is greatest in smokers
- Dehydration and hemoconcentration
- Fever
- Sickle cell anemia
- Pregnancy and the postpartum period
- Polycythemia vera
- Abrupt discontinuance of anticoagulants
- Sepsis
- Protein C, protein S, or antithrombin III deficiency
  Alterations in the vessel wall may result from the following:
- Trauma
- IV drug use
- Vascular changes of aging, including arteriosclerosis
- Vasculitis
- Varicose veins
- Diabetes mellitus
- Atherosclerosis
- An inflammatory process
  Venous stasis may result from the following:
- Prolonged bed rest or immobilization
- Obesity
- Advanced age
- Burns
- Pregnancy and the postpartum period
- Heart failure
- Myocardial infarction
- Bacterial endocarditis
- Recent surgery (especially of the legs, pelvis, or abdomen)
- Thrombus formation in the heart, such as mural thrombi in atrial fibrillation
- Cardioversion

4.22   Learning Activity

List three causes of pulmonary embolism in each of the following categories.

Hypercoagulability	Alteration in Blood Vessel	Venous Stasis

Answers to this activity can be found in the Answer Key.

Risk factors for fat embolism include long bone (e.g., femur) fracture, pelvic fracture, multiple fractures, orthopedic surgery with intramedullary manipulation, osteomyelitis, trauma to adipose tissue or the liver, liposuction, sickle cell crisis, burns, and

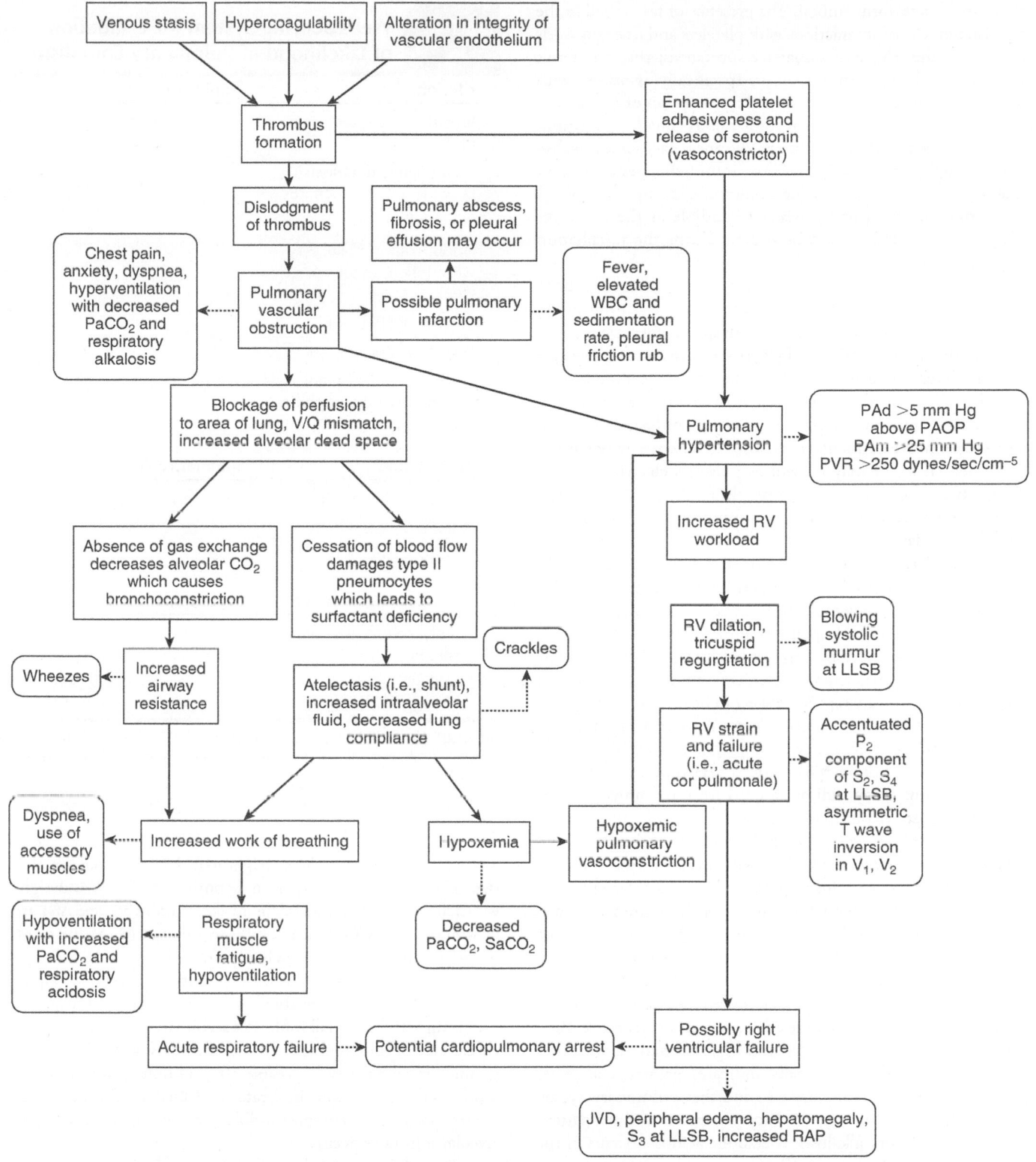

FIGURE 4-31 Pathophysiology of pulmonary embolism. Dotted lines connect pathology to the clinical presentation. (From Dennison, R. D. [2013]. *Pass CCRN!* [4th ed.]. St. Louis, MO: Elsevier.)

acute pancreatitis. Risk factors for air embolism include having had a recent surgical procedure, insertion of a deep vein catheter, cardiopulmonary bypass, hemodialysis, and endoscopy.

The pathophysiology of pulmonary embolism (Figure 4-31) begins with thrombus formation followed by dislodgement of the thrombus with movement into the pulmonary vascular system.

This obstruction causes V/Q mismatching with dead space and shunt resulting in hypoxemia, hypoxemic pulmonary hypertension with potential for acute cor pulmonale and acute respiratory failure.

Fat emboli are most likely to develop 1 to 3 days after injury, but may occur up to a week after injury. Fat globules enter the bloodstream and form emboli. The presence of fat emboli in the bloodstream causes interactions with platelets and free fatty acids along with the release of vasoactive substances; this may result in cerebral ischemia. Air emboli are specifically associated with activation of the clotting cascade and interruption of circulation.

A small PE may be asymptomatic. A small to medium embolus may manifest as anxiety, dyspnea, tachypnea, tachycardia, cough, and chest pain. Heart sound changes include an accentuated P_2 (the second [i.e., pulmonic] component of S_2) and a right-sided S_3 or S_4, which is audible at the left lower sternal border. Crackles may be audible during the auscultation of breath sounds.

A large to massive PE occurs with 50% occlusion of pulmonary artery bed. Patients may express a feeling of impending doom. The patient may complain of dyspnea, chest pain, mental clouding and/or syncope. Tachypnea, tachycardia, and cyanosis are likely to be evident. There may be clinical indications of RVF: JVD, hepatomegaly, murmur of tricuspid regurgitation (i.e., systolic murmur at left lower sternal border), and a right ventricular heave. Patients may also experience hypotension or sudden shock or may present as pulseless electrical activity (PEA). If pulmonary infarction develops, the patient will also have fever, pleuritic chest pain, hemoptysis, and pleural friction rub hours to days after embolism.

The patient's troponin I may be elevated, indicating right ventricular microinfarction. The brain natriuretic peptide (BNP) may be elevated in patients with right ventricular overload. The D-dimer will be elevated in almost all patients with PE because of endogenous fibrinolysis. This test has high sensitivity but low specificity with a 99% negative predictive value so patients with a negative D-dimer are highly unlikely to have a PE, but patients with a positive D-dimer do not necessarily have a PE. Age, surgery, immobility, malignancy, and pregnancy are all strongly associated with D-dimer positivity. Indeterminate V/Q and a positive D-dimer may indicate a need for a pulmonary angiogram or CT scan, but evidence-based literature supports the practice of determining the clinical pretest probability of pulmonary embolism before proceeding with invasive and/or expensive diagnostic testing (Boka, 2014). The Wells scoring system (Table 4-27) assigns points for criteria that have been identified as increasing the likelihood that a PE exists. The summative score is used to evaluate the likelihood that the patient has a PE and to plan additional diagnostic studies. Initial studies support the validity of this score (Penaloza, Verschuren, & Meyer, 2013).

If the PE is thrombotic, the ABGs will show decreased PaO_2 and SaO_2. A PaO_2 less than 50 mm Hg in a patient with previously normal ABGs generally indicates greater than 50% obstruction of the pulmonary tree and that pulmonary hypertension is present. Initially, the $PaCO_2$ decreases and the patient will have respiratory alkalosis. Metabolic acidosis occurs in the presence of severe hypoxemia. Respiratory acidosis may develop with significant atelectasis or fatigue.

If the case of a fat or air embolism, the PaO_2 and SaO_2 decreases and the $PaCO_2$ increases causing respiratory acidosis. Patients with severe hypoxemia will have metabolic acidosis.

An ECG will reveal dysrhythmias. Sinus tachycardia will be present. Atrial dysrhythmias, especially atrial fibrillation, are common. Ventricular dysrhythmias may occur in hypoxemia. A new right bundle branch block (RBBB) may occur. The presence of tall, peaked P waves in lead II indicate P-pulmonale

TABLE 4-27 Wells Scoring System for Evaluation of Likelihood of Pulmonary Embolism

Criterion	Point Value
Clinically suspected cases of DVT	3
An alternative diagnosis being less likely than PE	3
Tachycardia	1.5
Immobilization or surgery within the previous 4 weeks	1.5
A history of DVT or PE	1.5
Presence of hemoptysis	1
Treatment for malignancy within 6 months or palliative management	1

Interpretation	Summative Score
High probability of PE	>6
Moderate probability of PE	2-6
Low probability of PE	0-1

Testing Recommendations	Summative Score
PE likely, so consider diagnostic imaging	>4
PE unlikely, so consider D-dimer to rule out PE	<4

Adapted from Wells, P. S., & Ginsberg, J. S. (1995). DVT and pulmonary embolism: Choosing the right diagnostic tests for patients at risk. *Geriatrics, 50* (2), 29-32, 35-26.

and right atrial enlargement. Right axis deviation may be seen (i.e., QRS complex negative in I, positive in aVF) and right ventricular strain (i.e., ST-segment elevation in V_1 and V_2) are common. The ECG is also helpful to rule out MI as the cause of the patient's dyspnea and chest pain.

Initially, the chest x-ray is normal, but it may still be helpful to rule out other causes of the patient's symptoms. If the embolism is thrombotic, small infiltrates secondary to atelectasis with an elevated hemidiaphragm on the affected side and decreased pulmonary vascularity are visible after 24 hours. In the case of a pulmonary infarction, infiltrates and pleural effusion occur. In the case of a fat embolism, diffuse extensive interstitial and alveolar infiltrates occur.

Echocardiography will usually be normal but may show right ventricular dilation, hypokinesis, and tricuspid regurgitation. It may also show bulging of the interventricular septum into the LV, reducing the LV size with a D-shaped LV. An echocardiogram is also helpful to rule out cardiac tamponade, dissection of the aorta, and acute myocardial infarction.

A V/Q lung scan will show a perfusion defect with normal ventilation. The positive predictive value of high probability V/Q scan is 96% when supported by high clinical suspicion of PE. A negative predictive value of a negative V/Q scan is also excellent with a normal V/Q scan to accurately rule out PE

98% of the time. Unfortunately, 75% of patients fall within the indeterminate category. Intermediate or low probability V/Q scan with positive D-dimer is an indication for further pretest screening to determine the risk prior to invasive pulmonary angiography and or an expensive spiral CT scan.

A spiral (helical) CT is widely available and an easier study to perform than a V/Q scan or pulmonary angiogram. It is capable of demonstrating a variety of thoracic pathologies that can mimic PE. The generation of the scanner used affects the sensitivity of a spiral CT; the sensitivity is excellent with new scanners. However, in pregnant patients suspected of a pulmonary embolism, safety for the fetus has not been determined.

Gadolinium-enhanced magnetic resonance angiography allows high-resolution angiography through a single breath. It is a fast but accurate test that does not involve nephrotoxic contrast agents.

Pulmonary angiography shows the cutoff of a vessel or a filling defect within 24 to 72 hours. It continues to be the "gold standard," but it is not without risks. Pulmonary angiography is indicated in patients with a high probability of having a PE but have nondiagnostic noninvasive studies. It has excellent sensitivity and specificity; however, it comes with a significant risk of bleeding. Unfortunately, it provides a relative contraindication for fibrinolytic therapy because of the risk of bleeding from the puncture site.

In patients with a fat embolism, symptoms may not appear for 12 to 48 hours. Symptoms may include restlessness, agitation, irritability, confusion, dyspnea, and delirium. Objective findings include tachypnea; tachycardia; fever; petechiae on conjunctivae, anterior chest, neck, or axilla; and retinal hemorrhages with emboli present on the retina. Breath sound changes include stridor, wheezes, or crackles. Clinical indications of hypoxia (see Box 4-2) are likely. Altered consciousness or seizures may occur. ABGs show decreased SaO_2 and PaO_2. Serum analysis will show elevated lipase levels, elevated triglycerides, increased free fatty acids, elevated sedimentation rate, decreased hemoglobin or hematocrit, thrombocytopenia, and elevated fibrin split products. Fat globules will appear in the urine and sputum.

Patients with an air embolism complain of a feeling of impending doom, lightheadedness, weakness, nausea, chest pain, dyspnea, palpitations, and confusion. Objective findings include pallor, tachypnea, tachycardia, hypotension, and possibly a churning noise ("mill wheel murmur") audible over the precordium. Clinical indications of hypoxia (see Box 4-2) may be evident. Clinical indications of pulmonary edema, including S_3 and crackles, may be noted. Seizures may occur. ABGs show decreased SaO_2 and PaO_2 along with an increase in $PaCO_2$. Chest x-ray may show evidence of right ventricular failure and/or pulmonary edema. The V/Q scan may be similar to findings in thrombotic PE, but symptoms may resolve within 24 hours. Echocardiography will show air in the right ventricle, right ventricular dilation, and/or pulmonary hypertension.

Implement measures to prevent thrombus formation and pulmonary embolism for all patients because all hospitalized patients are at risk for pulmonary embolism, but some patients are at higher risk. Instruct patients to do deep breathing exercises; postoperative patients should do them hourly. Ambulate patients as soon as possible. Instruct patients who cannot ambulate to do leg exercises hourly. Perform passive range of motion of all extremities for patients who cannot do active exercises. Reposition patients who are not ambulatory at least every 2 hours, avoiding extreme knee or hip flexion. Instruct the patients not to cross their legs. Ensure that patients receive adequate fluid intake to prevent dehydration and hypercoagulability. Provide careful venipuncture and IV care, avoiding venipunctures in the legs. Provide atraumatic venipuncture, avoiding multiple sticks.

Patients with a moderate risk for deep vein thrombosis (DVT) also require elastic stockings or intermittent pneumatic compression devices. Take care to prevent constriction and a tourniquet effect when using elastic stockings. Intermittent pneumatic compression devices, also referred to as *sequential compression devices,* stimulate endogenous fibrinolytic activity in addition to the direct physical effect of increased venous blood return. Patients at high risk for DVT are likely to be prescribed subcutaneous low-dose unfractionated heparin (UFH) or low-molecular-weight heparin (LMWH), provided it is not contraindicated. Enoxaparin (Lovenox) 30 or 40 mg every 12 hours, unfractionated heparin 5000 units every 8 to 12 hours, or dalteparin sodium (Fragmin) 2500IU daily is likely to be prescribed. Patients with documented DVT require low-dose UFH or LMWH.

Monitor patients closely for clinical indications of DVT, such as low-grade fever, calf pain or tenderness, unilateral edema, erythema, warmth, or dilated collateral veins. Venography, venous duplex, and/or compression ultrasonography may be required to confirm the presence of a DVT. Prevent dislodgment of the clot if the patient has DVT. Instruct the patient how to avoid the Valsalva maneuver. Maintain steady IV flow rates; fluid boluses change the rate of blood flow and may dislodge the clot. Avoid massaging the patient's legs. Avoid bed rest in patients with DVT unless there is substantial pain and swelling (Kearon, Ahl, Comerata, et al., 2012).

Maintain adequate airway, ventilation, and oxygenation. Administer oxygen to maintain SpO_2 greater than 90%. Use a nasal cannula at 5 L/min unless contraindicated. High concentrations of O_2 via nonrebreathing mask may be required to maintain a SpO_2 greater than 90%. Administer analgesics as prescribed to prevent splinting and encourage deep breathing. Ensure that the patient has a quiet, restful environment. Provide intubation and mechanical ventilation if required. The primary initial problem in PE is diffusion due to a perfusion defect. Initially, the patient is generally ventilated adequately and frequently even excessively as evidenced by a low $PaCO_2$. Intubation and mechanical ventilation may be required as respiratory muscle fatigue occurs and the $PaCO_2$ increases causing respiratory acidosis. Progression to this condition requires a transfer to a higher-acuity level of care.

To restore normal V/Q matching, take measures to arrest thrombosis and reestablish perfusion. Obtain a baseline clotting profile and administer prescribed anticoagulants. Fibrinolytics are indicated for PE in the event of hypodynamic instability, acute right ventricular failure, and significant hypoxemia despite optimal oxygen therapy. Fibrinolytics dissolve clots promptly to speed pulmonary tissue reperfusion, reverse right ventricular failure, and improve pulmonary capillary blood volume. The most commonly used agent is tissue plasminogen activator (tPA), such as alteplase (Activase), 100 mg over 2 hours. Contraindications and nursing management are the same as patients with MI (see Chapter 3). The patient is transferred to a higher-acuity level of care to receive fibrinolytic.

Anticoagulation therapy will follow fibrinolytic therapy or be used alone if fibrinolytics are not indicated or contraindicated. Administer anticoagulants as prescribed to prevent extension of the clot and reocclusion. Maintain parenteral agents for 7 to 10 days. Fondaparinux (Arixtra), a factor Xa inhibitor, is administered subcutaneously and the dose is based on body weight. The advantage of fondaparinux is that there is a lower risk of heparin-induced thrombocytopenia (HIT) and a lower risk of major bleeding compared with heparin. LMWH, such as enoxaparin (Lovenox), is an indirect thrombin inhibitor. It is administered subcutaneously at 1 mg/kg every 12 hours. LMWH has a longer plasma half-life than UFH and the response to weight-adjusted doses is more predictable than UFH. The longer half-life is a potential disadvantage because it is less reversible than UFH. There is no need to monitor clotting studies with LMWH although monitoring is indicated in patients who are morbidly obese, have renal insufficiency, or who weigh less than 50 kg. There is a lower incidence of HIT with LMWH than with UFH. UFH is an indirect thrombin inhibitor. It is administered IV as a bolus dose 70 to 80 units/kg initially, followed by 15 to 20 units/kg/hr to maintain aPTT between 60 and 80 seconds. Higher doses may be necessary initially due to low antithrombin III levels after PE. For patients with HIT (also referred to as *heparin-associated thrombocytopenia* or *white clot syndrome*), lepirudin (Refludan) and argatroban will be prescribed. Warfarin is an oral agent. It is started 3 to 4 days before parenteral anticoagulants are discontinued and continued for up to 6 months. The usual starting dose is 5 mg daily. This is adjusted to maintain an INR between 2 and 3.

Prepare the patient for pulmonary embolectomy as requested. An embolectomy is indicated for patients with a massive PE with hemodynamic instability (e.g., cardiogenic shock) who cannot receive fibrinolytic therapy. Surgical pulmonary embolectomy has a relatively high complication rate and requires cardiopulmonary bypass. Catheter embolectomy may entail clot fragmentation using a pigtail catheter, rheolytic thrombectomy using a high-velocity saline jet (e.g., AngioJet), or clot aspiration (e.g., transluminal extraction catheter).

Prepare the patient for insertion of an inferior vena cava filter as requested. This procedure is indicated for patients who experience recurrent PE despite effective anticoagulation or when anticoagulants are contraindicated. Note that these are effective in protecting the lung from successive emboli, but they do not do anything about the current PE. There are several types of filters: a vena cava umbrella, the Greenfield filter, and the bird's nest filter. The advantage to the bird's nest filter is that it does not require precise axial orientation.

Provide treatment of pulmonary hypertension and acute right ventricular failure as prescribed. The first priority is elimination of the pulmonary vascular obstruction and reduction of pulmonary vascular resistance via fibrinolytics and embolectomy. Inotropes (e.g., dobutamine [Dobutrex]) and fluids may be required to ensure adequate left ventricular contractility and filling volume. If required, transfer to a higher acuity level of care. Administer antibiotics rather than fibrinolytics and anticoagulants as prescribed for septic emboli.

Monitor patients for complications, including pulmonary infarction, cerebral infarction, myocardial infarction, right ventricular failure, and dysrhythmias or blocks. Atrial dysrhythmias are common if RVF occurs. Ventricular dysrhythmias may occur in hypoxemia. RBBB may occur, but it is usually transient. Other complications include hepatic congestion and necrosis, pneumonia, pulmonary abscess, acute respiratory distress syndrome, disseminated intravascular coagulation, shock, and complications of therapy, such as bleeding related to fibrinolytic or anticoagulant therapy and oxygen toxicity related to high concentrations of oxygen.

TABLE 4-28	Mechanisms of Chest Trauma	
Blunt chest trauma	Rapid acceleration/deceleration	Shearing force causes stretching of tissue, organs, or blood vessels with resultant tearing, leaking, or rupture
	Direct impact	Object striking chest or chest striking object causes rib, sternal, or scapular fractures; injury to the heart or lung parenchyma
	Compression	Force of rapid deceleration as tissues hit a fixed object, such as the sternum or rib cage, causes concussion, contusion, bleeding, or rupture of an organ
Penetrating chest trauma	Penetration of lung, heart, great vessel, or diaphragm	Causes bleeding and injury to an organ or vessel

Assist in preventing fat embolism with early immobilization of long-bone fractures. If fat embolism does occur, provide oxygen via nasal cannula at 5 L/min unless contraindicated. A 100% nonrebreathing mask may be required to maintain SpO_2 of at least 90%. Intubation and mechanical ventilation may also be necessary. Administer steroids (e.g., hydrocortisone) as prescribed to decrease the inflammatory response; however, this is controversial. Provide adequate fluids to flush the fatty acids and prevent renal damage. Administer osmotic diuretics (e.g., mannitol [Osmitrol]) as prescribed if pulmonary edema is present. Replace red blood cells and/or platelets as prescribed.

To prevent an air embolism, prime IV tubing and central catheters with fluid to remove air before connection or insertion. Use IV pumps with air detectors and twist-lock connections on central venous catheters to prevent accidental disconnections. Position the patient in the Trendelenburg position to facilitate insertion of central venous catheters or treatment of chest trauma unless contraindicated (e.g., head trauma). Instruct the patient to hold his or her breath and bear down (i.e., Valsalva maneuver) during tubing changes and catheter removal. Upon the removal of the catheter, apply a pressure dressing to the central venous site.

Place a patient suspected to have an air embolism in the left lateral decubitus position with the head down (referred to as *Durant's maneuver*) Attempt to aspirate the air embolus Give external cardiac compressions to push air out of the right ventricle into the pulmonary circulation, fragmenting the air bolus into smaller air bubbles. Provide oxygen via a 100% nonrebreathing mask. Arterial embolization and patients who have deteriorated clinically may need hyperbaric oxygen therapy.

CHEST TRAUMA

There are several mechanisms of chest trauma (Table 4-28). Blunt trauma leaves the body surface intact; penetrating trauma disrupts the body surface. Perforating trauma leaves both entrance and exit wounds as an object passes through the body.

These types of trauma may occur from a motor vehicle collision, motorcycle collision, vehicle/pedestrian collision, a fall, assault, an explosion (e.g., a blast injury), or projectiles, including a bullet, knives, or impalement.

Pulmonary Contusion

Pulmonary contusion is damage to the lung parenchyma that causes localized edema and hemorrhage. It may occur when high-velocity blunt trauma disperses across the chest, or it may occur from crush injuries. Pulmonary contusion may also occur iatrogenically from chest compressions during cardiopulmonary resuscitation. Other chest injuries, such as flail chest, are frequently associated with pulmonary contusion.

Blunt trauma causes a deceleration injury to the chest wall and compression of the thoracic cavity. The diminished thoracic size compresses the lung tissue. Decompression then causes capillary rupture and subsequent hemorrhage. Initial hemorrhage may occur from bruising, pulmonary tears, and/or lacerations. Interstitial and alveolar edema occurs at the site of the contusion. Massive interstitial edema with general inflammation follows. Damaged or closed alveolar-capillary units cause V/Q mismatch and shunt, followed by increased PVR, decreased lung compliance, and decreased pulmonary blood flow. Atelectasis occurs and results in retained secretions and infection. Severe pulmonary lacerations may cause a concurrent hemothorax. Pulmonary contusion may accompany a flail chest and masked by the obvious ventilation difficulties seen in the flail chest.

Patients with pulmonary contusion may be asymptomatic for 24 to 48 hours after a precipitating event. Patients may complain of anxiety, dyspnea, and chest tenderness. They may exhibit tachycardia and tachypnea. They may also use accessory muscles of ventilation. Ecchymosis may appear at the site of impact. Patients may have an ineffective cough with guarding and hemoptysis. Crepitus or deformity may be noted on palpation if there are rib fractures. Subcutaneous emphysema suggests concurrent pneumothorax or upper airway injury. There may be dullness to percussion on the affected side. Crackles or wheezes may be heard during auscultation of breath sounds.

ABG changes may occur as pulmonary issues progress. These changes include a decrease in Pao_2 and changes in $Paco_2$. The $Paco_2$ may be normal or decreased depending on ventilation pattern; $Paco_2$ will be low due to hyperventilation or high if pain or fatigue causes hypoventilation.

Changes on the chest x-ray may take 2 to 24 hours to develop. Patchy or poorly defined areas of increased parenchymal density may reflect intraalveolar hemorrhage. Linear and irregular infiltrates may be detected in the bronchioles. If the trauma is severe, extensive areas of increased parenchymal density will be seen within one or both lungs. The diaphragm may be lower on the affected side owing to the enlarged injured lung. Differentiate a pulmonary contusion from ARDS; pulmonary contusion is usually localized and occurs near the site of external trauma; ARDS causes diffuse bilateral changes. A CT scan may be performed to assess damage to pulmonary parenchyma and the pleural cavity.

The priority of collaborative management is to establish and maintain airway, ventilation, and oxygenation. Provide oxygen therapy via a nasal cannula at 2 to 6 L/min to achieve a Spo_2 greater than 90% unless contraindicated. In patients with a history of COPD, administer oxygen to achieve an oxygen saturation of a by pulse oximetry. Position the patient "good lung down."

Provide analgesics in doses adequate to allow the patient to turn and breathe deeply. Suctioning may be necessary if the patient cannot adequately cough. Endotracheal intubation and mechanical ventilation may be required.

Exercise care when administering fluids to patients with pulmonary contusion to prevent pulmonary edema. Monitor CVP and maintain level at approximately 6 cm H_2O. Administer diuretics as prescribed. Steroids are no longer recommended due to the risk of resultant immunosuppression and infection.

Monitor the patient for complications. Pneumonia is a very common complication. Avoid prophylactic antibiotics; antibiotics are indicated only in the presence of infection, with symptoms such as fever and a cough with sputum production. Culture the sputum if indicated. Other complications include lung abscess, empyema, pulmonary edema, pulmonary embolism, and ARDS.

Closed (Noncommunicating) Pneumothorax

A closed pneumothorax (Figure 4-32) occurs when air enters the intrapleural space through the lung, causing partial or total collapse of the lung. A small pneumothorax occupies less than 15% of the pleural space, a medium pneumothorax occupies 15% to 60% of the space, and a large pneumothorax occupies more than 60% of the space.

There are many possible reasons for a closed pneumothorax. A primary cause is the presence of a congenital bleb, which is common in endomorphic males aged 20 to 40 years. Secondary causes include an emphysematous bullous, tuberculosis, or lung cancer. A closed pneumothorax may also occur from a non-penetrating blunt trauma related to a motor vehicle collision, a fall, blow to the chest, or a blast injury. Iatrogenic causes include central venous catheterization via subclavian or low jugular vein puncture, intracardiac injection, thoracentesis, cardiopulmonary resuscitation, or positive pressure ventilation.

Pneumothorax involves the disruption of normal negative intrapleural pressure as a result of lung laceration by rib fracture or needle, compression of the lung at the height of inspiration when the alveolar pressure is high, or rupture of a weak alveolus, bleb, or bullous. This disruption of the normal negative pressure causes the lung to collapse, which decreases the surface area for the exchange of gases. Acute respiratory failure may occur.

Patients will complain of dyspnea and chest pain, which may be sudden or sharp and referred to the corresponding shoulder, across the chest, or abdomen. Clinical findings may include tachycardia; tachypnea; a dry, nonproductive cough; asymmetric chest excursion with limited motion of the affected hemithorax; subcutaneous emphysema; hyperresonance to percussion on the affected side; diminished to absent breath sounds on the affected side; and clinical indications of hypoxia (see Box 4-2). If the patient is on a mechanical ventilator, there may be a dramatic increase in peak inspiratory pressures, causing the high-pressure alarm to sound.

ABGs may reveal a decreased Spo_2 and Pao_2 with increased Pco_2. Chest x-ray will reveal air in the pleural space and a collapsed lung on the affected side. There may be a mediastinal shift toward the affected side. A CT of the thorax is more effective in detecting very small or anterior pneumothorax, often missed on the chest x-ray.

The priority of collaborative management is to establish and maintain airway, ventilation, and oxygenation. Administer oxygen by nasal cannula at 1 to 5 L/min to achieve a Spo_2

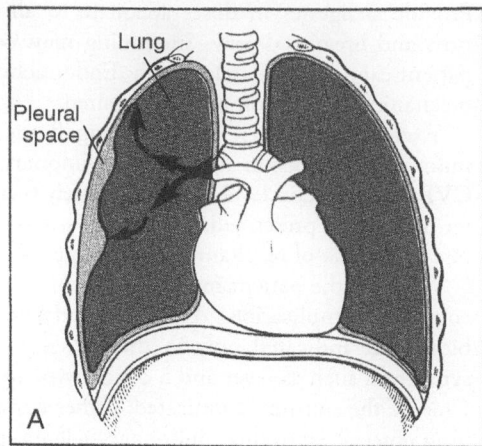
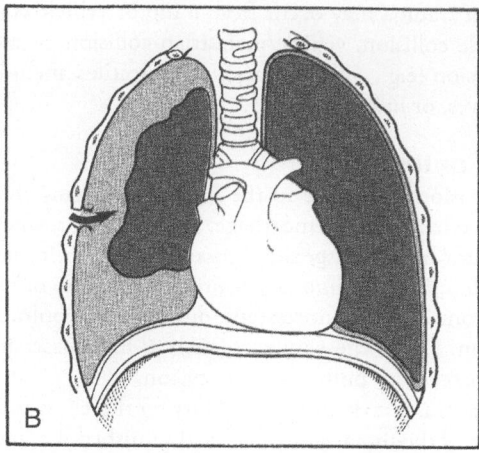
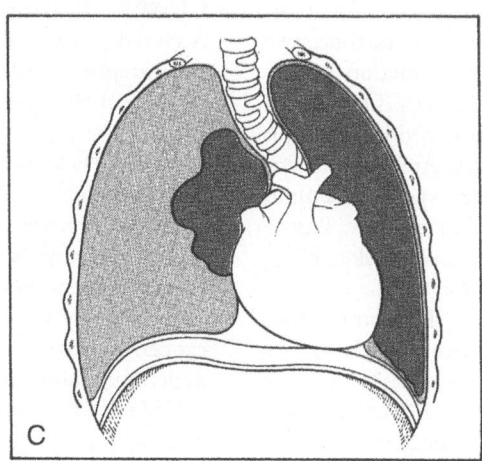

FIGURE 4-32 Pneumothorax. A, Closed. **B,** Open. **C,** Tension. (From Wilson, Thompson. [1990]. *Respiratory disorders [Mosby's clinical nursing series]*. St. Louis, MO: Mosby.)

greater than 95% unless contraindicated. In patients with a history of COPD, administer oxygen to achieve an oxygen saturation of approximately 90% by pulse oximetry. Provide adequate analgesics to allow the patient to breathe deeply and cough as indicated. Position the patient for optimal ventilation in the semi-Fowler's or Fowler's position. Position the patient "good lung down" or supine with regular turning. Encourage sustained inspiratory maneuvers, such as deep breathing and incentive spirometry; this should be all that is necessary for patients with small (less than 15%) pneumothorax. Insertion of a chest tube is not necessary if the pneumothorax is less than 15% and asymptomatic. Assist with insertion of a chest tube in patients with pneumothorax 15% or greater. Because the goal is to remove air, the provider inserts the tube into the fourth to fifth intercostal space at the midaxillary line and connects it to a Heimlich flutter valve or chest drainage system.

Monitor patients for complications, such as recurrent pneumothorax, atelectasis, and pneumonia or abscess. Decortication may be performed for patients with recurrent spontaneous pneumothorax.

Tension Pneumothorax

A tension pneumothorax (see Figure 4-32) occurs when air accumulates in the pleural space with no means of escape; this results in complete collapse of the lung and a potential mediastinal shift. Tension pneumothorax occurs from blunt or penetrating trauma or positive pressure mechanical ventilation, especially if the patient has emphysematous bullae or congenital bleb and is receiving large tidal volumes and/or PEEP. It may also occur from a nonfunctional (e.g., clotted or clamped) chest drainage system or an occlusive dressing on an open pneumothorax.

In tension pneumothorax, air rushes into, but not out of, the pleural space. This disrupts the negative intrapleural pressure and creates a positive pressure in the pleural space. Consequently, the ipsilateral lung collapses. If a tear does not seal, a one-way valve effect results, allowing air to enter during inspiration but not to escape during exhalation. Increasing positive intrapleural pressure may cause mediastinal shift leading to compression of the contralateral lung, thoracic aorta, vena cava, and heart, leading to decreased right ventricular filling and decreased cardiac output. Acute respiratory failure and shock may occur.

Patients with tension pneumothorax usually present with dyspnea and chest pain. Objective findings include tachycardia, tachypnea, asymmetric chest excursion with limited motion of affected hemithorax, possible subcutaneous emphysema, hyperresonance to percussion on the affected side (may even be tympanic), and diminished to absent breath sounds on the affected side. Clinical indications of hypoxia (see Box 4-2) may be present. If there is mediastinal shift, the trachea will shift away from the affected side, the point of maximal impulse (PMI) will be displaced, JVD will be noted, and there may be significant hypotension and even cardiac arrest.

The SpO_2 will be decreased, ABGs will reveal a decreased PaO_2, and the $PaCO_2$ may be increased. The chest x-ray will show an absence of lung markings and widening of the intercostal spaces on the affected side. Mediastinal shift away from the affected side may be present.

The priority of collaborative management is to establish and maintain airway, ventilation, and oxygenation. Administer oxygen by nasal cannula at 1 to 5 L/min to achieve a SpO_2 greater than 95% unless contraindicated. In patients with a history of COPD, administer oxygen to achieve an oxygen saturation of approximately 90% by pulse oximetry. Assist with emergency decompression: the provider inserts a large-bore needle (or IV catheter) perpendicularly into the second anterior interspace at the midclavicular line on the affected side until a chest tube can be inserted. Place a flutter valve (e.g., Heimlich valve, finger cot with a slit cut at the end) on the needle to allow air to escape while preventing atmospheric air from entering the pleural space. Maintain the chest tube and chest drainage system.

Provide adequate analgesics to allow the patient to breathe deeply and cough as indicated. Control pain with regularly scheduled narcotics or by patient-controlled analgesia. Position the patient for optimal ventilation in the semi-Fowler's or Fowler's position. Position the patient "good lung down" or supine with regular turning. Monitor the patient for complications including atelectasis, pneumonia, lung abscess, shock, and cardiopulmonary arrest.

Open (Communicating) Pneumothorax (Also Called Sucking Chest Wound)

An open (communicating) pneumothorax (see Figure 4-32) occurs when air enters the interpleural space through the chest wall. This may occur with penetrating trauma. Communication between the intrathoracic space and the atmosphere results in equilibrium between intrathoracic and atmospheric pressures. Air moves in and out of the opening in the chest wall. If there is an opening in the chest wall smaller than the diameter of the trachea, the patient may tolerate the condition well. However, if the opening is larger than the trachea, more air enters the pleural space than enters the lungs through the trachea so that during inspiration, the affected lung collapses, resulting in ineffective gas exchange and causing tension pneumothorax.

A patient with an open pneumothorax will complain of dyspnea and chest pain. Clinical findings include tachycardia and tachypnea. In addition, there will be an obvious wound with the audible sound of air moving in and out of the chest. Subcutaneous emphysema is usually present. Other findings are similar to those one would find with closed pneumothorax.

The priority of collaborative management is to establish and maintain airway, ventilation, and oxygenation. Administer oxygen by nasal cannula at 1 to 5 L/min to achieve a SpO_2 greater than 95% unless contraindicated. In patients with a history of COPD, administer oxygen to achieve an oxygen saturation of approximately 90% by pulse oximetry.

Close the open chest wound with gauze dressing taped on three sides so that air can escape during expiration. Assist with insertion of a chest tube and attach it to a chest drainage system. Prepare the patient for surgical intervention if requested; surgery may be needed to explore and debride the wound. Position the patient "good lung down" or supine with regular turning. Provide analgesics in doses adequate to allow the patient to breathe deeply and cough as indicated. Control the pain with regularly scheduled narcotics or by patient-controlled analgesia. Monitor the patient for complications such as tension pneumothorax, atelectasis, pneumonia, and/or abscess.

Hemothorax

Hemothorax involves the accumulation of blood in the pleural space, causing compression and collapse of the lung. It may occur from blunt or penetrating trauma to the chest wall, lung tissue, or mediastinum. It may also result from pleural or pulmonary neoplasm, anticoagulant therapy, and iatrogenic causes, including subclavian vein puncture (e.g., insertion of a deep vein catheter) or lung biopsy. The hemorrhage into the pleural space compresses and collapses the lung. This impairs ventilation and oxygenation. Hemorrhaging may lead to shock.

Patients with hemothorax complain of chest pain and dyspnea. Objective findings include tachycardia, hypotension, asymmetric chest excursion with limited motion in the affected hemithorax, dullness to percussion on the affected side, diminished or absent breath sounds on the affected side, and clinical indications of shock especially if the blood loss is greater than 400 mL. Diagnostic studies may reveal a decrease in hemoglobin and hematocrit, but those levels may be normal because it may take up to 6 hours after blood loss for changes in hemoglobin and hematocrit to occur. ABGs will reveal a decreased PaO_2 and the $PaCO_2$ may be increased. The chest x-ray will show fluid in the pleural space and lung compression, blunting of the costophrenic angle if the volume is greater than 250 mL, and a hazy appearance over the lower chest.

The priority of collaborative management is to establish and maintain airway, ventilation, and oxygenation. Administer oxygen by nasal cannula at 1 to 5 L/min to achieve a SpO_2 greater than 95% unless contraindicated. In patients with a history of COPD, administer oxygen to achieve an oxygen saturation of approximately 90% by pulse oximetry.

Assist with insertion of a chest tube with a chest drainage system as requested; this may prove adequate if the bleeding is self-limiting. Prepare a patient for surgery to isolate and repair the source of the hemorrhage, especially when initial drainage from chest tube is more than 1500 mL, drainage of blood occurs at a rate greater than 250 mL/hr for more than 2 hours after placement of the chest tube, or if there is hemodynamic instability despite fluid resuscitation. Maintain perfusion and adequate circulating volume by administering fluids and/or blood transfusion as prescribed. Blood loss greater than 400 mL is an indication for autotransfusion.

Position the patient for optimal ventilation in the semi-Fowler's or Fowler's position, unless the patient has significant hypotension with the head of the bed elevated. After thoracotomy, position the patient "good lung down" or supine with regular turning. Provide analgesics in doses adequate to allow the patient to breathe deeply and cough as indicated. Control the pain with regularly scheduled narcotics or by patient-controlled analgesia. Monitor patients for complications, such as atelectasis and/or shock.

4.23   Learning Activity

Match the clinical presentation to the type of chest trauma.

_____ 1. Pulmonary contusion
_____ 2. Closed pneumothorax
_____ 3. Hemothorax
_____ 4. Tension pneumothorax

a. Chest pain, dyspnea, diminished breath sounds on affected side, hyperresonance to percussion, tracheal shift away from affected side
b. Ecchymosis at site of impact, chest tenderness, dyspnea, hemoptysis
c. Chest pain, dyspnea, diminished breath sounds on affected side, hyperresonance to percussion, tracheal shift toward from affected side
d. Chest pain, dyspnea, diminished breath sounds on affected side, dullness to percussion

Answers to this activity can be found in the Answer Key.

4.24   Synthesis Learning Activity: Crossword Puzzle

Complete the following crossword puzzle to review pulmonary conditions and management.

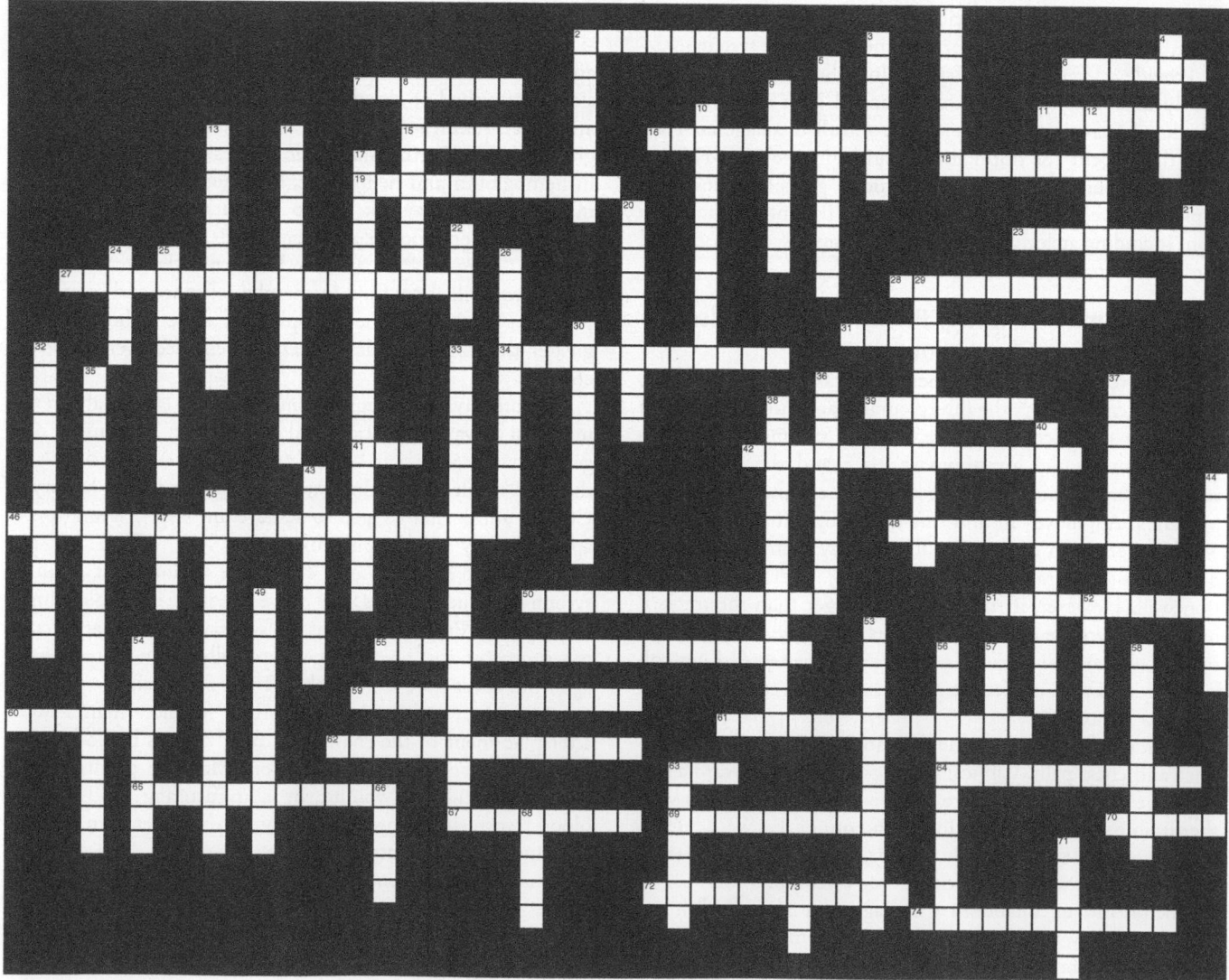

Answers to this activity can be found in the Answer Key.

ACROSS

2. A sedative frequently used in mechanically ventilated patients (generic)
6. Indicated when Sao_2 is less than 90%
7. _____ triad are three things that predispose to clot formation: hypercoagulability, venous stasis, and vascular injury
11. A drug used to prevent extension or recurrence of a clot in patients with pulmonary embolism (generic)
15. The most likely cause of ARDS
16. This is more likely to occur in the right lung
18. Testing sputum for _____ is a common method to check for aspiration of enteral feeding
19. This type of disorder is when expansion of the alveolus, lung, or chest wall is impaired and compliance is decreased
23. A feeling of impending doom is a symptom of massive pulmonary _____
27. This condition is characterized by an increase in the number and size of mucous and goblet cells
28. Inflammatory mediators including leukotrienes are released by _____ in ARDS
31. Bloody sputum; may be seen in lung cancer or tuberculosis
34. Pulmonary _____ is when the pulmonary vascular pressures are elevated
39. These sounds are heard when listening with a stethoscope to a patient with pneumonia or chronic bronchitis
41. This may be caused by pulmonary hypertension (abbrev.)
42. A steroid that is frequently given by inhalation in patients with asthma (generic)
46. This is caused by the decrease in Pao_2 in COPD, ARDS, and PE (2 words)
48. Results from release of erythropoietin in response to chronically low oxygen levels
50. A diagnostic study to obtain fluid from the pleural space for analysis

51. Drug used for stress ulcer prophylaxis that does not support gastric colonization (generic)
55. This diagnostic study is used to evaluate the adequacy of ventilation and oxygenation (3 words)
59. A procedure to view the bronchioles with a fiberoptic scope
60. Shift of this structure is seen with mediastinal shift
61. A drug that may be given in metabolic alkalosis; may cause metabolic acidosis
62. A xanthine bronchodilator; also dilates pulmonary vasculature (generic)
63. A decrease in surfactant would cause a decrease in compliance and an increase in _____ (abbrev.)
64. Collapse of alveoli; frequently seen in postoperative patients
65. The treatment of pneumonia includes oxygen, bronchial hygiene, and _____
67. These sounds are heard when listening with a stethoscope to a patient with atelectasis, pulmonary edema, and ARDS
69. This disorder is a chronic obstructive lung disease associated with the breakdown of elastic tissue, air trapping, and dyspnea
70. Two common symptoms of pulmonary conditions are dyspnea and _____
72. The complication caused by hyperventilation in asthma
74. Increased $Paco_2$

DOWN

1. This habit is the number one cause of COPD
2. Most community-acquired pneumonia is caused by gram-_____ bacteria
3. The term for shortness of breath
4. A gas that may be used in place of nitrogen in inspired air for patients with increased airway resistance
5. Airway _____ affects the work of breathing

8. Antibiotic _____ gram-positive bacterial strains have increased the mortality of health care–associated pneumonia
9. Chronic air _____ cause the shape of the thorax to change to be barrel-shaped
10. This type of pneumothorax is most often associated with rupture of a congenital bleb
12. Inflammation of the alveoli and bronchioles
13. This type of disorder is when airway resistance is increased
14. These receptors cause an increase in ventilation rate in response to body movement
17. This is caused by histamine
20. Patients with obstructive disease have prolonged _____
21. Type of heparin that may be administered subcutaneously to prevent deep vein thrombosis and pulmonary embolism (abbrev.)
22. The type of cell that secretes histamine
24. Patient position recommended to optimize V/Q matching in patients with ARDS
25. Surfactant is produced by the type II _____
26. An antibiotic that may be used to increase gastric motility (generic)
29. A pulmonary vasodilator (generic)
30. A muscle paralytic that may be administered by IV infusion in patients on mechanical ventilation (generic)
32. Impaired _____ is the risk factor most commonly associated with aspiration
33. Another term for type II acute respiratory failure (2 words)
35. Another term for type I acute respiratory failure (2 words)
36. This group of drugs should be administered to allow a patient to breathe deeply after thoracotomy
37. Another name for health care–associated pneumonia
38. A drug that breaks down the disulfide bonds in mucus (generic)
40. This type of airway provides a relative seal to allow mechanical ventilation without the surgical risks of tracheostomy

43. This type of chest pain is sharp pain that occurs with deep inspiration
44. A $beta_2$-stimulant that is administered orally or by inhalation
45. The cause of hypoxemia in myasthenia gravis is alveolar _____
47. A form of noncardiac pulmonary edema caused by inflammatory mediators and surfactant deficiency (abbrev.)
49. A $beta_2$-stimulant that may be given orally, subcutaneously, or by inhalation (generic)
52. Also referred to as *restrictive airway disease*; mucosal swelling and smooth muscle spasm causes wheezing and increased airway resistance
53. Fibrous exudate causes the _____ in pneumonia, which is manifested by crackles and bronchial breath sounds
54. A drug used in patients with pulmonary embolism with acute right ventricular failure or refractory hypoxemia to break down the clot (generic)
56. Pulmonary edema in ARDS is caused by increased capillary _____
57. The goal of oxygen therapy in this condition is to keep the Sao_2 at around 90% (abbrev.)
58. A pulmonary embolism would decrease _____ relative to ventilation
63. These sounds are heard when listening with a stethoscope to a patient with asthma (plural)
66. When deoxygenated blood comes in contact with non-ventilated alveoli; V<Q
68. The first treatment for asthma is the elimination of _____
71. Placing a patient with an air embolism in a left lateral decubitus position with his head down is referred to as _____ maneuver
73. $Paco_2$ of greater than 50 mm Hg and/or Pao_2 of less than 50 to 60 mm Hg (abbrev.)

4.25   Learning Activity

Match the patient characteristic with the appropriate description.

Criteria	Description
_____ 1. Resiliency—level 5	a. A 60-year-old woman with a history of diabetes and severe rheumatoid arthritis complaining of moderate chest pain and dyspnea shortly after arriving at the airport from a long international flight.
_____ 2. Vulnerability—level 1	b. A 30-year-old comatose man after a head injury, being weaned from tracheostomy before transfer to a skilled nursing facility.
_____ 3. Stability—level 5	c. A 74-year-old former smoker in whom pneumonia develops post influenza.
_____ 4. Complexity—level 3	d. A 92-year-old man recovering from community-acquired pneumonia who is eager to ambulate and use the incentive spirometer but requires assistance with ambulation and repeated instruction on proper use of the spirometer.
_____ 5. Resource availability— level 1	e. A 58-year-old man with chronic bronchiectasis admitted after an episode of hemoptysis. He has no health insurance, is estranged from his only sibling, and lives at a local shelter.
_____ 6. Participation in care— level 3	f. A 55-year-old man with a history of sleep apnea admitted for observation after a lap cholecystectomy.
_____ 7. Participation in decision making—level 1	g. A 30-year-old woman, height 5'2," weight 394 lbs., admitted for possible aspiration during extubation after an appendectomy.
_____ 8. Predictability—level 5	h. An 18-year-old woman admitted with a traumatic pneumothorax following a rib fracture from a fall.

Answers to this activity can be found in the Answer Key.

4.26   Synthesis Learning Activity: Clinical Vignette

A 28-year-old woman complains of shortness of breath and chest pain. The patient states that she is 38 weeks pregnant and on bed rest for the last 2 weeks. The patient states that the shortness of breath developed suddenly. The physical examination reveals crackles scattered throughout the lung fields and hyperpnea. She appears anxious and keeps asking the nursing staff if the baby will be okay.

Clinical findings include the following:

Vital signs: 98/54 mm Hg, 22 bpm with sinus tachycardia, and respirations 36 breaths/min.

ECG: sinus tachycardia with T wave inversions in V_1-V_4.

ABGs: Pao_2 70 mm Hg, $Paco_2$ 28 mm Hg, and pH 7.5.

1. When assessing the patient's relative risk for a pulmonary embolism, determine the clinical probability of pulmonary embolism. The patient's risk is low, moderate, or high? _____
2. Due to the pregnancy state, the recommended diagnostic test to confirm the diagnosis may include the following (identify all that apply):
   a. D-dimer assay
   b. Modified V/Q scan
   c. Spiral CT
   d. Ultrasound of peripheral veins
3. Treatment of choice for a pulmonary embolism in a pregnant patient is _____.
4. The drugs _____ and _____ are contraindicated in pregnancy.

Answers to this activity can be found in the Answer Key.

The Renal System

ANATOMY AND PHYSIOLOGY

Function

The renal system regulates the body's internal environment by maintaining homeostasis and hormone production and release. To maintain the body's environment, the renal system has an active role in the excretion of metabolic wastes and regulation of extracellular fluid osmolality, electrolyte balance, and acid-base balance in conjunction with the pulmonary system. Blood pressure regulation is influenced by aldosterone, released by the adrenal cortex, and antidiuretic hormone (ADH), released by the posterior pituitary. Hormone production and release stimulates the production of red blood cells (RBCs) via erythropoietin, improves glomerular filtration rate (GFR) through the synthesis and release of prostaglandins, and participates in activation of vitamin D.

Anatomy

The renal system consists of two kidneys, two ureters, the urinary bladder, and the urethra (Figure 5-1). The kidneys are bean-shaped organs with a convex lateral border and concave medial border. Approximately the size of a fist, the kidneys weigh 120 to 170 g, have a vertical long axis, and are located in the posterior abdominal wall behind the peritoneum opposite the last thoracic vertebra and first three lumbar vertebrae on each side of the spine. The right kidney is slightly lower than the left due to the location of the liver. The ureters are fibromuscular tubes located behind peritoneum. They extend from each kidney to the posterior part of the bladder floor. Ureter walls are composed of smooth muscle with mucosa lining and a fibrous outer coat. The ureters collect urine from the renal pelvis and propel it to the bladder by peristaltic waves. Ureters enter the superior posterior bladder at an oblique angle. The angle and the peristaltic action of the ureters prevent reflux of urine. The bladder is a collapsible bag of smooth muscle located behind the symphysis pubis, below the peritoneum. The bladder acts as a reservoir for urine until a sufficient amount accumulates for elimination, and then the urine leaves the body via the urethra. The urethra is located behind the symphysis pubis, anterior to the vagina in females, and extends through the prostate gland and penis in males. The urethra acts as a passageway for expulsion of urine from the urinary bladder to the urinary meatus and expelled from the body. Adults void approximately 100 to 300 mL of urine 5 to 9 times per day.

External Structures

External to the kidneys, essential structures provide circulation and protection of the kidneys including the hilum, renal capsule, perirenal fat, and fascia. The hilum is the concave notch of the medial aspect of the kidney. Both an entry site for the renal artery and nerves and an exit site for the renal vein and ureter, the hilum area is where circulation to and from the kidney occurs. The renal capsule is a thin, smooth layer of fibrous membrane that surrounds each kidney to act as a protective layer. The capsule prevents kidney swelling and contains pain receptors. The fat and renal fascia that surrounds the kidney helps to support, protect, and hold the kidney in place.

Renal Parenchyma

The cortex and medulla are the two divisions of the renal parenchyma. The cortex has a reddish-brown color and granular appearance and is approximately 1 cm wide. The cortex is the metabolically active portion of the kidney in which aerobic metabolism and the formation of ammonia and glucose occur. It is the site of the glomerulus and the proximal and distal tubules.

The medulla is darker than the cortex, striated, approximately 5 cm wide, and the site of the deepest part of the loop of Henle. Pyramids are triangular wedges of medullary tissue and are composed of collecting tubules and ducts; there are 6 to 10 pyramids. Columns are inward extensions of cortical tissue between the pyramids. Many of the kidney's blood vessels and nerves are in these columns. A renal lobe is composed of a pyramid and surrounding cortical tissue.

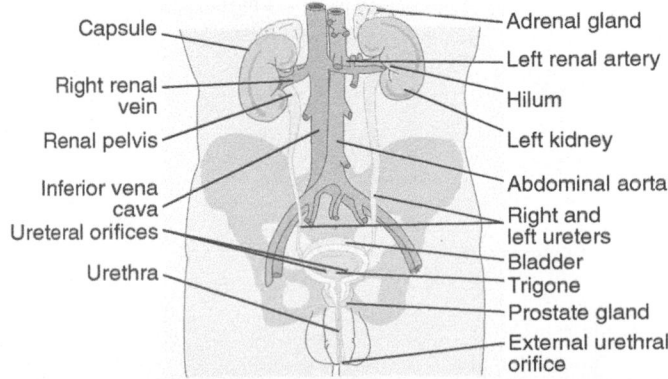

FIGURE 5-1 **The kidneys and other structures of the urinary tract.** (From Montague, S. E., Watson, R., & Herbert, R. [2005]. *Physiology for nursing practice* [3rd ed.]. Oxford: Bailliére Tindall.)

The renal sinus is a spacious cavity filled with adipose tissue, the renal pelvis, minor and major calyces, and the origin of the ureter. Calyces are cuplike structures that drain the papillae. Eight to 12 minor calyces open into 2 to 3 major calyces that form the renal pelvis. The renal pelvis papillae are at the apices of the renal pyramids. Collecting tubules drain into minor calyces at papillae. The union of several calyces, known as the renal pelvis, forms a small funnel that tapers into the ureter. Urine flows from the collecting duct to the renal pelvis and into the ureter (Figure 5-2).

Functional Units

The nephron is the microscopic functional unit of the kidney (Figure 5-3). There are approximately 1 million nephrons in each kidney. The nephron unit is able to compensate for a significant degree of nephron destruction by filtering a greater solute (i.e., dissolved substances) load and by hypertrophy of remaining functional nephrons. There are two types of nephrons: cortical (85%) and juxtamedullary (15%). Cortical nephrons contain short loops of Henle that dip into the outer edge of the medulla. The glomerulus is located in the outer and inner cortex. Juxtamedullary nephrons contain long loops of Henle that penetrate deep into the medulla. These nephrons are important in the kidney's ability to concentrate the urine.

The renal corpuscle is a functional segment that contains Bowman's capsule and the glomerulus. The glomerulus is a cluster of tightly coiled capillaries that produces an ultrafiltrate; a portion of the ultrafiltrate eventually becomes urine. Bowman's capsule is the funnel-shaped upper end of the proximal tubule.

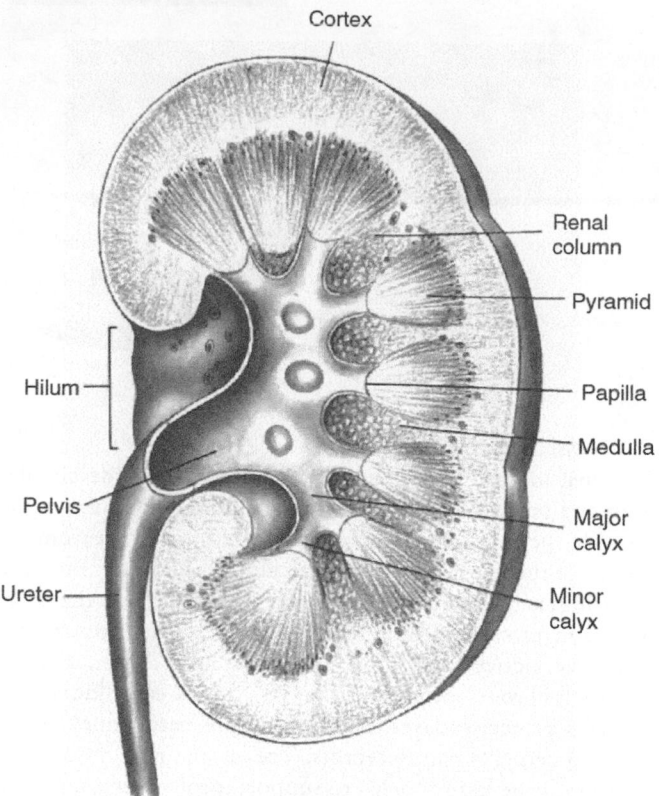

FIGURE 5-2   Cross-section of the kidney. (From Thompson, J. M., McFarland, G. K., Hirsch, J. E., & Tucker, S. M. [2002]. *Mosby's clinical nursing* [5th ed.]. St. Louis, MO: Mosby.)

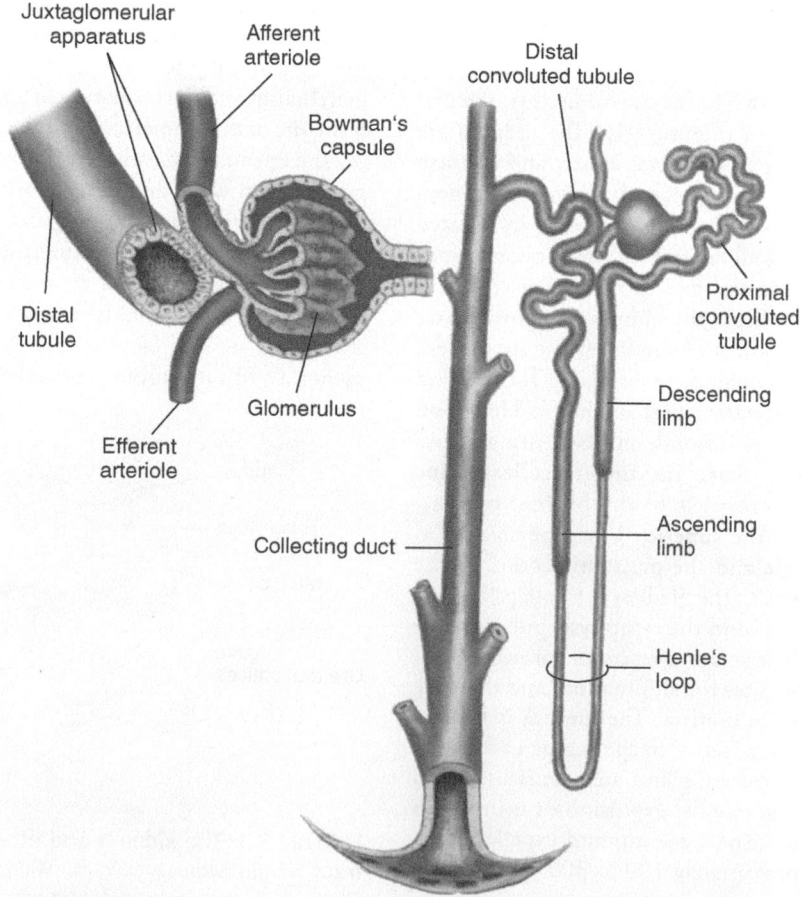

FIGURE 5-3 Components of the nephron. (From Urden, L. D., Stacy, K. M., & Lough, M. E. [2010]. *Critical care nursing: Diagnosis and management* [6th ed.]. St. Louis, MO: Mosby.)

Segments of the renal tubules are divided into the proximal convoluted tubule, loop of Henle, and distal convoluted tubule. The tubules are responsible for reabsorption and secretion, which alter the volume and composition of the ultrafiltration to form the final urine volume and composition. Several nephrons converge into a collecting duct. The collecting duct relays the urine from the tubules to the minor calyx.

5.1 Learning Activity

Number the structures according to the order of their involvement in urine formation.

__ Ureters
__ Glomerulus
__ Loop of Henle
__ Proximal convoluted tubule
__ Bladder
__ Bowman's capsule
__ Collecting ducts
__ Distal convoluted tubule
__ Urethra

Answers to this activity can be found in the Answer Key.

Renal Vasculature Pathway

Blood supply to the kidneys comes from the renal arteries that branch from the aorta. The renal arteries branch into the interlobar arteries to the arcuate arteries to the interlobular arteries. These interlobular arteries become the afferent arteriole that forms the glomerulus in each nephron. The efferent arteriole leads out of the glomerulus and forms the peritubular capillary network. The efferent arteriole from the juxtamedullary nephron forms a different capillary network called the *vasa recta*. The vasa recta is a complex of long straight capillary loops that run parallel to the ascending and descending loop of Henle. The anatomic area known as the vasa recta plays an important role in concentrating interstitial fluid found in the medulla. Blood flow through the vasa recta is sluggish. The peritubular capillary network leads to the interlobular vein that leads to the arcuate vein. The arcuate vein leads to the interlobar vein that leads to the renal vein. The renal vein empties into the inferior vena cava.

Renal Blood Flow. The kidneys receive 20% to 25% of the cardiac output, or approximately 1200 mL/min (600 mL/min for each kidney). Autoregulation is the process that maintains constancy in the glomerular filtration rate (GFR). Systemic arterial pressure between 80 and 180 mm Hg prevents large changes in GFR because of the ability of the afferent arteriole to constrict or dilate. Increases in mean arterial pressure (MAP) cause constriction of the afferent arteriole that prevents the increased arterial pressure from raising the pressure in the glomerulus. A decrease in MAP causes dilation of the afferent arteriole, allowing blood to flow into the glomerulus. Autoregulation fails at a MAP of 60 mm Hg or less, which may lead to prerenal acute kidney injury progressing to prolonged intrinsic acute kidney injury. The juxtaglomerular apparatus consists of the macula densa and the juxtaglomerular cells. The macula densa is a part of the distal tubule that lies close to the afferent and efferent arterioles. Juxtaglomerular cells produce and store the enzyme renin. Renin is secreted in response to hypotension.

Lymphatics. There is an abundant supply of lymphatics to the kidney. Lymphatics from the kidney drain into the thoracic duct. Lymphatics are abundant around the arteries and veins. Lymphatics are also present in the renal cortex and medulla.

Nervous Innervation. The autonomic nervous system (ANS) supplies the primary innervation of the kidney and the urinary tract. The superior splanchnic and inferior splanchnic nerves enter the kidney at the hilum, forming the renal plexus. The inferior mesenteric plexus, the hypogastric plexus, and the pubic nerve from the sacral region supply the bladder, ureters, and urethra.

Both the sympathetic nervous system (SNS) and the parasympathetic nervous system (PNS) innervate the kidney, but the SNS has the prominent effect on the kidney. Located in the afferent and efferent arterioles and in all sections of the tubule, the SNS fiber endings' effects on the kidney include the following:

* Low levels of innervation increase sodium reabsorption within the proximal tubule.
* Moderate levels of innervation decrease renal blood flow and glomerular filtration rate because of constriction of afferent and efferent arterioles.
* High levels of innervation cause extreme reduction in renal blood flow and potential cessation of glomerular filtration rate due to afferent arteriole constriction.

Physiology
Urine Formation

Formation of urine involves three processes: filtration, reabsorption, and secretion (Figure 5-4). Glomerular filtration occurs because the pressure of the blood within the glomerular capillaries filters blood into the Bowman's capsule, where it begins to pass down to the tubule. GFR is dependent on permeability of the capillary walls, vascular pressure, and filtration pressure. Filtration is the transfer of water and dissolved substances through a permeable membrane from a region of high pressure to a region of low pressure. Dependent on hydrostatic pressure, the process of filtration may be affected by the following:

* Diminished renal perfusion from hypovolemia
* Occlusion of the glomeruli from diabetic neuropathy

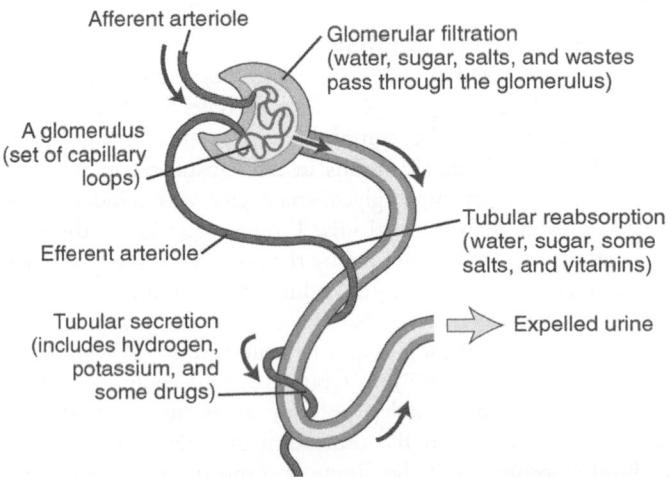

FIGURE 5-4 Major functions of each portion of the nephron.
(From Sole, M. L., Klein, D. G., & Moseley, M. J. [2005]. *Introduction to critical care nursing* [4th ed.]. Philadelphia, PA: Saunders.)

- Alteration in the plasma protein concentration from hypoproteinemia
- Alterations in the basement membrane from an autoimmune disorder
- Arteriolar constriction from SNS stimulation or vasopressors

Clearance is the complete removal of a solute from blood. Clearance of a solute equals GFR if the tubules neither reabsorb nor secrete the solute. Clearance of a substance is less than GFR if the tubules reabsorb the substance. Clearance of a substance is greater than GFR if the tubules secrete the solute. The creatinine clearance is the clinical test used to measure clearance. Creatinine is filtered by the glomeruli and not reabsorbed by the tubules. The formula for GFR is the urine concentration of x (i.e., creatinine) × the urine flow rate per minute divided by the plasma concentration of x (i.e., creatinine).

Creatinine clearance is a calculation of GFR by comparing serum creatinine with the amount of creatinine excreted in the urine over a 24-hour period. Autoregulation ensures the constant rate required to maintain the GFR. Systemic mean arterial pressure between 80 and 180 mm Hg maintains autoregulation.

The glomerular membrane is a porous but semipermeable membrane. Glomerular filtrate is similar in composition to blood except that it lacks blood cells, platelets, and large plasma proteins. Water, sodium, glucose, potassium, chloride, phosphate, urea, uric acid, creatinine, ammonia, phenol, calcium, and magnesium pass through the glomerular membrane. Glomerular filtrate volume is usually 120 mL/min, but 99% of the volume is reabsorbed in the renal tubule.

Reabsorption refers to the passage of a substance that the body needs from the lumen of the tubules through the tubular cells and into the capillaries. Reabsorption involves both active and passive transport processes. Active transport is the force used when the cell membranes must move molecules against a concentration gradient. Active transport requires the use of energy and a carrier substance. The substance combines with a carrier and diffuses through the tubular membrane where they reenter the bloodstream. Substances moved by active transport include glucose, protein, amino acids, and phosphate. Passive transport processes include diffusion and osmosis. Diffusion is the passive movement of solute from an area of higher concentration to an area of lower concentration. Diffusion is the process used to move urea and electrolytes. Osmosis is the passive movement of water from an area of lower solute concentration to an area of higher solute concentration.

The renal threshold of a substance, otherwise known as the maximal tubular transport capacity, reflects the maximum amount of a substance completely reabsorbed in 1 minute. Exceeding this threshold results in the substance's appearance in the urine. For example, glycosuria occurs with a blood sugar that is greater than 300 mL/dL. Tubular secretion is the passage of a substance not needed by the body from the capillaries through the tubular cells into the lumen of the tubule.

The countercurrent mechanism utilizes the juxtamedullary nephrons with their long loops of Henle and occurs within the renal medullary interstitium. Countercurrent multiplication is the mechanism that enables the body to excrete urine with an osmolality higher than the osmolality of serum. Transport of sodium chloride out of the filtrate as it moves up the ascending limb of the loop of Henle occurs, but water is not able to follow because this limb is impermeable to water. Some of the sodium chloride enters the peritubular capillaries and is removed from the kidney, but some reenters the descending limb of the loop of Henle, making the filtrate more concentrated than the blood from which it was derived. This process increases the osmotic pressure in the capillaries and tubules of the papillary region of the kidney until it is four times stronger than that of the blood in the afferent arteriole. Countercurrent exchange is the maintenance component of the countercurrent mechanism. The vasa recta tissue minimizes the loss of solute from the interstitium by passive diffusion, maintaining the osmotic gradient necessary for the countercurrent multiplication process. A total of 99% of the glomerular filtrate is reabsorbed from the tubules (especially the proximal tubule) and the remaining 1% is excreted as urine output.

Normal urine output is approximately 1500 mL/day. Urine is composed of water, nitrogenous wastes (urea, uric acid, creatinine, and ammonia), ions (potassium, sodium, calcium, chloride, bicarbonate, hydrogen, phosphate, and sulfate), hormones and their breakdown products, water-soluble vitamins, toxins, and drugs. In addition, abnormal constituents such as glucose, albumin, RBCs, calculi, casts, and pigments may be in the urine, but these signify dysfunction.

Excretion of Metabolic Waste Products

Urea is a protein that is broken down into amino acids and nitrogenous wastes. The end product of protein metabolism, urea nitrogen circulates in the bloodstream and is eliminated via urine excretion. Blood urea nitrogen (BUN) varies with protein intake and hydration status, so the BUN level is an unreliable evaluation of renal function. Creatinine is a waste product of muscle metabolism. The normal kidney excretes creatinine at a rate equal to the kidney's blood flow or GFR. Serum creatinine is a better test for evaluation of renal function than BUN. Urine creatinine clearance, which provides a comparison of serum creatinine and 24-hour urine creatinine, is an even better evaluation of renal function, especially for the elderly or people with low or high muscle mass destruction (e.g., heat stroke and rhabdomyolysis).

Acid-Base Regulation

In response to acidosis, the renal system will increase hydrogen ion secretion, increase bicarbonate reabsorption, and produce ammonia to accommodate hydrogen ion excretion. In response to alkalosis, the renal system will decrease hydrogen ion secretion, increase bicarbonate excretion, and decrease production of ammonia. In conjunction with the pulmonary system, the renal system helps to regulate acid-base balance by:

- Tubular excretion of H^+ ions in exchange for sodium reabsorption
- Bicarbonate reabsorption into the circulation, or excretion into the urine
- Excretion of H^+ ions in the urine, such as NH_4Cl, H_2PO_4, or H_2O

Fluid Balance

Body fluids are dilute solutions of water and solutes. The unit of measure for fluid volume is the milliliter (mL). The unit of measure for chemical combining activity of an electrolyte is a milliequivalent (mEq). The unit of measure for osmotic pressure based on the number of dissolved particles in solution is milliosmoles (mOsm).

The terms *osmolality* and *osmolarity* are fused interchangeably, although osmolality provides the basis for most calculations of body fluids. Osmolality is the number of osmoles per kilogram of solution. Expressed as mOsm/kg, osmolality can be measured in the blood or urine. The main constituent of normal blood is sodium and the osmolality equals 280 to 295 mOsm/kg. Normal urine constituents are urea and sodium and the normal osmolality level is 50 to 1200 mOsm/kg H_2O.

Osmolarity is defined as the number of osmoles per liter of solution. Isotonic solutions have the tonicity of body fluids with an osmolarity of 280 to 295 mOsm/L. Hypotonic solutions have lower tonicity than body fluids. Hypertonic solutions have higher tonicity than body fluids. The human body is mostly water. In adult males, 60% of total body weight is water. In adult females, slightly less than 55% of total body weight is water due to a higher percentage of body fat. Older adults have less water at 45% to 55% of total body weight as well as obese patients because the amount of water in the body decreases as body fat increases.

Distribution

Fluid is distributed into five different compartments: intracellular, extracellular, interstitial, intravascular, and transcellular compartments. Intracellular fluid contained within the cells accounts for 40% of total body weight. Extracellular fluid accounts for 20% of total body weight. Interstitial fluid surrounding the cells accounts for 15% of total body weight. Intravascular fluid contained within the blood vessels accounts for approximately 5% of total body weight. Transcellular fluid is contained within specialized cavities of the body (e.g., cerebrospinal, pericardial, pleural, synovial, intraocular, and digestive fluids) and accounts for approximately 1% of total body weight (Figure 5-5).

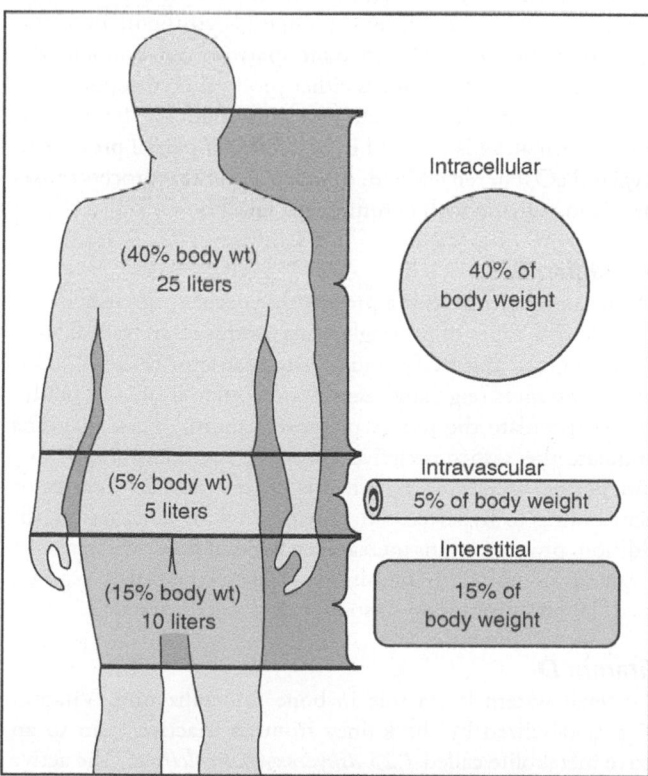

FIGURE 5-5 Distribution of body fluids. (From Urden, L. D., Stacy, K. M., & Lough, M. E. [2010]. *Critical care nursing: Diagnosis and management* [6th ed.]. St. Louis, MO: Mosby.)

Homeostasis

Homeostasis is the state of internal equilibrium within the body; therefore, fluid, electrolyte, and acid-base levels are in balance. Water and solutes are in constant movement and exchanged continuously. Most of the membranes of the body are semipermeable, which allows free movement of water and many nonelectrolytes and selective movement of electrolytes according to concentration gradients. Movement of fluids, electrolytes, and other solutes occurs by the following processes:

- Diffusion: Solutes move from an area of higher solute concentration to an area of lower solute concentration.
- Osmosis: Solutions move from an area of lower solute concentration to an area of higher solute concentration.
- Active transport: Use of an energy source to move solutes from an area of lower solute concentration to an area of higher solute concentration.
- Filtration: Use of the pushing force of hydrostatic pressure to move water and selective solutes through a semipermeable membrane.
- Movement into and out of the cell occurs by diffusion, osmosis, and active transport.
- Capillary hydrostatic pressure pushes fluid out of the capillary and into interstitium.
- Interstitial hydrostatic pressure pushes fluid out of the interstitium and into the capillary.
- Capillary colloidal oncotic pressure pulls and holds fluid in the capillary.
- Interstitial colloidal oncotic pressure pulls and holds fluid in the interstitium.

Fluid Movement

Starling's law of the capillaries describes the movement of fluid into and out of the capillaries. Pressure differences at the venous and arterial ends of the capillaries influence the direction and rate of water and solute movement. Pressures pushing fluid out of the capillary dominate at the arterial end, while pressures pushing fluid back into the capillary dominate at the venous end.

Third-spacing of fluid is the accumulation of fluid in any space that is not intravascular or intracellular (e.g., interstitial edema, ascites, pleural effusion, pericardial effusion). Fluid and peripheral edema accumulates with heart failure pathology. Venous congestion and excessive hydrostatic pressure at the venous end cause peripheral edema. Malnutrition decreases protein stores. The decrease in plasma proteins decreases capillary colloidal oncotic pressure and allows excessive fluid to leak out of the capillary. Fluid resuscitation with hypotonic solutions (e.g., D_5W) causes movement of fluid out of the vascular bed into the interstitium because the fluids have less osmolality than serum.

5.2 Learning Activity

Complete the following statements related to the movement of solutes and solutions.

Water moves by the process of _____.
Electrolytes move by the process of _____.
The sodium-potassium pump is an example of

_____

The use of a pushing force, such as hydrostatic pressure, is called _____.

Answers to this activity can be found in the Answer Key.

Normal functioning of cells requires constancy of the body's compartments. Imbalances disrupt homeostasis. Water exchanges occur continuously via the lungs (400 mL), skin (400 mL), kidneys (1500 mL), and intestines (100 mL) for a total loss of up to 2400 mL/24 hours. Loss of water occurs by any of the following:

• Increased respiratory rate
• Fever
• Hot, dry environment
• Injury to the skin (e.g., burns)

Gains of water intake total ~2400 mL/24 hr. Oral fluids account for 1500 mL and liquid in food accounts for 500 mL. Remember that the oxidation of food and body tissues also provides a 400 mL gain in water.

Thirst regulates body fluid. The thirst mechanism is located in the anterior hypothalamus. Osmoreceptor cells sense changes in serum osmolality and initiate impulses to produce the thirst sensation and the release of ADH.

The mechanism is stimulated by any of the following:

• Intracellular dehydration
• Hypertonic body fluids
• Extracellular fluid loss
• Hypotension or decreased cardiac output
• Angiotensin
• Dry mouth

The effect of thirst is the conscious desire to drink fluids. It is important to note that thirst is unreliable in the elderly or confused. The hypothalamus produces ADH and the hormone is stored in and released by the posterior pituitary gland. Intracranial processes (e.g., head injury, tumors, craniotomy) and extracranial processes (e.g., mechanical ventilation, tuberculosis, cancer) alter the release of ADH. Hyperosmolality of extracellular fluid, decrease in extracellular fluid volume, and hyperthermia stimulate ADH. ADH acts on distal and collecting tubules, resulting in more water pulled from the tubule back into the blood, which increases total volume of body fluid by decreasing urine volume.

Decreased blood pressure triggers stretch receptors in juxtaglomerular cells and the sympathetic nervous system along with the conditions of hyponatremia and hyperkalemia, and increased adrenocorticotropic hormone (ACTH) levels stimulate the renin-angiotensin-aldosterone (RAA) system. The RAA system causes the secretion of aldosterone. Angiotensin II causes vasoconstriction and secretion of aldosterone, a mineralocorticoid produced by the adrenal cortex. Aldosterone stimulates the renal tubules to reabsorb more sodium and water, which causes sodium retention, water retention, and decreased urine volume. Vasoconstriction, hypernatremia, and hypervolemia increase blood pressure, which decreases renin secretion (Figure 5-6).

Atrial natriuretic peptide (ANP) is a hormone-like substance synthesized and stored by specialized atrial muscle cells. ANP secretion is stimulated by volume expansion and elevated cardiac filling pressures. ANP increases excretion of sodium and water by the kidney, decreases the synthesis of renin, and decreases release of aldosterone. This countercurrent mechanism of the kidney is responsible for the concentration and dilution of urine.

Electrolyte Balance

Solutes are substances dissolved in a solution and may be nonelectrolytes or electrolytes. Nonelectrolytes (e.g., glucose, proteins, lipids, oxygen, carbon dioxide, urea, creatinine, and bilirubin) are solutes without an electrical charge. Nonelectrolytes stay intact in solution. Electrolytes (Table 5-1) are solutes that, when in solution, dissociate into positive or negative ions and will generate an electrical charge. Cations are positively charged ions. The major intracellular cation is potassium (K^+). The major extracellular cation is sodium (Na^+). Other cations important in body functions include calcium (Ca^{++}), magnesium (Mg^{++}), and hydrogen (H^+). Anions are negatively charged electrolytes. The major intracellular anion is chloride (Cl^-). The major extracellular anion is phosphate (PO_4^{3-}). Another anion important in body function is bicarbonate (HCO_3^-).

In each fluid compartment, the various cations and anions balance each other to achieve electrical neutrality. There is no net charge within a fluid compartment (Figure 5-7). The renal system regulates the excretion and/or retention of electrolytes. The kidneys filter and reabsorb about half of unbound serum calcium and activate vitamin D_3, a compound that promotes intestinal calcium absorption. In addition, the kidneys regulate phosphorus excretion.

Blood Pressure

The renal system has a role in regulation of blood pressure. The juxtaglomerular apparatus is a combination of specialized cells located near the glomerulus at the junction of the afferent and efferent arterioles. The juxtaglomerular cells contain granules of inactive renin. The release of renin, triggering the initiation of the RAA system, retention of sodium and water, and vasoconstriction and elevation of blood pressure, results from hypoperfusion to the juxtaglomerlular cells.

Red Blood Cells

Red blood cell (RBC) synthesis and maturation is dependent on erythropoietin secretion from the kidney. Erythropoietin stimulates production of RBCs in bone marrow and prolongs the life of RBCs. Normal kidneys either produce erythropoietin or synthesize an enzyme that catalyzes its formation. The stimulation for formation is believed to be decreased partial pressure of oxygen (PaO_2) in renal blood. Interference in this process causes anemia in patients with chronic renal failure.

Prostaglandins

Prostaglandin synthesis is a process that occurs primarily in the medulla. The types of prostaglandins produced are vasodilators (PGE_2, PGD_2, and PGI_2) and a vasoconstrictor (PGA_2). Vasoactive substances (e.g., angiotensin, norepinephrine, and bradykinins) stimulate the release of prostaglandins. Prostaglandins modulate the vasoconstrictive effects of angiotensin and norepinephrine. Interference with this process may be one factor contributing to hypertension in patients with renal failure. In addition, prostaglandins increase renal blood flow, which results in arterial vasodilation, inhibition of the distal tubule's response to ADH, and promotion of sodium and water excretion.

Vitamin D

The renal system has a role in bone mineralization. Vitamin D is metabolized by the kidney from an inactive form to an active metabolite called *1,25-dihydroxycholecalciferol*. The active vitamin D is necessary for the absorption of calcium and phosphorus from the intestine. Interference in this process causes low serum calcium levels and demineralization of calcium from

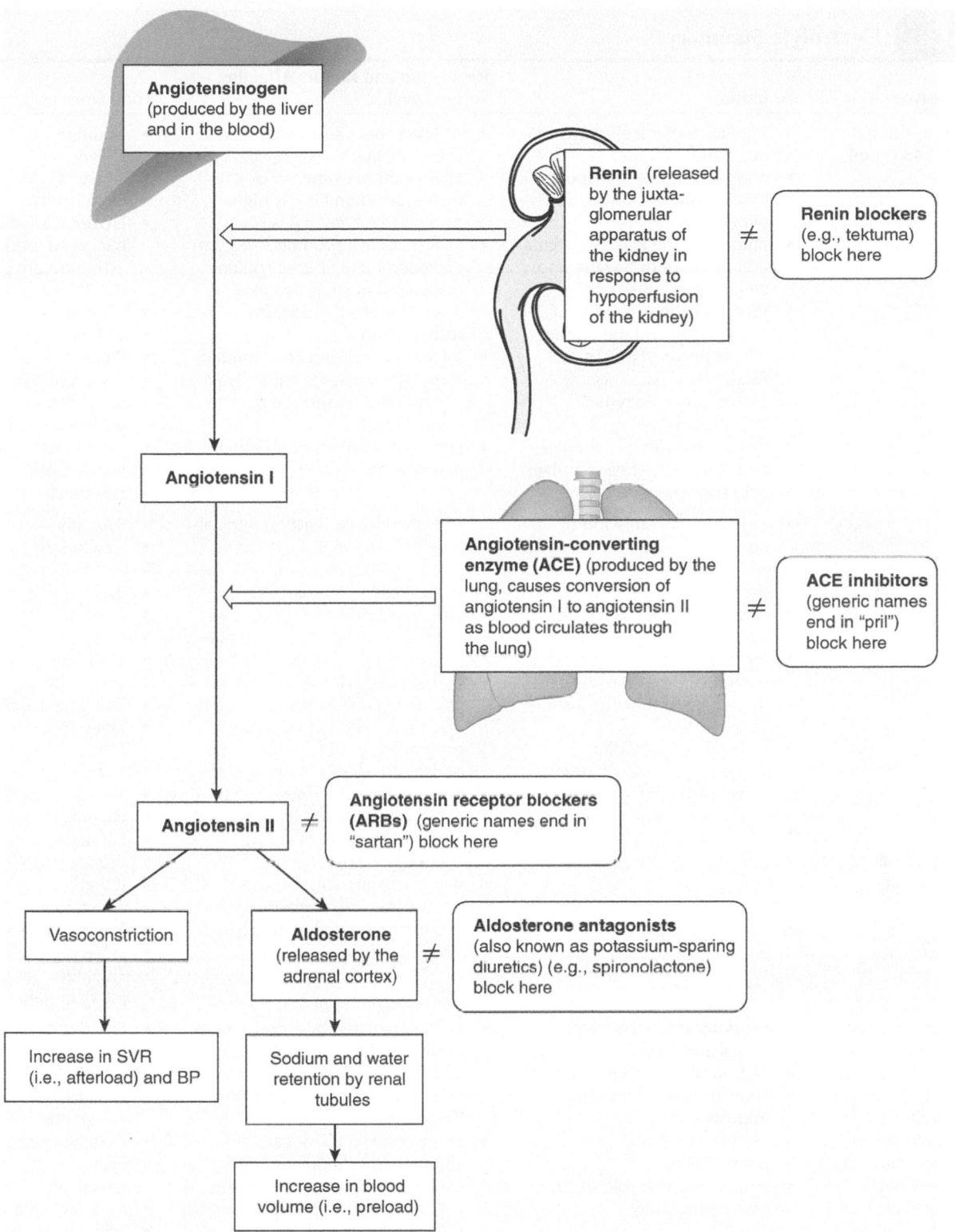

FIGURE 5-6 Renin-angiotensin system. (From Dennison, R. D. [2013]. *Pass CCRN!* [4th ed.]. St. Louis, MO: Elsevier.)

the bones, resulting in osteodystrophy in patients with chronic renal failure. Calcium and phosphorus have an inverse relationship; therefore, low serum calcium levels lead to the hyperphosphatemia seen in patients with renal failure.

Age-Related Changes

Renal function decreases with age. As early as 20 to 40 years of age, renal changes begin to occur, including a decrease in tubular length. By the age of 65, renal function decreases by 10% and diminishes further with aging. Due to a decrease in nephrons, renal mass and the GFR decrease. Age-related vascular changes impact renal blood flow. Decreased serum renin and aldosterone reduce the ability to conserve sodium, excrete water, and limit urinary concentration. As a person ages, there is diminished creatinine production (less muscle mass) and diminished ability to excrete creatinine; therefore, elevation

| TABLE 5-1 | **Electrolyte Summary** | | |

Electrolyte	Functions	Regulation and Factors Affecting Serum Level	Food Sources
Sodium: normal 136-145 mEq/L	• Maintains extracellular osmolality and volume • Maintains active transport mechanism in conjunction with potassium • Influences the kidney's regulation of the body's water and electrolyte status • Promotes the irritability of nerve tissue and the conduction of nerve impulses • Facilitates muscle contraction • Aids in some enzyme activities • Combines with bicarbonate and chloride to help regulate acid-base balance	• Aldosterone: causes sodium and water retention • GFR: sodium excretion is increased when GFR is high; decreased when GFR is low • "Third factor": promotes sodium excretion by inhibiting sodium reabsorption; suppression of this factor ensures sodium reabsorption • Increase in sodium concentration stimulates water retention by ADH release diluting sodium back to normal level • Some excretion through skin in perspiration	• Bouillon • Celery • Cheeses • Dried fruits • Frozen, canned, or packaged foods • Monosodium glutamate (MSG) • Mustard • Olives • Pickles • Preserved meat • Salad dressings and prepared sauces • Sauerkraut • Snack foods • Soy sauce
Potassium: normal 3.5-5.0 mEq/L	• Promotes transmission of nerve impulses • Maintains intracellular osmolality • Activates several enzymatic reactions • Helps regulate acid-base balance • Influences kidney function and structure • Promotes myocardial, skeletal, and smooth muscle contractility	• Aldosterone: increase in intracellular potassium or decrease in serum sodium causes aldosterone release and potassium excretion • GFR: potassium excretion is directly related to GFR in a normal kidney • Obligatory loss: the kidneys are unable to conserve potassium; it may be flushed out by diuresis even in the presence of a body deficit; 40-50 mEq lost each day • Renal failure: if kidneys fail to excrete potassium normally from the body (e.g., renal failure), toxic levels can occur • pH: potassium shifts into the cell in alkalosis (causing hypokalemia) and out of the cell in acidosis (causing hyperkalemia)	• Apricots • Artichokes • Avocado • Banana • Cantaloupe • Carrots • Cauliflower • Chocolate • Dried beans, peas • Dried fruit • Mushrooms • Nuts • Oranges, orange juice • Peanuts • Potatoes • Prune juice • Pumpkin • Spinach • Sweet potatoes • Swiss chard • Tomatoes, tomato juice, tomato sauce
Calcium: normal 8.5-10.5 mg/dL or 4.5-5.8 mEq/L (NOTE: Calcium is affected by albumin levels; to correct calcium, add 0.8 mg/dL for each 1 g/dL decrease in albumin)	• Hardens and strengthens bones and teeth • Aids in blood coagulation • Transmits neuromuscular impulses • Maintains cellular permeability • Serves essential role in cardiac contractility	• PTH: stimulated by a decrease in serum calcium; promotes calcium transfer from bone to plasma and aids in renal and intestinal absorption • Phosphorus: inhibits calcium absorption; calcium and phosphorus have an inverse relationship; if calcium goes up, phosphorus goes down and vice versa • Vitamin D: necessary for GI absorption; promotes calcium absorption • Calcitonin: aids transfer of calcium from plasma to bone, which directly lowers serum calcium • Albumin: 50% of serum calcium is bound to serum albumin; therefore, a decrease in serum albumin will lower the total calcium level but not the ionized calcium level and the patient will not have symptoms of hypocalcemia	• Brazil nuts • Broccoli • Cheese • Collard, mustard, turnip greens • Cottage cheese • Eggnog • Ice cream • Milk and cream • Milk chocolate • Molasses • Oat flakes • Rhubarb • Seafood, especially sardines with bones • Sesame seeds • Soy flour • Spinach • Yogurt

| TABLE 5-1 | Electrolyte Summary—cont'd | | | |

Electrolyte	Functions	Regulation and Factors Affecting Serum Level	Food Sources
		• pH: alkalosis increases binding between albumin and calcium so that the patient will exhibit symptoms of hypocalcemia, though total body calcium is normal; acidosis decreases binding between albumin and calcium so that the patient may exhibit symptoms of hypercalcemia • Corticosteroids: contribute to demineralization of the bone and calcium loss; large doses decrease calcium absorption in GI tract • Diuretic effect: calcium is lost, along with potassium and magnesium, in patients on diuretics	
Phosphorus: normal 3.0-4.5 mg/dL	• Aids in structure of cellular membrane • Essential for glucose metabolism in red cells; produces 2,3-DPG as an end product • Regulates the delivery of oxygen to the tissues; 2,3-DPG encourages unloading between hemoglobin and oxygen • Essential for ATP or high-energy phosphate formation • May be connected with DNA, RNA, genetic coding • Helps maintain bone hardness • Aids in enzyme regulation (ATPase) • Used by kidneys to buffer hydrogen ions (PO_4)	• PTH: inhibits renal reabsorption of phosphates; calcium and phosphorus have an inverse relationship; if calcium goes up, phosphorus goes down and vice versa • Alterations in GFR affect phosphate excretion; increased GFR decreases reabsorption of phosphorus; decreased GFR increases reabsorption of phosphorus	• Dried beans and peas • Eggs and egg products • Fish, poultry • Meats, especially organ meats • Milk and milk products • Nuts • Seeds • Whole grains
Magnesium: normal 1.5-2.5 mEq/L	• Aids in neuromuscular transmission • Aids in cardiac contractility • Activates enzymes for cellular metabolism of CHO and proteins • Aids in maintaining the active transport mechanism at the cellular level • Aids in the transmission of hereditary information to offspring	• Not completely understood • Factors that influence calcium and potassium balance also affect magnesium • Deficiencies of these electrolytes usually occur together (e.g., diuretics cause the loss of all three) • Availability of sodium: sodium is necessary for the absorption of magnesium • Diuretics: cause the loss of excessive magnesium • PTH: affects magnesium reabsorption as it does calcium	• Bananas • Chocolate • Coconut • Grapefruit • Green, leafy vegetables • Legumes • Milk • Molasses • Nuts and seeds • Oranges • Refined sugar • Seafood • Soy flour • Wheat bran
Chloride: normal 96-106 mEq/L	• Maintains serum osmolality (along with sodium) • Combines with major cations to form important compounds (e.g., NaCl, HCl, KCl, CaCl) • Helps maintain acid-base balance through HCl production	• Indirectly affected by aldosterone • Changes almost always linked to sodium • pH: acidosis causes bicarbonate to be reabsorbed while chloride is excreted; alkalosis causes bicarbonate to be excreted while chloride is reabsorbed	• Bananas • Celery • Cheese • Dates • Eggs • Fish • Milk • Spinach • Table salt • Turkey

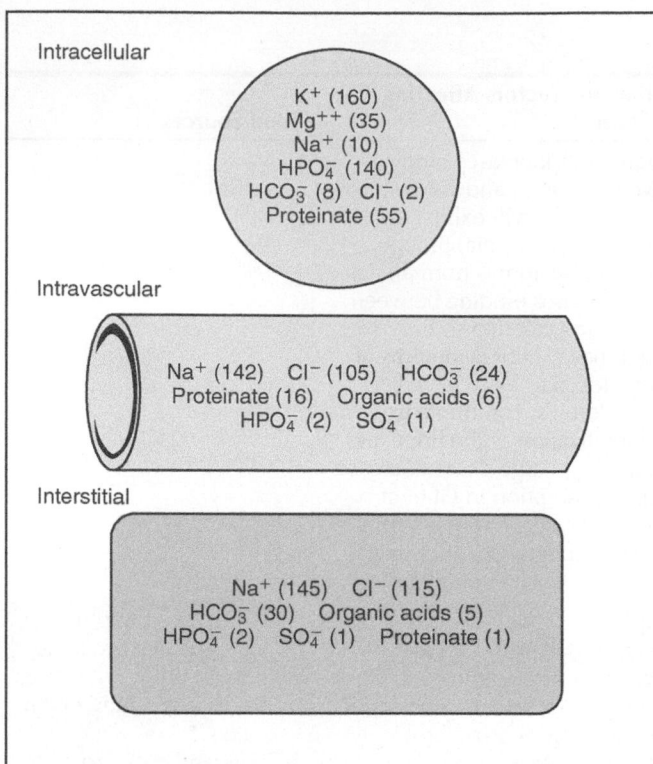

FIGURE 5-7 Electrolytes by fluid compartment. (From Urden, L. D., Stacy, K. M., & Lough, M. E. [2010]. *Critical care nursing: Diagnosis and management* [6th ed.]. St. Louis, MO: Mosby.)

of serum creatinine levels may not be demonstrated. Slightly elevated uric acid levels also occur with aging.

ASSESSMENT

The progressive care nurse requires skills to assess fluid, electrolyte, and renal status. This assessment begins with the patient interview, which includes the chief complaint, history of the present illness, medical and surgical history, family history, and psychosocial history. Accurate diagnosis is dependent on a good history.

Interview

The chief complaint is the condition for which the patient sought care and should be recorded in the patient's own words. Investigate the common symptoms of fluid, electrolyte, or renal conditions or other disease processes that affect the renal system.

Flank, groin, or costovertebral angle pain is a main reason patients will seek health care. The pain can be unilateral or bilateral, constant or intermittent, and intensity can range from a dull ache to a stabbing or throbbing pain relieved only by analgesics or treatment of underlying disease. Percussion of the costovertebral angle may aggravate and/or elicit pain. Hematuria, pyuria, and a change in urine volume may accompany the complaint of pain. Possible causes of flank pain are renal calculi, bladder cancer, bacterial cystitis, acute glomerulonephritis, obstructive uropathy, perirenal abscess, polycystic kidney disease, acute pyelonephritis, renal infarction, renal cancer, renal trauma, renal vein thrombosis, and acute pancreatitis.

Seek health care for changes in the pattern of urination. Common problems in the pattern of urination include:

- Frequency (frequent voiding)
- Nocturia (getting up at night to void more than twice)

- Dysuria (painful urination)
- Urgency (a feeling of the need to void immediately)
- Hesitancy (difficulty starting the flow of urine)
- Change in the stream of urine
- Retention (incomplete emptying of the bladder)
- Incontinence (inability to control urination)
- Enuresis (incontinence of urine in bed at night)

In addition, report and evaluate an increase or decrease in urine output and a change in the appearance of the urine. Examples of urine characteristics to report include:

- Dilution level: clear to light yellow
- Concentrated level: dark to amber
- Clarity: Clear to cloudy (pyuria)
- Hematuria: pink to red
- Bilirubinemia: orange to brown
- Myoglobinuria: tea-colored or cola-colored
- Hemoglobinuria: wine-colored

Neurologic symptoms that stem from renal problems are often the reason the patient is seeking care. Visual changes may be associated with uremia, fluid overload, or electrolyte imbalance. Paresthesias may be associated with hypocalcemia. Headaches may be associated with fluid overload, uremia, or renal-induced hypertension. Seizures may be associated with uremia, electrolyte imbalances, or fluid overload. Decreased ability to concentrate may be associated with uremia, electrolyte imbalance, or fluid overload. Uremia is also associated with a patient's demonstration of apathy.

Patients with fluid, electrolyte, or renal abnormalities may present with cardiovascular or pulmonary symptoms. Heart palpitations, dysrhythmias, and chest pain may occur due to uremia and electrolyte imbalance. Edema may be associated with uremia, fluid overload, or hypoproteinemia. Pericarditis and cardiac effusions are a complication of renal failure. Dyspnea may be seen in patients with renal failure due to left ventricular failure or pleural effusion. Goodpasture syndrome, which is an autoimmune disease that affects the kidneys and lungs, results in hemoptysis and hematuria.

Several gastrointestinal symptoms can indicate renal problems. A urine-like foul breath odor (halitosis) may be associated with uremia. Some patients may complain about a metallic taste in the mouth. Anorexia, nausea, or vomiting may be associated with uremia, electrolyte imbalance, or fluid overload. Fluid imbalance may result in constipation or diarrhea.

Musculoskeletal, dermatologic, and sexual problems may occur due to renal disease. Joint pain may accompany uremia, fluid imbalance, and electrolyte imbalance. Muscle weakness may be associated with electrolyte imbalance. Muscle pain or cramps may be associated with uremia or electrolyte imbalance. Dermatologic symptoms associated with uremia include pruritus, bruises, and delayed healing. Sexual issues related to uremia include impotence, decreased libido, and infertility.

Other symptoms related to problems with the renal system include fatigue, fever, thirst, and changes in body weight. Fatigue may be associated with uremia. Fever may be associated with infection or dehydration. Thirst may be associated with fluid imbalance. Change in body weight may be associated with uremia or fluid imbalance.

During the interview, it is important to elicit the history of present illness (HPI). Evaluate pain symptoms per the mnemonic OPQRST: onset, provocation or palliation, quality, region and radiation, severity, and time (history) or type. Discuss accompanying, aggravating, or ameliorating factors.

Learning the past medical history may give direction toward the current diagnosis. Ask if there has been a history of renal/urinary tract infection, calculi, renal insufficiency/failure, dialysis, renal transplantation, or surgical procedures. Determine whether the patient has a history of cardiovascular, pulmonary, endocrine, metabolic, immunologic, hematologic, and/or gynecologic problem. Cardiovascular disease such as hypertension, arteriosclerosis/atherosclerosis, heart failure, and/or bacterial endocarditis can result in abnormal renal function. Pulmonary or miliary tuberculosis may affect kidney function. Diabetes can cause the complication of diabetic nephropathy resulting in renal failure. Gout crystals can also lead to kidney stones, tubular obstructions, and hydronephrosis. Several immunologic disorders such as systemic lupus erythematosus (SLE), scleroderma, and Goodpasture syndrome may progress to the point of renal glomerulonephritis and failure. Hematologic conditions of hemophilia, disseminated intravascular coagulation (DIC), sickle cell disease, malignancy, and blood transfusion reactions also damage the kidneys. Gynecologic conditions such as toxemia of pregnancy, recent beta-hemolytic streptococcal infection, and urinary tract infection (UTI) can all lead to damaged kidneys.

Family history indicates a patient's risk factors for developing specific conditions. Renal diseases that have a genetic component include:
- Glomerulonephritis
- Polycystic disease
- Inherited nephritis (Alport syndrome)
- Inherited amyloidosis
- Malignancy

Specific genetically linked disease processes involving other body systems and having an effect on the renal system include:
- Cardiovascular: Hypertension and coronary artery disease
- Immunologic/hematologic: Hemophilia and sickle cell disease
- Endocrine: Diabetes mellitus

A patient's social history may identify several risk factors known to be involved in renal dysfunction. It is important for the nurse to elicit a patient's:
- Occupational exposure to toxins such as lead, mercury, pesticides, methanol, radiation, carbon tetrachloride, and phenol
- Exercise habits; strenuous exercise in an unconditioned person may cause rhabdomyolysis
- Fluid intake and type of fluids
- Smoking history; smoking increases the incidence of bladder cancer
- Use of saccharin; saccharin increases the incidence of bladder cancer

Medication History

Prescribed medications are a common source of acute kidney injury. In general, patients today are older, have more comorbidities, and are increasingly exposed to more diagnostic and therapeutic procedures with the potential to harm kidney function. Toxic effects of medications occur due to common pathophysiologic mechanisms. Drug-induced nephrotoxicity tends to be more common among certain patients and in specific clinical situations. Successful prevention requires knowledge

TABLE 5-2	Nephrotoxic Agents
Drug Classification	**Potential Injury**
Aminoglycosides	Tubular toxicity
Amphotericin B	Tubular toxicity
Cyclosporine	Altered glomerular hemodynamics
Nonsteroidal antiinflammatory	Interstitial nephritis; glomerulonephritis
Radiocontrast dye	Tubular cell toxicity
Antidepressants	Rhabdomyolysis
Antiplatelet aggregators	Thrombotic microangiopathy
Loop diuretics	Acute interstitial nephritis

of pathogenic mechanisms of renal injury, patient-related risk factors, drug-related risk factors, and preventative measures, together with close monitoring and early detection and treatment (Nguyen, 2010). Many common drugs are nephrotoxic (Table 5-2).

Physical Examination
Vital Signs
Various vital sign changes are present in patients with renal disease. Variation in blood pressure measurements occurs. Increased pressure is due to fluid overload and a history of hypertension. During dialysis, a decreased systolic reading may occur due to treatment. A fluid loss of 15% to 25% is required before systolic blood pressure falls. Frequently, a postural drop (tilt positive) occurs with a decrease of 15 mm Hg in systolic pressure when a patient sits or stands. This fall in pressure may occur even earlier if the patient is suffering from hypovolemia.

Increased pulse rates due to sympathetic nervous system (SNS) stimulation caused by fluid overload or dehydration may occur. It is important to remember that a blunted or absent response may occur in a patient taking beta-blockers. A postural heart rate change occurs when the pulse increases by 20 beats/min when the patient sits or stands. This postural pulse change may also occur earlier if the patient is suffering from hypovolemia.

Both respiratory rate and rhythm increase from SNS stimulation. Both fluid overload and dehydration stimulate the SNS. Kussmaul breathing, demonstrated by rapid, deep, gasping breaths, may occur due to metabolic acidosis. Dehydration may increase body temperatures. Various weight changes in a patient may be evident. A change of 1 lb. is equal to 500 mL of fluid; therefore, a change of 1 kg is equal to 1 liter (L). In renal patients, evaluate weight before and after hemodialysis or after drainage of dialysate in patients on peritoneal dialysis. Generalized debilitation results in weight loss in renal failure patients.

Inspection and Palpation
Skin color changes are noted in renal failure patients. Renal failure patients have a yellowish-gray color, and pallor may indicate anemia. Petechiae or bruising is often a result of platelet dysfunction in renal failure patients. Skin texture is rough and dry, and with untreated uremia, a filmy coating over the skin called uremic frost is often noted. This uremic frost causes extreme

pruritus, and lesions or scratch marks are evident. Normal skin turgor recoil should be immediate. A decrease in skin turgor indicates interstitial dehydration but is not an early sign. In addition, evaluation of skin turgor to determine hydration status is not reliable in elderly patients because of poor elasticity. Edema is a late change of overhydration because the patient may gain 3 to 4 kg before edema is actually noticeable. Edema in the face is frequently the initial location for patients with renal disease. Anasarca is a generalized, massive edema that does not pit and is an end-stage symptom in renal disease. In a mouth examination of a renal failure patient, halitosis is often present due to a uremic fetor (urine-like odor to the breath). When assessing for dehydration, use a tongue blade to assess stickiness. Stickiness of the oral mucous membranes and tongue is the preferred indicator of dehydration in the elderly. Nephrotic syndrome and other forms of renal disease may result in periorbital edema. Cataract formation is also common in renal failure as is nerve deafness.

Renal patients often have changes in neurologic status. A change in level of consciousness may indicate azotemia or electrolyte imbalance. Confusion may be indicative of uremia. Seizures may indicate electrolyte disturbance of hyponatremia or the presence of cerebral edema. Neuromuscular irritability and changes in muscle strength may reflect electrolyte imbalance.

Cardiovascular changes seen in renal patients include dysrhythmias and jugular venous distention (JVD). Dysrhythmias are common in electrolyte imbalance, particularly potassium imbalances. Neck vein distention of greater than 2 cm above the angle of Louis may be indicative of hypervolemia.

The abdomen assessment in a renal impairment patient may reveal generalized edema and/or ascites. In addition, the capture technique enables palpation of the kidney. To perform this assessment, put one hand under the patient's back, below the costal margin, and the other hand on the abdomen, below the costal margin. Ask the patient to take a deep breath and move your hands together to try to capture and feel the kidney. The liver pushes down on the right kidney; therefore, it is possible to palpate a normal right kidney. A normal left kidney is not palpable. If a kidney is palpable, evaluate the size. Normal size of the kidney is 10 × 5 × 2.5 cm or about the size of a fist. An acute kidney injury, polycystic disease, obstructive uropathy, pyelonephritis, renal abscess, or the presence of a tumor increases the size of a kidney, while chronic kidney disease decreases the size. Pain or discomfort during palpation may indicate infection, calculi, tumor, hydronephrosis, or glomerulonephritis. The bladder is palpable in the suprapubic area only when full. If palpable, the bladder is a smooth, round, firm organ that is sensitive to palpation.

Assessment of the extremities in a patient with renal failure may initiate asterixis. Asterixis is a hand-flapping tremor induced by extending the arm and dorsiflexion of the wrist. Asterixis is indicative of increased ammonia levels and seen in patients with renal failure and hepatic encephalopathy. A vascular access (e.g., fistula, AV graft) may be present in the extremity of a patient receiving dialysis. A thrill over the vascular access should be palpable because it would indicate patency.

Percussion

The assessment technique of percussion may elicit abnormalities in the lungs, abdomen, and bladder. Percussion of the thorax may elicit a sound of flatness at the lung bases, which may indicate pleural effusion, a frequent finding in renal failure patients. The percussed abdomen may indicate a fluid wave, revealing ascites. Tapping over the costovertebral angle (CVA) with the ulnar surface of the hand is a percussion technique used to elicit CVA tenderness. Conditions such as pyelonephritis, renal calculi, renal abscess or tumor, glomerulonephritis, or intermittent hydronephrosis elicit CVA tenderness. Bruising over the CVA may indicate renal trauma. Percuss over the bladder area. Dullness is audible above the symphysis pubis if the bladder has at least 150 mL of urine. Pain elicited during bladder percussion may indicate cystitis.

Auscultation

Assess vascular sounds, heart sounds, breath sounds, and bowel sounds with the auscultation assessment technique. A renal bruit may be audible to the left or right of midline in the periumbilical region in renal vascular disease or renal vascular trauma. With a vascular access (e.g., fistula, AV graft), a bruit over the access device indicates patency. Associated electrolyte imbalances precipitate rate and rhythm changes along with dysrhythmias. Renal patients suffer from several heart sound abnormalities. An S_3 indicates heart failure. Fluid overload may cause the flow murmur of mitral regurgitation, an asystolic murmur heard best at the apex with the diaphragm of the stethoscope. A pericardial friction rub may indicate pericarditis, a common complication of renal failure. Crackles, an adventitious breath sound, may indicate fluid overload. Crackles are heard initially at the base of the lung but move upward as the fluid overload progresses. Bowel sound changes may indicate a potassium electrolyte imbalance. Hypokalemia causes hypoactive bowel sounds, and hyperkalemia elicits active bowel sounds.

Urine Output

Urine output is an important indicator of GFR. Urine output decreases with diminished cardiac output or dehydration and increases in overhydration situations. Specific parameters define the amount of urine output (Table 5-3).

Bladder Scan Volume

Recent introduction of a portable ultrasound bladder scanner to patient care units has improved nursing care. The technology of the portable ultrasound bladder scanner automatically computes the bladder volume based on cross-sectional images of the bladder. The use of this new technology permits the nurse to differentiate between an empty bladder and urinary retention, thereby avoiding unnecessary catheterization. The scanner also provides an accurate measure to evaluate residual urine in the bladder after voiding.

TABLE 5-3	Urine Output Volume Parameters
Urine Output	**Volume Parameters**
Normal	1500 mL/24 hr or at least 0.5 mL/kg/hr
Polyuria	>2500 mL/24 hr
Oliguria	100-400 mL/24 hr
Anuria	0-100 mL/24 hr

The bladder scanner is a handheld ultrasound transducer and instrument box with a digital display screen of bladder volume. The nurse enters the patient's gender into the equipment keypad, washes the transducer tip and applies ultrasound gel, then positions the tip of the transducer above the symphysis pubis and toward the bladder. After proper positioning, the nurse presses the transducer button and holds the transducer tip still until the machine beeps, indicating that scanning is complete. Consistency is determined with repetition to obtain a reliable reading. Upon completion, the nurse washes the gel from the patient's abdomen and transducer tip. Bladder readings greater than 300 mL of volume indicate the need for urinary catheterization.

The Synergy Model guides the physical examination. Determine patient characteristic levels of resiliency, vulnerability, stability, complexity, resource availability, participation in care, participation in decision making, and predictability. Patients with acute, life-threatening renal problems have a wide variety of clinical characteristics. During hospitalization, the clinical status may resolve, improve, or deteriorate. Progressive care nursing has the responsibility to continually monitor, assess, intervene, and evaluate. To improve clinical outcomes, make every attempt to synergize the nursing care with the patient's characteristics.

Diagnostic Laboratory Studies

Diagnostic laboratory studies play an important role in evaluating renal function. Common diagnostic labs evaluated for renal function include serum osmolality, BUN, creatinine, BUN:creatinine ratio, anion gap, serum electrolytes, and chemistries. In addition, body weight is an indicator used to assess fluid balance when evaluating renal function.

Serum osmolality measures the osmolar concentration of plasma and correlates to the number of particles per kilogram of serum; it is expressed as mOsmol/kg. Serum osmolarity measures the osmolar concentration of plasma and correlates to the number of particles per liter of serum; it is expressed as mOsmol/L. Serum osmolality reflects the total body hydration level with normal levels at 280 to 295 mOsm/L. Increased osmolality occurs in dehydration, while fluid overload decreases osmolarity. Calculate osmolality with the formulas listed in the box below.

SIDEBAR 5-1

Serum Osmolality

A quick and easy way to calculate serum osmolality is to double the serum sodium, although this method is not accurate when the patient has an elevated BUN or glucose. For a more accurate calculation of the serum osmolality, use the following formula:

Serum sodium × 2 + (BUN/2.6) + (serum glucose/18).

Because the PCCN™ is a multiple-choice examination, you might want to use this formula:

Serum sodium × 2 + (BUN/3) + (serum glucose/20) because this is an easier calculation and will yield a value very close to the true value.

Normal is 280 to 295 mEq/kg; a value less than normal indicates too few solutes per liter (i.e., overhydration and hemodilution) and a value greater than normal indicates too many solutes per liter (i.e., dehydration and hemoconcentration).

5.3 Learning Activity

A 72-year-old woman admitted to the emergency department from a long-term care facility was recently started on enteral feedings. Nursing staff identified that the patient had a change in her level of consciousness. The serum sodium level is 150 mEq/L, BUN is 80 mg/dL, and serum glucose is 1000 mg/dL. Calculate the serum osmolality and identify what this serum osmolality indicates. What is the most likely cause of this abnormal serum osmolality? _____

_____

_____

_____

_____

Answers to this activity can be found in the Answer Key.

The BUN reflects the difference between rate of urea synthesis and its excretion by the kidneys. Formed in the liver through enzymatic breakdown of protein, the BUN is not as accurate an indicator of renal failure as is creatinine because BUN levels fluctuate greatly with protein intake. Creatinine levels are relatively unchanged by protein intake and hydration level. The normal range for BUN is 5 to 20 mg/dL and uremia is defined as an increased BUN. Abnormal values increase with decreased renal blood flow or urine production, dehydration, some neoplasms, and certain antibiotics. Decreased BUN occurs in pregnancy, overhydration, severe liver disease, and malnutrition states.

To determine whether problems are due to prerenal or intrinsic (i.e., intrarenal) factors, it is recommended to evaluate the BUN:creatinine ratio. This ratio is normally about 10:1. When BUN is elevated disproportionately to the creatinine (e.g., BUN:creatinine equals a 20:1 ratio), consider an extrarenal cause such as volume depletion, insufficient fluid intake, excessive fluid loss, diuresis, vomiting, poor renal perfusion, shock, sepsis, decreased cardiac output, renovascular disease, protein catabolism, starvation, blood in the GI tract, or corticosteroids. When the BUN and creatinine ratio are both elevated while maintaining the normal 10:1 ratio, consider an intrinsic renal cause such as acute or chronic renal failure. When the BUN:creatinine ratio is lower than normal, consider decreased protein intake or liver dysfunction.

Creatinine is a nonprotein end product of muscle metabolism. Creatinine is more accurate than BUN in evaluating renal function because creatinine is normally filtered by the glomerulus and not reabsorbed by the tubule. It is also unaffected by diet and fluid intake. The normal creatinine level is 0.7 to 1.5 mg/dL. Increased creatinine levels that are twice the normal (~3 mg/dL) suggest a 50% nephron loss. Creatinine levels greater than 10 mg/dL indicate end-stage renal disease with less than 10% of nephrons still functioning. Mean lower muscle mass caused by a disease, such as muscular dystrophy, or by aging produce low serum creatinine levels. Low levels can also mean some types of severe liver disease or a diet very low in protein. Pregnancy can also cause low blood creatinine levels.

5.4   Learning Activity

Identify three major reasons for the BUN to be elevated in a patient with a normal creatinine.
1. _____
2. _____
3. _____

Answers to this activity can be found in the Answer Key.

Serum electrolytes, blood glucose, hematology studies, clotting profiles, lipid profiles, and arterial blood gases are also routinely monitored to evaluate renal function. Arterial blood gases to determine the acid-base state and the anion gap can be used to determine the causes of acidosis. Refer to Appendix D for diagnostic laboratory parameters.

SIDEBAR 5-2

Anion Gap

The anion gap is the difference between cations (positive ions) and anions (negative ions). To calculate the anion gap, use the following formula:

(Serum sodium + serum potassium) − (serum chloride + carbon dioxide content [from venous blood]
OR bicarbonate [from arterial blood gases])

Normal anion gap is between 5 and 15. The anion gap is a useful tool to determine whether a metabolic acidosis is due to an acid gain or a bicarbonate loss. If the anion gap is normal, the metabolic acidosis is due to a bicarbonate loss, such as diarrhea. If the anion gap is above normal, the metabolic acidosis is due to a metabolic acid gain, such as lactic acidosis, renal failure, ketoacidosis, or toxins (e.g., ethylene glycol or methanol).

5.5   Learning Activity

Specify whether the following causes of metabolic acidosis would have a normal anion gap or an increased anion gap.

Condition	Normal Anion Gap	Increased Anion Gap
Shock		
Renal failure		
Diarrhea		
Diabetic ketoacidosis		
Salicylate overdose		
Renal tubular acidosis		
Rhabdomyolysis		

5.5   Learning Activity—cont'd

Condition	Normal Anion Gap	Increased Anion Gap
Carbonic anhydrase inhibitors		
Ethylene glycol poisoning		

Answers to this activity can be found in the Answer Key.

Urinalysis

The analysis of urine (Table 5-4) starts with a visual examination. Normal urine should be clear or light yellow. Microscopic evaluation of urine determines normal component levels such as pH level, osmolality, creatinine clearance, specific gravity, and spot electrolytes. Large amounts of or abnormal components such as glucose, ketones, protein, myoglobin, hemoglobin, bilirubin, and sediment or casts, erythrocytes, leukocytes, eosinophils, and epithelial renal cells may indicate certain conditions.

Other diagnostic assessments of renal function include radiologic tests and procedures (Table 5-5). Noninvasive tests such as x-rays and ultrasounds are inexpensive and can provide baseline data to guide more extensive diagnostic examinations. Computerized tomography (CT) scans and magnetic resonance imaging (MRI) are noninvasive but costly. Other procedures such as intravenous pyelograms, retrograde urograms, angiography, and biopsy are invasive; therefore, certain risks may be involved.

Specific Clinical Conditions Related to Renal Function

Nursing care of a patient with actual or potential renal dysfunction can be multifaceted and complex. Problems associated with renal disease involve issues related to hydration status, electrolyte imbalance, malnutrition, hypertension, metabolic acidosis, anemia, uremic syndrome, infection, altered medication metabolism and excretion, and psychosocial issues of the patient and family. The patient's response to each of these directs the patient's care. An intraprofessional collaborative team approach is the best method to achieve desired patient care goals. Team members may include the progressive care nurse, primary health care provider, advanced practice nurse or physician assistant, case manager, dietician, nephrologist consult, and hemodialysis nurse; these team members work collaboratively to identify the problem and etiologic factors, develop a plan, and evaluate the patient outcomes.

Hydration Status

Patients may present with overhydration or dehydration. With overhydration, the patient experiences fluid retention and edema because the kidneys cannot eliminate excess body water. On the opposite side of the spectrum, a patient with dehydration experiences vascular, cellular, or intracellular volume depletion due to active fluid loss. Emphasis of care is on identifying the cause, monitoring I&O and daily weights, assessing renal function with serum and urine tests, preparing and supporting patients through procedures, and administering or restricting fluid therapy, medications, and/or dietary recommendations. Stable vital signs, urine volume, specific gravity (SG), and hemodynamic parameters

| TABLE 5-4 | Urine Component Values and Indications |

Component	Normal Value	Indications
pH	4-8 with average of 6	Increased urinary acidity indicates that the body is retaining bicarbonate. Decreased urinary acidity (more alkaline) indicates that the kidneys are retaining sodium and acids. Alkaline urine may be associated with urinary tract infection. Alkaline urine and serum acidosis are associated with renal tubular acidosis.
Specific gravity	1.005-1.030	Increased specific gravity occurs with any condition causing hypoperfusion of kidneys leading to oliguria (e.g., shock, severe dehydration, proteinuria, glycosuria, contrast media). Decreased specific gravity is seen in diabetes insipidus, in overhydration, or when renal tubules lose their ability to reabsorb water and concentrate urine as in early pyelonephritis.
Osmolality	50-1200 mOsm/kg	Measures number of particles per unit of water in urine and is dependent on the circulating titer of ADH and the rate of urinary solute excretion. It should be 1.5 times that of serum osmolality. Osmolality is increased in fluid volume deficits and decreased in fluid volume excesses.
Creatinine clearance	85-135 mL/min	Estimates GFR. Urine specimen for 24-hour period and a serum creatinine are required.
Spot urine electrolytes	Sodium: 40-220 mEq/L Potassium: 25-120 mEq/L Chloride: 110-250 mEq/L	Evaluates the kidneys' ability to conserve sodium and concentrate urine. Measures sodium, potassium, and chloride concentrations in the urine.
Myoglobin	<20 ng/mL	Myoglobinuria indicates muscle breakdown.
Hemoglobin	Negative	Hemoglobinuria indicates free hemoglobin in the urine that occurs in hemolytic blood transfusion reaction, hemolytic or sickle cell anemia, fresh-water drowning, burns, and disseminated intravascular coagulation (DIC).
Bilirubin	Negative	Urobilinogen indicates biliary obstruction or liver disease.
Culture and sensitivity	No bacteria present	Identifies bacteria present and appropriate antibiotic for therapy.
Casts	Normally none or occasional	Precipitation from the kidney that takes the shape of the tubule where it was formed. • Hyaline casts: small amounts normal, but large amounts indicative of significant proteinuria • Erythrocyte casts: indicative of glomerulonephritis or vasculitis • Leukocyte casts: indicative of infectious processes • Granular casts: indicative of acute tubular necrosis, interstitial nephritis, acute or chronic glomerulonephritis, chronic renal failure • Fatty casts: indicative of lipoid nephrosis or nephrotic syndrome • Renal tubular casts: indicative of AKI
Bacteria	None	Abnormal in catheterized specimen.
Erythrocytes	Small numbers	Large amount indicates glomerulonephritis, interstitial nephritis, malignancy, infection, calculi, cystitis, or trauma.
Leukocytes	Small numbers	Large amount indicates infection or interstitial nephritis.
Eosinophils	None	Indicates allergic reaction in kidney.
Epithelial renal cells	None	Indicates acute tubular necrosis, glomerulonephritis, or interstitial nephritis.

along with the absence of edema, adventitious breath sounds (e.g., crackles), or hypertension are evaluation measures utilized to determine hydration status patient care outcomes.

Malnutrition

Malnutrition and hypoalbuminemia are associated with increased morbidity in patients with chronic kidney disease. To preserve kidney function, dietary protein intake is restricted in the early stages of chronic kidney disease, which can contribute to malnutrition. The collaborative health team members address malnutrition by identifying the causes, providing education on the renal diet, and teaching methods to enhance the patient's appetite, along with monitoring weight changes, nutritional intake, and adherence with dietary instructions. The desired goals of patient care aim to ensure that the patient's intake meets nutritional requirements, that the patient maintains a stable baseline weight and adequate muscle mass, and that the patient's serum protein, albumin, BUN, and creatinine levels improve or remain at baseline.

Hypertension

In renal failure, the hypertensive state (diastolic BP >90 mm Hg, systolic BP >140 mm Hg) is due to fluid retention and/or stimulation of the renin-angiotensin mechanism. Preexisting hypertension is also common because it is a major cause of renal

TABLE 5-5	Renal Diagnostic Studies		

Study	Purposes	Comments
Computerized tomography (CT) scan	• Provides a view of kidneys, retroperitoneal space, bladder, prostate • Evaluates kidney size • Evaluates the kidney for tumors, abscesses, and obstruction	• No special preparation required • Can be safely used in patients with renal failure • Contrast medium may be used
Cystometrogram	• Evaluates the pressure exerted against the wall of the bladder to evaluate bladder tone	• No special preparation required • Urinary catheter inserted and saline instilled into bladder Postprocedure • Monitor for clinical indications of urinary tract infection
Cystoscopy	• Visualizes bladder and urethra for identification of pathology	Preprocedure • NPO after midnight if general anesthesia is to be used • Administer sedative if prescribed • No special preparation required Postprocedure • Pink-tinged urine is normal but gross hematuria is abnormal; monitor urine output • Encourage fluids

Intravenous pyelogram (IVP)	• Evaluates position, size, shape, and location of kidneys
	• Provides visualization of internal kidney (parenchyma, calyces, pelvis)
	• Evaluates filling of renal pelvis
	• Outlines ureters and bladder
	• Identifies presence of cysts and tumors
	• Identifies obstruction, congenital abnormality
		• Also called *excretory urogram*
		• Contraindicated in renal insufficiency, multiple myeloma, pregnancy, congestive heart failure, sickle cell disease
		• Bowel preparation (e.g., cathartics as prescribed)
		• NPO for 8 hours before the test
		• Contrast media used
		  • Check for allergy to iodine before the study
		  • Monitor for allergic reaction postprocedure
		  • Ensure hydration postprocedure

Kidneys, ureters, and bladder (KUB)	• Outlines kidneys, ureters, and bladder • Evaluates size, shape, and position of kidneys • Identifies location of calculi	• Also called *flat plate of abdomen* • Bowel preparation (e.g., cathartics may be prescribed if to be followed by IVP)
Magnetic resonance imaging (MRI)	• Differentiation between cyst and solid mass • Identifies infarction, trauma, obstruction	• More specific than renal ultrasonography or CT scan because it shows subtle density changes • Cannot be used in patients with any implanted metallic device, including pacemakers • No special preparation required
Nephrotomogram	• Evaluates segments of the kidney at different levels • Differentiates cysts from solid masses	• Bowel preparation (e.g., cathartics as prescribed) • NPO for 8 hours before the test • Contrast media used • Check for allergy to iodine before the study • Monitor for allergic reaction postprocedure • Ensure hydration postprocedure

Renal angiography	• Evaluates renal vasculature
	• Identifies renal artery stenosis
	• Identifies cysts, tumors, infarction, trauma
		• Bowel preparation (e.g., cathartics) as prescribed
		• NPO for 8 hours before the test
		• Sedative is usually prescribed before the procedure
		• Contrast media used
		  • Check for allergy to iodine before the study
		  • Monitor for allergic reaction postprocedure
		  • Ensure hydration postprocedure
		Postprocedure
		• Keep extremity in which catheter was placed immobilized in a straight position for 6-12 hours
		• Monitor arterial puncture point for hemorrhage or hematoma
		• Monitor neurovascular status of affected limb
		• Monitor for indications of systemic emboli

TABLE 5-5	Renal Diagnostic Studies—cont'd	
Study	**Purposes**	**Comments**
Renal biopsy	• Obtains tissue specimen for microscopic evaluation	• May be performed open or closed • Clotting profile is evaluated preprocedure • Type and crossmatch for two units of blood preprocedure • Usually not performed if patient has only one functioning kidney (unless being done to evaluate possible transplant rejection) • Closed biopsy contraindicated in bleeding abnormalities, polycystic disease, hydronephrosis, neoplasm, urinary tract infection, and uncooperative patient Postprocedure • Pressure dressing is applied, and the patient is on bed rest for 24 hours • Observe for hematuria, flank pain, or hypotension
Renal radionuclide scan (renogram)	• Evaluates position, size, shape, and location of kidneys • Identifies obstruction, abscesses, cysts, tumors • Evaluates renal perfusion • Evaluates glomerular filtration, tubular function, and excretion • Assesses status of renal transplant	• Assure patient that the amount of radioactive material is minimal • Do not schedule within 24 hours after IVP • Ask patient to void before scan • Encourage fluids after the procedure

Retrograde pyelogram	• Evaluates position, size, shape, and location of kidneys
	• Outlines ureters and bladder
	• Identifies presence of cysts and tumors
	• Identifies obstruction
		• Does not require the kidney to excrete dye so may be used in patients with renal insufficiency
		• Bowel preparation (e.g., cathartics as prescribed)
		• NPO for 8 hours before the test
		• Contrast media used
		  • Check for allergy to iodine before the study
		  • Monitor for allergic reaction postprocedure
		  • Ensure hydration postprocedure
		• Monitor patient for clinical indications of urinary tract infection or sepsis

Ultrasonography	• Evaluates fluid versus solid mass
	• Identifies obstructions
	• Identifies cysts, abscesses, tumors, polycystic kidney disease
	• Identifies hemorrhage
	• Identifies urinary tract obstruction and leaks
		• No special preparation required
		• Can be safely used in patients with renal failure
		• Contrast media may be used
		  • Check for allergy to iodine before the study
		  • Monitor for allergic reaction postprocedure
		  • Ensure hydration postprocedure

Voiding cystourethrography	• Identifies abnormalities of lower urinary tract to determine presence of reflux and residual urine	• No special preparation required • Encourage fluids postprocedure

failure in the United States. Treating hypertension in an aggressive manner with a diuretic, ACE inhibitor, beta-blocker, and/or calcium channel blocker has the benefit of slowing down the progression of chronic kidney disease (see Chapter 3).

Metabolic Acidosis

Renal failure impairs the inability of the kidneys to excrete the hydrogen ion, which results in a condition known as metabolic acidosis (see Chapter 4). Metabolic acidosis is an increase in unmeasurable anions (high anion gap) caused by many conditions, including renal failure and uremia (see Chapter 4).

Anemia

The lack of erythropoietin synthesis and secretion, actual blood loss, and uremic syndrome causes anemia in renal failure patients. Treatment of anemia associated with renal failure is oral or intravenous iron supplement unless excess stores of iron exist in the patient. Vitamin replacement (B_6 and folic acid) are also very important because the dialysis procedure removes them. Epogen (recombinant human erythropoietin) stimulates erythropoietin production and prevents the anemia of chronic kidney disease. Because it takes 3 months for peak results, patients with acute kidney injury do not benefit from Epogen.

Uremic Syndrome

The kidney's inability to excrete toxic waste products results in uremic syndrome. Symptoms of uremia occur when BUN levels reach about 100 mg/dL or as the GFR falls below 10 to 15 mL/min. Uremic syndrome affects every organ in the body, producing a myriad of symptoms that can occur in any combination (Table 5-6). Maintaining the BUN to less than 100 mg/dL is the most common goal in the treatment of uremia. Each

TABLE 5-6   **Clinical Findings in Uremic Syndrome**

System	Findings
Neurologic	Sensorium changes: attention span deficit, lethargy, fatigue, coma, headache, peripheral neuropathy, tremors, seizures
Skin	Pale yellow-tinged color, pruritus, dryness, ecchymosis, edema, uremic frost
Hematologic and Immunologic	Platelet dysfunction, bleeding, decreased immune response, anemia
Gastrointestinal	Nausea and vomiting, anorexia, weight loss, stomatitis, uremic fetor, metallic taste (dysgeusia), gastritis, colitis, constipation
Metabolic	Carbohydrate intolerance, hyperkalemia, hypernatremia, hypocalcemia, hyperphosphatemia, hypermagnesemia
Musculoskeletal	Renal osteodystrophy (soft tissue calcification), bone pain, diminished mobility, decreased strength, gait changes, muscle atrophy, weakness, paralysis
Genitourinary	Flank pain, hematuria, proteinuria, dysuria, urinary frequency, polyuria, urine volume ranges from norm to oliguria or anuria, urinary tract infections, sexual dysfunction
Cardiac	Pericarditis, heart murmurs; accelerated atherosclerosis; hypertension; pulse rate changes: normal, bradycardia, or tachycardia; 12-lead ECG changes consistent with pericarditis, hyperkalemia, or hypocalcemia; chest pain: pleuritic, pericardial, or ischemic
Endocrine	Hyperparathyroidism (secondary)
Pulmonary	Pleuritis, pulmonary edema, Kussmaul breathing (deep, rapid), recent infections (Goodpasture syndrome or recent streptococcal), antineutrophil cytoplasmic antibody-related or Wegener's granulomatosis
Psychosocial	Altered self-image, diminished body image, depression, suicidal ideation
Sensory	Deafness (Alport syndrome)

patient's uremic symptoms occur at varying levels of BUN and creatinine; therefore it is important to identify these individual values and strive to maintain levels below that amount to minimize or eradicate uremic symptoms. Specific interventions for treating uremia include the following:

- Oral protein intake restriction
- GI tract blood removal to prevent metabolism to ammonia and urea
- Dialysis

Infection

A major problem for patients in renal failure is infection. An impaired immune system from uremic toxins and reduced phagocytosis increases mortality and morbidity. Careful monitoring and preventative strategies are necessary. Urinary tract infections may be asymptomatic; therefore, urine specimens for culture should be obtained on admission.

It is necessary to prevent introduction of microorganisms by avoiding indwelling urinary catheters and unnecessary invasive procedures. Maintaining the BUN less than 80 to 100 mg/dL will help to minimize susceptibility to infection. Implement isolation techniques for hepatitis antigen-positive patients receiving hemodialysis.

Altered Pharmacokinetics

Impaired kidneys are unable to metabolize or excrete pharmacologic agents, which results in the retention of active or toxic metabolites of a medication. Uremia may also cause increased sensitivity to drugs. All these things can lead to an elevation of metabolic wastes and increase azotemia along with drug toxicity. Health care providers need to ensure careful and astute

selection, administration, monitoring, and evaluation of drug therapy response to avoid untoward drug effects. Monitor the prescribed serum drug levels to make sure levels are adequate.

Renal failure causes many alterations in pharmacokinetics. Distribution of lipid-soluble drugs is impaired due to decreased body fat stores. Cardiac failure and low cardiac output reduce metabolism and excretion of drugs. Acidemia alters the tissue's ability to uptake the drugs. Increased body water causes dilution effects, and decreased protein binding causes competition by various drugs for tissue binding sites, which leads to a higher concentration of unbound drug. The decreased GI motility and altered gastric pH of uremia affect drug absorption. Uremic electrolyte imbalances may affect the GI tract.

Apply some general principles when dealing with any form of renal insufficiency or failure. Recommendations include drug dosage reduction and increased intervals between doses. Question prescriptions for drugs known to be nephrotoxic (NSAIDS, meperidine) and avoid if possible. Closely observe patients for toxicosis due to drug accumulation. To establish a stable concentration, administer initial loading doses of drugs that have a long half-life. Report any untoward signs, especially increased serum creatinine, to the provider. Discontinue, decrease, or replace the drug as ordered. Monitor serum drug levels, especially with drugs requiring special concentrations, with a narrow therapeutic index, and with a high risk for toxicity (antibiotics, digoxin). Evaluate the patient's ongoing tolerance to pharmacologic therapy.

Ineffective Patient and Family Coping

The patient may need to manage adaptive tasks related to the stress of renal failure. Insufficient and ineffective support may be an issue. Signs of maladaptive coping include verbalizations of inability to cope and asking for help. Patients often have an inability to meet role expectations and find problem solving difficult. Diminished communications and socialization compound the problem. Patients may demonstrate destructive behavior toward themselves and others. Ineffective coping is a major reason for failure to comply with the treatment regimen.

Family may also have some maladaptive coping issues. Patients may communicate concern about family's response to the disease and treatment plan. Family members may demonstrate preoccupation with their own personal reaction of fear, anticipatory grief, guilt, and anxiety. Inadequate understanding of the patient's condition or therapy may interfere with supportive behaviors. In addition, family members may withdraw from communications with the patient or demonstrate overprotective or underprotective behaviors.

The life-threatening nature of the disease, inability to perform activities of daily living, restrictions caused by dialysis treatments, access devices, diet, and procedures can lead to stress. The reversal of family roles that affect sexual activity, work, and day-to-day functioning all lead to stress as well. Nurses need to recognize the psychological consequences of renal disease and its treatment, including denial, depression, and dependency. The suicide rate of hemodialysis patients is believed to be 100% greater than the general public; therefore, it is vital that the nurse be able to assess the patient's ability to cope and provide specific interventions to support adaptation. Teach patients about the various treatment alternatives, encourage patient participation in the selection of treatment modalities, and link the patient and family with support systems. In addition, provide support for family members. Evaluation measures to ensure effective coping include patient participation in care, decreased levels of anxiety, use of support systems, and compliance with the treatment program.

PHARMACOLOGIC AGENTS USED IN PATIENTS WITH IMPAIRMENT IN RENAL FUNCTION

Diuretics

To treat the edema and hypertension associated with renal insufficiency and failure, administer diuretics (Table 5-7). Diuretics affect the renal system by enhancing the excretion of fluid and sodium. Give diuretics for treatment of hypertension, heart failure, edema, drug toxicity, and presence of renal pigments. Diuretics are classified as thiazide, loop, osmotic, potassium-sparing, and carbonic anhydrase inhibitors. In pulmonary edema, the diuretic used is usually a loop diuretic because it is potent and rapid acting. In more stable heart failure, thiazide, loop, and/or potassium-sparing may be used. Cerebral edema responds better to mannitol, an osmotic diuretic. In peripheral edema, both thiazide and loop diuretics are used depending on the extent of the problem. Because the edema in hepatic failure is associated with the inability of the liver to detoxify aldosterone, administer an aldosterone antagonist as ordered. Issues with toxicity or pigments require forced diuresis; therefore, an osmotic diuretic is the preferred agent.

Dopamine Stimulators

Dopamine stimulators (see Table 5-7) trigger the dopaminergic receptors in the renal and mesenteric artery bed. Low-dose dopamine targets the dopaminergic receptors. Results are often unpredictable, and dopamine can cause several alpha-induced and beta-induced side effects (Abay, Reyes, Everts, & Wisser, 2007). The inotropic effect of $beta_1$ stimulation causes the diuretic effect of dopamine. Fenoldopam mesylate (Corlopam) causes diuresis by dilating the arterial system, which decreases afterload and stimulating dopamine D1 receptors in the kidneys. This is the drug of choice for hypertension and renal protection when a patient is receiving nephrotoxic dyes.

FLUID IMBALANCES

Determine whether the fluid loss or gain includes the loss or gain of sodium when evaluating fluid imbalance. Fluid imbalances include hypovolemia (loss of sodium and water), water-loss syndrome (loss of water in excess of sodium), hypervolemia (gain of water and sodium), and water-gain syndrome (gain of water in excess of sodium) (Table 5-8).

Hypovolemia results from significant losses such as hemorrhage, GI losses (e.g., vomiting, diarrhea), renal losses (e.g., diuresis), increased insensible losses (e.g., tachypnea, perspiration), and intravascular to extravascular fluid shifts (i.e., third-spacing). Inadequate fluid replacement heightens hypovolemia. Water-loss syndrome, sometimes referred to as hypovolemic hypernatremia, is a hypertonic state caused by inadequate intake of water, excessive loss of hypotonic fluids (i.e., watery diarrhea), or the addition of hypertonic fluids, such as total parenteral nutrition, hypertonic saline, or enteral feedings. Several pathologic states cause hypovolemia. Hypovolemia results from the inadequate ADH secretion or response in diabetes insipidus. In addition, the inadequate insulin secretion or insulin resistance that occurs in diabetes mellitus will also result in hypovolemia.

Although hypovolemia and water-loss syndrome both present with clinical indications of dehydration and hypovolemia, there are some differences in the clinical presentation. Serum sodium and osmolality are the best indicators of whether the loss was isotonic or hypotonic. Collaborative management begins with the treatment of the cause, such as control of bleeding, antidiarrheals, or antiemetics. The key aspect of collaborative management is fluid replacement. If the fluid loss is blood, replacement of blood is necessary if the patient is showing clinical indications of hypoperfusion, such as chest pain or dyspnea. Oral fluids may be adequate for mild hypovolemia, but intravenous fluids are usually required. During fluid challenges, monitor the patient closely for clinical indications of fluid overload (e.g., S_3, crackles). Isotonic fluid, such as 0.9% saline, is a solution that has the same salt concentration as cells and blood and is used to replace volume. However, water-loss syndrome requires the replacement of more water than sodium, so 0.45% saline is indicated initially in most cases; patients with severe water-loss syndrome and hypernatremia, such as in diabetes insipidus, may even require D_5W initially. If the cause of the water-loss syndrome is hormonal, replace the hormones (e.g., insulin for diabetes mellitus, ADH for diabetes insipidus, or aldosterone for Addison disease).

Hypervolemia may result from the excessive intake of isotonic fluid, the retention of sodium and water, or an interstitial to intravascular shift of fluid. Examples of pathologic states that can cause hypervolemia include heart failure, liver failure, or renal failure. Endogenous (i.e., Cushing's syndrome) or exogenous

TABLE 5-7	Selected Diuretics and Dopamine Stimulants		
Drug	**Administration**	**Adverse Effects**	**Nursing Implications**
Furosemide (Lasix) (loop diuretic)	• PO: 20-80 mg daily • IV injection: 20-120 mg; administer at rate not to exceed 10 mg/min; if initial dose is ineffective, the next dose is usually double the original dose • IV infusion: mix 250 mg in 250 mL (1 mg/mL); usual dose is 0.1-0.75 mg/kg/hr; not to exceed 4 mg/min • Maximum: 1 g/day • Do not mix with acidic solutions Other loop diuretics • Torsemide (Demadex): PO 5-20 mg daily; IV 5-20 mg over 2 minutes • Bumetanide (Bumex): PO 0.5-2 mg daily; IV 0.5-1.0 mg, which may be repeated at 2- to 3-hour intervals	• Hypotension • Hypovolemia • Nausea, vomiting, abdominal pain • Rash • Electrolyte imbalance: hypocalcemia, hypokalemia, hypomagnesemia, hyponatremia • Acid-base imbalance: hypochloremic alkalosis • Increased uric acid and BUN • Renal failure • Hyperglycemia • Photosensitivity • Thrombocytopenia, agranulocytosis, leukopenia, neutropenia, anemia • Transient deafness (with rapid IV injection)	• Monitor HR, BP, urine output, serum electrolytes, BUN, creatinine, uric acid, CBC, daily weights • Monitor patients also on digitalis for clinical indications of digitalis toxicity • Monitor serum glucose in patients with diabetes mellitus • Monitor for clinical indications of gout • Note contraindications: known hypersensitivity to sulfonamides, anuria, hypovolemia, electrolyte depletion • Sulfonamide-sensitive patients may have allergic reaction to these drugs (furosemide, bumetanide, torsemide) because they are all sulfa derivatives • Use cautiously in diabetes mellitus, dehydration, severe renal disease, gout, hepatic disease • Do not administer if solution is yellow or if precipitate is present • Teach patient about potassium-rich foods
Mannitol (Osmitrol) (osmotic diuretic)	• IV infusion: 1-2 g/kg over 30-60 minutes; average dose 50-100 g • Use inline filter when administering mannitol	• Tachycardia • Nausea, vomiting • Fluid and electrolyte imbalance • Pulmonary edema • Thirst • Phlebitis • Seizures • Rebound cerebral edema 8-12 hours after diuresis	• Monitor BP, HR, urine output, serum osmolality, serum electrolytes, BUN, uric acid, daily weights • Note contraindications: known hypersensitivity, active intracranial bleeding, anuria, severe dehydration • Use cautiously in severe renal failure, HF, dehydration • Check bottle or ampule for crystallization: discard and replace • Monitor closely for rebound effect: return of clinical indications of intracranial hypertension 8-12 hours after mannitol
Hydrochlorothiazide (HydroDIURIL, Oretic) (thiazide diuretic)	• PO: 25-100 mg daily or twice daily • Older adult: 12.5-25 mg daily Other thiazide diuretics • Chlorothiazide (Diuril): PO 500-1000 mg daily or twice daily; IV 500 mg twice daily • Chlorthalidone (Hygroton): PO 25-100 mg daily	• Hypovolemia • Electrolyte imbalance: hyponatremia, hypokalemia, hypochloremia, hypercalcemia, hypomagnesemia, • Acid-base imbalance: hypochloremic alkalosis • Anorexia, nausea, vomiting • Dizziness, light-headedness, vertigo • Polyuria and nocturia • Increased uric acid and BUN • Hyperglycemia, glucosuria • Renal failure • Acute pancreatitis • Aplastic anemia, hemolytic anemia, leukopenia, agranulocytosis, thrombocytopenia, neutropenia • Anaphylaxis, photosensitivity, rash	• Monitor BP, HR, urine output, serum osmolality, serum electrolytes, BUN, uric acid, daily weights • Note contraindications: known hypersensitivity to thiazide diuretics or sulfonamide antibiotics; severe renal impairment or anuria; hepatic coma; hypomagnesemia • Use cautiously in renal disease, lupus erythematosus, liver disease, fluid and electrolyte imbalances, diabetes, gout, elevated serum lipids, asthma, CAD • Encourage patient to take with food or milk • Instruct patient to use sunscreen

TABLE 5-7 Selected Diuretics and Dopamine Stimulants—cont'd

Drug	Administration	Adverse Effects	Nursing Implications
Spironolactone (Aldactone) (potassium-sparing diuretic)	• PO: 25-200 mg daily Other potassium-sparing diuretics • Triamterene (Dyrenium): PO 100-300 mg daily in divided doses • Amiloride (Midamor): PO 5-20 mg daily	• Electrolyte imbalance: hyperkalemia • Hypovolemia • Anorexia, nausea, vomiting, diarrhea • Dry mouth • Dizziness, fatigue, headache • Gynecomastia • Jaundice, elevated liver enzymes • Elevated BUN and creatinine, azotemia, renal failure • Thrombocytopenia, megaloblastic anemia, agranulocytosis • Anaphylaxis, photosensitivity, rash	• Monitor BP, HR, urine output, serum osmolality, serum electrolytes (especially potassium), BUN, uric acid, daily weights • Note contraindications: known hypersensitivity, preexisting hyperkalemia, anuria, ESRD, hepatic failure • Use cautiously in renal disease, history of renal stones, diabetes, folic acid deficiency • Frequently used with loop or thiazide diuretic to minimize potassium loss and because they work synergistically • Encourage patient to take with food or milk • Instruct patient to use sunscreen • Instruct patient to avoid high-potassium foods and salt substitutes
Fenoldopam mesylate (Corlopam) (dopaminergic stimulator)	• IV infusion: mix 10 mg in 250 mL (40 mcg/mL); usual dose is 0.03-0.3 mcg/kg/min • Maximum: 1.7 mcg/kg/min	• Tachycardia, hypotension • Ventricular dysrhythmias • Dizziness • Anxiety • Headache • Flushing • Nausea, vomiting, abdominal pain • Hypokalemia • Increased intraocular pressure • Increased intracranial pressure	• Monitor HR, BP, urine output, neurologic status • Note contraindications: known hypersensitivity to fenoldopam or sulfite, intracranial hypertension • Use caution in patients with glaucoma or ocular hypertension and in patients on other drugs that may cause hypotension (e.g., beta-blockers)

(i.e., cortisol) glucocorticoids also cause the retention of sodium and water. Fluid remobilization after a burn, fluid resuscitation, and/or the administration of hypertonic or hyperosmolar solutions (e.g., 3% saline, albumin) are examples of fluid shifts from interstitial to intravascular spaces. Water-gain syndrome, sometimes referred to as hypervolemic hyponatremia, occurs when hypotonic fluids are used to replace isotonic body fluid losses due to the use of enemas with hypotonic fluid; excessive GI or GU loss of hypotonic fluid; excessive intake of ice chips; or psychogenic polydipsia, a psychiatric disorder. Syndrome of inappropriate antidiuretic hormone (SIADH), an excessive secretion or response to ADH, also causes water-gain syndrome.

Clinical presentation of hypervolemia and water-gain syndrome is typical of fluid overload. The most significant difference between hypervolemia and water-gain syndrome is the serum sodium and osmolality. Treatment of both of these fluid imbalances is to restrict fluids and remove excess fluid with diuretics or dialysis. Patients with water-gain syndrome who have severe hyponatremia will require the administration of hypertonic (e.g., 3%) saline. Administer hypertonic saline slowly. Maintain the infusion rate at 100 mL/hr and no more than 400 mL/24 hr. It is necessary to monitor the patient closely for clinical indications of fluid overload because 3% saline pulls fluid into the vascular space.

ELECTROLYTE IMBALANCES
Sodium Imbalances

Sodium has many important functions. It maintains extracellular osmolality and volume, maintains the active transport mechanism along with potassium, and influences the kidneys' regulation of water and electrolyte balance. Sodium also promotes conduction of nerve impulses and muscle contraction and aids in some enzyme activities. Sodium is also important in acid-base balance. Consider water when evaluating and treating serum sodium levels since water and sodium are closely linked in physiologic processes. Normal serum sodium is 136 to 145 mEq/L. Sodium imbalances include hyponatremia and hypernatremia (Table 5-9).

Hyponatremia

Hyponatremia is defined as a serum sodium less than 136 mEq/L. Sodium and water are decreased in the state of hyponatremia. This happens when there is a decreased sodium intake or increased sodium excretion. A decreased intake occurs with a sodium-restricted diet or malnutrition. Increased sodium excretion may be due to skin, GI, or renal losses. Skin loss occurs from diaphoresis or burns. Loss of sodium from the GI tract may occur from a number of factors, such as GI suctioning, vomiting, diarrhea, draining wound or fistula, or laxative abuse. The causes of a loss of

TABLE 5-8   Fluid Imbalances Summary

Etiology	Clinical Presentation	Collaborative Management
Hypovolemia		

• Excessive fluid losses
  • Hemorrhage
  • GI losses
  • Renal losses
  • Increased insensible losses
  • Draining wounds
• Inadequate replacement following excess fluid loss
• Intravascular to extravascular shift (also called third-spacing)
  • Ascites
  • Intestinal obstruction
  • Peritonitis
	• Tachycardia
	• Orthostatic hypotension
	• Weight loss >5% of body weight
	• Flat jugular veins
	• Weakness
	• Anorexia, nausea, vomiting, constipation
	• Flushed skin (fluid loss) or cool, clammy skin (blood loss)
	• Dry, sticky tongue and mucous membranes
	• Poor skin turgor
	• Thirst
	• Low-grade fever
	• Syncope
	• Lethargy, disorientation, coma
	• Oliguria
	• Decreased CVP
	• Urine specific gravity >1.030 if ADH osmoreceptor mechanism is intact
	• BUN increased with normal creatinine
	• Increased HCT and serum osmolality
		• Monitor I&O, daily weight
		• Replace fluids
		  • Oral fluids for mild deficits
		  • Parenteral fluids for moderate or severe deficits
		  • Replace fluids lost with similar fluids (e.g., blood for hemorrhage, normal saline with electrolytes for excessive diuresis)
		• Provide frequent oral and skin care

Water-Loss Syndrome (also referred to as Hyperosmolar Hypernatremia)		

• Water loss without sodium loss
• Inadequate water intake
• Watery diarrhea
• Hypertonic fluids or enteral feedings
• Excess TPN
• Addison's disease
• Diabetes insipidus
• Diabetes mellitus
	• Tachycardia
	• Hypotension
	• Flushed skin
	• Dry, sticky tongue and mucous membranes
	• Poor skin turgor
	• Thirst
	• Low-grade fever
	• Mental irritability, confusion
	• Oliguria to anuria (except DI)
	• Increased HCT, serum osmolality, serum sodium
		• Treat the cause
		  • Vasopressin for central diabetes insipidus; chlorpropamide (Diabinese) for nephrogenic diabetes insipidus
		  • Insulin for diabetes mellitus, hyperglycemia
		  • Antidiarrheals for diarrhea
		• Replace fluid with water in excess of sodium (e.g., D_5W or ½NS)
		• Provide frequent oral and skin care

Hypervolemia		

• Excessive intake of fluid
• Retention of sodium and water
  • Steroid therapy
  • Heart failure
  • Liver disease (e.g., cirrhosis)
  • Stress response via ADH secretion, renin-angiotensin-aldosterone system
  • Nephrotic syndrome
  • Acute or chronic renal failure
• Interstitial to intravascular shift
• Administration of hypertonic or hyperosmolar solutions (e.g., 3% NS, albumin)
	• Tachycardia, increased BP
	• Weight gain >5% of body weight
	• Jugular venous distention
	• Tachypnea, dyspnea, crackles
	• Peripheral edema
	• Ascites
	• Anasarca may be present
	• Increased urine output
	• Urine specific gravity <1.010 if ADH osmoreceptor mechanism is intact
	• Increased CVP
	• Muscle weakness
	• Lethargy, apathy, disorientation, coma
	• Decreased HCT
	• Decreased BUN
	• Clinical indications of pulmonary or cerebral edema
		• Monitor I&O, daily weight
		• Monitor IV fluids closely; volumetric or controller pumps should be used for patients predisposed to hypervolemia
		• Restrict fluids and/or sodium
		• Remove excess fluids
		  • Diuretics as prescribed
		  • Dialysis or CRRT may be utilized especially if renal failure is present
		• Provide frequent oral and skin care

TABLE 5-8	Fluid Imbalances Summary—cont'd	
Etiology	**Clinical Presentation**	**Collaborative Management**
Water Excess Syndromes (also referred to as Hypoosmolar Hyponatremia)		

• Water increased in excess of sodium
• Replacement of isotonic body fluids with hypotonic solution (e.g., D_5W)
• Excess use of tap water enemas
• Psychogenic polydipsia
• GI or GU irrigation with hypotonic fluids (e.g., tap water or distilled water)
• Excessive ice chips
• Syndrome of inappropriate antidiuretic hormone (SIADH)
• Administration of oral hypoglycemic agents, tricyclic antidepressants
	• Anorexia, nausea, vomiting
	• Abdominal and muscle cramps
	• Headache, confusion
	• Weakness
	• Edema
	• Lethargy
	• Muscle twitching, seizures
	• Decreased HCT, serum osmolality, serum sodium
		• Restrict fluid
		• Remove excess fluids
		  • Diuretics as prescribed
		  • Dialysis or CRRT may be utilized especially if renal failure is present
		• Administer hypertonic (3%) saline as prescribed for severe hyponatremia
		• Treat the cause: demeclocycline or lithium as prescribed for nephrogenic SIADH
		• Institute seizure precautions
		• Monitor for clinical indications of cerebral or pulmonary edema
		• Provide frequent oral and skin care

TABLE 5-9	Sodium Imbalances Summary	
Etiology	**Clinical Presentation**	**Collaborative Management**
Hyponatremia		

• Decreased sodium intake
  • Sodium-restricted diet
  • Alcoholism
• Increased sodium excretion
  • Skin losses
  • GI losses
  • Renal losses
  • Adrenal insufficiency
	• Tachycardia
	• Postural hypotension
	• Anorexia, nausea, vomiting, abdominal cramps, diarrhea
	• Weight loss
	• Decreased skin turgor
	• "Fingerprinting" over sternum
	• Apprehension
	• Headache, irritability
	• Weakness, fatigue
	• Personality changes
	• Mental confusion, disorientation
	• Lethargy progressing to coma
	• Muscle cramps, muscle twitching, increased DTRs
	• Tremors, seizures
	• Oliguria
	• Serum sodium <136 mEq/liter
		• Replace sodium
		  • High-sodium diet
		  • Normal saline or hypertonic (3%) NS solution parenterally as prescribed
		• Replace potassium as needed
		• Institute seizure precautions
		• Provide frequent oral and skin care

Hypernatremia		
• Excess/rapid administration of normal saline or hypertonic saline solution • Administration of sodium bicarbonate, sodium polystyrene sulfonate (Kayexalate) • Near-drowning with ingestion of salt water • Heart failure • Renal failure • Cirrhosis • Steroid therapy • Cushing's syndrome • Primary hyperaldosteronism	• Tachycardia • Hypertension • Weight gain • Edema • Thirst • Low-grade fever • Dry, sticky tongue and mucous membranes • Flushed, dry skin • Muscle rigidity and weakness • CNS irritability: restlessness, agitation • Mental confusion, disorientation • Altered level of consciousness • Muscle cramps, muscle twitching, increased DTRs • Tremors, seizures • Oliguria • Serum sodium >145 mEq/liter	• Treat precipitating factors • Restrict sodium and water • Administer diuretics as prescribed • Provide frequent oral and skin care • Institute seizure precautions • Monitor for indications of pulmonary edema or increased intracranial pressure

sodium from the kidneys include diuretics, cerebral salt-wasting syndrome, and adrenal insufficiency (i.e., Addison disease).

Subjective symptoms of hyponatremia include anorexia, nausea, vomiting, abdominal cramps, apprehension, headache, weakness, and fatigue. The patient has low serum sodium (<136 mEq/L) with normal serum osmolality. The objective signs and symptoms include clinical indications of hypovolemia, such as tachycardia, postural hypotension, weight loss, oliguria, and poor skin turgor. "Fingerprinting" may be seen over the sternum. Neurologic findings include personality changes, confusion, and level-of-consciousness changes. Seizures may occur especially if serum sodium is less than 110 mEq/L. Muscle cramping and twitching along with increased deep tendon reflexes (DTRs) may occur.

To properly manage a patient with hyponatremia, the collaborative patient care team monitors urine output, I&O, daily weight, and laboratory studies. Close observation for neurologic changes and implementation of seizure precautions are highly recommended. Patient care should include frequent oral and skin care along with restoring serum electrolyte levels, and preventing the complication of fluid overload. Restore serum sodium levels by increasing dietary sodium for mild deficiency. Administer prescribed parenteral solution of normal saline (NS) for a moderate to severe deficiency. Give hypertonic (3%) saline as prescribed for severe hyponatremia. Hypertonic solutions are to be administered at a slow rate, usually no more rapidly than 1 to 2 mL/kg/hr and no more than 400 mL/24 hr. Monitor for clinical indications of fluid overload because hypertonic solutions pull fluid into the vascular space. Also, replace potassium as needed.

Hypernatremia

The definition of hypernatremia is a serum sodium greater than 145 mEq/L. Hypernatremia is a state where both sodium and water are increased. Causes of hypernatremia include excessive administration of sodium, including sodium bicarbonate or sodium polystyrene sulfonate (Kayexalate) or consumption of sodium chloride; heart failure; renal failure; or hepatic failure. Excessive exogenous or endogenous corticosteroids also cause hypernatremia.

The relevant diagnostic value is a high serum sodium (>145 mEq/L) with normal serum osmolality. The patient suffering from hypernatremia may complain about thirst, muscle weakness, or muscle cramps. The typical clinical presentation includes tachycardia; hypertension; low-grade fever; edema; weight gain; dry, sticky tongue and mucous membranes; flushed, dry skin; muscle rigidity; twitching; and increased DTRs. CNS irritability with restlessness, agitation, mental confusion, and disorientation are common as levels increase. Seizures may occur.

Collaborative management of hypernatremia is focused on monitoring urine output, I&O, daily weight, and laboratory studies. Patient care should provide frequent oral and skin care. Closely observe for changes in neurologic status and the institute seizure precautions on patients with hypernatremia. Identifying and treating the cause of the condition is paramount along with restoring normal serum electrolyte levels. Administer diuretics as prescribed and implement sodium restriction to restore the electrolyte levels per the following recommended criteria:

- Mild restriction: 3 to 4 g/day; commonly referred to as a *"no added salt"* diet
- Moderate restriction: 2 g/day; consumption of only foods specifically "low sodium"
- Severe restriction: 500 mg/day; only low-sodium foods with avoidance of shellfish and limitation of dairy and meat

Potassium Imbalances

Potassium is crucial in the transmission of nerve impulses, maintenance of intracellular osmolality, activation of several enzymatic reactions, regulation of acid-base balance, and muscle, skeletal, and smooth muscle contraction. Potassium imbalances are the most potentially life-threatening of all electrolyte imbalances, primarily related to dysrhythmia potential. Normal serum potassium is 3.5 to 5.0 mEq/L. Potassium imbalances include hypokalemia and hyperkalemia (Table 5-10).

Hypokalemia

Hyperkalemia is defined as a serum potassium less than 3.5 mEq/L. Low serum potassium (<3.5 mEq/L) may be caused by inadequate potassium intake, increased potassium losses, or an extracellular to intracellular shift. Inadequate potassium intake is due to starvation, alcoholism, or inadequate potassium in fluids, nutrition, or dialysate. Increased potassium losses may be through the GI tract, the kidney, or excessive perspiration. Extracellular to intracellular shift of potassium may be related to acid-base imbalances or insulin administration. Alkalosis causes potassium to shift from the extracellular to the intracellular space, causing serum potassium to drop. Insulin facilitates the movement of potassium into the cell, so treatment of diabetic ketoacidosis with insulin reduces serum potassium levels.

The most significant effects of hypokalemia are cardiac, neuromuscular, and GI. Patients with hypokalemia may present with subjective symptoms of anorexia, nausea, vomiting, malaise, fatigue, dizziness, and muscle cramps.

Cardiovascular effects of hypokalemia include orthostatic hypotension, ECG changes, and dysrhythmias. ECG changes include flat T waves and prominent U waves, depressed ST segment, and prolonged QT and PR intervals. The dysrhythmias (e.g., PVCs, ventricular tachycardia, ventricular fibrillation, torsade de pointes) reflect ventricular irritability. Hypokalemia accentuates any digitalis effect and increases the likelihood of digitalis toxicity.

Muscle weakness progresses to decreased deep tendon reflexes and flaccid paralysis. The patient may exhibit irritability, confusion, and altered level of consciousness. Respiratory muscle weakness may progress to respiratory paralysis and respiratory arrest.

GI effects include decreased GI motility, paralytic ileus, and abdominal distention. Hypokalemia is a potential cause of postoperative paralytic ileus. Renal effects include polyuria, polydipsia, and an inability to concentrate urine.

Collaborative management focuses on monitoring urine output, I&O, daily weight, and laboratory studies. The first priority, as always, is to treat the cause, such as correcting alkalosis or treating diarrhea or diuresis. Next, the focus is on restoration of normal serum potassium levels. For mild hyperkalemia, teach the patient to regularly eat foods that are high in potassium and encourage use of a potassium chloride salt substitute. Administer oral potassium supplements as prescribed. Teach the patient about adequate potassium replacement if receiving diuretics; potassium-sparing diuretics may be used. Parenteral administration of potassium is given for severe hypokalemia with the following safety measures:

- Never administer potassium IV push and always use an infusion pump.

TABLE 5-10	Potassium Imbalances Summary	
Etiology	**Clinical Presentation**	**Collaborative Management**
Hypokalemia		

• Poor potassium intake (e.g., administration of potassium-deficient parenteral fluids or nutrition)
• Increased GI losses
• Increased renal losses
• Skin losses
• Extracellular to intracellular shift
  • Alkalosis
  • Insulin
  • Treatment of diabetic ketoacidosis
	• Orthostatic hypotension
	• Anorexia, nausea, vomiting
	• Decreased GI motility, paralytic ileus, abdominal distention
	• Malaise
	• Muscle cramps, muscle weakness to flaccid paralysis
	• Decreased DTRs
	• Dizziness
	• Apathy, mental confusion, drowsiness to coma
	• Respiratory muscle weakness causing shallow ventilation, dyspnea progressing to respiratory paralysis and respiratory arrest
	• Polyuria, polydipsia
	• Enhanced digitalis effect
	• ECG changes
	  • Flat T waves and prominent U waves
	  • Depressed ST segment
	  • Prolonged QT and PR intervals
	  • Dysrhythmias
	• Cardiac arrest
	• Serum potassium <3.5 mEq/liter
		• Replace potassium as prescribed (depending on how severely low the potassium level is)
		  • Dietary potassium; potassium chloride salt substitute
		  • Potassium supplements orally
		  • Potassium to IV solution (should not exceed 60 mEq/liter)
		  • Potassium "runs" IV usually via minibag (usual safe maximum 10 mEq/100 mL over 1 hour)
		   – May be administered at 20 mEq/hr if serum potassium is <2.5 mEq/liter
		   – Administer at no greater concentration than 10 mEq/100 mL if given via peripheral catheter or 20 mEq/100 mL if given via a central venous catheter
		• Correct alkalosis
		• Consider need for magnesium or calcium replacement
		• Assess for clinical indications of digitalis toxicity
		• Provide patient education regarding adequate potassium replacement if receiving diuretics

Hyperkalemia		

• Increased potassium intake
  • Excessive administration/ingestion of potassium: oral or parenteral
  • Excessive or too rapid potassium replacement
  • Transfusion of banked blood; the longer the blood has been stored, the higher the extracellular potassium content
• Decreased potassium excretion
  • Acute and chronic renal disease
  • Adrenal insufficiency (Addison's disease)
  • Potassium-sparing diuretics
  • ACE inhibitors or angiotensin-receptor blockers (ARBs)
• Cellular disruption with leak of intracellular potassium
  • Hemolysis (e.g., blood transfusion reaction)
  • Trauma or tissue ischemia/necrosis
  • Catabolism
  • Rhabdomyolysis
• Intracellular to extracellular shift
  • Acidosis
  • Hypertonic glucose with insulin deficiency
  • Muscle paralyzing agents (e.g., succinylcholine)
	• Tachycardia progressing to bradycardia and cardiac arrest
	• Nausea, vomiting, intestinal colic, diarrhea
	• Muscle weakness progressing to flaccid paralysis
	• Numbness, tingling of extremities
	• Increased DTRs
	• Fatigue
	• Lethargy, apathy, mental confusion
	• Respiratory muscle weakness may cause hypopnea, dyspnea
	• Respiratory distress
	• Oliguria
	• Decreased contractility, cardiac output
	• ECG changes
	  • Tall, peaked T waves
	  • Wide QRS complex
	  • Prolonged PR interval
	  • Flattened to absent P wave
	  • Bradycardia
	  • Dysrhythmias
	• Serum potassium >5.0 mEq/L
		• Restrict potassium intake
		  • Make sure that IV solution or TPN contains no potassium
		  • Check medications for potassium content
		• Evaluate BUN, creatinine levels for data about renal function
		• Provide treatments to shift potassium back into the cell if K > 6.5 or dysrhythmias present
		  • 50 mL of 50% dextrose and 10 units of insulin as prescribed
		  • Sodium bicarbonate if patient is acidotic
		• Provide treatment to cause the excretion or removal of potassium
		  • Sodium polystyrene sulfonate (Kayexalate), an exchange resin, orally or by retention enema and sorbitol, an osmotic diarrheal, as prescribed; this exchanges sodium for potassium and moves potassium out of the body via the GI tract
		  • Dialysis if due to renal failure
		• Correct hypomagnesemia and/or hypocalcemia
		• Administer calcium IV as prescribed for serum potassium levels of >6.5 mEq/liter to block the neuromuscular and cardiac effects; contraindicated if on digitalis

- Do not add to a preexisting infusion; if potassium is to be added to maintenance fluids, a new solution should be mixed to avoid uneven distribution of the potassium.
- The usual safe maximum is 10 mEq/100 mL minibag over 1 hour but may be administered at 20 mEq/100 mL over 1 hour if serum potassium is less than 2.5 mEq/L. (NOTE: It takes 100-200 mEq of potassium to increase serum potassium by 1 mEq/L.)
- Do not administer a concentration greater than 10 mEq/100 mL if given via peripheral catheter or 20 mEq/100 mL if given via a central venous catheter.
- Potassium is administered in NS unless contraindicated because dextrose may stimulate insulin secretion and intracellular shift of potassium.
- Close monitoring of ECG is required when administering high concentrations of potassium; also, clinical indications for digitalis toxicity are required if the patient is receiving a digitalis preparation.

Hyperkalemia

Hyperkalemia is defined as a serum potassium greater than 5 mEq/L. High serum potassium ranges from mild (>5.0 mEq/L) to moderate (>5.6 mEq/L) to severe (>7 mEq/dL). Causes of hyperkalemia include excessive potassium intake, decreased potassium excretion, cellular disruption with leak of intracellular potassium, and intracellular to extracellular shift. The patient may consume excessive potassium especially if there is coexisting renal insufficiency. Other causes of hyperkalemia include excessive parenteral potassium, including in medications such as potassium penicillin; or transfusion of banked blood, especially older banked blood because cell lysis causes the potassium level to be higher. Decreased potassium excretion is a major issue in patients with renal insufficiency or failure, but also occurs in Addison's disease or in patients receiving potassium-sparing diuretics, ACE inhibitors, or angiotensin-receptor blockers (ARBs). Conditions that cause cell lysis will cause hyperkalemia because it allows the leak of intracellular potassium into the extracellular, including intravascular, space. Blood transfusion reaction, tissue ischemia or necrosis, catabolism, and rhabdomyolysis are examples of conditions that cause cell lysis and hyperkalemia. Acidosis, hyperglycemia, and succinylcholine may all cause the shift on intracellular potassium into the extracellular, including intravascular, space causing hyperkalemia.

The patient with hyperkalemia presents with numerous complaints. As with hypokalemia, the clinical presentation will include primarily cardiovascular, neurologic, and gastrointestinal findings. Subjective complaints include GI symptoms of nausea, vomiting, abdominal cramping, and diarrhea. The patient may also complain of numbness, paresthesia of extremities, weakness, and fatigue.

Abdominal distention, hyperactive bowel sounds, and muscle weakness progressing to flaccid paralysis may be present. The patient's DTRs are initially increased but progressively decrease until absent. Respiratory muscle weakness may cause hypopnea and respiratory distress. In addition, the patient may present with lethargy, apathy, mental confusion, and oliguria.

The most life-threatening effects of hyperkalemia are on the cardiovascular system. Decreased contractility, decreased cardiac output, and hypotension may occur. Although tachycardia is present initially, bradycardia and cardiac arrest occur with severe hyperkalemia. On ECG, tall, narrow, peaked T waves and shortened QT intervals occur when serum potassium level is between 5.5 and 6 mEq/L. As the serum potassium level climbs to between 6 and 7 mEq/L, wide QRS complexes and prolonged PR intervals develop. P waves flatten until absent and the QRS complexes widen when the serum potassium level reaches between 7 and 8 mEq/L. A serum potassium level that reaches 8.0 mEq/L or greater results in fusion of QRS complexes and T waves, idioventricular rhythm, and asystole.

Collaborative patient care management includes the monitoring of urine output, I&O, daily weight, and laboratory studies. Identify potential causes of hyperkalemia by conducting a dietary history and checking BUN and creatinine levels for information regarding renal function. Treatment of the cause of the hyperkalemia might include dialysis for a patient in renal failure or insulin therapy for a patient with hyperglycemia. Correct acidosis and discontinue causative drugs such as potassium-sparing diuretics, ACE inhibitors, angiotensin receptor blockers, and NSAIDs.

Restore normal serum electrolytes by instituting the following interventions:

- Potassium restriction: Ensure that the IV solution or TPN contains no potassium and check medications for potassium content.
- Diuretics administered as prescribed: usually 40 to 80 mg furosemide (Lasix).
- Emergency treatment measures if serum potassium is greater than 6.5 mEq/L or dysrhythmias are present; however, patients with chronic renal failure may tolerate high levels of potassium and not be symptomatic until 7 mEq/L or greater.

Emergency treatment for severe and symptomatic hyperkalemia includes dextrose and insulin administration, sodium polystyrene sulfonate (Kayexalate) therapy, diuretic therapy, nebulized albuterol, bicarbonate, renal replacement therapy, or calcium administration. These measures (Table 5-11) remove potassium from the body, shift the potassium from the extracellular space to the intracellular space, and protect the heart.

Calcium Imbalances

Calcium is crucial in transmission of neuromuscular impulses, blood coagulation, cardiac contractility, and strength of bones and teeth. Normal serum calcium is 8.5 to 10.5 mg/dL. Calcium imbalances include hypocalcemia and hypercalcemia (Table 5-12).

Hypocalcemia

A serum calcium less than 8.5 mg/dL defines hypocalcemia. Because calcium binds to albumin, only the unbound (free or ionized) calcium is biologically active. Hypocalcemia is present if serum ionized calcium is less than 4.1 mg/dL.

The causes of hypocalcemia include decreased calcium intake or absorption, increased calcium excretion, and increased calcium binding with decreased ionized calcium. Conditions that cause decreased calcium intake or absorption include chronic inadequate dietary calcium intake, vitamin D deficiency or resistance, hypoparathyroidism, hypomagnesemia, renal failure, liver disease, postgastrectomy, malabsorption syndrome, Cushing's syndrome, and steroid therapy. Increased excretion of calcium occurs with diuretic therapy, chronic diarrhea, hyperphosphatemia, and the diuretic phase of acute kidney injury. Remember that due to the inverse relationship of calcium and

TABLE 5-11	Specific Emergent Interventions to Treat Life-Threatening Hyperkalemia
Intervention	**Rationale**
Insulin and dextrose	Moves potassium back into the cell and the effect lasts about 4-6 hours. The usual dosage is 50 mL of 50% dextrose and 10 units of insulin. Monitor the patient for increased or decreased serum glucose.
Sodium polystyrene sulfonate (Kayexalate)	Exchange resin that exchanges sodium for potassium and moves potassium out of the body via the GI tract. It is given orally or by retention enema, though oral administration is preferred. The usual dose is 15-50 g in 50-100 mL of 20% sorbitol orally or 50 g in 200 mL of dextrose as retention enema. Sorbitol, an osmotic laxative, produces a cathartic effect only when given orally and may contribute to intestinal necrosis when given by enema, so do not include sorbitol when given by enema.
Nebulized albuterol	Stimulates the Na-K ATPase pump resulting in intracellular K uptake. The usual dose is 10-20 mg nebulized over 15 minutes. Monitor for the adverse effect of tachycardia.
Bicarbonate	Corrects acidosis to move potassium back into the cell. The usual dose is 50 mEq IV over 5 minutes. This effect lasts approximately 1-2 hours. Closely monitor for the adverse effects of hypernatremia and hyperosmolality.
Continuous renal replacement therapy (e.g., continuous venous-venous hemodialysis)	Removes excess serum potassium.
10% Calcium chloride	Does not correct the hyperkalemia but protects the heart until other measures effectively reduce the serum potassium levels. Intravenous calcium blocks the neuromuscular and cardiac effects. The usual dose is 5-10 mL of over 2-5 minutes but is contraindicated if patient is receiving digitalis.

phosphorus, anything that increases phosphorus decreases calcium. Alkalosis increases the binding of calcium to albumin, which reduces ionized calcium, and citrated blood causes the binding of calcium to the citrate. Acute pancreatitis causes hypocalcemia by the binding of calcium in fat necrosis. Some drugs may also bind with calcium, causing hypocalcemia.

Hypocalcemia manifests symptoms primarily on the neuromuscular and cardiovascular systems. Patients may complain of abdominal cramps, biliary colic, muscle cramps, and paresthesia of fingertips and/or the circumoral area. The major clinical presentation of hypocalcemia is tetany. Tetany results in cramps, twitching of the muscles, sharp flexion of the wrist and ankle joints (i.e., carpopedal spasm), increased deep tendon reflexes, and possibly seizures. Both Chvostek's and Trousseau's signs may be noted. Chvostek's sign is a facial twitching in response to tapping on the facial nerve. Trousseau's sign is a carpal spasm after 3 minutes of inflation of a blood pressure cuff to a level above systolic pressure. Increased deep tendon reflexes are noted.

Hypocalcemia produces the ECG changes of prolonged QT intervals and dysrhythmias (e.g., torsades de pointes). Decreased cardiac contractility and cardiac output may be noted. Patients may also exhibit irritability, confusion, psychosis, and memory loss. They may also have laryngospasm with stridor. Renal calculi from urinary excretion of excess calcium can produce oliguria or anuria. Also, because calcium is a needed catalyst for each sequence of blood coagulation pathway, low levels can cause coagulation problems, resulting in bruising and bleeding.

The collaborative health care team needs to monitor the hypocalcemic patient's airway patency and ventilation. A cricothyroidotomy may be necessary for severe laryngospasm. The team must monitor urine output, I&O, daily weight, and laboratory studies along with treating the cause of the hypocalcemia by administering phosphate-binding antacids for

hyperphosphatemia, phosphate restriction, and phosphate-binding agents for renal failure. Normal serum calcium levels can be restored with a high-calcium, low-phosphorus diet; oral calcium with vitamin D supplements; and/or parenteral calcium. Calcium gluconate (10 mL) contains 4.5 mEq of calcium; calcium chloride (10 mL) contains 13.6 mEq of calcium. Calcium chloride produces higher ionized calcium; however, calcium gluconate is frequently preferred because it is less irritating to tissues. Administer parenteral calcium through a central venous catheter if possible. If a peripheral catheter access is used, implement measures to prevent extravasation because intravenous calcium may cause necrosis and sloughing. Dilute medication in 100 mL of D_5W and administer slowly over 10 to 30 minutes. Hypocalcemia unresponsive to treatment may indicate concurrent hypomagnesemia, so check levels and administer magnesium concurrently. Closely monitor blood pressure and cardiac rhythm during calcium administration. Monitor for and prevent neurologic seizure complications by instituting seizure precautions.

Hypercalcemia

A serum calcium greater than 10.5 mg/dL defines hypercalcemia. Hypercalcemia may be due to increased calcium intake or absorption, hypophosphatemia, increased mobilization of calcium from the bone, decreased calcium excretion, or an increased ionized calcium level. Increased calcium intake may result from excessive intake of calcium supplements or calcium antacids. Milk-alkali syndrome is an acquired condition in which there is hypercalcemia and a shift in the body's acid-base balance toward metabolic alkalosis. Milk-alkali syndrome is caused by drinking too much milk (which is high in calcium) and long-term intake of certain antacids, especially calcium carbonate or sodium bicarbonate (baking soda). Hypophosphatemia also

TABLE 5-12 Calcium Imbalances Summary

Etiology	Clinical Presentation	Collaborative Management
Hypocalcemia		

• Decreased calcium intake or absorption
  • Chronic insufficient calcium intake
  • Hypoparathyroidism
  • Hypomagnesemia
  • Acute and chronic renal failure
  • Liver disease
  • Postgastrectomy
  • Chronic malabsorption syndrome
  • Cushing's syndrome
  • Steroid therapy
• Increased calcium excretion
  • Diuretic therapy
  • Chronic diarrhea
  • Hyperphosphatemia
  • Diuretic phase of acute kidney injury
• Increased calcium binding, decreased ionized calcium
  • Citrated blood administration
  • Alkalosis
  • Acute pancreatitis
  • Drugs: aminoglycosides, heparin, theophylline
	• Abdominal cramps, biliary colic
	• Paresthesia of fingertips, circumoral area
	• Chvostek's sign: facial twitching in response to tapping on the facial nerve
	• Trousseau's sign: carpal spasm after 3 minutes of inflation of a blood pressure cuff to a level above systolic pressure
	• Muscle cramps, tremors
	• Increased DTRs, carpopedal spasm
	• Confusion, psychosis
	• Memory loss
	• Laryngospasm, stridor
	• Tetany (characterized by cramps, twitching of the muscles, sharp flexion of the wrist and ankle joints, seizures)
	• Hyperphosphatemia
	• Decreased contractility, cardiac output
	• Oliguria, anuria if renal calculi obstructive
	• Bruising, bleeding
	• ECG changes
	  • Prolonged QT interval
	  • Dysrhythmias
	• Serum calcium <8.5 mg/dL (4.5 mEq/liter)
		• Replace calcium depending on severity of deficit
		  • High-calcium, low-phosphorus diet
		  • Oral calcium with vitamin D supplements as prescribed
		  • Calcium gluconate or calcium chloride IV as prescribed
		  • 10 mL of calcium gluconate contains 4.5 mEq of calcium and 10 mL of calcium chloride contains 13.6 mEq of calcium; administer both no more rapidly than 1 mL/min
		• Administer phosphate-binding antacids as prescribed for hyperphosphatemia
		• Administer magnesium as prescribed: hypocalcemia unresponsive to treatment, may indicate concurrent hypomagnesemia
		• Evaluate airway patency; cricothyroidotomy may be necessary for severe laryngospasm
		• Institute seizure precautions

Hypercalcemia		

• Increased calcium intake
  • Milk-alkali syndrome
• Increased calcium absorption
• Hypophosphatemia
• Increased mobilization of calcium from bone
  • Hyperparathyroidism
  • Immobility
  • Malignancy especially bone, breast, lung, lymphoma, multiple myeloma
  • Granulomatous disease (e.g., sarcoidosis, TB, histoplasmosis)
  • Thyrotoxicosis
• Decreased calcium excretion
  • Thiazide diuretics
  • Adrenal insufficiency (Addison's disease)
  • Renal tubular acidosis
• Increased ionized calcium (e.g., acidosis)
	• Anorexia, nausea, vomiting, abdominal pain, constipation
	• Bone and/or flank pain: pathologic fractures may occur
	• Malaise, fatigue
	• Decreased DTRs
	• Neuromuscular weakness to flaccidity
	• Subtle personality changes progressing to psychosis
	• Confusion
	• Depression, lethargy, stupor, coma
	• Renal calculi
	• Polyuria, polydipsia
	• Azotemia
	• Enhanced digitalis effect
	• Dysrhythmias and/or blocks
	• ECG changes: shortened QT interval
	• Serum calcium >10.5 mg/dL (>5.8 mEq/L)
		• Restrict calcium: low-calcium, high-phosphorus diet
		• Provide therapies to increase calcium excretion
		  • Oral fluids
		  • Normal saline infusion and diuretics
		  • Calcitonin
		  • Phosphorus
		  • Corticosteroids
		  • EDTA
		  • Plicamycin
		• Administer calcium channel blockers to protect the heart from effects of hypercalcemia
		• Ambulate to increase bone resorption of calcium
		• Monitor for clinical indications of digitalis toxicity

causes hypercalcemia because it increases calcium absorption. Hypercalcemia due to increased mobilization from bone occurs in hyperparathyroidism, vitamin D excess, immobility, malignancies, granulomatous diseases, or thyrotoxicosis.

Increased ionized calcium occurs in the state of acidosis. Only 1% to 2% of total body calcium is in the exchangeable form in circulation, and the rest forms part of the skeleton. Only one-half of the exchangeable calcium is in the active ionized form with the remainder bound to albumin, globulin, and other inorganic molecules. The pH influences protein binding to calcium. Metabolic alkalosis leads to reduced ionized calcium from increased protein binding. Decreased calcium excretion that occurs with thiazide diuretics, adrenal insufficiency (Addison disease), or renal tubular acidosis also causes hypercalcemia.

Patients with hypercalcemia may complain of thirst, anorexia, nausea, vomiting, abdominal pain, malaise, fatigue, weakness, depression, and bone and/or flank pain due to pathologic fractures or kidney stones. They may have decreased bowel sounds, constipation, and paralytic ileus. They are likely to have neuromuscular weakness to flaccidity with decreased DTRs. Patients may be agitated, confused, lethargic, or comatose. They may have subtle personality changes progressing to psychosis. Cardiovascular effects include shortened QT interval on ECG, dysrhythmia and/or blocks, and increase in risk of digitalis toxicity. Renal effects may include polyuria, renal calculi, and azotemia.

Collaborative patient care management focuses on monitoring urine output, I&O, daily weight, and laboratory studies. Place emphasis on treating the cause and restoring normal serum electrolyte levels. Interventions related to treatment of the cause of hypercalcemia include discontinuance of causative drugs; surgery, radiation, and antineoplastic therapy for malignancy; and partial parathyroidectomy for hyperparathyroidism.

To restore normal serum electrolyte levels, provide a low-calcium, high-phosphorus diet and administer steroids to decrease calcium absorption. Facilitate calcium excretion by increasing oral fluids and administering a large volume (100 to 200 mL/hr) of intravenous isotonic saline. In addition, enhance excretion with the use of dialysis, loop diuretics (e.g., furosemide [Lasix]), calcitonin, phosphorus, or EDTA (disodium salt).

The nurse should also monitor for and prevent cardiac effects of hypercalcemia. Give calcium channel blockers as prescribed and monitor for clinical indications of digitalis toxicity.

Weight-bearing activities and medication will decrease bone resorption of calcium. Medications used to decrease bone resorption include etidronate (Didronel), pamidronate (Aredia), gallium nitrate, corticosteroids, plicamycin (formerly known as *mithramycin*) (Mithracin), or inorganic phosphate.

Employ strategies to prevent renal calculi while correcting hypercalcemia, such as increasing fluid intake and encouraging mobility. Administer agents to acidify the urine because acidification of urine increases solubility of calcium.

Phosphorus Imbalances

Phosphorus is essential for glucose metabolism in red blood cells, producing 2,3-diphosphoglyceric acid (2,3-DPG) as an end product and for ATP or high-energy phosphate formation. It helps maintain bone hardness and aids in enzyme regulation (ATPase), and the kidneys use phosphorus to buffer hydrogen ions (PO_4). Normal serum phosphorus is 3.0 to 4.5 mg/dL. Phosphorus imbalances include hypophosphatemia and hyperphosphatemia (Table 5-13).

Hypophosphatemia

A serum phosphate less than 3.0 mg/dL defines hypophosphatemia. The causes of hypophosphatemia include an inadequate intake of phosphorus, decreased GI absorption, increased intestinal loss, increased renal excretion, or extracellular to intracellular shifts of phosphorus. Inadequate intake of phosphorus is due primarily to malnutrition or inadequate phosphorus replacement with nutritional support (i.e., refeeding syndrome). Poor GI absorption or increased GI loss of phosphorus occurs with the excessive use of phosphate-binding gels, prolonged vomiting or diarrhea, gastric suction, sucralfate (Carafate), malabsorption syndrome, and vitamin D deficiency. Increased renal excretion of phosphorus occurs with thiazide diuretics, hypomagnesemia, hypokalemia, or

hyperparathyroidism. Fanconi's syndrome is a disease of the proximal kidney renal tubules in which glucose and bicarbonate pass into the urine instead of being reabsorbed, resulting in the increased renal excretion of phosphate. Extracellular to intracellular shift of phosphorus occurs with parenteral glucose, insulin and respiratory alkalosis, or beta-adrenergic drugs (e.g., albuterol [Proventil]).

Hypophosphatemia causes patients to complain of anorexia, nausea, vomiting, malaise, fatigue, paresthesia, bone pain, and chest pain. Cardiovascular effects may include tachycardia, hypotension, and heart failure. The neuromuscular effects of hypophosphatemia mimic the symptoms of hypercalcemia, especially muscle weakness. The patient may exhibit incoordination, ataxia, confusion, lethargy, coma, or seizures. Respiratory muscle weakness may result in respiratory failure. Hemolytic anemia, immunosuppression, and platelet dysfunction may occur.

Collaborative patient care management focuses on monitoring urine output, daily weight, I&O, and laboratory studies. Monitor for cardiovascular, pulmonary, and neurologic effects of hypophosphatemia. To treat the cause, discontinue phosphate-binding gels and correct hypercalcemia. Restore normal serum phosphate by a high-phosphorus, low-calcium diet and administering oral or parenteral phosphate supplements. Monitor for signs of hypocalcemia when giving oral or parenteral supplements and use a central venous catheter if possible. If phosphate is less than 1 mg/dL without adverse effects, the usual parenteral dose is 0.6 mg/kg/hr. If phosphate is less than 2 mg/dL with adverse effects, the usual parenteral dose is 0.9 mg/kg/hr. It is contraindicated to administer intravenous phosphate to patients with hypercalcemia.

Hyperphosphatemia

A serum phosphate greater than 4.5 mg/dL defines hyperphosphatemia. Causes of hyperphosphatemia include increased phosphorus intake, decreased phosphorus excretion, intracellular to extracellular shifts of phosphorus, and cell destruction. Increased phosphorus intake can occur with cathartic abuse of phosphate-containing laxatives and enemas, excessive vitamin D, transfusion of stored blood, and acute elemental phosphorus poisoning. Acute or chronic renal failure and hypoparathyroidism causes decreased phosphorus excretion. Acidosis, malignant hyperthermia, or severe hypothermia may result in intracellular to extracellular shift. Neoplastic disease treated with chemotherapy, catabolism, and rhabdomyolysis cause cell destruction and release of intracellular phosphates.

The clinical presentation of a patient with hyperphosphatemia is the same as one with hypocalcemia. The priority patient care focuses on airway patency. A cricothyroidotomy may be necessary for severe laryngospasm. The patient's urine output, I&O, daily weight, and laboratory studies need to be monitored. The treatments for the restoration of normal serum electrolyte levels include a low-phosphorus, high-calcium diet and sucralfate (Carafate) or aluminum antacids to bind with phosphate in the GI tract. Acetazolamide (Diamox) may be used.

Monitor for and prevent neurologic complications. Institute seizure precautions and correct hypocalcemia. Dialysis may be required if renal failure is the cause. Saline diuresis and urinary alkalization is the treatment for tumor lysis syndrome or rhabdomyolysis.

TABLE 5-13 Phosphorus Imbalances Summary

Etiology	Clinical Presentation	Collaborative Management
Hypophosphatemia		

• Inadequate intake of phosphorus
  • Malnutrition
  • Prolonged low-phosphorus or phosphate-free IV therapy or TPN therapy
• Decreased GI absorption or increased intestinal loss
  • Excessive use of phosphate-binding gels such as aluminum hydroxide
  • Prolonged vomiting or diarrhea
  • Gastric suctioning
  • Sucralfate (Carafate)
  • Chronic malabsorption syndrome
• Increased renal excretion of phosphorus
  • Thiazide diuretics
  • Hypomagnesemia
  • Hypokalemia
  • Hyperparathyroidism
  • Fanconi's syndrome
• Extracellular to intracellular shifts
  • Parenteral glucose or insulin administration
  • Respiratory alkalosis
  • Large amounts of carbohydrate
  • DKA (after treatment)
	• Tachycardia, hypotension
	• Anorexia, nausea, vomiting
	• Malaise, fatigue
	• Paresthesia, tremors
	• Nystagmus, anisocoria
	• Incoordination, ataxia
	• Seizures
	• Mental confusion, lethargy, coma
	• Memory loss
	• Muscle weakness especially respiratory muscles
	• Bone pain
	• Chest pain
	• Dyspnea, crackles
	• Weight loss
	• Hemolytic anemia
	• Immunosuppression
	• Platelet dysfunction: petechiae
	• Dysrhythmias
	• Heart failure
	• X-ray: skeletal abnormalities
	• Serum phosphorus <3.0 mg/dL
		• Discontinue phosphate-binding gels if indicated
		• Administer phosphorus
		  • High-phosphorus, low-calcium diet
		  • Dietary phosphate supplements as ordered and monitor for signs of hypocalcemia when giving supplements
		  • Potassium phosphate IV as ordered and monitor for signs of hypocalcemia
		• Correct hypercalcemia if cause of hypophosphatemia

Hyperphosphatemia		

• Increased phosphorus intake
• Decreased phosphorus excretion
  • Acute or chronic renal failure
  • Hypoparathyroidism
• Extracellular shifts
  • DKA (before treatment)
  • Respiratory acidosis
  • Malignant hyperthermia
  • Severe hypothermia
• Cellular destruction
  • Neoplastic disease treated with chemotherapy
  • Catabolism
  • Rhabdomyolysis
	• Same as hypocalcemia
	• Serum phosphorus >4.5 mg/dL
		• Restrict phosphorus: low-phosphorus, high-calcium diet
		• Administer treatments to cause elimination of phosphorus
		  • Aluminum or calcium antacids to bind with phosphate
		  • Acetazolamide (Diamox)
		  • Dialysis if renal failure is cause
		  • Correction of hypocalcemia: calcium
		• Maintain airway patency; cricothyroidotomy may be necessary for severe laryngospasm
		• Institute seizure precautions

Magnesium Imbalances

Magnesium aids in neuromuscular transmission, cardiac contractility, and active transport at the cellular level. It also activates enzymes for cellular metabolism of carbohydrates and proteins. Normal serum magnesium is 1.5 to 2.5 mEq/L. Magnesium imbalances include hypomagnesemia and hypermagnesemia (Table 5-14).

Hypomagnesemia

A serum magnesium less than 1.5 mEq/L defines hypomagnesemia. Potential causes of hypomagnesemia include decreased magnesium intake or absorption, increased magnesium loss, increased magnesium binding, and extracellular to intracellular shift. Potential causes of decreased magnesium intake include

malnutrition, starvation, or inadequate magnesium in total parenteral nutrition (TPN). Increased magnesium loss occurs with GI losses, the diuretic phase of acute kidney injury, hyperparathyroidism, hyperaldosteronism, steroids, diabetic ketoacidosis, or heart failure. Drugs associated with increased magnesium loss include diuretics, antimicrobials (e.g., aminoglycosides, pentamidine, amphotericin B), ethanol, cisplatin, or cyclosporin A. Citrated blood administration causes binding of magnesium and citrate. Concentrated glucose solutions, amino acid solutions, or insulin may cause the extracellular to intracellular shift of magnesium leading to decreased serum magnesium. Patients with hypomagnesemia often have concurrent hypocalcemia and hypokalemia. The clinical presentation of hypomagnesemia is the same as for hypocalcemia.

TABLE 5-14	Magnesium Imbalances Summary		
Etiology	**Clinical Presentation**	**Collaborative Management**	

Hypomagnesemia

Etiology	Clinical Presentation	Collaborative Management

• Decreased magnesium intake or absorption
  • Protein-calorie malnutrition
  • Starvation
  • Prolonged low-magnesium or magnesium-free IV therapy or TPN therapy
• Increased magnesium loss
  • Diuretics
  • Vomiting, gastric suction, fistula
  • Acute pancreatitis
  • Chronic diarrhea
  • Hyperparathyroidism
  • Hyperaldosteronism
  • Steroids
  • DKA
  • HF
  • MI
• Increased magnesium binding
  • Citrated blood administration
• Extracellular to intracellular shift
  • Concentrated glucose solutions
  • Amino acid solutions
  • Insulin
	• Tachycardia, hypotension
	• Anorexia, nausea, vomiting, abdominal distention
	• Paresthesia of fingertips, circumoral area
	• Chvostek's and Trousseau's signs
	• Muscle cramps, tremors
	• Increased DTRs, carpopedal spasm
	• Confusion, psychosis
	• Memory loss
	• Laryngospasm, stridor
	• Tetany
	• Seizures
	• Concurrent hypocalcemia, hypokalemia
	• Decreased contractility, cardiac output
	• Increased digitalis effect
	• ECG changes
	  • Prolonged QT interval
	  • Dysrhythmias especially torsades de pointes
	• Serum magnesium <1.5 mEq/liter
		• Replace magnesium depending on severity of deficit
		  • High-magnesium diet
		  • Magnesium supplements in the form of magnesium antacids
		  • Magnesium sulfate IV as prescribed
		• Monitor calcium levels closely and replace if indicated
		• Maintain airway patency; cricothyroidotomy may be necessary for severe laryngospasm
		• Institute seizure precautions
		• Monitor for clinical indications of digitalis toxicity

Hypermagnesemia

Etiology	Clinical Presentation	Collaborative Management

• Increased magnesium intake (e.g. magnesium antacids, magnesium sulfate IV, magnesium containing laxatives, enemas)
• Decreased magnesium excretion
  • Acute/chronic renal failure
  • Hypoparathyroidism
  • Hypoaldosteronism
• Intracellular to extracellular shift
  • Untreated DKA
  • Rhabdomyolysis
	• Bradycardia, hypotension
	• Facial flushing
	• Dialysis
	• Muscle weakness progressing to paralysis
	  • Respiratory muscle weakness may cause hypoventilation and dyspnea
	  • Respiratory muscle paralysis and apnea may occur with levels >10 mEq/liter
	• Decreased DTRs; loss of patellar reflex occurs at levels >8 mEq/liter
	• Confusion, lethargy, coma
	• Cardiopulmonary arrest
	• Serum magnesium >2.5 mEq/liter
		• Restrict and/or eliminate magnesium
		  • Low-magnesium diet
		  • Discontinuance of magnesium antacids or IV magnesium
		  • 0.45% saline and diuretics as prescribed if normal saline function
		  • Dialysis if renal failure is cause of hypermagnesemia
		• Administer calcium IV as prescribed to antagonize neuromuscular effects of hypermagnesemia
		• Monitor and maintain airway and ventilation; intubation and mechanical ventilation may be necessary

A priority in the collaborative patient care management is monitoring airway patency. A cricothyroidotomy may be necessary for severe laryngospasm. Closely monitor urine output, I&O, daily weight, and laboratory studies. Provide nutritional support for malnutrition, a high-magnesium diet, oral magnesium supplements in the form of magnesium antacids, and potassium-sparing diuretics because they spare magnesium.

Administer magnesium sulfate IV slowly to restore electrolyte levels. Administer 1 to 2 g diluted in 100 mL and administered over 1 hour unless critical level, then give a 4-g dose over 2 hours. When life-threatening dysrhythmias occur such as torsades de pointes, administer 1 to 2 g diluted in 10 mL over a 5- to 20-minute period. Many patients with hypomagnesemia are also hypocalcemic; therefore, during calcium replacement, monitor for and prevent neurologic complications and institute seizure precautions. In addition, monitor for clinical indications of digitalis toxicity for patients on digitalis preparations.

5.6   Learning Activity

Identify three electrolyte imbalances that enhance the digitalis effect and increase the chance of digitalis toxicity.

a. _____

b. _____

c. _____

Answers to this activity can be found in the Answer Key.

Hypermagnesemia

A serum magnesium greater than 2.5 mg/dL defines hypermagnesemia. Possible causes of hypermagnesemia include increased intake, decreased excretion, and intracellular to extracellular shift. Increased magnesium intake occurs with administration of a magnesium sulfate IV or magnesium-containing antacids, laxatives, or enemas. Decreased magnesium excretion occurs from acute or chronic renal failure, hyperparathyroidism, hypoaldosteronism, and hypothyroidism. Untreated ketoacidosis, burns, and rhabdomyolysis are the causes for intracellular to extracellular shift. Blood sample hemolysis can cause a pseudo-hypermagnesemia; therefore, it is important to verify abnormal values and correlate with clinical presentation.

Clinical presentation of hypermagnesemia is similar to the clinical presentation of hypercalcemia. Patients with hypermagnesemia complain about weakness, fatigue, nausea, vomiting, somnolence, and diplopia. Bradycardia, hypotension, and facial flushing may be noted. Muscle weakness progressing to paralysis and loss of deep tendon reflexes (DTRs) occurs as serum levels rise. Loss of the patellar reflex occurs at levels greater than 8 mEq/L. Respiratory muscle weakness may cause hypoventilation, dyspnea, respiratory muscle paralysis, and apnea with levels greater than 10 mEq/L. Confusion, somnolence, lethargy, coma, and cardiopulmonary arrest can also occur. Abnormal ECG parameters include prolonged PR, QRS, and QT along with bradycardias and conduction blocks.

Priority collaborative patient care management is to monitor and maintain airway and ventilation. Intubation and mechanical ventilation may be necessary. As with all renal problems, monitor urine output, I&O, daily weight, and laboratory studies. Treat the cause by discontinuance of magnesium-containing antacids or laxatives and oral and IV magnesium supplements. Restore normal serum electrolyte levels with a low-magnesium diet. If normal renal function is present, stimulate diuresis with NS or half-NS infusions and furosemide (1 mg/kg). Monitor for hypocalcemia and hypokalemia, which commonly occur with hypomagnesemia. Administer IV calcium as prescribed. The usual dose is 5 to 10 mL of 10% calcium chloride over 2 to 5 minutes. Calcium will block the neuromuscular and cardiac effects, but in patients receiving digitalis it is contraindicated. Consider dialysis if renal failure is the cause of hypermagnesemia.

5.7   Learning Activity

Identify whether these signs and symptoms are indicative of electrolyte deficit or excess.

Sign/Symptom	Excess (Hyper)	Deficit (Hypo)
Sodium		
Weight gain		
Abdominal cramps		
Flushed, dry skin		
Postural hypotension		
Headache		
Hypertension		
Potassium		
Flat T waves, prominent U waves		
Decreased GI motility, paralytic ileus		
Intestinal colic, diarrhea		
Muscle cramps → flaccid paralysis		
Decreased cardiac contractility		
Tall, peaked T waves, widened QRS complex		
Calcium		
Tetany		
Decreased deep tendon reflexes		
Neuromuscular weakness, flaccidity		
Seizures		
Bone or flank pain		
Laryngospasm		

5.7 Learning Activity—cont'd

Sign/Symptom	Excess (Hyper)	Deficit (Hypo)
Phosphorus		
Tetany		
Fatigue		
Chest pain		
Dyspnea		
Increased deep tendon reflexes		
Abdominal cramps		
Magnesium		
Decreased deep tendon reflexes		
Anorexia, nausea, vomiting		
Cardiopulmonary arrest		
Lethargy		
Dysrhythmias, especially torsades de pointes		
Facial flushing		

Answers to this activity can be found in the Answer Key.

5.8 Learning Activity

Identify the electrolyte or electrolytes that the statement describes.
a. Serum levels of this electrolyte go up in acidosis and down in alkalosis. _____

b. These three electrolytes frequently go down together. _____
_____

c. Serum levels of this electrolyte go down in hypoalbuminemia. _____
d. These two electrolytes have an inverse relationship: When one goes down, the other goes up. _____

e. These two electrolytes are frequently deficient in malnourished patients. _____

f. Loss of either of these electrolytes causes hydrogen ions to move into the cell, resulting in metabolic alkalosis.
_____

Answers to this activity can be found in the Answer Key.

5.9 Learning Activity

Identify the fluid, electrolyte, or acid-base imbalances to which these patients would be predisposed:
a. A patient receiving regular doses of furosemide _____
b. A patient with persistent vomiting _____
c. A patient with acute kidney injury (oliguric phase) _____
d. A patient with diabetic ketoacidosis (before treatment) _____
e. A patient receiving multiple units of banked blood _____

Answers to this activity can be found in the Answer Key.

RENAL FAILURE

Renal failure refers to temporary or permanent damage to the kidneys resulting in the loss of normal kidney function. There are two different types of renal failure: acute and chronic. Acute renal failure, now called acute kidney injury (AKI), has an abrupt onset, developing rapidly over a few hours or a few days. AKI is most common in people who are already hospitalized, particularly in critically ill patients. AKI may be reversible with intensive treatment, but it may be fatal. Chronic kidney disease (CKD) progresses slowly over at least 3 months and leads to end-stage renal disease (ESRD) that requires lifelong dialysis treatment or a renal transplant for survival.

Acute Kidney Injury

Acute kidney injury occurs when the kidneys suddenly become unable to filter waste products from the blood.

When the kidneys lose their filtering ability, dangerous levels of wastes accumulate. The sudden decline in kidney function results in fluid, electrolyte, and acid-base imbalances caused by decreased GFR and impaired clearance of small solutes.

AKI is classified by etiology: prerenal, intrinsic (also referred to as intrarenal), or postrenal. Prerenal AKI is due to disrupted blood flow to the kidney that can occur from decreased intravascular volume, decreased cardiac output, severe vasodilation, or renovascular changes. Damage to the cortical and medullary renal tissue occurs with intrinsic AKI. Cortical damage results from glomerulonephritis, vasculitis, and interstitial nephritis. Medullary damage, also known as acute tubercular necrosis (ATN), is associated with nephrotoxic agents, rhabdomyolysis, or hemolysis. Disrupted urine flow occurs in postrenal AKI due to either mechanical or functional forces.

5.10   Learning Activity

Categorize the following causes of acute renal failure as prerenal, intrinsic, or postrenal.

Condition	Prerenal	Intrinsic	Postrenal
Acute pyelonephritis			
Aminoglycosides			
Benign prostatic hypertrophy			
Contrast dyes			
Diuretics			
Aminoglycosides			
Glomerulonephritis			
Goodpasture syndrome			
Hemorrhage			
Hepatorenal syndrome			
Hypersensitivity reactions			
Intraabdominal tumor			
Malignant hypertension			
Neurogenic bladder			
Prolonged hypotension			
Renal calculi			
Rhabdomyolysis with myoglobinuria			
Septic shock			

Answers to this activity can be found in the Answer Key.

The pathophysiology of AKI (Figure 5-8) varies depending on whether prerenal, intrinsic, or postrenal. The two types of intrinsic AKI, medullary and cortical, also vary from one another. All pathophysiologic sequences result in a decrease in GFR.

The RIFLE classification (Table 5-15) is an evidence-based practice tool used for the diagnosis of AKI. The diagnosis of AKI can be the result of changes in the serum creatinine level, a change in the urinary output, or both. The RIFLE tool assesses the degree of the following criteria: risk of renal dysfunction, injury to the kidney, failure of kidney function, loss of kidney function, and end-stage kidney disease.

Clinical presentation of patients with AKI varies depending on the stage of the illness and other organ systems affected.

Patients may complain of flank pain, dyspnea, pruritus, headache, or decreased libido. Uremic syndrome (i.e., uremia) is a serious complication of AKI that occurs when urea and other waste products build up in the blood because the kidneys are unable to eliminate them. These substances can become toxic to the body if they reach high levels. Prolonged or severe edema may make the uremic syndrome worse.

The patient may have a decrease in urine volume or an inability to concentrate the urine. Nonoliguria is dilute urine output greater than 400 mL/24 hr. Oliguria is urine output less than 400 mL/24 hr. Anuria is urine output less than 100 mL/24 hr. Although rare, complete postrenal obstruction results in anuria. Bladder distention often occurs with postrenal failure. Due to

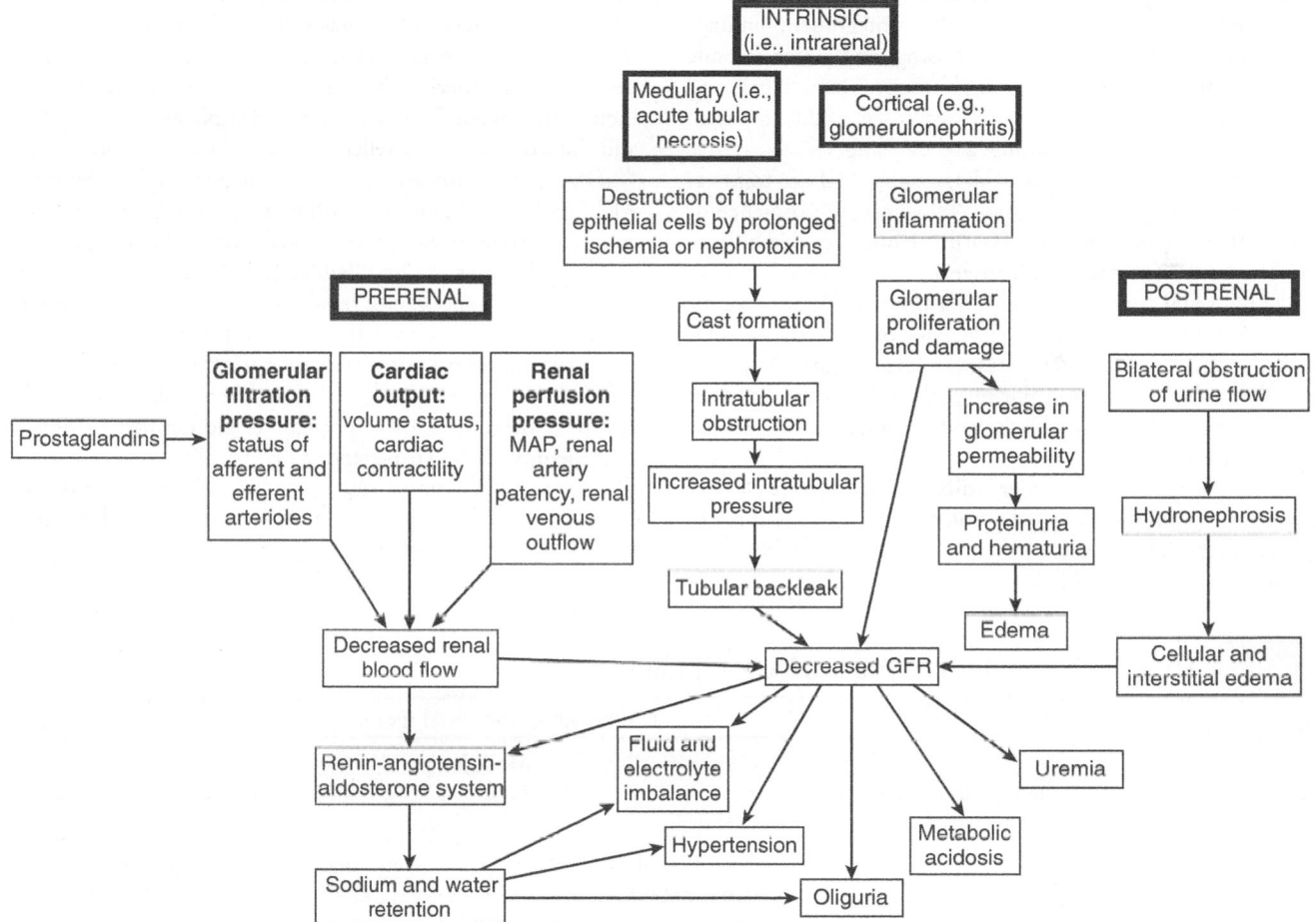

FIGURE 5-8 Pathophysiology of acute kidney injury. (From Dennison, R. D. [2013]. *Pass CCRN!* [4th ed.]. St. Louis, MO: Elsevier.)

| TABLE 5-15 | **RIFLE Classification System** |

Grades of Severity	Serum Creatinine	Glomerular Filtration Rate	Urine Output
Risk	1.5 × normal	Decreased by greater than 25%	Less than 0.5 mL/kg for 6 hours
Injury	2 × normal	Decreased by greater than 50%	Less than 0.5 mL/kg for 12 hours
Failure	3 × normal or greater than mg/dL	Decreased by greater than 75%	Less than 0.5 mL/kg for 24 hours or anuria for 12 hours
Loss	Complete loss of renal function for greater than 4 weeks		
End-stage kidney disease	Complete loss of renal function with need for renal replacement therapy for greater than 3 months		

Adapted from Bellomo, R., Ronco, C., Kellum, J. A., Mehta, R. L., & Pavelsky, P. (2004). Acute renal failure—Definition, outcome measures, animal models, fluid therapy and information technology needs: The Second International Consensus Conference of the Acute Dialysis Quality Initiative (ADQI) Group. *Crit Care, 8*(4), R204-212.

renal damage, altered excretion of drugs may produce toxic drug levels. Neurologic findings may include a change in behavior, confusion, changes in level of consciousness, focal neurologic deficits, tremors, twitching, increased DTRs, asterixis, and seizures. Gastrointestinal findings may include bleeding gums, uremic breath, abdominal distention, malnutrition, GI bleeding, melena, constipation, or diarrhea. The patient may have a paralytic ileus. Abnormal respiratory findings may include deep, rapid breathing (i.e., Kussmaul breathing) associated with metabolic acidosis, bilateral crackles associated with pulmonary edema, or hemoptysis associated with Goodpasture syndrome. Cardiovascular findings may include tachycardia, dysrhythmias, hypertension, and friction rub associated with pericarditis. The presence of a vascular access device requires assessment for thrills, bruits, and neurovascular checks peripheral to the access. Musculoskeletal findings include muscle weakness and impaired mobility. Integument findings include dry skin, pruritus, edema, bruising, and pallor. Uremic frost would only be present in terminal stages. Hematologic and immune findings may include increased susceptibility to infection and sepsis, petechiae, bruising, and bleeding.

The conventional methods of diagnosing AKI are to assess urine output, creatinine, and urea. However, the presence or absence of urine does not necessarily denote renal malfunction. The output is more indicative of renal hemodynamics than actual renal function. The excretion of sodium and urea is not a sensitive indicator in early AKI because the tubular functions may remain intact unless clinical conditions such as sepsis alter tubular function. Urine protein is present in other diseases such as diabetes, shock, and chronic kidney disease (Kosinski, 2009).

AKI can be diagnosed earlier utilizing the following newer biomarkers in addition to the conventional markers listed previously: Cystatin C, Interleukin 18 (IL 18), Neutrophil Gelatinase-Associated Lipocalin (NGAL), and Kidney Injury Molecule (KIM-1). Cystatin C is a marker of the GFR and is independent of age, sex, and muscle mass. Cystatin C is freely filtered at the glomerulus because it has a small molecular mass. Interleukin 18 is an inflammatory cytokine that enters urine in the proximal tubule. NGAL propagates with injured endothelium of the lungs, stomach, colon, and kidneys and rises with acute infections. KIM-1 is a transmembrane protein excreted in the proximal tubule and detected in ischemic kidney disease. Cystatin C is measured in the serum. IL-18 and KIM-1 are measured in the urine. NGAL is measured in both the plasma and urine.

Routine diagnostic blood levels reflect an elevated BUN and creatinine. Electrolyte imbalances include hyperkalemia, hyperphosphatemia, hypocalcemia, and hypermagnesemia. The sodium level is dependent on water balance; therefore, normal or dilutional hyponatremia exists. Hyperuricemia is present. The arterial blood gas state is metabolic acidosis with an increased anion gap. Hematologic studies usually reflect a decreased hematocrit or hemoglobin, but dehydration causes an increase in prerenal failure. A decreased platelet count is likely, and the clotting profile reflects increased bleeding time.

Diagnostic urine test results vary depending on the type of AKI (Table 5-16), but there will be a decreased creatinine clearance consistent with the decreased GFR. Radiologic studies such as a kidneys, ureter, bladder (KUB) (also referred to as a flat plate of the abdomen); renal ultrasonography; or computed tomography may indicate the cause of postrenal failure. Chest x-ray may show the presence of a pericardial effusion, pleural effusion, and/or pulmonary edema. A renal biopsy is the most definitive diagnostic test, especially for glomerulonephritis.

Patients with AKI experience a rapid decline in renal function. The stages include onset, oliguric-anuric, diuretic, and recovery. Some patients do progress from AKI to chronic kidney disease (CKD), but if reversal occurs, the recovery period is approximately 8 days for nonoliguric acute tubercular necrosis (ATN)

TABLE 5-16   **Diagnostic Findings of Types of Acute Kidney Injury**

| | Prerenal: disrupted blood flow to the kidney | Intrinsic: damage to the renal tissue | | Postrenal: disrupted urine flow |
		Cortical	Medullary (acute tubular necrosis [ATN])	
Diagnostics	• Oliguria • Urinary sodium <20 mEq/liter • Increased BUN with BUN:creatinine ratio >10:1 (usually 20:1) • Urine specific gravity >1.020 • Urine osmolality increased except with metabolic acidosis or diuretics • Urine pH <6.0 • No protein in urine or only minimal amount of protein in urine • Sediment in urine: hyaline casts, finely granular casts	• Urine output may be normal (nonoliguria), oliguria, or polyuria • Urine sodium <20 mEq/liter • BUN:creatinine increased with 10:1 ratio • Urine specific gravity varies • Urine pH >6.0 • Moderate to heavy proteinuria • Sediment in urine: RBCs, WBCs, casts	• Urine output may be normal (nonoliguria), oliguria, or polyuria • Urine sodium >20 mEq/liter • Urine specific gravity 1.010 • BUN:creatinine elevated with 10:1 ratio • Urine specific gravity 1.010-1.015 • Urine pH >6.0 • Minimal to moderate proteinuria • Sediment in urine: tubular epithelial cells, tubular casts, rare RBC	• Oliguria with partial obstruction; anuria with complete obstruction • Urine sodium >20 mEq/liter • BUN:creatinine elevated with 10:1 ratio • Urine specific gravity 1.010-1.015 • Urine pH > 6.0 • Sediment in urine: RBCs, WBCs, calculi, uric acid crystals, hyaline casts • KUB, IVP may show obstruction and/or ureteral dilatation • May have positive culture for bacteria

and approximately 2 weeks to 3 months for oliguric ATN. Some patients, especially with nephrotoxic AKI, go through only three phases: onset, nonoliguric, and recovery (Table 5-17).

Prevention, early recognition, and fast, competent treatment are the priority focus for collaborative patient care management of AKI. Acetylcysteine (Mucomyst) and/or fenoldopam (Corlopam) along with adequate hydration prevents dye-related acute tubular necrosis. In cases of rhabdomyolysis with myoglobinuria, fluids, diuretics (usually mannitol), and sodium bicarbonate are usually prescribed. When patients are receiving nephrotoxic agents (e.g., aminoglycosides, amphotericin B, and vancomycin), it is crucially important to maintain adequate hydration and monitor drug levels and serum creatinine. Prevent and treat abdominal hypertension and abdominal compartment syndrome in patients with abdominal surgery or trauma.

The focus of treatment for AKI is to support renal perfusion and improve GFR through appropriate interventions. Administer volume to improve preload in patients with hypovolemia. Inotropic agents improve contractility in patients with decreased contractility, and vasopressors increase afterload in patients with massive vasodilation. There is no benefit to low-dose dopamine in patients with acute oliguric renal failure and this can predispose the patient to bowel ischemia through splanchnic vasoconstriction; therefore, it is no longer recommended for the management of acute oliguric renal failure. Administer fenoldopam (Corlopam), a dopaminergic stimulator, as prescribed to increase renal blood flow. It is controversial, but if the patient is not anuric, a diuretic trial may be prescribed. Agents used for diuresis are typically loop diuretics (e.g., furosemide [Lasix] and bumetanide [Bumex]). Rhabdomyolysis treatment often includes osmotic diuretics (e.g., mannitol [Osmitrol]), but these are contraindicated in heart failure and pulmonary edema. For an immune-mediated cause of AKI (e.g., Goodpasture syndrome), administer immunosuppressants and initiate plasmapheresis to remove antibodies.

A major focus of AKI treatment is to maintain fluid, electrolyte, and acid-base balance. Monitor clinical indications of fluid overload. Patients are encouraged to maintain sodium and fluid restrictions for 24 hours. The 24-hour fluid restriction is usually determined by adding 500 mL (for insensible loss) to the previous day's urine output. Space fluid allowances over the entire 24-hour period. Treat the patient's thirst with ice chips (must be included as intake), wet washcloths, and misting the mouth and provide frequent oral care.

Electrolyte imbalances, especially sodium, potassium, calcium, phosphorus, and magnesium, are common. Monitor the patient closely for clinical indications of imbalances and serum levels. Sodium restriction is usually 1 to 2 g/day. Potassium restriction is usually 40 mEq/day. Avoid salt substitute (KCl) and do not permit it on dietary trays. Elevated potassium levels may be life-threatening in AKI. Initiate emergency treatment for life-threatening dysrhythmias (see Table 5-11). Treatment of hyperphosphatemia includes dietary restrictions and phosphate-binding agents (e.g., Basaljel and Amphojel). Because these aluminum-containing phosphate-binding agents may contribute to dialysis encephalopathy due to accumulation of aluminum, administer calcium carbonate (Caltrate) or calcium acetate (PhosLo) instead.

As phosphorus goes up, calcium goes down. Treat hypocalcemia with calcium administration and increasing serum calcium will decrease serum phosphorus. Maintain dietary magnesium restrictions and do not administer magnesium-containing medications (e.g., Maalox, magnesium sulfate, and magnesium citrate).

Monitor arterial blood gases for acid-base imbalance. Initiate dialysis to eliminate the nitrogenous waste causing the metabolic acidosis. Administer sodium bicarbonate or Carbicarb only for severe metabolic acidosis (pH less than 7.1).

A very important goal in the treatment of AKI is to diminish the accumulation of nitrogenous wastes. Protein intake is restricted to 0.6 g/kg/day initially but may be as high as 1 to 1.5 g/kg/day if on hemodialysis or continuous renal replacement therapy (CRRT) and 1.5 to 2 g/kg/day if on peritoneal dialysis. Provide protein of high biologic value that contains all the essential amino acids. Also, it is important to provide adequate

TABLE 5-17   Stages of Acute Kidney Injury

	Onset	Oliguric-Anuric	Diuretic	Recovery
Definition	Period of time from the precipitating event to the beginning of oliguria or anuria	Period of time when urine output is <400 mL/24 hr	Period of time between urine output of >400 mL/24 hr until when laboratory values stabilize	Period of time between when the laboratory values stabilize until they are normal
Duration	Hours to days	1-2 weeks	1-2 weeks	3-12 months
BUN/creatinine	Normal or slight increase	Increased	Begins to decrease	Almost normal
Urine output	Decreased; about 20% of normal	<400 mL/24 hr; about 5% of normal	May exceed 3 L/24 hr; about 150%-200% of normal	Back to 100% of normal
Mortality	5%	50%-60%	25%	10%-15%
Other characteristics		• Metabolic acidosis • Water gain with delusional hyponatremia • Hyperkalemia • Hypocalcemia • Hyperphosphatemia • Hypermagnesemia • Azotemia	• Metabolic acidosis • Sodium may be normal or decreased • Hyperkalemia continues	• Uremia, acid-base imbalances, and electrolyte imbalances gradually resolve

caloric intake to prevent catabolism and utilization of dietary protein for energy needs. Indications for dialysis in the patient with AKI generally include the following:

- Volume overload (especially with pulmonary edema)
- Uncontrollable hyperkalemia
- Uncontrollable hyperphosphatemia
- Uncontrollable acidosis
- Symptomatic uremia (e.g., neurologic changes)
- Pericarditis
- Seizures or coma
- BUN 80 to 100 mg/dL or greater but may be initiated at BUN greater than 50 to 60 mg/dL
- Serum creatinine 10 mg/dL or greater

Since dialysis is contraindicated in hemodynamic instability, an alternative treatment is CRRT. Other contraindications to dialysis include the inability to tolerate anticoagulation and lack of vascular access.

Hemodialysis requires a vascular access. Maintenance of the patency and prevention of infection of the vascular access are very important. Palpate the fistula or AV graft for a thrill and auscultate for a bruit. Also, palpate pulses and check capillary refill distal to the access. Do not allow venipuncture, IV cannulation, injections, or blood pressure measurements in a limb with the access. Monitor for constrictive clothing or dressing in the limb with the access. Also, monitor for bleeding and use a pressure dressing to stop bleeding if it occurs. Note any redness, induration, or purulent drainage around the access and culture any purulent drainage. Change the dressing as for a central venous catheter. Instruct the patient not to disturb scabs at the puncture sites from hemodialysis.

Peritoneal dialysis is another type of treatment. With peritoneal dialysis, a trocar is inserted into the abdomen and the peritoneum is the semipermeable membrane utilized. Maintenance of patency and prevention of infection of the peritoneal access are the top priorities. Note any redness, induration, or purulent drainage around the access and culture any purulent drainage. Provide aseptic catheter care by washing with antibacterial soap. Dress with light gauze dressing and use aseptic technique with catheter manipulation. There is a need to periodically culture the peritoneal dialysate outflow fluid as indicated.

It is important to prevent further damage to the kidney by nephrotoxic agents. Decrease the dosages of drugs eliminated by the kidney and increase the interval between doses in patients with renal impairment. Monitor the peak and trough serum drug levels when appropriate (e.g., aminoglycosides) and monitor urine creatinine clearance when the patient is receiving nephrotoxic agents. Prevent contrast-dye-related nephrotoxicity by increasing oral and/or parenteral fluids. Administer acetylcysteine (Mucomyst) as prescribed; this drug acts as an oxygen free radical scavenger. The usual dose is 600 mg orally every 12 hours the day before and the day of a radiologic procedure that requires contrast. Administer fenoldopam (Corlopam) as prescribed; this drug acts as a dopaminergic stimulator to improve renal blood flow. The usual dose is an intravenous infusion of 0.05 to 0.1 mcg/kg/min for 60 to 90 minutes before the injection of the contrast material and for hours after the injection if no adverse reactions occur. Monitor for changes in urine color, which can indicate the presence of heavy pigments that may cause acute tubular necrosis. Myoglobinuria has a tea or cola color; hemoglobinuria appears wine colored.

It is important to provide the patient adequate nutrition while maintaining dietary restrictions. Provide high biological protein within protein restriction parameters ordered. Provide

enough calories to prevent catabolism of somatic protein stores. To prevent electrolyte imbalances, increase dietary calcium and decrease dietary sodium, potassium, and phosphorus.

During the diuretic phase, the focus of care is to prevent fluid volume deficit. Monitor for clinical indications of fluid volume deficit. Replace volume hourly during this phase by replacing the last hour's urine output during the following hour plus the insensible loss.

When BUN levels are greater than 70 to 100 mg/dL, place increased emphasis on preventing infections and injuries. Impaired safety is due to neurologic changes and high BUN levels are associated with increased risk of infection and injury. To prevent infection, initiate dialysis when the BUN level is greater than 80 to 100 mg/dL because BUN values above this level are associated with an increased risk of infection.

Impaired renal function causes anemia and platelet dysfunction. Monitor hemoglobin, hematocrit, platelets, and RBCs. Treat anemia with folic acid, iron, and vitamin B_{12}. Recombinant erythropoietin (Epogen) will improve anemia by stimulating RBC production, but it takes at least 3 months; therefore, it is not effective for AKI. Recombinant erythropoietin is also dialyzed out so it is ineffective for CRRT patients. Administer packed RBC transfusion as prescribed if the patient is symptomatic of anemia (e.g., dyspnea, chest pain, syncope, and hypotension). Monitor patients for clinical indications of platelet dysfunction (e.g., petechiae, ecchymosis, and bleeding). Administer desmopressin (DDAVP) as prescribed for platelet dysfunction.

Skin care can be a challenge. Administer antipruritics and utilize emollient or cornstarch baths to provide comfort.

Monitor for further progression to chronic kidney disease and complications in other body systems. The complications of AKI include the following:

- Renal: chronic kidney disease will develop in 25% to 30% of AKI patients.
- Cardiovascular: dysrhythmias, hypertension, pericarditis, cardiac tamponade, and pulmonary edema
- Neurologic: coma and seizures
- Metabolic: Electrolyte imbalances (e.g., hyperkalemia, hyperphosphatemia, hypermagnesemia, hypocalcemia) and acid-base imbalance (i.e., metabolic acidosis)
- Gastrointestinal: Peptic ulcer disease and GI hemorrhage
- Hematologic: Anemia and uremic coagulopathies
- Infection: Increased susceptibility to pneumonias, septicemias, urinary tract infections, and wound infections
- Miscellaneous: Drug toxicity

Chronic Kidney Disease and End-Stage Renal Disease

Chronic kidney disease (CKD) is defined as a progressive and irreversible destruction of kidney structures. CKD progresses through specific stages (Table 5-18). The loss of function usually takes months or years to occur. In the early stages, there may be no clinical indications of renal impairment. Symptoms do not appear until kidney function is less than one-tenth of normal. End-stage renal disease (ESRD) is the final stage of CKD. At this stage, the kidneys are no longer able to remove wastes and excess fluids from the body. The patient needs dialysis or a kidney transplant. CKD and ESRD affect more than 2 out of every 1000 people in the United States.

There are many causes of CKD. The major causes are diabetes mellitus, hypertension, glomerulonephritis, polycystic

| TABLE 5-18 | Stages of Chronic Kidney Disease |

Stage	Severity	GFR (mL/min)	Progression	Symptoms	Intervention
1	Kidney damage but normal or increased GFR	Greater than 90	None apparent	Usually none but may be hypertensive	Screening for risk factors
2	Mild: decreased GFR	60-89	• Increasing PTH • Early bone disease • Increasing BUN and creatinine	Subtle • Hypertension	Screening/ reduction of risk factors
3	Moderate: decreased GFR	30-59	• Anemia • Increasing BUN and creatinine	Mild • Anemia • Hypertension	Treatment and prevention of progression
4	Severe: decreased GFR	15-29	• Increased triglycerides • Metabolic acidosis • Electrolyte imbalance • Increasing BUN and creatinine	Moderate • Anemia • Hypertension • Hyperphosphatemia • Hyperkalemia • Edema	Treatment of complications and preparation for renal replacement therapy
5	End-stage kidney disease	Less than 15	Uremia requiring dialysis for survival	Severe • Anemia • Hypertension • Hyperphosphatemia • Hyperkalemia • Edema	Renal replacement therapy; possible renal transplant

| TABLE 5-19 | Etiology of Chronic Kidney Disease |

Condition	Etiology
Diabetes	Leading cause of kidney failure in the United States, approximately 35%-40% lose their kidney function. Good control may slow the progression, but research suggests that even diabetics with good lifelong control can develop kidney failure.
Hypertension	Second most common cause of kidney disease. Hypertension (HTN) may cause no symptoms until it is very advanced. Many people are not treated for HTN until damage to kidneys, heart, blood vessels, and/or eyes has already occurred.
Glomerulonephritis	Diseases of glomeruli may be slow and progressive or have a rapid onset. Some glomerulopathies may be caused by autoimmune responses (e.g., streptococcal infections, systemic lupus erythematosus [SLE]).
Polycystic kidney disease	Inherited disease that causes large fluid-filled cysts to develop and progressively destroys function, usually by the time the individual reaches middle age.
Drug toxicity	Damaging drugs: anesthetics, antimicrobials, antiinflammatory drugs, chemotherapy, diuretics, and organ transplant antirejection agents. Radiocontrast dye. Biological substances: heme pigments, hemoglobin, and myoglobin. Environmental agents: pesticides and fungicides. Heavy metals: lead, gold, and mercury. Plant and animal substances: mushrooms and snake venom.
Interstitial nephritis	Damage done to the supporting structure of a kidney, such as an allergic reaction to an antibiotic or AKI.
Obstruction	Malformed structures of the lower urinary tract caused from congenital anomalies or scarring from infections can cause backup, hydronephrosis, and injury. Renal failure caused by obstructive processes may heal if the cause of obstruction is removed.

kidney disease, drug toxicity, interstitial nephritis, obstruction, and the progression of irreversible AKI (Table 5-19).

A normal kidney contains approximately 1 million nephrons, each of which contributes to the total GFR. In the face of renal injury, the kidney has an innate ability to maintain GFR, despite progressive destruction of nephrons, as the remaining healthy nephrons manifest hyperfiltration and compensatory hypertrophy. The hyperfiltration and hypertrophy of residual nephrons, although beneficial for the reasons noted, represent a major cause of progressive renal dysfunction. The increased glomerular capillary pressure may damage the capillaries, leading initially to secondary focal and segmental glomerulosclerosis (FSGS) and eventually to global glomerulosclerosis (Figure 5-9).

The patient care collaborative management for CKD is the same as for AKI. The priorities of care are maintaining ventilation, oxygenation, and circulation. Also significant are the

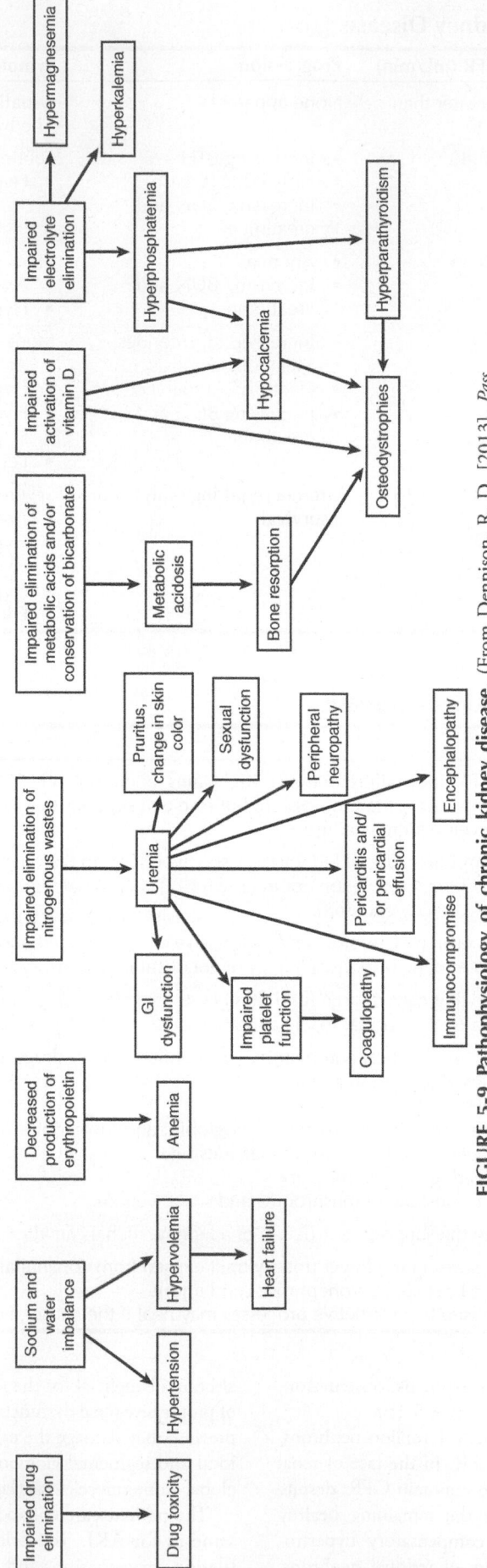

FIGURE 5-9 Pathophysiology of chronic kidney disease. (From Dennison, R. D. [2013]. *Pass CCRN!* [4th ed.]. St. Louis, MO: Elsevier.)

monitoring and treatment of the patient for clinical indications of pericarditis; heart failure; hypertension; and life-threatening fluid, electrolyte, and/or acid-base imbalances. In CKD, treatment with renal replacement therapy and/or a transplant is required to sustain life. With the addition of renal replacement therapy, the collaborative health care team has a responsibility to maintain safety and to provide patient and family education.

To maintain safety, adjust drug dosages and monitor the patient for delirium due to uremic encephalopathy. Provide mobility assistance to prevent fractures due to osteopathy. Avoid invasive procedures and monitor for bleeding due to the hematologic and coagulation problems associated with CKD. Patient and family education helps reduce anxiety and promotes participation in care and decision making. Provide patient and family education about dietary restrictions and how to prevent complications.

RENAL REPLACEMENT THERAPY

Renal replacement therapies include hemodialysis, continuous ambulatory peritoneal dialysis (CAPD), acute peritoneal dialysis, and renal transplant. Continuous renal replacement therapy (CRRT) is a form of dialysis usually reserved for patients with AKI and performed in the critical care unit. The concept behind CRRT is to provide dialysis to patients in a more physiologic way, slowly over 24 hours, just like the kidney. Acutely ill patients tolerate CRRT since the procedure does not have fluid swings that occur with intermittent hemodialysis.

Progressive care nurses need to be knowledgeable regarding the basic care of patients receiving hemodialysis. Specially trained hemodialysis nurses perform the hemodialysis procedure; however, the preprocedure and postprocedure care are the responsibility of the staff nurse. A progressive care nurse is responsible to be knowledgeable and skilled at doing acute peritoneal dialysis. In addition, a patient who does CAPD at home admitted for other conditions requires CAPD maintenance. The purposes of dialysis are to eliminate excess body fluids, maintain or restore electrolyte balance, maintain or restore acid-base balance, and eliminate nitrogenous wastes and toxins from the blood. Dialysis separates solutes by differential diffusion through a semipermeable membrane that is placed between the two solutions (Figure 5-10). The dialysis procedure is indicated for acute or chronic renal failure, symptomatic uremia, uremic pericarditis, severe water intoxication, severe electrolyte imbalance, drug intoxication (drug must be dialyzable [e.g., alcohol, salicylates, lithium, barbiturates, and some poisons]), and hepatic encephalopathy/coma.

The components of the dialysis procedure include a dialysate concentration, semipermeable membrane, and the patient's blood. The dialysate concentrate is a solution of water, electrolytes (sodium, chloride, magnesium, and bicarbonate), nonelectrolytes (glucose), and a buffer (acetate, lactate, or bicarbonate). Adjust the electrolyte concentration in the dialysate to the patient's needs. The semipermeable membrane is the peritoneum in peritoneal dialysis and an extracorporeal membrane in hemodialysis. The patient's blood must be in contact with the membrane.

The dialysis procedure employs the principles of osmosis, diffusion, filtration, and convection (Figure 5-11). A hypertonic dialysate solution moves water across the semipermeable membrane in osmosis. In diffusion, the dialysate solution contains a concentration of selected solutes lower than the blood

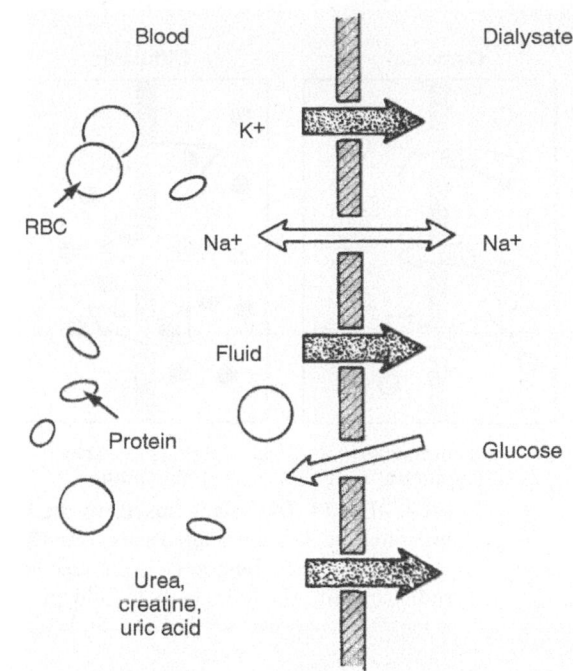

FIGURE 5-10 Osmosis and diffusion in dialysis. Net movement of major particles and fluid is illustrated. (From Long, B. C., Phipps, W. J., & Cassmeyer, V. L. [1993]. *Medical-surgical nursing: A nursing process approach* [3rd ed.]. St. Louis, MO: Mosby.)

concentration so that these solutes will move across the semipermeable membrane and into the dialysate solution. In some forms of dialysis, there is a pressure difference between the sides of the semipermeable membrane with the highest pressure on the forward side of the membrane to act as a hydrostatic force pushing against the membrane to provide a filtration effect. CRRT uses the principle of convection, which is the transfer of solutes and solutions simultaneously moving across the semipermeable membrane. Renal replacement therapy is effective, but there are some variables that will affect efficiency, such as:

- Size and number of the pores in the semipermeable membrane
- Surface area of the semipermeable membrane
- Thickness of the semipermeable membrane
- Size of the solute molecules
- Concentration of solutes in the blood
- Osmotic concentration
- Pressure gradients
- Temperature of the solution
- Rate of blood flow

The different types of renal replacement have advantages and disadvantages. The types need to be examined and discussed with the patient and family to help them make the right choice. Progressive care nurses perform peritoneal dialysis on the unit; therefore, the nurses are required to have the knowledge and skill necessary to safely manage care during peritoneal dialysis. Specially trained nurses perform hemodialysis, which may be performed in the progressive care unit. Patients requiring CRRT are generally transferred to a critical care unit The progressive care nurse may care for a patient pending the initiation of treatment or hospitalized for other conditions and should be knowledgeable about all the types of renal replacement therapies. Intermittent hemodialysis is the therapy of choice for hemodynamically stable patients in a hospital setting. Peritoneal dialysis is suited for hemodynamically stable patients with an intact peritoneum but has low efficiency. CRRT is

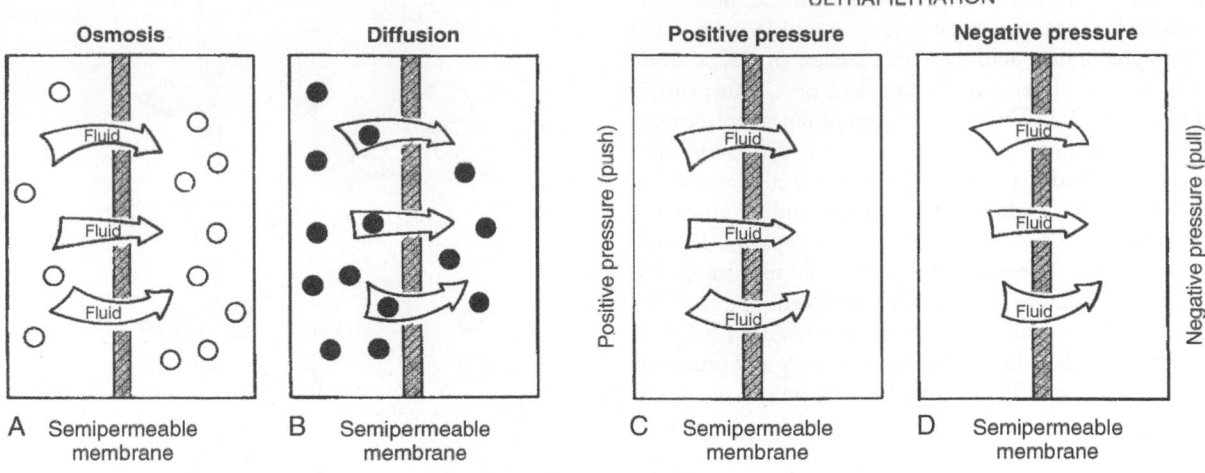

FIGURE 5-11 **Dialysis is based on the following principles. (A)** Osmosis and **(B)** diffusion and ultrafiltration. Ultrafiltration occurs when either positive pressure **(C)** or negative pressure **(D)** is placed on the system. Ultrafiltration is maximized by exerting both positive and negative pressure on the system simultaneously. (From Long, B. C., Phipps, W. J., & Cassmeyer, V. L. [1993]. *Medical-surgical nursing: A nursing process approach* [3rd ed.]. St. Louis, MO: Mosby.)

suitable for critically ill or hemodynamically unstable patients and has a higher efficiency than peritoneal dialysis (Table 5-20).

Peritoneal Dialysis

Peritoneal dialysis requires an insertion of a peritoneal catheter (Figure 5-12, A). Explain the procedure to the patient and ask the patient to void or insert a urinary catheter before abdominal puncture. Weigh the patient before treatment and daily after draining dialysate. The dialysate is infused through a gravity system dwelled inside the peritoneum and then drained by gravity (Figure 5-12, B).

There are two methods of peritoneal dialysis. With continuous ambulatory peritoneal dialysis (CAPD), dialysis solution is instilled into the peritoneal cavity, allowed to dwell for a designated period, and then allowed to flow out of the peritoneal cavity by gravity. There are usually 3 to 4 exchanges per day, with a longer exchange during sleep time. Continuous cycling peritoneal dialysis (CCPD) is instituted using an automated cycler that performs 3 to 5 exchanges during sleep time. CCPD allows more flexibility during waking hours but does require attachment to the automated cycler for 10 to 12 hours during sleep time.

Before the peritoneal dialysis procedure, it is necessary to warm dialysate to body temperature. Ensure that prescribed medications, such as heparin, potassium chloride, antibiotics, and/or lidocaine, are added to the dialysate. During the inflow phase, infuse 1 to 3 L of dialysate concentrate volume at a rate of 2 L in 10 to 20 minutes. On the first exchange, do not allow dialysate to dwell as you would the subsequent runs. Drain this run immediately to ensure catheter patency and placement. On subsequent runs, allow the volume to dwell in the intraperitoneal space for 20 to 30 minutes. After the dwell time, the outflow phase begins by draining the peritoneum of dwell fluid. Measure dialysate outflow and assess the appearance of the dialysate. Normal outflow appearance should be clear, pale yellow, or straw colored. If the outflow is cloudy, suspect infection and obtain a culture and sensitivity (C&S). With bloody outflow, suspect intraabdominal bleeding or coagulopathy. Some blood during the first four exchanges is due to insertion of trocar, but

after that all bleeding is abnormal. Outflow drainage that is amber colored is suspicious of bladder perforation; brownish outflow may indicate bowel perforation.

Promote adequate outflow drainage. If the outflow amount is less than the amount instilled, turn the patient side to side and apply gentle pressure to the abdomen. Do not continue the fluid runs unless fluid is being eliminated ±100 mL of inflow volume. Keep meticulous cumulative I&O records. For example, if the amount drained is 300 mL less than the amount instilled (+300 mL) during one exchange but the next exchange yields a drain volume of 400 mL more than the amount instilled (–400 mL), the cumulative volume is –100 mL.

Monitor for hypotension and respiratory distress, especially during the inflow phase. Monitor vital signs during the outflow phase. Monitor serum glucose levels in all patients because hyperglycemia occurs in diabetic patients or with a 4.25% dialysate concentration. It is also important to provide peritoneal catheter site care and closely observe for signs and symptoms of infection such as erythema, warmth, swelling, and drainage.

Hemodialysis

Specially trained nurses perform the hemodialysis procedure. Weigh the patient having hemodialysis before the procedure. The weight is done before the dialysis nurse's arrival and is usually the responsibility of the nursing staff on the unit. The nursing staff must also hold medications that may cause hypotension before hemodialysis such as antihypertensives, antiemetics, narcotics, beta-blockers, or calcium channel blockers. In addition, hold any medications that are dialyzed out during the procedure till after the completion of hemodialysis.

The hemodialysis nurse starts the procedure by cannulation of the vascular access and connecting the tubing to the dialyzer (Figure 5-13). Monitor blood chemistries throughout the treatment and maintain anticoagulation. Check and record vital signs frequently for evaluation of hemodynamic stability and tolerance. Monitor hematocrit for changes that may indicate rapid fluid removal. Observe the vascular access and the hemofilter for indications of clotting.

TABLE 5-20	**Types of Dialysis**	
	Hemodialysis	**Intermittent Peritoneal Dialysis**
Principles	• Osmosis • Diffusion • Filtration	• Osmosis • Diffusion • Filtration
Treatment requirements	• Vascular access • Membrane: extracorporeal membrane or high coefficient membrane • Blood pump • Dialyzer • Dialysate • Anticoagulation	• Membrane: peritoneum • Dialysate: 1.5%, 2.5%, 4.25% • Access: peritoneal catheter
Specific indications	• Need for rapid treatment • Hemodynamically stable patient • Fluid overload unresponsive to diuretics • Electrolyte imbalance • Acute or chronic renal failure • Drug overdose or poison intoxication with dialyzable agent • Pulmonary edema refractory to diuretics	• Fluid overload • Electrolyte imbalance • Acute or chronic renal failure • Drug overdose or poison intoxication with dialyzable agent • Intact peritoneum • Inability to anticoagulate • Hemodynamic instability
Contraindications	• Hemodynamic instability • Hypovolemia • Inadequate vascular access • Coagulopathy	• Rapid treatment required • Acute peritonitis • Recent abdominal surgery • Known abdominal adhesions • Abdominal trauma • Intraperitoneal hematoma • Recent vascular anastomosis of abdominal vessels • Respiratory distress • Sepsis • Extreme obesity • Coagulopathy
Advantages	• Rapid and efficient; only 3-4 hours per session (usually 3 times weekly) unless overdose treatment, which may require 8-16 hours • Very efficient for small molecules; corrects biochemical disturbances quickly for time on therapy	• Equipment is easily and readily assembled • Fairly simple, requiring less staff and patient education • Relatively inexpensive • Minimal danger of acute electrolyte imbalance or hemorrhage • Dialysate can be individualized easily • Anticoagulation not required
Disadvantages	• Complex procedure requiring extensive staff training • Expensive equipment • Machine availability may be limited • Requires anticoagulation • Vascular access necessary	• Relatively slow to alter biochemical imbalances, usually requiring 36 hours for therapeutic effect • May cause protein loss • May be difficult to gain and maintain peritoneal access

Complications	• Access complications: bleeding, clotting, infection
	• Acute fluid and electrolyte imbalances
	• Hemorrhage
	• Hypovolemia
	• Air embolus
	• Disequilibrium syndrome caused by too rapid removal of waste products
	• Allergic reaction to membrane
	• Hepatitis
	• Dialysis encephalopathy (related to accumulation of aluminum from water used to prepare dialysate)
	• Infection
	• Dysrhythmias
		• Access complications: infection, dialysate leak, bleeding, and peritonitis
		• Too rapid fluid removal causing the following:
		  • Hypovolemia
		  • Hypernatremia
		• Hypervolemia caused by dialysate retention
		• Hypokalemia caused by potassium-free dialysate usage
		• Alkalosis caused by alkaline dialysate usage
		• Disequilibrium syndrome caused by too rapid removal of waste products
		• Hyperglycemia caused by high glucose concentration of dialysate
		• Protein loss
		• Respiratory distress

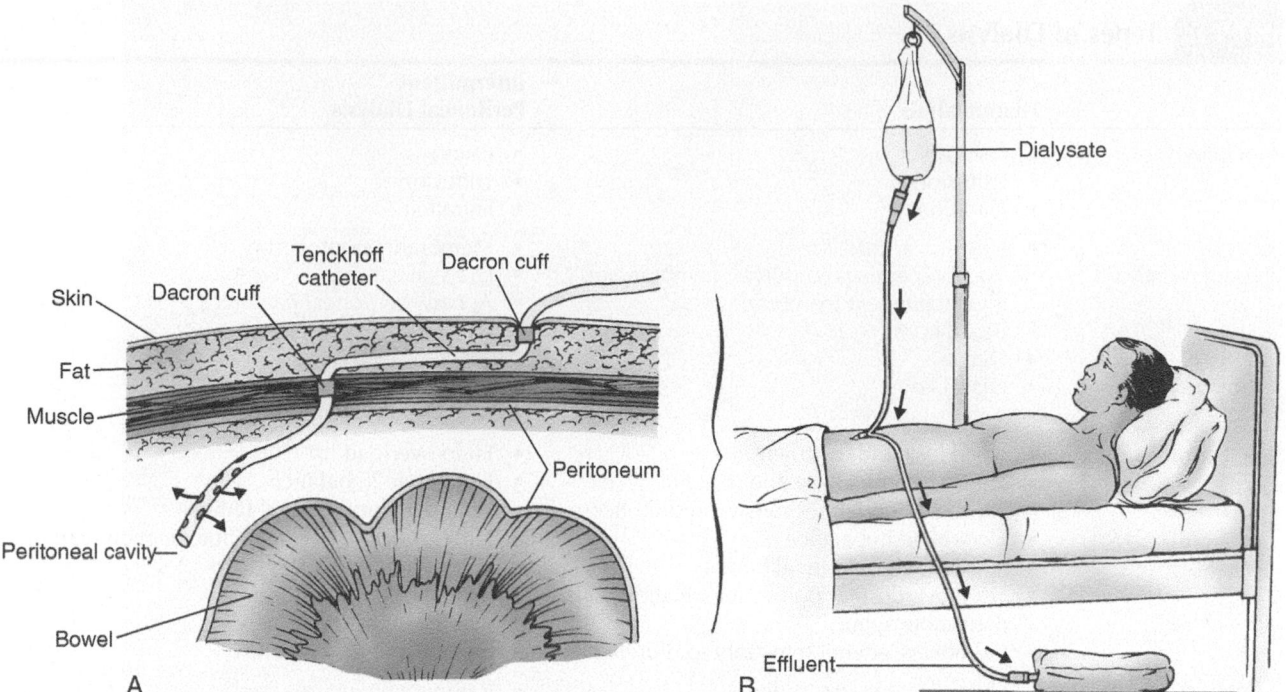

FIGURE 5-12 Manual peritoneal dialysis via an implanted Tenckhoff catheter. A, Catheter position in peritoneal cavity. **B,** Manual peritoneal dialysis process. (From Ignatavicius, D. D., & Workman, M. L. [2006]. *Medical-surgical nursing: Critical thinking for collaborative care* [5th ed.]. Philadelphia, PA: Saunders.)

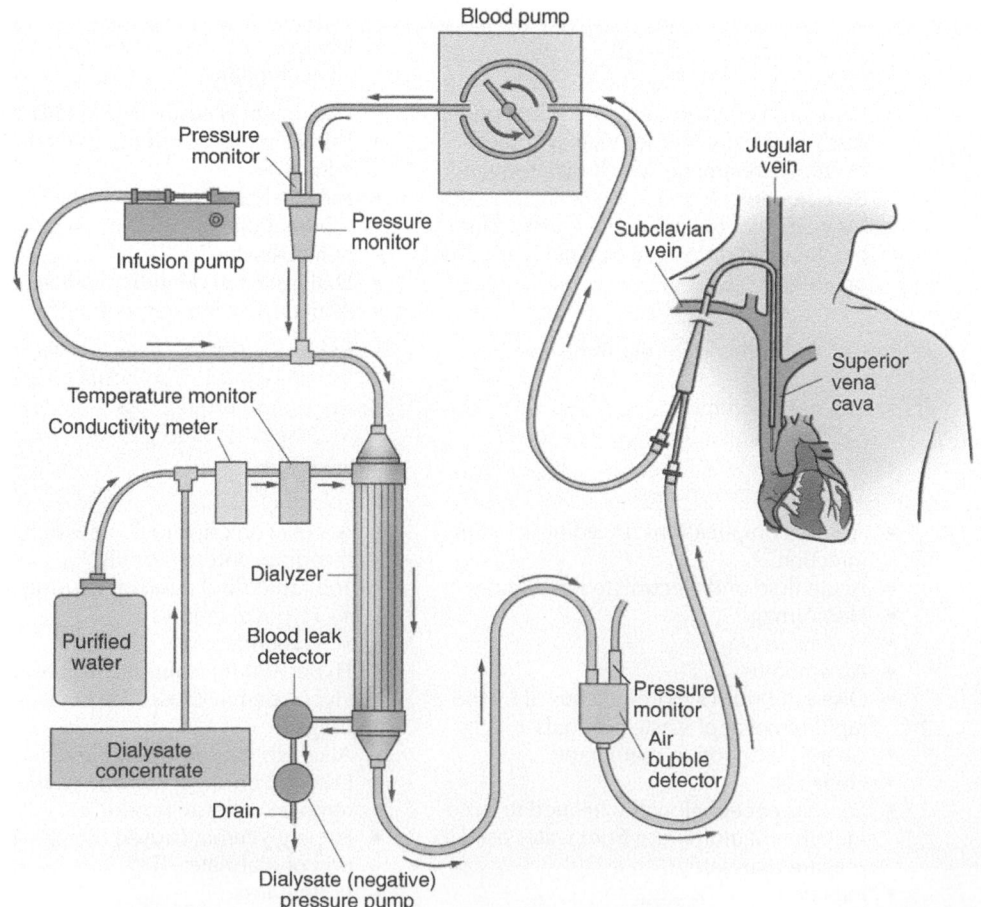

FIGURE 5-13 Components of a hemodialysis system. (From Urden, L. D., Stacy, K. M., & Lough, M. E. [2010]. *Critical care nursing: Diagnosis and management* [6th ed.]. St. Louis, MO: Mosby.)

TABLE 5-21 Vascular Access for Dialysis

Access	Advantages	Disadvantages	Management
Double-lumen vascular catheter inserted into subclavian, jugular, or femoral vein; may be tunneled (see Figure 5-14)	• Easy insertion • Immediate use • High flow rates are achieved • No venipuncture required for access	• Externally located • Can be easily dislodged • Prone to infection and thrombosis • Femoral catheters are associated with a higher incidence of infection	• Monitor site daily and provide site care • Restrict use of this catheter to dialysis only • Administer heparin into catheter if prescribed • A fibrinolytic may be used to reestablish patency of an occluded catheter
Fistula (see Figure 5-15, A)	• Located internally • Greater longevity • Lower clotting and infection rates than external devices • No danger of disconnect	• Requires 4-6 weeks to mature before use • Requires venipuncture for access • May result in ischemia to affected limb (referred to as "vascular steal syndrome") • May thrombose	• Do not use limb for BP or venipuncture • Listen for bruit, feel for thrill: indicate patency • Assess neurovascular status of affected limb frequently • Teach patient exercises to increase blood flow in fistula (e.g., squeezing a ball) • Warn patient not to wear constrictive clothing
AV graft (see Figure 5-15, B)	• Same as for fistula • May be used for patients with vessels inadequate for fistula formation • Can be used earlier than traditional fistula	• Same as for fistula • Infection is more serious than with traditional fistula due to risk of disintegration and hemorrhage • May cause aneurysm formation	• Same as for fistula • Rotating puncture sites and applying pressure on needle removal aids in prevention of aneurysm and pseudoaneurysm

Procedure-specific complications that occur with hemodialysis are disequilibrium syndrome and cramping. Toxins cause these complications. Hemodialysis rapidly removes urea from the blood, but it does not happen in the cerebrospinal fluid (CSF) as quickly. The higher concentration of toxins in the CSF shifts fluid into the brain cells, which results in cerebral edema. Clinical indications may include nausea, vomiting, headache, hallucinations, and seizures. To prevent or manage the syndrome, the hemodialysis nurse may use a smaller dialyzer, reduce the blood pump speed, shorten the time and increase the frequency, and treat any seizures with diazepam and Dilantin. The patient may suffer from muscle cramps caused by rapid water removal and sodium shifts. Administer quinine before the procedure to prevent and reduce the occurrence of cramps. In addition, administer hypertonic saline during the procedure to reduce cramps.

Vascular Access for Hemodialysis
The dialysis procedure removes and returns continuous high-volume blood via the vascular access site. A vascular access should be prepared weeks or months before starting dialysis. The early preparation of the vascular access will allow easier and more efficient removal and replacement of blood with fewer complications. The three basic kinds of vascular access for hemodialysis are an arteriovenous (AV) fistula, an AV graft, and a double-lumen central venous catheter (Table 5-21). The AV fistula is a connection between an artery and a vein. The AV fistula is useful because it causes the vein to grow larger and stronger for easy access to the blood system. The best long-term vascular access for hemodialysis because it provides adequate blood flow, lasts a long time, and has a lower complication rate than other types of access is the AV fistula. If the creation of an AV fistula is not possible, an AV graft or venous catheter is used (Figures 5-14 and 5-15).

Renal Transplant
Renal transplantation has become the treatment of choice for most patients with ESRD. At present, more than 82,000 patients are waiting for kidney transplants in the United States. Immunosuppression therapy has improved the results of transplantation. Acute rejection and complications associated with steroid therapy remain, but the improvements in early graft survival and long-term graft function have made kidney transplantation a more cost-effective alternative to dialysis.

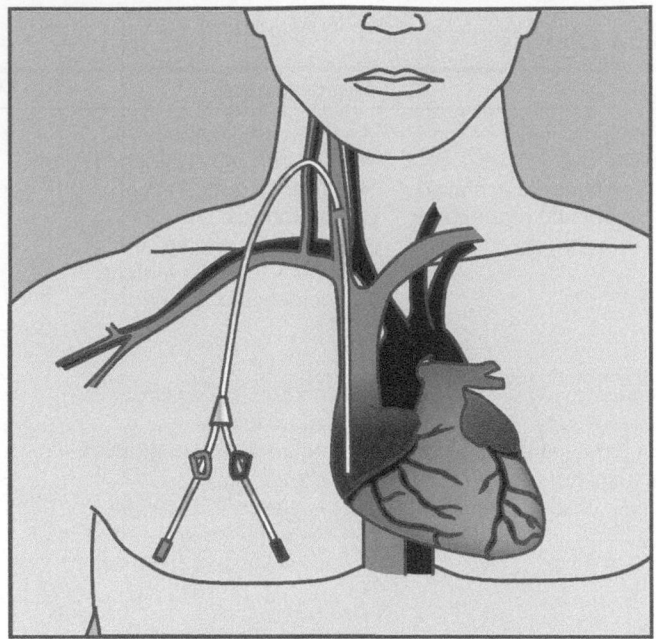

FIGURE 5-14 Double-lumen vascular catheter used as access for dialysis. (From Phillips, N. [2013]. *Berry & Kohn's operating room technique* [12th ed.]. St. Louis, MO: Elsevier.)

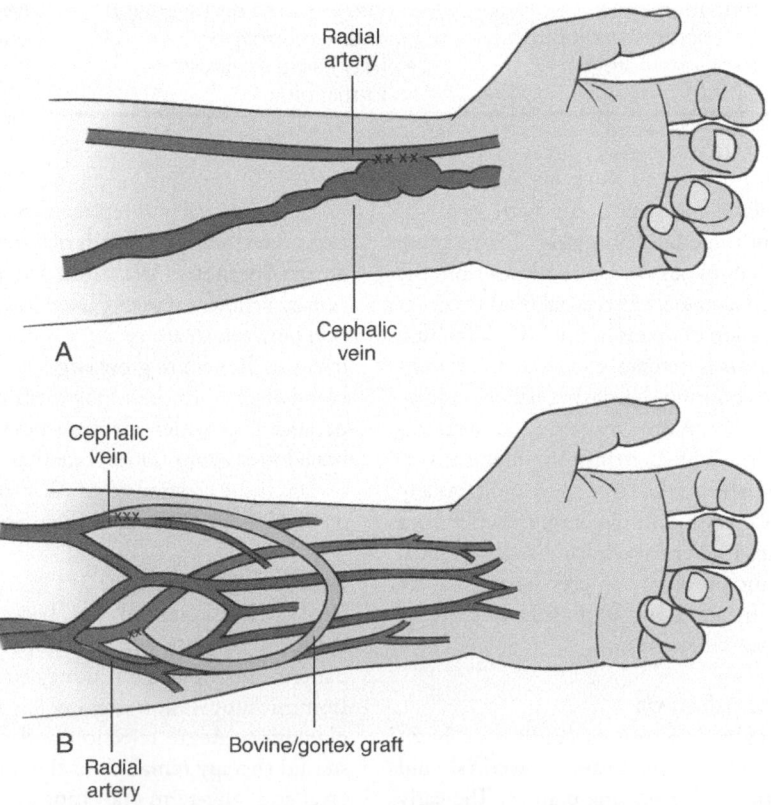

FIGURE 5-15 Permanent vascular accesses. A, AV fistula. **B,** AV graft. (From Urden, L. D., Stacy, K. M., & Lough, M. E. [2010]. *Critical care nursing: Diagnosis and management* [6th ed.]. St. Louis, MO: Mosby.)

5.11   Synthesis Learning Activity: Crossword Puzzle

Complete the following crossword puzzle related to anatomy and physiology of the renal system.

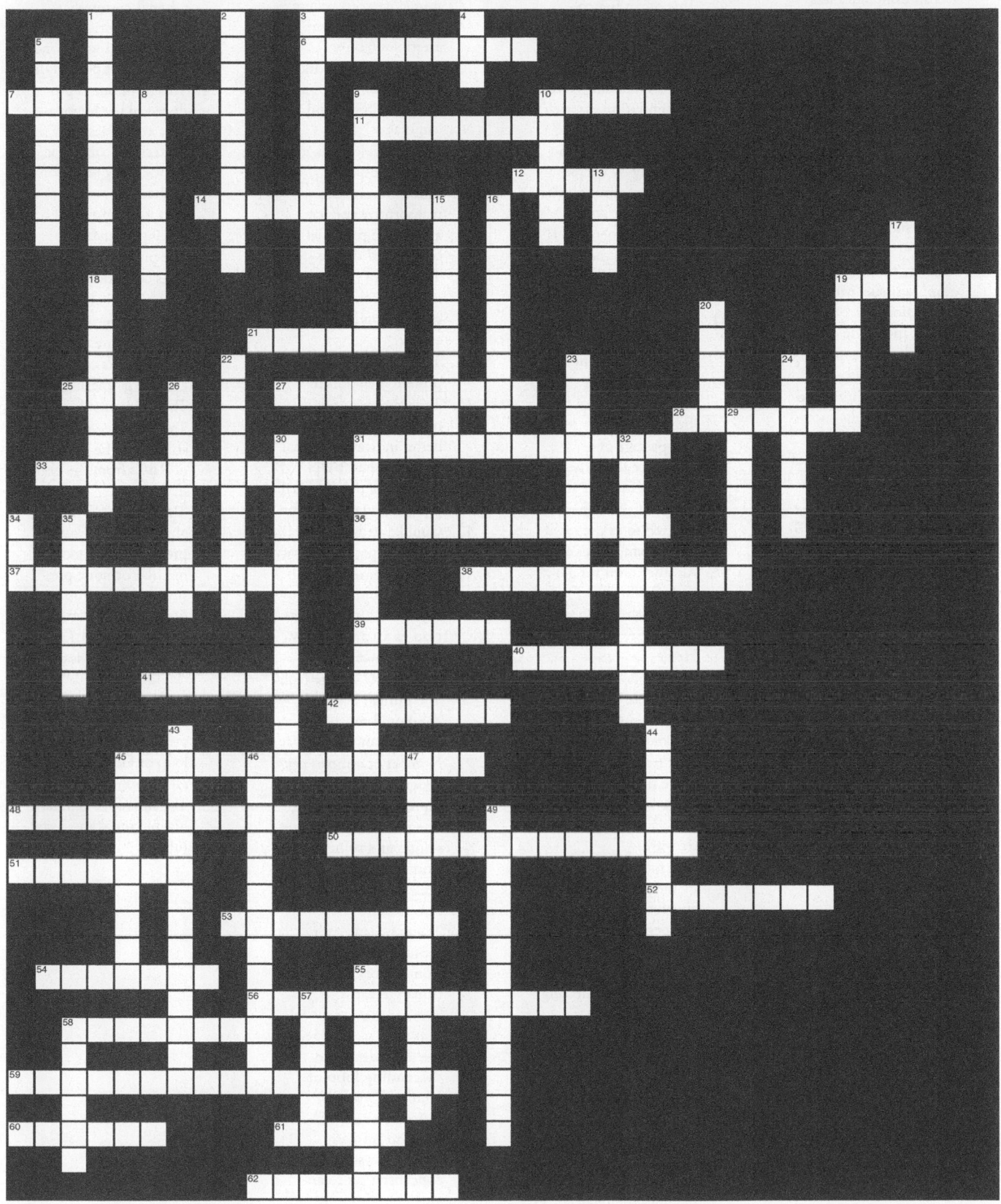

Answers to this activity can be found in the Answer Key.

ACROSS

6. Indicates that the fluid has an osmolality less than body fluids; such as ½ (0.45%) NS

7. An estimate of a known substance in the plasma compared with the amount in the urine

10. A negatively charged ion

11. Indicates that the fluid has approximately the same osmolality as body fluids, such as (0.9%) NS

12. A cavity filled with adipose tissue, minor and major calyces, renal pelvis, and is the origin of the ureter

14. Indicates that the fluid has an osmolality more than body fluids, such as 3% saline

19. The inward extension of cortical tissue between the pyramids

21. A small funnel tapering into the ureter

25. This laboratory value reflects protein metabolism and is normally 10 times the creatinine value (abbrev.)

27. The type of fluid loss (or gain) that cannot be measured

28. Urea is the result of the breakdown of this macronutrient

31. The fluid between cells

33. This substance is made by the kidney and modulates the vasoconstrictive effects of angiotensin and norepinephrine

36. The movement of substances from the tubule back into the capillaries

37. This pressure is a pushing force

38. The state of internal equilibrium within the body

39. The primary extracellular cation; reabsorbed primarily in the proximal convoluted tubule

40. The concentration of this ion determines pH

41. Vitamin D is necessary for the absorption of this mineral

42. This organ is a collapsible bag of smooth muscle

45. A complex physiologic process that allows for concentration of urine

48. The kidney aids in acid-base regulation primarily by excreting and retaining this extracellular anion

50. This type of nephron is important in the kidney's ability to concentrate urine

51. The thin layer of fibrous membrane that surrounds each kidney

52. The microscopic functional unit of the kidney

53. The passage of a substance from the capillary into the tubule

54. The endocrine gland referred to as the *suprarenal gland*

56. Another term for glomerular filtrate

58. This type of nephron has a short loop of Henle

59. This hormone is secreted in response to atrial stretch; causes excretion of sodium (2 words)

60. This structure collects urine from the renal pelvis and propels it to the bladder by peristaltic waves

61. This substance is secreted by the juxtaglomerular apparatus in response to low perfusion

62. Triangular wedges of medullary tissue; composed of collecting tubules

DOWN

1. The primary intracellular cation; reabsorbed primarily in the collecting duct

2. This area of the kidney includes the renal cortex and medulla

3. This electrolyte is crucial for cellular energy

4. This branch of the autonomic nervous system controls the afferent arterioles (abbrev.)

5. This electrolyte works with sodium to maintain body fluid osmolality

8. This arteriole leads into the glomerulus

9. These increase the reabsorptive surface area in the proximal convoluted tubule

10. This type of transport is against concentration gradients and requires energy

13. The end product of protein metabolism

15. The waste product of muscle metabolism; better indicator of renal function than BUN

16. A cluster of tightly coiled capillaries in the nephron

17. Cuplike structures that drain the papillae

18. The movement of solutes from an area of high solute concentration to an area of low solute concentration

19. A positively charged ion

20. The human body is composed mostly of this substance

22. Number of osmoles per kilogram of solution; expressed as mOsm/kg

23. The movement of solutes and solutions from an area of high pressure to an area of low pressure

24. The passageway for expulsion of urine from the bladder to the urinary meatus

26. The capillary network that runs parallel to the ascending and descending loop of Henle (2 words)

29. The movement of solution from an area of low solute concentration to an area of high solute concentration

30. The fluid inside cells

31. The fluid inside vessels

32. The hormone of the adrenal cortex that causes retention of sodium and water and excretion of potassium

34. This hormone is produced in the hypothalamus and released by the posterior pituitary; it causes water retention in the renal tubule

35. This is composed of 6 to 10 pyramids

43. The process that maintains constancy in GFR

44. This arteriole leads out of the glomerulus

45. This structure consists of Bowman's capsule and the glomerulus

46. The fluid outside cells

47. The hormone that stimulates the release of RBCs from the bone marrow

49. This pressure is the glomerular hydrostatic pressure minus glomerular osmotic pressure AND hydrostatic pressure in Bowman's capsule (2 words)

55. This electrolyte is crucial for neuromuscular transmission

57. This structure includes proximal convoluted, loop of Henle, and distal convoluted segments

58. The site of the glomerulus, proximal and distal tubules

5.12   Synthesis Learning Activity: Fluid Replacement

A. A 70-year-old woman is admitted to your unit with severe dehydration. She has a history of heart failure. Her blood pressure is 90/60 mm Hg. A prescription for 0.45% NS @ 75 mL/hour is given. Would you hang it?
Yes ( ) No ( )
Why? _____

B. A 45-year-old man is admitted to your unit with a history of hypertension. Blood pressure upon admission is 220/120 mm Hg. He has been on furosemide therapy and has severe intracellular dehydration. A prescription for D5% NS at 50 mL an hour is given. Would you hang it?
Yes ( ) No ( )
Why? _____

C. A 40-year-old woman is admitted to your unit after abdominal surgery. She has a nasogastric tube to low suction, which is draining approximately 1000 mL/shift. She is losing gastric acids, and thus her pH is 7.58. Because she is also losing a large amount of electrolytes through her nasogastric tube, a prescription for lactated Ringer's solution at 150 mL/hour is given. Would you hang it?
Yes ( ) No ( )
Why? _____

Answers to this activity can be found in the Answer Key.

5.13   Synthesis Learning Activity: Pharmacology

A. A 50-year-old woman has a history of hypertension but she admits that she doesn't take her antihypertensive because she is concerned about not being near a restroom when she needs one. She comes to the emergency department with complaints of swollen ankles and shortness of breath. Which type of diuretic is most likely to be prescribed?
a. thiazide
b. loop
c. potassium-sparing
d. osmotic

B. A 56-year-old man is on your unit with hepatic failure. He has peripheral edema and ascites. Which type of diuretic is most likely to be prescribed?
a. thiazide
b. loop
c. potassium-sparing
d. osmotic

C. A 42-year-old man was seen in a primary care clinic 3 months ago. He was noted to have a BP of 180/100 mm Hg at that time. Despite sodium restriction and an exercise program, his BP is still 176/108 mm Hg. Which type of diuretic is most likely to be prescribed?
a. thiazide
b. loop
c. potassium-sparing
d. osmotic

D. A 66-year-old woman with an elevated creatinine is required to have a diagnostic study requiring dye. Which of the following drugs would most likely be prescribed for nephroprotection?
a. furosemide
b. fenoldopam
c. mannitol
d. dopamine

Answers to this activity can be found in the Answer Key.

CHAPTER 6

The Gastrointestinal System

ANATOMY AND PHYSIOLOGY

The general functions of the gastrointestinal (GI) system include digestion and absorption of nutrients, elimination of waste material, and detoxification and elimination of bacteria, viruses, chemical toxins, and drugs. The processes of ingestion, digestion, absorption, and elimination categorize each function (Figure 6-1).

Ingested material travels from the mouth and esophagus to the stomach. Secretion of enzymes from the salivary glands transforms the material to chyme in the stomach. Additional secretion of enzymes continues and the digestion process begins as material enters the small intestine. Secretion of enzymes from the liver, pancreas, intestinal wall, and small intestine continues the digestion process. It is in the small intestine where absorption to blood and lymph takes place. Upon entering the large intestine, formation of feces occurs. The feces is ultimately excreted through the rectum and anus, where the alimentary canal ends (Figure 6-2). Each area of the GI tract performs a specific important function (Table 6-1). Various digestive enzymes are necessary for proper functioning of digestion (Table 6-2).

The alimentary canal begins in the oropharynx and travels through the esophagus, stomach, small intestine, and large intestine. The small intestine divides into three areas: duodenum, jejunum, and ileum. The cecum, ascending colon, transverse colon, descending colon, sigmoid colon, and rectum make up the large intestine. In addition, the liver, gallbladder, and pancreas are accessory organs of digestion.

Most areas of the GI tract are composed of the same three cellular layers. The serosa is the outermost layer that is frequently continuous with the peritoneum. The muscularis and submucosa make up the middle layers. The mucosa is the innermost layer lined with the mucous membrane and exposed to dietary material.

The abdominal viscera are covered by the peritoneum. The parietal layer of the peritoneum lines the abdominal cavity wall. The visceral layer covers the abdominal organs. The peritoneal cavity is a potential space between the parietal and visceral layers. There are two folds of the peritoneum: the mesentery and the omentum. The mesentery contains blood and lymph vessels and attaches the small intestine and part of the large intestine to the posterior abdominal wall. The omentum contains fat and

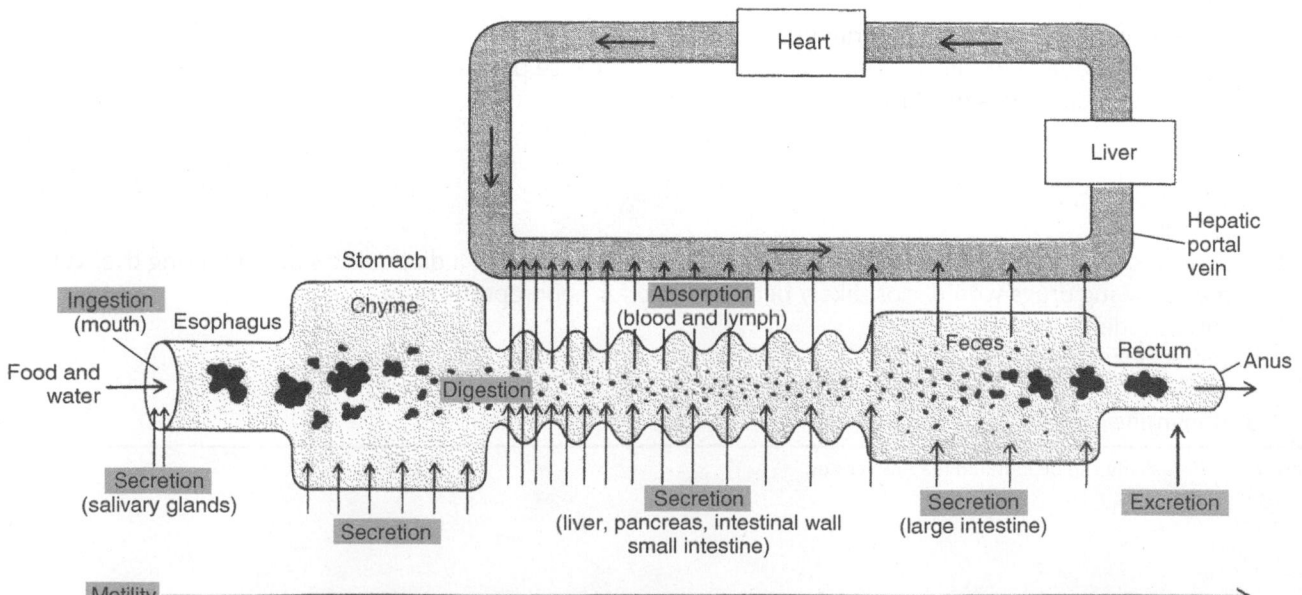

FIGURE 6-1 Summary of processes of the gastrointestinal system. (From Kinney, M., Dunbar, S., Brooks-Brunn, J. A., Molter, N., & Vitello-Cicciu, J. [1998]. *AACN clinical reference for critical care nursing* [4th ed.]. St. Louis, MO: Mosby.)

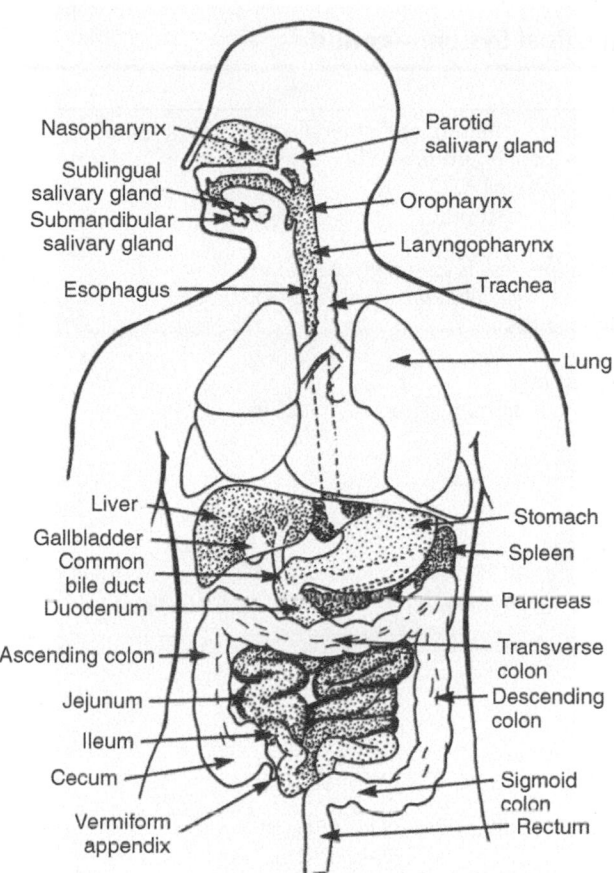

lymph nodes. The lesser omentum extends from the lesser curvature of the stomach and upper duodenum to the liver. The greater omentum extends from the stomach over the intestines.

Oral Cavity

The oral cavity includes the lips, gums, teeth, inner structures of the cheeks, soft and hard palate, tongue, and salivary glands. Chewing prepares food by softening and moving it around and mixing it with saliva to form a bolus. The cranial nerves V, VII, IX, X, XI, and XII control and coordinate the skeletal muscles for chewing.

Approximately 570 mL/day of secreted saliva aids in swallowing. The salivary, parotid, submandibular, parotid, and sublingual glands secrete the saliva mix. The mix is 99% water and 1% solids and includes electrolytes and organic protein molecules. The saliva mix consists of ptyalin (i.e., amylase), which begins the breakdown of polysaccharides (i.e., starches) to disaccharides. Mucus provides lubricant to the mix. The volume produced is about 1500 mL/day. Thought, sight, smell, or taste of food stimulates these secretions.

The process that occurs is that the teeth break up the food into smaller pieces to increase surface area for digestive enzymes to act. Cranial nerve V (trigeminal) innervates the masseter muscles. The tongue moves the food around in the mouth for better chewing and moves the food to the back of the throat to begin the process of swallowing. Chewing and digestive enzymes (see Table 6-2) facilitate the formation and movement of a food bolus along the alimentary tract.

FIGURE 6-2 Structures of the gastrointestinal system. (From Kinney, M., Dunbar, S., Brooks-Brunn, J. A., Molter, N., & Vitello-Cicciu, J. [1998]. *AACN clinical reference for critical care nursing* [4th ed.]. St. Louis, MO: Mosby.)

Pharynx

The pharynx divides into three regions: nasopharynx, oropharynx, and laryngopharynx. It extends from the nose entry past the cricoid cartilage to the level of the sixth cervical vertebra.

TABLE 6-1	Functions of the Components of the Gastrointestinal System
Component	**Function**
Oropharynx	• Salivation • Ingestion • Mastication • Lubrication and moistening of food • First and second stage of swallowing
Esophagus	• Third stage of swallowing • Lubrication of food • Provision of vent for increased gastric pressures
Stomach	• Secretion of gastric enzymes • Mixing of food with gastric enzymes • Reduction of osmolality of food • Absorption of water • Movement of food through the pylorus
Small intestine	• Receipt of chyme from the stomach and moves chyme forward to facilitate proper absorption of proteins, carbohydrates, fats, electrolytes, vitamins, minerals, drugs, and water • Receipt of bile and pancreatic fluid to aid in digestion • Movement of chyme via peristalsis and segmentation • Bacteria in the small intestine help break down and digest protein and, to some degree, fat
Large intestine	• Secretion of mucus to lubricate and protect intestinal lining • Movement of chyme through colon to rectum and initiates urge to defecate • Storage of feces • Elimination of digestive wastes: defecation • Absorption of water and electrolytes • Synthesis of vitamins (folic acid, riboflavin, vitamin K, nicotinic acid) • Metabolism of blood urea to ammonia

Continued

| TABLE 6-1 | Functions of the Components of the Gastrointestinal System—cont'd |

Component	Function
Liver	• Secretion of bilirubin, bile salts, cholesterol, fatty acids, calcium, and other electrolytes into bile • Storage of amino acids, glucose, vitamins, minerals (copper, iron), and blood • Vitamins: riboflavin, nicotinic acid, pyridoxine, vitamins A, D, E, K, B_{12} • Conversion of complex sugars to simple sugars • Conversion of carbohydrates to fats • Conversion of stored glucose (glycogen) to glucose (process is called *glycogenolysis*) • Conversion of amino acids and fats to glucose (process is called *gluconeogenesis*) • Conversion of amino acids to fatty acids and triglycerides • Formation of phospholipids and cholesterol • Formation of lipoproteins from triglycerides and peptides • Conversion of amino acids to plasma proteins (e.g., albumin, fibrinogen, globulins) • Phagocytosis of old RBCs • Formation of clotting factors and heparin • Conversion of ammonia to urea • Conversion of creatine to creatinine • Conversion of vitamin D_3-25-hydroxycholecalciferol • Detoxification of bacteria • Biotransformation of drugs to active and/or inactive metabolites • Deactivation of certain hormones
Gallbladder	• Collection, concentration, and storage of bile • Passageway for bile from liver to intestine • Regulation of bile flow • Release of bile

Pancreas	• Exocrine function
	   • Secretion of pancreatic juice for digestion of carbohydrates, proteins, and fats
	   • Secretion of bicarbonate to neutralize chyme
	• Endocrine function
	   • Secretion of insulin and glucagon

| TABLE 6-2 | Digestive Enzymes |

Source	Enzyme	What It Acts On	What Is Produced
Salivary glands (saliva) (1500 mL/day)	• Ptyalin (amylase)	• Polysaccharides (starches)	• Disaccharides
Stomach (gastric juice) (2500 mL/day)	• Pepsin	• Proteins	• Polypeptides
	• Gastric lipase	• Emulsified fats	• Fatty acids • Glycerol
	• Renin	• Soluble milk protein	• Insoluble form
Liver (bile) (500 mL/day)	• None	• Nonemulsified fats	• Emulsified fats
Pancreas (pancreatic juice) (1500 mL/day)	• Trypsin	• Denatured proteins • Polypeptides	• Peptides • Amino acids
	• Chymotrypsin	• Proteins • Polypeptides	• Peptides • Amino acids
	• Pancreatic lipase	• Emulsified fats	• Fatty acids • Glycerol
	• Pancreatic amylase	• Disaccharides	• Polysaccharides
	• Nucleases	• Nucleic acids	• Nucleotides
	• Carboxypeptidase	• Polypeptides	• Smaller polypeptides
Small intestine (1000 mL/day)	• Enterokinase	• Trypsinogen	• Trypsin
	• Aminopeptidase	• Polypeptides	• Smaller polypeptides
	• Dipeptidase	• Dipeptides	• Amino acids
	• Sucrase	• Sucrose	• Glucose • Fructose
	• Lactase	• Lactose	• Glucose • Galactose

TABLE 6-2	Digestive Enzymes—cont'd		
Source	Enzyme	What It Acts On	What Is Produced
	• Maltase	• Maltose	• Glucose
	• Nucleotidase	• Nucleotides	• Nucleosides • Phosphoric acid
	• Nucleosidase	• Nucleosides	• Purine • Pentose
	• Intestinal lipase	• Fat	• Glycerides • Fatty acids • Glycerol

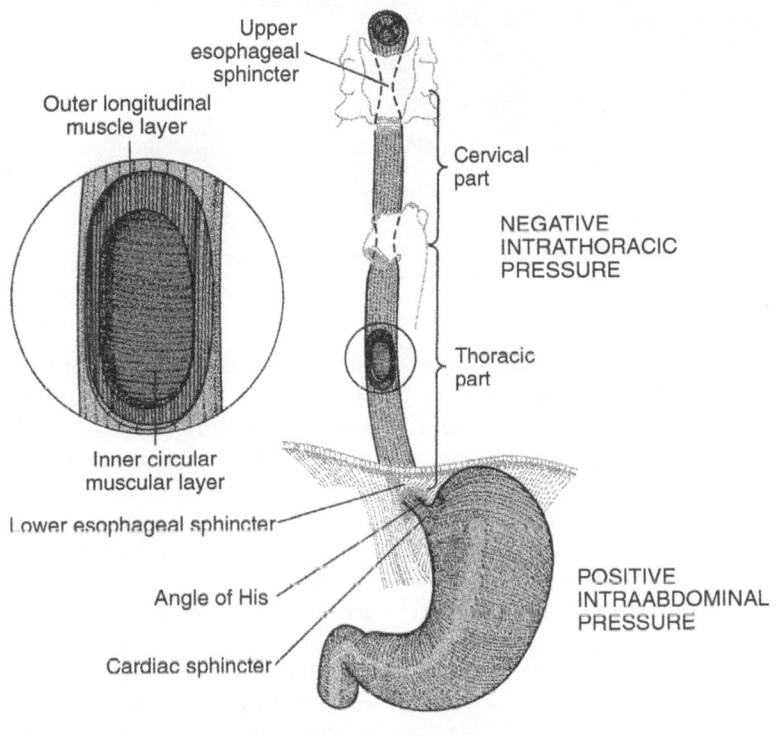

FIGURE 6-3 Anatomy of the esophagus. (From Beare, P. G., & Myers, J. L. [1994]. Principles and practice of adult health nursing [2nd ed.]. St. Louis, MO: Mosby.)

The autonomic nervous system stimulates the swallowing receptors when a food bolus moves toward the back of the mouth. Cranial nerves V, IX, X, and XII transmit the motor impulses to swallow. Swallowing (i.e., deglutination) consists of three stages: voluntary, pharyngeal, and esophageal. Only stage one, the voluntary stage, occurs in the mouth. The voluntary stage is where the tongue forces the bolus of food into the pharynx. In the pharyngeal stage, the bolus of food passes from the pharynx to the esophagus and the epiglottis closes to protect the larynx. During the esophageal stage, the bolus of food passes from the esophagus to the gastroesophageal sphincter.

Esophagus

The esophagus (Figure 6-3) is located behind the trachea. It passes through the thoracic cavity and the diaphragm. The esophagus passes through the diaphragm at the diaphragmatic hiatus. The esophagus is a hollow, collapsible tube from the pharynx to the stomach and is approximately 25 cm in length

and 2 cm in diameter. The esophagus transports food from the mouth to the stomach and prevents retrograde movement of the stomach contents.

The esophagus does not have a serous layer but does have both skeletal and smooth muscle. The upper one-third of the esophagus is striated skeletal muscle and the lower two-thirds is smooth muscle. The esophagus begins at the level of the sixth cervical vertebra and extends down through the diaphragm to the level of the first thoracic vertebrae. The vagus nerve mediates the motor and sensory impulses for swallowing and food passage. The splanchnic and sympathetic neurons innervate the lower esophagus. Two directions of muscle movement occur in the esophagus. The inner area has circular motion, whereas the outer area uses longitudinal movement to create peristalsis. The upper esophageal sphincter (UES), also known as the hypopharyngeal, is made of cricopharyngeal muscle and prevents air from entering the esophagus during inspiration. The lower esophageal sphincter (LES), also known as the gastroesophageal,

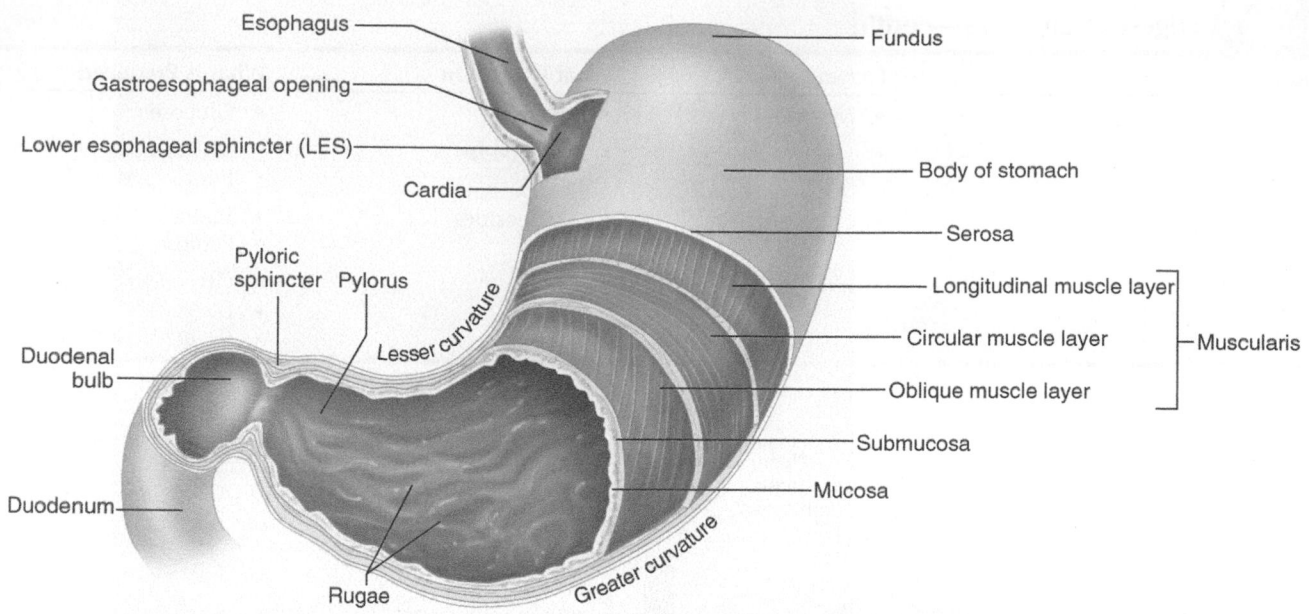

FIGURE 6-4 Anatomy of the stomach. (From Thompson, J. M. et al. [1993]. *Mosby's clinical nursing* [3rd ed.]. St. Louis, MO: Mosby.)

prevents gastric reflux into the esophagus. This last 2 to 4 cm of the esophagus is a physiologic rather than anatomic sphincter. The mucous membrane of the submucosa and mucosa secretes a protective mucoid substance, creating a lubricant.

The final phase of swallowing is involuntary. When a bolus of food enters the esophagus, the hypopharyngeal sphincter opens. Food moves through the esophagus by gravity and peristaltic action. Peristalsis is the alternating contraction and relaxation of muscle fibers, which propels the substance in a wavelike motion through the esophagus, stomach, and intestines. The gastroesophageal sphincter opens and food enters the stomach. The process takes 5 to 10 seconds.

Stomach

The stomach lies inferior to the diaphragm with approximately 80% to 85% of the organ to the left of midline. The stomach is the largest dilation of the GI tract and is approximately 25 to 30 cm in length and 10 to 15 cm at its maximal diameter. The stomach has relatively little muscle tone, which permits increased distention. The stomach is a food storage reservoir with normal storage capacity of 100 to 1500 mL but enlarges up to 6000 mL.

The structure of the stomach divides into anatomic divisions (Figure 6-4). The cardia portion of the stomach immediately adjoins the esophagus. The fundus is a dome-shaped portion of the stomach that extends left of the cardia. The greater curvature is on the lateral, convex side. The body is the major area (i.e., belly) of stomach. The lesser curvature is on the medial, concave side. The antrum is the lower portion of the stomach close to the pylorus. The stomach has two sphincters. The cardiac sphincter is between the esophagus and stomach. The pyloric sphincter is between the stomach and duodenum.

The serosa cell layer is continuous with the visceral layer of the peritoneum. The muscularis outer layer has longitudinal muscle fibers. The middle layer consists of circular muscle

fibers, whereas the inner layer has transverse muscle fibers. The muscles help in the modification of foods into a liquid consistency and move it along the GI tract. Movement is tonic and rhythmic, occurring every 20 seconds. The lamina propria contains lymphocytes and is the site of the gut immunologic response. The muscularis mucosae contain a thin smooth muscle layer. Blood vessels, lymph vessels, connective tissue, and fibrous tissues are within the submucosa and are responsible for secreting gastric enzymes.

Cells in the mucosa produce mucus that lubricates and protects the inner surface. Cell replacement occurs every 4 to 5 days, and these cells receive the majority of the blood supply to the stomach. The mucosa contains rugae, which are thick folds on the interior of the stomach. The rugae do all of the following:

- Increase surface area for exposure
- Allow for distention
- Contain the openings of the gastric glands

The stomach has several types of gastric glands (see Table 6-2). The epithelium of the stomach contains the gastric, cardiac, fundic, and pyloric glands. The cardiac glands are just distal to the gastroesophageal junction and secrete pepsinogen and mucus. The mucous neck cells secrete mucus. The oxyntic glands are in the fundic area and contain chief and parietal cells. The chief cells secrete pepsinogen. The oxyntic (also referred to as parietal) cells secrete hydrochloric acid and intrinsic factor. Hydrochloric acid lowers the pH and kills bacteria. The intrinsic factor is a glycoprotein necessary for vitamin B_{12} absorption. Pyloric glands are located in the antral area where G-cells secrete gastrin and enterochromaffin cells secrete serotonin.

The hormone gastrin is stimulated when a bolus of food enters the upper portion of the stomach. It stimulates the secretion of hydrochloric acid by the parietal cells and the secretion of pepsin by the chief cells. The mast cells secrete histamine in response to the presence of food. Histamine stimulates gastric acid and pepsin secretion, initiates the contraction of the gallbladder, relaxes the sphincter of Oddi, and increases GI motility. Gastric secretions are clear and contain water, salts, enzymes, and hydrochloric acid. Histamine, acetylcholine, and gastrin stimulate the 1500 to 3000 mL of daily gastric secretions and mix with food entering the stomach. The function of the secretions is to denature protein and break intermolecular bonds, activate a number of enzymes secreted by stomach, and kill bacteria.

Hydrochloric acid activates pepsinogen to form pepsin, which is a catalyst that splits the bonds between particular types of amino acids in protein chains. The intrinsic factor is a mucoprotein that is necessary for intestinal absorption of vitamin B_{12} in the ileum; deficiency of vitamin B_{12} causes pernicious anemia. Mucus contributes to the maintenance of the gastric mucosal barrier.

The control of gastric secretions has two phases. The parasympathetic nervous system (PNS), when stimulated by thought, sight, smell, or taste of food, releases hydrochloric acids, which mediate the cephalic phase. The gastric phase enhances acid secretion. Distention of the stomach and digestion products of food stimulate the gastric phase. The intestinal phase is a continuation of gastric acid secretion but in lesser amounts. The distention, hypertonic solution, acid, and fat within the duodenum stimulate the intestinal phase.

As food moves toward the pyloric sphincter at the distal end of the stomach, peristaltic waves increase in force and intensity. The food bolus becomes a substance known as chyme. The quantity and pH of the stomach contents, the degree of mixing, and peristalsis control gastric motility. The sympathetic and parasympathetic nervous systems, reflexes, and gastric hormones control the ability of the duodenum to accept the chyme.

Stomach peristalsis pumps the chyme through the pyloric sphincter into the duodenum. The stomach empties as chyme travels through the pyloric channel. The rate of gastric emptying is proportional to the volume of the stomach's contents. The consistency of the fluid chyme and receptiveness of the duodenum regulate the gastric emptying. Liquids selectively move through the pylorus before solids. Other factors that accelerate gastric emptying include a large volume of liquids, and insulin. In addition, factors inhibiting gastric emptying include chyme with high lipid, protein, and fat content; high acidity in the antrum; and the duodenal hormones of secretin and cholecystokinin. Emotions such as pain, anxiety, sadness, and hostility can also inhibit gastric emptying. Food usually stays in the stomach for 2 to 6 hours after ingestion.

The vomiting center in the medulla coordinates vomiting in response to afferent impulses throughout the body. Stimuli that induce vomiting include tactile irritation in the back of the throat, increased intracranial pressure, intense pain, dizziness, anxiety, and/or pathogens or toxins ingested. Autonomic nervous system symptoms such as diaphoresis, increased heart rate, increased salivation, and muscular force of the diaphragm and abdomen often precede vomiting.

Small Intestine

The small intestine extends from the pylorus to the ileocecal valve and has a length of 7 m and diameter of 2.5 cm. The structure divides into three sections. The duodenum is a short segment only 30 cm long. The jejunum makes up the next two-fifths after the duodenum and is about 250 cm long. The ileum is the last three-fifths after the duodenum and is approximately 350 cm long. The intestine has four cell layers. The serosa is continuous with the peritoneum, and beneath that the intestine has muscular, submucosal, and mucosal layers. The intestine has two sphincters. The pylorus sphincter lies between the stomach and the duodenum, controls the flow of contents into the duodenum, and prevents reflux back into the stomach. The ileocecal sphincter controls the flow of contents into the large intestine and prevents reflux from the large intestine back into the ileum.

The small intestine has many villi in the duodenum and jejunum. Villi are fingerlike projections of mucosa and submucosa. Villi increase surface area. They contain a single lymph vessel called a *lacteal* and a dense capillary bed to aid in absorption. The villi contain many types of cells to absorb fat, carbohydrates, or protein and secrete enzymes and mucus. Brunner's glands are cells that are primarily in the duodenum and secrete mucus; goblet cells also secrete mucus. The Crypts of Lieberkühn are cells that produce watery mucus called *succus entericus*, a carrier substance for absorption of nutrients when the villi contact the chyme. The function of Paneth's cells is uncertain but they may regulate intestinal flora. Peyer's patches are lymphoid follicles in the mucosa and submucosa; they carry out antibody synthesis.

Small intestine digestive enzymes are integral components of the mucosa. The gallbladder secretes bile and the pancreas secretes pancreatic enzymes into the duodenum. Food is digested and absorbed in the jejunum and ileum. Up to 3000 mL/day of digestive enzymes (i.e., lipase, amylase, maltase, lactase) facilitates the digestive process. The presence of chyme in the duodenum and the release of gastric hormones (see Table 6-2) stimulate intestinal secretions.

Intestinal movement of chyme is an involuntary process. During fasting and sleeping states, the muscle contraction moves from the antrum to the ileum to sweep the gut of its contents. While eating, concentric, segmenting contractions take place in the jejunum to help mix secretions of the small intestine with the chyme particles. Slow, propulsive contractions (i.e., peristalsis) slowly push the chyme in the direction of the large intestine. The continuous shortening and lengthening of the villi constantly stirs the intestinal contents. The gastroileal reflex and increased contractions in the ileum as the chyme nears the large intestine regulate the movement of chyme from the small intestine to the large intestine. Movement of chyme through the small intestine takes approximately 3 to 10 hours.

Almost all nutrient absorption occurs in the small intestine. Four mechanisms of active transport, passive diffusion, facilitated diffusion, and nonionic transport are the mechanisms involved with absorption. Vitamins, water, electrolytes, iron, carbohydrates, proteins, and fats are absorbed in the small intestine.

Large Intestine

The large intestine (also referred to as the colon) (Figure 6-5) extends from the ileum to the anus. Its length is about 90 to 150 cm and the diameter is 4 to 6 cm. Anatomic divisions of the colon include the cecum, ascending colon, transverse colon, descending colon, and sigmoid colon, which is inclusive of the rectum. The cecum is a blind pouch attached to the appendix. It is about 2.5 cm from the ileocecal valve. The ascending colon extends from the cecum to the lower border of the liver, where it forms the right hepatic flexure. The transverse colon crosses the upper half of the abdominal cavity and curves

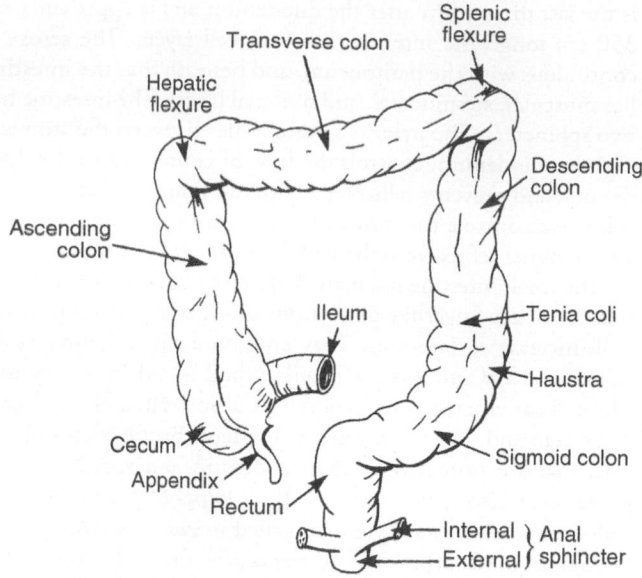

FIGURE 6-5 Anatomy of the large intestine. (From Kinney, M., Dunbar, S., Brooks-Brunn, J. A., Molter, N., & Vitello-Cicciu, J. [1998]. *AACN clinical reference for critical care nursing* [4th ed.]. St. Louis, MO: Mosby.)

downward at the lower end of the spleen at the left splenic flexure. The descending colon extends from the splenic flexure to the sigmoid colon. The sigmoid colon is an S-shaped curve extending from the descending colon to the rectum. The rectum extends from the sigmoid colon to the anus. The ileocecal valve is located at the junction of the small intestine and the cecum. Internal and external anal sphincters control stool evacuation.

The layers of the large intestine wall are similar to the small intestine in that they consist of a serosa, muscularis, submucosa, and mucosa; however there are no villi and no secretion of digestive enzymes. The large intestine walls have an epithelial surface that contains cells that absorb water and electrolytes. They also have crypts covered by epithelial cells that produce mucus.

Movement of intestinal contents in the large intestine occurs by a process known as Haustral shuttling, characterized by periodic uncoordinated tonic contractions or segmentations of both the longitudinal and circular muscles. Weak peristaltic contractions move the chyme through the large intestine by phasic, random, nonpropulsive contractions lasting 30 seconds to 2 minutes. The contents are displaced short distances in both directions to mix the stool material and help in the absorption of liquid contents without advancement toward the anus.

Spontaneous mass movements push fecal contents forward and typically occur only a few times each day. Gastrocolic reflexes initiated when food enters the duodenum from the stomach, especially after the first meal of the day, stimulate mass movements. These movements move feces into the rectum. The defecation reflex occurs as feces enter the rectum and peristaltic waves in the rectum and relaxation of the internal and external anal sphincter occur. Afferent impulses transmitted to the sacral segment of the spinal cord transmit reflex impulses back to the colon and rectum and initiate relaxation of the internal anal sphincter.

The Valsalva maneuver facilitates the evacuation of the colon. Factors that enhance colonic motility include a high-residue diet, hyperosmolality, fluids, irritation of the colon (e.g.,

spicy foods), bacterial endotoxins, viral infections of the gut, regional enteritis, ulcerative colitis, increased bile salts, osmotic overload, and irritant laxatives. Factors that inhibit colonic motility include a low-residue diet, parenteral nutrition, bed rest, dehydration, paralytic ileus, fasting, anticholinergic drugs, and opiates. Poor motility through the colon results in increased absorption of water and the development of hard feces in the transverse colon causing constipation. Aging causes a reduction in peristalsis and decreased GI motility. Movement of fecal contents through the intestine takes approximately 18 hours.

The major function of the colon is the absorption of water and electrolytes (Table 6-1). Approximately 500 mL of chyme (i.e., the byproduct of digestion) enters the colon daily, and the colon reabsorbs 400 mL of water and electrolytes. Another major function of the large intestine is the breakdown of cellulose by enteric bacteria. Enteric bacteria also play a role in the synthesis of vitamins (e.g., folic acid, vitamin K, riboflavin, and nicotinic acid). The colon stores and then expels the fecal mass.

The colon also has a major role in gut defense protection. The gut encounters a variety of potential harmful substances daily. The GI tract has a number of mechanisms to protect the integrity of the gut. B lymphocytes bear surface immunoglobulin A (IgA) that prevents antigens from binding to mucous cells. Lymphoid tissues and macrophages are present in the submucosa (i.e., lamina propria and Peyer's patches). Glutamine, a primary fuel of the gut, maintains the gut mucosal barrier. Gastric acid keeps the pH below 4.0, which prevents bacteria from entering the intestine. Natural gut flora is stable and protective in a healthy person by competing with pathogenic species for nutrients, attachment sites, and production of inhibitory substances. Dietary intake is a major factor in determining intestinal flora. Any impairment of gut protection facilitates bacteria transfer across the mucosal barrier and into the lymphatic and portal circulation, potentially causing sepsis.

Accessory Organs of Digestion

The digestive system is composed of more than the alimentary canal. In addition to the tubular organs in which actual digestion takes place, there are a number of accessory organs vital to normal function. These accessory organs include the liver, gallbladder, and pancreas (Figure 6-6).

Liver

The liver is located in the right upper quadrant (RUQ) of the abdomen. It fits snugly against the right inferior diaphragm. The liver is the largest organ in the body (1.5 kg). The liver attaches to the abdominal wall by the falciform ligament, which also divides the left and right lobes. The right lobe is larger than the left. The four main lobes of the liver include the right, left, caudate, and quadrate. A thick capsule of connective tissue called *Glisson's capsule*, which contains blood vessels and lymphatics, covers the liver. Covered by a layer of serosa, the capsule is continuous with the peritoneum.

The lobes subdivide into lobules, the functioning units of the liver. There are over 1 million lobules. Hepatic cells (i.e., hepatocytes) are arranged in chains around a central vein. Blood flows through sinusoids, which separate the hepatic chains. The sinusoids receive oxygenated blood from branches of the hepatic artery and nutrient-rich blood from branches of the hepatic portal vein. The hepatic cells remove oxygen, nutrients, and toxins from the blood. Each lobule has its own hepatic artery,

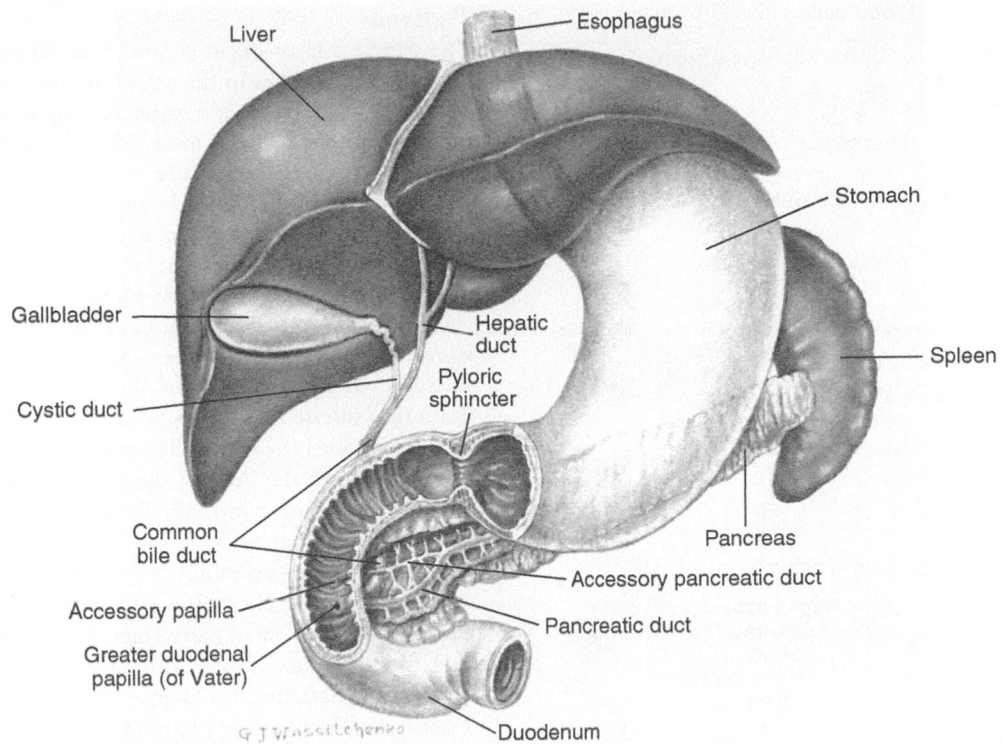

FIGURE 6-6 Accessory organs of the gastrointestinal system. (From Doughty, D. B., & Jackson, D. B. [1993]. *Gastrointestinal disorders: Mosby's clinical nursing series.* St. Louis, MO: Mosby.)

portal vein, and bile duct, collectively called the *portal triad.* The lobule is composed of branching plates of liver cells radiating out to the periphery. Kupffer cells, which are responsible for phagocytosis, line the sinusoids. Kupffer cells are a part of the reticuloendothelial system (RES); they destroy old or defective red blood cells and remove bacteria and foreign particles from the blood.

Bile canaliculi are located between the hepatic cells and empty bile into the small bile ducts. Small bile ducts join to form the right and left hepatic ducts. The left and right hepatic ducts merge to form the common hepatic duct. The cystic duct from the gallbladder joins the common hepatic duct to form the common bile duct. The pancreatic duct joins the common bile duct and together they empty into the duodenum through the ampulla of Vater. The sphincter of Oddi is a valve in the common bile duct, which regulates the passage of bile from the common bile duct into the duodenum (Figure 6-7).

The liver is a metabolically complex organ with interrelated digestive, metabolic, exocrine, hematologic, and excretory functions. The digestive functions include a role in the synthesis, metabolism, and transport of carbohydrates, fats, and proteins. The liver maintains normal serum glucose, bile secretion for fat digestion, lipid synthesis and metabolism, production of proteins, and metabolism of amino acids (see Table 6-1).

Gallbladder

The gallbladder attaches to the undersurface of the liver and connects to the upper portion of the duodenum by the common bile duct. The gallbladder is a saclike organ about 7 to 10 cm in length and 3 cm in diameter. It stores bile and has a storage capacity of 50 to 70 mL. The serous layer of the gallbladder is

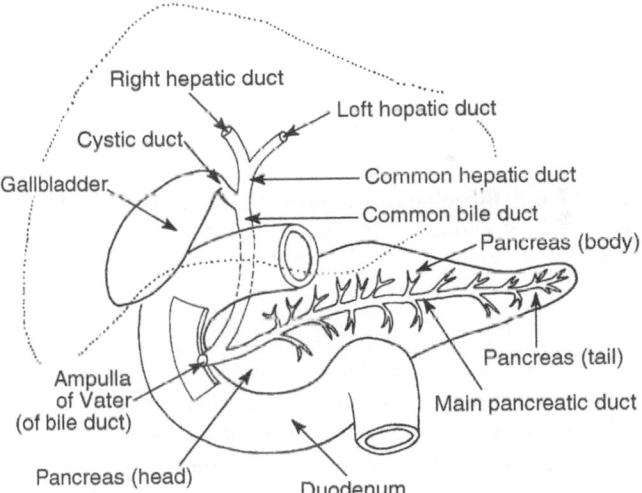

FIGURE 6-7 Ductal systems of the gastrointestinal tract. (From Kinney, M., Dunbar, S., Brooks-Brunn, J. A., Molter, N., & Vitello-Cicciu, J. [1998]. *AACN clinical reference for critical care nursing* [4th ed.]. St. Louis: Mosby.)

continuous with the peritoneum. The gallbladder has a smooth muscle layer. The mucous membrane layer has rugae, which allow an increase in gallbladder size.

There are four anatomic divisions of the gallbladder: fundus, body, infundibulum, and neck. The fundus is the distal portion of the body that forms a blind sac. The body connects the fundus to the infundibulum. The infundibulum connects the body to the neck, which narrows into the cystic duct. The cystic duct merges with the common hepatic duct to form the common bile duct, which joins with the pancreatic duct to form the ampulla of Vater. The sphincter of Oddi is at the terminal end of the

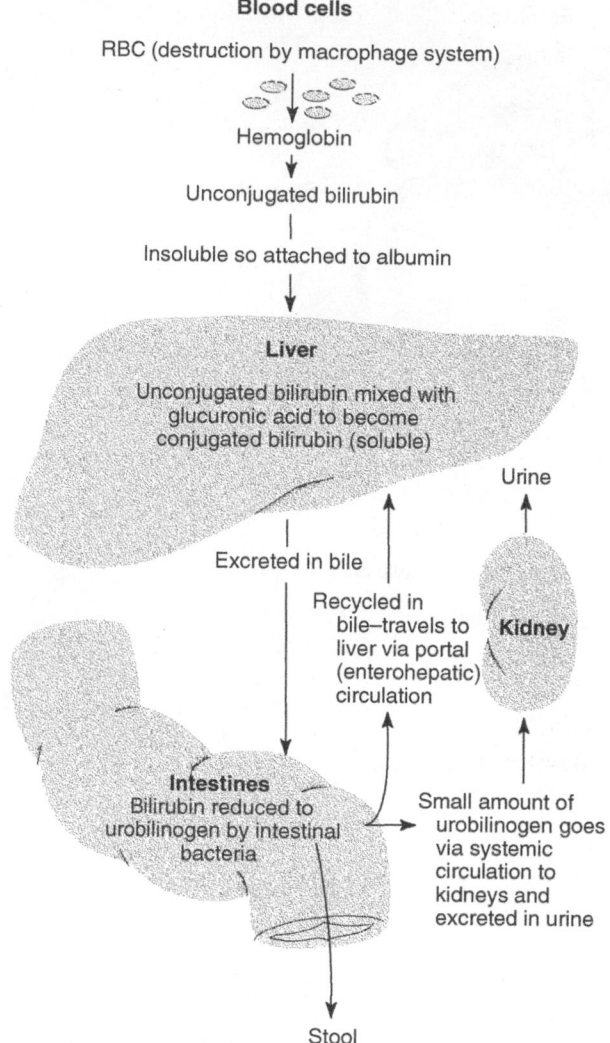

Blood cells

RBC (destruction by macrophage system)

Hemoglobin

Unconjugated bilirubin

Insoluble so attached to albumin

Liver
Unconjugated bilirubin mixed with glucuronic acid to become conjugated bilirubin (soluble)

Urine

Excreted in bile

Recycled in bile—travels to liver via portal (enterohepatic) circulation

Kidney

Intestines
Bilirubin reduced to urobilinogen by intestinal bacteria

Small amount of urobilinogen goes via systemic circulation to kidneys and excreted in urine

Stool

FIGURE 6-8 Bilirubin metabolism. (From Lewis, S. M., Heitkemper, M. M., & Dirksen, S. R. [2000]. *Medical-surgical nursing. Assessment and management of clinical problems* [5th ed.]. St. Louis, MO: Mosby.)

common bile duct, located at the entrance into the duodenum. This sphincter regulates the flow of bile and pancreatic juices into the intestine. It also inhibits the entry of bile into the pancreatic duct and prevents reflux of intestinal contents into the duct.

Produced by the liver and stored in the gallbladder, bile is composed of water, bile pigments, bile salts, a high concentration of cholesterol, and some neutral fat, phospholipids, and inorganic salts. The major bile pigment is bilirubin, a breakdown product of hemoglobin. The heme portion of the hemoglobin molecule is converted to bilirubin by reticuloendothelial cells, released into the bloodstream, and binds to albumin as fat-soluble, unconjugated (i.e., indirect) bilirubin. In the liver, indirect bilirubin is bound to glucuronic acid to form water-soluble conjugated (i.e., direct) bilirubin, which is excreted into the hepatic ducts (Figure 6-8).

The release of the hormone cholecystokinin is stimulated when fatty food is present in the small intestine; cholecystokinin causes contraction of the gallbladder, facilitates the delivery of bile to the duodenum, and relaxes the sphincter of Oddi. The action of bile is to assist in the absorption of fats by emulsifying the fat and breaking down large fat droplets into small droplets (see Table 6-2).

Pancreas

The pancreas is an organ about 15 to 20 cm in length and 5 cm in width and lies in the posterior curvature of the stomach behind the duodenum and spleen (see Figure 6-6). The pancreas has three anatomic divisions called the head, body, and tail. The head lies over the vena cava in the C-shaped curve of the duodenum. The body lies behind the duodenum and extends across the abdomen behind the stomach. The tail is under the spleen. The pancreas is not encapsulated.

The pancreas consists of lobes formed by lobules of clustered cells with the acini arranged around a small central lumen. They secrete their enzymes into the central lumen, which drain into ductules. The ductules drain into intralobular ducts, which drain into interlobular ducts, which empty into the pancreatic duct (also called the *duct of Wirsung*). The pancreatic duct runs from the tail to the head of the pancreas and unites with the common bile duct to form the ampulla of Vater, which empties into the duodenum.

The cells have exocrine and endocrine functions. Acinar cells have exocrine (i.e., through a duct) functions. Alpha and beta cells of the islets of Langerhans have endocrine (i.e., ductless) functions (see Table 6-2). Alpha cells secrete glucagon. Beta cells secrete insulin. Delta cells secrete somatostatin (see Table 6-2). The presence of undigested food in the small intestine triggers the release of pancreatic secretions. Acinar cells secrete a high concentration of sodium bicarbonate, water, sodium, potassium, and digestive enzymes (lipase, amylase, trypsin, ribonuclease, and deoxyribonuclease). Secreted in the inactive form, trypsinogen and chymotrypsinogen become activated when in contact with bile salts (Table 6-3). The vagus nerve and parasympathetic nervous system control the secretions.

Blood Supply

Arterial branches from the abdominal aorta supply blood to the GI system (Figure 6-9). The main vessels are the celiac, superior mesenteric, inferior mesenteric, and hepatic arteries. The celiac artery branches into several arteries: left, hepatic, and splenic arteries. The left gastric artery supplies the stomach and esophagus. The right gastric and the gastroduodenal arteries are branches from the common hepatic artery. The right gastric artery supplies the stomach. The gastroduodenal artery supplies the stomach and duodenum. The proper hepatic artery is a branch of the common hepatic artery, and the cystic artery is a branch of the common hepatic artery. The cystic artery supplies the gallbladder and the splenic artery supplies the stomach, pancreas, and spleen. The superior mesenteric artery supplies the jejunum, ileum, cecum, ascending colon, and part of the transverse colon. The inferior mesenteric artery supplies the transverse, descending, and sigmoid colon, along with the rectum. The hepatic artery and vein supply the liver.

The portal vein collects and delivers blood from the entire venous drainage of the GI tract to the liver branches: gastric, splenic, superior mesenteric, and inferior mesenteric. The portal vein subdivides into liver sinusoids, which then unite with branches from the hepatic artery. Blood flows from branches of the hepatic artery and mixes in the sinusoids to supply the hepatocytes with oxygen. This mixture permeates through the sinusoids. A liver sinusoid serves as a location for the oxygen-rich blood from the hepatic artery and the nutrient-rich blood from the portal vein. Partially metabolized digestive products

TABLE 6-3   Gastrointestinal Hormones

Hormone	Source	Stimulus for Release	Action
Gastrin	Gastric mucosa of the antrum of the stomach and the pylorus	Partially digested proteins in pylorus	• Stimulates release of gastric juices
Secretin	Duodenal mucosa	Partially digested proteins, fats, and acids in intestine	• Inhibits gastric motility and acid secretions • Secretes pancreatic bicarbonate
Cholecystokinin	Duodenal mucosa	Fats in duodenum	• Increases gallbladder contraction • Decreases stomach tone
Gastric inhibitory peptide	Small intestine mucosa	Fat and carbohydrate in duodenum	• Stimulates secretion of insulin • Decreases motor activity of the stomach • Slows emptying of gastric contents into the small intestine
Vasoactive intestinal peptide	Small intestine mucosa	Acid in the duodenum	• Stimulates intestinal juice • Inhibits gastric secretion
Enterogastrone	Small intestine mucosa	Partially digested proteins, fats, and acids in intestine	• Inhibits gastric secretion and motility • Relaxation of sphincter of Oddi and contraction of gallbladder
Villikinin	Small intestine mucosa	Chyme in intestine	• Stimulates movement of intestinal villi
Pancreozymin	Duodenal mucosa	Partially digested proteins, fats, and acids in duodenum	• Stimulates pancreatic juice

brought to the liver sinusoids for hepatocytes complete the next stage of metabolism (see Figure 6-9).

Nervous Innervation

The GI system receives both extrinsic and intrinsic innervation from the nervous system. The extrinsic innervation involves the parasympathetic nervous system (PNS) and sympathetic nervous system (SNS). The PNS, innervated by the vagus nerve, increases the activity of the GI tract. The sympathetic nervous system, innervated by SNS fibers, which run parallel to the major blood vessels of the GI tract, decreases the activity of the GI tract. The intrinsic nerve cells are located inside the wall of the GI tract; they consist of extensions from extrinsic nerves of the autonomic nervous system (ANS) that form two major and three minor networks of plexuses.

FUNCTIONS OF THE GASTROINTESTINAL SYSTEM

The major functions of the GI system are ingestion, secretion, digestion, absorption, synthesis, and fluid and electrolyte balance. Ingestion begins with the sensation of hunger, controlled by the feeding center of the hypothalamus. Ingestion ends with the sensation of satisfaction provided by the satiety center, also in the hypothalamus. Food and liquids enter the alimentary tract at the mouth. The cells of the gastrointestinal system secrete substances (e.g., hormones and enzymes) to aid in digestion (see Table 6-2).

Digestion of the body's nutrient requirements (i.e., carbohydrates, proteins, fats) is a major function of the gastrointestinal system. Carbohydrate digestion begins in the mouth where polysaccharides (i.e., starch) are broken down to disaccharides (e.g., sucrose, lactose, maltose) by the action of ptyalin (i.e., amylase). The process continues when the disaccharides break down to monosaccharides (e.g., glucose, galactose, fructose) by the action of pancreatic amylase and intestinal enzymes (e.g., sucrose, lactase, maltase). Carbohydrates provide 4 kcal of energy/gram.

Digestion of protein begins in the stomach where pepsin breaks down proteins into polypeptides. The process continues when the polypeptides are broken down into peptides and amino acids in the small intestine by the action of trypsin, chymotrypsin, carboxypeptides from the pancreas, and aminopeptidases and dipeptidase from the intestinal villi. Proteins provide 4 kcal of energy/gram.

Digestion of fat that is already emulsified (e.g., cream, butter) begins in the stomach by lipase. Digestion of nonemulsified fat occurs in the small intestine with emulsification of the fat by bile and pancreatic lipase. Fat is broken down into glycerol and fatty acids. Fats provide 9 kcal of energy/gram.

Absorption of nutrients by the GI systems occurs by the basic mechanisms of active transport, passive diffusion, facilitated diffusion nonionic transport, and solvent drag. Active transport requires an energy source (i.e., ATP) to move substances into and out of the cell. Substances absorbed by active transport include proteins, glucose, sodium, and potassium. Passive diffusion is passive movement from an area of high solute concentration

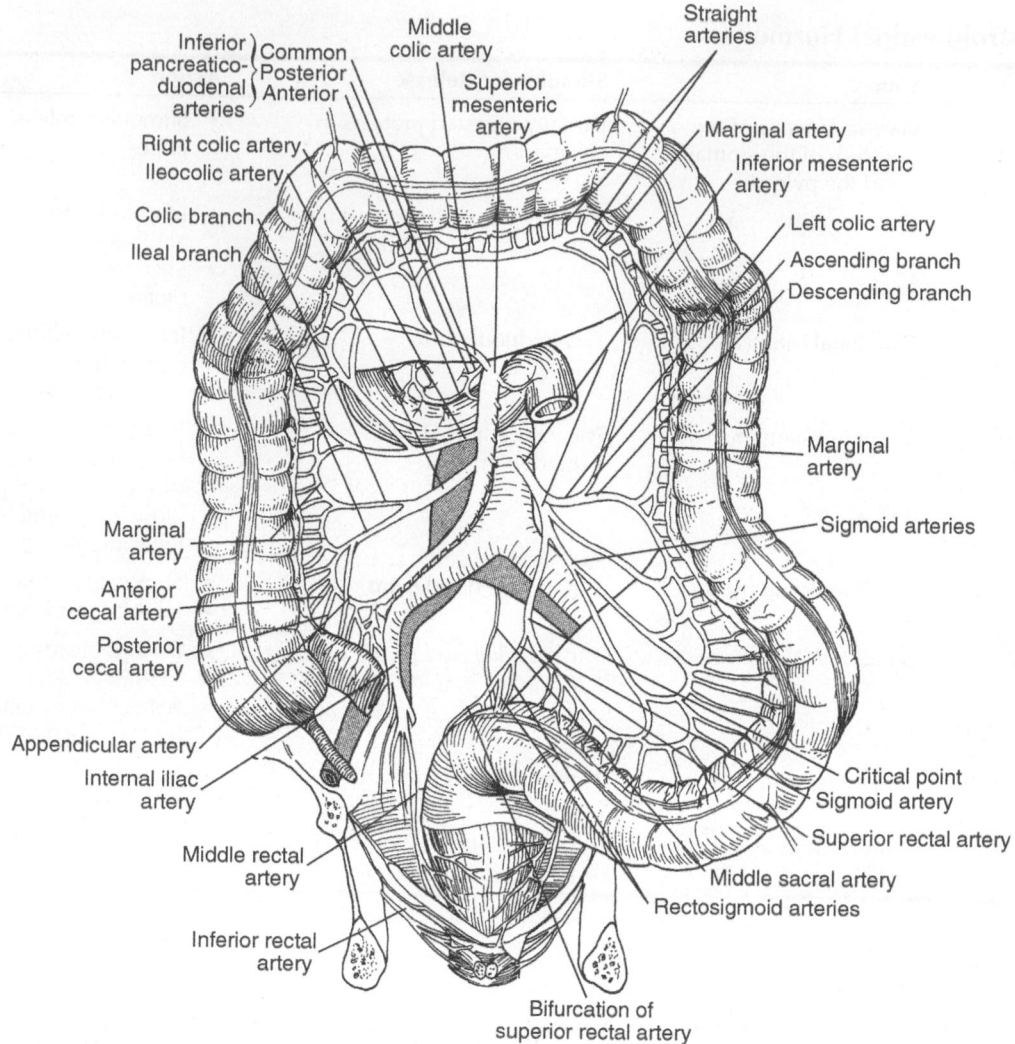

FIGURE 6-9 Arterial blood supply of the gastrointestinal system. (From Society of Gastroenterology Nurses and Associates SGNA [1993]. *Gastroenterology nursing: A core curriculum.* St. Louis, MO: Mosby.)

to an area of low solute concentration. Substances absorbed by passive diffusion include free fatty acids and water. Facilitated diffusion is movement that requires a carrier that moves into the cell, but energy is not required. An example of a substance absorbed by facilitated diffusion is fructose. Nonionic transport is movement of solutes freely into and out of the cell. Substances absorbed by nonionic transport include unconjugated bile salts and drugs. Solvent drag is the flow of water to higher osmotic concentration. It contributes to absorption and reduction in osmolality that occurs in the jejunum.

In the small intestine, specific absorption of substances occurs. Electrolyte absorption occurs from active transport from all areas of the intestine. Water absorption occurs in the small and large intestine. A person ingests approximately 2 L of fluid daily, and the GI tract secretes approximately 7 L of fluid daily. Of these 9 L, the intestines reabsorb 7500 mL, with only 1500 mL reaching the cecum. Additional fluids are reabsorbed in the large intestine, with only 200 mL lost in the stool.

Carbohydrate (CHO) absorption occurs by both facilitated diffusion and active transport. Fructose absorption occurs by facilitated diffusion. Glucose and galactose absorption occur by active transport. The protein absorption of amino acids occurs by active transport in the ileum and jejunum.

Fat absorption occurs with micellar solubilization of fatty acid with bile salt to form micelle, which diffuses into jejunal cells. The delivery of fatty acids to the circulation is via the lymphatic system.

Water-soluble vitamin absorption occurs in all areas of the small intestine by passive diffusion. The absorption of vitamin B_{12} requires the intrinsic factor. Fat-soluble vitamin absorption occurs in the jejunum and requires bile salts. Calcium absorption occurs mainly in the duodenum and requires vitamin D. Iron absorption also occurs in all areas of the intestine, but predominantly in the duodenum by active transport. Iron is stored as protein-bound iron.

Another function of the GI system involves the production of vitamin K and antibody synthesis. Bacteria in the large intestine produce vitamin K. Peyer's patches in the small intestine play a role in antibody synthesis. The GI system also has an effect on fluid and electrolyte balance. Gastric losses are acidic; therefore, increased gastric losses (e.g., nasogastric suction, vomiting) cause metabolic alkalosis, hypokalemia, hyponatremia, and hypovolemia. Intestinal losses are alkaline; therefore, increased intestinal losses (e.g., biliary losses, pancreatic fistula, intestinal suction, diarrhea) cause metabolic acidosis, hypokalemia, hyponatremia, and hypovolemia.

6.1   Synthesis Learning Activity: Crossword Puzzle

Complete the following crossword puzzle related to gastrointestinal anatomy and physiology.

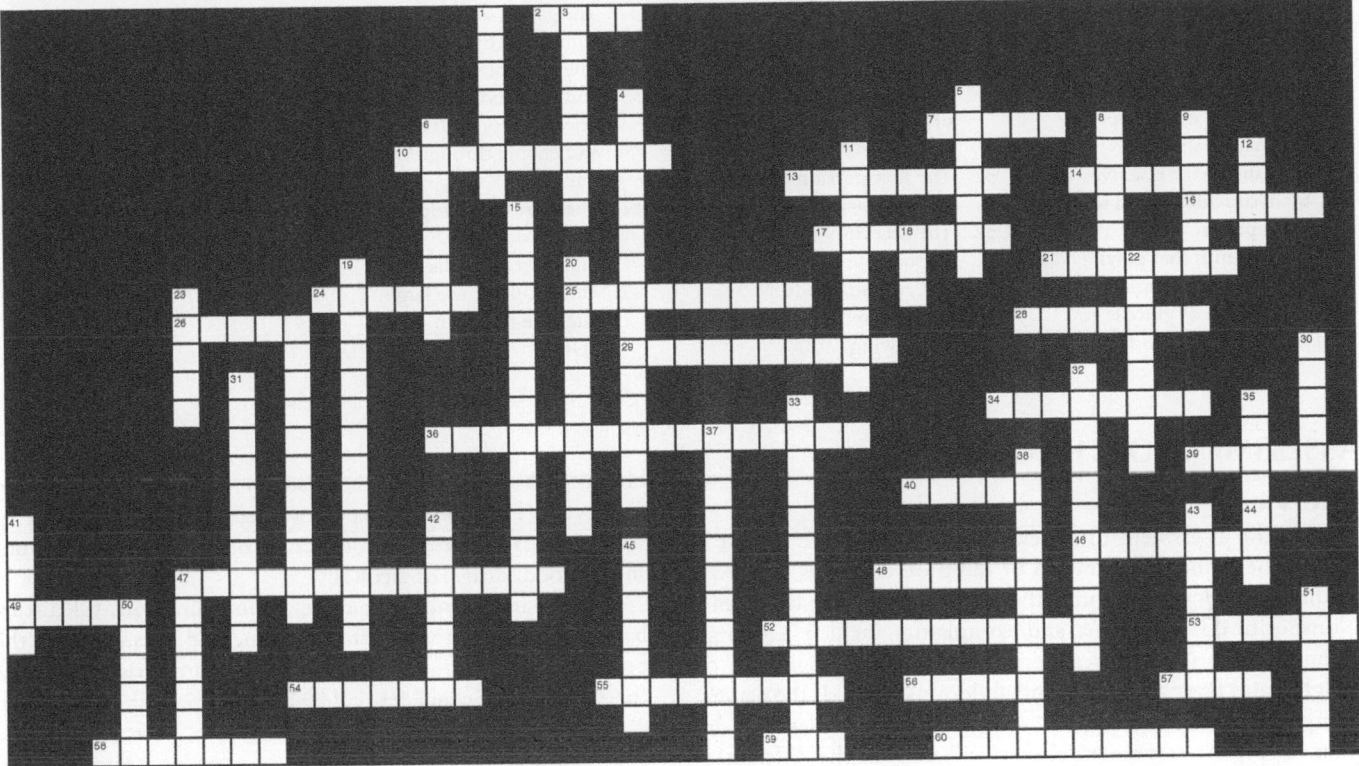

Answers to this activity can be found in the Answer Key.

ACROSS

2. The sphincter of _____ is a valve in the common bile duct that regulates passage of bile

7. _____'s patches are lymphoid follicles in the intestines

10. The membrane that covers the abdominal viscera

13. The accessory organ with both endocrine and exocrine functions

14. The accessory organ responsible for the conversion of ammonia to urea

16. These cells in the pancreas secrete somatostatin

17. The enzyme responsible for the breakdown of protein into amino acids

21. One of these lymph vessels is located in each villus

24. This duct comes from the gallbladder and joins the common hepatic duct to form the common bile duct

25. The hollow tube that passes through the thoracic cavity and the diaphragm

26. The last section of the small intestine

28. Absorption of this mineral requires vitamin D; it goes down if phosphorus goes up

29. This structure protects the airway by closing during swallowing

34. Intestinal losses are _____ so significant losses cause metabolic acidosis

36. The sphincter that is also referred to as the lower esophageal sphincter

39. This enzyme breaks down lipid

40. The term for the viscous, semifluid stomach contents that move through the pylorus into the small intestine

44. The nutrient source that is broken down into fatty acids

46. The enzyme in saliva that begins the breakdown of polysaccharides to disaccharides

47. The process of breaking down stored carbohydrate

48. The dome-shaped portion of the stomach that extends left of the cardia

49. These cells in the pancreas secrete glucagon

52. The nutrient source that is broken down into glucose, fructose, and galactose

53. These cells are in the pancreas and are responsible for exocrine function

54. The largest dilation of the GI tract

55. The major bile pigment; this is a breakdown product of hemoglobin

56. GI secretions are controlled by this nerve and the parasympathetic nervous system

57. These cells in the pancreas secrete insulin

58. The fold of the peritoneum that contains fat and lymph nodes

59. This branch of the autonomic nervous system slows gastric emptying (abbrev.)

60. Absorption of this type of vitamin requires the presence of bile salts; examples are ADEK (2 words)

DOWN

1. These glands are also referred to as parietal cells; they secrete hydrochloric acid and intrinsic factor

3. The shortest segment of the small intestine

4. The process of converting fat and protein to glucose

5. The flexure of the large intestine that is in the RUQ

6. The phase of gastric secretion that is stimulated by the thought, sight, smell, or taste of food

8. Gastric losses are ____ so significant losses cause metabolic alkalosis

9. The upper portion of the stomach

11. This factor is necessary for the intestinal absorption of vitamin B_{12}

12. This fluid is produced by the liver and stored in the gallbladder

15. The hormone that stimulates contraction of the gallbladder

18. The branch of the autonomic nervous system that speeds gastric emptying (abbrev.)

19. The sphincter that is also referred to as the upper esophageal sphincter

20. This substance is activated by hydrochloric acid to form pepsin

22. The vitamin that plays a chief role in the metabolic breakdown of glucose to yield energy in body tissue

23. These are fingerlike projections of mucosa and submucosa in the duodenum and jejunum that increase surface area (plural)

27. Another term for chewing

30. This substance is important in maintaining protection of the gastric mucosa from the effects of acid

31. The first portion of the alimentary canal

32. The accessory organ responsible for the storage and release of bile

33. Another term for swallowing

35. The cells that line the sinusoids of the liver and are responsible for phagocytosis

37. The gastric acid that is stimulated by gastrin

38. The alternate contraction and relaxation of muscle fibers that propels food and chyme through the GI tract

41. These are thick folds on the interior of the stomach that increase surface area

42. The flexure of the large intestine that is in the LUQ

43. The enzyme that breaks down lactose

45. The nutrient source that is broken down into amino acids

47. The hormone responsible for the secretion of hydrochloric acid

50. The lower portion of the stomach, close to the pylorus

51. The oral secretion stimulated by the thought, sight, smell, or taste of food

ASSESSMENT OF THE GI SYSTEM

Interview

During the assessment interview, determine why the patient is seeking help and the duration of the problem. This is known as the chief complaint and is the reason for seeking treatment. Nonspecific GI problems and complaints include a change in appetite, fatigue or weakness, unintentional weight loss or weight gain, fever and chills, and abdominal pain. If the patient complains of abdominal pain, ask him or her to describe the pain. Complete assessment of pain will assist in the differentiation of abdominal pain (Table 6-4).

Ask the patient to describe the pain using the OPQRST pneumonic. The **O** stands for onset of symptoms. The **P** stands for provocation or palliation. Provocation is the relationship of the pain to food, drugs, activity, position, bowel movements, breathing, and stress. Palliation refers to the ineffectiveness or effectiveness of treatments. Try to elicit what alleviates the pain (e.g., positioning). The **Q** stands for quality description. Elicit if the pain is sharp, dull, tearing, cramping, burning, gnawing, stabbing, aching, or colicky. Visceral pain is dull, poorly localized, and caused by organic lesions or functional disturbance within the GI tract. Somatic pain is sharp and well localized. Somatic pain may be caused by inflammation of abdominal organs, which causes peritoneal irritation. Referred pain is pain experienced at a distance from the disease process and related to the embryologic origins of the structures involved. The **R** stands for the region or location, which may be poorly localized because of referred pain. Pain may be felt in a remote area that is supplied by the same nerve as the diseased or damaged organ or may radiate to another location. This pain is usually sharp and localized but not over the area of injury. The **S** stands for severity and is measured according to a 0 to 10 scale. The **T** stands for the timing of the pain, which involves the duration and whether it is constant or intermittent.

Bloating is a subjective feeling of abdominal fullness versus abdominal distention, which is an objective increase in abdominal girth. Abdominal volume increase by at least 1 L needs to occur for measurable enlargement. Patients with GI disturbances may report a change in bowel elimination. A change in the color of stools may occur. Clay-colored stools indicate biliary obstruction. Tarry stools (i.e., melena) indicate upper GI bleeding. Bloody stools (i.e., hematochezia) indicate lower GI bleeding. A change in the consistency or shape of stools may also occur. Patients may report a change in the frequency of stools, excessive flatus, use of laxative or enemas, or a relationship to food, drugs, or alcohol.

Nausea and vomiting may be a complaint with GI disturbances. Ascertain the onset, duration, and frequency of the problem. It is important to note any characteristics such as the consistency, character, color, and/or presence of blood in vomitus (i.e., hematemesis). Ask the patient what palliates the problem. Search for the ineffective or effective treatments and alleviating factors. Investigate when the nausea and vomiting occurs, such as the time of day and if there is any relationship to food, odors, drugs, alcohol, activity, or bowel movements. Find out if there are any aggravating factors or associated pain.

Abdominal trauma is a major cause of GI disturbances. Motor vehicle accidents, falls, and violence are major causes of abdominal trauma. With gunshot wounds, look for both the entrance and exit sites. In addition, due to the velocity of the bullet, massive damage can occur to abdominal organs from tearing and shearing forces beyond the damage of what the bullet hits. Knife wounds, burns, or abrasions may be the cause of abdominal trauma. The appearance of ecchymotic areas across the abdomen often signifies blunt trauma has occurred. Penetrating wounds require exploratory surgery and repair.

Dentition issues and problems can be a major cause of GI disturbance. Caries, gingivitis, and poor-fitting dentures can affect eating habits and cause pain. In addition, odynophagia (painful swallowing), dysphagia (difficulty swallowing), and dyspepsia (impaired digestion) may be manifested by indigestion, nausea, abdominal pain, bloating, belching, and/or early satiety. GI problems may result in eructation (belching), flatulence, edema, abnormal bruising or bleeding, and jaundice. A change in urine color to dark brown or orange may indicate biliary obstruction. GI patients may complain of pruritus, fecal incontinence, rectal bleeding, or anal discomfort or pressure.

Determine whether the patient's past medical history indicates any past illnesses related to GI problems. Investigate whether the patient has ever had any jaundice or anemia. A history of obesity and the use of liquid diets or bariatric surgery would be important to know as well as any history of eating disorders (e.g., bulimia, anorexia nervosa). Elicit if there is a

TABLE 6-4	Differentiation of Abdominal Pain	
Condition	Description of Pain	Associated Signs/Symptoms
Abdominal aortic aneurysm	• Abdominal • Ripping or tearing • May radiate to back	• Pulsatile mass in abdomen • If ruptured, clinical indications of hypoperfusion and shock
Appendicitis	• Epigastric or periumbilical pain; later localizes to RLQ • Dull to sharp • May be referred to right shoulder • McBurney sign: pain with palpation at McBurney's point (i.e., point at ⅓ the distance between the right anterior iliac crest and the umbilicus) • Rovsing sign: pain in RLQ with palpation of LLQ indicates peritoneal irritation • Iliopsoas sign: abdominal pain caused by hyperextension of right hip	• Anorexia, nausea, or vomiting • Fever • Diarrhea • Leukocytosis • Clinical indications of peritoneal irritation if ruptured
Cholecystitis	• Epigastric or RUQ • Cramping • May be referred to below right scapula • Murphy sign: pain with deep breath while the nurse palpates under the right costal margin	• Nausea and vomiting, especially after fatty foods • Abdominal tenderness in RUQ • Leukocytosis
Diverticulitis	• LUQ • Cramping • Tenderness over descending colon	• Vomiting, diarrhea • Fever, chills • Bloating
Gastritis	• Epigastric or slightly left of midline • May be described as indigestion	• Nausea and vomiting • May have hematemesis • Abdominal tenderness
Intestinal obstruction	• Epigastric or periumbilical • Sharp if small intestine; dull if large intestine	• Change in bowel habits • Melena or hematochezia • Hyperactive to hypoactive bowel sounds
Mesenteric ischemia	• Diffuse midabdominal • Severe	• Nausea and vomiting may occur • Diarrhea or constipation
Pancreatitis	• Epigastric or periumbilical LUQ • Boring; worsened by lying down • May be referred to back, left flank, or left shoulder	• Nausea and vomiting • Mild fever • Abdominal tenderness • May have Cullen sign (i.e., bluish discoloration at umbilicus) indicating intraperitoneal bleeding or Grey-Turner sign (i.e., bluish discoloration at flanks) indicating retroperitoneal bleeding • May be jaundiced
Peptic ulcer	• Epigastric or RUQ • Gnawing or burning • May be referred to back	• Abdominal tenderness • Hematemesis (gastric) or melena (duodenal) • Clinical indications of peritoneal irritation if perforated
Strangulated hernia	• Localized • Severe • Generalized if bowel obstruction	• Distention if bowel obstruction

history or current issue with substance abuse of nonprescribed drugs or alcohol. Investigate the chronic use of potentially hepatotoxic agents such as acetaminophen. Identify any past or current history of GI disease. Query the patient on a history of the following:

• Peptic ulcer disease
• Gastroesophageal reflux disease (GERD)
• GI hemorrhage
• Cholelithiasis
• Hepatic disease
  • Cirrhosis
  • Hepatitis
  • History of blood transfusion
• Pancreatitis
• Cancer
• Irritable bowel syndrome
• Inflammatory bowel disease
  • Ulcerative colitis
  • Crohn disease
  • Antibiotic-associated colitis, *Clostridium difficile* colitis

- Diverticulitis
- Polyps
- Hemorrhoids
- Renal disease
- Cardiovascular disease
- Diabetes mellitus
- COPD (high incidence of peptic ulcer disease)
- Past injury: abdominal trauma
- Past surgical procedures
- Past diagnostic studies
  - Endoscopy
  - X-rays
  - Stool examination for occult blood
- Food intolerances or allergies; type of reaction if allergy

Question the patient about his or her family history. Often, many GI conditions have a familial tendency, and this knowledge can help determine a patient's risk. Determine whether the family history includes any of the following:

- Eating disorders (e.g., obesity, anorexia nervosa, bulimia)
- Anemia
- Peptic ulcer disease
- Pancreatic disease (e.g. pancreatitis, pancreatic cancer)
- Diabetes mellitus
- Liver disease (e.g., cirrhosis, hepatitis)
- Malabsorption syndrome
- Inflammatory bowel disease (e.g., ulcerative colitis, Crohn disease)
- Irritable bowel syndrome
- Alcoholism
- Cancer

Social history is also a very important part of a patient's history. Ask the patient about the current relationship with his or her spouse or significant other along with the current family structure. To develop the appropriate plan of care, seek knowledge about the patient's occupation, educational level, stress level, and usual coping mechanisms, along with individual recreational, exercise, and dietary habits.

The patient's appetite is an important clue to GI disorders. Ask the patient about the usual foods eaten and the number and timing of meals and snacks. Determine the patient's fluid intake. Find out if there are any food allergies, intolerances, prescribed restrictions, or religious restrictions. Ask whether there has been a change in eating habits. Determine the patient's caffeine intake, tobacco use, and alcohol use. Record tobacco use as pack-years (number of packs per day times the number of years of smoking). Record alcoholic beverages as consumed per month, week, or day.

Determine whether there has been recent travel and/or exposure to toxins or infectious disease. Finally, ask if there has been any change in bowel habits.

Medication history is vital to assessment. Find out about prescribed drugs, dosage, frequency, and time of last dose. Ask about intake of nonprescribed drugs, including over-the-counter drugs, herbal drugs and remedies, and substance abuse. Assess the patient's understanding of drug actions and side effects. Determine whether the patient is taking any of the following common drugs known to cause potential problems for patients with GI problems: antibiotics, aspirin, nonsteroidal antiinflammatory drugs (NSAIDs), corticosteroids, and acetaminophen. Many drugs have anorexia, nausea, or vomiting as side effects. Many drugs are potentially hepatotoxic (Box 6-1).

Many drugs treat GI problems. Antacids, H_2 receptor antagonists, and proton pump inhibitors treat indigestion and symptoms of GERD; these drugs are available over the counter. To regulate stool evacuation, the drugs that may be recommended include probiotics, antidiarrheals, stool softeners, laxatives, and cathartics. Many of these drugs are available over the counter. Anticholinergic medication treats abdominal cramping and spasms. Corticosteroids decrease inflammation and are effective for inflammatory bowel diseases. Antiemetic drugs treat nausea and vomiting. In addition, tranquilizers, sedatives, and barbiturates may be prescribed for severe irritable bowel syndrome, anxiety-induced GI symptoms, and nervous system disorders affecting the GI system.

Vital Signs

Vital signs including heart rate (HR), respiratory rate (RR), and temperature (T) along with blood pressure (BP) may indicate abnormalities. A blood pressure taken while the patient is sitting, lying, and standing is especially important to evaluate volume status. A systolic BP reading that is less than 100 mm Hg and an HR greater than 100 beats per minute (BPM) may indicate at least a 20% reduction in blood volume. An orthostatic change of 20 mm Hg in BP and/or 10 BPM in HR is also suggestive of hypovolemia. Current measurement of height and weight is important to note nutrition status and fluid balance. The body mass index (BMI) takes into account not just weight but also height to indicate body fat. A goal for most people is a BMI of 18 to 25 kg/m^2.

Inspection

Anatomic landmarks determine the location and documentation of assessment findings. Important landmarks of the abdomen include the xiphoid process, costal margin (along ribs), midline (center), umbilicus, anterior superior iliac crest, and symphysis pubis (Figure 6-10). The abdomen divides into four main quadrants (Figure 6-11) where the horizontal and vertical lines intersect at the umbilicus. In addition, the abdomen divides further into nine regions (Figure 6-12).

The general survey includes an assessment of the patient's apparent health status. Areas of assessment include whether the patient's apparent age is relative to the chronologic age, level of consciousness, presence of any gross deformity, nutritional status, body stature, gait, and posture. In a patient with abdominal pain, determine whether the patient is flexing his or her knees while supine. This position relieves abdominal tension frequently seen in peritonitis. A patient with pancreatitis leans forward to relieve abdominal pain. Inspect the patient's mouth. Note the lips for color, texture, lesions, swelling, and symmetry. Assess the gums for inflammation, retraction, hypertrophy, bleeding, and lesions. Examine the teeth for caries, state of repair, and the presence of an occlusion. Ascertain whether the patient has dentures and if they fit properly. Note if there is any gum ulceration caused by ill-fitting dentures. Check the tongue for swelling, lacerations, lesions, and the presence of any coating. Also, note moisture, lesions, and color of the oral mucosa. Assess mouth odor. Fetor hepaticus is a sweet fecal odor caused by hepatic failure. A feculent breath odor stems from a severe bowel obstruction. Poor dental hygiene or neoplasms of the esophagus or stomach result in severe halitosis.

Inspect the patient's skin color over the entire abdomen; the color should be homogenous and consistent with race.

BOX 6-1

Hepatotoxic Agents

- 6-Mercaptopurine (Purinethol)
- Acetaminophen (Tylenol)
- Acetylsalicylic acid (ASA)
- Allopurinol (Zyloprim)
- Amiodarone (Cordarone)
- Amitriptyline (Elavil)
- Ampicillin (Polycillin)
- Carbamazepine (Tegretol)
- Carbon tetrachloride
- Chlorambucil (Leukeran)
- Chloramphenicol (Geopen)
- Chlordiazepoxide (Librium)
- Chlorpromazine (Thorazine)
- Chlorpropamide (Diabinese)
- Cimetidine (Tagamet)
- Clindamycin (Cleocin)
- Cyclosporine (Sandimmune)
- Dantrolene (Dantrium)
- Diazepam (Valium)
- Doxepin (Sinequan)
- Erythromycin estolate (Ilosone)
- Ethanol
- Ethrane
- Ferrous sulfate
- Fluothane
- Haloperidol (Haldol)
- Halothane
- Hydrochlorothiazide (HydroDIURIL)
- Imipramine (Tofranil)
- Indomethacin (Indocin)
- Isoniazid (Isoniazid)
- Ketoconazole (Miconazole)
- Meprobamate (Equanil)
- Methotrexate (Methotrexate)
- Methyldopa (Aldomet)
- Monoamine oxidase (MAO) inhibitors
- Nicotinic acid
- Oral contraceptives
- Oxacillin (Prostaphlin)
- Penicillin (Pen Vee K)
- Erythromycin estolate (Ilosone)
- Penthrane
- Phenazopyridine (Pyridium)
- Phenobarbital (Luminal)
- Phenylbutazone (Butazolidin)
- Phenytoin (Dilantin)
- Probenecid (Benemid)
- Prochlorperazine (Compazine)
- Promethazine (Phenergan)
- Propylthiouracil (PTU)
- Quinidine
- Rifampin (Rifadin)
- Sulfonamides (Bactrim, Septra, Gantrisin)
- Tetracyclines (Achromycin)
- Tolbutamide (Orinase)
- Trimethobenzamide (Tigan)
- Tripelennamine (Pyribenzamine)

Pallor of skin indicates the presence of anemia, which can be from a GI source. Jaundice of the skin occurs when bilirubin is greater than 3 mg/dL and can be associated with liver disease, biliary obstruction, and excessive hemolysis. A bluish hue is due to infiltration of the abdominal wall with blood. Specific location of this bluish color is a sign of either retroperitoneal or intraperitoneal bleeding. Grey-Turner sign is ecchymosis to flanks and is indicative of retroperitoneal bleeding (e.g., pancreas, duodenum, kidneys, vena cava, aorta). Cullen sign is ecchymosis around the umbilicus indicative of intraperitoneal bleeding (e.g., liver, spleen). The major causes of intraperitoneal bleeding are hemorrhagic pancreatitis, infarcted bowel, and a ruptured ectopic pregnancy.

Note any lesions or discoloration of the abdomen. It is important to be knowledgeable about potential assessment findings and the relative effect of each discovery. There may be scars noted from trauma or prior surgical procedures. A stoma may be present from a prior surgery. If a stoma is present, note the stoma's location, color, drainage, and condition of peristomal skin. Striae (i.e., stretch marks) are usually vertical. Initially, striae are pinkish or bluish, but become silvery with time. Striae results from pregnancy, obesity, or ascites. Cushing's syndrome causes purplish striae. Additional assessment findings of the abdomen may include the presence of a rash, ecchymosis, abrasions, spider angiomas, and palmar erythema. Spider angiomas may be associated with vitamin B_{12} deficiency, liver disease, or pregnancy. Palmar erythema occurs in patients with cirrhosis and hepatic failure. A shiny, edematous abdomen indicates the

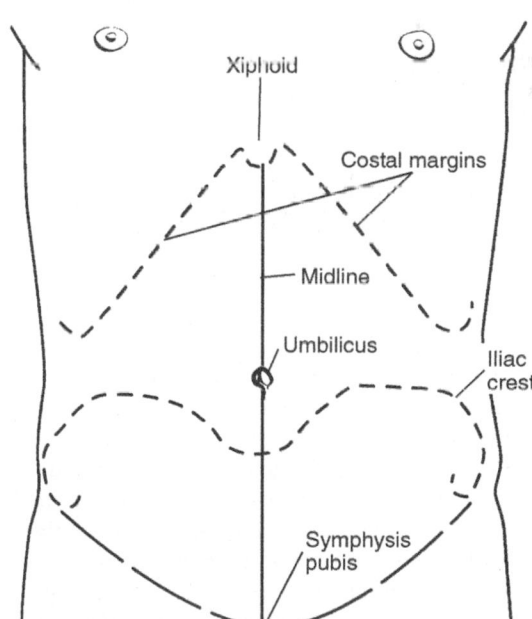

FIGURE 6-10 Abdominal landmarks.

presence of ascites or anasarca. Ascites is intraperitoneal fluid frequently associated with cirrhosis, intraabdominal malignancy (e.g., liver or ovarian), or right ventricular failure. Anasarca is entire body edema. Patients in end-stage heart failure or chronic kidney disease suffer from anasarca. Superficial vascularity of the abdomen occurs from obstruction of the inferior vena cava

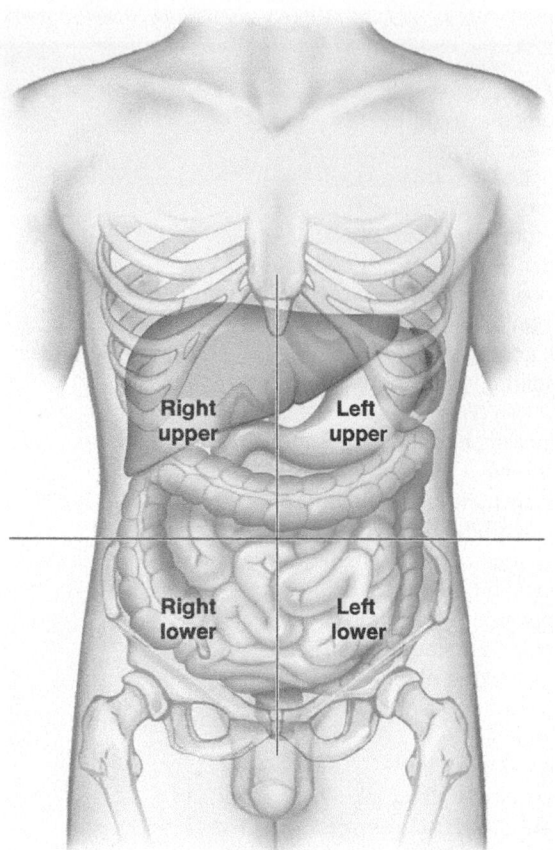

FIGURE 6-11 The abdomen divided into four quadrants. (From Patton, K. T., & Thibodeau, G. A. [2013]. *Anatomy & physiology* [8th ed.]. St. Louis, MO: Mosby.)

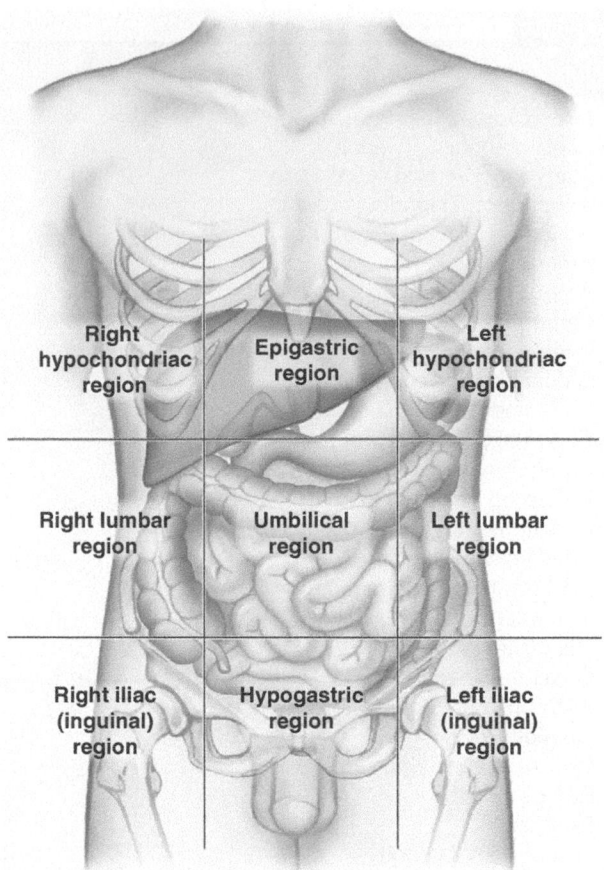

FIGURE 6-12 The abdomen divided into nine regions. (From Patton, K. T., & Thibodeau, G. A. [2013]. *Anatomy & physiology* [8th ed.]. St. Louis, MO: Mosby.)

or portal vein. Caput medusa is a pronounced dilation of the periumbilical veins radiating from the umbilicus seen in severe portal venous hypertension. In addition, it is important to note the presence and location of any draining wounds and/or fistulas. Assess the drainage and condition of surrounding skin.

Examine the contour of the abdomen. Note if the abdomen profile is normal, scaffold, or distended. A normal profile is flat from the xiphoid process to the pubic symphysis. A scaffold abdomen is concave and often seen in malnutrition. Distention or protuberance may be diffuse and symmetric. This contour profile is seen with obesity, flatus, pregnancy, fecal obstruction, ascites, malignancy, or fibroids. Abdominal distention in the upper quadrants tends to be from gastric dilation, pancreatic cyst, or malignancy. Distention in the lower quadrants is due to pregnancy, uterine fibroids, distended bladder, or ovarian tumors. Distention in one quadrant indicates a hernia, tumor, cyst, obstruction, or organomegaly. Measure abdominal girth at the largest area of the abdomen. Mark on either side of the abdomen with a tape measure so that measurements are consistently at same location. A one-inch increase is equal to an increase in intraabdominal volume of 500 to 1000 mL. Note any abdominal, umbilical, or inguinal hernia.

Movement of the abdomen occurs and is visualized with breathing, peristalsis, and aortic pulsations. Movement with breathing is normal. Visualization of abdominal movement with peristalsis is abnormal and when seen it is generally associated with intestinal obstruction. Aortic pulsation may be normally visible at the end of expiration in a supine patient, especially if the patient is thin. A pulsatile swelling in the

epigastrium suggests an abdominal aortic aneurysm or an epigastric solid tumor overlying the aorta.

Examine the color and contour of the umbilicus. A bluish color around the umbilicus (i.e., Cullen sign) is due to infiltration of the abdominal wall with blood. Poor hygiene results in inflammation and redness of the umbilicus area. The contour of the umbilicus may be inverted or everted. The umbilicus may be deeply inverted in obese patients. An everted umbilicus is seen with pregnancy or ascites. A nodule in the umbilicus, known as Sister Mary Joseph's nodule, may indicate intraabdominal carcinoma, especially in the stomach, with metastasis to the navel.

6.2   Learning Activity

List three general causes of jaundice.
1. _____
2. _____
3. _____

Answers to this activity can be found in the Answer Key.

Auscultation

Perform auscultation before percussion or palpation to prevent "stirring up" the abdomen. The order for physical assessment of the abdomen is inspection, auscultation, percussion, and palpation. Prepare the patient for the examination. It may be helpful to put a pillow under the patient's knees to relax abdominal muscles. Drape the patient to provide privacy. Make an effort to keep the patient warm and comfortable during the examination.

Auscultate bowel sounds using the diaphragm with light pressure for 1 minute in each of the four abdominal quadrants. If the patient is on nasogastric suction, disconnect the suction during the examination. If bowel sounds are hypoactive, 5 minutes of auscultation without audible bowel sounds is required before documenting the absence of bowel sounds. Normal bowel sounds are bubbling or soft gurgling noises heard every 5 to 20 seconds in an irregular pattern and auscultated in all quadrants.

Return of bowel motility after surgery is expected to occur in the small intestine first, usually within 4 to 24 hours. The sounds from the stomach occur in 2 to 4 days; sounds from the colon may not return until 3 to 7 days. Feeding before return of bowel sounds after surgery is now considered safe and bowel sounds are not considered an indication of expected feeding tolerance.

Very infrequent or absent bowel sounds indicate an abnormality. There can be a functional obstruction, such as a paralytic ileus, or an advanced mechanical intestinal obstruction.

Hyperperistalsis (e.g., diarrhea, catharsis caused by GI bleeding) results in loud, hyperactive, but normal pitched bowel sounds. High-pitched "rushing" bowel sounds indicate an early mechanical small intestinal obstruction. Low-pitched "rushing" bowel sounds indicate an early mechanical large intestinal obstruction. Roll the patient from side to side to assess for a succussion splash, which is indicative of a pyloric obstruction.

Auscultate vascular sounds using the bell of the stethoscope over specified areas of the abdomen. The presence of a bruit indicates turbulent blood flow. Listen for bruits over the midline and the renal and femoral arteries. If a bruit is noted, check the circulation to the extremities. If decreased blood flow is noted, suspect an aneurysm and notify the physician, keep the patient quiet, and do not palpate the abdomen. Also, assess for a venous hum and a peritoneal friction rub. Blood flow in a large, engorged vascular organ such as the liver or spleen creates the medium-toned venous hum. A peritoneal friction rub is a scratchy sound heard over inflamed spleen or neoplastic liver.

Percussion

Percussion is a technique valuable in assessment of the abdomen. The percussion tones normally heard over the abdomen are dull, flat, or tympanic. Dull percussion tones are heard at the liver, full sigmoid colon, and full bladder. Flat sounds are heard over bone. Tympany is heard at the gastric bubble and over empty bowel areas.

Tests for ascites include the fluid wave, shifting dullness, and midline dullness. To test for a fluid wave, tap one side of the abdomen and feel the wave sensation hit the hand on the other side of the abdomen. Have a colleague or the patient place the ulnar surface of his or her hand at the abdomen's midline to stop skin transmission. To conduct the test for shifting dullness, percuss dullness indicating fluid at flanks while the patient is supine. Mark the fluid level and turn the patient on one side, and determine if the line shifts from the previous marked area. To test for midline dullness, have the patient lean forward in a standing position and percuss the abdomen for dullness at the midline. A positive finding on any of these tests indicates intraabdominal fluid.

Determine the location of organ borders and organ size using percussion. The liver span is the area of dullness between right lung resonance and bowel tympany. Normal span is 6 to 12 cm in the right midclavicular line. Patients with right ventricular failure (RVF), hepatitis, and mononucleosis present with an enlarged and tender span. The liver may be large or small in cirrhosis. Absence of liver dullness may indicate free air in the peritoneum from bowel perforation. In some instances, the spleen can be percussed as dullness under the left diaphragm. If percussible, it should be less than 7 cm at the left midaxillary line. The percussion tone of the stomach is tympany under the left costal margin. Percussed dullness above the symphysis pubis detects an enlarged bladder due to volume or excess mass. Otherwise, the bladder is not percussible. Tympanic tones over the intestines signify empty lumen, while dullness occurs over the left lower quadrant (LLQ) if the sigmoid colon is full.

Palpation

Warm your hands before performing palpation. Carry on a conversation with the patient to keep him or her relaxed, which will relax the abdominal muscles as well. Place a pillow under the patient's knees and another pillow under the head. Keep the patient warm and properly draped. Examine each quadrant. Always palpate any tender areas last.

Perform light palpation first. Use your fingertips to depress 1 to 2 cm and note the skin temperature and moisture level. Determine whether guarding is voluntary or involuntary. With voluntary guarding, the patient may voluntarily splint abdominal muscles, especially when a sensitive spot is touched. Watch for nonverbal indicators of pain during palpation. Diffuse involuntary guarding or rigidity suggests an infectious, neoplastic, or inflammatory process in the peritoneal cavity. A rigid, boardlike abdomen is associated with acute perforation of a viscus with spillage of air or GI contents into the peritoneal cavity. Note any tender areas or large masses. If a mass is pulsatile, refrain from additional abdominal palpation because this may be an abdominal aortic aneurysm. If the mass is not pulsatile, describe the size, location, consistency, contour, tenderness, and mobility.

Avoid deep palpation in patients with aneurysms or polycystic kidneys, after renal transplant or recent surgery, and in the presence of a malignant tumor (may cause seeding). Perform deep palpation using one hand on top of the other to depress 4 to 5 cm. Note direct tenderness and rebound tenderness. Direct tenderness is associated with local inflammation of the abdominal wall, the peritoneum, or a viscus. Perform rebound (or indirect) tenderness (also referred to as *Blumberg's sign*) by pressing into the tender area and then letting go. If the pain occurs when pressure is released, rebound tenderness is present and peritoneal inflammation is suspected. Rebound tenderness is especially significant when it occurs at a site away from the area of direct tenderness.

Organ size and tenderness can also be estimated using deep palpation. The liver edge may be palpable. Ask the patient to take a deep breath and move your hand in and up to check for tenderness and the smoothness of edge. Tenderness is frequently caused by hepatitis or engorgement caused by RVF. A hard, lumpy liver may be associated with cancer or cirrhosis. A normal size liver may be palpable especially in patients with COPD due to hyperinflation of the lungs so hepatomegaly exists only if the liver span by percussion is greater than 12 cm. The gallbladder can be palpable only if enlarged with stones. If it is palpable, it is located under the liver edge in the right upper quadrant. The spleen is palpable only if significantly enlarged (e.g., injury, leukemia, mononucleosis, portal hypertension). Palpate in the spleen area to note tenderness. Palpate the left side of the abdomen with the patient in the lateral decubitus position. Check any aortic pulsation for lateral expansion, which may indicate an aneurysm. Ballottement is the gentle repetitive bouncing of tissues against the hand used to evaluate organ enlargement.

Diagnostic Studies

Routine serum chemistry analysis helps evaluate a patient's GI status. Examine electrolyte levels. Some specific alterations are associated with GI problems. The serum sodium level is elevated in dehydration from severe diarrhea or intestinal obstruction. The serum potassium level is decreased in GI losses from the upper or lower GI tract. The serum chloride level may be elevated in dehydration, yet decreased in patients who suffer from vomiting, diarrhea, or intestinal obstruction. Serum calcium level decreases in acute pancreatitis. Serum phosphorus level is elevated in intestinal obstruction but decreased with malnutrition or malabsorption syndromes. Chronic diarrhea causes the serum magnesium to decrease. Fasting serum glucose levels are elevated in diabetes mellitus, in pancreatitis, and during acute stress. The BUN and creatinine remain relatively stable in GI disturbances unless there is compromise to the renal function.

The complete blood count (CBC) evaluates any variations from normal with the hemoglobin, hematocrit, and white blood cell count with differential. In addition, the erythrocyte sedimentation rate (ESR) and a clotting profile are useful to examine any associated impact of GI disturbances on normal and therapeutic values.

Other serum analyses evaluated in GI problems include gastrin, ammonia, iron, iron-binding capacity, lactate, carcinoembryonic antigen (CEA), and bilirubin. The gastrin level is elevated in Zollinger-Ellison syndrome (i.e., gastrin-producing pancreatic tumor) or G-cell hyperplasia that may cause peptic ulcer disease. Ammonia is a byproduct of protein metabolism, and serum ammonia level is elevated in hepatic failure, acute kidney injury or chronic kidney disease, and heart failure. GI problems may affect iron, iron-binding capacity, and lactate levels. CEA is elevated in cancer of the colon, lung, pancreas, stomach, breast, head, neck, and prostate. Total bilirubin is elevated in hepatic disease, biliary obstruction, or excessive hemolysis. Direct (i.e., conjugated) bilirubin is elevated in biliary obstruction, and indirect (i.e., unconjugated) bilirubin is elevated in hepatic disease or excessive hemolysis.

Serum proteins are important to evaluate in GI disturbances. The major serum protein is albumin. Because the half-life of albumin is 19 to 20 days, it is a poor indicator of acute changes in nutritional status. However, the half-life of prealbumin is only 2 to 3 days, so it is a better indicator of changes in nutritional status. Transferrin has a half-life of 8 to 10 days, so it also indicates changes in nutritional status better than albumin but not as promptly as prealbumin. The albumin/globulin ratio (A/G) is normally 1.5:1 to 2.5:1; this ratio is reverse in chronic hepatitis and chronic liver disease. Evaluate serum lipids and pepsinogen in GI disturbances. Serum pepsinogen is elevated in any situation of hemoconcentration and decreased with poor nutrition or hemorrhage.

A major function of the GI system is the secretion of enzymes to aid the digestion process; therefore, the enzyme evaluation is crucial in the diagnostic process of GI disturbances. Serum alkaline phosphatase is elevated in cirrhosis, rheumatoid arthritis, biliary obstruction, liver tumor, and hyperparathyroidism. Serum amylase is elevated in acute pancreatitis, pancreatic cancer, pancreatic pseudocysts, perforated peptic ulcer, mesenteric thrombosis, ectopic pregnancy, acute kidney injury or chronic kidney disease, and the mumps. Serum lipase level is elevated in acute or chronic pancreatitis, duodenal ulcer, biliary obstruction, cirrhosis, and hepatitis. The serum lipase level also stays elevated longer than the amylase level in pancreatitis. Serum alanine aminotransferase (ALT) level, formerly called the serum glutamic-pyruvic transaminase (SGPT), measures the amount of a substance called glutamate pyruvate transaminase (GPT), an enzyme that is concentrated in the liver and released into the blood when liver cells are damaged. ALT is elevated in hepatitis, cirrhosis, liver tumor, hepatotoxic drugs, cholestasis, and infectious mononucleosis. Serum aspartate aminotransferase (AST) level, formerly called serum glutamic oxaloacetic transaminase (SGOT), is an enzyme found in the liver, muscles (including the heart), and red blood cells and is released into the blood when these cells are damaged. AST is elevated in hepatitis, cirrhosis, acute pancreatitis, skeletal muscle disease or trauma, and liver tumors. Gamma-glutamyl transferase (GGT) is elevated in hepatitis, cirrhosis, liver tumor, cholestasis, alcohol ingestion, and myocardial infarction. Lactate dehydrogenase (LDH) is elevated in hepatitis, hemolytic anemia, pancreatitis, muscular dystrophy, pulmonary infarction, myocardial infarction, pernicious anemia, and renal disease. Serum analysis may include serology for viral hepatitis.

A urinalysis may show abnormalities in urobilogen level. Urobilogen is elevated in hepatic disease and decreased in complete biliary obstruction. Gastric analysis examines acids and other secretions found in the stomach. Gastric analysis provides diagnostic information and determines effectiveness of surgical or medical treatments. This study begins with insertion of a nasogastric tube. The patient receives a histamine or insulin injection to stimulate acid production. Gastric secretions collected are analyzed for hydrochloric acid. It is important to have diphenhydramine (Benadryl) available if histamine is used or 50% dextrose available if insulin is used.

The evaluation of gastric pH determines the tube placement. The stomach pH is 1 to 3, whereas the intestine pH is 6.5 or greater. Analysis of the pH also determines effectiveness of proton pump inhibitors, H_2 receptor antagonists, and/or antacid therapy. A pH of 3.5 to 5 is desirable.

Stool examination includes checking for fecal occult blood and the presence of ova or parasites. Freshly collected specimens should be taken to the lab within 1 hour if formed stool and within 30 minutes if liquid stool. Normal results would be a negative for presence of blood, ova, and parasites. Fecal fat content is elevated in cystic fibrosis, Crohn disease, biliary tract obstruction, and pancreatic duct obstruction. This type of specimen requires a wax-free container. Fecal urobilinogen decreases in biliary obstruction. The specimen requires a light-resistant container. A stool culture should demonstrate normal intestinal flora, but no pus should be present. An assay for *Clostridium difficile* toxin A or B in the stool may be positive in diarrhea if caused by *C. difficile,* an opportunistic infection associated primarily with suppression of normal flora by anti-biotic therapy.

The findings of the basic assessment and baseline diagnostic tests guide further diagnostic workup. Other diagnostic studies for GI disturbance include more invasive and costly procedures and diagnostic examinations. These diagnostic examinations provide a more definitive diagnosis but are associated with an increased complication risk, increased preparation time, and more complex preprocedure and postprocedure care (Table 6-5).

PHARMACOLOGY

Several classifications of medications treat various GI disorders. One major indication for pharmacologic treatment is the need to decrease gastric acidity and/or to protect the gastric mucosa. This action will prevent and/or treat a peptic ulcer. Antacids such as aluminum-magnesium complex (Riopan), magnesium hydroxide and aluminum hydroxide (Maalox), or calcium carbonate (TUMS) will buffer gastric acid and increase pH to decrease the activity of pepsin. Another drug classification used to decrease gastric acidity and protect the gastric mucosa is histamine (H_2) receptor antagonists. H_2 blockers cimetidine (Tagamet), ranitidine (Zantac), famotidine (Pepcid), and nizatidine (Axid) block the action of histamine on parietal cells to inhibit volume and concentration of gastric secretions.

Proton pump inhibitors (PPIs) inactivate the hydrogen pump, preventing formation of hydrochloric acid by parietal cells. Examples of PPIs include omeprazole (Prilosec), lansoprazole (Prevacid), and pantoprazole sodium (Protonix). Misoprostol (Cytotec) is a prostaglandin E1-analog drug that enhances the body's normal gastric mucosal protective mechanisms, increases mucosal blood flow, and decreases gastric acid secretion. A muscle protectant, sucralfate (Carafate), combines with gastric acid forming an adhesive protective coating over an ulcer crater and absorbs pepsin.

Controversies exist regarding the prophylactic treatment with medications to decrease gastric acidity and/or to protect the gastric mucosa. Costs of prophylaxis are considerable, and the number needed to treat or prevent even one case of GI bleeding is significant. There are associated risks of changing the pH of the gastric secretions. The action may impair digestion and absorption of drugs normally absorbed in the acidic environment of the stomach. These drugs may also increase the risk of pneumonia because bacteria killed in the acid medium of the stomach live, proliferate, and ascend the esophagus and are silently aspirated. Due to these risks, reserve prophylaxis treatment for the following patients:

- Patients already exhibiting GI bleeding
- Patients with a history of GI bleeding
- Patients with head injury
- Patients with burns

The medications vasopressin (Pitressin) and octreotide acetate (Sandostatin) treat GI bleeding. The indication for octreotide acetate (Sandostatin) includes severe diarrhea associated with carcinoid tumors or vasoactive intestinal peptide tumors. It has been also used off-label for GI bleeding and GI or pancreatic fistula and after partial pancreatectomy (Whipple procedure). Octreotide acetate inhibits the release of vasodilatory hormones to cause vasoconstriction of the viscera and decrease portal vein flow and portal hypertension. The drug also suppresses the secretion of serotonin, gastroenteropancreatic peptides, and growth hormones and stimulates fluid and electrolyte absorption from the GI tract and prolongs GI transmit time. Another drug indicated to treat GI bleeding but currently less commonly used is vasopressin. The action of this drug is to constrict the mesenteric arterioles and decrease portal circulation and pressure.

GI patients may be taking a complex regimen of medications. Their individual conditions and health status may dictate the need for several alternatives. Shorter-acting drugs and dosing patterns may be required. Medications administered may relate to the treatment of the primary cause of disorder and/or the prevention and treatment of complications. Close monitoring and caution are required (Table 6-6).

6.3 Learning Activity

List four classifications of drugs used to prevent ulcers and an example of each one.

Type	Example
1.	
2.	
3.	
4.	

Answers to this activity can be found in the Answer Key.

GENERAL PATIENT CARE FOR PATIENTS WITH GI CONDITIONS

Priorities of patient care for GI patients in the progressive care unit focus on maintaining a patent airway; managing fluid, electrolyte, and/or acid-base imbalances; and ensuring adequate nutrition. With acute hemorrhage or encephalopathy, the patient may be unable to maintain the airway because of altered levels of consciousness or possible aspiration due to vomiting. The goal of care for the health care team in the progressive care unit is to closely monitor airway compromise and to reestablish and maintain a patent airway. If airway problems occur, arrange to transfer the patient to a higher level of care. To manage fluid, electrolyte, and acid-base imbalances, assess the patient values and restore deficits of circulating fluid volume, replace electrolytes, and normalize pH. To maintain nutritional status, perform accurate monitoring and recording of the patient's weight, intake and output, and calorie count and ensure the patient's intake meets minimum daily requirements for both calories and nutrients.

MALNUTRITION

Malnutrition exists when the dietary intake of essential nutrients is insufficient to meet the metabolic demands of the body. Both macronutrients and micronutrients are required to sustain body functions. Macronutrients come from the carbohydrate, protein, and fat intake. Micronutrients include vitamins, minerals, and water.

TABLE 6-5	Gastrointestinal Diagnostic Studies	
Study	**Evaluates**	**Comments**

Angiography: celiac or mesenteric	• Evaluates portal vasculature
	• Identifies source of gastrointestinal bleeding
	• Evaluates cirrhosis, portal hypertension, vascular damage resulting from trauma, intestinal ischemia, tumors
	• May be used to treat GI bleeding using vasopressin
		• Bowel preparation (e.g., cathartics) as prescribed
		• NPO for 8 hours before the study
		• Sedative is usually prescribed before the procedure
		• Contrast media used
		  • Check for allergy to iodine before the study
		  • Monitor for allergic reaction following procedure
		  • Ensure hydration following procedure
		Postprocedure
		• Keep extremity in which catheter was placed immobilized in a straight position for 6-12 hours
		• Monitor arterial puncture point for hemorrhage or hematoma
		• Monitor neurovascular status of affected limb
		• Monitor for indications of systemic emboli

Barium enema (also called lower GI series) NOTE: Meglumine diatrizoate (Gastrografin) may be used especially if bowel perforation is suspected	• Visualizes the movement, position, and filling of various segments of the colon after instillation of barium by enema • Diagnoses colorectal lesions, diverticulitis, inflammatory bowel disease, strictures, and fistulas • Evaluates colon size, length, and patency	• Low-fiber diet for 1-3 days before the study • Bowel preparation with bowel irrigation (e.g., GoLYTELY) and cathartics • NPO for 8-12 hours before study • Cathartics must be given after study • Contraindicated if bowel perforation or obstruction exists
Barium swallow, upper GI series, and small bowel follow-through NOTE: Ordered according to which area or areas need to be evaluated (e.g., upper GI with small bowel follow-through means stomach, pylorus, or duodenum; barium swallow with upper GI means esophagus, stomach, or pylorus) NOTE: Meglumine diatrizoate (Gastrografin) may be used especially if bowel perforation is suspected	• Visualizes the position, shape, and activity of the esophagus, stomach, duodenum, and jejunum • Diagnoses esophageal lesions, varices, or esophageal motility disorders; hiatal hernia; gastric ulcers and tumors, small bowel obstruction; small bowel lesions; Crohn disease • Evaluates gastric and small bowel motility	• Bowel preparation with bowel irrigation (e.g., GoLYTELY) and cathartics • NPO for 8-12 hours before study • Cathartics must be given after study • Contraindicated if bowel perforation or obstruction exists

Cholecystography (oral, intravenous, percutaneous transhepatic, or common bile duct)	• Assesses gallbladder function, patency of the biliary system, and presence of gallstones
	• Diagnoses extrahepatic or intrahepatic jaundice, biliary calculi, biliary obstruction, and common bile duct injury
		• Percutaneous transhepatic cholangiography is contraindicated in patients with bleeding disorders
		• Fatty meal the day before the study, but the evening meal is fat-free
		• Enema may be given the evening before the study
		• NPO 8-12 hours before the study
		• Contrast medium is administered orally the evening before the study, administered intravenously immediately before the study, injected percutaneously into the bile duct, or injected directly into the common bile duct during surgery
		  • Check for allergy to iodine before the study
		  • Monitor for allergic reaction following procedure
		  • Ensure hydration following procedure
		• Monitor for clinical indications of bile leakage, hemorrhage, or peritonitis after percutaneous transhepatic cholangiography

TABLE 6-5	Gastrointestinal Diagnostic Studies—cont'd	
Study	**Evaluates**	**Comments**

Computed tomography (CT) scan of abdomen	• Identifies tumors, pancreatic cancer or cysts, pancreatitis, biliary tract disorders, obstructive versus nonobstructive jaundice, cirrhosis, liver metastases, ascites, lymph node metastases, aneurysm
	• Evaluates vasculature and focal points found on nuclear scans
	• Used to direct biopsy of tumors or aspiration of abscess
		• No special preparation required
		• If contrast medium is used:
		  • Check for allergy to iodine before the study
		  • Monitor for allergic reaction postprocedure
		  • Ensure hydration postprocedure

Endoscopic retrograde cholangiopancreatography (ERCP)	• Identifies biliary stones, ductal stricture, ductal compression, and neoplasms of the pancreas and biliary system • Evaluates patency of biliary and pancreatic ducts, jaundice, pancreatitis, cholecystitis, and hepatitis	• Same as for EGD • Contraindicated if patient is uncooperative or if bilirubin is greater than 3.5 mg/dL • Monitor for clinical indications of pancreatitis (most common complication) after study • Monitor for clinical indications of sepsis
Endoscopy • EGD • Colonoscopy • Proctosigmoidoscopy	• Directly visualizes mucosa of areas of the GI tract • EGD can be extended to visualize the pancreas and gallbladder • EGD is used to diagnose esophagitis, esophageal ulcers, esophageal strictures, esophageal varices, hiatal hernia, gastritis, gastric ulcers, pyloric obstruction, pernicious anemia, foreign bodies, duodenal inflammation or ulcers, and to evaluate esophageal or gastric motility, bleeding, lesions, and status of surgical anastomoses • Esophagoscopy or gastroscopy may also be used therapeutically for sclerosis of varices • Proctosigmoidoscopy diagnoses rectosigmoid cancer, strictures, polyps, inflammatory processes, and hemorrhoids and evaluates bleeding from rectosigmoid and surgical anastomoses • Colonoscopy diagnoses diverticular disease, obstruction, strictures, radiation injury, polyps, neoplasms, bleeding, and ischemia • Colonoscopy or sigmoidoscopy may be used therapeutically for removal of polyps • Biopsies may be taken during any endoscopy	• Sedation may be prescribed, especially for colonoscopy • Bowel preparation with gastric irrigation (e.g., GoLYTELY) and cathartics required before lower GI endoscopy • NPO 4-8 hours before study • Keep NPO until gag reflex returns if sedation used • Monitor closely after procedure for clinical indications of perforation or hemorrhage
Flat plate of abdomen (may also be referred to as *KUB*)	• Diagnoses perforated viscus, paralytic ileus, mechanical obstruction, and intraabdominal mass • Evaluates the distribution of visceral gas (and identifies free air in the peritoneum, indicative of bowel perforation) • Evaluates organ size	• No preparation required

Continued

TABLE 6-5	Gastrointestinal Diagnostic Studies—cont'd		
Study	**Evaluates**	**Comments**	

Liver biopsy	• Obtains tissue specimen for microscopic evaluation
	• Diagnoses liver disease or malignancy
		• May be performed open or closed
		  • Open is done in surgery
		  • Closed biopsy may be done at bedside
		• Clotting profile is evaluated preprocedure
		  • Closed biopsy is contraindicated if platelet count is less than 100000/mm³
		• Patients must be cooperative because they must hold their breath during closed biopsy
		• Type and crossmatch for two units of blood preprocedure
		• NPO for 4-8 hours before study
		Postprocedure
		• Position patient on right side for 2 hours
		• Pressure dressing is applied, and the patient is on bed rest for 24 hours
		• Observe for:
		  • Hemorrhage: hypotension or dyspnea (subphrenic hematoma)
		  • Pneumothorax: dyspnea, chest pain, diminished breath sounds on right, and hypoxemia
		  • Sepsis: fever, leukocytosis, rebound tenderness	

Liver scan	• Identifies cirrhosis, hepatitis, tumors, abscesses, cysts, and tuberculosis	• No preparation required	
Magnetic resonance imaging (MRI)	• Evaluates liver, biliary tree, pancreas, and spleen • Differentiation between cyst and solid mass • Diagnoses hepatic metastasis • Evaluates abscesses, fistulas, and source of GI bleeding • Used for staging of colorectal cancer	• Cannot be used in patients with any implanted metallic device, including pacemakers • No special preparation required • Cannot be done on a patient being mechanically ventilated • Must be able to lie flat and still for ~30-60 minutes during the scan; sedation may be necessary	
Paracentesis	• Analysis of fluid removed during peritoneal tap • Diagnoses intraperitoneal bleeding with diagnostic peritoneal lavage	• Monitor for peritoneal leakage after tap • Monitor for clinical indications of infection or peritonitis after tap	
Percutaneous transhepatic cholangiography	• Identifies extrahepatic or intrahepatic jaundice, biliary calculi, bile duct obstruction, and bile duct injury • Evaluates the patency of the biliary ductal system	• Contraindicated in uncorrected coagulopathy, allergy to iodine, severe ascites, and cholangitis • Monitor closely for clinical indications of bleeding or peritonitis	
Percutaneous transhepatic portography	• Identifies esophageal varices and visualizes portal venous circulation	• As for angiography	
Radionuclide imaging (hepatobiliary scintigraphy) • Hepatobiliary iminodiacetic acid (HIDA) scan • Paraisopropyl iminodiacetic acid (PIPIDA) scan	• Identifies hepatocellular disease, hepatic metastasis, biliary disease, lower GI bleeding, gastric reflux	• NPO 2 hours before study • Must be able to lie flat and still for 60 minutes during the scan	
Schilling test	• Evaluates ileal absorption of vitamin B_{12} • Identifies pernicious anemia caused by intrinsic factor and inadequate ileal absorption of intrinsic factor-vitamin B_{12} complex	• Intramuscular (IM) vitamin B_{12} and oral radioactive B_{12} are given and 24-hour urine specimen is collected	

TABLE 6-5	Gastrointestinal Diagnostic Studies—cont'd	
Study	**Evaluates**	**Comments**
Ultrasound of abdomen	• Evaluates the pancreas, biliary ducts, gallbladder, and liver • Identifies tumor, abdominal abscesses, hepatocellular disease, splenomegaly, and pancreatic or splenic cysts • Differentiates obstructive from nonobstructive jaundice	• All barium must have been cleared from the GI tract before ultrasonography • NPO for 8 hours before study • If for evaluation of gallbladder: fat-free meal the evening before study • Must be able to lie flat and still for 30 minutes during the procedure

TABLE 6-6	Selected GI Drugs		
Drug	**Administration**	**Adverse Effects**	**Nursing Implications**
Octreotide acetate (Sandostatin)	For GI hemorrhage • SC: 50-150 mcg bid or tid • IV injection (for GI bleeding): 25-50 mcg followed by IV infusion • IV infusion (for GI bleeding): 25-50 mcg/hour for 48 hours	• Orthostatic hypotension • Anorexia, nausea, vomiting, and abdominal pain • Diarrhea, constipation, and steatorrhea • Abdominal bloating, flatulence • Increase in liver enzymes • Anxiety • Dizziness • Drowsiness • Heartburn • Hypoglycemia or hyperglycemia • Rectal spasm	• Monitor HR, BP • Monitor for GI complaints and/or bleeding and serum glucose • Note contraindication: known hypersensitivity • Note that this drug is tolerated better than vasopressin for GI bleeding, especially in patients with CAD • Note pain or burning at injection site • Do not administer if precipitation or discoloration occurs
Prototype PPI Pantoprazole sodium (Protonix)	• IV injection: 40 or 80 mg over 2 minutes; may also be diluted in 100 mL and infused over 15 minutes; followed by infusion • IV infusion: 8 mg/hour • PO: 40 mg twice daily	• Headache • Diarrhea, abdominal pain, flatulence • Rash • Hyperglycemia	• Monitor for GI complaints and/or bleeding and serum glucose • Note contraindications: known hypersensitivity
Prototype H$_2$ receptor antagonist Ranitidine (Zantac)	• PO: 150 mg twice daily with 300 at bedtime • IM: 50 mg every 6-8 hours • IV injection: 50 mg in 20 mL slowly every 6-8 hours or 50 mg in 100 mL over 15-20 minutes • IV infusion: mix 300 mg in 250 mL (1.2 mg/mL); usual dose 6.25-12.5 mg/hour	• Dizziness • Elevated liver enzymes, hepatotoxicity • Headache • Malaise	• Monitor heart rate, BP, liver enzymes, gastric pH • pH is maintained 3.5 or greater • Note contraindications: known hypersensitivity • Use cautiously in liver disease, renal disease
Vasopressin (Pitressin)	For GI hemorrhage • IV infusion: mix 100 units/100 mL (1 IU/mL) and administer at 0.1-0.8 IU/minute (concurrent nitroglycerin is recommended with doses higher than 0.4 IU/minute) • Administer through central venous catheter	• Bradycardia • Hypertension • Fever • Water intoxication (SIADH), hyponatremia • Nausea, abdominal cramps • Tremor • Headache • Seizures • Coma • Constriction of cardiac arteries, resulting in chest pain and myocardial ischemia	• Monitor heart rate, BP, daily weight, serum sodium • Note contraindications: known hypersensitivity, nephritis • Use cautiously in coronary artery disease • Administer NTG as prescribed concurrently with IV vasopressin infusion to prevent potential complications related to cardiac ischemia • Prevent extravasation as necrosis may occur; treat with phentolamine (Regitine)

There are three types of malnutrition: marasmus, kwashiorkor, and mixed marasmus and kwashiorkor. Marasmus is a gradual wasting of body fat and somatic muscle with preservation of visceral proteins as seen in prolonged starvation and chronic illness. Visceral protein wasting with preservation of fat and somatic muscle defines kwashiorkor malnutrition and this type of malnutrition is seen in cases of poverty. The patient may appear well nourished, overweight, or obese, and edema may be present. Hospitalized patients suffer a mixed marasmus and kwashiorkor type of malnutrition that is associated with the highest mortality and morbidity rates. Conditions that decrease nutrient intake, decrease absorption, increase nutrient loss, or increase nutrient requirements cause malnutrition and occur in hospitals for various medical reasons (Table 6-7).

Without nutrient intake in individuals with even minor acute illness or injury, atrophy occurs. Atrophy of mucosal cells in the small bowel can occur in as little as 72 hours. This cell atrophy is a major facilitator for bacterial translocation, a common cause of sepsis, and multiple organ dysfunction syndrome (MODS) in acutely ill patients. Inadequate calories cause glycogenolysis and gluconeogenesis to occur. The stress of illness stimulates the stress hormones of cortisol and glucagon. These hormones have catabolic functions, which result in hypermetabolism, glycogenolysis with increased glucose utilization, gluconeogenesis with increased protein and fatty acid utilization, insulin resistance, and depletion of lean body tissue. Glycogenolysis, gluconeogenesis, and stress hormones all lead to hyperglycemia. The serum glucose level relates to the degree of illness/injury. Hyperglycemia requires treatment with insulin to keep serum glucose within normal levels because hyperglycemia interferes with immune function.

Malnutrition causes immunodeficiency, poor wound healing, and/or eventually organ failure. Patients with malnutrition may complain of anorexia, diarrhea, weakness, fatigue, apathy, irritability, and headache. Clinical assessment findings of malnutrition are varied. The patient may have brittle, dry hair or hair loss. The integumentary changes include pale, dry, flaky skin; poor skin turgor; poor wound healing; peripheral edema; and transverse ridging of the fingernails. Fissures at the angles of the lips (i.e., cheilosis), hyperemic tongue, and hypertrophic or atrophic tongue papillae are oral changes seen with malnutrition. In addition, gum and teeth problems are evident. There may be a loss of teeth, dental caries, and bleeding or receding gums. Patients with malnutrition may also demonstrate muscle wasting and ascites. Hepatomegaly and splenomegaly may be present and neurologic changes such as altered mental status and loss of balance and coordination may occur.

Unintentional weight loss may be an indicator of malnutrition. The degree of loss determines the extent of the problem. A significant loss is 10%, whereas a 20% loss indicates malnutrition. The loss of more than 1 kg/week is primarily associated with protein loss. The body mass index (BMI) is a measure of body fat based on height and weight. It is a way to begin to determine whether the patient's weight is healthy. For most people, BMI is a reliable indicator of body fatness and calculated using the following formula: Weight (kg)/Ht (m) × Ht (m). An optimal BMI is 18.5 to 25. Obesity is defined as a BMI greater than 30; underweight is defined as a value less than 18.5.

Although rarely used in acute care, diminished skinfold and arm circumference measurements determine a patient's

TABLE 6-7	Etiology of Malnutrition	
Etiology	**Related Conditions**
Decreased nutrient intake	• Recent weight loss • Recent change in diet; fad or limited diet • Eating disorder (e.g., obesity, bulimia, or anorexia nervosa) • Anorexia • Nausea • Difficulty chewing or swallowing (e.g., stomatitis or dysphagia) • Depression • Alcoholism or drug addiction • Social history of poverty, disability, or living alone • Loss of the sense of taste or smell • Use of drugs known to alter dietary intake or food utilization (e.g., antacids, antibiotics, laxatives, and antineoplastics)

Decreased absorption	• Decreased nutrient intake
	• Decreased absorption
	• Diseases of the GI tract:
	  • Malabsorptions (e.g., diarrhea or steatorrhea)
	  • Parasites
	  • Pernicious anemia
	  • Intestinal bypass or resection
	• Drugs (e.g., antacids, cholestyramine, neomycin, or alcohol)

Increased nutrient losses	• Recurrent vomiting or diarrhea • GI disease: peritonitis or inflammatory bowel disease • Diabetes mellitus • Hemorrhage • Peritoneal dialysis or hemodialysis

Increased nutrient requirements	• Recent surgery or trauma
	• Chronic illnesses such as malignancy or renal, liver, lung, or heart disease, or diabetes mellitus
	• Prolonged hypercatabolic state:
	  • Multiple trauma
	  • Major surgery
	  • Sepsis
	  • Burns
	• Hyperthyroidism
	• Hypoxia

Iatrogenic malnutrition	• NPO status for diagnostic studies or postoperatively
	• Feedings not advanced
	  • Wait and see attitudes
	  • If appetite improves
	  • If nausea, vomiting resolves
	  • If ileus resolves

nutrition status. Measure the triceps skinfold thickness with calipers. This procedure reflects the measurement of the subcutaneous fat reserves of the body. The normal value is 7.5 to 16.5 mm. A value less than 3 mm indicates severely depleted fat stores. Midarm muscle circumference of the middle of the upper nondominant arm reflects the measurement of the body's muscle stores.

Utilize laboratory test results to evaluate visceral protein measurements, including protein levels, albumin, prealbumin, transferrin, retinol-binding protein, hemoglobulin, hematocrit, and immune compromise. Decreased albumin occurs with malnutrition. Decreased albumin reflects changes in nutritional status slowly because its half-life is 10 to 20 days. In addition, decreased albumin may be secondary to liver disease, nephrotic syndrome, or hypercatabolism and/or be a reflection of overhydration. Designate the depletion of albumin levels by the following parameters:

- Normal: 3.5 to 5 g/dL
- Mild depletion: 2.8 to 3.4 g/dL
- Moderate depletion: 2.1 to 2.7 g/dL
- Severe depletion: less than 2.1 g/dL

A decreased prealbumin is a more reliable test than albumin for monitoring overall protein status in the acute care setting because the half-life is less than 48 to 72 hours. Other laboratory tests that may be used because they have a shorter half-life than albumin are a decreased transferrin (half-life: 8 to 10 days) and decreased retinol-binding protein (half-life: 10 hours). Retinol-binding protein decreases with even minor stress; yet the significance is not fully understood. The patient's hemoglobin and hematocrit may decrease. Conduct an evaluation for immunocompetence. If compromised, the total lymphocyte count (TLC) decreases. This can be determined by the following formula: TLC = WBC (in mm^3) × % of lymphocytes. Designate depletion of TLC by the following parameters:

- Normal: 1500 to 2500/mm^3
- Mild depletion: less than 1500/mm^3
- Moderate depletion: less than 1200/mm^3
- Severe depletion: less than 800/mm^3

6.4 Learning Activity

Why is serum prealbumin a better assessment tool than albumin to evaluate improvement from nutritional support?

_____
_____
_____
_____
_____

Answers to this activity can be found in the Answer Key.

Stress, steroids, and/or acute kidney injury or chronic kidney disease may decrease the TLC. Increased TLC occurs from infection, leukemia, and/or myeloma. In addition, cell-mediated immunity skin tests for *Candida albicans,* mumps, and the purified protein derivative (PPD) of tuberculin are completed. Failure to elicit a response to a skin test may suggest anergy and a decreased immune response.

To determine somatic (skeletal) protein measurements, the midarm muscle circumference is measured. A 24-hour urine specimen for creatinine should be collected. Examination of nitrogen balance may show a negative value. This requires a 24-hour dietary record to evaluate nitrogen intake and a 24-hour urine collection to measure urea nitrogen and evaluate nitrogen loss. The test is only reliable when renal function is normal.

A priority in the collaborative management of a patient with malnutrition focuses on the prevention and detection of a negative nitrogen balance and improvement in nutritional status. Weigh the patient daily at the same time, on the same scale. Monitor diagnostic studies reflective of visceral protein stores (e.g., albumin, transferrin, prealbumin). Ensure adequate delivery of appropriate nutrients and assess the need for nutritional support when the patient is required to be NPO for greater than 5 days or if the patient is unable to meet nutritional needs with oral feedings. It is important to be aware that 1 L of 5% dextrose provides only 170 kcal. Although this provides fluids and delays gluconeogenesis for a short period, catabolism occurs after approximately 5 days at basal metabolic rate and earlier in a hypermetabolic patient. Nutritional support within 48 hours of injury or acute illness may lessen the hypercatabolic state. Nutritional support does the following:

- Promotes anabolism to prevent negative nitrogen balance and loss of visceral and somatic protein stores
- Provides needed nutrients for cellular energy
- Supports healing and the immune system
- Enhances feeling of well-being

Calculate nutritional requirements on all acutely ill patients. Attention to protein, caloric intake, fluids, and distribution and balance of protein, fats, and supplements should be considered. The basal protein requirement is 0.8 g/kg/day. Most acutely ill patients require approximately 1.5 g/kg/day. Patients with direct protein loss (e.g., crush injuries, burns, hemorrhage) require 2 to 3 g/kg/day. It is important to note that too much protein is associated with azotemia.

The number of calories required ranges from 25 to 80 kcal/kg/day. This requirement varies according to age, activity level, metabolic rate, nutritional status, severity of illness, and other factors. Basal need or minimal illness requirements are 25 kcal/kg/day. A patient with a moderate illness may require a caloric intake of 35 kcal/kg/day. A patient suffering from sepsis or extensive trauma may require a caloric intake of 45 kcal/kg/day, whereas a burn victim may need up to 80 kcal/kg/day. Adequate caloric intake is important but it is necessary to avoid overfeeding. Overfeeding is associated with electrolyte imbalance, especially hypophosphatemia.

Administer fluids to deliver 25 to 35 mL/kg/day plus additional amounts in the presence of a fever. Administer 150 mL/day for each degree of body temperature above 37° C. The distribution of nutrients to ensure adequate nonprotein calories is also needed to prevent protein catabolism. The recommended distribution balance is the following:

- Protein: 15% to 20%
- Carbohydrate: 50% to 60%
- Fats: 20% to 30%

Glutamine is a nonessential neutral amino acid that plays an important role in maintaining normal intestinal structure and function. Glutamine may be "conditionally" essential in patients with acute illness and stress to support the integrity of the gut and decrease the rate of protein catabolism. Glutamine deficiency causes gut mucosal atrophy and eventually intestinal necrosis, leading to bacterial translocation and sepsis. Glutamine supplementation provides enterocytes their preferred energy source and prevents gut-induced systemic inflammatory response syndrome (SIRS). Use of glutamine in patients with intracranial pathology is questionable, especially if seizures are occurring, because glutamine is a predominant stimulatory neurotransmitter.

Arginine is a semiessential amino acid. Providing arginine is thought to promote nitrogen retention and improve protein turnover; therefore, it is being used to improve wound healing and enhance immune function. Arginine aids in the production of nitric oxide, a potent regulator of vascular tone and cardiac contractility. Arginine supplementation reduces the risk of infection and sepsis and promotes wound healing.

Nucleotides play a role in energy transfer. Provision of nucleotides enhances natural killer (NK) cell activity and supports growth and function of metabolically active cells, such as lymphocytes and macrophages. Branched-chain amino acids such as leucine, isoleucine, and valine have beneficial effects on nitrogen balance in patients under stress. These are especially helpful in patients with hepatic failure or encephalopathy, but temporarily lowering daily protein intake is likely to produce the same effect. Medium-chain triglycerides (MCTs) are less irritating and more easily absorbed by the small bowel mucosa.

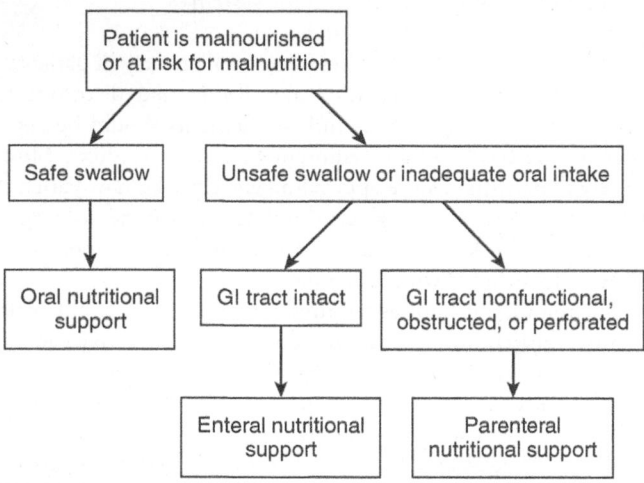

FIGURE 6-13 **Criteria for nutritional support.** (From Dennison, R. D. [2013]. *Pass CCRN!* [4th ed.]. St. Louis, MO: Elsevier.)

They may be better than long-chain triglycerides (LCTs) for patients with compromised GI function, SIRS, or sepsis. Essential polyunsaturated fatty acids (PUFAs), such as omega-6 (e.g., linoleic acid) and omega-3 (e.g., α-linolenic acid), facilitate efficient functioning of the immune system. Dipeptide/tripeptide formulas may be useful for patients with malabsorption (e.g., severe Crohn disease, bowel edema, inflammation, or ischemia).

Nutritional support can be provided either through a feeding tube (enteral nutrition) or, when the digestive tract cannot be used, through an intravenous tube called a catheter that is inserted directly into the veins (parenteral nutrition) (Figure 6-13). Tailor the amount, type, and route of nutrition specifically to each patient with the goal being to improve patient outcomes, minimize infections, and allow patients to live their lives as normally as possible.

Enteral nutrition is the provision of nutrition beyond that provided by normal food intake using oral supplementation, or enteral tube feeding. Administer enteral nutritional support (Table 6-8) to patients with a functioning GI tract requiring nutritional support. Always remember that "if the gut works, use it."

Parenteral nutrition (Table 6-9) refers to the administration of nutrients via a dedicated central or peripheral line. Indications for parenteral nutrition include GI tract dysfunction such as an ileus or other obstruction, severe dysmotility, fistulae, surgical resection, or severe malabsorption that precludes adequate nutrient absorption. Contraindication of parenteral nutrition includes when the GI tract is functional, except when enteral nutrition is impossible or impractical because of tube access. Correct hyperglycemia (serum glucose level of 300 mg/dL or greater), electrolyte abnormalities, or severe fluid overload before initiation of parenteral nutrition.

Parenteral nutritional support in conjunction with oral or enteral nutrition increases the amount of nutrients provided in hypermetabolic patients. Ensure a smooth transition from

TABLE 6-8	**Enteral Nutritional Support**
Indication	Patient has functioning GI tract but unable to consume adequate nutrients

Advantages	• Preferred route for patients with functional GI tract
	  • Maintenance of gut structure and absorptive ability
	  • Reduced incidence of sepsis by prevention of translocation of GI bacteria into blood or lymph
	  • Fewer complications than parenteral route
	  • Lower cost than parenteral route
	  • Early enteral

Disadvantages	Decreased gastric and intestinal motility often accompanies critical illness, which may lead to an inability to achieve adequate caloric intake as well as increase the risk of gastroesophageal reflux with resultant aspiration and pneumonia

Contraindications	• Absolute contraindications
	  • Diffuse peritonitis
	  • Intestinal obstruction
	    — Functional obstruction (e.g., paralytic ileus)
	    — Structural obstruction (e.g., tumor, volvulus, or adhesion)
	  • Intestinal perforation
	• Relative contraindications
	  • Gastrointestinal ischemia
	  • Enterocutaneous fistula
	  • Severe acute pancreatitis especially if hemorrhagic
	  • Severe malabsorption

TABLE 6-8	**Enteral Nutritional Support—cont'd**

Routes and choice of tubes	Routes
	• Gastric
	  • Advantages
	    — Maintains natural bacteriocidal quality of acid environment
	    — Provides some protection from stress ulceration
	  • Disadvantage
	    — Increases risk of aspiration especially in patients with gastric atony, which is common in critically ill patients
	      • Percutaneous endoscopic gastrostomy (PEG) may decrease this risk because the tube does not cause gastroesophageal sphincter incompetence
	• Intestinal
	  • Advantage: reduces risk of gastroesophageal regurgitation and microaspiration of gastric contents
	  • Disadvantage: placing tube is frequently difficult because critically ill patients frequently have delayed gastric motility; placement methods may include the following:
	    — Blind insertion
	      • Turn patient to right side and twist tube during advancement after gastric confirmation
	      • Air insufflation technique: instillation of 350-500 mL of air into the stomach
	      • Use of metoclopramide (Reglan)
	    — Fluoroscopic or endoscopic placement (e.g., percutaneous endoscopic jejunostomy [PEJ])
	    — Surgical (needle jejunostomy tube)
	Choice
	• Small-gauge tube that is placed below the gastroesophageal sphincter (such as percutaneous endoscopic gastrostomy [PEG] or jejunostomy tube [including needle jejunostomy which may be done at the conclusion of a laparotomy]) is preferred especially in patients with potential for impaired gastric motility and high risk of aspiration (Bourgault et al., 2007)
	• Short-term (<6 weeks)
	  • Nasogastric or orogastric tube
	  • Nasointestinal or orointestinal tube (this may be advanced to the duodenum or jejunum)
	  • Needle jejunostomy
	• Long-term (>6 weeks)
	  • Gastrostomy
	  • Jejunostomy

Types of formulas	• Monomeric (also referred to as *elemental*) diets (e.g., Vivonex, Vivonex HN, Criticare HN, Vital HN, Travasorb NH, Impact, Stresstein) contain predigested nutrients; required when feeding is delivered distal to presence of digestive enzymes (distal jejunum); hyperosmolar
	• Polymeric formulas contain intact protein and require a functional GI system
	  • Intact protein and lactose-free enteral diets (e.g., Sustacal, Ensure, Enrich, Osmolite)
	  • Intact protein, lactose-free, high-density enteral diets (e.g., Magnacal, Isocal HCN, Sustacal HC, Ensure Plus, Ensure Plus HN)
	  • Blenderized meat-based enteral diets (e.g., Vitaneed, Compleat B)
	  • Specialized enteral diets
	    — Immune-boosting formulas (e.g., Immune-Aid, Impact, Perative, Replete): contain glutamine, arginine, and/or nucleotides
	    — Trauma (e.g., TraumaCal, Traum-Aid HBC, Vivonex TEN)
	    — Hepatic (e.g., Travasorb Hepatic, Hepatic-Aid): increased branched-chain amino acids
	    — Pulmonary (e.g., Pulmocare): higher proportion of fats, less CHO to reduce CO_2 production
	    — Renal (e.g., Travasorb Renal, Amin-Aid): essential amino acids
	    — Diabetic (e.g., Glucerna, Suplena)
	    — Fiber-containing formulas (e.g., Ensure with fiber, Jevity, Sustacal with fiber)
	• Modular
	  • CHO (e.g., Polycose, Nutrisource Modular System [carbohydrate])
	  • Protein (e.g., ProMod, Nutrisource Modular System [protein])
	  • Lipid-Medium Chain Triglycerides (e.g., MCT oil, Nutrisource Modular System [lipid])
	  • Lipid-Long Chain Triglycerides (e.g., Nutrisource Modular System [lipid LCT])
	• Note calorie concentration (most 1 kcal/mL but some critical care solutions have 2 kcal/mL; Pulmocare, which is higher in fat, has 1.5 kcal/mL)
	• Note osmolality (isotonic is 250-350 mOsm/liter; hypertonicity contributes to dehydration and diarrhea)

Pattern of delivery	• Intermittent (cannot be used below the pylorus) • Continuous; provides more protection from stress ulcers • Cyclic; feeding may be discontinued for periods of time during the 24-hour period; infusion frequently initiated during nighttime hours

Continued

TABLE 6-8	**Enteral Nutritional Support—cont'd**

Monitor	• Position of the feeding tube
	  • X-ray is the only reliable method for confirming placement of enteral tubes; x-ray should be obtained to confirm desired placement before administering formula or medication by the tube for the first time
	  • Other nondefinitive methods include:
	    — pH of aspirate may be helpful but not definitive: pH 1-3 in stomach without pH-altering drugs, 3-5 in stomach with pH-altering drugs, >7 in small intestine
	    — Color of aspirate may be helpful but not definitive
	    — Stomach: green, cloudy, or colorless
	    — Intestine: yellow or brown
	    — Tracheobronchial: tan, white, pale yellow, or clear
	  • Auscultation over stomach when air is injected through the tube (air insufflation) is NOT recommended due to poor sensitivity
	• GI tolerance of enteral feeding
	  • Abdominal distention or complaints of discomfort or fullness
	  • Vomiting
	  • Excessive residual volumes
	• Intake and output totaled every 8-12 hours
	• Weight daily
	• Bedside glucose testing by fingerstick every 6 hours; serum glucose by laboratory daily
	• Electrolytes daily
	• BUN daily
	• Proteins, trace elements, and liver function studies weekly

General guidelines	• Start feedings within 24-48 hours of admission or when fully resuscitated and hemodynamically stable
	• Use an infusion pump for continuous infusion
	• Do not add blue food coloring (or methylene blue) to the enteral feeding; it is no longer recommended to add blue food coloring to enteral feedings for the following reasons:
	  • May result in generalized absorption of the dye from the GI tract; more likely in patients with multiple organ failure
	    — Discoloration of body fluids and tissues
	    — May cause fatal liver toxicity
	    — Causes questionable specificity because discoloration of tracheal secretions may have occurred by systemic route
	  • May result in infection due to contamination of the food coloring
	  • Interferes with occult blood testing
	  • Causes allergic reactions in some people due to presence of FD&C yellow No. 5
	  • Has relatively low sensitivity as an indication of aspiration
	• Keep HOB elevated 30-45 degrees during and 30-60 minutes after intermittent feeding and continuously for continuous feeding
	• Give formula full-strength but start at 25 mL/hour; increase rate by 25 mL/hour every 4 hours if tolerated until desired rate achieved
	• Check for residual volume every 4-6 hours or before next intermittent feeding; checking residuals is not recommended with small-lumen tubes because they tend to collapse and aspiration of gastric contents can cause clogging (Kenny & Goodman, 2010)
	  • If residual is >200 mL (Kenny & Goodman, 2010):
	    — The aspirate should be reinstilled in the absence of abdominal pain or distention; flush with water after reinstillation of aspirate
	    — The feeding should be continued and rechecked in 1 hour
	      • If the residual is still >200 mL, the infusion should be stopped for 4 hours and then rechecked
	        o If the residual is still >200 mL, notify physician
	        o If the residual is <200 mL, restart feeding at 50% the original rate and monitor
	      • Note that frequent interruptions may compromise adequacy of nutritional support
	  • If large residual volumes continue to limit feeding and impair nutritional support, consider the following interventions:
	    — Place the patient on the right side for 20 minutes before recheck
	    — Consult with the physician regarding the use of a drug to increase gastric motility (e.g., metoclopramide [Reglan], erythromycin); erythromycin has the potential risk of bacterial resistance
	    — Advance the tube to below the pylorus (intestinal motility is usually not affected by the same factors as gastric motility)
	    — Consult with the dietician regarding a more calorie-dense formula in order to reduce required volume
	    — Monitor and treat hyperglycemia to avoid gastroparesis
	• Use strict aseptic technique in administration of enteral feedings; discard feeding system after 24 hours if an open system or after 48 hours if a closed system
	• Administer free water in volumes of 1 mL/kcal to prevent hyperosmolality

TABLE 6-8	**Enteral Nutritional Support—cont'd**

Complications of enteral alimentation	• Clogged feeding tube
	  • Recognize factors that increase risk of clogging the tube
	    — Calorie-dense formula
	    — Protein formulas
	    — Instillation of crushed medications
	    — Small-bore feeding tube
	    — Gravity drip
	  • Prevent clogging
	    — Use an infusion pump for continuous feedings and by flushing with water when indicated
	      • Flush with 30 mL of water before and after medication administration via tube
	      • Flush with 30 mL of water before and after intermittent feedings or every 4 hours with continuous feedings
	      • Flush with 30 mL of water after checking for residuals
	      • Flush with 30 mL of water every 4 hours
	    — Use liquid-form medications when possible
	  • Attempt to reestablish patency of a clogged tube by flushing with warm water (note that cranberry juice or cola have not been shown to be more effective than water); if warm water is not successful in unclogging the tube, a physician's order for pancreatic enzymes or pancreatic enzyme–sodium bicarbonate suspension may be requested (note that proper tube placement confirmation is crucial before using pancreatic enzymes); tube replacement may be required
	• Tube displacement
	  • Tape tube securely and monitor for a change in external length
	  • Prevent vomiting with antiemetics
	• Nausea/vomiting
	  • Slow feeding
	  • Allow feeding to come to room temperature before infusion
	  • Reduce osmolality of the feeding by diluting with water
	  • Decrease amount of fat in feeding
	  • Administer lactose-free formula
	  • Consider the use of drugs to increase gastric motility (e.g., metoclopramide [Reglan], erythromycin)
	  • Consider the need to move the tube from the stomach into the duodenum
	• Endotracheal aspiration of tube feeding
	  • Elevate head of bed 30-45 degrees at all times if feeding is continuous; elevate during feeding and for 30-60 minutes after intermittent feeding
	  • Keep cuff inflated during feeding if patient is intubated or has a tracheostomy
	  • Check for residual volumes every 4-6 hours if administering gastric feedings through a large-bore tube
	• Diarrhea
	  • Caused by decreased plasma colloidal oncotic pressure (COP) due to low serum proteins
	    — Maintain adequate nutritional support; diarrhea will resolve when plasma proteins are more normal
	    — Administer intravenous albumin as prescribed
	  • Bacterial contamination
	    — Wash hands before manipulation of equipment and use clean technique; wipe top of formula cans with an alcohol wipe
	    — Utilize a closed system if possible
	    — Change administration system daily or according to policy
	    — Do not allow solutions to hang at room temperature for more than 4 hours if an open system or 24 hours if a closed system
	    — Avoid antidiarrheals, which slow peristalsis and increase the risk of sepsis
	  • Hypertonicity
	    — Initiate enteral feedings at a slow rate and/or half-strength; gradually increase rate and/or strength
	    — Use isotonic solutions if possible; dilute hyperosmolar feeding with free water
	  • Alteration in normal flora from antibiotics and proliferation of *Clostridium difficile*
	    — Administer metronidazole (Flagyl) or vancomycin
	    — Encourage yogurt (with active cultures) or *Lactobacillus acidophilus* to restore normal flora
	  • Other considerations for diarrhea
	    — Consider the addition of fiber (e.g., Jevity)
	    — Use only lactose-free formulas
	    — Consider discontinuance of causative medications (e.g., elixirs containing sorbitol, antacids)
	    — Administer pancreatic enzymes for pancreatic insufficiency

Continued

TABLE 6-8	Enteral Nutritional Support—cont'd

Complications of enteral alimentation—cont'd	• Constipation
	  • Add fiber
	  • Increase free water
	  • Increase activity if possible
	  • Administer laxative as prescribed
	• Dehydration
	  • Monitor daily weight and intake and output
	  • Administer free water as indicated
	• Electrolyte imbalance
	  • Treat the cause (e.g., diarrhea)
	  • Monitor serum electrolytes
	  • Replace electrolytes as prescribed
	  • Consult with the physician and dietician regarding modification of formula
	• Hyperglycemia
	  • Monitor serum glucose every 6 hours
	  • Consult with the physician and dietician regarding modification of formula
	  • Administer insulin as prescribed
	• Overfeeding
	  • Monitor renal and liver function studies
	  • Monitor for fluid overload, hyperglycemia, hyperlipidemia, and electrolyte imbalance
	  • Consult with the physician and dietician regarding caloric and protein prescriptions
	• Refeeding syndrome
	  • Start feedings slowly, especially in high-risk patients (e.g., NPO for several days, existing malnutrition, alcoholism, sepsis); may take 24-48 hours to get intake to recommended level of nutrition
	  • Monitor glucose, potassium, and phosphorus; insulin and electrolyte replacement may be required
	• Inadequate feeding (Bourgault et al., 2007)
	  • Minimize interruptions
	  • Stop feedings immediately before minor procedures and then restart within 1 hour after procedures
	  • Stop feedings no more than 4 hours before major procedures

TABLE 6-9	Parenteral Nutritional Support
Indications	• When the enteral route is contraindicated (see Table 6-8) • When the enteral route is ineffective (high caloric needs or shock)

Routes	• Central vein: referred to as total parenteral nutrition (TPN)
	  • Allows the administration of hypertonic glucose solutions because of rapid dilution by blood as the solution enters the great vessel
	  • Subclavian or internal jugular usually used; percutaneously inserted central catheter (PICC) may also be used
	• Peripheral vein: referred to as peripheral parenteral nutrition (PPN)
	  • Used for patients who cannot take in sufficient nutrition enterally for 5-7 days but are not hypermetabolic
	  • Not usually adequate to provide sufficient calories for critically ill patients because of osmolality (and therefore calorie) limitations

Type of catheter	• Short-term: peripheral (for PPN) or central venous catheter (for TPN); multilumen catheter usually used to provide lumen for parenteral nutrition, lumen for blood and/or fluids, and lumen for parenteral drugs • Long-term: Hickman, Broviac, or Groshong catheter; Infuse-a-Port; Port-a-Cath

Solution: 1 L of standard TPN formula (25% dextrose and 8.5% amino acids) provides approximately 1000 kcal (1 kcal/mL)	• CHO: hypertonic dextrose
	  • Concentrations
	    — TPN: usually 25% but may be as high as 35% dextrose
	    — PPN: no more than 10% dextrose
	  • CHO and fats provide enough calories for maximal protein-sparing effect
	  • Dextrose provides 3.4 cal/g
	• Protein: crystalline amino acids 2.5% to 8.5%; includes essential and nonessential (note that no more than 5% amino acid solution via parenteral line [i.e., PPN]) amino acids providing 4.3 cal/g
	  • Specialized formulas are available for specific diseases
	    — Hepatic failure (e.g., HepatAmine, Branch Amin): branched-chain amino acids
	    — Acute kidney injury or chronic kidney disease (e.g., RenAmin, NephrAmine): essential amino acids

TABLE 6-9	**Parenteral Nutritional Support—cont'd**

Solution: 1 L of standard TPN formula (25% dextrose and 8.5% amino acids) provides approximately 1000 kcal (1 kcal/mL)—cont'd	• Fats: oil-in-water emulsions composed of soybean oil or a combination of soybean oil and safflower oil that provide fatty acids as long-chain triglycerides
	  • 30-50% of nonprotein calories should be supplied by lipids, not exceeding 2.5 g/kg/day
	    — Linoleic acid, the only essential fatty acid, should provide at least 4% of the total calorie intake to prevent deficiency of essential fatty acid
	    — Excessive amounts of lipids may have a detrimental effect on pulmonary function and the reticuloendothelial system
	  • Concentrations
	    — 10% lipids provide 1.1 kcal/mL
	    — 20% lipids provide 2 kcal/mL
	    — 30% lipids provide 3 kcal/mL
	  • Medium-chain triglycerides are immediately oxidized for fuel and may be preferred in SIRS and sepsis
	• Electrolytes: sodium chloride, potassium, calcium, magnesium, and phosphate
	• Buffer: acetate or bicarbonate
	• Minerals: iron, zinc, copper, manganese, cobalt, iodine, chromium, and selenium
	• Vitamins: multivitamins 1 ampule daily
	  • Vitamin K (10-20 mg) should be administered every week; may be given IM or subcutaneously or added to TPN solution as phytonadione (AquaMEPHYTON)
	  • Thiamine replacement should be considered especially when chronic alcohol ingestion is known or suspected to prevent Wernicke's encephalopathy
	• 3-in-1 admixture has everything in one infusion rather than lipid piggybacked in separately
	  • Advantages: lower cost with less equipment, waste, and nursing time
	  • Disadvantage: risk of solution instability; monitor closely for a cream-colored layer (also referred to as *creaming*) or a complete emulsion crack with a separation of the oil and water and return to pharmacy if separation noted

Possible additives	• Regular insulin (note that sliding-scale insulin still must be administered as needed) • Heparin • H_2 receptor antagonists • Metoclopramide (Reglan) • Note: all additives should be added under laminar hood (in the pharmacy department) rather than on nursing unit
Monitor	• Vital signs and infusion rate at least every 4 hours (depending on the acuity of the patient) • Intake and output totaled every 8-12 hours • Weight daily • Bedside glucose testing by fingerstick every 6 hours; serum glucose by laboratory daily • Electrolytes daily • BUN daily • CBC, proteins, trace elements, liver function studies, triglycerides, cholesterol, platelet count, and prothrombin time weekly • Catheter site

General guidelines	• Utilize strict sterile technique during catheter insertion and management
	• Assess patient for central venous catheter insertion complications (pneumothorax, hemothorax, chylothorax, and arterial puncture); request chest x-ray after insertion of central venous catheter; do not initiate fluids at a rate faster than keep vein open (KVO) until chest x-rays confirms placement
	• Ensure a dedicated catheter or lumen of a multilumen catheter for TPN infusion (note: this is not universally adhered to, and CDC makes no recommendation regarding the need for a dedicated lumen)
	  • Do not use a catheter or lumen that has been previously used for CVP measurements or for the prolonged administration of crystalloid solution or blood products
	  • Do not use the catheter (or lumen) for drawing blood samples or infusing any other fluids
	• Assess the solution before infusion
	  • Examine expiration date and discard any expired solutions
	  • Do not hang cloudy solutions
	  • Monitor closely for emulsion crack if hanging 3-in-1 solution (also called *total nutrient admixture* [TNA]); do not hang solution if a layer of fat is seen separated at top of bag
	• Initiate at 1200-2400 cal/day and increase to desired caloric intake as prescribed
	• Remove from refrigerator 30 minutes before infusing
	• Keep rate constant (volumetric pump required)
	• Utilize an inline filter; 0.22 micron if lipids are piggybacked in distal to filter; 1.2 micron if TNA used as smaller filter will not allow lipids to flow through

Continued

TABLE 6-9	Parenteral Nutritional Support—cont'd
General guidelines—cont'd	• Change dressing every 48 hours or according to hospital policy or anytime the dressing becomes soiled • Use gauze and tape or a semipermeable transparent dressing (e.g., Op-Site, Tegaderm); note that semipermeable transparent dressings have been associated with a higher rate of catheter-related infection and sepsis than standard gauze and tape, probably because of inadequate permeability and infrequency of dressing changes; they should not be used in patients with oily skin or acne near the catheter insertion site • Change tubing every 24-72 hours or according to hospital policy; lipid tubing (including TNA tubing) should be changed every 24 hours • Do not allow a bag to hang more than 24 hours

Complications	• Allergic reaction (especially to lipids)
	  • Note fever, chills, shivering, or chest or back pain
	  • Stop infusion
	• Infection and sepsis
	  • Utilize meticulous aseptic technique with all aspects of catheter care; change dressing every 48 hours or whenever soiled; change tubing every 24-72 hours; minimize number of entries into the system
	  • Monitor for clinical indications of catheter-related sepsis: fever, leukocytosis, glucose intolerance, redness, swelling, tenderness, and purulent drainage at insertion site
	  • Obtain blood cultures (not through this catheter); remove catheter and culture tip
	• Hyperglycemia
	  • Monitor serum glucose levels
	  • Administer insulin therapy; usually administered as insulin drip if serum glucose >500 mg/dL
	• Hyperosmolar nonketotic dehydration
	  • Monitor serum glucose levels
	  • Administer insulin therapy; usually administered as insulin drip if serum glucose >500 mg/dL
	  • Administer 5% dextrose and hypotonic saline (¼ or ½) or D_5W (depending on patient's serum osmolality) to correct free water deficit
	  • Discontinue TPN until patient is stable as prescribed
	• Hypoglycemia
	  • Prevent interruption of TPN infusion (e.g., catheter occlusion or accidental removal)
	  • Use infusion pump (mandatory)
	  • Never discontinue TPN abruptly unless for hyperglycemic hyperosmolar state (HHS)
	• Electrolyte imbalances: hyperchloremic metabolic acidosis, hyponatremia, hypokalemia, hypocalcemia, hypomagnesemia, and hypophosphatemia
	  • Adjust TPN solution concentration and/or alteration of infusion rate as prescribed
	• Refeeding syndrome: fluid imbalance, hypokalemia, hypophosphatemia, hypoglycemia, or hyperglycemia
	  • Monitor fluid, electrolyte, and glucose levels especially during the first 24-48 hours after TPN initiated
	  • Adjust TPN solution concentration and/or alteration of infusion rate as prescribed
	• Increased CO_2 production
	  • Monitor closely for clinical indications of hypercapnia; request arterial blood gases (ABGs) as indicated
	  • Decrease the percentage of calories supplied by CHO and increase percentage of calories supplied by fats if hypercapnia occurs, or during weaning
	• Air embolism
	  • Prevent air embolus by doing the following:
	    — Ask the patient to hold their breath or perform the Valsalva maneuver during catheter insertion, tubing changes, and catheter removal
	    — Purge all air from tubings before attachment to catheter
	    — Use air-eliminating filters on central line tubings
	    — Use Luer-Lok connections
	  • Note dyspnea, hypotension, churning murmur over precordium, and/or confusion
	  • If clinical indications of air embolism do occur:
	    — Place patient in Trendelenburg position on left side
	    — Aspirate air with a syringe attached to the central venous catheter
	    — Administer oxygen
	• Subclavian thrombosis (rare)
	  • Monitor for swelling of involved arm, face, or neck; erythema; fever
	  • Remove catheter
	  • Administer fibrinolytic or anticoagulation therapy as prescribed

enteral or parenteral feedings to oral nutrition. Consult with the dietitian and the physician regarding plans for this transition. Routinely, cut the total parenteral nutrition (TPN) rate in half when one-half to one-third of the patient's total caloric requirements are met by enteral feeding. Discontinue TPN when the patient has met the total caloric requirements by enteral feedings. When transitioning to an oral diet, start with clear liquids and advance to full liquids while observing for aspiration. Advance to solid food after 2 to 3 days of liquids, and when at least 500 kcal is consumed, decrease the TPN by one-half. Discontinue nutritional support when the patient is able to tolerate sufficient oral nutrition for 2 to 3 days.

High-protein and high-calorie drinks, shakes, and puddings may be used as nutritional supplements to augment small, frequent meals. When transitioning from an enteral diet to an oral diet, monitor oral intake and utilize nutritional supplements to boost caloric intake if needed. Consider cyclic enteral feeding if calorie intake is consistently inadequate. Administer these cyclic feedings at night. Continue to monitor daily weight and food intake during transition times. Provide frequent oral hygiene. Brush teeth before meals to avoid aspiration of harmful bacteria. Prevent skin breakdown and implement the following precautions:

- Monitor for changes in edema.
- Keep skin clean and dry.
- Turn every 2 hours.
- Use special mattresses as indicated.

6.5 Learning Activity

Calculate the caloric intake for a patient receiving TPN with daily intake of 42 g of protein, 250 g of carbohydrate, and 140 g of fat. _____

Answers to this activity can be found in the Answer Key.

GASTROESOPHAGEAL REFLUX DISEASE

Gastroesophageal reflux disease (GERD) is a disorder that exposes the esophagus mucosa to gastric secretions. A weakened LES or hiatal hernia may contribute to the esophageal insult; however, any factor that delays the time for gastric emptying (i.e., gastric ulcers or stricture) can also cause the problem. Over time, continual damage to the esophageal mucosa can lead to erosions, ulcerations, basal cell hyperplasia, and Barrett's esophagus (McCance & Huether, 2015).

Patients with GERD may complain of heartburn and upper abdominal discomfort. Often the patient complains of chest pain. Initially, rule out a cardiac problem first. The pain may be worse when the patient lies down, coughs, or vomits. The patient may also complain of chronic cough, asthma, hoarseness, and chronic sore throat (Chen & Hsu, 2013).

GERD is diagnosed based on history and symptom presentation. Diagnostic studies include gastroscopy, barium upper GI series, and a 24-hour ambulatory pH study. Gastroscopy and barium upper GI series identify areas of damage (i.e., erosion). The 24-hour ambulatory pH study is the most accurate study for the diagnosis of GERD; however, the test is expensive and invasive.

The collaborative patient care plan focuses on lifestyle changes and medication therapy. Lifestyle changes include smoking cessation, elevating the head of bed for sleep, avoidance of alcohol, weight loss, and the avoidance of fatty and spicy foods. Medications that are used include antacids, H_2 receptor antagonists, proton pump inhibitors, and promotility agents (metoclopramide [Reglan]). It is often necessary to combine these therapies. The patient should avoid food and liquids before bedtime. If the patient is unresponsive to medication therapy, antireflux surgery may be required. Education of the patient and family should include information about causes of GERD, risks of untreated GERD, lifestyle modifications, and medication treatments Chen & Hsu, 2013.

UPPER GI HEMORRHAGE

Upper GI hemorrhage is most likely to result from gastritis, peptic ulcer, Mallory-Weiss tear, or esophageal varices. Some instances of GI hemorrhage are life-threatening; others may cause chronic blood-loss anemia.

Gastritis is an inflammation, irritation, or erosion of the lining of the stomach. It can occur suddenly (i.e., acute) or gradually (i.e., chronic). Gastritis can be caused by irritation due to excessive alcohol use; dietary intolerances, especially milk intolerance; chronic vomiting; stress; or the use of certain medications, such as aspirin or other antiinflammatory drugs. Bacterial and viral infections, pernicious anemia, and bile reflux may also cause gastritis. Pernicious anemia is a form of anemia that occurs when the stomach lacks a naturally occurring substance (intrinsic factor). To properly absorb and digest vitamin B_{12} requires the intrinsic factor. Certain clinical conditions such as uremia and systemic diseases like hepatitis also cause gastritis. Bile reflux is a backflow of bile into the stomach from the common bile duct. Ingestion of strong acids or alkalis will cause a corrosive type of gastritis. If left untreated, gastritis can lead to ulcers with a severe loss in blood and may increase the risk of developing stomach cancer.

Peptic ulcer is a sharply defined erosion in mucosa, which may involve the submucosa and muscular layers of the esophagus (~5%), stomach (~15%), or duodenum (~80%). A gastric ulcer is a peptic ulcer located in the stomach. A duodenal ulcer is located in the duodenum.

A bacterial infection, *Helicobacter pylori* (*H. pylori*), lives in the mucous lining of the stomach and has been identified as the most common cause of ulcer disease. Eighty percent of stomach ulcers and 90% of duodenal ulcers develop because of infection with *H. pylori*. Other predisposing factors include genetic predisposition, smoking, or a diet that has a high intake of coffee or tea, carbonated beverages, and beer. Drugs that are ulcer-producing culprits include drugs that alter the mucosal barrier (antineoplastics, alcohol, NSAIDs); drugs that decrease gastric mucosal renewal (corticosteroids, phenylbutazone); and drugs that increase acid stimulation. The peptides in coffee, nicotine, reserpine, and hormones (e.g., estrogen) stimulate acid production. Any high physiologic stress situation may induce peptic ulcer formation; therefore, the following conditions are known causes:

- COPD
- Multiple traumas
- Major surgery
- Myocardial infarction
- Hepatic failure
- Acute kidney injury or chronic kidney disease

- Burns: referred to as *Curling ulcer*
- Neurologic trauma: referred to as *Cushing ulcer*
  - Cerebral trauma
  - Spinal cord injury
  - Neurosurgery
- Acute respiratory distress syndrome
- Mechanical ventilation for more than 5 days
- Coagulopathy
- Sepsis
- Shock
- Multiple organ dysfunction syndrome

Normally, the lining of the stomach and small intestines protects against the irritating acids produced in the stomach. If this protective lining stops working correctly and the lining breaks down, it results in inflammation (i.e., gastritis) and development of an ulcer. Most ulcers occur in the first layer of the inner lining. A perforation is a hole that goes all the way through the stomach or duodenum. A perforation is a medical emergency and results in an acute abdomen (Table 6-10).

6.6   Learning Activity

List five classic indications of an "acute abdomen" seen in GI perforation.

1. _____
2. _____
3. _____
4. _____
5. _____

Answers to this activity can be found in the Answer Key.

A Mallory-Weiss tear occurs in the mucous membrane of the lower part of the esophagus or upper part of the stomach, near where they join. A Mallory-Weiss tear likely occurs due to a large, suddenly occurring, and transient transmural pressure gradient across the region of the gastroesophageal junction. Forceful retching and vomiting seen with alcoholism, particularly binge drinking, or bulimia are the major causes of a Mallory-Weiss tear; however, this tear may occur after any event that provokes a sudden rise in intragastric pressure or gastric prolapse into the esophagus. Precipitating factors include retching, vomiting, straining, hiccupping, coughing, screaming, blunt abdominal trauma, and cardiopulmonary resuscitation. The presence of a hiatal hernia is a predisposing factor found in many patients with Mallory-Weiss tears. During retching or vomiting, the transmural pressure gradient is greater within the hernia than the rest of the stomach and if the shearing forces are high enough, a longitudinal laceration eventually occurs. Within the hernia, the tear is more likely to involve the lesser curvature of the gastric cardia, which is relatively immobile compared with the remainder of the stomach. Another potential mechanism for Mallory-Weiss tears is the violent prolapse or intussusception of the upper stomach into the esophagus, as can be witnessed during forceful retching with endoscopy. A Mallory-Weiss tear may also be associated with other mucosal lesions because these abnormalities may potentially contribute to bleeding

TABLE 6-10	Acute Abdomen
Also known as	• Surgical abdomen • Hot belly
Possible causes	• Peptic ulcer perforation • Ruptured appendix • Intestinal perforation or rupture • Intestinal infarction with perforation • Penetrating abdominal trauma
Consequences	• Leakage of bowel contents • Peritonitis • Sepsis
Clinical indications	• Abdominal pain • Abdominal distention • Rigid, boardlike abdomen • Rebound tenderness • Diminished or absent bowel sounds • Nausea and vomiting • Fever • Leukocytosis
Immediate actions	• Immobilize the patient to localize leakage • Prepare the patient for surgery • Administer IV antibiotics as prescribed; antibiotic lavage may be used during surgery • Treat pain with analgesics • Position the patient with knees flexed

or actually cause retching and vomiting that would induce these tears. An acute distention of the nondistensible lower esophagus can also produce a linear tear in this region. In some cases, no apparent precipitating factor can be identified. Mallory-Weiss tears account for an estimated 1% to 15% of cases of upper GI bleeding. Although the age range varies widely, affected individuals are generally in middle age (40s to 50s), and men reportedly have a higher incidence than women do.

Esophageal varices are dilation of the submucosal esophageal veins. The vessels may leak blood or even rupture, causing life-threatening bleeding. Esophageal varices occur most often in people with serious liver diseases (e.g., cirrhosis or scarring of the liver caused by many forms of liver diseases and conditions, such as hepatitis and chronic alcohol abuse). Esophageal varices develop when normal blood flow to the liver is obstructed by scar tissue in the liver or by a clot. Seeking a way around the blockages, blood flows into smaller blood vessels that are not designed to carry large volumes of blood. The liver carries out several essential functions, including detoxifying harmful substances in your body, cleaning your blood, and making vital nutrients. Cirrhosis occurs in response to damage to your liver over many years. As cirrhosis progresses, more and more scar tissue forms, making it difficult for the liver to function. Advanced cirrhosis can be life-threatening. The most prominent cause of cirrhosis is alcohol abuse. Viral or toxic hepatitis, chronic biliary obstruction, and chronic right ventricular heart failure may also lead to cirrhosis. Rarer etiologies of cirrhosis stem from portal vein thrombosis, hepatic venous outflow obstruction, congenital hepatic fibrosis, and a parasitic infection called schistosomiasis.

6.7 Learning Activity

List five possible reasons for upper GI hemorrhage.

1. _____
2. _____
3. _____
4. _____
5. _____

Answers to this activity can be found in the Answer Key.

The pathophysiology of upper GI hemorrhage (Figure 6-14) is complex. The pathophysiologic sequence varies depending on the cause of the GI hemorrhage.

The clinical presentation of a patient with a peptic ulcer includes both subjective and objective findings. Subjectively, the patient will report a history of epigastric pain, previous ulcer, previous GI bleeding, alcoholism, and liver disease. Their chief complaints will be epigastric pain, fatigue, weakness, thirst, and anxiety. Objective evidence will include hyperactive bowel sounds and evidence of bleeding. If the bleeding is gradual, the patient may present with faintness, fatigue, and pallor.

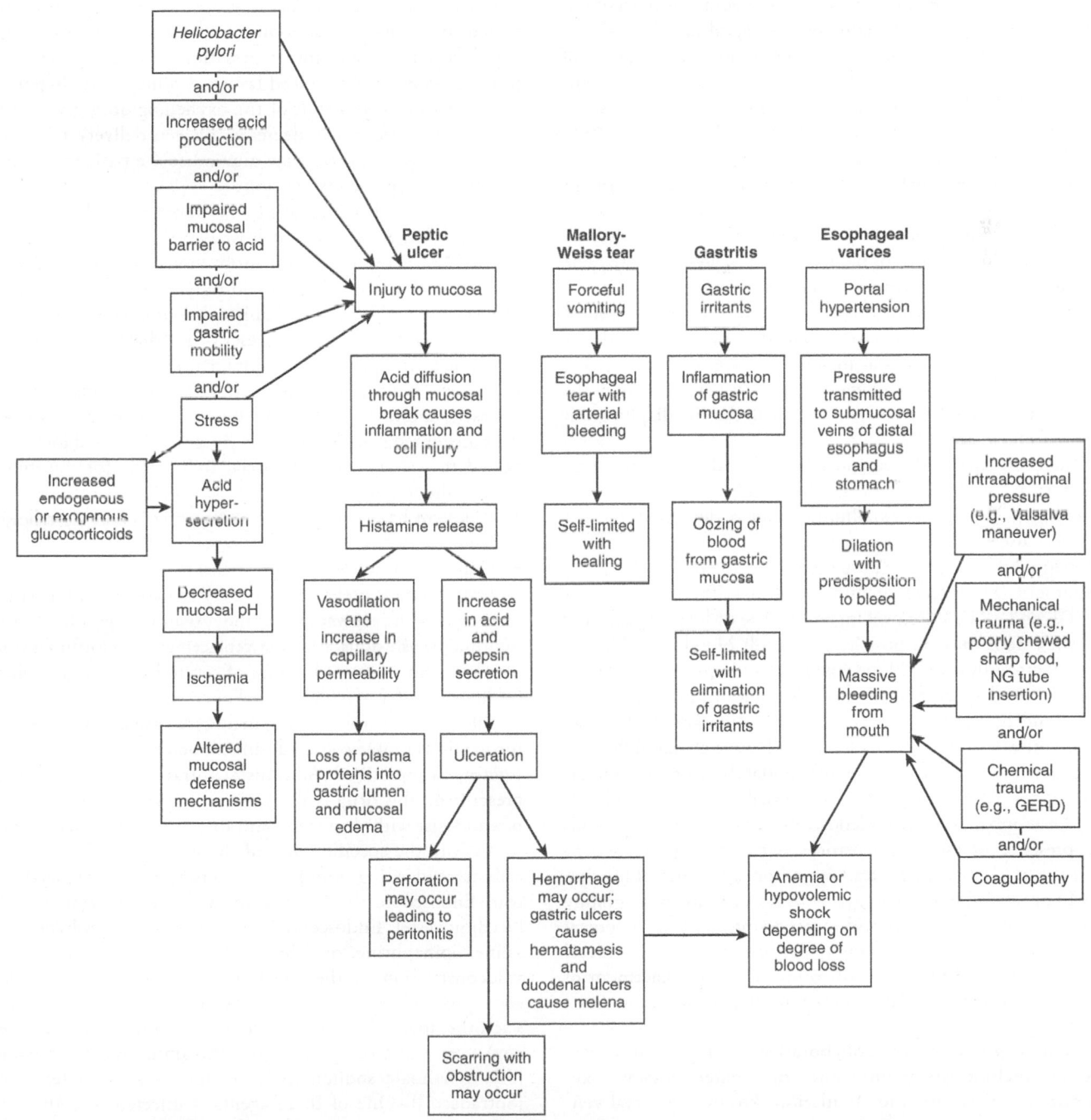

FIGURE 6-14 Pathophysiology of upper GI hemorrhage. (From Dennison, R. D. [2013]. *Pass CCRN!* [4th ed.]. St. Louis, MO: Elsevier.)

The bleeding characteristics seen are dependent on the location of the problem. Blood or coffee-ground–like material appears in vomitus if the problem is a gastric ulcer. Black stools are present if the problem is in the duodenal area.

Patients with esophageal varices will report a history of precipitating causes (i.e., excessive chronic alcohol intake) and reports of sudden, painless hemorrhage. The most obvious objective assessment finding is bright red blood gushing from the mouth. The average blood loss from esophageal varices is 10 units. Patients with esophageal varices may also have jaundice, abdominal distention, hyperactive bowel sounds, melena, hepatomegaly, and splenomegaly. The patients also demonstrate the clinical indications of hypoperfusion: tachycardia; tachypnea; hypotension; cool, clammy skin; decreased urine output; agitation; and confusion. The clinical presentation of a patient with a Mallory-Weiss tear is similar to the presentation of esophageal varices.

A workup for gastrointestinal bleeding includes a variety of diagnostic studies. These diagnostic tests include serum chemistries, CBC, clotting profile, radiologic studies, and some invasive procedures. Evaluate the CBC for decreases in RBC and hemoglobin. Assess clotting studies, PTT, and aPTT for coagulopathy that may be contributing to the bleeding. Patients with ulcers may have an elevated serum gastrin level. If there is perforation with pancreatitis, the serum amylase level will be elevated. Evaluate stools for blood. Gastric analysis may be done to determine whether there is hyperacidity or presence of blood in gastric secretions. Gastroscopy allows direct visualization of the esophagus and stomach to evaluate the mucosa and to determine whether there are local areas of bleeding. Upper GI series, angiography, and/or biopsy may be necessary. A flat plate of the abdomen (i.e., KUB) will show free air under the diaphragm if perforation occurs.

There are many diagnostic laboratory abnormalities that occur with esophageal varices. The BUN and bilirubin may be elevated. The patient's albumin level is decreased because of liver disease. Liver enzymes (i.e., AST, ALT, and LDH) are frequently elevated. The patient's hemoglobin (Hgb) and hematocrit (Hct) decrease with blood loss. The clotting studies (PT and aPTT) are prolonged because of liver disease. The patient's stool may be positive for occult blood. In addition, in patients with severe blood loss from esophageal varices, the arterial blood gases may reveal metabolic acidosis related to shock and hypoperfusion. The electrocardiogram (ECG) may show indications of ischemia (e.g., ST-T wave changes). Several GI procedures are used in the differential diagnosis of esophageal varices. A barium swallow will reveal the presence of varices. An esophagogastroduodenoscopy (EGD) not only reveals the presence of esophageal varices but also may be used to treat the active bleeding sites with esophageal variceal ligation (EVL) or sclerotherapy. Percutaneous transhepatic portography reveals esophageal varices and measures pressure in the portal circulation. Angiography is rarely performed, but it will reveal bleeding sites and may be used to introduce the placement of a catheter for intraarterial administration of vasopressors (e.g., vasopressin).

Priority goals in the collaborative management of GI patients include the maintenance of a patent airway, oxygenation, ventilation, and circulation. Promote optimal ventilation and prevent aspiration by positioning the patient. Elevate the head of the bed 30 to 45 degrees and keep the patient turned to the left. Administer oxygen as necessary to maintain SpO_2 at 95% unless contraindicated. In patients with COPD, administer oxygen to achieve a SpO_2 of ~90%. Ensure availability of oropharyngeal suctioning equipment at the bedside. If indicated, intubate before endoscopy. Facilitate transfer to a higher level of care if it is necessary to protect the airway with endotracheal intubation to reduce risk of aspiration.

Monitor blood loss and maintain hemodynamic stability. Insert a large-bore orogastric or nasogastric tube and perform gastric lavage. Note that new evidence reveals that gastric lavage does not truly aid in clotting and may actually dislodge clots. The recommendations for gastric lavage include monitoring bleeding, allowing visualization during endoscopy, and removing nitrogenous materials (i.e., blood) out of the gut. Removal of nitrogenous material prevents it from being converted to ammonia. Use room temperature saline for lavage. Iced lavage is less effective in cessation of bleeding because it prolongs clotting times. Iced lavage also may cause hypothermia that will cause a shift of the oxyhemoglobin dissociation curve to the left, which decreases oxygen delivery to the tissues. In addition, iced lavage may cause the patient to shiver, increasing oxygen consumption.

Insert an indwelling urinary catheter to evaluate hourly urine output. Also, insert at least two short (1¼-inch) large-gauge (16 or 18) peripheral intravenous catheters and draw blood for laboratory analysis and blood type, and crossmatch for two units of blood. Administer isotonic crystalloids, usually 0.9% saline, initially as prescribed. Administer colloids as prescribed. The goal is to maintain urine output of 0.5 to 1 mL/kg/hr. Avoid lactated Ringer's (LR) in patients with liver disease. Administer blood and blood products as prescribed. Administer red packed cells early if significant blood loss is suspected to prevent tissue hypoxia. Indications for transfusion include the following:

- Persistent hemodynamic instability after 2 L of crystalloid
- Hematocrit less than 25%
- Clinical indications of hypoperfusion

Fresh blood is preferred, especially in patients with liver disease, because it is lower in ammonia than banked blood. After multiple transfusions, consider replacement of clotting factors, platelets, and calcium. In cases of severe hemorrhage, quickly facilitate transfer to a higher level of care.

Efforts to control bleeding include invasive procedures and medications (Table 6-6). Administer octreotide acetate (Sandostatin) as prescribed. Administer intravenous vasopressin as prescribed. This drug is also used to control bleeding but less often. Assist with diagnostic and therapeutic gastroendoscopy to identify the specific cause of the bleeding and therapeutically treat bleeding from peptic ulcers and/or a Mallory-Weiss tear. Endoscopic thermal therapy uses heat to cauterize the bleeding vessel. Endoscopic injection therapy uses hypertonic saline, epinephrine, or dehydrated alcohol to cause localized vasoconstriction of the bleeding vessel. Therapeutic endoscopy procedures for esophageal varices include ligation and sclerotherapy. Endoscopic injection therapy (i.e., sclerotherapy) uses a sclerosing agent (ethanolamine oleate [Ethamolin], morrhuate sodium [Scleromate], or sodium tetradecyl [Sotradecol]). One of these agents is injected into the varix and surrounding tissue. The sclerosing agent causes variceal inflammation, venous thrombosis, and eventually scar tissue. Repeated injections may be necessary to completely

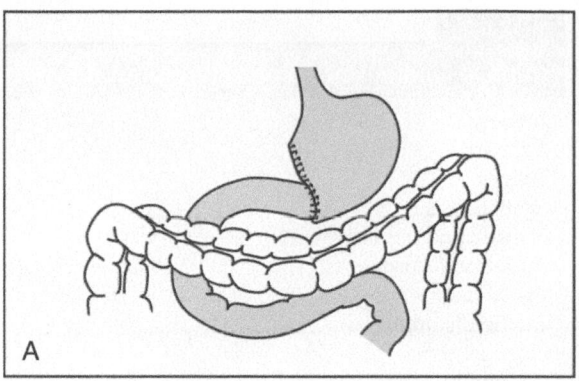
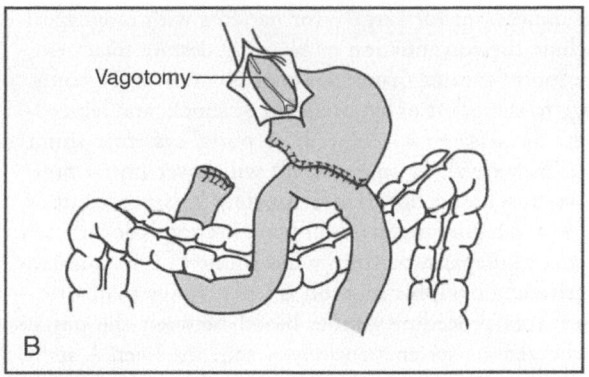
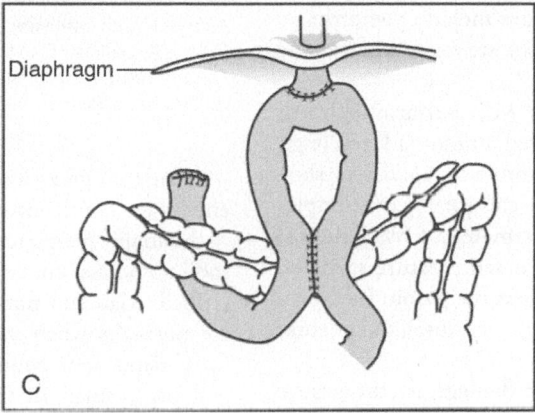

FIGURE 6-15 Gastric resection procedures. A. Billroth I; **B.** Billroth II; **C.** Total gastrectomy. (From Dennison, R. D. [2013]. *Pass CCRN!* [4th ed.]. St. Louis, MO: Elsevier.)

decompress the bleeding varix and decrease the risk of recurrent hemorrhage. Varices are categorized as I to IV by their size. Class III and IV are at high risk to bleed if not already bleeding. Sclerosing is repeated 4 to 7 days after the initial treatment and every 6 to 8 months thereafter. Monitor closely for complications of sclerotherapy:

- Retrosternal pain
- Transient fever
- Transient dysphagia
- Local ulceration
- Pulmonary symptoms including diminished breath sounds
- Bleeding
- Stricture
- Perforation
- Sepsis

Esophageal variceal ligation (EVL) is another invasive procedure performed to treat varices. Rubber bands or O-rings are placed on the target vessels at the gastroesophageal junction. Administer beta-blockers (e.g., propranolol) as prescribed to lower venous pressure to stop bleeding in esophageal varices.

Coagulopathy is frequently significant in patients with esophageal varices and liver disease. Administer vitamin K and recombinant clotting factors (e.g., rFVIIa) as prescribed. Monitor clotting studies and for evidence of bleeding. Avoid invasive procedures and injections if possible.

It may be necessary to prepare the patient for surgery to control bleeding. The indications for surgery in a patient with a peptic ulcer include the continuation of bleeding despite treatment, the need to administer greater than 8 units of blood over 24 hours, hemorrhage to the point of hypotension or shock, rebleeding after homeostasis is achieved, and perforation with evidence of pneumoperitoneum.

There are several possible surgical interventions. If the ulcer is prepyloric, the surgical procedure performed is an oversewing of the bleeding point along with a vagotomy. A vagotomy divides the vagus nerve along the esophagus and decreases acid secretion in the stomach. A vagotomy and pyloroplasty is a surgical procedure in which the pylorus is cut, then resutured to relax the muscle and widen the opening into the duodenum. A vagotomy and antrectomy is the surgical removal of the antrum to decrease acidity. Billroth procedures are used for gastroduodenal (Figure 6-15, A) and gastrojejunal reconstruction (Figure 6-15, B). A total gastrectomy involves the anastomosis of the esophagus to the duodenum or jejunum (Figure 6-15, C).

Monitor the patient postoperatively for early dumping syndrome. This syndrome occurs from a hyperosmolality effect related to a hyperosmolar bolus of food being "dumped" into the duodenum because of absence of the pyloric valve and normal, more gradual gastric emptying. This occurs within 30 minutes after eating and symptoms include dizziness, weakness, tachycardia, and cool, clammy skin. Late dumping syndrome can also be a complication of these procedures. This syndrome occurs from a hyperinsulinism effect related to an increase in insulin production by the pancreas in response to a large bolus of food causing an increase in blood glucose. This syndrome occurs 2 hours after a meal and patients complain of dizziness, weakness, and restlessness. Patients may also suffer from malabsorption and tachycardia along with cool, clammy skin. Pernicious anemia may also occur due to the removal of parietal cells that make intrinsic factor necessary for the absorption of vitamin B_{12} in the ileum.

Typical indications for surgery for patients with esophageal varices include the continuation of bleeding despite treatment, administration of greater than 8 units of blood over 24 hours, hemorrhage to the point of hypotension or shock, and rebleeding after homeostasis was achieved. A portal-systemic shunt (portacaval, mesocaval, or splenorenal) will lower portal pressure by diverting blood flow. Unfortunately, this procedure is associated with a higher incidence of hepatic encephalopathy. A transjugular intrahepatic portosystemic shunt (TIPS) inserted by an invasive angiographic method is less invasive than a surgical shunt. This procedure shunts blood between the portal and systemic venous systems entirely within the liver. A stent is placed in the tract between the hepatic and portal vein connection. Complications of this procedure include hemorrhage, acute kidney injury, septic shock, shunt stenosis, and hepatic encephalopathy.

It is necessary to monitor patients with portacaval shunts closely for clinical indications of elevated ammonia levels (e.g., confusion, irritability, decreased attention span, apathy, or slurring of speech). In addition, to prevent encephalopathy, implement measures to remove nitrogenous materials from the GI tract. Perform gastric lavage with room temperature saline so that bacteria in the GI tract cannot digest the globin (i.e., protein). Administer osmotic laxatives (e.g., lactulose) and enemas as prescribed.

It is important to prevent further damage to the gastric mucosa caused by gastric irritants, hyperacidity, and/or an impaired mucosal barrier. Discontinue any gastric irritants and decrease the gastric pH to between 3.5 and 5 (normal pH of gastric secretions is 1 to 3). Administer pharmacologic agents that decrease gastric acidity and/or protect gastric mucosa (see Table 6-6). To decrease acid, administer antacids, histamine (H_2) receptor antagonists, and proton pump inhibitors. In addition, provide agents to improve the mucosal barrier to acid such as prostaglandin E_1-analog (e.g., misoprostol [Cytotec]) and a mucosal protectant (aluminum hydroxide, sulfated sucrose, and sucralfate [Carafate]).

Employ additional measures to prevent mucosal damage. Provide required nutritional support by the enteral route if possible. A gastric tube may increase acid production by stimulating gastric secretion; therefore, remove any nasogastric or orogastric tube after lavage is completed and/or enteral nutritional support is not required. Administer drug therapy for *H. pylori*. Administer any of the following combinations of medication as prescribed:

- Bismuth subsalicylate + metronidazole + tetracycline + H_2 receptor antagonist
- Omeprazole + clarithromycin
- Ranitidine bismuth citrate + clarithromycin
- Lansoprazole + amoxicillin + clarithromycin
- Lansoprazole + amoxicillin

Maintain a calm and reassuring approach to decrease anxiety. Administer anxiolytics as prescribed and indicated. Avoid hepatotoxic agents if the patient has liver disease. Keep the patient and family informed regarding patient status and encourage discussion of fears and concerns. Institute the Clinical Institute Withdrawal Assessment of Alcohol (CIWA) Scale for patients with a history of chronic alcohol use. Monitor for clinical indications of alcohol withdrawal (Box 6-2). If alcohol withdrawal syndrome is present, begin treatment. Administer benzodiazepines (e.g., lorazepam

---

BOX 6-2

Clinical Findings of Alcohol Withdrawal Syndrome

Anxiety
Agitation
Tremor
Diaphoresis
Nausea and possibly vomiting
Auditory disturbances
Visual disturbances
Tactile disturbances
Headache
Change in orientation and sensorium

Adapted from Sullivan, J. T., Sykora, K., Schneiderman, J., Naranjo, C. A., & Sellers, E. M. (1989). Assessment of alcohol withdrawal: The revised clinical institute withdrawal assessment for alcohol scale (CIWA-Ar). *British Journal of Addiction, 84*(11), 1353–1357.

[Ativan]) as prescribed. Reorient the patient frequently and encourage family attendance.

Maintain the patient's fluid and electrolyte balance. Evaluate sodium, potassium, calcium, and magnesium, and replace as prescribed. Maintain nutritional status by administering appropriate nutrients when appropriate. Nutritional recommendations for patients with peptic ulcer include providing bland proteins and fats in small, frequent meals and avoidance of stimulants of gastric secretions, which include things like coffee, tea, cola, spicy foods, and alcohol. Progress the patient to a full diet as soon as possible. Dietary recommendations for patients with esophageal varices include giving clear liquids initially and to progress diet as indicated. Be careful to avoid alcohol-containing mouthwash and medications. Encourage thorough chewing of foods, especially hard, sharp foods like crackers as they may mechanically injure varices causing a recurrence of bleeding. Monitor the patient for the following postsurgical complications:

- Aspiration pneumonitis
- Recurrent bleeding, hemorrhage
- Perforation
- Peritonitis
- Penetration into surrounding tissues (e.g., acute pancreatitis)
- Gastric outlet syndrome related to ulcer inflammation and mucosal edema
- Obstruction due to ulcer scarring at the pylorus
- Myocardial infarction
- Cerebral infarction
- Disseminated intravascular coagulation (DIC)
- Sepsis
- Shock: hypovolemia or septic

6.8 Learning Activity

List four interventions for any patient with acute hemorrhage (regardless of location).

1. _____
2. _____
3. _____
4. _____

Answers to this activity can be found in the Answer Key.

6.9 Learning Activity

List four methods to control bleeding in esophageal varices.

1. _____
2. _____
3. _____
4. _____

Answers to this activity can be found in the Answer Key.

HEPATIC FAILURE/ENCEPHALOPATHY

Hepatic failure is the inability of the liver to perform organ functions. Acute liver failure (ALF) (previously referred to as *fulminant hepatic failure*) is defined as the onset of coagulopathy (INR greater than or equal to 1.5) and any degree of encephalopathy within 25 weeks of the appearance of liver failure symptoms in the absence of underlying liver disease (Larson, 2010). Hepatic encephalopathy is the neurologic failure that results from hepatic failure.

A common cause of acute liver failure is hepatotoxic drugs. Hepatotoxic drugs (see Box 6-1) include agents such as acetaminophen, halothane, methyldopa, isoniazid (INH), 3,4-methylenedioxymethamphetamine (Ecstasy), or toxins such

as *Amanita* mushrooms, carbon tetrachloride, and a sea anemone sting. An additional major cause of acute liver failure is fulminant viral hepatitis (Table 6-11).

Other viruses that may cause liver compromise and failure include herpes simplex, herpes zoster, Epstein-Barr, adenovirus, and cytomegalovirus. Ischemia from shock and MODS, trauma, Reye's syndrome, Budd-Chiari syndrome (i.e., hepatic vein obstruction), acute fatty liver of pregnancy, and acute hepatic vein occlusion may also cause chronic liver disease, resulting in ultimate liver failure. Chronic liver failure with an acute situation (e.g., peritonitis, GI hemorrhage, catabolism) may occur with cirrhosis, Wilson disease, and primary or metastatic tumors of the liver.

In cirrhosis, the liver parenchymal cells are progressively destroyed and replaced with fibrotic tissue. This results in impaired hepatic function. Three-quarters of the liver can be destroyed before symptoms appear. Distortion, twisting, and constriction of the central section causes impedance of portal blood flow and portal hypertension. In fulminant hepatitis, the liver cells fail to regenerate and necrosis occurs. The pathophysiology process of liver failure is complex and involves portal hypertension, impaired metabolism, inability to make plasma proteins, inability to inactivate hormones or detoxify drugs, and impaired protection from invading organisms. The failure of these processes results in coagulopathy, encephalopathy, and death (Figure 6-16).

TABLE 6-11 Types of Viral Hepatitis

Type	Route	Incubation Period	Onset/Chronicity	Comments
A (HAV, infectious hepatitis, enteric hepatitis)	• Fecal-oral	2-6 weeks	• Acute onset • Chronicity does not develop	• 99% resolves but 1% becomes fulminant • Treatment is supportive
B (HBV; serum hepatitis)	• Parenteral • Sexual • Perinatal	4-24 weeks	• Insidious onset • Chronicity develops in less than 5%	• 1% becomes fulminant • 15-25% develop liver cancer • Treatment includes Interferon alfa-2b (Intron A); antivirals such as lamivudine (Epivir) or famciclovir (Famvir) may also be prescribed
C (HCV; non-A, non-B hepatitis; posttransfusion hepatitis)	• Parenteral • Sexual • Perinatal	2-20 weeks	• Insidious onset • Chronicity develops in 50-60%	• 20-50% develop cirrhosis • 20% develop liver cancer • 20% develop liver failure • Treatment includes interferon alfa-2b (Intron A) or peginterferon alfa-2b (PegIntron) and ribavirin (Virazole); may also include corticosteroids
D (HDV; delta virus)	• Superinfection or coinfection in patient with chronic hepatitis B	4-24 weeks	• Acute onset • Chronicity common with superinfection	• Up to 30% become fulminant • Most have worsening active hepatitis • Treatment is as for hepatitis B
E (HEV; enteric non-A, non-B hepatitis)	• Fecal-oral • Perinatal	2-8 weeks	• Acute onset • Chronicity does not develop	• Generally benign and self-limiting; however, 10-20% mortality when it occurs during pregnancy
F (HFV)	• Parenteral • Sexual • Perinatal			• Now considered a variant of hepatitis B
G (HGV)				• Very little known

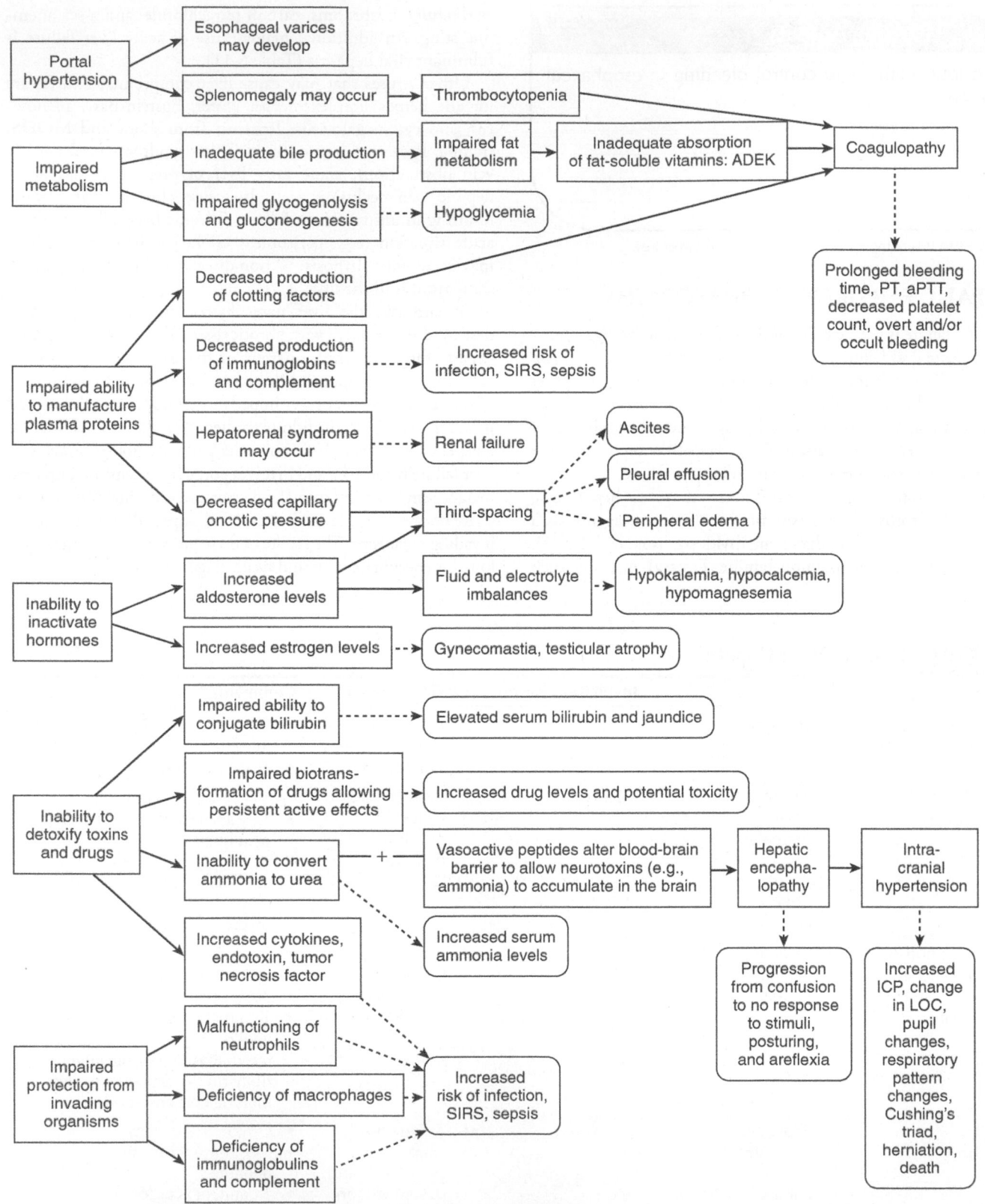

FIGURE 6-16 Pathophysiology of liver failure. Dashed lines connect pathology to clinical presentation. (From Dennison, R. D. [2013]. *Pass CCRN!* [4th ed.]. St. Louis, MO: Elsevier.)

The patient's history of present illness may include a precipitating event. The patient often complains of irritability, personality change, disorientation, weakness, fatigue, and GI symptoms of anorexia, nausea, and vomiting. The patient may also complain of dull pain in the right upper quadrant, abdominal fullness, a change in bowel habits, and weight loss.

The patient may present with general emaciation and cachectic appearance. Cardiovascular findings include tachycardia, dysrhythmias, bounding pulses, hypertension or hypotension, flushed skin, and spider angiomas on the upper trunk, face, neck, and arms. In addition, the patient may demonstrate jugular venous distention and distended superficial vessels on the abdomen (i.e., caput medusae). Pulmonary findings include tachypnea or hyperpnea and decreased respiratory excursion.

TABLE 6-12	Diagnostic Abnormalities in Liver Failure
Electrolytes	• Decreased or normal sodium • Decreased potassium, calcium, and magnesium
BUN	• Elevated due to dehydration, hepatorenal syndrome, or GI bleeding
Glucose	• Frequently decreased
Creatinine	• Elevated due to hepatorenal syndrome
Cholesterol	• Elevated
Liver enzymes	• Elevated ALT, AST, and LDH • AST/ALT ratio >1 in chronic liver failure or tumor and <1 in hepatitis • Elevated alkaline phosphatase
Bilirubin	• Elevated
Ammonia	• Elevated in encephalopathy
Total protein, serum albumin	• Decreased
Fibrinogen	• Decreased
Hemoglobin and hematocrit	• Decreased if hemorrhage or hypersplenism
WBC count	• Decreased; if normal or elevated, infection may be present
Platelets	• Decreased in splenomegaly
Arterial blood gases	• Respiratory alkalosis and hypoxemia
Urinalysis	• Decreased sodium • Elevated bilirubin in biliary obstruction • Elevated urobilinogen in hepatocellular disease; decreased in complete biliary obstruction

Neurologically, the patient frequently exhibits peripheral neuropathy; slow, slurred speech; asterixis; hyperactive reflexes; and seizures. The patient may have a positive Babinski's reflex, extreme lethargy, or coma in encephalopathy. GI symptoms include fetor hepaticus, ascites, and hematemesis. In the early stages, the patient has hepatomegaly, but liver atrophy occurs later. Esophageal varices and/or hemorrhoids may be present. The patient may also have splenomegaly. Bowel sounds are diminished and stools are clay-colored (i.e., pale) if biliary obstruction is present. Steatorrhea, which is a condition of excessive fat in the stool, may also occur. Oliguria and/or dark amber urine are likely. Abnormal bruising and bleeding along with an increased susceptibility to infection and poor wound healing are hematologic and immunologic system findings. In liver failure, effects on the integumentary system include the appearance of jaundice, which is usually noted in the sclera first. In addition, the patient's skin has evidence of palmar erythema, petechiae, bruises, edema, pruritus, and spider angiomas. Endocrine findings in men include testicular atrophy, reduced testosterone levels, and gynecomastia. Both males and females often have altered hair distribution.

Liver failure causes many alterations to serum laboratory tests, arterial blood gases, and urinalysis (Table 6-12). A chest x-ray may show pleural effusion or atelectasis. A flat plate of the abdomen may reveal hepatosplenomegaly, and abdominal haziness if ascites is present. An abdominal ultrasound may reveal intraabdominal fluid if ascites is present. Barium swallow or EGD may be done to identify presence of esophageal varices. A liver scan may show diffuse changes of cirrhosis, whereas a liver biopsy determines fatty infiltration in early stages or severe degeneration and scarring in the advanced stage. To identify biliary obstruction, an endoscopic retrograde cholangiopancreatography will be performed. A paracentesis with cytologic examination may be done to rule out malignancy. Ascites fluid in a paracentesis sample has low specific gravity, low protein concentration, and low cell counts. The patient's EEG may be abnormal and show generalized slowing in patients with encephalopathy. Sometimes a lumbar puncture may be done to rule out a neurologic cause of altered consciousness. The CSF sample shows an increase in glutamine.

The severity of hepatic encephalopathy is judged and staged according to the presence of symptoms; stages of hepatic encephalopathy are classified as stage I through IV based on the level of deterioration (Box 6-3). The last stage of hepatic encephalopathy manifests as a loss of consciousness.

6.10 Learning Activity

Match the following clinical manifestations of hepatic failure with the pathophysiologic change (answers may be used more than once).

_____ 1. Splenic engorgement
_____ 2. Stretching of the liver capsule
_____ 3. Decrease in the metabolism of testosterone
_____ 4. Decrease in metabolism of aldosterone
_____ 5. Decrease in production of plasma proteins
_____ 6. Decrease in metabolism of estrogen
_____ 7. Decrease in production of clotting factors
_____ 8. Decrease in conjugation and excretion of bilirubin

a. Petechiae, purpura, bleeding
b. Jaundice
c. Third-spacing
d. Testicular atrophy
e. Gynecomastia
f. Anemia, leukopenia, thrombocytopenia
g. Abdominal tenderness

Answers to this activity can be found in the Answer Key.

BOX 6-3

Stages of Encephalopathy

Stage I

- Mild confusion
- Decreased attention span
- Difficulty performing simple arithmetical computations (e.g., count backward from 100 by 7s)
- Decreased response time
- Forgetfulness
- Mood changes
- Slurred speech
- Personality changes
- Irritability
- Disruption in sleep-wake patterns
- EEG normal

Stage II

- Lethargy
- Confusion
- Apathy
- Aberrant behavior
- Tremor and asterixis (also referred to as *liver flap*)
- Inability to reproduce simple designs (constructional apraxia)
- Slowing of normal EEG

Stage III

- Somnolent with diminished responsiveness to verbal stimuli
- Severe confusion and incoherence following arousal
- Incomprehensible speech
- Tremor and asterixis
- Hyperactive deep tendon reflexes
- Hyperventilation
- EEG abnormal

Stage IV

- No response to stimuli or abnormal posturing (e.g., decorticate or decerebrate) to stimuli
- Areflexia except for pathologic reflexes
- Positive Babinski's reflex
- Fetor hepaticus
- EEG abnormal

The collaborative management of a patient in hepatic failure starts with the identification and treatment of the cause of hepatic failure. Administer N-acetylcysteine (Mucomyst) for acetaminophen toxicity within 24 hours of acetaminophen ingestion. Administer antivirals (e.g., acyclovir, ganciclovir) as prescribed for viral causes. Interferon may also be prescribed.

The second priority in collaborative management is to prevent further injury to the liver. Avoid hepatotoxic drugs and alcohol-containing mouthwash or medications. Monitor the patient's liver function studies closely.

During treatment, it is important to maintain the airway, oxygenation, and ventilation. Elevate the head of the bed 30 to 45 degrees especially if ascites restricts diaphragmatic excursion. Monitor the patient for and prevent aspiration. Utilize artificial airways as necessary in patients with altered consciousness and airway protective mechanisms (e.g., gag reflex). Intubation is usually required

at stage III hepatic encephalopathy. Administer oxygen as necessary to maintain SpO_2 at 95% unless contraindicated. In patients with COPD, administer oxygen to achieve a SpO_2 of ~90%. Assist in the management of ascites that cause decreased diaphragmatic excursion and ventilation difficulties. Monitor closely for clinical indications of atelectasis. Assist with a paracentesis procedure as necessary. A patient may need a paracentesis if extremely dyspneic.

Fluid and electrolyte balances need to be maintained and monitored. Administer aldosterone antagonists (also referred to as *potassium-sparing diuretics*) (e.g., spironolactone [Aldactone]) as prescribed. Loop diuretics may also be required as aldosterone antagonists tend to lose their effectiveness over time. Restrict sodium to 500 mg/daily and restrict fluids to 1500 mL/day as prescribed. Maintain vigilance and be alert to clinical indications of hypovolemia.

Surgical procedures that shunt ascites fluid into the superior vena cava may be needed. A LeVeen or Denver shunt may be performed when the patient is stable. A LeVeen shunt uses positive abdominal pressure caused by the descent of the diaphragm during inspiration to open an intraperitoneal valve to shunt fluid from the peritoneum to the superior vena cava. A Denver shunt adds a subcutaneous pump that can be compressed manually to irrigate the intraperitoneal tubing.

Close observation of arterial blood gases is important in the management of these patients. Monitor the patient closely for early signs of acute respiratory distress syndrome (ARDS) and clinical indications of respiratory distress and low SpO_2. Take care of and control respiratory alkalosis associated with hyperammonemia. Muscle paralysis, sedation, and mechanical ventilation may be required to control $Paco_2$ levels; this therapy requires transfer to a higher level of care.

Maintain adequate circulating volume and fluid and electrolyte balances. Maintain the circulating blood volume by administering colloids as prescribed to improve capillary oncotic pressure and to reduce third-spacing. Avoid protein-containing colloids (e.g., albumin) in hepatic encephalopathy. Administer crystalloids as prescribed. Avoid the administration of lactated Ringer's solution because the liver is responsible for converting lactate to bicarbonate. Invasive hemodynamic monitoring and vasopressors may be necessary to maintain vascular tone, especially in stage III and IV hepatic encephalopathy. Facilitate the transfer to a higher level of care if these invasive treatments are necessary.

Monitor closely for indications of fluid and electrolyte imbalances. Monitor vital signs and hemodynamic status. Weigh the patient daily at the same time on the same scale and measure abdominal girth daily for patients with ascites. Monitor serum osmolality, sodium, potassium, calcium, and magnesium. Administer electrolyte replacement as needed.

Observe the patient's urine output closely and note the following clinical indications of hepatorenal syndrome:

- Oliguria (less than 0.5 mL/kg/hr)
- Low urinary sodium
- Elevated BUN, serum creatinine
- Low serum sodium (i.e., dilutional hyponatremia)
- Moderately reduced GFR (less than 50 mL/min) as evaluated by 24-hour urine

Administer diuretics as prescribed and monitor closely for clinical indications of intravascular depletion and azotemia. Avoid thiazide diuretics and utilize aldosterone antagonists (also frequently referred to as potassium-sparing diuretics) (e.g., spironolactone [Aldactone]). Administer loop diuretics after albumin. Albumin pulls fluid back into the intravascular space. Furosemide (Lasix) then eliminates the fluid by preventing reabsorption of sodium and water in the renal tubules. Prepare the patient for transfer to a critical care unit if CRRT is required. CRRT is preferred over hemodialysis because it is less likely to precipitate rapid osmolar shifts that can cause intracranial hypertension. Unfortunately, patients with hepatorenal syndrome transferred to a higher level of care for these procedures are frequently unresponsive to treatment.

Maintain gastric pH to reduce the risk of stress ulcers, GI hemorrhage, and accumulations of toxins. Administer H_2 receptor antagonists and/or antacids as prescribed to maintain pH between 3.5 and 5 to reduce the risk of stress ulcer and GI hemorrhage. Prevent and reduce elevated levels of toxins, including ammonia. Stop nitrogen-containing drugs such as ammonium chloride and urea. Administer lactulose (combination of galactose and fructose) orally, via NG tube, or rectally as prescribed.

Lactulose acts as a chelating (bonding) agent of ammonia by changing gut pH, which results in ammonia excretion. The drug changes gut flora to foster growth of non-ammonia-forming bacteria and acts as an osmotic laxative. Adjust the dose of lactulose to produce two semiformed stools/day. The nurse may administer an antibiotic to kill the bacteria that convert nitrogenous wastes to ammonia as prescribed. Rifaximin (Xifaxan) is a nonabsorbable antibiotic that is now preferred over neomycin. Neomycin has been traditionally used and may be prescribed by oral or NG tube. If neomycin is used, monitor for auditory or renal toxicity. Administer magnesium citrate orally and/or tap water enemas as prescribed to remove nitrogenous wastes from the GI tract. The nurse needs to help prevent patient constipation with fiber, stool softeners, and enemas.

Patients in hepatic failure may require the use of liver support systems. Many of these procedures are done in a higher level of care unit; however, sometimes the patient may remain on the progressive care unit and the specialist will come to the unit to do the procedure. The patient may transition back and forth from the progressive care unit to the critical care unit. Both of these situations create the need for the progressive care nurse to be somewhat knowledgeable about the procedures to aid in the identification of the need for treatment and to monitor for and treat potential complications.

The liver support system may include hemodialysis, CRRT, therapeutic plasma exchange, and the use of a bioartificial liver or an extracorporeal liver in vitro. In hemodialysis, the blood is circulated through a porous filter for rapid removal of fluid and solutes. In CRRT, the blood is circulated through a porous filter for slow removal of fluid and solutes. Hemoperfusion may also occur with hemodialysis or CRRT with a charcoal or resin exchange filter added. Therapeutic plasma exchange is a treatment where the plasma removal is replaced by donor plasma. Bioartificial liver support involves the blood flowing through a hollow fiber cartridge loaded with either cultured human or porcine hepatocytes. In extracorporeal liver perfusion the blood is circulated through a human or animal liver in vitro. Although the progressive care nurse may not be directly involved with these procedures, it is important that he or she understand the concepts related to them.

In caring for a liver failure patient, a priority in care involves the prevention, assessment, and treatment for intracranial

hypertension and progression of hepatic encephalopathy. Perform frequent neurologic checks. Avoid activities that increase intracranial pressure (ICP) (see the intracranial hypertension section of Chapter 9). For the patient with hepatic encephalopathy, maintain bed rest. Teach the patient to avoid the Valsalva maneuver and other activities that increase intraabdominal or intrathoracic pressure. Maintain the patient's $Paco_2$ at a normal range and avoid hypoxemia. Both hypercarbia and hypoxemia will increase ICP. Institute seizure precautions to keep the patient safe. Administer hypertonic saline or mannitol (Osmitrol) and/or drainage of cerebrospinal fluid (if ICP catheter in place) to decrease cerebral edema. ICP monitoring is frequently utilized, especially in grade III and IV hepatic encephalopathy. Recognize if invasive ICP monitoring is required and facilitate a transfer to a higher level of care.

Medication management can be complex while caring for liver failure patients. Avoid the use of hepatotoxic agents (see Box 6-1). Avoid sedatives and analgesics and/or check to see if it is necessary to reduce dosage. Administer diphenhydramine (Benadryl) or oxazepam (Serax) as prescribed for restlessness because they can safely be eliminated.

Administer beta-blockers as prescribed to decrease portal hypertension. Prepare the patient for a shunt as requested. An interventional radiologic procedure, TIPS, may be done. A surgical procedure (e.g., portacaval shunt) may also be done, but this is associated with a higher incidence of hepatic encephalopathy than the TIPS procedure.

During care, it is important to maintain normal serum glucose and nutritional status. Monitor serum glucose every 4 to 6 hours. Administer IV dextrose solution continuously. To prevent hypoglycemia, it may be necessary to administer D_{10}. Increase dietary protein (0.6 to 1 g/kg/day) for patients with cirrhosis and hepatic failure, but restrict dietary protein to less than 0.5 g/kg/day in hepatic encephalopathy. Provide adequate carbohydrate intake to prevent muscle catabolism and muscle wasting (caloric requirements from 35 to 40 kcal/kg/day). Add protein in 20-g increments during recovery from encephalopathy.

Use the appropriate route for nutritional support: oral, enteral, or parenteral. With oral nutritional support, administer antiemetics as prescribed before each meal and whenever indicated to prevent nausea. Nausea is a significant impairment to oral nutritional intake in these patients. The use of enteral nutrition is necessary in patients with altered consciousness. Elemental formulas (e.g., Vivonex) are frequently used while maintaining protein restrictions if indicated (i.e., hepatic encephalopathy). In administering nutrition via a parenteral route, use branched-chain amino acid formulas in encephalopathy. Dextrose and lipids prevent the metabolism of parenteral amino acids or somatic protein (i.e., catabolism) for energy requirements. It is also important to administer vitamins and minerals. These patients need fat-soluble (i.e., A, D, E, K) vitamins, thiamine, and other B vitamins.

Prevent and monitor for injury, infection, and skin breakdown. Alleviate pruritus with cornstarch baths and lotions. Place the patient's hands in cotton gloves at night to prevent scratching during sleep. Administer cholestyramine (Questran) as prescribed to reduce bile pigment accumulation in skin. Monitor the patient closely for clinical indications of infection and sepsis and administer antibiotic and antifungal microbials as prescribed.

Because coagulopathy is an issue, prevent and monitor for bleeding. Avoid aspirin and NSAIDs. Avoid invasive procedures, including injections, if possible. Administer vitamin K, fresh frozen plasma, platelets, and aminocaproic acid (Amicar) as prescribed.

Institute the Clinical Institute Withdrawal Assessment of Alcohol (CIWA) Scale for patients with a history of chronic alcohol use. Monitor for clinical indications of alcohol withdrawal (see Box 6-2). If alcohol withdrawal syndrome is present, begin treatment. Administer benzodiazepines (e.g., lorazepam [Ativan]) as prescribed. Avoid alcohol-containing mouthwash and medications. Reorient the patient frequently and encourage family attendance.

Participate in consideration of long-term treatment of hepatic failure, such as early evaluation of candidacy for liver transplantation. Monitor for the following complications:
- Malnutrition resulting in immunosuppression, poor wound healing, and edema
- Coagulopathy
- Hemorrhage, which may be due to:
  - Esophageal varices
  - Coagulopathy
  - Disseminated intravascular coagulation (DIC)
- Hypoglycemia
- Electrolyte imbalance
- Acute respiratory failure related to intrapulmonary shunt or noncardiac pulmonary edema
- Pancreatitis
- Infection or sepsis
- Acute kidney injury related to hepatorenal syndrome, acute tubular necrosis, or hypovolemia
- Seizures
- Cerebral edema

6.11   Learning Activity

List one type of diuretic that is indicated and one type of diuretic that is contraindicated for ascites in hepatic failure.

Indicated	Contraindicated

Answers to this activity can be found in the Answer Key.

ACUTE PANCREATITIS

Acute pancreatitis is an acute inflammation of the pancreas. There are two forms of acute pancreatitis: mild and severe. Mild acute pancreatitis (previously referred to as *interstitial pancreatitis*) results in an edematous pancreas with little necrosis damage. Hypovolemia results from a fluid leak into the peritoneal cavity. Mild acute pancreatitis usually resolves within approximately 7 days. Severe acute pancreatitis (previously referred to as *necrotizing pancreatitis)* causes extensive necrosis of the pancreas, peripancreatic tissue, and fat along with erosion into the blood vessels with hemorrhage. SIRS frequently occurs and there is a high incidence of complications and death.

Pancreatitis occurs when digestive enzymes produced in the pancreas are activated while inside the pancreas, causing inflammation and damage to the organ. There are several causes of pancreatitis. Obstruction of the common bile duct may occur from cholelithiasis and postendoscopic retrograde cholangio-pancreatography. Chronic alcohol intake leads to secretory and structural changes in the pancreas, which contributes to duct obstruction. Alcohol also increases the amount of trypsinogen, a pancreatic enzyme normally secreted into the intestine. Other causes of pancreatitis include peptic ulcer with perforation, cancer of the lung or pancreas, hypertriglyceridemia, and drugs. Drugs known to cause pancreatitis are as follows:
- Thiazide diuretics
- Furosemide
- Estrogen
- Procainamide
- Tetracycline
- Sulfonamides
- Corticosteroids
- Azathioprine (Imuran)
- Opiates

Injury to the pancreas from trauma along with certain gastric, biliary, and duodenal surgeries can also cause pancreatitis. Pancreatitis can occur from radiation injury, during an ectopic pregnancy, or during the third trimester. Other known causes include ovarian cysts, hyperparathyroidism or other causes of hypercalcemia, lupus erythematosus, and infections. Infections known to cause pancreatitis include the following:
- Mumps
- Coxsackievirus B
- *Mycoplasma*
- Infectious mononucleosis
- Viral hepatitis
- Human immunodeficiency virus (HIV)
- Intestinal parasites (e.g., *Ascaris*)

Risk factors for pancreatitis include ischemia due to shock and multiple organ dysfunction syndrome, postcardiopulmonary bypass, sepsis, hereditary factors, and idiopathic factors (20% of cases).

The pathophysiologic process (Figure 6-17) that occurs with the development of pancreatitis is from the activation of pancreatic enzymes, which cause edema, necrosis of the pancreas, or necrosis of the fat in the pancreas. Activation of trypsin, elastase, and kallikrein leads to edema and necrosis of the pancreas. This will lead into erosion into the vessels, damage to the islet cells, and release of toxins and mediators. The end-result can be bleeding, hemorrhage, hypovolemia, hyperglycemia, SIRS, ARDS, sepsis, and/or hypovolemic and septic shock. Activation of the other pathway of pancreatitis occurs from the activation of phospholipase A. The release of phospholipase A leads to necrosis of the fat in the pancreas, which results in the precipitation of calcium and high albumin exudate causing hypocalcemia, hypoalbuminia, and ascites.

Patients with pancreatitis complain of abdominal pain and associated symptoms. A heavy (especially if fatty) meal or a drinking binge may precipitate the abdominal pain. The pain may be eased or palliated by leaning forward or by assuming the fetal position. The patient may describe the pain quality as a "boring" sensation that is diffusely located in the region of the epigastrium, but it may also appear in the left upper quadrant. The pain often radiates to the back or flank area. The patient often describes the pain severity as moderate to severe and usually states it came on suddenly and is constant. The patient may

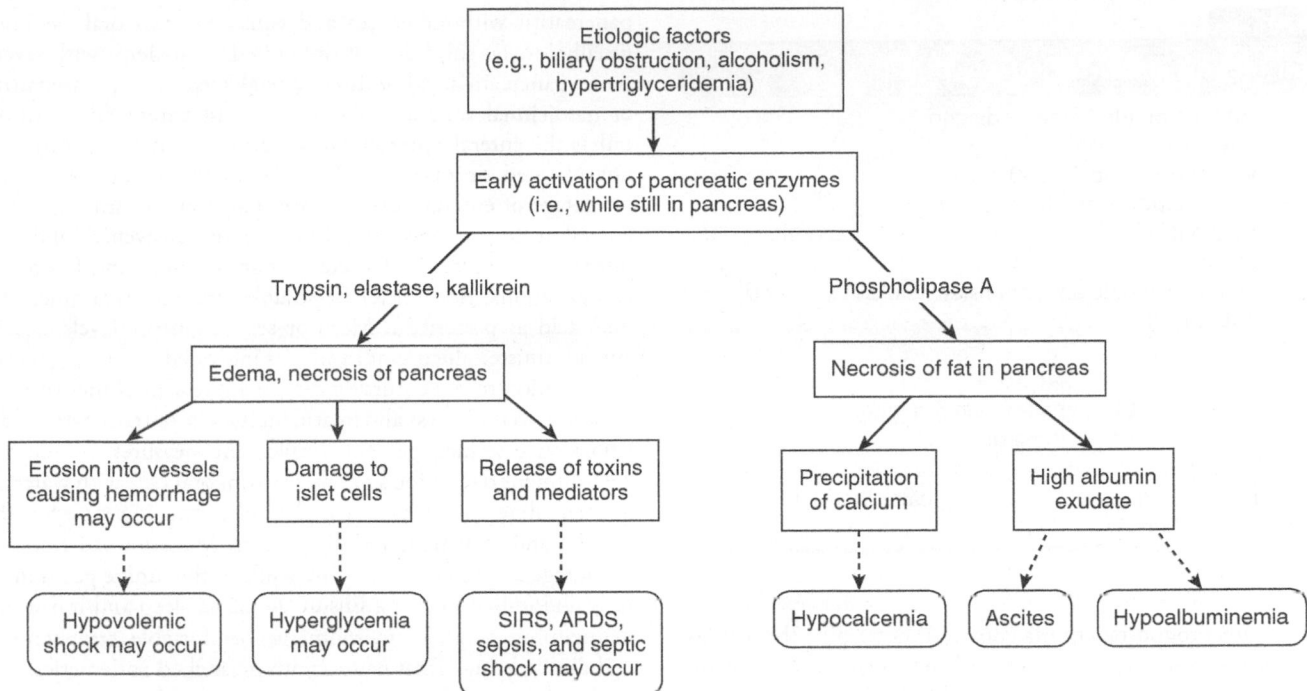

FIGURE 6-17 Pathophysiology of pancreatitis. Dashed lines connect pathology to clinical presentation. (From Dennison, R. D. [2013]. *Pass CCRN!* [4th ed.]. St. Louis, MO: Elsevier.)

also complain of the associated symptoms of abdominal tenderness, guarding, nausea, vomiting, retching, dyspepsia, flatulence, diarrhea, weight loss, and weakness.

Objective findings include tachycardia and hypotension due to decreased circulating volume related to effusion, hemorrhage, or septic shock. A low-grade (e.g., 37.8 to 39° C) fever may be present. If biliary obstruction is present, jaundice will be evident. Additional assessment findings include vomiting, hematemesis, Grey-Turner sign or Cullen sign seen with hemorrhage, and abdominal distention. Bowel sounds will be decreased or absent on auscultation. Patients may have indications of peritoneal irritation such as involuntary guarding during palpation of the abdomen and rebound tenderness. An epigastric mass may be palpable especially if there is a pseudocyst and ascites may be present. The patient may have steatorrhea: bulky, pale, foul-smelling, and floating stools. Breath sounds may be diminished or adventitious crackles auscultated due to atelectasis, pleural effusion, or ARDS. Chvostek sign or Trousseau sign may be positive in pancreatitis-related hypocalcemia.

The serum potassium, calcium, and magnesium are decreased in pancreatitis, while the glucose and triglyceride levels are elevated. The liver enzymes are also elevated. The amylase level is usually elevated to greater than 3 times the normal level. The levels peak at 4 to 24 hours after onset of symptoms and usually return to normal within 4 days. The amylase level may remain normal when pancreatitis is due to hypertriglyceridemia. The lipase level is elevated and stays elevated longer than amylase. The lipase elevation is more specific than amylase. In patients with pancreatitis, the albumin level decreases. The BUN may be elevated due to hypovolemia. The liver function tests of AST, ALT, LDH, alkaline phosphatase, and bilirubin are elevated in liver or biliary disease. The hematocrit is decreased with hemorrhage, but it is elevated with hemoconcentration due to third-spacing. The WBC is usually elevated with a shift to the left noted. The routine arterial blood gas derangement is metabolic

acidosis. In addition, respiratory complications may cause respiratory acidosis and hypoxemia.

The urine amylase is usually elevated. Fecal fat is increased. An ECG may show ST-T wave changes suggestive of a myocardial infarction (MI). Radiology examination of the chest (x-ray) may show bilateral or only left pleural effusion, elevated left hemidiaphragm, and left atelectasis; it may also show pulmonary complications of pancreatitis such as atelectasis, pneumonia, ARDS, and pleural effusion. A flat plate of the abdomen may show the cause of the pancreatitis (e.g., cholelithiasis); it may also show ileus and bowel dilation or calcified pancreatic stones. An upper GI series may show delayed gastric emptying, enlargement of the duodenum, and presence of a dilated loop of smooth bowel adjacent to the pancreas. An abdominal ultrasound may show pancreatic swelling, edema, gallstones, pseudocyst, and/or peripancreatic fluid collections. A CT scan with contrast may show enlargement, edema, and necrosis of the pancreas and/or complications of pancreatitis (e.g., pancreatic pseudocyst or abscess). Frequently, the grade of pancreatitis is determined using the CT scan by following Balthazar and Ranson's system:

- Grade A: Normal pancreas
- Grade B: Focal or diffuse enlargement of the pancreas
- Grade C: Mild peripancreatic inflammatory changes
- Grade D: Fluid collection in a single location
- Grade E: Multiple fluid collections or gas within the pancreas or peripancreatic inflammation

An MRI will show inflammatory changes within the pancreas. The procedure called endoscopic retrograde cholangiopancreatography (ERCP) is contraindicated in acute pancreatitis. It is used more often in chronic pancreatitis to identify ductal changes or calculi. A hepatobiliary iminodiacetic acid scan (HIDA), also referred to as cholescintigraphy, may identify hepatocellular disease from biliary obstruction as the cause of pancreatitis. In hemorrhagic pancreatitis, a peritoneal lavage is positive for blood.

BOX 6-4

Ranson's Prognostic Criteria

- At the time of admission or diagnosis
  - Age over 55 years
  - WBC count over 16000/mm³
  - Serum glucose greater than 200 mg/dL
  - Serum lactate dehydrogenase (LDH) greater than 350 units/L
  - Serum aspartate aminotransferase (AST) greater than 250 units/L
- After 48 hours
  - Hct drop greater than 10%
  - Increase in BUN greater than 5 mg/dL
  - Calcium less than 8 mg/dL
  - Base deficit greater than 4 mEq/L
  - Estimated fluid sequestration greater than 6 L
- PaO_2 less than 60 mm Hg

Ranson's prognostic criteria (Box 6-4) determine the severity and risk for mortality associated with pancreatitis. Each of the criteria increases the severity and risk for death. Mild pancreatitis scores only 1 to 2 criteria and the mortality rate is approximately 1%. More than 6 criteria indicate severe pancreatitis with a predicted mortality rate greater than 60%.

The priority focus of collaborative management for a patient with pancreatitis is to maintain airway, oxygenation, ventilation, and circulation. Elevate the head of the bed 30 to 45 degrees, especially if ascites restricts diaphragmatic excursion. Administer oxygen as necessary to maintain SpO_2 at 95% unless contraindicated. In patients with COPD, administer oxygen to achieve a SpO_2 of ~90%. Monitor SpO_2 closely and evaluate the work of breathing in detection of development of atelectasis and/or ARDS. To maintain adequate circulating volume and fluid and electrolyte balances, administer crystalloids and colloids as prescribed to restore circulating blood volume. Monitor closely for clinical indications of fluid overload; fluid overload is associated with increased risk of pulmonary edema, acute respiratory distress syndrome, and abdominal hypertension or abdominal compartment syndrome. Monitor sodium, calcium, potassium, magnesium, and phosphate levels. Administer calcium replacement orally or intravenously as prescribed. Administer potassium replacement as prescribed. Restrict sodium to 500 mg/daily for patients with ascites. Also, measure the patient's abdominal girth daily to assess for ascites and weigh daily at the same time on the same scale.

Decreasing the release of and destruction by pancreatic enzymes begins with treatment of the cause:
- Alcohol cessation if alcohol-related
- A cholecystectomy after resolution of pancreatitis if the cause is cholelithiasis
- Discontinuance of the offending drug if drug-induced
- Statins, niacin, fibrates, or omega-3 fatty acids given if the cause is hypertriglyceridemia

Also, administer drugs IV or subcutaneously as prescribed to decrease secretion of pancreatic enzymes, such as octreotide acetate (Sandostatin) and/or H_2 receptor antagonists IV (see Table 6-6).

Maintain NPO status during the acute phase if the patient has nausea and vomiting. In patients with mild acute pancreatitis without nausea and vomiting, start oral feedings, usually low-fat solid diet, as prescribed. In patients with severe acute pancreatitis, administer enteral feedings by nasogastric or nasojejunal tube as prescribed. Avoid parenteral nutrition unless the enteral route is contraindicated, enteral feedings are not tolerated, or it is required to meet caloric requirements. The advantage of enteral nutrition over parenteral nutrition is that enteral nutrition maintains immune responsiveness and gut integrity, reduces risk of bacterial translocation, and has fewer complications. Administer fat-soluble vitamins, thiamine, and folic acid as prescribed. Monitor serum glucose levels closely and administer glucose or insulin as indicated.

Attention to basic nursing care to address all of the patient's responses to the illness and treatment is an important part of collaborative care management. Implement measures to keep the environment free of food odors. Perform oral care with water or normal saline only. Do not use alcohol-containing mouthwash. Prevent and treat pain and discomfort. Maintain bed rest and encourage a knee flexion posture while in the supine position to relax abdominal muscles. Ensure adequate sleep and rest while maintaining a quiet environment, comfortable temperature, and dim lighting. Treat nausea with prescribed antiemetics.

Administer opiate analgesics (e.g., morphine, hydromorphone), preferably by patient-controlled analgesia (PCA). Although for years meperidine (Demerol) has been considered the analgesic of choice in acute pancreatitis, recent studies show no significant difference between morphine and meperidine in the degree of spasm of the sphincter of Oddi, and morphine has less toxicity. Consider a neurolytic block of the celiac plexus for severe persistent pain. Also, utilize nonpharmacologic pain relief methods such as imagery, distraction, and music.

Prevent and monitor for infection. Administer antibiotics as prescribed that effectively penetrate the pancreatic tissue and provide good coverage against gram-negative enteric and anaerobic organisms (e.g., imipenem/cilastatin [Primaxin], ofloxacin [Floxin], metronidazole [Flagyl]). If there is no improvement after 1 week, a CT-guided aspiration may be performed. Bacteria found present in the aspirate suggests pancreatic necrosis with infection and indicates the need for surgery. Monitor the patient for the clinical indications of abscess formation (e.g., increase in abdominal pain, vomiting, fever, and leukocytosis).

Prepare the patient for possible surgical measures for the relief of pancreatitis when absolutely necessary. A cholecystectomy may be performed if bile reflux is the cause of pancreatitis. An abscess or pseudocysts need to be drained. A pancreatic resection/total pancreatectomy is done if the pancreas and/or other organs are necrotic. After surgical débridement of necrotic tissue, the abdomen incision may be left open and packed, or closed with drains in place. A total pancreatectomy results in diabetes and other metabolic difficulties. The surgeon attempts to reimplant any viable pancreatic tissue following a total pancreatectomy. Islet cell autotransplantation and/or a segmental pancreatic autotransplantation can help to maintain metabolic function. Monitor and maintain normal serum glucose levels. Administer insulin as indicated and prescribed. Maintain constant infusion of TPN solution or enteral feedings.

Because pancreatitis is often a result of alcohol abuse, institute the Clinical Institute Withdrawal Assessment of Alcohol (CIWA) Scale for patients with a history of chronic alcohol use. Monitor for clinical indications of alcohol withdrawal (see Box 6-2). If alcohol withdrawal syndrome is present, begin treatment.

Administer benzodiazepines (e.g., lorazepam [Ativan]) as prescribed. Avoid alcohol-containing mouthwash or medications. Reorient the patient frequently and encourage family attendance.

Monitor patients with pancreatitis for general complications of fluid and electrolyte imbalances, and hypoglycemia or hyperglycemia. Pancreatitis can cause multisystem problems such as SIRS, pleural effusion, ARDS, GI bleeding, disseminated intravascular coagulation (DIC), sepsis, acute kidney injury, and perforation. Clinical presentation includes tachycardia, hypotension, oliguria, and other indications of hypoperfusion. Collaborative management includes volume resuscitation, including crystalloids; colloids; and blood administration for hemorrhagic pancreatitis. Specific pancreas complications include pseudocysts, abscesses, and fistulas.

The collection of inflammatory debris, pancreatic secretions, and necrotic tissue in the pancreatic tissue causes the formation of pseudocysts. The cysts may cause compression of the portal vein or bile duct or rupture and cause peritonitis and sepsis. Clinical presentation includes pain or ache in the abdomen, a feeling of bloating, or poor digestion of food. Complications related to the pseudocyst include infection of the pseudocyst with a pancreatic abscess, bleeding into the pseudocyst, or intestinal obstruction of the intestine by the pseudocyst. Collaborative management includes nothing for small cysts or drainage by a surgical, endoscopic, or percutaneous approach for larger cysts.

The accumulation of pus in or near the pancreas causes the formation of a pancreatic abscess. Clinical presentation includes fever, palpable mass, abdominal tenderness, nausea, vomiting, and leukocytosis. Collaborative management includes surgery for drainage.

A pancreatic fistula is another complication caused by a communication between the pancreas and the skin. Clinical presentation includes drainage of extremely alkaline pancreatic secretions onto the skin and severe excoriation. Collaborative management depends on the presence of symptoms (e.g., abdominal pain, fever, chills, jaundice, early satiety), the characteristics and location of the fluid collection on imaging (e.g., presence of pancreatic necrosis, proximity to the bowel lumen), and the presence of associated complications (e.g., infection of pancreatic fluid). Treatment includes suppression of pancreatic enzymes by restricting the patient's oral intake of food in conjunction with the use of long-acting somatostatin analogues and maintaining nutrition with TPN. Continue medical treatment for 2 to 3 weeks, and observe the patient for improvement. If no improvement is seen, the patient may receive endoscopic, ERCP, and surgical treatment.

INTESTINAL INFARCTION/OBSTRUCTION/PERFORATION

An intestinal infarction is the necrosis of the intestinal wall resulting from ischemia. An intestinal obstruction is a failure of the intestinal contents to progress forward through the lumen of the bowel. An obstruction may be partial or complete. The loss of peristalsis causes a functional obstruction referred to as paralytic ileus. A structural (i.e., mechanical) obstruction is caused by factors that occlude the bowel lumen. Grade obstructions based on severity, extent, and location. A simple obstruction occurs when the luminal obstruction does not compromise the blood supply. A strangulated obstruction occurs when the luminal obstruction also compromises the blood supply. The extent of the obstruction determines whether it is partial or complete. The location is defined as proximal versus distal. An obstruction can lead to a perforation. An intestinal perforation occurs when there is penetration of the lumen of the intestine with resultant spillage of intestinal contents into the peritoneal cavity.

Intestinal infarction occurs as an end-result of arteriosclerosis, vasculitis, mural thrombus, emboli after a myocardial infarction (MI), atrial fibrillation ventricular aneurysm, or endocarditis. Hypercoagulability states such as polycythemia or postsplenectomy increase the risk for intestinal infarction. Surgical procedures that involve aortic clamping (e.g., abdominal aortic aneurysm repair) may also cause an infarction. The use of vasopressors may also cause an infarction. The vasopressors can be endogenous due to sympathetic nervous system stimulation (e.g., shock) or exogenous (e.g., norepinephrine, high-dose dopamine). A strangulated intestinal obstruction, intraabdominal infection, and cirrhosis are also conditions that can cause intestinal infarct.

Functional obstruction (i.e., paralytic ileus) is the most common type of intestinal obstruction. Conditions that can cause a functional obstruction are abdominal surgery, hypokalemia, intestinal distention, peritonitis, intestinal ischemia, severe trauma, spinal cord injury, ureteral distention, pneumonia, pleuritis, subphrenic abscess, pancreatitis, acute cholecystitis, pelvic abscess, opioids (e.g., morphine), and sepsis. Structural (mechanical) obstruction occurs most often in the small bowel, especially at the ileum. The most common cause of mechanical obstruction occurs from postoperative adhesions. Other causes of mechanical obstruction are incarcerated hernia, volvulus, a foreign body, neoplasm, and Crohn disease. In the large bowel, mechanical obstruction occurs most often in the sigmoid colon. A neoplasm is the most common cause of obstruction in the large bowel. A stricture, intussusception, diverticulitis, and a fecal or barium impaction can obstruct the large bowel.

A perforation of the GI system is a medical emergency. GI perforation is a hole that develops through the whole wall of the esophagus, stomach, small intestine, large bowel, rectum, or gallbladder. This condition is a medical emergency. The major causes of a perforated bowel are a peptic ulcer, bowel obstruction, appendicitis, diverticulitis, and a penetrating wound.

Pathophysiology of intestinal obstruction, infarction, or perforation (Figure 6-18) is complex. In a simple mechanical obstruction, blockage occurs without vascular compromise. Ingested fluid and food, digestive secretions, and gas accumulate above the obstruction. The proximal bowel distends, and the distal segment collapses. The normal secretory and absorptive functions of the mucosa are depressed, and the bowel wall becomes edematous and congested. Severe intestinal distention is self-perpetuating and progressive, intensifying the peristaltic and secretory derangements and increasing the risks of dehydration and progression to strangulating obstruction. A strangulating obstruction is obstruction with compromised blood flow. A strangulating obstruction can progress quickly; the bowel becomes edematous and infarcts, leading to gangrene and perforation. An ischemic segment of the bowel (typically the small bowel) or marked dilation may result in perforation. Perforation of a tumor or a diverticulum may also occur at the obstruction site.

A patient with small bowel obstruction may give a history of a precipitating event. The chief complaint will be abdominal pain. Pain reported to be colicky and of shorter duration with bilious vomiting may be a more proximal obstruction. Pain that is progressive and lasting for several days with

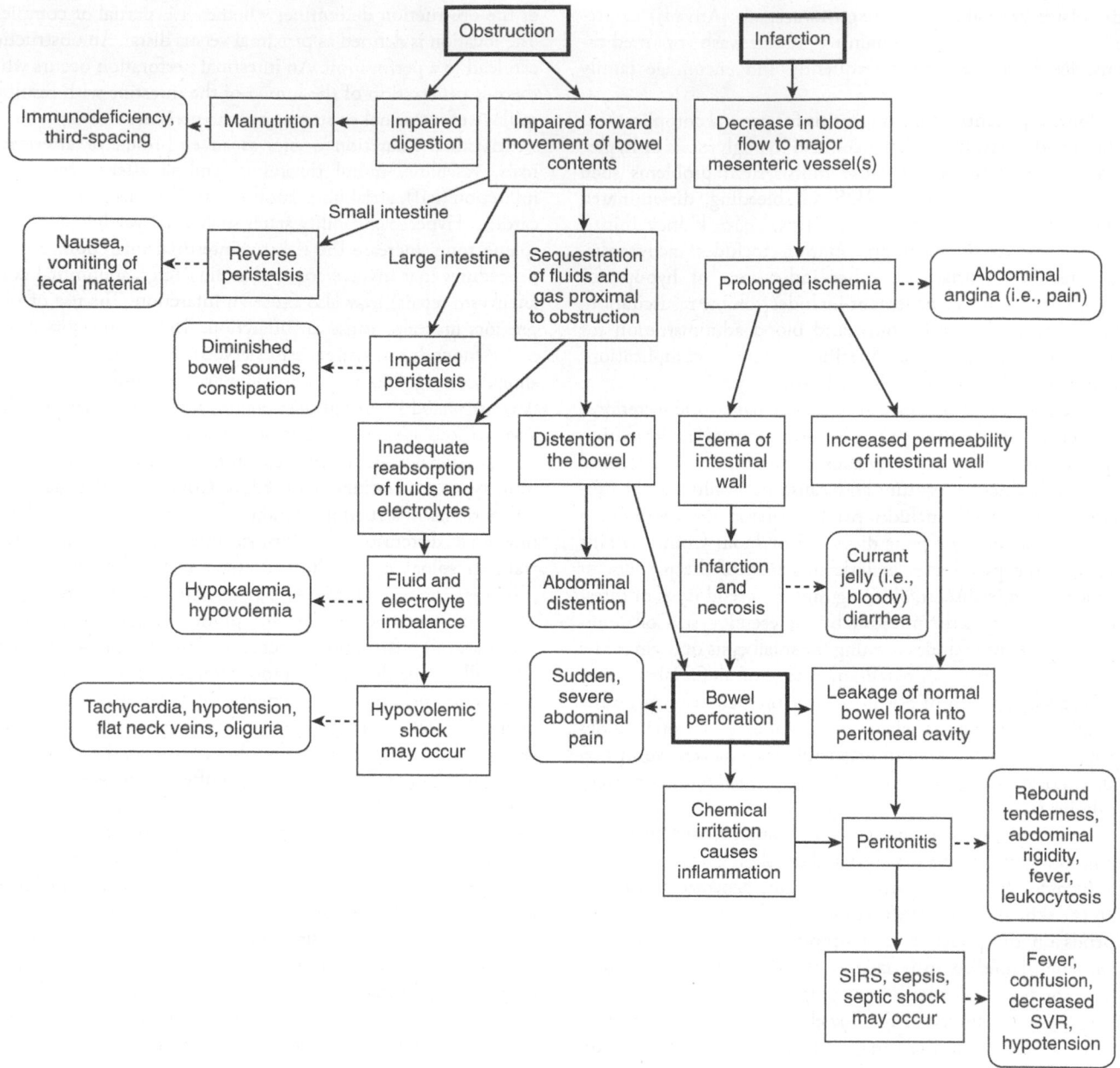

FIGURE 6-18 Pathophysiology of intestinal obstruction/infarction/perforation. Dashed lines connect pathology to clinical presentation. (From Dennison, R. D. [2013]. *Pass CCRN!* [4th ed.]. St. Louis, MO: Elsevier.)

abdominal distention may be a more distal obstruction. Steady, severe, localized pain may indicate strangulation. The patient may also report a change in bowel habits. In early or partial obstruction, the stools are normal or diarrhea is present. In late or complete obstruction, constipation or absence of stools predominates. Vomiting and the type of emesis indicate the stage and the obstruction's location. In the early stage, the vomiting may be projectile in nature. If the obstruction is at the pylorus, the emesis will be clear gastric fluid. When emesis contains gastric contents and bile, the obstruction is in the proximal small intestine and/or a paralytic ileus exists. Brown fecal emesis indicates that the obstruction is in the distal small intestine. In addition, the patient with an obstruction has abdominal distention, clinical indications of dehydration, and high-pitched bowel sounds. Increased bowel sounds are in the early stage and decreased bowel sounds occur in the later

stage of obstruction. Serum electrolyte abnormalities are present with obstructions. The sodium level may be decreased, increased, or normal depending on hydration level and serum osmolality, whereas a decrease in the potassium and chloride levels occurs. Due to dehydration, the BUN level is elevated. Hematology studies may also be abnormal. The hematocrit and WBC count are usually elevated. The acid-base state is usually metabolic acidosis, but metabolic alkalosis may occur with proximal obstruction and gastric losses. Radiology studies provide a more definitive diagnosis of the obstruction. An upper GI series may show the point of obstruction. A flat plate radiology examination of the abdomen will show dilated loops of gas-filled bowel. A CT and/or MRI aid in the differentiation of cause and location of obstruction.

A patient with a large bowel obstruction may report a history of the precipitating event, dull pain, and change in bowel habits. The patient may report a decrease in the ability to pass flatus and thin, ribbon like stools progressing to constipation, then to an absence of stools with a watery discharge. Physical findings include abdominal distention, vomiting in the later stage, and low-pitched bowel sounds. There is an increase in low-pitched bowel sounds during the early stage and a decrease in the later stage. In a large bowel obstruction due to ulcerative colitis, cancer, or diverticulitis, melena may occur. Serum electrolyte abnormalities also occur with large bowel obstruction. Serum sodium may be decreased, increased, or normal depending on hydration level and serum osmolality, whereas serum potassium and chloride are decreased. The BUN is elevated due to dehydration. If the cause of the obstruction is cancer, the carcinogen embryonic antigen (CEA) will be elevated. Hematology studies will also be abnormal with large bowel obstruction. The hematocrit may be elevated due to dehydration or decreased due to hemorrhage. A large intestinal tumor frequently causes slow bleeding. The WBC count is often elevated. The acid-base state is predominantly metabolic acidosis. The patient's stools may be positive for occult blood due to ulcerative colitis, cancer, or diverticulitis. Radiologic studies determine a more definitive diagnosis. A flat plate of the abdomen shows dilated loops of gas-filled bowel. A barium enema may show the point of obstruction. Endoscopy procedures (i.e., sigmoidoscopy or colonoscopy) permit actual visualization of the obstruction.

A patient with a bowel infarction frequently reports a precipitating event. The patient may also complain of anorexia, pallor, abdominal tenderness, urgency to have a bowel movement, and abdominal pain. The patient describes the abdominal pain as severe cramping, periumbilical, or nonspecific and diffuse. Abdominal pain related to mesenteric ischemia is referred to as *abdominal angina*. Clinical findings include tachycardia, hypotension, tachypnea, fever, and weight loss. Clinical indications of dehydration are evident, such as dry mucous membranes, low urine output, and poor skin turgor. The patient may have persistent vomiting, which may be bloody, and a distended abdomen with evidence of guarding and rigidity. The patient may have urgent and bloody diarrhea, frequently described as currant jelly diarrhea. Bowel sounds may be hypoactive or absent. With bowel infarction, serum laboratory abnormalities include an elevated BUN due to dehydration. The alkaline phosphatase, amylase, hematocrit, and white blood cell count are elevated. Metabolic acidosis is the predominant acid-base state. Stool samples are positive for occult blood. Invasive diagnostic examinations provide specific evidence of the infarct. An angiography will show the occlusion of the arterial supply. With a sigmoidoscopy, direct visualization of a dusky, ischemic bowel is possible.

When perforation occurs, the patient reports abdominal pain, tenderness, anorexia, and nausea. The patient appears acutely ill with tachycardia, tachypnea, fever, and vomiting. The abdomen is rigid and "boardlike" with rebound tenderness. There may be an absence of liver dullness due to free air in the peritoneum and diminished or absent bowel sounds. Abnormal diagnostic findings include an elevated WBC count and visualization of free air in the peritoneum with the flat plate of the abdomen radiology study. In cases of perforation, an upper GI series is contraindicated.

Priority collaborative care for all of these conditions includes maintaining airway, oxygenation, ventilation, and circulation. Elevate the head of the bed 30 to 45 degrees. Administer oxygen as necessary to maintain SpO_2 at 95% unless contraindicated. In patients with COPD, administer oxygen to achieve a SpO_2 of ~90%. Administer crystalloids and colloids as prescribed to restore circulating blood volume. Administer blood and blood products as needed. If significant bleeding is suspected, give whole blood or packed cells early. After multiple transfusions, consider replacement of clotting factors, platelets, and calcium. Monitor sodium, calcium, potassium, and phosphate levels; administer electrolyte replacement as indicated. Discontinue any vasopressors if the drugs are the cause of ischemia. If hemodynamic monitoring is required during fluid resuscitation, arrange a transfer to a higher level of care.

Prevent and treat the patient's pain and discomfort. Maintain bed rest and provide a quiet environment with a comfortable temperature and dim lighting. Administer analgesics (e.g., morphine) as prescribed, but until the diagnosis is confirmed, it may be necessary to withhold analgesics. Encourage knee flexion while supine to relax abdominal muscles. Utilize nonpharmacologic pain relief methods (e.g., imagery, distraction, and music). Treat nausea with prescribed antiemetics and perform oral care after emesis.

Prevent perforation of the bowel if obstruction is present. Discontinue all oral intake and insert a nasogastric tube or orogastric tube as prescribed to decompress the stomach, prevent vomiting, and reduce the risk of aspiration. Administer erythromycin, metoclopramide hydrochloride (Reglan), and/or octreotide acetate (Sandostatin) drugs as prescribed to enhance GI motility in partial intestinal obstruction. Insert a rectal tube as prescribed to reduce trapped air in a complete large bowel obstruction. Prepare the patient for a therapeutic colonoscopy, air insufflation for intussusception, and cecal dilation or endoscopic balloon duodenal dilation for small bowel obstruction. Assist with palliative procedures to enhance quality of life in patients with terminal disease associated with bowel obstruction. These procedures include the insertion of distal gastric or jejunal tubes, colonic dilation, and/or the insertion of intestinal stents.

Prepare the patient for surgery if indicated for a vascular obstruction, complete bowel obstruction, or bowel perforation. A strangulated obstruction is a surgical emergency. Do not give a cathartic or enema to a patient with a complete obstruction. To decrease the occurrence of infection, administer bowel preparation with cathartics, enemas, and sterilization before surgery. For bowel sterilization, administer a nonabsorbable aminoglycoside (e.g., neomycin).

The surgical procedures indicated for an infarction include an exploratory laparotomy and embolectomy and/or arterial reconstruction with resection of the irreparably damaged bowel. In cases of obstruction, surgical procedures correct the cause of the obstruction. A laparoscopic adhesiolysis relieves obstruction caused by adhesion. A herniorrhaphy will reduce a hernia, but reduction of volvulus or intussusception may require a bowel resection, which may require temporary or permanent bowel diversion with colostomy. A right hemicolectomy is the surgical procedure used for tumors in the cecum and ascending colon, whereas a left hemicolectomy is the procedure used for tumors of the descending and sigmoid colon. A transverse colectomy is the procedure used for tumors of the middle or left transverse colon. With these types of surgical procedures the patient must be prepared for the possibility of a temporary or permanent colostomy. For proximal and midrectal tumors, a low anterior resection is performed. An abdominoperineal resection is required for malignant lesions of the lower sigmoid colon, rectum, and anus, and this surgical procedure requires a permanent colostomy. In conditions where perforation has occurred, repair of perforation may require bowel resection. A temporary bowel diversion permits time for the anastomosis to heal. At a later date, a reversal of the temporary diversion occurs. During surgery, treatment with an antibiotic lavage may occur.

Answer all the patient's questions about the planned procedures. Prepare the patient for adjuvant therapy if required for colon cancer. There may be a need for chemoembolization. Chemoembolization involves the infusion of a concentrated dose of an antineoplastic agent into the hepatic artery to create an embolized agent. Cryosurgery, a freezing technique, is a treatment used for liver metastasis. The patient may need external beam radiation or brachytherapy. Brachytherapy is a type of radiation treatment where there is placement of radioactive seeds in the area of tumor location and removal. Treatment of a neoplasm may require chemotherapy, the administration of an antineoplastic agent, before, during, or after surgery.

A major focus of collaborative care is to prevent and monitor for infection. A concerted effort to reduce leakage of intestinal bacteria and reduce the risk of peritonitis and sepsis if perforation has occurred is a priority. Keep the patient immobilized to reduce the chemical irritation to the peritoneum. During surgery, treatment with an antibiotic lavage may occur. Administer antibiotics as prescribed preoperatively, during the surgery, and postoperatively. Monitor the patient closely for clinical indications of infection and sepsis. Measure temperature every 4 hours, assess HR and BP hourly, and note changes in mental status. Note changes in color and character of wound drainage. Monitor changes in WBC count. Clean around drains aseptically and protect skin around drains postoperatively.

Administer appropriate nutritional support considering the individual patient's restrictions. Administer parenteral nutritional support during the acute phase. Provide oral feedings and advance the diet when the patient's condition and postoperative paralytic ileus have resolved. Administer vitamin and mineral supplements as prescribed.

Monitor the patient for complications of fluid and electrolyte imbalances, hemorrhage, and sepsis. These surgical patients are at risk for peritonitis and respiratory distress secondary to abdominal distention. They also require close observation for clinical indicators of hypovolemic shock or septic shock along with perforation.

ABDOMINAL TRAUMA

Abdominal trauma is any injury that occurs between the nipple line to midthigh level due to penetrations, blunt force, and/or iatrogenic diagnostics or treatments. Common causes of penetrating trauma include motor vehicle collision, assault, and sharp instruments like knife or gunshot wounds and impalement injuries. Common causes of blunt trauma include motor vehicle collision, assault, falls, and sport injuries. The causes of iatrogenic trauma include invasive diagnostic procedures or treatments such as a peritoneal tap, endoscopy, biopsy, and cardiopulmonary resuscitation (CPR).

Abdominal trauma is seldom a single-organ injury. In incidences involving high-velocity penetrating trauma (i.e., gunshot wound), there is extensive destruction of contact tissue and severe associated blast effect on the surrounding tissues. The liver is the internal organ most often affected by penetrating trauma. Blunt trauma is due to direct injury from a crushing force between two objects and acceleration/deceleration forces that cause shearing, twisting, and pressure. The spleen is the internal organ most often affected by blunt trauma and the pancreas is the organ frequently injured along with the spleen.

The patient with abdominal trauma may complain of poorly localized or referred abdominal tenderness or pain. The patient may complain of left shoulder pain (i.e., Kehr sign). The Kehr sign is referred pain to the left shoulder indicative of splenic rupture and is caused by blood below the diaphragm that irritates the phrenic nerve. The Rovsing sign is pain elicited in the right lower quadrant (RLQ) upon palpation of the left lower quadrant (LLQ) and indicates peritoneal irritation.

Clinical findings of the patient with abdominal trauma include the following: seat belt sign, hematomas, Cullen sign, Grey-Turner sign, Coopernail sign, rigid abdomen, and Ballance sign. The seat belt sign is the presence of ecchymosis across the lower abdomen caused by a seat belt. Note the presence and location of any hematomas. A hematoma in the flank area indicates a renal injury. Examine the patient for entrance and exit wounds. Other signs of trauma include periumbilical ecchymosis (i.e., Cullen sign) or flank ecchymosis (i.e., Grey-Turner sign). The Coopernail sign, ecchymosis of the scrotum or the labia, is indicative of a fractured pelvis. A rigid abdomen may indicate intraabdominal bleeding. The Ballance sign is dullness to percussion in the left flank or LUQ and indicates a ruptured spleen. Other objective findings seen with abdominal trauma include the following:

- Diminished femoral pulses, which may be seen in vascular injury
- Loss of liver dullness, which indicates perforation with free air in the peritoneum
- Clinical indications of hypoperfusion or shock
- Clinical indications of perforation (e.g., severe abdominal pain, fever, nausea, and vomiting)
- Clinical indications of peritonitis (e.g., involuntary guarding, abdominal rigidity, and rebound tenderness)
- Specific assessment findings related to the organ(s) injured (Table 6-13)

Important and specific serum diagnostic tests used to assess patients with abdominal trauma include glucose levels, liver enzymes, hematology, and clotting profiles. The serum glucose level may be elevated due to stress. Due to the nature of trauma from various types of accidents and/or violence, perform drug and alcohol screens. Injury to the pancreas or bowel increases the amylase level. Damage to the liver will increase the liver enzymes of ALT, AST, and LDH. Decreased Hgb and Hct result from bleeding and/or hemorrhage. If the spleen ruptures or an infection is present, the WBC count will be elevated. Platelets will also elevate if the spleen is injured. Prolonged clotting profile studies (i.e., PT, aPTT) occur with abdominal trauma. A urinalysis may show hematuria if renal trauma has occurred or myoglobinuria may be present if a crush injury has occurred. Trauma may cause the stool to be positive for occult blood.

TABLE 6-13	Clinical Indications of Organ Injury		
Organ	**Suspect Injury to This Organ if**	**Clinical Indications of Injury**	**Complications**
Liver	• Seat belt sign • Local sign of injury (RUQ) • Lower right rib fracture • Blunt or penetrating trauma • Acceleration/deceleration MVC • Presence of other abdominal injuries	• RUQ pain, tenderness, and guarding • Referred pain to right shoulder • Increase in abdominal girth and rigidity • Increased pain on inspiration • Clinical indications of shock • Leukocytosis • Elevated ALT, AST, or LDH • Decreased Hgb and Hct • Abnormal clotting studies • Chest x-ray: elevated diaphragm on right side • Injury evident on FAST • Positive peritoneal lavage if performed	• Shock • Infection, sepsis • Subdiaphragmatic abscess • Clotting abnormalities • Atelectasis, pneumonia, or ARDS • Hepatic failure
Spleen	• Seat belt sign • Local sign of injury (LUQ) • Lower left rib fracture • Left pneumothorax • Blunt or penetrating trauma to abdomen • Acceleration/deceleration MVC • Presence of other abdominal injuries	• LUQ pain, tenderness, and guarding • Increased abdominal girth and rigidity • Kehr sign • Ballance sign • Increased pain on inspiration • Clinical indications of shock • Decreased Hgb and Hct • Injury evident on FAST • Positive peritoneal lavage • Shock	• Shock • Atelectasis, pneumonia, or ARDS • Infection, sepsis especially if splenectomy performed • Subdiaphragmatic abscess
Pancreas	• Seat belt sign • Presence of other abdominal injuries • MVC • Blunt or penetrating trauma to abdomen	• Epigastric, back, or shoulder pain • Abdominal tenderness and guarding • Increased abdominal girth • Diminished bowel sounds • Clinical indications of shock • Hyperglycemia or hypoglycemia • Elevated serum lipase • Leukocytosis • Positive peritoneal lavage for amylase but unreliable because the pancreas is located retroperitoneally	• Shock • Diabetes • Pancreatitis • Pancreatic abscess or pseudocyst • Pancreatic fistula • Atelectasis, pneumonia, or ARDS
Stomach	• Penetrating trauma to abdomen • Presence of other abdominal injuries	• Epigastric or LUQ pain and tenderness • Hematemesis or bloody aspirate from NG tube • Rebound tenderness • Clinical indications of shock • Leukocytosis • Positive peritoneal lavage • Free air on flat plate of abdomen	• Atelectasis, pneumonia, or ARDS • Gastric fistula
Intestine	• Seat belt sign • Presence of other abdominal injuries • Blunt trauma with deceleration • Penetrating injury	• Local sign of injury (e.g., ecchymosis, abrasion) • Nausea and vomiting • Abdominal pain: may be referred or rebound • Absent bowel sounds • Leukocytosis • Positive peritoneal lavage for blood and fecal matter • Free air on flat plate of abdomen • Positive fecal occult blood test	• Ileus • Peritonitis or sepsis • Abscess • Intestinal ischemia, infarction, obstruction, or perforation • Fistula
Abdominal vessels	• Other abdominal injuries • Blunt or penetrating abdominal injury • Sudden deceleration in MVC or fall	• Clinical indications of shock • Abdominal distention and guarding • Increased abdominal girth and rigidity • Abdominal bruit • Diminished femoral pulses if aorta or iliac injury • Mottled lower extremities • Cullen sign • Decreased Hgb and Hct • Shock	• Shock • Mesenteric ischemia or infarction • Infection or sepsis

Trauma usually affects more than one organ system. Obtain a chest x-ray to rule out concurrent thoracic injury and identify free air under the diaphragm. A flat plate of the abdomen may show free air in the peritoneum if the stomach or bowel is perforated. If hematuria is present, an intravenous pyelogram (IVP) will be performed to look for renal trauma. To identify areas of injury, a CT scan or MRI is performed. An angiography procedure may show a vascular injury.

A focused abdominal sonography for trauma (FAST) detects fluid or blood in the pericardium, abdomen, or pelvis and allows visualization of the spleen and liver. Although this cannot reliably identify injury to intraabdominal organs (requires CT), FAST can accurately predict the need for laparotomy in trauma patients with very good sensitivity and excellent specificity. The advantages of a FAST over a diagnostic peritoneal lavage (DPL) is that it is generally completed in less than 5 minutes, requires no preparation, is noninvasive, and has no contraindications.

A DPL assesses the patient for intraabdominal bleeding, though FAST is usually the preferred screening study. A major limitation of DPL is that it does not detect diaphragmatic or retroperitoneal injuries. The nurse will assist with placement of the peritoneal catheter and instills 1 L of normal saline over 15 to 20 minutes. The nurse then moves the patient from side to side after fluid instillation to distribute the lavage fluid, then drains the fluid and sends it to the lab for analysis. The appearance of gross blood upon catheter insertion in the abdominal cavity indicates a need for an immediate exploratory laparotomy. A positive test result is obtained if the lavage fluid is grossly bloody, a newsprint cannot be read through the lavage fluid (i.e., newsprint sign), or the fluid contains the following:

- RBC greater than $100000/mm^3$
- WBC greater than $500/mm^3$
- Amylase greater than 175 units/dL
- Bile, bacteria, or intestinal content

Priority collaborative management for trauma includes interventions to maintain the patient's airway, oxygenation, and ventilation status. Protect and stabilize the spine until a cervical injury is ruled out. Elevate the head of the bed 30 to 45 degrees to allow for optimal diaphragmatic excursion. Administer oxygen as necessary to maintain SpO_2 at 95% unless contraindicated. In patients with COPD, administer oxygen to achieve a SpO_2 of 90% by pulse oximetry. Place an oropharyngeal or nasopharyngeal airway in patients with altered consciousness and assist with endotracheal intubation if required.

Another major focus of collaborative care management is to detect bleeding and maintain adequate circulating volume. Detect bleeding by performing a head-to-toe assessment and assisting with peritoneal lavage. Peritoneal lavage is especially important in an unconscious patient because subjective report of tenderness or pain is absent. Insert an indwelling urinary catheter to evaluate hourly urine output unless the patient has the following contraindications:

- Blood around the urinary meatus
- Perineal or scrotal hematoma
- Displacement of the prostate gland noted during rectal examination by provider

The nurse inserts two short (1¼-inch) large-gauge (16 or 18) peripheral intravenous catheters and draws blood samples for laboratory analysis and type and crossmatch for blood. Administer intravenous fluids to restore circulating blood volume.

The types of fluids expected to be infused include crystalloids, colloids, blood, and blood products. Administer whole blood or packed cells early if significant bleeding is suspected. Consider replacement of clotting factors, platelets, and calcium after multiple transfusions. Apply direct pressure to an overt bleeding site. Interventions to control bleeding are also an important facet of care; therefore, collaborative care management includes preparing the patient for an exploratory laparotomy as indicated for the following conditions:

- Penetrating injury invading the peritoneum
- Clinical indications of perforation (e.g., acute abdomen)
- Free air in the peritoneum on x-ray
- Shock
- GI hemorrhage
- Massive hematuria
- Evisceration
- Positive peritoneal lavage
- Surgical indications on CT scan or angiography

The trauma patient with hemodynamic instability may require the insertion of an arterial catheter and pulmonary artery catheter. In this situation, the collaborative management includes stabilization efforts, assistance with insertion of hemodynamic catheters, and facilitation of a transfer to a higher level of care.

Prevent and treat the patient's pain and discomfort. Maintain bed rest and a quiet environment with a comfortable temperature and dim lighting. Administer analgesics (e.g., morphine) as prescribed, but recognize that until diagnoses are confirmed, it may be necessary to hold analgesia. Encourage the patient to use knee flexion while in a supine position to relax abdominal muscles. This is especially important for patients who may have peritoneal irritation. Nonpharmacologic pain relief methods such as imagery, distraction, and music are also helpful in a trauma patient's pain management.

Maintain fluid and electrolyte balances. Monitor sodium, calcium, potassium, magnesium, and phosphate levels and administer electrolyte replacement as indicated. Decompress the GI tract by insertion of a nasogastric tube. Use an orogastric tube for patients suffering from facial fractures. Monitor the nasogastric output for color, amount, and odor of drainage.

Administer appropriate nutritional support considering individual restrictions. Administer parenteral nutritional support during the acute stage. Provide oral feedings and advance the diet when the patient's condition is surgically resolved. Administer vitamin and mineral supplements.

Prevent and monitor the patient for infection and complications of the trauma and surgical interventions. Cover any eviscerated organs with saline-soaked pads. Observe for signs of peritonitis such as fever, peritonitis, and leukocytosis. Administer antibiotics as prescribed. Measure the patient's abdominal girth. The occurrence of bowel perforation necessitates an antibiotic lavage. Maintain asepsis of wounds and drains. Monitor bowel sounds. Evaluate tetanus immunization status and administer tetanus toxoid if indicated for penetrating trauma, abrasion, cuts, etc. Monitor the patient frequently for the following complications:

- Obstruction
- Perforation
- Peritonitis
- Pancreatitis

- Infection, abscess, and sepsis
- Hemorrhage
  - Retroperitoneal
  - Intraperitoneal
- Shock: hypovolemic or septic

- DIC
- Atelectasis, pneumonia, ARDS
- Organ failure
- Abdominal compartment syndrome
- GI surgery

6.12   Learning Activity

Describe the following "signs" and identify what they indicate.

Sign	Description	Indicates
Ballance		
Grey-Turner		
Cullen		
Coopernail		
Kehr		
Chvostek		
Trousseau		

Answers to this activity can be found in the Answer Key.

Collaborative care after GI surgeries requires extensive nursing care. Often, these patients require critical care nursing immediately after the procedure. Progressive care nurses need to be knowledgeable and skilled to care for these patients having these GI surgical procedures (Table 6-14 and Figures 6-19 through 6-23). The progressive care nurse needs to be able to prepare patients for surgery, support the families, and care for the patients once stabilized in recovery and transitioned back to the progressive care unit.

The focus of collaborative care in the postoperative period of care for patients undergoing GI surgery is to maintain airway, oxygenation, ventilation, and circulation status. The initial postoperative nursing care priority is to monitor airway patency and utilize artificial airways as indicated. Many of these patients will remain intubated and on mechanical ventilation in the critical care unit for a few days. Short-term breathing trials evaluate the patient's ability to maintain spontaneous breathing so that weaning and extubation are initiated as soon as possible. Once successfully weaned from mechanical ventilation and extubated, the patient is transferred to progressive care. Monitor SpO_2 and administer oxygen to maintain SpO_2 at 95% unless contraindicated. Encourage the patient to use deep breathing techniques and use incentive spirometry every 2 hours. Position the patient with the head of the bed elevated between 30 and 40 degrees unless contraindicated. The side-lying position is frequently more comfortable for patients who have had rectal or perineal procedures. Maintain the patient's hydration status, encourage leg exercises, and have the patient ambulate as soon as possible to prevent deep vein thrombosis (DVT) and pulmonary embolism.

The prevention of and monitoring for fluid volume deficit and/or electrolyte imbalance is a collaborative care priority. Monitor vital signs, hemodynamics, urine output, daily weights, and laboratory values. Utilize a CVP catheter when in place to evaluate fluid status. Weigh the patient daily at the same time.

Administer crystalloids and/or colloid fluids as prescribed. If drains are present, evaluate the site and the amount or character of drainage. In these types of surgeries, expect the mobilization of third-spaced fluids and an increase in urine output on the second or third postoperative day. Monitor the patient for changes in electrolyte levels. Monitor serum glucose and administer insulin to keep serum glucose within normal limits for both patients with and patients without diabetes. Elevated blood glucose impairs wound healing and increases morbidity and mortality. Observe the patient for complications of bleeding. Monitor for petechiae, ecchymosis, and changes in clotting profile, along with frank bleeding that may indicate a coagulopathy, such as disseminated intravascular coagulation (DIC).

Prevent and/or treat the patient's pain with opioids (e.g., morphine, hydromorphone, or fentanyl). It is best to administer the pain medications by PCA. Epidural analgesia may also be utilized to manage acute surgical pain. Adequate pain management may also require the administration of NSAIDs as prescribed to augment the analgesic effect of opioids by reducing inflammation. Initially, administer parenteral ketorolac (Toradol) as prescribed postoperatively until the patient is able to take drugs by mouth, and then convert to oral agents (e.g., acetaminophen [Tylenol], ibuprofen [Motrin], naproxen [Naprosyn, Anaprox]). Provide noninvasive pain control measures such as teaching the patient and the family how to splint the incision during deep breathing. Administer antiemetics for nausea; provide oral care and assess positioning of the nasogastric tube if still in place after each episode of vomiting.

An important aspect of postsurgical care is the close monitoring of the patient for clinical indications of infection. Evaluate the patient's temperature at least every 4 hours. Assess color, character, and odor of drainage from the incision line, drains, and tubes. Assess for clinical indications

TABLE 6-14	GI Surgical Procedures	
Surgical Procedure	**Description**	**Indication**
Billroth I (also referred to as *gastroduodenostomy*) (Figure 6-15, A)	• Resection of the antrum of the stomach and anastomosis of the remainder of the stomach to the duodenum	• Ulcer or malignancy
Billroth II (also referred to as *gastrojejunostomy*) (Figure 6-15, B)	• Resection of the antrum of the stomach and anastomosis of the remainder of the stomach to the jejunum leaving the duodenal stump and accompanied by a vagotomy	• Ulcer or malignancy
Complete gastrectomy (Figure 6-15, C)	• Removal of the stomach with anastomosis of the esophagus to the jejunum leaving the duodenal stump	• Ulcer or malignancy
Whipple procedure (also referred to as *radical pancreaticoduodenectomy*) (Figure 6-19)	• Removal of the lower stomach and duodenum with anastomosis of the remaining stomach to the jejunum with partial or total pancreatectomy and a possible splenectomy	• Cancer of the pancreas • May also be performed for resection of necrotic tissue as a result of pancreatitis
Esophagogastrectomy (Figure 6-20)	• Removal of all or a portion of the esophagus, possibly with a portion of the stomach, with anastomosis to the remaining portion of the stomach	• Cancer of the lower third and middle third of the thoracic esophagus • Corrosive esophagitis
Esophagoenterostomy (may also be referred to as *esophagogastrectomy with a colon interposition*) (Figure 6-21)	• Removal of all or a portion of the esophagus along with replacement with a segment of the colon	• Cancer of the esophagus • Corrosive esophagitis
Colon resection with end-to-end anastomosis; may include colostomy	• Removal of a portion of the colon; may include formation of a colostomy • Temporary colostomy may be developed to temporarily divert bowel contents to allow for healing of the anastomosis • May be performed laparoscopically	• Tumor, bleeding, inflammation, necrosis, or trauma of the large intestine
Total colectomy and ileostomy	• Removal of the entire large intestine and the formation of a stoma from the end of the ileum • May also include surgical formation of a continent ileostomy (i.e., Kock pouch) or ileoanal reservoir	• Ulcerative colitis
Abdominoperineal resection	• Removal of the anus, rectum, and sigmoid colon with creation of a permanent colostomy	• Malignancy of the rectum
Restrictive Procedures for Morbid Obesity		
Vertical banded gastroplasty (VBG)	• Partitioning of the stomach near the gastroesophageal junction to create a small gastric pouch and outlet • Less commonly performed today due to lack of sustained weight loss	• Morbid obesity (e.g., BMI greater than 40 kg/m^2 or BMI of greater than 35 kg/m^2 with serious medical problems)
Gastric banding (Figure 6-22)	• Placement of a prosthetic device around the gastric cardia to limit oral intake • May be done laparoscopically	• Morbid obesity (e.g., BMI greater than 40 kg/m^2 or BMI of greater than 35 kg/m^2 with serious medical problems)
Malabsorptive Procedures for Morbid Obesity		
Intestinal bypass	• Formation of an anastomosis between the upper small intestine and the lower small intestine or large intestine • Less commonly performed today due to high complication rate	• Morbid obesity (e.g., BMI greater than 40 kg/m^2 or BMI of greater than 35 kg/m^2 with serious medical problems)

TABLE 6-14	**GI Surgical Procedures—cont'd**	
Malabsorptive Procedures for Morbid Obesity		
Roux-en-Y gastric bypass (RYGB) (Figure 6-23)	• Combines gastric restriction and malabsorption; in addition to creating a gastric pouch, the small bowel is resected so that the upper jejunum is connected to the pouch and the lower jejunum is anastomosed to the biliopancreatic limb; digestive juices do not come into the small bowel until the lower jejunum, so absorption is decreased • Usually performed via laparoscopic technique	• Morbid obesity (e.g., BMI greater than 40 kg/m^2 or BMI of greater than 35 kg/m^2 with serious medical problems)

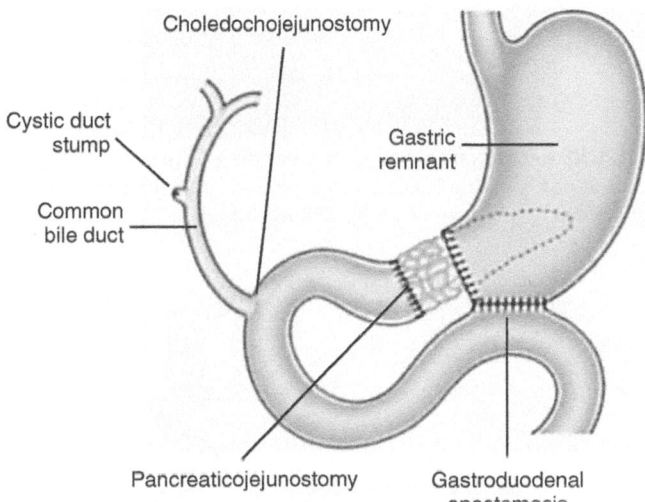

FIGURE 6-19 Whipple procedure (also referred to *radical pancreaticoduodenectomy*). (From Lewis, S. M., et. al. [2011]. *Medical-surgical nursing.* [8th ed.]. St. Louis, MO: Mosby.)

of peritonitis, which can be a result of an anastomosis leak. Symptoms to observe for include abdominal pain, abdominal distention, rebound tenderness, nausea, vomiting, fever, leukocytosis, diminished or absent bowel sounds, and a rigid boardlike abdomen. Also, monitor the patient for the clinical indications of an intraabdominal abscess (e.g., abdominal pain, fever, and leukocytosis).

Administer antibiotics prophylactically and therapeutically as prescribed and provide aseptic incisional and drain care. Assess the approximation of wound edges for indications of possible dehiscence or evisceration. Give focused attention to the patient's skin. Protect the skin from excoriation and change the incisional dressing, packing, and dressings around drains as indicated. Some patients may have wounds open and packed with saline-soaked dressings. Do not allow dressings to become dry (i.e., wet to dry). The dressings should be still moist (i.e., wet to moist) at the time of removal and replaced to prevent disruption of granulating tissue. Irrigate with saline as prescribed. Avoid the use of packing soaked with iodine because iodine on open wounds is toxic to fibroblasts, decreases epithelialization, and increases susceptibility to infection. In addition, the iodine may be absorbed and cause nephrotoxicity. Avoid the use of

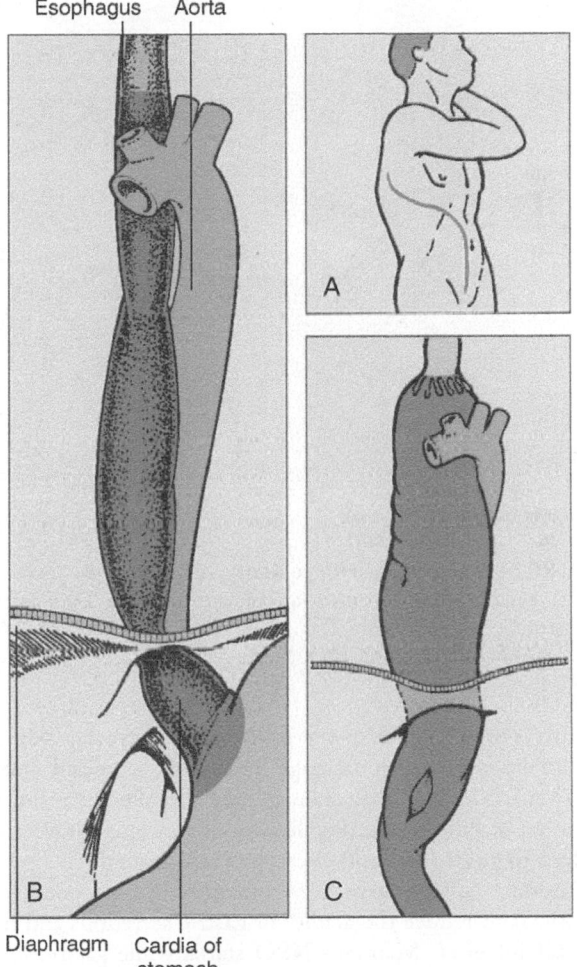

FIGURE 6-20 Esophagogastrectomy. A, Incision. **B,** Shaded portion to be resected. **C,** Completed reconstruction. (From Beare, P. G., & Myers, J. L. [1998]. *Adult health nursing* [3rd ed.]. St. Louis, MO: Mosby.)

hydrogen peroxide because it is damaging to new epithelium. Provide instruction to the patient and family regarding wound care, pharmacologic agents prescribed for home use, and signs or symptoms to report to the physician.

Monitor the patient closely for a fistula tract. Look for small openings along or near the incision or drain site. The output of

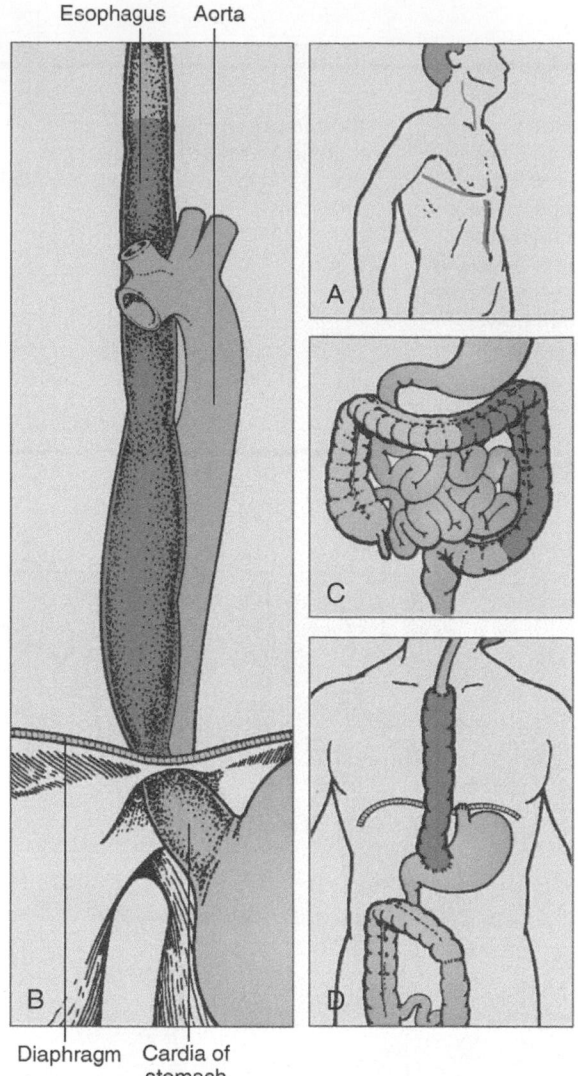

FIGURE 6-21 Esophagoenterostomy. **A,** Incision. **B,** Shaded portion to be resected. **C,** Portion of colon to be used. **D,** Completed reconstruction. (From Beare, P. G., & Myers, J. L. [1998]. *Adult health nursing* [3rd ed.]. St. Louis, MO: Mosby.)

a fistula is usually green or yellow in color. Protect the skin from potentially excoriating drainage by placing a wound drainage bag over the fistula. This drainage bag also allows for the measurement of fluid loss and collection of a sample for electrolyte analysis to guide fluid and electrolyte replacement.

Another collaborative care priority in postoperative GI patients is to reduce the acidity of gastric secretions and maintain GI integrity. Maintain NPO status while gastric suction is required for the patient. Administer antacids, H_2 receptor antagonists, and/or proton pump inhibitors as prescribed. Administer octreotide acetate (Sandostatin) as prescribed to suppress secretion of pancreatic peptides after a Whipple procedure. Decompression maintains GI integrity and function. Monitor and maintain NG tube decompression until the return of bowel sounds. Ensure the proper placement of the tube. Do not manipulate a tube placed during surgery without consulting the surgeon. Monitor the patient closely for indications of an anastomosis leak, the return of bowel sounds, flatus, and bowel movement (BM). Assess and provide bowel diversion care as indicated, such as with bowel resection with formation

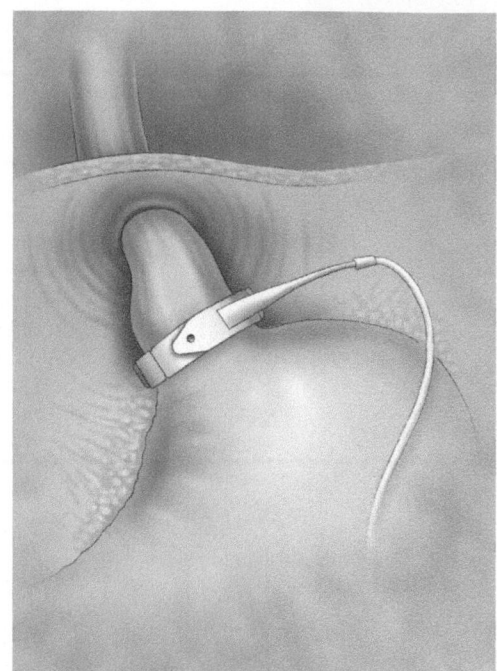

FIGURE 6-22 **Example of gastric banding.** (From American Association of Operating Room Nurses. [2004]. AORN bariatric surgery guideline. *AORN Journal, 79*[5], 1026-1052.)

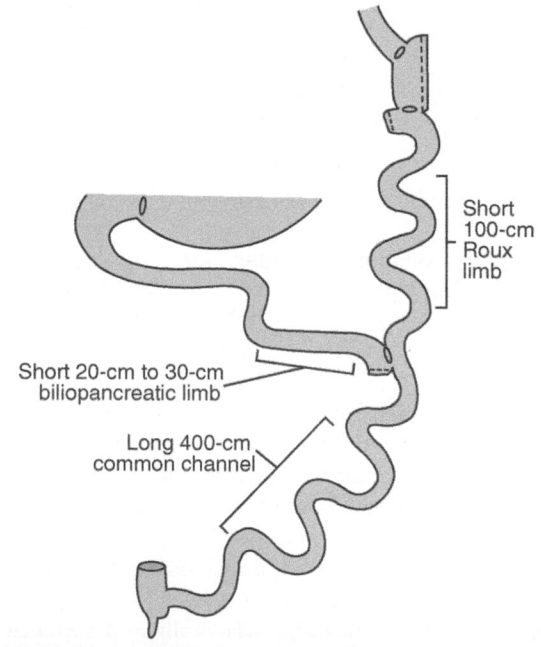

FIGURE 6-23 **Example of gastric bypass: Roux-en-Y proximal gastric bypass.** (From American Association of Operating Room Nurses. [2004]. AORN bariatric surgery guideline. *AORN Journal, 79*[5], 1026-1052.)

of a temporary or permanent bowel diversion. Keep a bowel diversion appliance intact and keep the peristomal skin clean and dry. Report any change in the drainage from the ileostomy/colostomy. Ileostomy drainage is watery, excoriating, and continuous. In an ascending colostomy, the drainage is watery or semisolid, excoriating, and continuous. In a patient with a transverse colostomy, the stool is pastelike or semisolid and occurs at unpredictable intervals. A patient with a descending or sigmoid colostomy will have formed stools that may be at predictable intervals (e.g., after breakfast), especially with an irrigation routine. Drainage may not appear for 3 to 5 days after the GI procedure resulting in bowel diversion. Assess the color of the stoma and report any indications of ischemia. The color of the stoma should be the same color as the oral mucosa and it should be moist. Report signs of a prolapse or retraction of the stoma and darkening of the tissue to a burgundy or black color.

Maintain or improve the patient's nutritional status. Assess the nutritional status parameters of weight, BUN, serum albumin, total protein, hemoglobin, and hematocrit. Administer TPN initially as prescribed and progress the diet as prescribed. Patients tolerate small frequent meals better than larger meals. Administer enteral feedings as prescribed. Place a jejunostomy tube for nutritional support access. Monitor the patient for diarrhea. Administer oral pancreatic enzymes (Creon, Pancrease, Viokase, and Cotazym) with each meal as prescribed after a Whipple procedure.

Patients with obesity deserve size-sensitive care. Ensure that appropriate bariatric equipment is available to provide safe, quality care. Avoid derogatory terms such as "big boy bed." Collaborative care team members should recognize and discuss prejudice based on size and weight. Provide obese patients privacy, dignity, and confidentiality. Weigh the patient in private and close doors and curtains when examining the patient.

Assist the patient and family with adjustment to the diagnosis of cancer if malignancy is present. Provide accurate information and clarification about the diagnosis, prognosis, and treatment plan. Be realistic but do not eliminate hope. Give the patient and family members the time to discuss their feelings and concerns. Encourage expression of feelings and understanding of the goals for treatment. Refer the patient and family to support groups or for counseling as indicated. Prepare the patient and family for additional treatments for malignancy such as radiation therapy, antineoplastic drug therapy, palliative care, and/or hospice care.

Monitor the patient for general postoperative complications. Hemodynamic stability, respiratory impairment, and infection are routine postoperative problems. Observe patients with GI surgery for an anastomosis leak, atelectasis, pneumonia, ARDS, DVT, pulmonary embolism, infection, sepsis, prolonged ileus, GI bleeding, stenosis or stricture, fistula, and cardiac, hepatic, pulmonary, and/or renal organ failure.

Observe for specific complications of gastric resections that include pernicious anemia, diarrhea, chronic gastritis, and dumping syndromes. Early dumping syndrome is from hyperosmolality and causes a hypovolemic effect. Late dumping syndrome results in hypoglycemia caused by a hyperinsulinemic response. Complications that are specific to a Whipple procedure include delayed gastric emptying, pancreatic fistula, intraabdominal abscess, and hemorrhage usually due to injury to the portal vein or vena cava. Wound infection, diabetes, pancreatic exocrine insufficiency, pancreatitis, and a marginal ulceration are also complications related to a Whipple procedure.

Observe a patient after esophagogastrectomy for esophageal stenosis or anastomotic stricture. Also, monitor for chylothorax, a type of pleural effusion that may result from lymphatic fluid leakage. Additionally, observe for the complications of myocardial ischemia and dysrhythmias in these patients.

Bariatric surgical patients are being treated for morbid obesity. Closely monitor patients after bariatric procedures for complications. These procedures have a high risk for pulmonary embolism, so monitor the patient closely for clinical indications of pulmonary embolism, such as decreased SpO_2, chest pain, and dyspnea. Also, observe closely for stoma outlet stenosis, severe gastroesophageal reflux, erosive esophagitis, and band erosion. Additionally, a herniation of the stomach upward inside the band and band migration can occur along with regaining of weight. Specific complications to the malabsorptive procedures used for morbid obesity include pulmonary embolism, gastric pouch outlet stricture, jejunojejunostomy obstruction, dumping syndrome, prolonged nausea and vomiting, cholelithiasis, anemia, electrolyte imbalance, and lactose intolerance. The patient may suffer from offensive, foul-smelling soft bowel movements and flatus. Vitamin (A, D, E, K, and B_{12}) and mineral (calcium, folic acid, and iron) deficiencies also occur.

INFLAMMATORY BOWEL DISEASE

Inflammatory bowel disease (IBD) is an immunologically related disorder. Diseases of this type of disorder include ulcerative colitis and Crohn disease characterized by chronic, recurrent inflammation of the intestinal tract. Clinical manifestations of IBD vary, with long periods of remission interspersed with episodes of acute inflammation. Both Crohn disease and ulcerative colitis can be debilitating. The cause to both is unknown, but possible causes include infectious agents, autoimmune responses, food allergies, and heredity factors.

In ulcerative colitis, there is an idiopathic inflammation involving the mucosa of the colon. The inflammation is continuous and circumferential and begins in the rectum progressing proximally toward the cecum. The inflammation begins at the base of the crypts of Lieberkuhn. Small erosions form and coalesce into ulcers. This process is followed by abscess formation, necrosis, and ragged ulcerations of the mucosa.

The onset of ulcerative colitis usually occurs at about 10 years of age, but can occur as late as 40. There is a higher incidence of ulcerative colitis in women and it is more common in Jewish, upper middle class. The etiology is unknown, but genetic and immunologic factors are suspected along with infections. Patients with ulcerative colitis often have other concurrent autoimmune disorders.

Patients with ulcerative colitis complain of a sensation of rectal urgency. Crampy abdominal pain and tenderness are usually present. The abdomen may be hypertympanic upon assessment. The predominant symptoms the patient will have are copious amounts of bloody, purulent, and watery diarrhea. The patient may have up to 30 stools per day, suffers from weight loss, and appears cachectic. The patient will also have vomiting, dehydration, and fever, which leads to fluid loss and orthostatic difficulties. Extra manifestations include anemia, arthritis, and hepatic dysfunction.

In Crohn disease, there is transmural inflammation of the digestive tract that can involve one or more areas of the GI tract from the mouth to the anus. The ileum, colon, and perianal areas are the most common sites of inflammation. In addition, extraintestinal organs may be affected. The tissue has a cobblestone tissue appearance under the microscope. The inflammation of the intestinal mucosa spreads inward and outward to involve the mucosa and serosa. The bowel becomes congested, thickened, and rigid with the development of adhesions. There is edema, thickening of the muscularis, and stricture of the lumen of the colon resulting in obstruction. Fistulas, abscesses, and perforation may occur from Crohn disease.

The onset of Crohn disease is most often between the ages of 10 and 30. Prevalence of Crohn disease is equal in men and women. The overall incidence of Crohn disease is lower than ulcerative colitis. Crohn disease is associated with cigarette smoking, NSAID use, and other autoimmune disorders. The exact etiology is unknown but possible causes include bacterial, viral, allergic, autoimmune, and hereditary factors. There is a familial predisposition to the disease and patients have increased suppressor T-cell activity along with alterations in IgA production.

The onset of Crohn disease is often insidious with diarrhea, fatigue, pain, weight loss, and fever. The initial pain the patient with Crohn disease complains of is a constant right-sided pain that may mimic appendicitis. Later in the disease process, the patient complains of pain that is more cramplike in description and is often associated with eating. Patients often avoid meals to avoid pain, resulting in weight loss, malnutrition, and cachexia. Predominant symptoms of Crohn disease include nausea and vomiting, watery diarrhea, steatorrhea, anal excoriation, and/or fistula. The patient also complains of arthralgia, malaise, and fever. Aphthous ulcers of the lips and mouth occur. When the ileum is involved, the patient will have a vitamin B_{12} deficiency. In addition, the patient may also have metabolic bone disease due to the malabsorption deficiencies of the colon in this disease process. There are similarities and differences between ulcerative colitis and Crohn disease (Table 6-15).

Laboratory findings in both ulcerative colitis and Crohn disease include decreased hemoglobin, hematocrit, potassium, and serum albumin levels. The WBC count and alkaline phosphatase levels are increased. Stool specimens detect occult blood along with overt bleeding. Other diagnostic examinations used in the differential diagnosis are proctosigmoidoscopy and colonoscopy procedures, barium enema (BE), radiology examinations, biopsy, and a stool culture and sensitivity test. In ulcerative colitis, the abdominal radiograph will reveal crypt abscesses, mucosal alterations, and dilated loops of bowel. The proctosigmoidoscopy will show diffuse erythema, mucosal inflammation, loss of vascular network, and mucosal bleeding. In Crohn disease, a narrowing of the distal ileum known as the "string sign" appears on the abdominal radiograph. With a sigmoidoscopy, direct visualization occurs. The inflammation of the intestinal mucosa and surrounding musculature, lumen stenosis, and longitudinal and transverse ulcers (cobblestoning) are seen. A colonoscopy determines the extent of the disease.

Biopsies are performed on the intestinal mucosa and surrounding musculature. The goals of care for ulcerative colitis are to minimize complications, restore and maintain nutritional status, and relieve symptoms. The goals of treatment for Crohn disease are to optimize GI function, restore and maintain nutritional status, and relieve symptoms. These are both chronic diseases with exacerbations; therefore, the care team should anticipate the patient's disease trajectory. Patients have nursing care needs in positioning, skin care, pain management, nutrition, infection control, discharge planning, pharmacology, psychosocial issues, and ethical issues. Position the patient for comfort, usually with the head of the bed raised. Provide interventions to prevent skin breakdown due to diarrhea. Keep the patient clean and dry. The patient's pain management needs to be individualized. To ease cramping, administer antidiarrheal agents and anticholinergics. Each patient will have varying nutritional intake; therefore, administer vitamin supplements as prescribed. Provide high-fiber, low-sugar diet and adjust for food allergies such as milk and yeast allergies.

The chronicity of these conditions results in frequent rehospitalization for exacerbations. Discharge planning is a very important aspect of the collaborative patient care plan. The chronic nature of these diseases and their impact on the patient's social structure may lead to isolation and may significantly affect the family unit and increase stress. The collaborative plan of care should include interventions to address individual and family psychosocial issues and problems. Discuss ethical issues, such as an advanced directive, and include in the plan of care.

An important aspect of collaborative care management is to monitor the patient for potential complications. A complication of ulcerative colitis is a toxic megacolon, due to the loss of contractility and massive dilatation of the colon, especially with the presence of fulminant disease. The colon tissue becomes friable, causing bleeding, and increases the risk of colon cancer. Total body system problems such as SIRS and sepsis can develop if the colon perforates. Complications of Crohn disease commonly include both GI and extra-GI issues. Fistulas are a cardinal feature. Urinary tract infections, impaired absorption, gluten intolerance (i.e., protein found in barley, wheat, and rye), kidney stones, and arthritis are comorbid with Crohn disease. A bowel obstruction, perforation, and/or GI hemorrhage may also occur. Monitor for clinical indications of an acute abdomen. Chronic complications of Crohn disease include extraintestinal disorders such as rheumatoid arthritis, sclerosing cholangitis, urinary calculi, and iron-deficiency anemia.

TABLE 6-15   **Comparison of Crohn Disease and Ulcerative Colitis**

Characteristic	Crohn Disease	Ulcerative Colitis
Bloody diarrhea	Rare	Common
Fistula and/or abscess formation	Very likely	May occur but rare
Abscess formation	Very likely	May occur but rare
Transmural involvement	Yes	No; limited to mucosa
Lesions	Discontinuous (i.e., "skip" lesions)	Continuous
Location of involvement	Any part of GI tract but most commonly distal small intestine and proximal large intestine	Most severe in rectum and sigmoid colon
Clinical course	Remissions and exacerbations	Remissions and exacerbations

Collaborative care management of mild to moderate ulcerative colitis includes a low-roughage diet, no dairy products, antimicrobial agents, steroids, anticholinergic agents, and antidiarrheal agents. Monitor the patient for exacerbation of symptoms. Keep accurate intake and output measurements along with close monitoring of electrolyte and hemoglobin levels. Optimize the patient's nutritional status and administer medications as ordered. In severe cases (fulminant disease), the patient will need IV fluids and electrolyte replacement, and blood transfusions. Maintain NPO status for fulminant stage patients, and have a nasogastric tube to low wall intermittent section. Provide parenteral nutrition to maintain the nutritional status during this stage. Prepare and educate the patient and family if a colon resection with ileostomy is required.

Collaborative care management of patients with Crohn disease includes close monitoring for infections or peritonitis. Check the stool for pus and/or blood. Keep an accurate record of intake and output to optimize nutritional status. Optimize bowel function and minimize episodes of diarrhea and abdominal pain. Administer medications as ordered. A diet high in calories, vitamins, and protein; low in residues; and that is milk-free is recommended along with supplementary parenteral and/or elemental feedings. Use antimicrobial agents and steroids. Promote physical and emotional rest. There may be a need for surgical procedures to drain abscesses, repair fistulas, seal perforations, relieve hydronephrosis and obstructions, and remove carcinogenic tumors.

6.13   Learning Activity

Complete the following table. You may include more than one condition for each but include only conditions discussed in this chapter.

Clinical Finding	Condition(s)
Elevated lipase, amylase	
Sudden, painless hematemesis	
Decreased protein	
Rebound tenderness	
Jaundice	
Hypocalcemia	
Bleeding tendencies	
Elevated ammonia	
Bloody diarrhea	
Hyperbilirubinemia	
Fetor hepaticus	
High-pitched rushing bowel sounds	
Succussion splash	
Management	**Condition(s)**
Irrigate NG tube until clear	
Neomycin and lactulose	
Sclerosis during endoscopy	
Aldosterone antagonist diuretics	
NPO status	
Sengstaken-Blakemore tube	
Volume and blood replacement	
Billroth I or II	

Answers to this activity can be found in the Answer Key.

6.14   Learning Activity

Synergy Model Application

Patients in progressive care units with acute GI problems have conditions that vary in complexity. Match the level of complexity to the situation described:

Situation	Level I Minimally Stable	Level III Moderately Stable	Level V Highly Stable
34-year-old married businessman who has had a small bowel resection for Crohn disease.			
36-year-old mechanic with cirrhosis and newly diagnosed liver cancer who is on the transplant list. He is separated from his wife and lives with his parents.			
18-year-old man with abdominal trauma due to MVA in which his girlfriend was killed.			

Answers to this activity can be found in the Answer Key.

6.15   Synthesis Learning Activity: Case Study

Mr. M. is a 57-year-old man admitted yesterday to the progressive care unit after starting to pass black, tarry stools. He has a 2-day history of severe stomach pains and has complained of severe indigestion the past few months. The patient is a life-long smoker, and has a 2-year medical history of mild chronic cardiac failure for which he has been taking enalapril 5 mg twice daily. He also recently started taking naproxen 500 mg twice daily for arthritis. Yesterday his hemoglobin was reported as 10.3 g/dL and his platelets as 162,000 mc/L, and his INR was 1.1. The urinalysis, electrolytes, and liver function studies were normal. He was mildly tachycardic (90 BPM) and had a slightly low blood pressure of 115/77 mm Hg. He was given 1.5 L of saline. An endoscopy procedure this morning determined the presence of a bleeding duodenal ulcer.

1. Which item(s) listed are a known risk factor for a peptic ulcer? (Select all that apply.)
   a. Enalapril
   b. Naproxen
   c. History of smoking
   d. Age
2. A proton pump inhibitor (PPI) has been ordered for Mr. M. The drug classification includes the following medication:
   a. Gaviscon
   b. Metoclopramide (Reglan)
   c. Omeprazole (Prilosec)
   d. Ranitidine (Zantac)

Answers to this activity can be found in the Answer Key.

6.16   Synthesis Learning Activity: Crossword Puzzle

Complete the following crossword puzzle related to GI assessment and diagnostics.

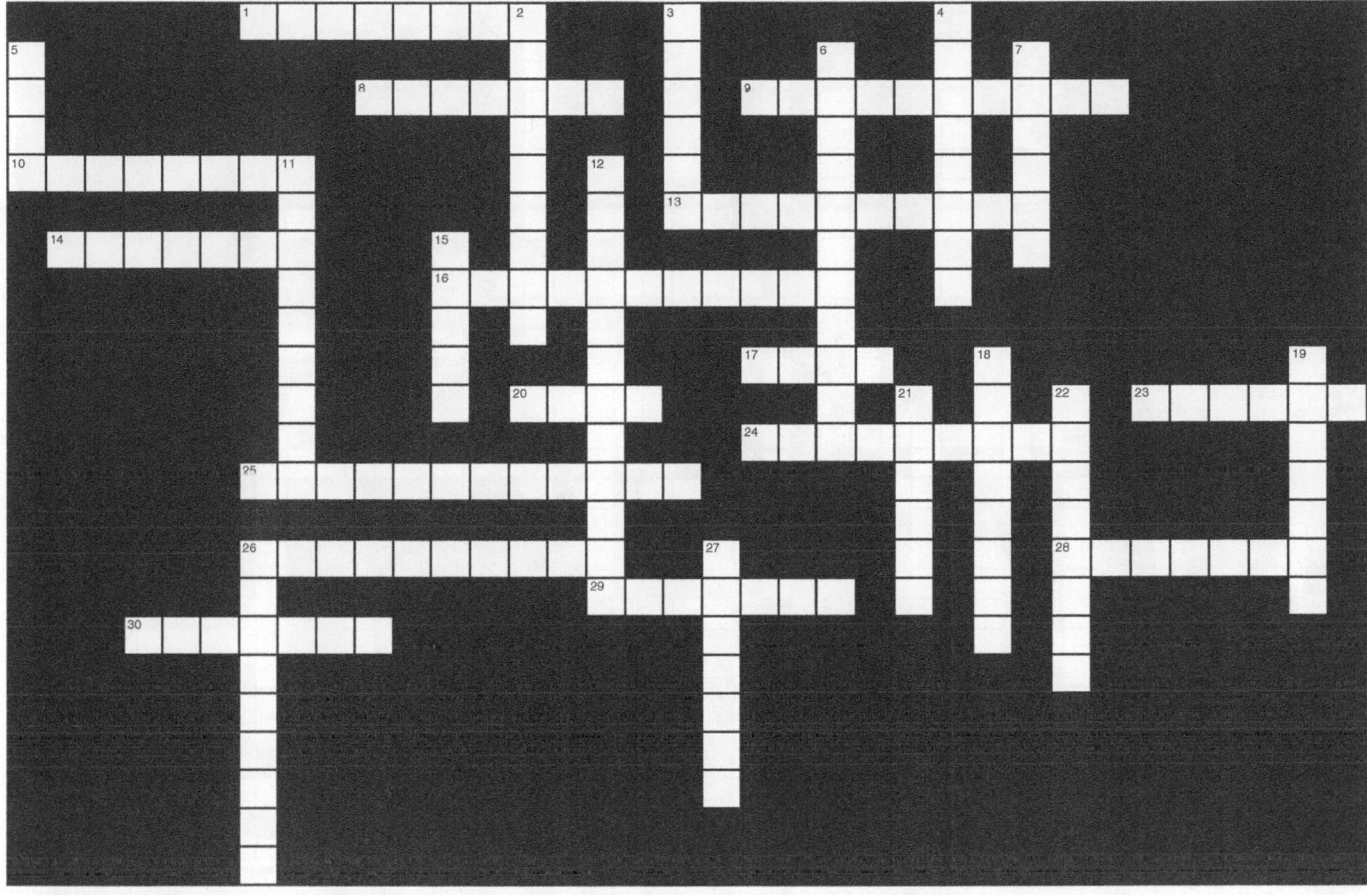

Answers to this activity can be found in the Answer Key.

ACROSS

1. Term for generalized, massive edema
8. An abnormal accumulation of fluid in the peritoneal cavity
9. _____ sign is a bluish tint to the flanks that is indicative of retroperitoneal bleeding (2 words)
10. This type of pain is experienced at a distance from the disease process
13. The term for belching
14. An obstruction here is manifested by vomiting and a succussion splash
16. The location of pain in acute pancreatitis
17. The acronym for a screening echo used in abdominal trauma (abbrev.)
20. This test may cause pancreatitis (abbrev.)
23. _____ sign is a bluish discoloration around the umbilicus; indicative of intraabdominal bleeding
24. The term for impaired digestion
25. The gentle repetitive bouncing of tissues against the hand; used to evaluate organ enlargement
26. The term for loud, hyperactive bowel sounds
28. The plasma protein most significant in maintaining capillary oncotic pressure
29. An elevated _____ level causes neurologic changes in patients with hepatic encephalopathy
30. Serum _____ is elevated in acute pancreatitis

DOWN

2. A flapping tremor seen in hepatic encephalopathy
3. Serum _____ is elevated in acute pancreatitis and is more specific than serum amylase
4. This physical finding may be caused by biliary obstruction, liver disease, or excessive hemolysis
5. _____ sign is caused by phrenic nerve irritation by subphrenic blood
6. The term for vomiting blood
7. Abdominal pain experienced with mesenteric ischemia is frequently described as abdominal _____
11. The term for difficulty swallowing
12. The term for bright red blood per rectum
15. A small bowel obstruction causes reverse peristalsis and vomiting that is ___
18. This type of pain is dull and poorly localized
19. _____ tenderness is when pain is more severe on release than with the direct pressure
21. The term for tarry stools
22. The _____ sign is indicative of splenic rupture
26. Jaundice occurs in hepatic failure due to the inability of the liver to convert fat-soluble _____ to water-soluble ___ (i.e., conjugation)
27. This type of pain is sharp and well localized

6.17 Synthesis Learning Activity: Crossword Puzzle

Complete the following crossword puzzle related to GI conditions and management.

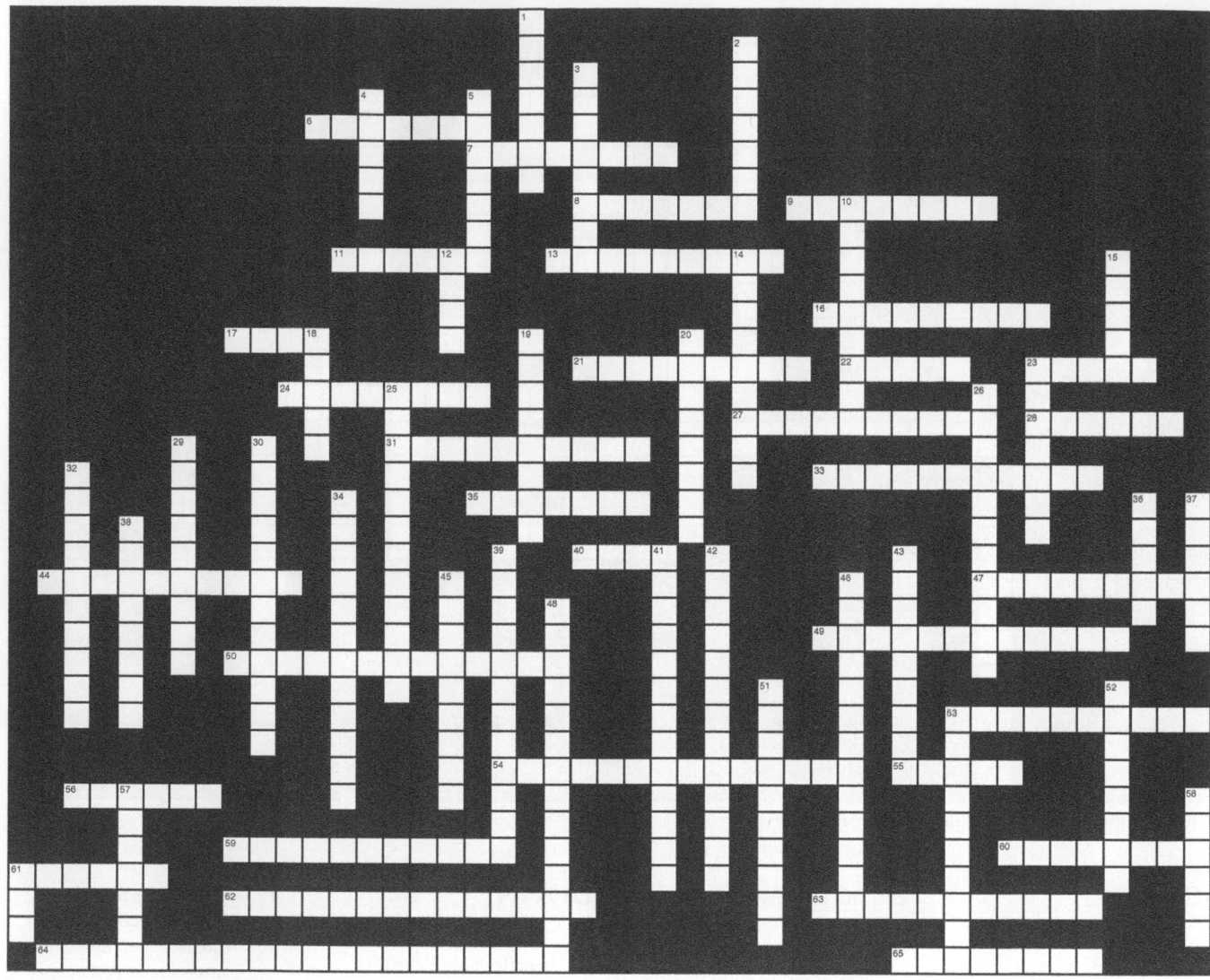

Answers to this activity can be found in the Answer Key.

ACROSS

6. This macronutrient is restricted in hepatic encephalopathy

7. A deficiency of this vitamin is commonly seen in alcoholism

8. _____ ulcer is a stress ulcer associated with cerebral trauma

9. This procedure divides the vagus nerve along the esophagus to decrease acid secretion in the stomach

11. Hypertension of this circulation system is seen in cirrhosis

13. One controversy regarding the use of drugs that alter the pH of the gastric secretions is the increased incidence of _____

16. An osmotic laxative frequently used in hepatic encephalopathy (generic)

17. This procedure is now preferred over intestinal bypass for weight reduction for patients with morbid obesity (abbrev.)

21. This treatment for esophageal varices is performed during endoscopy

22. The term for functional obstruction of the bowel

23. _____ disease is an inflammatory bowel disease that can affect any area of the GI tract from the mouth to the anus

24. The analgesic of choice in pancreatitis is _____ or hydromorphone

27. A drug used in GI hemorrhage to suppress gastrin (generic)

28. ___ of gastric contents can cause damage to the esophagus; associated with GERD

31. A collection of inflammatory debris, pancreatic secretions, and necrotic tissue in the pancreas

33. This condition may be caused by ulcer, appendicitis, diverticulitis, or intestinal obstruction; causes peritonitis

35. A _____ procedure is also called a pancreatoduodenectomy

40. A stent is placed between the hepatic and portal veins in this procedure performed in patients with esophageal varices (abbrev.)

44. An H_2 receptor antagonist (generic)

47. This type of enteral formula is required if feeding is delivered distal to the jejunum

49. This diuretic is frequently used for fluid retention in hepatic failure; blocks aldosterone (generic)
50. *Clostridium difficile* is usually initially treated with _____ (generic)
53. This type of anemia is caused by a deficiency of intrinsic factor
54. The term for abnormal function of the brain; may be caused by elevated ammonia levels
55. Hepatitis B is sometimes referred to as _____ hepatitis
56. A type of shunt that is used for ascites
59. This condition occurs as a result of a disruption in the integrity of the GI tract; causes an acute abdomen
60. This osmotic diuretic may be used for cerebral edema in hepatic encephalopathy
61. This type of ulcer causes erosion in the mucosa of the esophagus, stomach, or duodenum
62. A common cause of acute pancreatitis
63. This drug may be used for GI hemorrhage but it may cause myocardial or mesenteric ischemia (generic)
64. The spore-producing bacterium that is a common cause of diarrhea in critically ill patients (2 words)

65. A "maneuver" that facilitates evacuation of the colon

DOWN

1. Hepatitis A and E are sometimes referred to as _____ hepatitis
2. This syndrome may occur after gastric resection; may be classified as early or late
3. This antibiotic is used in hepatic encephalopathy to kill intestinal bacteria that convert nitrogenous wastes to ammonia (generic)
4. Ulcerative colitis is an inflammatory bowel disease that affects the _____
5. The preferred method of nutritional support; should be used unless contraindications exist
10. A conditionally essential amino acid that aids in maintaining the integrity of the gut to prevent bacterial translocation
12. A serious pulmonary complication of acute pancreatitis (abbrev.)
14. A bowel diversion that is most likely to cause skin erosion if excellent containment not achieved
15. A complication of vasopressin therapy that causes water intoxication (abbrev.)

18. The form of fluid replacement that is indicated for acute GI hemorrhage
19. An IV proton pump inhibitor (brand name)
20. A semiessential amino acid that enhances the immune system and promotes wound healing
23. _____ is a stress ulcer associated with burns
25. An electrolyte imbalance seen in acute pancreatitis
26. A syndrome of acute kidney injury associated with hepatic failure
29. This condition causes coffee-ground–like hematemesis
30. A common description of the appearance of the stool seen with mesenteric infarction (2 words)
32. A drug that acts as a mucosal barrier used to protect the gastric mucosa (generic)
34. This antibiotic may be used to stimulate peristalsis
36. An intestinal perforation causes an _____ abdomen and requires surgical intervention
37. Enteral feeding administration may be intermittent, continuous, or _____
38. A type of parenteral catheter
39. This type of esophageal tear is caused by forceful retching and vomiting (2 words)

41. A complication of hernia that may cause bowel ischemia or infarction
42. A drug commonly used for suicide that is a major cause of hepatic failure in adolescents (generic)
43. Inflammation and then fibrosis of the liver frequently associated with alcoholism
45. The term for inflammation of the liver
46. This may be an indication of diabetes mellitus in a patient with chronic pancreatitis
48. This drug is used for acetaminophen toxicity; must be administered within 24 hours of acetaminophen ingestion (generic)
51. An exploratory _____ may be necessary to localize organ injury and/or hemorrhage in trauma patients
52. The type of drug frequently prescribed for patients with ascites
53. The route of nutritional support used in functional or structural obstruction
57. Esophageal _____ causes sudden, painless hemorrhage by mouth; caused by portal hypertension
58. Helicobacter _____ is a bacteria associated with peptic ulcer
61. A gastric feeding tube that is endoscopically placed (abbrev.)

CHAPTER 7

The Endocrine System

ANATOMY AND PHYSIOLOGY

The overall function of the endocrine system is to maintain stability despite constant changes in the external and internal environment. In response to specific stimuli, endocrine organs use hormones to talk to target cells throughout the body. The endocrine system influences every cell in the human body. The metabolic body functions regulated by the endocrine system include:

- Chemical reactions and transport of chemicals across cell membranes
- Growth and development
- Metabolism
- Fluid and electrolyte balance
- Acid-base balance
- Adaptation
- Reproduction

Glands

The endocrine system consists of glands or glandular tissue (Figure 7-1) that synthesize, store, and secrete hormones. An endocrine gland is ductless but highly vascular.

Hormones

Specialized cells synthesize and secrete complex chemical substances called hormones, which are released into the blood, exerting biochemical effects on target cells away from the site of origin. In essence, hormones are a set of commands produced by endocrine organs and secreted in response to the body's needs. Endocrine glands release hormones in response to specific signals (e.g., low target gland hormone levels, low serum calcium, sympathetic nervous system innervation).

There are three types of hormones: single amino acids, proteins, and steroids. Chemically, hormones are categorized by their physiologic action (Table 7-1). Examples of single amino acids include epinephrine, dopamine, and thyroid hormones. Growth hormone and follicle-stimulating hormone are examples of protein hormones. Androgens, aldosterone, and cortisol are examples of steroid hormones.

Although not normally considered part of the endocrine system, the gastrointestinal (GI) system, heart, and kidneys also secrete hormones. Gastrin, cholecystokinin, somatostatin, gastric inhibitory peptide, secretin, and vasoactive intestinal peptide are hormones secreted by the GI system. The heart secretes atrial natriuretic hormone. The kidneys secrete erythropoietin, renin, and calcitriol.

Hormones are released directly into the bloodstream and distributed throughout the body to activate receptors on a target gland or target organ. Receptor cells, otherwise known as

target cells, are located in an organ or a group of cells in another part of the body. The hormone triggers the receptor to initiate a response. The specific receptors on or in the target cell determine hormone specificity. For example, protein hormones react with receptors on the cell surface, while steroid hormones react with receptors inside the cell. The receptors distinguish different hormones from each other and translate the hormonal signal into a cellular response. The hormone receptor complex initiates intracellular events that lead to the metabolic activity on the target cells via activation of cyclic adenosine monophosphate (cAMP) or activation of genes.

Regulation of Hormones

The hypothalamus regulates the hormone levels through secretion of releasing factors. The pituitary gland is stimulated by

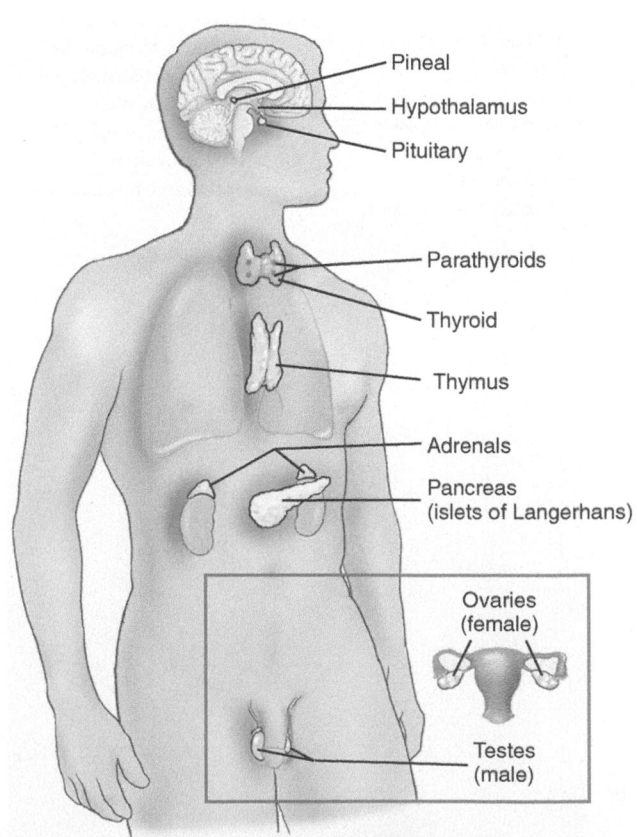

FIGURE 7-1 Location of endocrine glands. (From Shiland, B. J. [2010]. *Mastering healthcare terminology* [3rd ed.]. St. Louis, MO: Mosby.)

these releasing factors from the hypothalamus to secrete stimulating factors. The target gland is then stimulated to secrete the hormone into circulation where receptor binding occurs in the target cells.

The concentration of the hormone present in the circulation determines the self-regulation of hormone production and release (Figure 7-2). Electrolyte levels, metabolites, osmolality, fluid status, and other hormones also influence regulation. Regulation by negative feedback is most common; high hormone levels inhibit the release of the releasing factor from the hypothalamus or stimulating factor from the pituitary gland or secretion of the hormone from the gland. Positive feedback regulation is less common. A hormone stimulates

TABLE 7-1   Hormone Chemical Classification

Physiologic Action Category	Examples
Peptide or protein hormones	• Vasopressin (antidiuretic hormone [ADH]) • Thyrotropin-releasing hormone (TRH) • Insulin • Growth hormone (somatotropin [GH]) • Follicle-stimulating hormone (FSH) • Luteinizing hormone (LH) • Corticotropin (adrenocorticotropin [ACTH]) • Calcitonin
Steroids	• Glucocorticoids (i.e., cortisol) • Mineralocorticoids (i.e., aldosterone) • Estradiol • Progesterone • Testosterone
Amines and amino acid derivatives	• Norepinephrine • Epinephrine • Triiodothyronine (T_3) • Thyroxine (T_4)

continued secretion until a specific level is reached. Neural regulation and the release of epinephrine are a result of stress and the stimulation of the sympathetic division of the autonomic nervous system (SNS); when stress occurs, the SNS is no longer stimulated and results in reduction of epinephrine release. Several types of classification systems exist for endocrine dysfunction. The level of hormone activity determines one type of classification. Hyperfunction is an increase in hormonal activity, whereas hypofunction is a decrease in hormonal activity. The location of the gland or response also determines a classification of endocrine dysfunction. Primary disorders are a condition of the target gland (e.g., adrenal or thyroid). A secondary disorder is one where the problem occurs from the stimulating gland (e.g., pituitary). A tertiary disorder stems from a problem with the hypothalamus. The acuity and time of occurrence of the endocrine dysfunction can determine the classifications. Acute problems begin abruptly with marked intensity. Chronic disorders develop slowly and persist for a long time, often for the remainder of the lifetime of the individual. Finally, the cause of the problem such as dysfunction of a particular gland, altered secretion of the stimulating hormones for that gland, and/or altered response to the hormone itself at the target cell determines the classification.

Most endocrine glands and hormones are significant in the care of acutely ill patients (Table 7-2). Somatostatin is a hormone present in the islet cells, the hypothalamus, and the GI tract. The physiologic action of somatostatin is that of an inhibitor. It inhibits the secretion of insulin, glucagon, GH, TSH, and the GI hormones gastrin and secretin. The gonadal hormones, testosterone, estrogen, and progesterone are not typically significant in progressive care, so for the purpose of the exam, do not focus on these hormones.

ASSESSMENT OF THE ENDOCRINE SYSTEM

Interview

Endocrine disorders are often insidious and chronic in nature, and delay of diagnosis is common. The thyroid gland is the only endocrine gland that is palpable and available for direct examination. Endocrine dysfunction often underlies an admitting

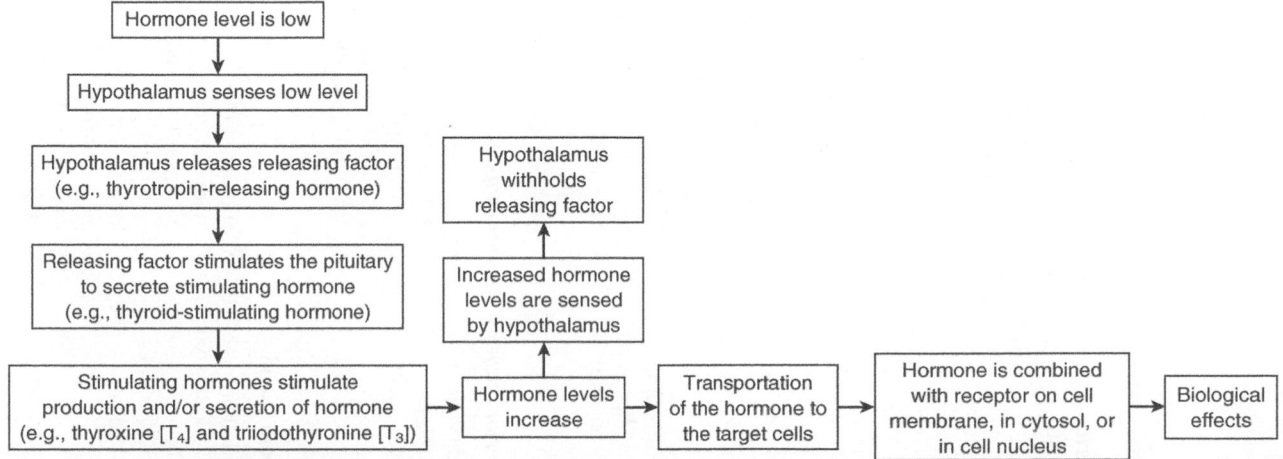

FIGURE 7-2 Process of hormone synthesis, secretion, effect, and suppression of endocrine dysfunction. (From Dennison, R. D. [2013]. *Pass CCRN!* [4th ed]. St. Louis, MO: Elsevier.)

TABLE 7-2 Endocrine Glands and Hormones Significant in the Care of Acutely Ill Adults

Hormone	Actions	Releasing Factors	Target	Hypersecretion	Hyposecretion
Pituitary (Hypophysis)					
		Hypothalamus: Controls the release of pituitary hormones			
Anterior Pituitary (Adenohypophysis)					
Growth hormone (somatotropin)	• Stimulates protein anabolism • Mobilizes fatty acids • Conserves carbohydrates • Stimulates growth of bone, muscle, and cartilage	• Growth hormone-releasing hormone (GHRH) from hypothalamus in response to exercise, starvation, decreased amino acid levels, stress, hypoglycemia	• All body cells capable of growth, especially muscle, bone, and cartilage cells	• Giantism in children; acromegaly in adults	• Dwarfism in children; possible decrease in organ weight in adults
Adrenocorticotropic hormone (ACTH)	• Stimulates growth and function of adrenal gland • Controls production and release of glucocorticoid hormones • Stimulates mineralocorticoid production • Stimulates androgen production	• Corticotropin-releasing hormone (CRH) from hypothalamus in response to hypoglycemia, decrease in cortisol levels, hypoxia, trauma, surgery, physical and/or psychological stress	• Cells of adrenal cortex	• Cushing disease	• Adrenal insufficiency (chronic) and/or adrenal crisis (acute)
Thyroid-stimulating hormone (thyrotropin)	• Increases size and growth of thyroid cells • Increases synthesis of thyroid hormones • Releases stored thyroid hormones	• Thyrotropin-releasing hormone (TRH) from the hypothalamus in response to cold temperature or a decrease in thyroid hormone levels	• Cells of the thyroid gland	• Hyperthyroidism	• Hypothyroidism
Posterior Pituitary (Neurohypophysis)					
Antidiuretic hormone (vasopressin)	• Increases water reabsorption (inhibits diuresis) by kidney tubules and collecting ducts • Vasoconstriction of arterioles • Abdominal cramping	• Increase in serum osmolality; hypernatremia; hypovolemia; hypoxia; hypotension; pain; trauma; stress; nausea; pharmacologic agents	• Distal renal tubules and collecting ducts; smooth muscle of arterioles and GI tract	• Syndrome of inappropriate antidiuretic hormone (SIADH)	• Diabetes insipidus
Thyroid Gland					
Triiodothyronine (T_3) and thyroxine (T_4) NOTE: T_3 is more biologically active	• Stimulates metabolic rate • Increases protein synthesis • Increases carbohydrate and fat metabolism • Increases bone growth • Increases oxygen consumption • Increases metabolism and clearance of drugs	• Thyroid-stimulating hormone (TSH) from anterior pituitary; thyrotropin-releasing hormone (TRH) from hypothalamus; cold temperature	• Most body cells	• Hyperthyroidism (chronic); thyroid storm or crisis (acute)	• Hypothyroidism (chronic); myxedema coma (acute)

Hormone	Actions	Stimulus for Secretion	Target	Hypersecretion	Hyposecretion
Thyrocalcitonin (calcitonin)	• Reduces plasma calcium levels by inhibiting bone lysis and decreasing calcium resorption by the kidney	• Increase in serum calcium, magnesium, or glucagon	• Bone cells, kidney cells	• Not significant	• Not significant
Parathyroid Gland					
Parathyroid hormone (parathormone)	• Increases serum calcium by accelerating bone breakdown with release of calcium into the blood, increasing calcium reabsorption from intestine, and decreasing kidney tubule reabsorption of calcium • Decreases blood phosphate levels by increasing phosphate loss in urine • Increases resorption of magnesium by the renal tubules	• Low serum calcium or high serum phosphate level; catecholamines; cortisol	• Bone cells, cells of GI tract and kidney	• Hypercalcemia and hypophosphatemia; osteoporosis and possibly renal calculi; decreased neuromuscular irritability and muscle weakness	• Hypocalcemia and hyperphosphatemia; neuromuscular irritability and tetany
Adrenal Cortex					
Glucocorticoids (i.e., cortisol) **SUGAR**	• Increases blood glucose by stimulating gluconeogenesis in the liver • Inhibits glucose utilization by the cell • Inhibits protein anabolism • Promotes fatty acid mobilization • Inhibits inflammatory response	• CRH from hypothalamus; ACTH from anterior pituitary	• Most body cells	• Cushing syndrome	• Addison disease (chronic); adrenal crisis (acute)
Mineralocorticoids (i.e., aldosterone) **SALT**	• Increases sodium and water reabsorption and potassium excretion	• ACTH from anterior pituitary (minor effect); primary stimulus is renin-angiotensin system; decrease in serum sodium; increase in serum potassium	• Distal and collecting tubules of kidney; sweat glands; salivary glands; intestines	• Hyperaldosteronism	• Addison disease (chronic); adrenal crisis (acute)
Androgens (e.g., testosterone) **SEX**	• Not of significance on this exam				

Continued

TABLE 7-2   Endocrine Glands and Hormones Significant in the Care of Acutely Ill Adults—cont'd

Hormone	Actions	Releasing Factors	Target	Hypersecretion	Hyposecretion
Adrenal Medulla					
Catecholamines (i.e., epinephrine, norepinephrine)	• Dilates pupils • Increases heart rate and contractility • Dilation of blood vessels to heart, brain, and skeletal muscle • Constriction of blood vessels to nonessential organs (i.e., skin, kidneys, GI tract) • Bronchodilation • Increases in respiratory rate and depth • Increases in perspiration, peristalsis, and secretion in GI tract • Increases in blood sugar	• Sympathetic nervous system innervation; insulin; histamine; anxiety; fear; pain; trauma; exercise; temperature extremes; hypoxia; hypotension; hypovolemia; excess thyroid hormone	• Most body cells, vascular beds, smooth muscle	• Exaggeration or prolongation of normal effects; may be caused by adrenal medulla tumor called *pheochromocytoma*	• May have decrease in stress response or no noticeable effect
Pancreas					
Glucagon (from alpha cells)	• Stimulates glycogenolysis and gluconeogenesis to increase blood glucose • Inhibits glycolysis • Increases lipolysis	• Decrease in blood glucose; elevated blood amino acids; catecholamines; exercise; starvation	• Most body cells, especially liver cells	• Hyperglycemia	• Hypoglycemia
Insulin (from beta cells)	• Enables glucose to move into the cell • Aids in muscle and tissue oxidation of glucose • Enhances storage of glycogen • Increases protein synthesis • Inhibits lipolysis	• Increase in blood glucose; gastrin; increase in growth hormone; ACTH; glucagon	• Most body cells, especially liver cells	• Hypoglycemia	• Hyperglycemia (DM)

diagnosis and profoundly affects treatment and recovery. The patient interview has paramount importance because history of increased risk is the best indicator to accurate diagnosis. Hormones affect every body tissue; therefore, numerous symptoms may indicate endocrine dysfunction.

The assessment of the endocrine system starts with eliciting the patient's chief complaint. Determine what the reason was that the patient sought help and the duration of the problem. The patient may present with a number of general symptoms in addition to specific signs and symptoms attributed to every body system (Table 7-3).

During the interview process, the nurse needs to determine the history of present illness. Use OPQRST format (onset, provocation or palliation, quality, region and radiation, severity, and time [history] or type) to elicit the history and occurrence of the signs and symptoms of the present problems. Determine the past medical history, as some conditions may result in endocrine dysfunction, such as the following:

- Trauma
- Ischemia or infarction
- Neoplasm
- Inflammation, infection
- Autoimmune conditions
- Acquired immunodeficiency syndrome (AIDS)
- Irradiation, antineoplastic drugs
- Surgical removal of an endocrine gland
- Interruption of a prescribed pharmaceutical agent for treatment of a preexisting chronic endocrine dysfunction

Family history is also important to elicit. It is important to distinguish problems from inherited traits. Endocrine disorders often have an inherited tendency. Question the patient's family history of diabetes mellitus (DM), cardiovascular disease, cerebrovascular disease, and cancer.

In addition to medical history, assess the patient's social history, focusing on his or her occupation and education level. Determine the relationship with the patient's spouse or significant other including family structure and current stress level and usual coping mechanisms. Also, include an assessment of the patient's recreational, exercise, and dietary habits. Address the patient's usual nutritional intake along with compliance to prescribed dietary limitations. Determine the patient's normal fluid intake. Query the patient about caffeine, tobacco, alcohol, and recreational drug usage. Record tobacco use as pack-years (number of packs per day times the number of years the patient has been smoking). Document the alcoholic beverages consumed per month, week, or day. Also, question the patient to identify recent travel and potential toxin exposure.

Pharmacologic agents may alter endocrine function by either stimulating or inhibiting hormone release or interfering with hormone action at the target tissue. Individual pharmacologic agents used to treat chronic endocrine dysfunction will be discussed in detail with each condition but generally involve hormone replacement, hormone suppressive agents, agents that trigger release of a hormone or potentiate the effect of the hormone, and vitamins or minerals necessary for body synthesis of hormones.

In addition to being aware of the appropriate endocrine pharmacologic treatment, investigate the patient's medication history of prescribed drugs. Note the drug, dose, frequency, and time of last dose of each medication. It is important to elicit the patient's compliance with prescribed therapy along with his or

TABLE 7-3 Subjective and Objective Findings of Endocrine Disorders

Body System	Subjective and Objective Findings
Generalized	Fatigue; lethargy; sleep disorders; cold or heat intolerance; weight loss or gain, or rapid fluctuations in weight; and increase in size of head, hands, or feet
Dermatologic	Pruritus, hair loss, changes in distribution and hair quality, changes in skin color or pigmentation, changes in skin moisture and striae
Eye	Visual changes
Neck	Jugular neck vein distention and enlarged lymph nodes
Cardiovascular	Palpitations and syncope
Pulmonary	Dyspnea
Neurologic	Voice changes, tremors, nervousness, visual changes, loss of the sense of smell, headache, sensory changes, memory loss, personality changes, confusion, agitation, delusions, paranoia, depression, muscle twitching, and seizures
Gastrointestinal	Nausea, vomiting, change in appetite, abdominal pain, constipation or diarrhea, involuntary stool, polyphagia, and polydipsia
Genitourinary	Polyuria, oliguria, nocturia, incontinence, decreased libido, and menstrual irregularities
Musculoskeletal	Muscle or joint pain, or aching muscles or joints; muscle weakness; muscle cramping; muscle wasting; twitching; and fractures

her understanding of drug actions, side effects, and appropriate sick day management. Investigate the use of over-the-counter drugs, supplements, and herbs. Ask about substance abuse including drug, route, and frequency.

Inspection and Palpation
Vital Signs
Measure the blood pressure (BP) to evaluate for orthostatic changes while the patient is lying, sitting, and standing. Orthostatic BP changes may occur with endocrine problems due to hypovolemia (i.e., diabetes insipidus [DI] or DM). Heart and respiratory rate abnormalities may also be detected.

Bradycardia occurs frequently in patients with hypothyroidism. Tachycardia may be associated with hyperthyroidism, infection (which may be a cause of diabetic ketoacidosis [DKA] or hyperosmolar hyperglycemic state [HHS]), hypovolemia (which may occur in DKA, HHS, or DI), and hypervolemia (which may occur in syndrome of inappropriate antidiuretic hormone [SIADH]). A decreased respiratory rate (i.e., bradypnea) occurs in hypothyroidism. Tachypnea may be associated with hyperthyroidism, infection (which may be a cause of DKA or HHS), hypovolemia (which may occur in DKA, HHS, or DI), and hypervolemia (which may occur in SIADH).

Temperature alterations are quite common in endocrine disorders. Hypothermia may be associated with hypothyroidism. Hyperthermia may be associated with hyperthyroidism, with extreme hyperthermia during thyroid crisis, sometimes referred to as *thyroid storm*. Hyperthermia may also indicate infection that may be a cause of DKA or HHS. Changes in weight are common. Weight increase may be associated with hypothyroidism or Cushing syndrome. Weight decrease may be associated with hyperthyroidism.

During the general survey, determine the patient's apparent health status. The presence of a Medic-Alert bracelet may indicate chronic endocrine condition or steroid dependency. An altered level of consciousness may occur due to changes seen in cerebral function. Other factors to determine regarding health status include whether the apparent age is consistent with the patient's chronologic age, gross deformity or asymmetry, nutritional status, stature and posture, and mobility.

Specific to the endocrine system evaluation, the redistribution of body fat may cause a "buffalo hump," "moon face," and a thick trunk with thin arms and legs (e.g., Cushing syndrome). Gynecomastia occurs in males due to hypogonadism, hyperthyroidism, or Cushing syndrome. Specific signs and symptoms of several body systems may be present (Table 7-4).

Percussion

The only percussion technique used in assessment of the endocrine system is eliciting deep tendon reflexes (DTRs). Neurologic

TABLE 7-4   Endocrine Dysfunction Objective Findings

System	Objective Findings

Head, neck, eyes, ears, and throat	• Protruding eyeballs (exophthalmos): frequently seen in hyperthyroidism; lid lag frequently seen in patients with exophthalmos
	• Sunken eyes: may be seen in hypothyroidism or dehydration
	• Strabismus: may be seen with hyperthyroidism
	• Periorbital edema: frequently seen in Cushing syndrome; may also be seen in hypothyroidism
	• Changes in visual acuity and visual fields: may be related to pituitary tumor
	• Facial bone structure: facial changes including protruding forehead and prominent jaw seen in acromegaly
	• Facial edema
	• Enlargement and protrusion of tongue: may be seen in hypothyroidism or acromegaly
	• Thyroid gland
	  • Enlargement or palpable mass or nodule
	  • Tenderness
	  • Presence of thrill

Integument	• "Bronzing" of the skin with Addison disease • Gray-brown pigmentation around neck and axillae may be seen in Cushing syndrome • Yellowish skin discoloration may be seen in hypothyroidism • Temperature changes frequently seen in thyroid conditions • Warm, moist, paper-thin skin may be seen in hyperthyroidism • Dry, scaly skin may be seen in hypothyroidism • Decreased skin turgor may be seen in dehydration, which may be seen in DI, DKA, and HHS • Lesions: acne; spider angiomas • Scars: e.g., on the neck area due to prior thyroid surgery • Bruising: increased bruising may be seen in Cushing syndrome • Striae: purplish striae on abdomen may be seen in Cushing syndrome • Alopecia: may be seen in hyperthyroidism, hypothyroidism, and hypopituitarism • Coarse hair: frequently seen in hypothyroidism • Thin, silky hair: frequently seen in hyperthyroidism • Increased body or facial hair: may be seen in acromegaly or Cushing syndrome • Brittle nails: frequently seen in hypothyroidism
Cardiovascular	• Point of maximal impulse (PMI) displacement: may indicate cardiomegaly, which may be seen in hypothyroidism • Heave: may be associated with heart failure, which may be seen in hyperthyroidism • Peripheral pulses: increased or decreased quality
Pulmonary	• Odor of breath: acetone (fruity) breath noted in DKA • Changes in respiratory rate, depth, and rhythm • Kussmaul breathing pattern associated with metabolic acidosis such as DKA
Neurologic	• Level of consciousness or mental status changes: may be related to intracranial mass (e.g., pituitary tumor), cerebral edema, or dehydration (e.g., ADH disorders) • Pupil size, shape, and reactivity: Changes may be related to intracranial mass (e.g., pituitary tumor) or cerebral edema
Gastrointestinal	• Abdominal mass or organ enlargement
Genitourinary	• Suprarenal mass may indicate adrenal tumor (e.g., pheochromocytoma)

TABLE 7-5	Common Diagnostic Laboratory Studies and Normal Values	

Diagnostic Examination	Normal Value
Thyroid-stimulating hormone (TSH)	2-10 mU/mL
T3	0.2-0.3 mcg/dL
T4	6-12 mcg/dL
Antithyroglobulin antibody	normal <1:100
Radioactive iodine uptake	8-35%
ACTH	AM 15-100 pg/mL PM <50 pg/mL
Cortisol	6-28 mcg/dL at 8 AM 2-12 mcg/dL at 4 PM
ADH	1-5 pg/mL

changes such as an increase or decrease in the DTRs due to serum sodium changes occur in the conditions of DI or SIADH.

Auscultation

Auscultation may detect a thyroid gland bruit. A bruit is a sign of increased blood flow detected in hyperthyroidism. An S_3 heart sound, indicative of heart failure may be present in patients with hyperthyroidism. A systolic murmur may also be present because of the high cardiac output state related to hyperthyroidism. Auscultation detects crackles in the lungs due to fluid overload and pulmonary edema related to the heart failure brought on by hyperthyroidism. In patients with hypoparathyroidism, low calcium levels may produce stridor. The endocrine system also can affect the GI system; therefore hyperactive or hypoactive bowel sound changes may be auscultated.

Diagnostic Studies

As discussed earlier, the endocrine system affects every cell in the body. Hormone levels (Table 7-5) are frequently relevant to a diagnosis or treatment. Provocative tests assess the ability of an endocrine gland to respond to a stimulus, assess reserve capacity, and confirm either hypo- or hyperfunction of an endocrine gland. Fluid and electrolyte imbalances are very common in endocrine disorders.

Other diagnostic tests used in the diagnosis and management of endocrine disorders include radiology studies. Radiologic studies such as skull series, chest x-ray, and flat plate of the abdomen (KUB) are routinely used. Some diagnoses require more sophisticated examinations such as computerized tomography (CT) or magnetic resonance imaging (MRI) of the head or abdomen. Thyroid and abdominal ultrasound examinations and specific organ scans such as a brain, thyroid, or pancreatic scan may be used. When needed, the patient may require invasive diagnostic studies such as a biopsy or an adrenal angiography. Other diagnostics relied on are an electrocardiogram (ECG) and electroencephalogram (EEG). A multitude of different diagnostics are relevant to use with endocrine disorders primarily because the endocrine system affects all body cells.

Data retrieved from patient assessment is the basis for patient characteristic appraisal. The provision of quality patient care requires addressing individual patient characteristics outlined in the Synergy Model (see Chapter 2). The patient level (graded 1 minimally resilient through 5 highly resilient) is determined in each of the categories: resiliency, vulnerability, stability, complexity, resource availability, participation in care, participation in decision making, and predictability.

7.1 Learning Activity		

Identify the patient characteristic and level that characterizes the described situation.

Situation	Patient Characteristic	Level
A 36-year-old patient with type 1 DM was admitted with DKA. This is the fourth occurrence of DKA this past year. She is a smoker and was recently diagnosed with COPD.	Resiliency Vulnerability Stability Complexity Resource availability Participation in care Participation in decision making Predictability	1 2 3 4 5
A 76-year-old is admitted with adrenal insufficiency (Addison). The patient has durable power of attorney for health care and living will. The family is present and knowledgeable about the disease. They have provided history and treatment authorization and will aid in care when the patient is discharged.	Resiliency Vulnerability Stability Complexity Resource availability Participation in care Participation in decision making Predictability	1 2 3 4 5

Continued

7.1   Learning Activity—cont'd

Situation	Patient Characteristic	Level
A patient is newly diagnosed with type 2 DM. The patient resides in an assisted living facility and receives Medicare. She has a niece who lives nearby and visits often.	Resiliency Vulnerability Stability Complexity Resource availability Participation in care Participation in decision making Predictability	1 2 3 4 5
A 78-year-old man is admitted with DKA. He has two necrotic toes and an open wound on his right hip from a fall. The patient is confused, speaks only German, and has no family nearby.	Resiliency Vulnerability Stability Complexity Resource availability Participation in care Participation in decision making Predictability	1 2 3 4 5
An 83-year-old man is admitted with hypoglycemia after 3 days of nausea, vomiting, and diarrhea. He reported feeling sweaty and shaky. He now appears agitated and confused.	Resiliency Vulnerability Stability Complexity Resource availability Participation in care Participation in decision making Predictability	1 2 3 4 5
A 52-year-old woman in a chronic vegetative state after a head injury is admitted to a nursing home with DM. No family is nearby.	Resiliency Vulnerability Stability Complexity Resource availability Participation in care Participation in decision making Predictability	1 2 3 4 5

Answers to this activity can be found in the Answer Key.

ENDOCRINE PHARMACOLOGY

The treatment of endocrine disorders includes drugs from several drug categories, and it is important to recognize that drugs used for other problems may also have an effect on the endocrine system. A good example of this is glucocorticoids used for lung disease and autoimmune problems. The exogenous intake of corticosteroids can have a significant impact on the endocrine system.

Insulin

Diabetes mellitus (DM) is a disease of metabolism. Patients with type 1 or type 2 DM require medication to control their metabolism of protein, fats, and carbohydrates. The disease prevents glucose from entering the body cells due to a lack of insulin, ineffective insulin, or tissues not responding to insulin. In essence, the tissues suffer glucose starvation. In type 1 DM,

there is an absence of insulin; therefore, the pharmacologic treatment is administration of subcutaneous insulin. With diabetes type 2, there is an insulin deficiency, insulin insensitivity, or insulin resistance. In type 2 DM, the pharmacologic treatment is an oral hypoglycemic agent, and in some cases, administration of subcutaneous insulin.

Insulin dosage recommendations include short-acting insulin at meal times with basal long-acting insulin taken before bed. The long-acting insulin at bedtime provides a constant basal level of insulin, except at meal times when the short-acting insulin counters the increased glucose intake. Another regimen could include medium-acting and short-acting insulin combined at meals that address peaks to counter the increased glucose intake and provide basal insulin requirements. There are currently many insulin preparations (Table 7-6).

TABLE 7-6	Characteristics of Insulin Preparations				
Generic Name	Brand Name	Onset (min)	Peak (hr)	Duration (hr)	
Short Duration/Rapid Acting					
Insulin lispro (SC)	Humalog	15-30	0.5-2.5	3-6.5	
Insulin aspart	NovoLog	10-20	1-3	3-5	
Insulin glulisine	Apidra	10-15	1-1.5	3-5	
Short Duration/Slower Acting					
Human regular (IV)	Humulin R	Immediate	0.25-0.5	1-2	
Human regular (SC)	Humulin R, Novolin R	30-60	1-5	6-10	
Human regular (SC)	Exubera	15-30	0.5-1.5	6.6	
Intermediate Duration					
Human NPH (SC)	Humulin N, Novolin N	60-120	6-14	16-24	
Insulin detemir	Levemir	—	6-8	12-24*	
Long Duration					
Insulin glargine	Lantus	70	No discernible peak	24	

*Duration is dose dependent: At 0.2 unit/kg, duration is 12 hours, but at 2.5 units/kg, duration is 20 to 24 hours.
Adapted from Blair, E. (2014). Insulin A to Z: A guide on different types of insulin. *Joslin Diabetes Guidelines*. Retrieved from www.joslin.org/info/insulin_a_to_z_a_guide_on_different_types_of_insulin.html.

The health care provider determines the best regimen based on desired goals and individual patient self-care abilities. The regimen that provides a close match to intrinsic needs is preferred but is dependent on patient and/or family cognitive capabilities.

Oral Hypoglycemics

Oral hypoglycemic agents, along with behavioral changes to diet and exercise regimens, are preferred to help control type 2 diabetes. The varying oral hypoglycemic agents (Table 7-7) have different mechanisms of action and sites of action; therefore, the agents are often used in combination to gain better blood glucose control.

Glucagon

Hypoglycemia is an indication for the use of glucagon. To increase serum glucose levels, administer glucagon to promote the breakdown of glycogen, reduce glycogen synthesis, and stimulate biosynthesis of glucose. To work effectively, adequate glycogen stores are required, so this treatment is ineffective if hypoglycemia is due to starvation. The 0.5- to 1-mg dose is administered via the intramuscular (IM), subcutaneous (SC), or intravenous (IV) route. The IV route is preferred in patients with severe hypoglycemia. Expect the return to consciousness within 20 minutes of administration if the condition is due to hypoglycemia. Following the administration of glucagon, the patient should be given oral carbohydrate and protein.

DIABETES MELLITUS

Diabetes mellitus (DM) is a group of metabolic diseases characterized by hyperglycemia and confirmed by a fasting serum glucose of greater than or equal to 126 mg/dL. DM results from defects in insulin secretion, insulin action, or both. Characterized

by beta cell destruction, type 1 DM results in absolute insulin deficiency and was previously known as juvenile onset, type I, insulin-dependent DM (IDDM). Characterized by insulin resistance, type 2 DM results in a relative (rather than absolute) insulin deficiency. Previously, type 2 was known as age-onset, type II, and non–insulin-dependent DM (NIDDM). Note that current terminology uses Arabic rather than Roman numeral for the types of DM.

Hyperglycemia

Hyperglycemia is the technical term for high serum glucose (blood sugar). High serum glucose happens when the body has too little insulin or when the body cannot use insulin properly. The condition of DM is the most common cause of chronic hyperglycemia; however, hyperglycemia also can occur in patients without diabetes. Causes of hyperglycemia in patients without diabetes include other diseases, pregnancy, critical illness, and certain drugs. Known diseases that may cause hyperglycemia are Cushing syndrome, hyperthyroidism, and pancreatitis. Gestational diabetes may occur in pregnancy. The stress of critical illness, trauma, and/or surgery may increase the incidence of hyperglycemia. Hyperglycemia causes increased morbidity and mortality of these conditions. Several drugs are also known to cause hyperglycemia and include glucocorticoids (e.g., prednisone), thiazide diuretics (e.g., hydrochlorothiazide), phenytoin (Dilantin), sympathomimetics (e.g., epinephrine), and diazoxide (Hyperstat).

Patients with diabetes can suffer from two types of hyperglycemic crises: diabetic ketoacidosis (DKA) or a hyperglycemic hyperosmolar state (HHS), previously referred to as hyperglycemic hyperosmolar nonketotic (HHNK) condition. Insulin deficiency is the cause of DKA, resulting in a hyperglycemic

TABLE 7-7	Mechanism, Site of Action, and Efficacy of Oral Hypoglycemic Agents			
Classification	Mechanism of Action	Site of Action	Reduction FBS	Reduction in HgbA1c
Sulfonylureas • Glyburide (Micronase, DiaBeta, Glynase Prestab) • Glipizide (Glucotrol)	Stimulates insulin release	Pancreas	3.34-3.88	1.0-2.0
Biguanides • Metformin (Glucophage, Glucophage XR, Glumetza, Fortamet, Riomet)	Stimulates hepatic glucose production Increases insulin sensitivity	Liver Peripheral tissues	3.34-3.88	1.0-2.0
Thiazolidinediones • Pioglitazone (Actos)	Stimulates hepatic glucose production Increases insulin sensitivity	Liver Peripheral tissues	1.90-2.20	0.7-1.0
Alpha-glucosidase inhibitors • Acarbose (Precose) • Miglitol (Glycet)	Delays carbohydrate absorption	Small Intestine	1.38-1.66	0.5-1.0
Dipeptidyl peptidase-4 inhibitors (DDP-4 inhibitors) • Sitagliptin (Januvia) • Exenatide (Bydureon, Byetta) • Liraglutide (Victoza)	Enhances endogenous GLP-1	β cells Stomach, liver	0.5-1.0	0.73-1.2
Sodium-glucose cotransporter 2 (SGLT-2) inhibitors • Canagliflozin (Invokana)	Inhibits renal proximal tubular reabsorption Increases glucose excretion	Renal tubules SGLT-2 Receptor	0.6-1.2	0.37-0.72

Adapted from Oral diabetes medication summary chart. *Joslin Diabetes Guidelines.* Retrieved from www.joslin.org/info/oral_diabetes_medications_summary_chart.html.

crisis associated with metabolic acidosis and elevated serum ketones. DKA is the most serious metabolic disturbance of type 1 DM. Relative insulin deficiency causes HHS. This hyperglycemic crisis is associated with the absence of ketone formation, because the presence of some insulin prevents the glyconeogenesis that causes the ketoacidosis associated with the absence of insulin in DKA. HHS is the most serious metabolic disturbance in type 2 DM.

SIDEBAR 7-1
Metabolic Syndrome

Metabolic syndrome is the name for a group of five metabolic risk factors that raises the risk for diabetes and heart disease. The presence of metabolic syndrome is determined in a patient who has at least three of the following metabolic risk factors:
• Abdominal obesity or having an apple shape
• A high triglyceride level or being treated with medication to lower triglycerides
• A low HDL cholesterol level or being treated with medication to raise HDL cholesterol
• High BP or being treated with medication to control high BP
• High fasting blood sugar or being treated to control blood sugar

Diabetic Ketoacidosis

Twenty percent of DKA cases occur with undiagnosed or new onset of type 1 DM. The patient is unaware of the diagnosis until he or she becomes acutely ill. Several conditions can precipitate DKA in patients with known diabetes. The most likely causes of DKA in known type 1 DM patients are illness, infection, omission of exogenous insulin, trauma, surgery, and dietary noncompliance.

Every cell in the human body needs energy in order to function. The body's primary energy source is glucose, a simple sugar resulting from the digestion of foods containing carbohydrates (i.e., sugars and starches). Glucose from the digested food circulates in the blood as a ready energy source for any cells that need it. Insulin is a hormone produced by beta cells in the pancreas. Insulin bonds to a receptor site on the outside of a cell and acts like a key to open a doorway into the cell through which glucose can enter. Some of the glucose converts to a concentrated energy source like glycogen or fatty acids and is saved for later use.

The pathophysiology of DKA (Figure 7-3) begins when there is not enough insulin produced or when the doorway no longer recognizes the insulin key. Glucose stays in the blood rather than entering the cells, resulting in cell starvation and elevated serum glucose. The body will attempt to dilute the high level of glucose in the blood by drawing water out of the cells and into the bloodstream and excrete it in the urine. Symptoms reported by people with undiagnosed diabetes include constant thirst causing them to drink large quantities

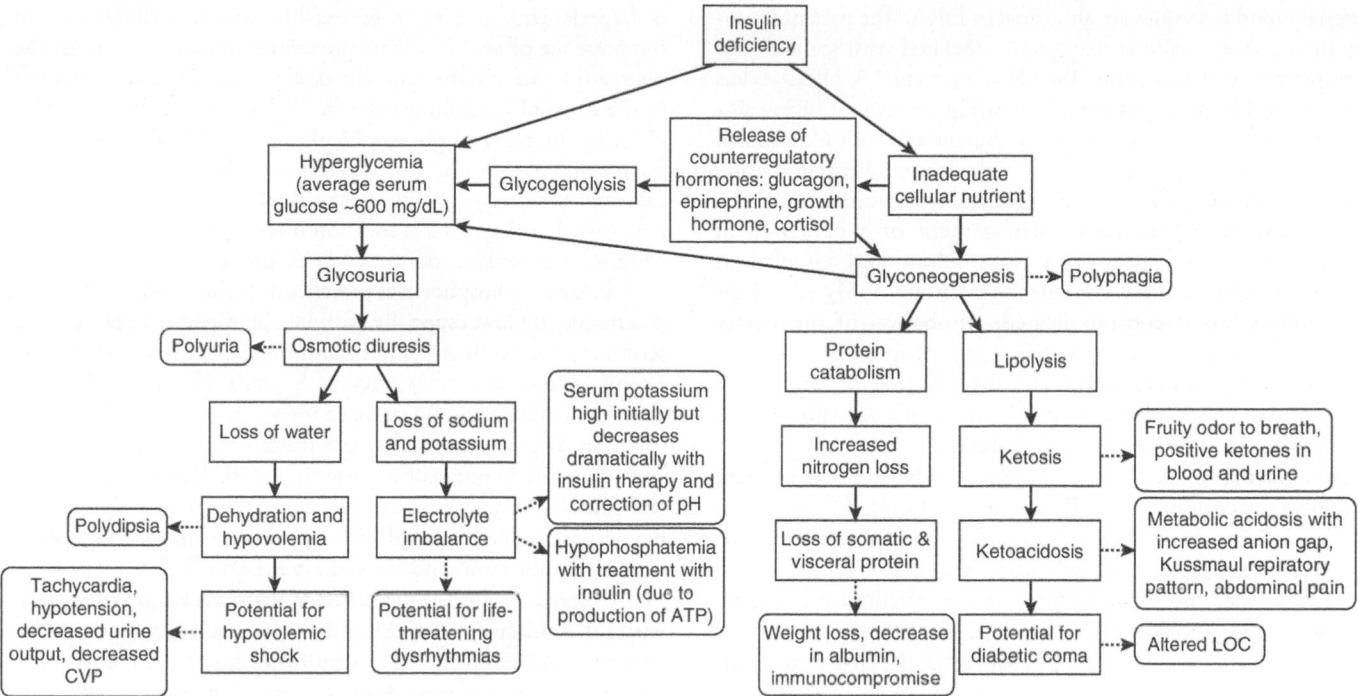

FIGURE 7-3 Pathophysiology of diabetic ketoacidosis (DKA). Dotted lines connect pathology to clinical presentation. *ATP,* Adenosine triphosphate; *CVP,* central venous pressure; *LOC,* level of consciousness. (From Dennison, R. D. [2013]. *Pass CCRN!* [4th ed]. St. Louis, MO: Elsevier.)

of water (i.e., polydipsia) and to have excessive urinary volume and urinary frequency (i.e., polyuria) because their bodies try to get rid of the extra glucose. This creates high levels of glucose in the urine.

At the same time that the body is trying to get rid of glucose from the blood, the cells are starving for glucose and sending signals to the body to eat more food, thus making patients extremely hungry (i.e., polyphagia). To provide energy for the starving cells, the body also tries to convert fats and proteins to glucose. The breakdown of fats and proteins for energy causes acid compounds called ketones to form in the blood. Excretion of ketones occurs in the urine. As ketones build up in the blood, a condition called ketoacidosis can occur; it is life threatening and if left untreated leads to coma and death.

DKA results in a clinical presentation reflecting changes in most body systems. Subjectively, the patient will often complain about GI symptoms. Although polyphagia is present initially, this usually progresses to anorexia, nausea, and abdominal pain as the patient develops metabolic acidosis. The patient complains of increased thirst despite drinking large quantities. Fatigue and weakness, headache, visual disturbances, and weight loss are common. Objective findings are associated primarily with dehydration including flushed, warm, dry skin; poor skin turgor; and sunken eyeballs. The patient may experience either hypothermia or hyperthermia.

Patients with insulin deficiency have significant dehydration caused by the osmotic effect of the hyperglycemia and resultant polyuria. This results in weak and thready pulses, tachycardia, orthostatic hypotension, and a decrease in CVP. The patient's breathing patterns may change. Kussmaul breathing, the classic pattern seen in diabetic ketoacidosis, consists of rapid, deep breathing. In response to metabolic acidosis, Kussmaul breathing is the body's attempt to blow off CO_2 to buffer a fixed acid such as ketones.

In addition, the exhaled breath of a DKA patient may have an acetone (i.e., fruity) odor. Peristalsis is impaired, resulting in vomiting and hypoactive bowel sounds. In the early stages of DKA, polyuria predominates, but this eventually leads to oliguria in the later stages as the patient becomes increasingly dehydrated. Diminished DTRs occur. The patient is likely to be lethargic and can quickly progress to coma and death.

Diagnostic laboratory studies important to assess and monitor in the patient with a diagnosis of DKA are serum electrolytes and serum glucose levels, arterial blood gases, and urinalysis. Serum glucose levels are usually elevated to between 300 and 800 mg/dL with the average DKA level being 600 mg/dL. The serum sodium level may be normal, elevated, or decreased depending on hydration status. The serum potassium levels are elevated initially due to the effect of acidosis; acidosis causes potassium to move out of the cell and into the serum. Once the correction of pH occurs, the potassium moves back into the cell. Serum potassium usually plummets because total body potassium is low due to losses with diuresis. Serum calcium decreases due to osmotic diuresis. The serum phosphorus level is normal initially, but decreases with treatment of insulin and fluids. Magnesium levels are also elevated initially and then decrease. Because of the ketoacids in the blood, calculation of the anion gap results in an elevated level, usually greater than 15. Ketones and glucose are both elevated in the urine. An ECG may show changes associated with potassium levels (e.g., T wave changes) and sinus tachycardia.

The BUN and creatinine are elevated with the BUN:creatinine ratio greater than 10:1. Lipids may also be elevated. Severe dehydration is evident with serum osmolality elevated, usually between 295 and 330 mOsm/kg. The hematocrit is also elevated due to dehydration. The WBC count may be elevated but it is an unreliable indication of infection in DKA. Urine testing indicates the presence of glucose and ketones.

Arterial blood gas values are abnormal in DKA. The patient is usually in metabolic acidosis frequently associated with some degree of respiratory compensation. The pH is less than 7.3, HCO_3 is less than 15, and $Paco_2$ is less than 35 mm Hg. In areas of higher altitude (i.e., Colorado), use the Denver norms as a basis for acidosis. Normal $Paco_2$ tends to be lower at high altitudes because ventilation is stimulated, and local norms must be established.

Initially, the collaborative management of a patient with DKA focuses on oxygenation, ventilation, and circulation. Deliver oxygen by nasal cannula to maintain SpO_2 of at least 95% unless this is contraindicated. Intubation of the airway may be required if the patient's consciousness is impaired. Implement measures to correct the fluid volume deficit. Closely monitor the clinical and laboratory indications of hypovolemia, hypoperfusion, and electrolyte imbalance.

Establish an IV access with at least one large-gauge catheter and administer appropriate IV solution. During the first hour, the rate is 10 to 30 mL/kg. After the first hour, a 500- to 1000-mL/hr rate is appropriate depending on cardiovascular status, volume deficit, and urine output. To correct the total volume deficit requires approximately 4 to 8 L.

Administer normal (i.e., 0.9%) saline for the first 1 to 2 L or until the patient is hemodynamically stable and continue if the serum sodium level returns to normal or if serum osmolality is less than 320 mOsm/kg. If the patient is hypernatremic or serum osmolality is more than 320 mOsm/kg, then administer half-normal (i.e., 0.45%) saline. The hypotensive patient may require colloids such as albumin or plasma protein fraction. Normalize the serum glucose level gradually. Monitor serum glucose every hour initially. Rapid correction of serum glucose is associated with hypoglycemia, hypokalemia, and cerebral edema. The goal of insulin therapy is to decrease serum glucose by 50 to 100 mg/dL each hour. Dextrose 5% is added to intravenous fluid (e.g., D_5NS or $D_5\frac{1}{2}NS$) when serum glucose reaches more than 250 mg/dL. Administer dextrose 10% if serum glucose falls to 150 mg/dL or less.

In DKA, administer IV regular insulin injection as prescribed. The usual dose is 10 to 20 units (i.e., 0.15 units/kg). Follow this injection with the initiation of a continuous IV regular insulin infusion at 0.1 unit/kg/hr or 5 to 10 units/hr. Insulin is mixed in normal saline, and the IV tubing is flushed with 50 mL of insulin solution to saturate binding sites on the IV tubing before administration. Start to decrease the insulin infusion to 3 to 5 units/hr when serum glucose is less than 250 mg/dL. Start subcutaneous insulin 1 to 2 hours before discontinuing the infusion. When serum glucose is less than 250 mg/dL, pH is greater than 7.2, and bicarbonate is greater than 18 mEq/L, administer subcutaneous insulin as prescribed

Another priority in the collaborative management for DKA includes correction of any electrolyte imbalance. Monitor the patient for clinical, laboratory, and ECG indications of hyperkalemia initially and hypokalemia, hypophosphatemia, and hypomagnesemia with correction of pH and hydration with insulin and fluids. The treatment for these electrolyte losses is replacement. Patients with DKA are prescribed potassium replacement; monitor potassium levels every 1 to 2 hours. If the patient is dehydrated and potassium is severely low, replace the potassium intravenously prior to initiating an insulin infusion because starting an insulin drip in a dehydrated patient will cause serum potassium levels to drop quickly. Severe total body potassium depletion occurs in DKA, but serum levels show a normal level

or hyperkalemia due to an intracellular-to-extracellular shift in the presence of acidosis. Start potassium replacement when the potassium level is at the upper level of normal. Replace potassium in the form of potassium chloride (KCl), but a portion may be given in the form of potassium phosphate (KPO_4), depending on phosphorus levels. Refractory hypokalemia suggests hypocalcemia and/or hypomagnesemia. Replace serum magnesium if low, with 1 to 2 g of 10% solution if renal function is adequate. Monitor and replace sodium and calcium as needed.

Administer phosphorus as prescribed for this condition because it is frequently low, especially with insulin therapy. Replace if the serum level is less than 1 mg/dL or if the patient has heart failure, pneumonia, or any other cause of hypoxia. Hypophosphatemia shifts the oxyhemoglobin curve to the left and impairs tissue oxygenation. Replace one-half to two-thirds of potassium with KCl, and one-third to one-half of potassium with KPO_4. Phosphorus and calcium have an inverse relationship. To prevent episodes of hypocalcemia due to phosphorus replacement therapy, phosphate administration should not exceed 1.5 mEq/kg/24 hr.

Metabolic acidosis is the primary acid-base abnormality seen with DKA. Correction of this imbalance requires adequate rehydration and insulin therapy. Administer sodium bicarbonate if the patient is in severe acidosis (i.e., pH 7 or less). Discontinue sodium bicarbonate as soon as pH is 7.2. In addition to the metabolic acidosis caused by accumulation of ketones, monitor the patient for hyperchloremic acidosis caused by NaCl and KCl administration.

Implement general safety precautions to protect patients from harm and ensure patient safety. Prevention of aspiration due to paralytic ileus commonly seen in DKA includes interventions such as keeping the head of the bed elevated 30 degrees. If indicated, insertion of a nasogastric tube may be required to prevent the problem of aspiration. Institute and maintain seizure precautions. There is an increased risk of seizure due to electrolyte imbalances and abnormal serum glucose.

To treat the DKA appropriately, it is important to identify and treat the cause of the condition. The main causes of DKA are new onset of type 1 DM, lack of diabetes control, and infection. To identify the cause of DKA, assess for a source of infection, including early indications of sepsis. Obtain indicated cultures and administer antibiotics as prescribed. Assess the patient's knowledge level related to self-care. Be alert to possible drug therapy errors, noncompliance with diet, and drug interactions.

The condition of DKA can result in major body system complications. The condition may cause comorbid conditions related to the cardiovascular, neurologic, pulmonary, and endocrine systems. Monitor for the cardiovascular complications of hypovolemic shock, dysrhythmias, thromboembolism, myocardial infarction, and pulmonary edema. Neurologic conditions to be alert for include cerebral edema, seizures, and coma. The pulmonary system may be compromised by the occurrence of acute respiratory distress syndrome (ARDS) and pulmonary embolism. Labile conditions and response to treatment can bring on hypoglycemia reactions that need constant vigilance. Injury to the renal system (i.e., diabetic nephropathy) can cause acute renal failure. Monitor urine output and indications of renal involvement (e.g., elevated BUN and creatinine). Careful monitoring of potassium, sodium, phosphorus, and magnesium is also a priority to prevent further complications. In the case of infection, assist in localization of the site of infection, provide prescribed antibiotics and other methods of treatment, and monitor closely for sepsis. Development of sepsis may lead to multisystem organ failure and death.

To prevent the reoccurrence of DKA, provide instruction and counseling regarding lifestyle modification and the need for pharmacologic therapy. Nonpharmacologic therapies include weight management, dietary modifications, tobacco use cessation, alcohol avoidance, moderate aerobic exercise, stress reduction, and immunizations. Patients with diabetes must be able to recognize indications of hyperglycemia and hypoglycemia and know when it is appropriate to call the physician.

Determine the patient's ideal weight and encourage the patient to achieve this ideal weight and self-monitor his or her weight. Dietary modifications include a low-saturated-fat and American Dietetic Association (ADA) diet for control of serum glucose. Stress can elevate blood sugar, so employing strategies to reduce stress are beneficiary. Complementary therapies such as relaxation, imagery, and biofeedback reduce stress.

Diabetes is a chronic disease and therefore warrants a pneumococcal vaccine and an annual flu vaccine to prevent infection. The patient should be knowledgeable of all the pharmacologic agents prescribed to control not only diabetes but also associated hypertension, hyperlipidemia, and thyroid disorders. Patients should comply with the treatment regimen to prevent DKA and diabetes complications. Education and knowledge of insulin therapy including sick-day management is a priority to prevent DKA.

Hyperglycemic Hyperosmolar State

Hyperglycemic hyperosmolar state (HHS) is a hyperglycemic crisis associated with the absence of ketone formation and is the most common severe metabolic disturbance in type 2 DM. HHS is usually seen in patients over 50 years old with glucose intolerance or type 2 DM with some form of concomitant illness that leads to reduced fluid intake. It is less common than DKA and can be a life-threatening emergency. The cause of HHS is noncompliance with diet or drug therapy in a patient with known type 2 DM. In addition, the physical stress of acute illness, trauma, surgery, and infection can potentiate the occurrence of HHS. Several disease processes predispose a patient with type 2 DM to HHS. These disorders include pancreatitis, acute burn injury, hepatitis, Cushing syndrome, and hyperthyroidism. Certain clinical procedures can also precipitate HHS, including peritoneal dialysis, hemodialysis, and the use of hypertonic nutrition therapy (e.g., enteral and total parenteral nutrition). The use of alcohol and several medications can also be a factor in the development of HHS (Box 7-1).

Infection is the most common preceding illness. Once HHS has developed, it may be difficult to differentiate it from the antecedent illness. The concomitant illness may not be identifiable. HHS was previously termed hyperosmolar hyperglycemic nonketotic coma (HHNK); however, because coma is rare in patients with HHS, a change in terminology occurred. HHS is characterized by hyperglycemia, hyperosmolarity, and dehydration without significant ketoacidosis (Figure 7-4).

A patient with HHS complains about weakness and fatigue. In general, objective findings include weight loss; flushed, warm, dry skin; poor skin turgor; polydipsia; and fever. In addition, specific cardiovascular, pulmonary, renal, and neurologic symptoms are evident during HHS. The patient often has

BOX 7-1

Common Drugs That May Precipitate HHS

Beta-blockers (e.g., propranolol)
Calcium channel blockers
Chlorpromazine (Thorazine)
Cimetidine (Tagamet)
Diazoxide (Hyperstat)
Glucocorticoids (e.g., prednisone)
Immunosuppressive drugs
Loop diuretics (e.g., furosemide)
Mannitol (Osmitrol)
Phenytoin (Dilantin)
Sympathomimetic drugs (e.g., epinephrine)
Thiazide diuretics (e.g., hydrochlorothiazide)
Thyroid preparations

tachypnea, tachycardia, orthostatic hypotension, and decreased CVP. Polyuria occurs in the early stage and oliguria in the late stage. Neurologic assessment indicates sensory deficits (i.e., paresthesia) and motor deficits (i.e., paresis, plegia). Other neurologic symptoms seen in HHS are aphasia, decreased DTRs, and seizures. Lethargy can progress quickly to coma and death.

The major diagnostic tests used to identify and monitor treatment response for HHS include serum analysis, arterial blood gases, urinalysis, and an ECG. Serum analysis includes a complete blood count (CBC) and a chemistry panel inclusive of glucose, electrolytes, ketones, BUN, creatinine, and osmolality. The CBC may show an elevated hematocrit and WBC count. The hematocrit may be elevated due to dehydration, while the WBC count would elevate with the presence of infection. Arterial blood gas values determine the extent of metabolic acidosis to differentiate between HHS and DKA. Mild metabolic acidosis may be present in HHS, but significant metabolic acidosis indicates DKA. A urinalysis determines the presence of glucose and ketones. Glucose is present in the urine, but ketones are either not present or minimal. The ECG will show tachycardia and there may be changes associated with hypokalemia (e.g., PVCs, torsades de pointes) (Table 7-8).

The collaborative management priorities for HHS are mostly the same as for DKA, but there are some differences. As with DKA, the main priority is to maintain oxygenation, ventilation, and circulation. IV fluid replacement is vital. In fact, because the HHS total volume deficit is more significant (i.e., usually 8 to 15 L), the appropriate volume required is usually greater. Another difference is that even though HHS causes higher serum glucose levels, the condition requires smaller amounts of insulin to normalize serum glucose. Discontinue the IV insulin infusion when subcutaneous insulin is initiated. There is usually no overlap required in HHS. As with DKA, electrolyte imbalances can be significant. Monitor for clinical, laboratory, and ECG indications of hypokalemia, hypophosphatemia, and hypomagnesemia, especially with insulin therapy. Ensure patient safety due to the same concerns as with DKA.

It is very important to identify and treat the cause of HHS. Assess for the source of infection by obtaining cultures and administering antibiotics as indicated and prescribed. Regularly monitor the serum glucose in patients on enteral and parenteral nutrition, glucocorticoids, dialysis, and diuretics. Treat elevations in glucose due to these factors per a protocol (e.g., sliding scale insulin). Assess the patient's and family's knowledge level related to self-care management and be alert to possible drug therapy errors, noncompliance with diet, and drug interactions. Instruction and reinforcement of teaching and counseling regarding lifestyle modification and the need for pharmacologic therapy is a priority intervention. Lastly, the health care team must monitor for complications associated with HHS (Box 7-2).

7.2   Learning Activity

Complete the clinical presentation findings in each type of hyperglycemic crises associated with DM.

Clinical Presentation	DKA	HHS
Type of diabetes mellitus		
Onset		
Typical serum glucose range		
Presence of ketosis		
pH		
Anion gap		
Respiratory pattern		
Breath odor		
Serum osmolality		
Serum sodium		
Serum potassium		
BUN		
Average fluid deficit		

Answers to this activity can be found in the Answer Key.

7.3   Learning Activity

Identify the following clinical indications as DKA, HHS, or both.

Indicator	DKA	HHS	Both
Serum glucose greater than 300 mg/dL			
Serum glucose greater than 600 mg/dL			
pH less than 7.3			
Positive serum and urine ketones			
Abdominal pain			
Dehydration			
Lethargy → coma			
Kussmaul breathing			

Answers to this activity can be found in the Answer Key.

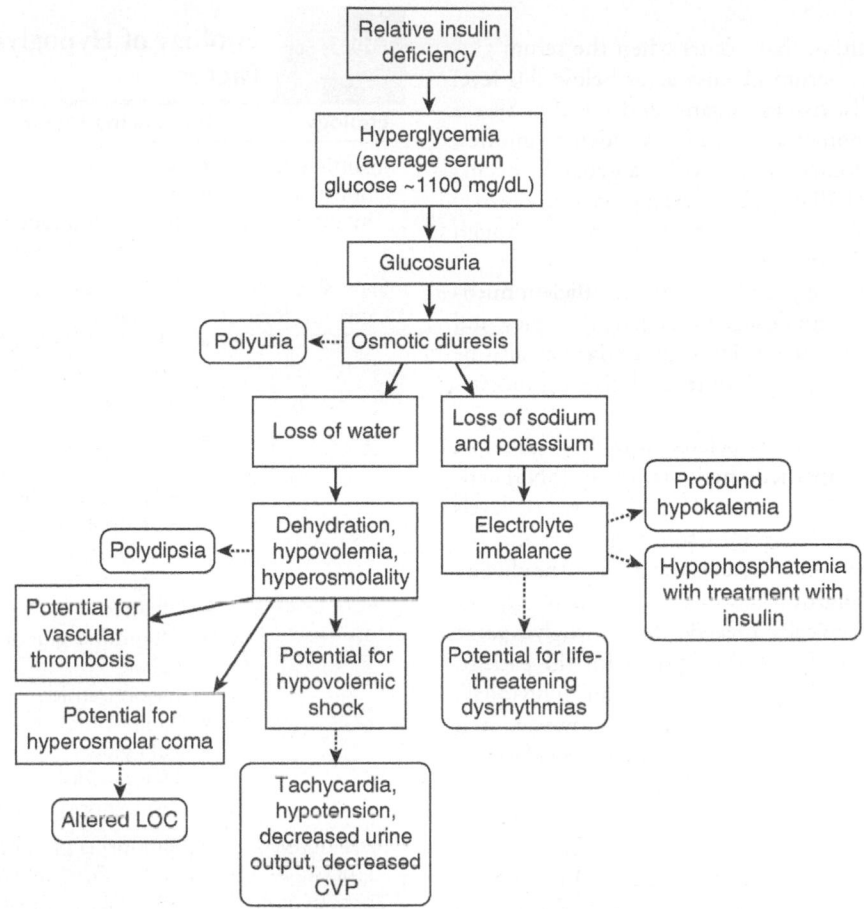

FIGURE 7-4 Pathophysiology of hyperglycemic hyperosmolar state (HHS). Dotted lines connect pathology to clinical presentation. *CVP,* Central venous pressure; *LOC,* level of consciousness. (From Dennison, R. D. [2013]. *Pass CCRN!* [4th ed]. St. Louis, MO: Elsevier.)

TABLE 7-8	Common HHS Diagnostic Values
Diagnostic Test	**Value**
Glucose	600-2000 mg/dL; average 1100 mg/dL
Electrolytes	Sodium: normal or elevated Potassium: decreased Calcium: may be decreased Phosphorus: decreased Magnesium: decreased
Ketones	Normal or only mildly elevated
BUN, creatinine	Elevated
BUN:creatinine ratio	Greater than 10:1
Serum osmolality	Greater than 330 mOsm/kg; may be as high 450 mOsm/kg
Complete blood count	Hematocrit (Hct) elevated WBC count elevated
Urinalysis	Glucose positive Ketones negative or trace
Arterial blood gas (ABG)	Normal pH or only mildly acidotic; if acidosis present, it is lactic acidosis related to hypoperfusion instead of ketoacidosis
Electrocardiogram	Sinus tachycardia Ventricular dysrhythmias related to hypokalemia

BOX 7-2

Complications of HHS

Cardiovascular
- Hypovolemic shock
- Dysrhythmias
- Thromboembolism
- Myocardial infarction
- Pulmonary edema

Neurologic
- Intracranial hypertension
- Cerebral edema
- Cerebral infarction
- Coma

Pulmonary
- ARDS
- Pulmonary embolism

Endocrine
- Hypoglycemia
- Labile hyperglycemia

Renal
- Acute renal failure
- Electrolyte imbalances: potassium, sodium, phosphorus, and magnesium

Sepsis

Multisystem organ failure

Hypoglycemia

Hypoglycemia is a condition that occurs when the serum glucose is below 70 mg/dL. Serum glucose at or below this level can harm the body's cells, tissues, organs, and systems. Severe hypoglycemia has the potential to cause accidents, injuries, coma, and death. Symptomatic hypoglycemia generally occurs at a serum glucose level of 50 mg/dL or less, but symptoms may occur if a sudden decrease in serum glucose occurs even though the level is not less than 50 mg/dL.

Causative factors of hypoglycemia include insufficient nutrient intake, an excessive insulin dose, certain drug therapies, and inadequate production of glucose. Hypoglycemia may also be precipitated by various clinical procedures and disease processes (Table 7-9).

The pathophysiologic events associated with hypoglycemia are primarily related to sympathetic nervous system (SNS) activation and cerebral dysfunction secondary to decreased levels of glucose (Figure 7-5). A decrease in serum glucose and the cerebral dysfunction occurs and activates the SNS as the glucose levels decrease below 40 mg/dL.

The SNS symptoms typically precede the neuroglycopenic symptoms, providing an early warning system for the patient. Previous blood glucose levels can influence an individual's response to a particular level of blood sugar. However, it is important to note that a patient with repeated hypoglycemia can have almost no symptoms (hypoglycemic unawareness). The threshold at which a patient feels the hypoglycemic symptoms decreases with repeated episodes of hypoglycemia.

A patient with activation of the SNS caused by hypoglycemia will complain of palpitations, anxiety, nausea, and weakness. Objective indications of SNS activation caused by hypoglycemia include diaphoresis, pallor, cool skin, tremors, piloerection, tachycardia, and tachypnea. As the serum glucose continues to decrease, the patient may complain of hunger, anxiety, paresthesia, blurred vision and/or diplopia, headache, irritability, difficulty with concentration, and fatigue. The neuroglycopenic indicators of hypoglycemia include a vasomotor change resulting in hypotension, slurred speech, agitation, confusion, and a staggering gait. Sensory changes such as paresthesias, and motor changes such as paresis, hemiplegia, and or paraplegia may occur with hypoglycemia, along with seizures and coma.

Nocturnal hypoglycemia can be extremely dangerous. Nocturnal hypoglycemia is common in patients with type 1 DM and is usually asymptomatic, but the patient may complain of a restless sleep, nightmares, and early morning headache. The problem not only interferes with a patient's sleep but also, due to the sleep state, the patient may be unaware of the problem, allowing it to progress to dangerous levels. Almost 50% of all episodes of severe hypoglycemia occur at night during sleep. Such episodes can cause convulsions and coma and have been implicated as a precipitating factor in cardiac arrhythmias resulting in sudden death. Nocturnal hypoglycemia seems to have no immediate detrimental effect on cognitive function; however, on the following day, mood and well-being may be adversely affected. Recurrent exposure to nocturnal hypoglycemia may impair cognitive function and precipitate the development of acquired hypoglycemia syndromes, such as impaired awareness of hypoglycemia.

The primary diagnostic study for hypoglycemia is serum glucose. A serum glucose of 50 mg/dL or less is diagnostic.

TABLE 7-9 **Etiology of Hypoglycemia-Influencing Factors**

Etiology	Influencing Factors
Insufficient nutrient intake	• Missed or delayed meal • Nausea and vomiting • Interrupted tube feeding • Interrupted parenteral nutrition
Excessive insulin dose	• Poor visual acuity causing dose inaccuracy • Change from pork or beef insulin to human insulin (Humulin) • Injection in area of improved absorption

Drugs	• Sulfonylurea (e.g., glyburide, glipizide, glimepiride) therapy
	  • Renal insufficiency potentiates effects
	  • Hepatic insufficiency delays metabolism and excretion and impairs gluconeogenesis and glycogenolysis
	• Ethanol
	• Quinidine gluconate and quinidine sulfate
	• Disopyramide
	• Alpha-blockers
	• Salicylates
	• Haloperidol
	• Trimethoprim-sulfamethoxazole

Inadequate glucose production	• Strenuous physical exercise or stress with inadequate adjustment of food intake and/or insulin dosage • Excessive alcohol intake ingested without adequate food intake • Glucagon deficiency
Procedures	• Postgastrectomy

Disease processes	• Pancreatic islet cell necrosis: may occur with pentamidine therapy causing an acute increase in insulin release
	• Adrenal insufficiency
	• Severe liver disease
	• Beta-cell tumors (i.e., insulinomas)
	• Non–beta-cell tumors
	  • Malignant: sarcoma, mesothelioma, hepatomas, lymphoma, leukemia, adrenal carcinoma
	  • Benign: carcinoid and carcinoidlike tumors, pheochromocytoma

Pregnancy	• Gestational diabetes • Inadequate calorie consumption (e.g., morning sickness) • Hormonal influence on the way body uses insulin

Glucose levels of 20 to 40 mg/dL are associated with seizures. A serum glucose level of less than 20 mg/dL is associated with coma. An ECG often shows sinus tachycardia. BUN, creatinine, and liver function studies may be elevated. A drug screen for a possible drug cause is indicated in some cases.

The priority in the collaborative management of hypoglycemia is to restore the normal serum glucose level. Measure the serum glucose level immediately when clinical indications of hypoglycemia occur. Administer 15 g (60 calories)

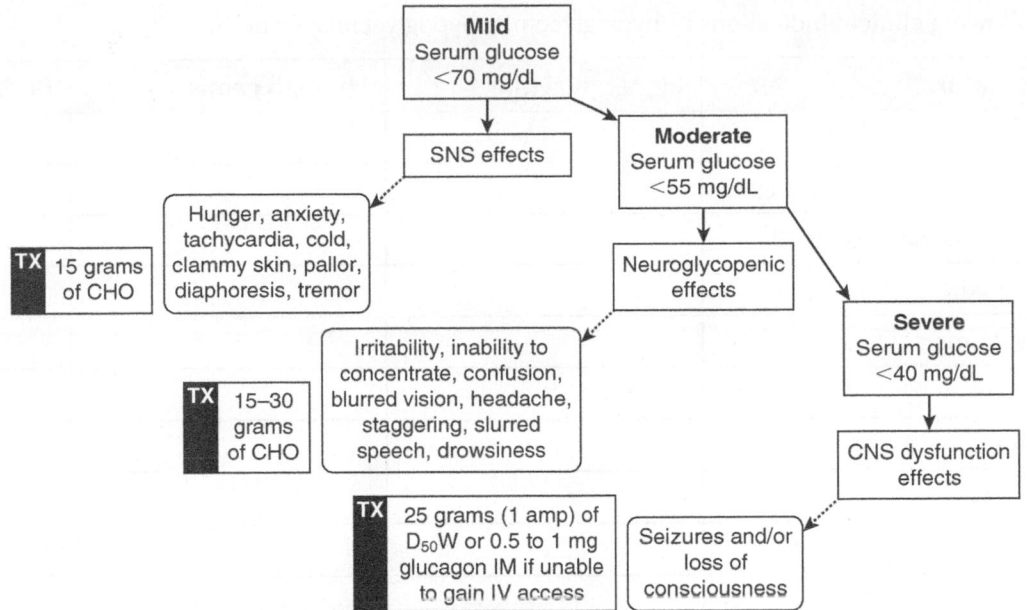

FIGURE 7-5 Pathophysiology of hypoglycemia. Dotted lines connect pathology to clinical presentation. *CHO,* Carbohydrate; *CNS,* central nervous system; *IM,* intramuscular; *IV,* intravenous; *SNS,* sympathetic nervous system; *TX,* treatment. (From Dennison, R. D. [2013]. *Pass CCRN!* [4th ed]. St. Louis, MO: Elsevier.)

BOX 7-3

Foods Providing 15 Grams of Carbohydrates for Treatment of Hypoglycemia

3 (5 g) glucose tablets or gel
6 oz of apple or orange juice
6 oz of nondiet carbonated beverage
8 oz of skim or 1% milk
4 cubes or 2 packets of sugar

---

of carbohydrates for conscious patients (Box 7-3). Glucose tablets or gel is **required** if the patient has been prescribed an alpha-glucosidase inhibitor (e.g., acarbose [Precose], miglitol [Glyset]) because these agents block the conversion of carbohydrates to glucose.

Administer parenteral glucose if the patient is unconscious, usually 50 mL (i.e., 25 g) of $D_{50}W$ injection over 3 to 5 minutes. Give thiamine 100 mg IV as prescribed before dextrose administration, especially in alcoholics, to prevent Wernicke's encephalopathy. Administer $D_{10}W$ or D_5W infusion following the $D_{50}W$ injection as prescribed. Administer glucagon 0.5 to 1 mg IM as prescribed to unconscious patients if IV access cannot be obtained. Provide a longer-acting carbohydrate source (i.e., milk, cheese, or crackers) or the regularly scheduled meal to avoid recurrence. Reassess serum glucose 15 minutes after treatment and every 15 minutes until serum glucose is within normal range. An additional 50 mL of $D_{50}W$ may be required for refractory hypoglycemia.

Prevent patient injury. Maintain the airway if the patient is unconscious. Monitor closely for seizures and maintain seizure precautions.

It is very important to identify and treat the cause of the hypoglycemia. Assess serum glucose by laboratory or by a bedside glucose-monitoring device as indicated. Anticipate times when the patient is most likely to exhibit hypoglycemia. Be aware of peak times for administered insulin therapy. Be aware of missed or late meals or snacks that predispose the patient to hypoglycemia. Be aware of excessive exertion that may predispose the patient to hypoglycemia. Note any drugs that the patient is receiving that may potentiate insulin.

Assess the patient's and family's knowledge level related to self-care. Be alert to possible drug therapy errors, noncompliance with diet, and drug interactions. Be aware and make the patient and family aware that beta-blockers block the SNS (i.e., early) symptoms of hypoglycemia. Test serum glucose frequently in patients on beta-blockers.

Consider Somogyi phenomenon (i.e., insulin-induced posthypoglycemic hyperglycemia) as a cause of early morning hyperglycemia. This is a result of counterregulatory hormone secretion in response to hypoglycemia, which results in early morning hyperglycemia after nighttime hypoglycemia (Figure 7-6). Determine the occurrence of Somogyi phenomenon by taking serum glucose at 3 AM. Treat the syndrome with a decrease in insulin dose and/or a bedtime snack. It is recommended to administer hydrocortisone if adrenal insufficiency is suspected. The Somogyi phenomenon needs to be differentiated from dawn phenomenon, in which hyperglycemia is caused by nocturnal elevations in growth hormone.

Monitor patients who have hypoglycemia for complications. Potential complications include myocardial ischemia or infarction, seizures, coma, and irreversible neurologic damage. Provide patients and their families with instruction and counseling regarding lifestyle modification and the need for pharmacologic therapy. Place an emphasis on the importance of not skipping meals, recognition of symptoms of hyperglycemia and hypoglycemia, and when to call the physician. Patients must be knowledgeable of insulin and/or oral hypoglycemic agents, including sick-day management along with an understanding of the importance to control associated hypertension, hyperlipidemia, and thyroid disorders.

7.4 Learning Activity

Identify the following clinical indications as hyperglycemia, hypoglycemia, or both.

Clinical Indicator	Hyperglycemia	Hypoglycemia	Both
Headache			
Serum glucose greater than 300 mg/dL			
Serum glucose less than 50 mg/dL			
Cold, clammy skin			
Nervousness, tremors			
Polyuria			
Lethargy → coma			
Seizures → coma			
Glycosuria			
Tachycardia			
Agitation, difficulty with concentration			
Weakness, fatigue			
Fruity breath			
Abdominal pain			

Answers to this activity can be found in the Answer Key.

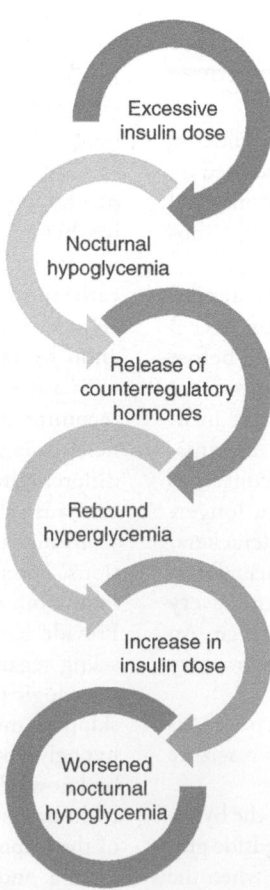

Excessive insulin dose

Nocturnal hypoglycemia

Release of counterregulatory hormones

Rebound hyperglycemia

Increase in insulin dose

Worsened nocturnal hypoglycemia

FIGURE 7-6 Somogyi effect. (From Dennison, R. D. [2013]. *Pass CCRN!* [4th ed]. St. Louis, MO: Elsevier.)

7.5 Learning Activity

Match the following endocrine conditions with appropriate pharmacologic therapy. More than one therapy may be listed for each condition.

_____ 1. DKA
_____ 2. HHS
_____ 3. Hypoglycemia

a. 50% dextrose
b. Parenteral fluids
c. Insulin
d. Potassium

Answers to this activity can be found in the Answer Key.

7.6 Synthesis Learning Activity: Crossword Puzzle

Complete the following crossword puzzle.

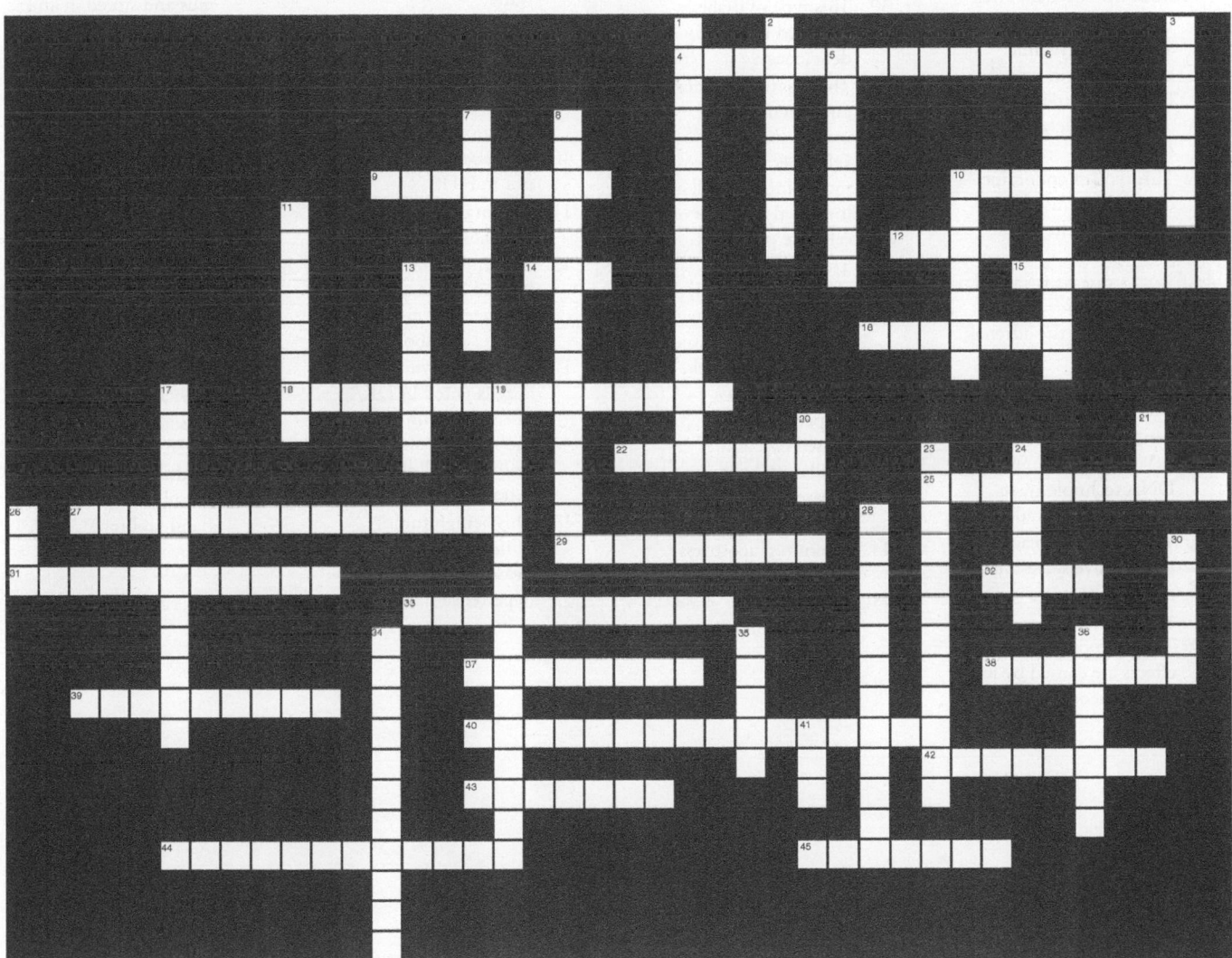

Answers to this activity can be found in the Answer Key.

ACROSS

4. This is most likely the result of insulin deficiency but also may be caused by stress, steroids, or insulin resistance
9. This type of diabetes is caused by insulin deficiency
10. _____ breathing is seen in DKA due to the metabolic acidosis
12. This hormone is produced by the anterior pituitary gland and causes the production and release of hormones from the adrenal cortex (abbrev.)
14. This hyperglycemic crisis occurs in type 2 DM or in patients with glucose intolerance (abbrev.)
15. This type of endocrine disorder is caused by a problem in the target gland
16. _____ disease is caused by a deficiency of hormones from the adrenal gland
18. Another term for the anterior pituitary
22. Insulin manufactured using recombinant DNA technology, so nonantigenic (trade)
25. This disorder is caused by excessive secretion of growth hormone in an adult
27. These hypoglycemic effects are caused by low brain glucose

29. This type of endocrine disorder is caused by a problem with the pituitary gland
31. This electrolyte imbalance is noted in DKA as the acidosis is corrected and in HHS
32. These cells produce insulin
33. This is another name for ADH
37. This hormone is considered a stress hormone and is produced by the adrenal cortex
38. This hormone enables glucose to move into the cell
39. This type of diabetes is caused by ADH deficiency
40. This electrolyte imbalance occurs with insulin therapy in DKA because glucose moves into the cell and increased amounts of ATP are produced
42. This is given with glucose for hypoglycemia in patients with substance abuse issues to prevent Wernicke encephalopathy
43. Hyperglycemia caused by counter regulatory hormones released in response to hypoglycemia
44. A serum glucose less than normal
45. This endocrine gland is located on top of the kidney

DOWN

1. A complication in HHS caused by severe dehydration
2. This type of regulation controls the release or retention of hormones
3. This area of the adrenal gland produces epinephrine and norepinephrine
5. This hormone triggers glycogenolysis and gluconeogenesis
6. This hormone is secreted by the adrenal cortex and causes the retention of sodium and water
7. The change in urine output that occurs in DKA and HHS
8. Another term for the posterior pituitary
10. This occurs in DKA but not in HHS
11. This organ produces glucagon and insulin
13. This endocrine gland is located in the neck and produces hormones that control metabolic rate
17. This electrolyte imbalance is noted in DKA due to acidosis causing the shift of potassium from intracellular to extracellular
19. This benign tumor of the adrenal medulla causes labile hypertension

20. The initial symptoms of hypoglycemia are caused by stimulation of the ___ (abbrev.)
21. This hyperglycemic crisis occurs in type 1 DM (abbrev.)
23. The treatment for hypoglycemia in a conscious patient is 15 g of ____
24. The hormones from this area of the adrenal gland can be remembered as sugar (i.e., cortisol), salt (i.e., aldosterone), and sex (i.e., androgen)
26. This hormone is produced by the hypothalamus and stored in and released by the posterior pituitary (abbrev.)
28. In HHS the serum becomes _____
30. DKA causes an increase in this "gap"
34. This type of drug blocks the early symptoms of hypoglycemia
35. These cells produce glucagon
36. _____ syndrome is caused by an excess of hormones from the adrenal cortex
41. This hormone is produced by the anterior pituitary gland and stimulates the thyroid gland (abbrev.)

The Hematologic and Immunologic Systems

ANATOMY AND PHYSIOLOGY

The anatomic structures involved in the hematologic system include the bone marrow and the liver. The bone marrow is the spongy center of the bones where the hematologic and immunologic cells develop and mature before released into the circulation. Though the bone marrow is present throughout the bones of the body, the majority of the hematologic and immunologic cells are produced in the vertebrae, ribs, sternum, pelvis, and proximal epiphyses of the femur and humerus. The liver synthesizes various plasma proteins, including clotting factors and albumin. In addition, the liver has a role in clearing damaged and nonfunctioning red blood cells (RBCs) from the circulation. The liver receives 27% of cardiac output with approximately 1350 mL of blood flowing through the liver via the hepatic artery and portal vein every minute.

The hematologic system provides the medium for transportation of oxygen, carbon dioxide, and nutrients to the tissues. The system is involved in maintaining homeostasis and the internal environment, including participation in regulation of temperature and acid-base balance.

The components of the immunologic system include the bone marrow, thymus, spleen, liver, lymph tissue, and blood plasma cells. The immunologic system protects the body's internal environment against invading organisms and against the development, growth, and dissemination of abnormal cells. The system maintains homeostasis by removing damaged cells from the circulation.

Components

Bone Marrow

Adults have 30 to 50 mL of bone marrow per kilogram of body weight. The bone marrow produces erythrocytes (red blood cells) and leukocytes (white blood cells), including granulocytes (neutrophils, eosinophils, basophils), agranulocytes (monocytes), lymphocytes, and thrombocytes (platelets). The bone marrow recognizes and removes senescent cells and has a role in the participation of cellular and humoral immunity.

Thymus

The thymus is a lymphoid organ located in the mediastinum below the thyroid. During fetal development and throughout the toddler years, the thymus grows rapidly and is the place that lymphocytes from the bone marrow mature into T cells. Unlike most organs that grow until the age of maturity, the thymus enlarges throughout childhood but slowly shrinks from the onset of puberty and throughout adulthood. As the thymus shrinks, adipose tissue replaces the thymus tissue. The immune system produces most of its T cells during childhood and acquires very few new T cells after puberty. The thymus also secretes a hormone, thymosin, which is thought to stimulate immune function.

Spleen

The spleen is a lymphoid organ located in the upper left quadrant of the abdomen. The spleen clears damaged or nonfunctioning RBCs and filters antigens from the blood for evaluation by the lymphocytes. The white pulp of the spleen primarily supports humoral immunity and performs the following functions:

- Produces lymphocytes
- Stimulates B cell activity to produce immunoglobulins; therefore, patients who have had a splenectomy have a greatly increased risk of sepsis with encapsulated microorganisms
- Stores splenic reticuloendothelial tissue and immunoglobulins

The red pulp of the spleen contains reticuloendothelial tissue that stores and releases RBCs into the circulation. Contraction of smooth muscle in the capsule surrounding the spleen and in the invaginations of the capsule, called the *trabeculae*, cause the release of RBCs. When stimulated by the sympathetic nervous system (SNS), as much as 100 mL of concentrated RBCs releases into the circulation, raising the hematocrit by 1% to 2%. The red pulp is also responsible for the culling of damaged or old erythrocytes by phagocytosis. The bone marrow reuses the iron when the spleen destroys the RBCs and releases hemoglobin. The spleen's red pulp is also responsible for filtering and trapping foreign material, including bacteria and viruses, and the storage and release of platelets along with the destruction of damaged or senescent platelets.

Liver

The liver is responsible for the filtering of blood as it comes from the gastrointestinal (GI) tract. The Kupffer cells lining the sinusoidal beds of the liver remove foreign material, including microorganisms, damaged or old RBCs, and other degradation products. The destruction of RBCs produces bilirubin, which the liver converts to bile; bile is necessary for fat digestion. Additional functions of the liver include the elimination of immune complexes (e.g., antigen-antibody complexes) from the blood, detoxification of toxic substances that enter the blood, manufacture of some clotting factors (i.e., vitamin K-dependent factors II, VII, IX, X) along with antithrombin, and the storage of blood (e.g., in heart failure the liver becomes engorged with blood).

Lymphatic System

Lymph is a pale yellow fluid that contains lymphocytes, granulocytes, enzymes, and antibodies. Lymph is deficient in platelets and fibrinogen, so it coagulates very slowly. The function of lymph is to facilitate the return of proteins and fat from the GI tract, excess interstitial fluid, and certain hormones to the blood. Filtered and returned to the circulatory system, lymph fluid maintains normal pressures and prevents edema. The lymph system is a separate vessel system that collects plasma and leukocytes. Lymph circulation is composed of lymphatic capillaries that are somewhat larger than blood capillaries and are irregular in diameter. Lymphatic vessels are formed by lymphatic capillaries and the lymph ducts drain into subclavian veins. The right lymphatic duct collects lymph from the right side of the head, neck, and thorax and from the right arm, right lung, right side of the heart, and right upper surface of the diaphragm. The thoracic duct collects lymph from all other parts of the body.

Lymph nodes are small, spongy, bean-shaped organs located along lymph vessels. Lymph nodes are multichanneled and line the inside of the lymph vessel. They are the sites of B cell and T cell lymphocyte production and maturation before distribution. The function of the lymph nodes is to filter and allow white blood cells (WBCs) to consume the bacteria and foreign materials carried by the lymph. Granulocytes, macrophages, and lymphocytes pass through the lymph node to return to the blood. Enlargement of lymph nodes occurs with inflammation, infection, or malignancy. Enlargement of superficial nodes can be palpated, but enlarged deep nodes can only be visualized on x-ray or computed tomography (CT).

Additional lymphoid tissue synthesizes the immunoglobulins. There are five major types of immunoglobulins: IgM, IgG, IgA, IgE, and IgD. Mucosa-associated lymphoid tissues (MALTs) are clusters of T-lymphocytes and B-lymphocytes, macrophages, and phagocytes dispersed in the mucosal linings of the respiratory, GI, and genitourinary tracts. Gut-associated lymphoid tissues (GALTs), called Peyer's patches, are in the intestinal tract.

Glial cells are located in the white matter of the brain. These cells are rich in lymphocyte tissue and destroy foreign matter that crosses the blood-brain barrier.

Blood Plasma

Blood plasma makes up 55% of total blood volume. The plasma is composed of serum and plasma proteins, including prealbumin, albumin, serum globulins, fibrinogen, prothrombin, and plasminogen. The hematocrit (Hct) expresses the percentage of red blood cells in the total blood volume. The fluid component of the blood affects the Hct. Increased Hct may indicate polycythemia or hemoconcentration and decreased Hct may indicate anemia or hemodilution.

Pluripotent Stem Cells

All blood cells originate from self-renewing pluripotent stem cells that differentiate into myeloid and lymphoid lineage cells. The erythroid stem cells (i.e., pronormoblasts) develop into reticulocytes and finally into erythrocytes. The myeloid stem cells (i.e., myeloblasts or monoblasts) develop into granulocytes and monocytes. The lymphoid stem cells (i.e., lymphoblasts) develop into B-lymphocytes and T-lymphocytes. The thrombocytic stem cells (i.e., megakaryoblasts) develop into thrombocytes.

Red Blood Cells

Erythrocytes, also referred to as red blood cells or RBCs, are nonnucleated, round biconcave disk-shaped cells with a tough, flexible membrane. The inner part of RBCs (referred to as *stoma*) is the location of hemoglobin attachment. The cell membrane contains the genetic antigens that determine ABO and Rh blood type. RBCs are highly permeable to hydrogen, chloride, and bicarbonate ions and water. RBCs perform the following functions:

- Transport oxygen from lungs to tissues
- Participate in maintenance of the acid-base balance
- Provide insulation and weight to the blood

Reticulocytes are immature RBCs and evaluation of reticulocyte count in the blood is useful in assessing erythrocyte production. An elevated reticulocyte count (i.e., greater than 25% of total RBC count) means that production of new RBCs is greater than normal. These reticulocytes will mature in 1 to 4 days after release and function like normal RBCs but may have a shortened life span. The release of reticulocytes occurs after sudden blood loss, such as hemorrhage. Repeated challenges to this compensatory mechanism lead to exhaustion of reticulocyte reserves. The mature erythrocytes' (RBCs) life span is approximately 120 days. The spleen acts as an RBC reservoir and contains 1% to 2% of circulating RBCs.

The relationship of the cellular oxygen requirement and general metabolic activity determines erythropoiesis regulation. Increased muscle mass and androgen hormones increase RBC production. Decreased estrogen hormone levels decrease RBC production. The hormone erythropoietin stimulates the bone marrow to make more RBCs. The kidney secretes erythropoietin in response to hypoxemia.

RBC and hemoglobin (Hgb) production have nutritional requirements. The required nutrients to produce RBCs and Hgb include adequate iron and iron precursors such as ferritin, vitamin B_{12}, folic acid, and the essential elements of zinc, selenium, and copper. The RBC process begins with a stem cell that forms the erythroblast. Hemoglobin synthesis takes place in bone marrow. Hemoglobin consists of four globin chains and four heme groups per hemoglobin molecule. The heme portion of hemoglobin molecules contains iron. More than two-thirds of the body's iron is contained in hemoglobin and myoglobin.

Oxygen binds to the heme protein within the erythrocyte. The binding affinity of oxygen to hemoglobin is dependent on acid-base balance, temperature, and levels of 2,3-DPG. Alkalosis, hypothermia, and decreased levels of 2,3-DPG cause the oxyhemoglobin dissociation curve to shift to the left, increasing the affinity between oxygen and hemoglobin. This facilitates the pickup of oxygen at the lung but impairs drop-off of oxygen at the tissues. Acidosis, hyperthermia, and increased levels of 2,3-DPG cause the oxyhemoglobin dissociation curve to shift to the right, decreasing the affinity between oxygen and hemoglobin. This impairs the pickup of oxygen at the lung but facilitates drop-off of oxygen at the tissues.

Destruction (hemolysis) of old and immature RBCs occurs in the liver and spleen. Destruction of immature RBCs occurs primarily because they are misshapen or damaged. The spleen, liver, or bone marrow removes old and damaged RBCs from the circulation because of the following reasons:

- RBC membrane abnormalities
- Hemoglobin abnormalities
- Abnormal metabolic functions
- Physical trauma to the RBC
- Antibodies
- Infectious agents and toxins

Hemoglobin (Hgb) and iron are returned to the bone marrow. Hgb and iron are reused after the destruction of the RBCs. Heme is bound to haptoglobin for recirculation and iron is bound to transferrin for recirculation. Erythrocyte destruction increases bilirubin production. The bilirubin is transported to the liver attached to albumin.

Indirect bilirubin is unconjugated, which means the liver has not converted it to a water-soluble substance. Indirect bilirubin can become elevated in hemolytic states that overwhelm the liver's ability to conjugate or when the liver is unable to conjugate adequately as occurs in liver disease. Direct bilirubin is conjugated after the liver converted it to a water-soluble substance and is excreted into the bile. Direct bilirubin becomes elevated in biliary obstruction. The excretion of bilirubin occurs via the GI tract or as urobilinogen in the urine.

Leukocytes

Leukocytes are white blood cells (WBCs) that are involved with phagocytic and immunologic processes. Cytokines are proteins synthesized by the various leukocytes that act as chemical mediators of immunity and inflammation; they are important in regulation of normal immune and inflammatory responses. Cytokines are causative factors in systemic inflammatory response syndrome (SIRS) and multisystem organ failure. There are several types of cytokines. Mononuclear phagocytes synthesize monokines; lymphocytes synthesize lymphokines. Macrophages secrete nonspecific cytokines such as tumor necrosis factor (TNF), interleukins, and interferons.

Granulocytes are active phagocytes. Neutrophils (also known as *polymorphonuclear leukocytes [PMNs]*) are the largest component of granulocytes and the circulating WBC mass (40% to 80% of WBCs). The neutrophils leave the blood vessel, migrate through the tissues, and search for microorganisms or damaged body cells to engulf, kill, and digest through the process of phagocytosis. Neutrophils are attracted to inflammation and bacterial microorganisms, and are the most actively phagocytic of granulocytes. After phagocytosis, the neutrophil dies and pus is the end-product of neutrophil death. Neutrophils exhibit a burst of oxygen consumption during phagocytosis known as a *respiratory burst*. This burst produces superoxide, hydrogen peroxide, and hydroxyl radicals. These oxygen-derived radicals normally function in destruction of microorganisms but may be injurious to normal body tissue.

Neutrophils contain cytoplasmic granules, which include lysosomal enzymes that aid in killing microorganisms. Neutrophils after maturation have a half-life of 4 to 10 hours. Bands are phagocytic immature neutrophils and in acute bacterial infections, an increase in bands, called a *shift to the left*, occurs. Phagocytic-segmented neutrophils (i.e., *segs*) are mature neutrophils. An increase in mature segmented neutrophils is seen in inflammation, liver disease, and pernicious anemia. The increase in segs is referred to as a *shift to the right*. Microorganisms or antigen-antibody reactions stimulate the recruitment of neutrophils and the movement into the tissues. When the body needs more neutrophils for phagocytosis, the bone marrow speeds maturation and release. The GI tract, pulmonary or oral secretions, and urinary excretion remove neutrophils from the blood.

Eosinophils make up 0% to 5% of WBC mass. Eosinophils have some phagocytic activity, but their main function is to ingest immune complexes (i.e., antigen-antibody complexes) and inactive mediators of the allergic response. Eosinophils are most important during parasitic infections and allergic reactions. They are especially vital in helminth infections because these parasitic worms are too large to be phagocytized and eosinophils secrete chemicals that destroy the surface of the helminth. Eosinophils are also elevated in pulmonary and dermatologic inflammation and infection. After maturation, the half-life of eosinophils is approximately 30 minutes in circulation and 12 days in the tissues. Tissue eosinophils are present in large numbers on mucosal surfaces of the respiratory and GI systems and the skin because these locations are common entry points for foreign material.

Basophils make up 0% to 2% of WBC mass. Like mast cells, basophils degranulate during acute local or systemic allergic reactions and release heparin and histamine. Mast cells stay in the tissue, and basophils stay in the circulatory system. If a basophil leaves the circulatory system to stay in the tissue, it becomes a mast cell. Basophils do not participate in phagocytic activity. The life span of basophils after maturation is unknown.

Agranulocytes include mononuclear phagocytes called monocytes. Monocytes make up 3% to 8% of WBC mass and differentiate into macrophages as they migrate into the tissues. The half-life after maturation of circulating monocytes is 8 to 10 hours. The WBC count does not include macrophages because they are located in the tissues. Macrophages have greater phagocytic ability than neutrophils or monocytes. Macrophages are especially involved in the removal of damaged or senescent cells, cellular debris, and mutant or cancer cells. They produce the cytokine interleukin-1 (IL-1), which increases proliferation of T cells, stimulates the growth and development of B-lymphocytes, causes fever, and stimulates the release of prostaglandin. They also produce interleukin-6, interleukin-8, TNF, and the cytokine alpha interferon, which is important in the body's defense against viruses and tumors. Macrophages can be fixed or mobile. Fixed (or tissue) macrophages stay in one organ and phagocytize live and dead debris in the following tissues:

- Lung (alveolar macrophages)
- Brain (microglia)
- Liver (Kupffer cells)
- Bone (osteoclast)
- Peritoneum (peritoneal macrophages)
- Kidney (mesangial cells)
- Spleen (splenic mononuclear cells)

Mobile macrophages are located primarily at the sites of inflammation and in peritoneal, pleural, and synovial spaces. They migrate through the circulatory system as monocytes and have a life span of months or years.

Lymphocytes. Lymphocytes make up 10% to 40% of WBC mass and are also called T cells or B cells. The T cells comprise approximately 70% to 80% of lymphocytes. T cells develop in the bone marrow and then mature and differentiate in the thymus and the lymph nodes. The T cell is involved with cellular immunity. B cells comprise approximately 10% to 20% of lymphocytes. The B cells develop and mature in the bone marrow (i.e., bursa) and migrate to lymph nodes and lymphoid tissue for differentiation and antibody production or plasma cell differentiation. B cells are involved with the production of immunoglobulins and humoral immunity.

Helper T cells (also referred to as *CD4 T lymphocytes, T4 lymphocytes,* or T_H) detect foreign cells and produce lymphokines to stimulate the production or activation of other cells to fight infection.

Lymphokines are soluble proteins that function as chemical communicators to transmit instructions to macrophages, lymphocytes, and tissue cells. Cytotoxic T cells (also referred to as *killer cells* or T_c) emit chemicals that dissolve the foreign cell's membrane to kill the cell before the invader can use it as a base for multiplication. Suppressor T cells (also referred to as *CD8 T lymphocytes, T8 lymphocytes,* or T_S) modulate the overall immune system by signaling B cells and T cells to slow down or stop their activity. Memory T cells circulate in blood and lymph after the initial infection to allow ready response to subsequent invasion by the same organism. Helper T cells typically carry the CD4 surface molecule. Suppressor and cytotoxic T cells typically carry the CD8 surface molecule. Normally, there are twice as many CD4 cells as CD8 cells.

Once activated, B cells become plasma cells that recognize specific foreign material and develop specific immunoglobulins to that antigen. Memory B cells circulate in blood and lymph after the initial infection to allow ready response to subsequent invasion by the same organism.

Natural killer (NK) cells (also referred to as *null cells*) comprise approximately 10% of lymphocytes. The NK cells are large granular cytotoxic lymphocytes that are neither T cells nor B cells (no surface marker exists on these lymphocytes). NK cells kill nonspecifically and do not need prior exposure for activation. They are involved in surveillance against tumors, some parasites, and viruses.

Thrombocytes

Thrombocytes, also called platelets, are nonnucleated cell fragments of megakaryocytes produced in the bone marrow. Platelets activate the blood clotting system when injury occurs. Platelets travel to the damaged vessel or tissue and clump together to form a platelet plug. Released cytokines recruit more platelets and clotting factors to the site. The platelet's life span is approximately 8 to 10 days; they are very fragile and susceptible to injury.

Clotting Factors

Clotting factors are proteins and other substances, numbered I to XIII. Clotting factors are responsible to form a fibrin matrix at a site of injury. To achieve and maintain hemostasis, the clotting factors respond to injury in a sequential cascade-type process through the interaction of three pathways known as the intrinsic, extrinsic, and common pathways. Calcium, coenzymes, or phospholipids are required to proceed through the enzymatic reactions of each step in the cascade.

INFLAMMATION

Inflammation is a sequential physiologic response the body makes to injuries, immunologic processes, or foreign substances in the body. The inflammation process may be acute or chronic and occurs at sites of tissue damage irrespective of the etiology. Inflammation may occur locally or can become systemic, known as systemic inflammatory response syndrome (SIRS).

The inflammatory process has three stages. Stage I is called the vascular stage. In this stage, there is an immediate but temporary vasoconstriction caused by trauma to vascular smooth muscle. Warmth, redness, swelling, pain, and loss of function are the five classic indications of inflammation. Injured tissues and cells secrete chemical mediators (Table 8-1) with the predominant effects of vasodilation and

TABLE 8-1	Chemical Mediators of the Inflammatory Process
Chemical Mediator	**Actions**
Bradykinin	• Causes vasodilation • Increases capillary permeability • Enhances chemotaxis • Causes pain • Converts plasminogen to plasmin • Produces smooth muscle contraction (e.g., bronchospasm)
Collagenase	• Degrades clots
Complement cascade	• Triggers neutrophil aggregation • Increases capillary permeability • Activates mast cells and basophils
Elastase	• Degrades clots
Endorphin	• Causes vasodilation • Produces analgesia
Fibrinolysin	• Digests fibrin
Histamine	• Causes vasodilation • Increases capillary permeability • Increases heart rate and contractility • Produces bronchospasm • Increases secretion of mucus and gastric acid • Inhibits T cells
Interleukin-1 (IL-1)	• Stimulates protein catabolism • Causes fever • Activates lymphocytes • Stimulates fibroblasts
Interleukin-2 (IL-2)	• Activates B lymphocytes to make antibodies • Activates macrophages
Leukotriene	• Causes vasoconstriction • Increases capillary permeability • Produces smooth muscle contraction (e.g., bronchospasm)
Lipase	• Degrades fat
Plasminogen	• Degrades clots when activated to plasmin
Prostacyclin	• Causes vasodilation • Inhibits platelet aggregation • Increases capillary permeability
Prostaglandin (PGD_2, PGF_{2a})	• Vasoconstriction • Bronchoconstriction
Prostaglandin (PGE_2, PGI_2)	• Causes vasodilation • Produces smooth muscle relaxation (e.g., bronchodilation) • Promotes platelet aggregation • Increases capillary permeability • Activates lysosomal enzymes • Potentiates leukotrienes • Causes pain
Serotonin	• Causes vasodilation • Increases capillary permeability • Causes pulmonary vasoconstriction • Produces smooth muscle contraction (e.g., bronchospasm)

TABLE 8-1	Chemical Mediators of the Inflammatory Process—cont'd	
Chemical Mediator	**Actions**	
Thromboxane	• Causes vasoconstriction and endothelial damage • Causes pulmonary vasoconstriction • Acts as a potent platelet aggregator	
Tumor necrosis factor (TNF)	• Causes necrosis of bacteria or tissue • Stimulates muscle catabolism • Induces fever	

an increase in capillary permeability, causing warmth, redness, and swelling.

During the inflammatory process, enhanced healing occurs due to an increased mobilization of nutrients to the area. A decrease in the actual tissue injury occurs from dilution of the toxins or microorganisms that enter the area. Tissue stretching and release of histamine and prostaglandin cause the pain associated with inflammation. Tissue swelling and pain cause the loss of function that accompanies inflammation. The major leukocyte in stage I of inflammation is the tissue macrophage. The response is immediate because the tissue macrophage is already in the tissue. The macrophage secretes granulocyte colony-stimulating factor (G-CSF) to stimulate the bone marrow to speed up the maturation and release of leukocytes. Cytokines secreted by the macrophage attract neutrophils to the area of injury or invasion.

In stage II, called the cellular stage, the neutrophil attacks and destroys foreign material and removes necrotic tissue. In addition, thromboxane (a procoagulant) and prostacyclins (anticoagulants) act to wall off the site of injury. Repair and/or replacement of damaged tissue occur in stage III of the inflammatory process, but it is important to remember that this stage begins at the time of injury. Repair is the replacement of lost cells with connective tissue cells to form scar tissue. Regeneration is the replacement of lost cells with the same type of cells. Some loss of function occurs with the degree of loss. This loss of function is dependent on the percentage of previously functional tissue replaced by scar tissue.

8.1 Learning Activity

If a patient has a localized inflammation, what are the five major clinical indications that you would expect?

a. _____

b. _____

c. _____

d. _____

e. _____

Answers to this activity can be found in the Answer Key.

IMMUNITY

Immunity is defined as the protection of the body against pathogenic organisms or other foreign material. Immunity is dependent on the ability to recognize self from nonself. Self is determined genetically and includes anything synthesized by a person's own particular DNA code. Nonself describes anything that is different in its chromosome structure and evokes a response from the immune system. Antigens are chemical substances, which are usually protein and viewed by the body as foreign (i.e., nonself). Nonself proteins may be normally pathogenic and warrant an immunologic response (e.g., foreign microbes). Nonself antigens/proteins are not pathogenic but precipitate an immunologic response, known as a hypersensitivity reaction. Allergens such as animal dander and plant pollens trigger this type of reaction. When the body perceives an existing body cell as foreign due to surface markers or cellular changes and mounts a response against it, the response is called an autoimmune reaction.

The body's immunity has three lines of defense. The first line of defense is innate immunity involving the skin and mucous membranes, acid secretions and enzymes, and natural immunoglobulins. The second line of defense is the team of macrophages and neutrophils. The third line of defense is composed of the cellular and humoral immunity.

Innate immunity is the body's inherent immune mechanisms, is present at birth, and does not require prior exposure to antigen for activation. Anatomically, the skin and mucous membranes provide a barrier. Chemical secretions also aid in protection. Acid secretions in the stomach, vagina, and mouth; digestive enzymes in the GI tract; tears and perspiration; lysosomes; and natural immunoglobulins, cytokines, and pyrogen produced by granulocytes to cause an increase in body temperature all play a part in the body's defenses.

Cellular defense includes the normal bacterial flora in the GI tract, vagina, and respiratory tract. Tissue macrophages, leukocytes, and mobile macrophages along with the inflammatory process are part of the second line of defense. In this line of defense, the body recognizes foreign or nonself substances and attacks, but cannot tell what the agent is. There is no memory or prior exposure recognized.

Acquired immunity develops when the body produces antibodies. In response to exposure to foreign material (i.e., antigens), the body creates the antibodies and forms T memory cells and B memory cells. Passive acquired immunity is produced by the injection of antibodies or sensitized lymphocytes. Natural exposure to an antigen (e.g., exposure to a microorganism) or administration of live attenuated vaccines (e.g., influenza "FluMist") that trigger a direct response from the body produces active acquired immunity.

Cell-mediated immunity is particularly effective against viruses, parasites, some fungi, and bacteria harbored inside of cells. Cell-mediated immunity is responsible for delayed hypersensitivity, transplant rejection, and malignancy surveillance and possibly destruction. T cells that are induced and regulated primarily through the production and activity of cytokines mediate cell-mediated immunity.

In the cell-mediated immunity process, the macrophage is the first cell to detect most antigens. The macrophage processes the antigen and "presents" it to both T cells and B cells. The T cells recognize the antigen as foreign when it is on the

TABLE 8-2 Immunoglobulins (Igs)

Ig	Actions	Comments	Examples of Related Conditions
IgG	• Coats microorganisms (primarily bacteria and viruses) to enhance phagocytosis • Activates complement system	• Most abundant immunoglobulin (75%-80% of total) • Present in intravascular and extravascular spaces • Crosses the placental barrier and provides natural immunity	• IgG low levels: Nephrotic syndrome, leukemia • IgG high levels: Chronic infection, AIDS, multiple myeloma, hepatitis
IgA	• Protects epithelial surfaces against antigen adhesion and invasion • Protects against entry via the respiratory tract, GU tract, and GI tract • Activates the complement system	• Present in many body secretions (e.g., saliva, tears, sweat, mucus, breast milk) • 10%-15% of total	• IgA low levels: Leukemia, high-risk blood transfusion reactions, intestinal enteropathy • IgA high levels: Multiple myeloma, autoimmune disease, SLE, hepatitis
IgM	• Kills bacteria in the bloodstream • Activates complement system	• First responder to bacterial or viral invasion • Present mostly in intravascular space • 5%-10% of total immunoglobulins	• IgM low levels: Multiple myeloma, inherited immune disorder, leukemia • IgM high levels: Viral hepatitis, mononucleosis, rheumatoid arthritis, kidney damage
IgD	• Not well understood • May activate B cells	• 1% of total immunoglobulins	• IgD low levels: Unknown • IgD high levels: Multiple myeloma
IgE	• Attaches to mast cells and basophils and causes them to release their contents (e.g., histamine) in response to contact with specific antigens	• Present in serum, interstitial space, and exocrine secretions, and on basophils and mast cells • Very small (0.002) percentage of total immunoglobulins	• IgE low levels: Muscle coordination disorder (rare) • IgE high levels: Atopic conditions, allergies, asthma, dermatitis

macrophage cell membrane. The antigen binds with an antigen receptor on the surface of the T cell, sensitizing the T cell. The sensitized T cells secrete lymphokines, which regulate and coordinate the immune response to combat foreign cells, protect the body against mutant or cancer cells, and destroy foreign tissue. Interleukin-8 is secreted by the macrophage and stimulates T cell division. T cells are programmed to recognize the body's own tissue (i.e., self) from antigen (i.e., nonself). Autoimmune diseases occur when the immune system cannot recognize self-tissue and the body is damaged by the immune system. NK cells also contribute to cellular immunity, especially in relation to cancer cell surveillance.

Humoral-mediated immunity is primarily effective against bacteria and viruses and is mediated by B cells. In the humoral immunity process, the B cells become plasma cells and make antibodies called immunoglobulins to recognize specific foreign cells or antigens on subsequent exposures.

Immunoglobulins (i.e., antibodies) are serum proteins that bind to specific antigens. They begin the process that causes lysis or phagocytosis of an offending antigen. The immunoglobulins include IgG, IgA, IgM, IgD, and IgE, with each having a specific role in the immune system (Table 8-2).

One end of the immunoglobulin (Ig) molecule has a constant fragment with a fixed sequence of amino acids that is constant within the category of the immunoglobulin (e.g., IgG, IgM, etc.). The other end of the molecule has an antigen-binding fragment with an amino acid sequence specific to the antigen for which the antibody was formed. The first exposure to an antigen is followed by a latent phase in which no antibody levels are detected. The primary response follows as serum antibody levels rise rapidly. Maximal antibody response takes 3 to 5 days, and then levels plateau and finally decline. Subsequent exposure to the antigen results in more rapid production of antibodies to that antigen and higher concentrations of the antibody. This primary and secondary immune response (Figure 8-1) is the basis for immunizations as well as the consequence of increasing severity of allergic reactions.

Inflammation occurs because antigen-antibody complexes referred to as *immune complexes* attracts WBCs. Immune complexes activate the complement cascade. Complement is a group of more than 20 serum proteins. Complement proteins act sequentially and in concert to lyse microorganisms and/or infected cells. When activated, complement functions as mediators to enhance various aspects of the inflammatory response. Complement attracts and stimulates PMNs and kills microorganisms by punching holes in the cell membranes of the offending agent and allowing intracellular fluid to leak out. Mononuclear phagocytes and monocytes then clear the debris from the bloodstream. Complement also causes the agglutination of the bacteria and activates basophils and mast cells. Complement deficiencies may be congenital or acquired and result in unusual infections and abnormal hypersensitivity reactions.

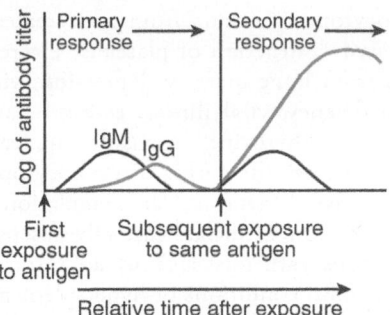

FIGURE 8-1 Primary and secondary immune responses. The introduction of antigen induces a response dominated by two classes of immunoglobulins, IgM and IgG. IgM predominates in the primary response, with some IgG appearing later. After the host's immune system is primed, another challenge with the same antigen induces the secondary response, in which some IgM and large amounts of IgG are produced. (From Lewis, S. M. et al. [2014]. *Medical-surgical nursing: Assessment and management of clinical problems* [9th ed.]. St. Louis, MO: Mosby.)

Activation of complement occurs with or without previous exposure to the antigen. In an anaphylactoid reaction, there is no previous exposure to the antigen and no true antigen-antibody interaction. In an anaphylactic reaction, there is previous exposure to the antigen and an antigen-antibody interaction.

Hypersensitivity (i.e., allergic) reactions can also occur and there are five types: Type I is called an immediate hypersensitivity reaction, ranging from mild reaction with localized response to a severe systemic reaction referred to as *anaphylaxis*. This reaction usually occurs within 5 to 20 minutes of exposure to even a miniscule amount of the antigen. A type I hypersensitivity reaction is caused by IgE specific to the antigen. The antigen binds to one end of IgE. IgE is bound to a mast cell or basophil and when the antigen attaches, the mast cell or basophil degranulates and histamine release occurs. Slow-reacting substance of anaphylaxis (SRS-A) and eosinophil chemotactic factor of anaphylaxis (ECF-A) are also released to recruit eosinophils to the site. An example of a type I hypersensitivity reaction is an anaphylactic reaction to a penicillin, insect venom, foods, or pollen.

A type II hypersensitivity reaction is a cytotoxic hypersensitivity. This reaction usually occurs within minutes or days and is caused by the combination of IgG, IgM, or IgA antibody and antigenic receptors on membranes of cells. An activated complement cascade and NK cells are involved in the destruction of the immune complex attached to a cell. Macrophages may phagocytize the immune complexes. An example of the type II cytoxic hypersensitivity occurs with a mismatched blood transfusion reaction.

In a type III hypersensitivity reaction, an immune complex-mediated reaction occurs usually within hours as a result of large quantities of antigen-antibody (IgG, IgM, or IgA) complexes that cannot be quickly and efficiently cleared by the reticuloendothelial system. In this type of response, activation of both the complement cascade and neutrophils occurs. Stimulation of the inflammatory process releases mediators. An example of a type III immune complex-mediated reaction is vasculitis and renal damage caused by immune complexes due to rheumatoid arthritis.

A type IV hypersensitivity reaction is a delayed or cell-mediated hypersensitivity and the reaction occurs within one or more days. This delayed reaction is poorly understood but is presumed to be that cells require time to migrate to the site and is probably caused by previously sensitized lymphocytes and lymphokines that activate the inflammatory response at the site. Some examples of this type of reaction include skin testing for tuberculosis, contact dermatitis, and latex allergy.

8.2 Learning Activity

Identify which type of hypersensitivity reaction (I, II, III, or IV) the following situations demonstrate.

Example	Type
Skin testing for tuberculosis	
Poststreptococcal glomerulonephritis	
Anaphylaxis to penicillin	
Hemolytic blood transfusion reaction	

Answers to this activity can be found in the Answer Key.

HEMOSTASIS

Hemostasis is the termination of bleeding by a complex process that involves integrated interactions among blood vessels, platelets, clotting factors, and the fibrinolytic system. Hemostatic mechanisms include a vascular response, platelet aggregation, coagulation, and fibrinolysis.

Vascular Response

Disruption of vascular integrity causes vasoconstriction. The SNS response to an insult results in a vasospasm and blood vessel constriction in the injured vessel. Thromboxane A_2, endothelin, the alpha-adrenergic system, and serotonin mediate this response.

Platelet Aggregation

Platelets (i.e., thrombocytes) aggregate during the second step in the process to maintain hemostasis. The bone marrow produces platelets and their life span is approximately 10 days. It is postulated that thrombopoietin, a hormone-like substance, is secreted to increase production and release of thrombocytes. Thrombopoiesis requires iron and thrombocytes are stored in and destroyed by the spleen.

Endothelial damage exposes the basement membrane of the subendothelial collagen, which stimulates the platelet aggregation process. Damaged tissues release chemicals (e.g., thromboplastin) to activate platelets. The activated platelets swell and develop hairlike projections. The swelling increases the surface area of the platelets for platelet adhesion and makes platelets more likely to aggregate. Platelets release granules and components necessary for the clotting process. The adenosine diphosphate (ADP) released by degranulation of the platelets enhances adhesiveness and aggregation. The adhesiveness aids in the platelets' ability to stick to vessel walls. The circulating von Willebrand factor (vWF), collagen, and endothelial collagen–specific glycoprotein Ia/IIb surface receptors also enhance platelet aggregation. Additional glycoprotein receptors, such as IIb, IIIa, IV, and V, progress the adhesive reaction to aggregation.

Drugs That Decrease Platelet Aggregation

- Alcohol
- Aminoglycosides (e.g., gentamicin)
- Aspirin (ASA)
- Catecholamines (e.g., epinephrine, norepinephrine, dopamine)
- Clopidogrel (Plavix)
- Dextran 40 (i.e., low-molecular-weight dextran)
- GP IIb/IIIa platelet receptor blockers (e.g., abciximab [Reo-Pro], eptifibatide [Integrilin], tirofiban HCl [Aggrastat])
- Heparin
- Herbs such as ginkgo biloba, Chinese ginseng, chamomile, and ginger
- Loop diuretics (e.g., furosemide) and thiazides (e.g., hydrochlorothiazide)
- Nonsteroidal antiinflammatory agents (e.g., phenylbutazone [Butazolidin], ibuprofen [Motrin])
- Phenothiazines
- Quinidine
- Ticlopidine (Ticlid)
- Vitamin E

Disorders That Alter Platelet Quality

- Catecholamine release
- Diabetes mellitus
- Hepatic cirrhosis
- Hyperthermia/hypothermia
- Malignant lymphomas
- Sarcoidosis
- Scleroderma
- Systemic lupus erythematosus (SLE)
- Thyrotoxicosis

Aggregation is the process of platelets adhering or clumping together to form the platelet plug. Activated platelets become adhesive and aggregate. Platelet aggregation becomes large enough to form a platelet plug (sometimes referred to as a *white clot*) that seals the damaged blood vessel. This platelet plug lasts 2 to 5 hours and dissolves as fibrin clots replace the platelets. During aggregation of the platelets, platelet factor III (PFIII), an important contributor in the intrinsic pathway, is released. Platelets contain factor XIII (fibrin-stabilizing factor), which is essential in the formation of a stable fibrin clot. Drugs (Box 8-1) or health disorders (Box 8-2) may affect the number or function of the platelets.

Thrombocytopenia and thrombocytosis are quantitative changes that occur with platelets. The significance of thrombocytopenia is determined by the level of impairment. Mild thrombocytopenia occurs when the platelet counts are greater than 50,000/mm^3 but less than normal. Surgery can generally be tolerated with this level. Moderate thrombocytopenia occurs when the platelet count is 20,000/mm^3 to 30,000/mm^3. The occurrence of spontaneous bleeding is unlikely unless vascular injury occurs. In severe thrombocytopenia, the platelet counts are less than 10,000/mm^3. Spontaneous intracranial hemorrhages are likely with a high risk of bleeding without provocation.

Thrombocytopenia occurs from a decreased production or an increased destruction of platelets. Decreased production occurs from bone marrow depression, vitamin B_{12} or folic acid deficiency, viral illness, estrogen, and metabolic hormones (e.g., thyroxine, cortisol). Increased destruction may result from idiopathic thrombocytopenic purpura (ITP), disseminated intravascular coagulation (DIC), heat stroke, hypertension, artificial heart valves, sepsis, and large-bore intravenous catheters such as an intraaortic balloon pump. The clinical conditions of hypersplenism from portal hypertension, heparin-induced thrombocytopenia (HIT), and dilutional thrombocytopenia caused by large volumes of fluids that do not contain platelets are other causes of thrombocytopenia.

On the other end of the spectrum, thrombocytosis or an increase in platelets may cause excessive thrombosis or bleeding, depending on the quality of the platelets. The causes of thrombocytosis include malignancy, granulomatous disease, polycythemia vera, leukemia, postsplenectomy, rheumatoid arthritis, trauma, and vitamin E deficiency.

Coagulation

Coagulation is the formation of a clot. Coagulation is dependent on presence of clotting factors, active ionized calcium, and functioning of the coagulation pathways (Figure 8-2). Blood coagulation factors consist of proteins, lipoproteins, and calcium, which are critical in the intrinsic, extrinsic, and common pathways. These inactive factors circulate and then activate in a cascade fashion.

The pathways are cascades in which one action is dependent on a preceding action or interaction. A fibrin clot may be produced through activation of either the intrinsic or extrinsic pathway, although the factor VII-initiated extrinsic pathway is a more potent and significant initiator of clotting.

Damage to red blood cells or platelets initiates the intrinsic pathway. The time from activation through the intrinsic pathway and common pathway to a clot is 2 to 6 minutes. The diagnostic tests aPTT or factor Xa detect problems or monitor the intrinsic pathway. Injured tissue and subsequent release of tissue thromboplastin initiates the extrinsic pathway. The time from activation through the extrinsic pathway and common pathway to a clot is 15 to 20 seconds. The PT/INR tests this pathway. In the common pathway, platelet factor III and tissue thromboplastin combine to become a prothrombin activator. Prothrombin converts to thrombin and fibrinogen converts to fibrin, forming a fibrin clot. The aPTT, factor Xa levels, PT/INR, fibrinogen level, and thrombin time test the common pathway. Other prothrombotic mechanisms also exist. Inflammation triggers thromboxane. Cancer procoagulants, such as cancer procoagulant (CP) or heat shock proteins (HSPs), enhance coagulability.

Fibrinolysis

Fibrinolysis is the anticoagulant mechanism in the normal body system. It exists to balance the clotting process (Figure 8-3). The reticuloendothelial system clears activated clotting factors. Clot-lysing activities maintain blood in a fluid state. The process of clot breakdown takes approximately 7 to 10 days.

Blood (i.e., intrinsic pathway) or tissue (i.e., extrinsic pathway) plasminogen activators stimulate the conversion of plasminogen to plasmin; therefore, development of a clot initiates

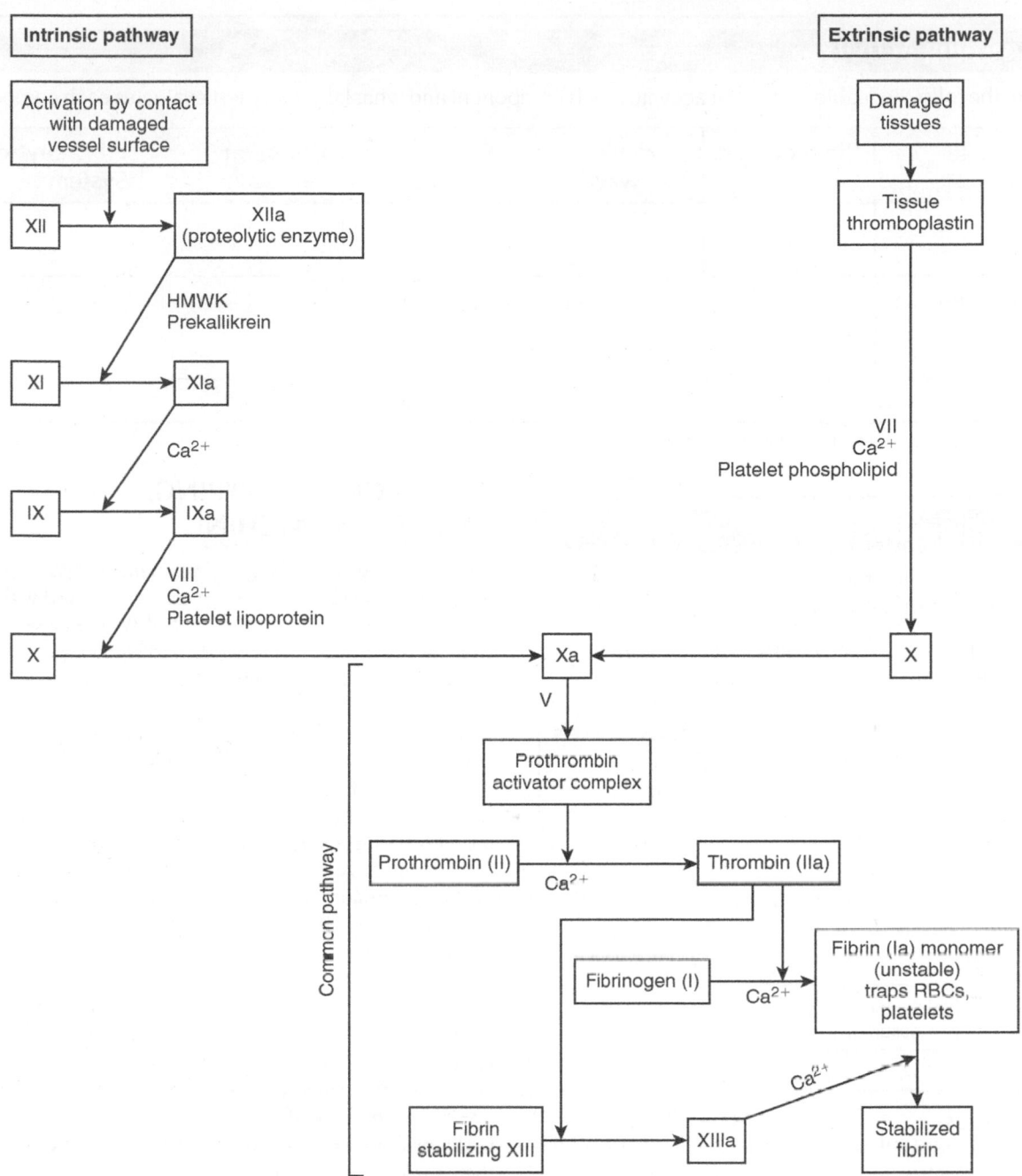

FIGURE 8-2 The clotting pathways: intrinsic, extrinsic, and common. (From Lewis, S. M. et al. [2014]. *Medical-surgical nursing: Assessment and management of clinical problems* [9th ed.]. St. Louis, MO: Mosby.)

a process to eliminate the clot. Plasmin works to lyse fibrin clots producing fibrin degradation products (FDPs), which are also referred to as *fibrin split products (FSPs)*. FDPs have anticoagulant properties and increased amounts of FDPs enhance the potential for patients to bleed. Fibrinolytics speed up this process by either directly providing tissue plasminogen activator (e.g., alteplase [Activase], reteplase [Retavase]) or tenecteplase (TNKase), or by triggering the process by adding a complex to cause the activation of the fibrinolytic system (streptokinase [Streptase]).

Different mechanisms control fibrinolysis. Plasminogen activator inhibitor type 1 (PAI-1) inactivates tissue plasminogen activator. Alpha$_2$-antiplasmin is an inhibitor of plasmin. Antithrombin is a serum protease that degrades the coagulation factors IXa, Xa, and XIIa. The antithrombin system defends

against excessive clotting by the release of antithrombin III (ATIII) from mast cells. This neutralizes the clotting capability of thrombin. In addition, an extrinsic infusion of antithrombin III can provide anticoagulant effects.

There are also regulators of coagulation. Calcium is required for activation of factors. Tissue factor pathway inhibitor (TFPI) inhibits excessive tissue factor activity. Protein C and thrombomodulin enhance degradation, but an absence leads to thrombophilia and excess clotting.

The intrinsic or extrinsic administration of heparins affects ATIII degradation. Plasmin is cleaved by tissue plasminogen activator (tPa). Prostacyclin (PGI$_2$) released by damaged endothelium or extrinsic administration inhibits platelet aggregation (Table 8-3).

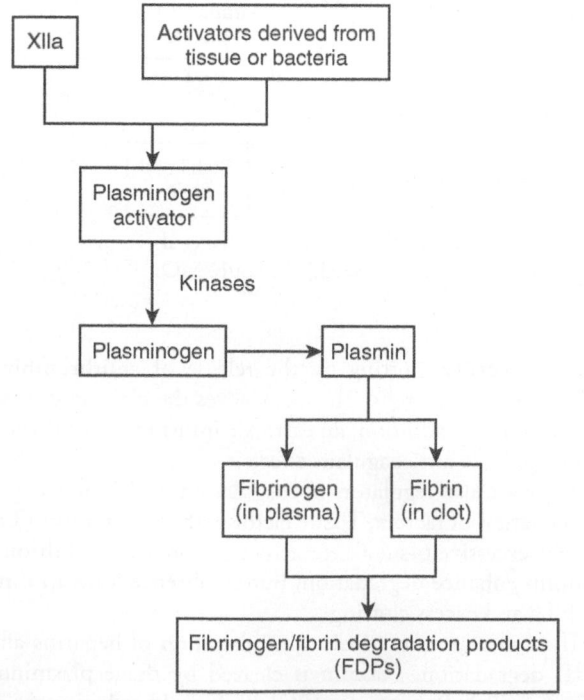

FIGURE 8-3 The fibrinolytic process. (From Lewis, S. M. et al. [2011]. *Medical-surgical nursing: Assessment and management of clinical problems* [8th ed.]. St. Louis, MO: Mosby.)

BLOOD GROUPS, TYPING, AND CROSSMATCHING

Three systems describe the most important antigens on RBCs, tissues, and other cells. The ABO system is concerned with antigens on the RBC that are designated A and B. The presence of these antigens is genetically controlled. The blood type is named for the antigen that is present on the RBC. Antibodies are present in the plasma for the antigen or antigens that are not present (e.g., B antibodies are found in group A blood because B antigens are absent). Blood that contains both A and B antigens is termed *type AB blood*. Blood that contains neither A nor B antigens is termed *type O blood*. Agglutination that occurs in mismatched blood is the basis for typing and crossmatching. Blood typing detects the major antigens: A, B, and Rh. Crossmatching detects the presence of major or minor RBC antigens in donor blood that can lead to reactions for a specific recipient (Table 8-4).

The Rh system (Table 8-5) is composed of a series of six common types of Rh antigens, each called an Rh factor. Each person has one of each of three pairs so they have three of these Rh factors designated c, C, d, D, e, and E. Only C, D, and E are antigenic enough to cause significant development of anti-Rh antibodies; therefore, these have the potential to cause a blood transfusion reaction if nonmatched blood is administered. If C, D, or E antigens are present, the person is Rh+. If none of these three antigens is present, the person is Rh−. Most (85%) of Americans are Rh+.

Rh antibodies do not develop spontaneously. They only occur after exposure to Rh antigen. On second exposure, a reaction can occur (i.e., second exposure to non–Rh-matched blood or an Rh− mother pregnant with a second Rh+ fetus). A delayed mild transfusion reaction can occur even after the first exposure to Rh+ blood. Administration of Anti-Rh globin (Rho-gam) to Rh− mothers prevents this complication.

Another known red cell antigen is cold agglutinins. Cold agglutinins are antibodies that cause erythrocytes to coagulate when blood plasma temperature is below normal body temperature. Before giving blood to a patient who has cold agglutinins, warm the banked blood to normal body temperature (37° C). Cold agglutinins more commonly occur in non-Caucasians, elderly patients, or patients with autoimmune disease or after viral infection. This may be a temporary or permanent condition.

The Coombs test determines the presence of hemolyzing antibodies. A direct Coombs detects antibodies attached to

TABLE 8-3	Blood Coagulation Factors	
Factor	**Name(s)**	**Comments**
I	Fibrinogen	• Synthesized in liver • Precursor to fibrin (Ia)
Ia	Fibrin	• Activated fibrinogen (I) becomes fibrin (Ia)
II	Prothrombin	• Synthesized in liver • Vitamin K dependent • Precursor to thrombin (IIa)
IIa	Thrombin	• Activated prothrombin becomes thrombin
III	Tissue thromboplastin Tissue factor	• First factor of extrinsic pathway
IV	Calcium	• Acts as an enzyme cofactor for most of the activation steps in intrinsic, extrinsic, and common pathways
V	Proaccelerin Labile factor Ac globulin	• Synthesized in liver • Combines with Xa and phospholipid to accelerate conversion of prothrombin (II) to thrombin (IIa)
VI	There is no designated factor VI	
VII	Proconvertin Stable factor	• Synthesized in liver • Vitamin K dependent • Part of extrinsic pathway • Complexes with tissue thromboplastin (III) to activate X
VIII	Antihemophiliac factor A	• Part of intrinsic pathway • Complexes with IXa and platelet phospholipid to activate X
IX	Plasma thromboplastin component Christmas factor Antihemophiliac factor B	• Synthesized in liver • Vitamin K dependent • Associated with factors VIII, XI, and XII in the intrinsic pathway
X	Stuart-Prower factor	• Synthesized in liver • Vitamin K dependent • Part of intrinsic and extrinsic pathways • Complexes with V and phospholipid to accelerate prothrombin (II) conversion
XI	Plasma thromboplastin antecedent	• May be synthesized in liver • May be vitamin K dependent • Part of intrinsic pathway • Associated with factors VIII, IX, and XII in the intrinsic pathway
XII	Hageman factor Contact factor	• First factor in intrinsic factor • Indirectly activates plasmin and complement cascades
XIII	Fibrin-stabilizing factor Fibrinase Laki-Lorand factor	• May be synthesized in liver • Activated by thrombin (IIa) • Produces a stronger, insoluble clot; stabilizes clot formation

NOTE: "a" after the factor indicates an activated factor.

TABLE 8-4	ABO Blood Groups				
Patient's ABO Group	**Percentage of Population**	**Antigen on RBC**	**Antibodies in Plasma**	**Compatible RBCs**	**Compatible Plasma**
O	47%	None	Anti-A, Anti-B	O	O, A, B, AB
A	41%	A	Anti-B	O, A	A, AB
B	9%	B	Anti-A	O, B	B, AB
AB	3%	A and B	None	O, A, B, AB	AB

TABLE 8-5	Rh Compatibility	
Patient's Rh Type	**RBC Rh Type for Transfusion**	**Plasma Rh Type for Transfusion**
Positive	Positive or negative	Positive or negative
Negative	Negative	Positive or negative

the RBCs. An indirect Coombs detects antibodies in serum. Other tests for RBC antigens include the Kell test, which is the third most common test; the Duffy test; and the Kidd test.

Uncrossmatched type O negative packed red blood cells may be used in exsanguinating patients. Avoid whole blood to decrease the risk of reaction caused by anti-A and anti-B antibodies in type O plasma. Blood antigen-antibody complexes may complicate later crossmatching and may cause future blood transfusion reaction to one's own blood type unless it is O negative. Type-specific blood may be preferable, and type matching takes only 5 to 15 minutes. Therefore, the ideal is typed and crossmatched blood, next best is type-specific blood, and the universal donor blood, O negative, is only given in an extreme emergency.

Human leukocyte antigen (HLA) is a group of antigenic substances found on many cell types (including WBCs and platelets but not on erythrocytes). Cytotoxicity assays serologically test for HLAs. HLA-A, HLA-B, and HLA-C are found on all nucleated cells, but HLA-D and HLA-DR antigens are only located on B-lymphocytes, monocytes, epidermal cells, and endothelial cells. The human leukocyte antigen is very important in organ transplantation.

ASSESSMENT OF THE HEMATOLOGIC AND IMMUNOLOGIC SYSTEMS

Interview

First, ascertain the patient's chief complaint. Elicit why the patient is seeking help now and what is the duration of the problem. Ask the patient to describe the symptoms. The symptoms of hematologic or immunologic conditions are both general and system specific (Table 8-6).

History

Assess the patient's past medical, surgical, and family history along with a social history to provide information in regards to actual and potential hematologic and immunologic problems (Box 8-3). Check to see if the patient has any known allergies and the type of any reaction to food, environment, or medications. Address all types of medications: inhalants, dermal contact agents, injected drugs, and ingested medications. Ascertain if the patient has ever had a reaction to a transfusion with blood or blood products. Note the patient's immunization record, recording the types, dates, and any adverse reactions.

Social history is also very important to elicit from the patient during the interview process. Ask the patient about the relationship with the spouse or significant other and the family structure. Knowledge of the patient's occupation and military service may give insight to occupational exposure to radiation and/or exposure to toxins and chemicals (e.g., lead, benzene, ethylene oxide, insecticides, or vinyl chloride). Additional information to seek includes the patient's educational level, stress level, and usual coping mechanisms. Ask about any lifestyle changes,

recreational habits, and exercise habits, and if there has been any recent foreign travel. Dietary habits are important to assess for potential or actual etiologies of deficiencies in iron, folic acid, and vitamin B_{12}. Record the patient's caffeine intake and alcohol and tobacco use. Record the alcoholic beverages consumed per month, week, or day and the date of the last drink. Record pack-years of tobacco use, which is the number of packs per day times the number of years the patient has been smoking.

Address sexuality and question the patient about safe sex practices. Determine whether he or she has multiple sexual partners or has sexual activity with prostitutes, homosexuals, or bisexuals that would increase the risk of sexually transmitted disease.

Medication History

Elicit a detailed medication history from the patient. Examine the drugs the patient takes to treat existing hematologic and immunologic conditions as well as those drugs that may exert a negative effect on these systems. Question the patient regarding nonprescribed drugs and use of over-the-counter drugs such as vitamins, minerals, and herbs. Ask if a substance abuse exists with injectable drug use, especially if needles are shared. While intravenous drug use is a concern, intramuscular steroid use and intradermal "poppers" also represent significant risk.

Ask about drugs that are used to treat various hematologic conditions such as coagulation disorders, inflammation, cancer, autoimmune disease, or viral disease and those used to augment the immune system. Drugs used for erythropoiesis include iron, vitamin B_{12}, pyridoxine, folic acid, and recombinant human erythropoietin. Drugs used for bleeding or clotting disorders include aspirin, nonsteroidal antiinflammatory drugs (NSAIDs), aminocaproic acid (Amicar), cryoprecipitate, and anticoagulants. Antineoplastic agents treat cancer and/or autoimmune disease. Antiviral agents and antiretroviral medications attack various viruses that affect the immune system. Other drugs that augment the immune system include interferon, interleukin-2, and colony-stimulating factors. Antibody preparations targeting autoimmune disorders (e.g., infliximab for Crohn disease, rituximab for rheumatoid arthritis) are also important to note.

Drugs that patients are receiving for other health problems may also exert a negative effect on the hematologic or immunologic system. Allergy medication, analgesics, and antiinflammatory agents may decrease platelets and/or cause hemolytic anemia. Opiates such as heroin and morphine sulfate may decrease platelets. Antigout drugs (e.g., colchicine) may cause aplastic anemia. Aspirin inhibits platelet aggregation and decreases macrophage activity. Corticosteroids (e.g., prednisone) suppress the immune/inflammatory process. Nonsteroidal drugs such as ibuprofen (e.g., Motrin) inhibit platelet aggregation and depress bone marrow. NSAIDs may cause aplastic anemia; lyse T, B, and NK cells; and inhibit interferon, IL-1, and IL-2 production. Antibiotics can also affect the hematologic and immunologic systems. Always examine medication usage to see if they are the cause of any health problems. Common drug classifications (Table 8-7) may have a negative effect.

Physical Examination

Begin the physical examination by taking the patient's vital signs and weight. Often weight loss occurs with hematologic and immunologic problems. Anemia, blood loss, and infection often cause tachycardia. Blood loss may cause hypotension.

TABLE 8-6	Hematologic and Immunologic Disorders: Subjective and Objective Findings
System	**Subjective Report or Objective Finding**

General	• Fatigue, weakness, chills, fever, weight loss, night sweats, apathy, lethargy, and malaise
	• Abnormal bleeding, bruising, or swelling
	• Chronic or recurrent infections
	• Lymph node swelling or tenderness (>2 cm for longer than 2 weeks)
	   • Benign or inflammatory lymph nodes: regular borders, movable, and tender
	   • Malignant lymph nodes: irregular shape, lack of movability, and nontender

Skin, hair, and nails	• Dry and rough skin (i.e., xeroderma) • Petechiae or ecchymosis • Bleeding from skin wounds or puncture • Poor wound healing • Color changes: jaundice, pallor, cyanosis, or flushing of mucous membranes and palmar creases • Presence of a rash, pruritus, lesions, or inflammation • Presence of lesions, wounds, rashes, excoriations, and leg ulcers • Moisture-related skin breakdown and fungal infections at skin folds (e.g., axillae, groin, and perineal areas) • Pitting edema • Alopecia • Pallor of nail beds, spoon nails, or clubbing
Eyes	• Visual disturbances: blurring or diplopia • Blindness related to retinal hemorrhage • Scleral hemorrhage may be noted • Conjunctival pallor and/or inflammation
Ears	• Vertigo • Tinnitus
Nasopharynx, mouth, and neck	• Epistaxis • Gingival bleeding • Dryness of the mouth (i.e., xerostomia) • Gingival and mucosal ulceration • Swollen, reddened, bleeding gums • Painful lesions on mouth and lips • Cracks in corners of mouth (i.e., angular cheilitis) • Sore or red, beefy tongue • Purplish lesions on tongue • White coating on tongue (e.g., candidiasis, also called *thrush*) • White, irregular lesions on lateral surfaces of tongue (i.e., oral hairy leukoplakia frequently seen in HIV-positive patients) • Sore throat • Persistent hoarseness • Dysphagia • Nuchal rigidity
Cardiovascular	• Chest pain • Sternal and rib tenderness • Palpitations • Dysrhythmia • Extra heart sounds: S_3 and/or S_4 • Murmur • Rub • Bruits over carotids or aorta
Pulmonary	• Exertional dyspnea or orthopnea • Cough • Hemoptysis • Respiratory tract infections • Crackles • Pleural rub

Continued

TABLE 8-6	Hematologic and Immunologic Disorders: Subjective and Objective Findings—cont'd
System	**Subjective Report or Objective Finding**
Gastrointestinal	• Anorexia, abdominal pain or tenderness, cramping, bloating, or eructation • Ulcers: oral, esophageal, or gastric • Vomiting of blood or coffee-ground material • Change in bowel habits: diarrhea or constipation • Bloody or black stools • Rectal pain or bleeding • Hepatomegaly • Splenomegaly • Peritoneal friction rub
Genitourinary	• Hematuria • Pyuria • Abnormal menstrual flow: menorrhagia or amenorrhea • Incontinence, dysuria, hesitancy, or frequency • Urinary retention • Pelvic or flank pain
Neurologic	• Confusion, irritability, or change in level of consciousness • Memory loss • Headache • Ataxia, syncope • Sensory changes: paresthesia or anesthesia • Pupil changes • Decreased deep tendon reflexes
Musculoskeletal	• Pain and/or tenderness in joints, back, shoulder, or bone • Joint stiffness or swelling • Muscle weakness

BOX 8-3

Patient History Related to Hematologic and Immunologic Problems

Surgical
- Splenectomy
- Thymectomy
- Tonsillectomy
- Tumor removal
- Total or partial gastrectomy
- Surgical excision of duodenum
- Organ or tissue transplant
- Prosthetic heart valves
- Prolonged/excessive bleeding

Medical
- Anemia
- Asthma
- Autoimmune disease (e.g., SLE)
- Deep vein thrombosis
- Pulmonary embolus
- Diabetes mellitus
- HIV/AIDS
- Liver disease
- Malabsorption syndrome
- Malignancy
- Leukemia
- Lymphoma
- Multiple myeloma
- Mononucleosis
- Poor wound healing
- Prolonged or excessive bleeding
- Radiation therapy
- Recent viral illness exposures
- Coxsackie virus
- Epstein-Barr virus
- Recurrent infections
- Renal failure
- Sexually transmitted disease
- Spleen disorders
- Vitamin K deficiency

Family
- Congenital
  - Immune deficiency
  - Hemophilia
  - Sickle cell anemia
  - Thalassemia
- Asthma
- Allergies
- Anemia
- Jaundice
- Malignancies
- Autoimmune disease
  - SLE
  - Rheumatoid arthritis

TABLE 8-7	Medication Effects on the Hematologic and Immune systems	
Classification	**Drug**	**Negative Effect**
Anesthetics	• Halothane • Nitrous oxide • Cyclopropane	• Decrease phagocytosis • Inhibit T cell function
Antibiotics	• All	• Kill vitamin K-producing bacteria • May cause opportunistic infection by altering normal flora in GI tract (i.e., *Clostridium difficile*)
	• Tetracycline	• Inhibits chemotaxis • Inhibits activation of lymphocytes
	• Sulfonamides	• Inhibit chemotaxis • Inhibit activation of lymphocytes • May cause aplastic anemia or thrombocytopenia
	• Chloramphenicol	• Depresses WBC production • May cause aplastic anemia
Anticoagulants	• Heparin	• May cause thrombocytopenia
Anticonvulsants	• Phenytoin (Dilantin)	• Inhibits the effects of corticosteroids • May cause lymph node hyperplasia • May cause anemia or thrombocytopenia
	• Phenobarbital	• May cause aplastic anemia
Antidysrhythmics	• Procainamide	• May cause hemolytic anemia • May cause thrombocytopenia • Decreases production of WBCs
	• Quinidine	• May cause hemolytic anemia • May cause thrombocytopenia • Decreases production of WBCs
	• Propranolol	• Inhibits platelet aggregation
Antifungals	• Amphotericin B	• May cause anemia • May cause thrombocytopenia
Antihypertensives	• Captopril (Capoten)	• May cause pancytopenia
	• Methyldopa (Aldomet)	• May cause thrombocytopenia • May cause anemia
Antituberculins	• Para-aminosalicylic acid (Isoniazid)	• May cause anemia • May cause thrombocytopenia • Decreases WBC production • May cause lymphadenopathy
Diuretics	• Chlorothiazide (Diuril) • Furosemide (Lasix)	• May cause anemia • May cause thrombocytopenia
Histamine receptor antagonists	• Ranitidine (Zantac)	• May cause thrombocytopenia
Immunosuppressives	• Steroids • Methotexate	• Suppress inflammation • Suppress immune processes
Oral contraceptives	• Diethylstilbestrol • Estrogen	• May cause anemia
Oral hypoglycemic	• Chlorpropamide	• May cause anemia • May cause thrombocytopenia
Sympathomimetics	• Epinephrine	• Decreases chemotaxis • Decreases WBC production • Decreases response to antigens • Alters antibody production

Infection causes hyperthermia, but remember that elderly patients often do not develop a fever. Anemia may cause hypothermia. Hematologic and immunologic conditions cause various abnormalities noted on physical examination in patients (see Table 8-6).

Diagnostic Studies

Hematology blood tests are used to diagnose and monitor hematologic and immune disorders. The normal level for RBCs is 4.4 to 5.9×10^6/mL for males, and 3.8 to 5.2×10^6/mL for females. The quantity of RBCs is elevated in dehydration, chronic hypoxemia, or high altitudes. The count may also temporarily increase after a cold shower or with intense emotions. Bone marrow suppression, hemorrhage, anemia, leukemia, or hypothyroidism causes a decrease in RBCs. Determine the quality of the RBC by examination of the size and color. Microcytic RBCs are too small and macrocytic RBCs are too large. The color of the RBC depends on the hemoglobin concentration. In a hypochromic RBC, the hemoglobin concentration is too low; in a hyperchromic RBC, the hemoglobin concentration is too high.

The normal mean corpuscular volume (MCV), which is an average of the size of the RBC, is 80 to 100 fL. The MCV is decreased in iron deficiency and pernicious anemia and increased in folic acid deficiency and high reticulocyte count. The mean corpuscular hemoglobin (MCH), which is an average of the weight of hemoglobin in an RBC, has a normal value of 26.6 to 34 pg. The MCH is decreased in iron deficiency and sickle cell anemia while increased in polycythemia. The normal value of the mean corpuscular hemoglobin concentration (MCHC) is 31.4 to 36.3 g/dL.

The color, size, and mean red blood cell indices help to determine the following anemia diagnoses:

- Macrocytic, normochromic: pernicious anemia, folate deficiency
- Microcytic, hypochromic: iron deficiency anemia
- Normocytic, normochromic: aplastic anemia, posthemorrhagic anemia, hemolytic anemia, sickle cell anemia, and anemia of chronic illness; note that the RBCs are normal in size and color but the numbers are insufficient

A reticulocyte is an immature RBC and the normal count is 0.5% to 1.5% of the total RBC count. The reticulocyte count assesses the responsiveness and potential of the bone marrow to respond to bleeding or hemolysis.

The erythrocyte sedimentation rate (ESR or sed rate) is normally 1 to 13 mm/hr for males and 1 to 20 mm/hr for females. The ESR is a nonspecific test that measures the amount of RBCs that settle in 1 hour. The ESR is elevated in inflammatory processes (e.g., rheumatoid arthritis, malignancy, rheumatic fever, hemolytic anemia, thyroid disorders, autoimmune disorders, nephrotic syndrome). The rate is decreased in polycythemia vera, hypofibrinogenemia, sickle cell anemia (not crisis), and heart failure. The ESR may be used to monitor trends in patients with chronic inflammatory diseases undergoing treatment

The normal hemoglobin (Hgb) is 13 to 18 g/dL for males and 12 to 16 g/dL for females. Hemoglobin is elevated in polycythemia, which may occur in chronic hypoxia or at high altitudes. Anemia and hemorrhage cause a decrease in Hgb. The normal hematocrit (Hct) is 40% to 52% for males and 35% to 47% for females. The Hct is elevated in dehydration or polycythemia and decreased with anemia, leukemia, or normal Hgb and water overload.

A peripheral smear is an evaluation of blood cell size, shape, and composition to provide insight but not confirmation of medical disorders. Heinz bodies are evident in the peripheral smear of patients with hemolytic anemia and portal hypertension. Schistocytes are present with disseminated intravascular coagulation and spherocytes occur after massive transfusion. Target cells are present with iron deficiency and liver disease.

The WBC count is normally 3500 to 11,000/mm³. WBCs increase in inflammation, infection, trauma, surgery, acute

TABLE 8-8 Lymphocyte Assays

Lymphocyte Type	Percentage of Lymphocytes
Total T cells	70-80%
CD4 (helper T cells)	29-60%
CD8 (suppressor T cells)	18-42%
CD4:CD8 (helper/suppressor ratio)	0.8:2.9
Total B cells	10-20%

leukemia, and stress and decrease in bone marrow depression (e.g., aplastic anemia, agranulocytosis, chronic leukemia, sepsis, chronic illness, autoimmune disorders).

The differential is a breakdown percentage of the different types of WBCs. Neutrophils normally make up 40% to 80% of the count. Neutrophils are elevated in infection, stress, inflammatory processes, malignancy, trauma, hemorrhage, burns, tissue necrosis (e.g., myocardial infarction), and ketoacidosis. Overwhelming infection, bone marrow depression, vitamin B₁₂ or folic acid deficiency, and hypersplenism decrease the neutrophil count. The presence of excessive bands rather than mature neutrophils signifies a bacterial infection (termed a *left shift*). The presence of *blasts,* grossly immature or malformed cells, is indicative of leukemia.

Eosinophils are normally 0% to 5% of the count and are elevated in allergic and inflammatory conditions; asthma; eczema; eosinophilic leukemia; autoimmune disorders; skin rashes; parasitic infections, especially helminthic infections; and pulmonary disorders such as pneumonia. Adrenocortical stimulation, stress, Cushing syndrome, and systemic lupus erythematosus (SLE) decrease eosinophils.

The basophil normal percentage is 0% to 2%. Basophils are elevated in allergic conditions, inflammatory processes, graft rejection, acute leukemia, and recent splenectomy and decreased in hyperthyroidism and long-term corticosteroid therapy.

A normal monocyte percentage of the count is 3% to 8%. Chronic inflammatory conditions, viral infections, tuberculosis, ulcerative colitis, and parasitic infections cause an increase in monocytes. Immunodeficiency disorders cause a decrease in monocytes.

Lymphocytes usually make up 10% to 40% of the count. Lymphocytes are elevated in acute or chronic lymphocytic leukemia, chronic bacterial and viral infections, multiple myeloma, mononucleosis, and Cushing syndrome. In immunodeficiency disorders (e.g., AIDS, systemic lupus erythematosus, leukemia, antineoplastic drugs, steroids), prolonged critical illness or malnutrition, burns, and sepsis, lymphocytes cause a decrease in lymphocytes. Lymphocyte assays of T cells, B cells, and NK cells are also performed (Table 8-8).

A shift to the left is an increased percentage of bands (i.e., immature neutrophils) seen in bacterial infection. A shift to the right is an increased percentage of segs (i.e., segmented neutrophils) seen in inflammation, pernicious anemia, viral illness, or hepatic disease. A regenerative shift (i.e., shift to the left) is an elevated WBC count with increased percentage of bands. A regenerative shift is indicative of stimulation of bone marrow. A degenerative shift is a decreased WBC count with increased percentage of bands. A degenerative shift is indicative of bone marrow depression.

A normal platelet count is 150,000 to 400,000/mm³. Systemic lupus erythematosus (SLE), HIV infection, idiopathic thrombocytopenic purpura, sepsis, and disseminated intravascular coagulation (DIC) decrease the platelet count. With a platelet count of 50,000 to 100,000/mm³, prolonged bleeding times and an increased risk of bleeding after severe trauma or surgery are present. Platelet counts that are below 50,000/mm³ increase the risk of bleeding after minor trauma. Spontaneous bleeding, including intracranial bleeding, occurs with platelet counts below 20,000/mm³. Transfuse platelets as prescribed for active bleeding or in preparation for an invasive procedure that would cause bleeding. A prophylactic transfusion prevents spontaneous bleeding. Transfuse actively bleeding patients with thrombocytopenia with platelets immediately to keep platelet counts above 50,000/mm³ in most bleeding situations, and above 100,000/mm³ if there is DIC or central nervous system bleeding.

Additional hematology diagnostic tests include erythropoietin, ferritin, iron, total iron-binding capacity, transferrin, haptoglobin, and hemoglobin variant/fetal hemoglobin levels. The erythropoietin level is normally greater than 5 to 35 IU/L. Anemia, chemotherapy, AIDS, and renal cell carcinoma cause an increase in erythropoietin, and polycythemia vera or chronic kidney disease cause a decrease in erythropoietin. A normal ferritin level is 20 to 200 ng/mL. Ferritin is an iron precursor that stores iron and has the ability to make new RBCs. Iron-deficient anemia, nutritional deficiencies, and some bone marrow suppression decreases ferritin. A normal iron level is 50 to 150 mcg/dL, which reflects total iron but not the ability to create new iron. Use this test in conjunction with ferritin level and iron-binding capacity or transferrin saturation. The normal total iron-binding capacity (TIBC) is 250 to 410 mcg/dL and reflects iron binding to hemoglobin. Decreased TIBC occurs with abnormal hemoglobin or anemia. The transferrin saturation is normally greater than 20% and provides an indication of available iron. A normal haptoglobin level is 60 to 270 mg/dL in a fasting state. Decreased haptoglobin occurs in hemolytic anemia. The hemoglobin variant/fetal hemoglobin is normally less than 1% of RBCs and determines or monitors the level of hemolysis in sickle cell disease.

One of the diagnostic clotting profile studies is the prothrombin time (PT). The normal PT is 12 to 15 seconds and assesses the extrinsic coagulation pathway and the common pathway. The international normalized ratio (INR) is a mathematical calculation that accounts for the differences in sensitivity between reagents and standardizes the PT values. A therapeutic INR is usually 2 to 3 but may be higher, depending on indications for anticoagulant therapy.

Activated partial thromboplastin time (aPTT) is the diagnostic laboratory test that assesses the intrinsic coagulation pathway. The normal value is 25 to 38 seconds, but therapeutic goals of treatment are set at 1½ to 2 times the control depending on the indication for anticoagulant therapy.

Activated clotting time (ACT) is the therapeutic diagnostic test done during procedures that require anticoagulation (e.g., percutaneous coronary intervention [PCI]). The normal time is 300 to 350 seconds. The ACT is a bedside test used to monitor heparin-induced anticoagulation. Delay a sheath removal until ACT is less than 150 seconds.

Thrombin time assesses the time for thrombin to convert fibrinogen to a fibrin clot. The normal time is 10 to 15 seconds.

Use the thrombin time to monitor fibrinolytic therapy (e.g., r-PA and rt-PA). Thrombin is highly sensitive to minimal exposure to anticoagulants, and thus used for trending value rather than a precise medication dose adjustment. A bleeding time assesses platelet function, and the normal time is 1 to 4 minutes. A rarely used nonspecific test for clotting abnormalities is a Lee White clotting time, which is normally 6 to 12 minutes.

The normal fibrinogen level is 200 to 400 mg/dL. Fibrinogen is elevated in hypercoagulable states and inflammatory conditions. Lymphoma, acute leukemia, and autoimmune diseases increase fibrinogen levels. A decreased level of fibrinogen occurs in hypocoagulable states with a propensity to bleed. Chronic liver disease may cause increased or decreased fibrinogen levels. Fibrin degradation products (FDPs) (also referred to as *fibrin split products [FSP]*) are normally 0 to 10 mcg/dL. These products are elevated in excessive fibrinolysis (e.g., DIC). The D-dimer is a diagnostic test that differentiates DIC from abnormal fibrinogen produced by a failing liver. The normal level of the D-dimer is 250 ng/mL or less. The D-dimer is elevated in DIC and used to detect pulmonary embolism in some patients without factors that may falsely increase D-dimer such as recent surgery, solid malignancies, autoimmune disease, and heart failure.

Specific factor assays of antithrombin III, Protein C, and Protein S measure amounts of each factor in the blood. Antithrombin III levels are normally greater than 50% of control and decreased in clotting disorders such as DIC. Protein C levels are normally 60% to 130% of baseline activity and decreased by heparin, DIC, and liver disease. Protein S levels are usually 70% to 150% of normal activity and decreased by heparin, DIC, and liver disease.

The serum proteins used in the diagnostic evaluation process are total protein, albumin, and a C-reactive protein. The normal total protein level is 6 to 8 g/dL and the normal albumin level is 3.5 to 4.5 g/dL. The normal C-reactive protein level is less than 0.8 mg/dL. C-reactive protein is a nonspecific test for evaluating severity and course of inflammatory conditions. Other diagnostic studies include a serum protein electrophoresis to provide an immunoglobulin analysis (Table 8-9).

In addition, a complement assay provides information relative to numerous conditions. The major components examined are the total complement, C1 esterase inhibitor, C3, and C4. The normal total complement has 41 to 90 hemolytic units. The normal C1 esterase inhibitor is 16 to 33 mg/dL. The C3 normally is 88 to 252 mg/dL in men and 88 to 206 mg/dL in women. The normal C4 is 12 to 72 mg/dL in men and 13 to 75 mg/dL in women. Both increased and decreased complement levels occur in disease processes (Box 8-4).

The blood chemistry parameters examined in hematologic and immune disorders include calcium and both indirect and direct bilirubin laboratory tests. The normal calcium level is 8.5 to 10.5 mg/dL. The normal total bilirubin level is 0.3 to 1.3 mg/dL. The normal level for indirect bilirubin, which is bilirubin before being conjugated by the liver, is normally 0.1 to 1 mg/dL. Direct bilirubin, which is bilirubin after being conjugated by liver, is normally 0.1 to 0.3 mg/dL.

In addition, agglutination studies determine the type and crossmatch of blood and tissues. These studies determine the Rh factor. The Coombs test detects immune antibodies important in crossmatching. The direct Coombs is normally negative and measures antibodies (IgG) attached to RBCs. The indirect

TABLE 8-9	Immunoglobulin Analysis	
Immuno-globulin	Increased	Decreased
IgG	• Infection • Hepatitis A • Glomerulonephritis • Rheumatoid arthritis • Systemic lupus erythematosus (SLE) • AIDS • IgG myeloma	• Agammaglobulinemia • Chronic lymphocytic leukemia
IgM	• Hepatitis A and B • Chronic infections • SLE • Rheumatoid arthritis • Sjögren syndrome • AIDS	• Hypogammaglobulinemia • Chronic lymphocytic leukemia • IgG myeloma • IgA myeloma • Agammaglobulinemia
IgA	• SLE • Rheumatoid arthritis • IgA myeloma	• IgA deficiency • Acute and chronic lymphocytic leukemia • Agammaglobulinemia • IgG myeloma • Chronic infections
IgE	• Allergic rhinitis • Allergic asthma • Parasitic infection	• IgA deficiency • Intrinsic asthma
IgD	• Eczema • Skin disorders	• Unknown

BOX 8-4

Conditions with Complement Alterations

Increased Complement
- Obstructive jaundice
- Thyroiditis
- Acute rheumatic fever
- Rheumatoid arthritis
- Acute myocardial infarction
- Ulcerative colitis
- Diabetes mellitus

Decreased Complement
- Systemic lupus erythematosus (SLE)
- Acute poststreptococcal glomerulonephritis
- Acute serum sickness
- Cirrhosis of the liver
- Multiple myeloma
- Severe immunodeficiency
- Rapidly rejecting allografts

Coombs is also normally negative and measures antibodies (IgG) in the serum. The human leukocyte antigens (HLAs) evaluate tissue compatibility with a complement-dependent cytotoxic assay, mixed lymphocyte culture, and crossmatching.

An immune profile determines the CD4 count and the CD4:CD8 ratio. The normal CD4 cell count is 800 cells/mm³.

The level varies with age and measures helper T cells. HIV infection and AIDS cause a decrease in the CD4 cell count. The diagnostic result of a CD4 count assists in staging HIV infection. Chronic corticosteroid therapy or immunosuppressive treatment causes a decrease in CD4. The T4:T8 (CD4:CD8) is the ratio between helper cells and suppressor/cytotoxic cells. The normal ratio is 1.8 with more CD4 cells than CD8 cells. There is a reverse ratio in HIV infection or AIDS.

HIV antibody screening is normally negative. The screening detects antibodies to HIV that are present with exposure to HIV. Absence of antibodies does not indicate immunity, nor does it eliminate patient exposure. Time is required for development of antibodies. There are two types of antibody screening tests. The enzyme-linked immunosorbent assay (ELISA) screening test is subject to error and has up to 10% false-positive results. The Western blot test is a more specific test than ELISA. Screening of HIV with a polymerase chain reaction (PCR) can detect the virus itself and is normally negative. The HIV viral load testing may range from imperceptible (i.e., less than 25 to 5000 copies of HIV/mL) to 1 million or more copies of HIV/mL. The higher the viral load, the more rapid the damage from HIV. The HIV viral load test evaluates the effectiveness of antiretroviral therapy.

Culture and sensitivity testing on various body secretions (e.g., blood, urine, and wound secretions) determines the infective organism and the effectiveness of antibiotics to treat the infection. A gram stain identifies gram-positive or gram-negative bacteria. The culture identifies the microorganism. The sensitivity determines the minimum inhibitory concentration (MIC) of the antibiotic needed. The MIC is the smallest concentration of antibiotic that effectively inhibits bacterial growth. The MIC reports the antibiotic concentration per mL of solution necessary for growth inhibition and then compares it with the achievable blood level of the antibiotic. If this level is less than the MIC, the bacterium is resistant to that antibiotic. If this level is greater than the MIC, the bacterium is sensitive to that antibiotic. Certain antimicrobials are dosed to achieve a specific MIC level (e.g., vancomycin), whereas other blood levels are used to assess toxicity (e.g., aminoglycosides). Other factors, such as known adverse effects of the antibiotic, are also considered.

Urine and stool analysis will also provide information about certain hematologic and immunologic conditions. A normal level of RBCs in the urine is 0 to 2/low power field. RBCs in the urine may indicate trauma (e.g., renal calculi), severe thrombocytopenia, or bleeding disorder (e.g., DIC). WBCs in the urine should be no more than 0 to 4/low-power field. WBCs in the catheterized urine specimen indicate urinary tract infection. There should be no bilirubin in the urine. Urobilinogen indicates biliary obstruction or liver disease. In the stool, the specimen may be grossly bloody or guaiac positive in bleeding disorders. A clostridial toxin assay should be negative. A positive finding indicates the presence of a toxin released by *Clostridium difficile*.

Several radiologic and radioisotope studies may reveal diagnostic data to make a differential diagnosis. A chest x-ray may show infiltrates indicative of infection or bleeding. A flat plate of the abdomen may show gross bleeding or hematoma. Visualization of the lymph system after injection of a dye with a lymphangiography assists in node assessment. An isotopic lymphangiography uses technetium-99m and is less invasive than radiographic lymphangiography. Computed tomography (CT) scans of the chest, liver, or spleen detect enlarged lymph nodes. The positron emission tomography (PET) scans demonstrate metabolic activity and glucose uptake that can indicate the presence of malignancy and abnormal lymph nodes.

Biopsy results provide a definitive diagnosis. A bone marrow aspiration reveals cell numbers and maturation to diagnose bone marrow suppression. A biopsy of the bone marrow is necessary for diagnosis of leukemia. An open, direct-visualization lymph node biopsy requires a surgical procedure performed in the operating room. A closed or needle aspiration is performed at the bedside. Assessment for transplant organ rejection requires a biopsy. Synovial fluid, chest drainage, and cerebrospinal fluid examinations are other methods used to evaluate certain conditions.

Anergy panel testing detects immunosuppression. Conduct anergy testing by administering an antigen for observation of a delayed inflammatory skin reaction. Tuberculosis, mumps, *Candida,* and trichophytin are the most frequently used antigens. The mumps antigen is contraindicated for patients allergic to chicken or eggs. A normal response is a negative response to tuberculosis (unless the patient has been previously exposed to tuberculosis) and a positive reaction to several of the other antigens within 24 to 72 hours. Anergy is the abnormal response that occurs when there is a failure to respond to any of the injections. Immunosuppression prevents a response to an antigen. For example, immunodeficiency is present when the induration from tuberculin antibody is less than 5 mm in diameter.

BLOOD, BLOOD COMPONENTS, AND PHARMACOLOGIC AGENTS

Blood and Blood Component Administration

Blood and blood component transfusions replace circulating volume, blood, or blood components. Transfusions improve oxygen-carrying capacity (RBCs, whole blood), replenish clotting factors (fresh frozen plasma, cryoprecipitate) and platelets, and replenish granulocytes. The administration of blood components (Table 8-10) is more common; however, an exsanguinating patient may need to receive whole blood.

Administer blood safely following the institution's policy and procedures. Insert or ensure patency of an intravenous (IV) catheter; do not use a catheter (or lumen) smaller than 20 gauge as this is likely to damage fragile RBCs. Ensure that the type and crossmatch have been done and blood or blood component is available. Assess vital signs before administration and notify the physician if the patient's temperature is 37.8° C (100° F) or higher. Request the blood or blood component from the blood bank when ready to administer. If you cannot begin the transfusion within 30 minutes after receiving the blood, return it to the blood bank. Check all of the following before administration of blood or blood component:

- Physician prescription for blood or blood component
- Consent form signed by the patient (according to hospital policy)
- Confirm the following with another registered nurse:
  - Patient's name and hospital number on patient ID bracelet
  - Type of blood component
  - Patient's blood group and Rh type
  - Donor's blood group and Rh type
  - Unit number of blood or blood component
  - Expiration date of the blood or blood component

- Sign the transfusion record, along with the RN who confirmed the information.

To set up the administration of the blood product, prime the blood administration set with normal (0.9%) saline. Allow the normal saline to cover the filter. Use only normal saline—do not use dextrose-containing solutions or lactated Ringer's solution. Warm the blood if indicated. Blood may be warmed to avoid hypothermia in the patient receiving 4 or more units over 6 hours or in the patient who has tested positive for cold agglutinins. Warm the blood to 32° to 37° C using a blood-warming device in these situations.

Clamp off the saline and start the blood or blood component. Adjust the rate to administer slowly: 25 to 50 mL within the first 15 minutes. Remain with the patient during this time. Ask the patient to notify you if he or she develops chills, low back pain, nausea, sweating, itching, hives, anxiety, and shortness of breath. Monitor for transfusion reaction and assess for clinical indications of transfusion reaction (Table 8-11 and Box 8-5). Take appropriate action for transfusion reactions if they occur (Box 8-6).

Monitor vital signs every 15 minutes for the first hour and then every 60 minutes until transfusion is complete or according to hospital policy. Adjust the rate to infuse packed RBCs within 4 hours of initiating the infusion. Administer FFP, platelets, and granulocytes rapidly. If the blood rate slows, do the following:

1. Ensure that the roller clamp is open.
2. Increase the height of the blood bag.
3. Gently squeeze the bag several times to agitate the blood cells.
4. Gently squeeze the tubing and flashbulb.
5. Remove the dressing and check the site.
6. Close the blood and open the saline to allow 50 to 100 mL to irrigate the line, and then restart the blood.
7. Flush administration set tubing with saline after the transfusion is complete.
8. Disconnect the empty blood bag from the administration set and dispose of these according to hospital policy.

Collaborative care requires the knowledge of the clinical indications and prevention and treatment for the adverse effects of hypocalcemia, hyperkalemia, deficiency in 2,3-DPG, hypoxia, ammonia intoxification, dilutional coagulopathy, and hypothermia (Table 8-12). Monitor the patient receiving blood and blood component therapy for complications.

The major complications (Table 8-11) of blood and blood product administration include hepatitis, HIV, cytomegalovirus (CMV), and acute respiratory distress syndrome (ARDS). Mandatory testing of all donor blood for hepatitis B surface antigen has reduced hepatitis B transmission. Non-A and non-B hepatitis (also referred to as type C hepatitis) accounts for 90% of transfusion-related hepatitis. Screening for HIV antibody, which started in 1985, and careful history taking of potential donors for risk factors for HIV have greatly reduced HIV transmission through blood transfusions. CMV is usually not a problem for immunocompetent patients but may be life threatening in immunodeficient patients. Clinical indications of CMV infection include mild fever, mild splenomegaly, and atypical serum lymphocytes. Immunodeficient patients require administration of CMV-negative blood products. ARDS and transfusion reaction acute lung injury (TRALI) are potential transfusion-related lung injuries that may occur.

TABLE 8-10   Blood and Blood Components

Product	Contents	Compatibility Required	Uses	Volume/Unit	Comments
Whole blood	RBCs, WBCs, platelets, plasma, and clotting factors	ABO, Rh specific. NOTE: In emergency situations, type-specific blood or O⁻ blood may be used	Restores blood volume and oxygen-carrying capacity	Approximately 500 mL	• Must be fresh (less than 4 hours old) to preserve platelet function • Administer over 2-4 hours • Best for hemorrhagic shock
Packed red blood cells	RBCs and 20% plasma	ABO, Rh specific preferred; ABO, Rh compatible required	Restores oxygen-carrying capacity	Approximately 250 mL	• Increases Hgb by 1 g/dL/unit and Hct by 2%-3%/unit; this change takes at least 6-12 hours • Administer over 2-4 hours
Washed red blood cells	RBCs and 20% plasma with fewer WBCs and platelets than packed RBCs	ABO, Rh specific preferred; ABO, Rh compatible required	Restores oxygen-carrying capacity in patients previously sensitized by transfusions	Approximately 250 mL	• As for packed RBCs • Must be administered within 24 hours of washing
Leukocyte-poor RBCs	RBCs, plasma but no leukocytes	ABO, Rh specific preferred; ABO, Rh compatible required	Restores oxygen-carrying capacity in patients susceptible to febrile reactions	Approximately 250 mL	• As for packed RBCs
Platelets	Platelets, WBCs, and plasma	ABO, Rh specific or compatible	Corrects low platelet levels to aid in clotting	Approximately 50 mL	• Administer 1 unit over 10 minutes • Will increase platelet count by 5000-10,000/mm³ • Agitate often as platelets tend to settle
Fresh frozen plasma (FFP)	Water, plasma proteins, and clotting factors	Rh compatibility required; ABO compatibility preferred	Expands blood volume; Restores clotting factor deficiencies; Contains no platelets	Approximately 250 mL	• Takes 20 minutes to thaw • Must be given within 6 hours of thawing • Administer 1 unit over 1-2 hours or more rapidly if for hemorrhage
Granulocytes	WBCs and small amount of plasma	ABO, Rh compatible; HLA (human leukocyte antigen) compatible if possible	Restores granulocytes in life-threatening granulocytopenia	Approximately 300 mL	• Administer rapidly • Chills and fever may occur; steroids and antihistamines may be given; meperidine may be used for shivering • Administer over 2-6 hours
Cryoprecipitate	VIII, XIII, fibrinogen, and fibronectin	ABO specific or compatible	Replaces clotting factors	Approximately 10 mL; usually 10 bags pooled	• Administer rapidly immediately after thawing • May administer 30 units at one time
Albumin	Albumin from plasma	No compatibility required	Provides volume expansion (no clotting factors)	5%: 200 mL or 500 mL 25%: 50 mL or 100 mL	• Administer 1 mL/min or more rapidly if patient is in shock • Chemically processed so no risk of hepatitis
Plasma protein fraction (PPF)	Albumin and globulin in saline solution	No compatibility required	Provides volume expansion (no clotting factors)	5%: 200 mL-500 mL	• Administer 10 mL/min • Chemically processed so no risk of hepatitis

TABLE 8-11   Types of Transfusion Reactions

Type of Reaction	Cause	Clinical Indications	Timing	Treatment
Febrile (nonhemolytic) NOTE: Most common type of transfusion reaction	Antigen-antibody reaction to WBCs, platelets, or plasma proteins in the blood product	• Fever (rise in temperature greater than 1° C) • Chills • Headache • Nausea, vomiting • Flushing • Anxiety • Muscle pain	Immediately or up to 6 hours after transfusion	• Stop transfusion • Keep vein open with saline • Notify physician and blood bank • Send blood specimens to blood bank • Antipyretics as indicated • Steroids may be prescribed • Washed blood or leukocyte-poor blood should be considered for future transfusions
Mild allergic (type I hypersensitivity reaction)	Allergic reaction to plasma-soluble antigen in blood product	• Flushing • Itching • Urticaria • Hives	During transfusion or up to 1 hour after transfusion	• If febrile, stop transfusion • If afebrile, slow transfusion to keep vein open until advised by physician • Notify physician and blood bank • Monitor vital signs • Antihistamines as prescribed
Anaphylaxis (type I hypersensitivity reaction)	Allergic reaction in patients with IgA deficiency sensitized to IgA through previous transfusion or pregnancy	• Anxiety • Urticaria • Facial edema • Dysphagia • Abdominal cramps, diarrhea • Urinary incontinence • Dyspnea • Stridor • Wheezing • Cyanosis • Chest pain or pulmonary edema may occur • Shock may occur • Cardiopulmonary arrest may occur	Immediately; after transfusion of only a few mL of blood	• Stop transfusion • Keep vein open with saline • Notify physician and blood bank • Oxygen • Antihistamines, steroids, and/or aqueous epinephrine as prescribed • Emergency airway and/or CPR may be necessary • Washed blood or leukocyte-poor blood or blood from IgA-deficient donor should be considered for future transfusions

Continued

TABLE 8-11   Types of Transfusion Reactions—cont'd

Type of Reaction	Cause	Clinical Indications	Timing	Treatment

Acute hemolytic (type II hypersensitivity reaction)	ABO group incompatibility; antibodies in recipient's plasma attach to antigens in transfused RBCs, causing RBC destruction	• Burning sensation along vein
		• Lumbar pain
		• Chills
		• Fever
		• Flushing
		• Nausea, vomiting
		• Tachycardia and/or tachypnea
		• Hypotension (may be the only sign in unconscious patient)
		• May have:
		  • Dyspnea
		  • Chest pain
		  • Hemoglobinemia or hemoglobinuria
		  • Anuria
		  • Disseminated intravascular coagulation
		• Shock may occur
		• Cardiopulmonary arrest may occur
			Usually within 15 minutes after initiation of transfusion, but may occur anytime during transfusion; may be delayed if Rh incompatibility	• Stop transfusion
				• Keep vein open with saline
				• Notify physician and blood bank
				• Send blood unit and blood sample from the patient to the blood bank immediately
				• Monitor vital signs and urine output
				• Fluids for shock as prescribed
				• Diuretics (usually mannitol) may be prescribed especially if hemoglobinuria occurs
				• Monitor for acute renal failure and shock
				• Request new crossmatch

Delayed hemolytic	Alloimmune response causes slow hemolysis	• Fever • Mild jaundice • Purpura • Anemia	Days to weeks after completion of transfusion	• Monitor urine output and Hgb and Hct levels
Noncardiac pulmonary edema (ARDS)	Donor antibodies react with recipient HLA antigen	• Fever, chills • Dyspnea • Cough • Crackles • Hypoxemia • Shock	During transfusion or shortly after the transfusion	• Stop transfusion • Administer oxygen • Intubation and mechanical ventilation may be necessary • Steroids may be prescribed

Reaction	Pathophysiology	Onset	Signs and Symptoms	Nursing Interventions
Transfusion reaction–acute lung injury (TRALI)	Unclear but postulated to be two mechanisms: an antibody-mediated and a soluble mediator-mediated	4-6 hours post plasma containing blood component administration	• Fever • Hypotension • Chills • Cyanosis • Nonproductive cough • Dyspnea	• Stop transfusion • Administer oxygen • Intubation and mechanical ventilation may be necessary • Steroids may be prescribed • Mild cases of TRALI may not be recognized. • Approximately 80% of patients improve both clinically and physiologically within 2 or 3 days with adequate supportive care.
Circulatory overload	Fluid administered faster than the cardiovascular system can accommodate	During transfusion or shortly after the transfusion	• Tachycardia • Hypertension • Headache • Jugular venous distention • Increased CVP • Dyspnea • Cough • Crackles	• Administer RBCs no more rapidly than 4 mL/kg/hr unless severe hemorrhage occurring • Slow or stop transfusion • Continue IV saline slowly if transfusion discontinued • Position the patient upright with legs over the side of bed • Oxygen as indicated • Diuretics or venous vasodilators as indicated
Sepsis	Transfusion of contaminated blood components (blood should be infused within 4 hours)	During or after transfusion	• Chills • Fever • Vomiting • Abdominal pain • Diarrhea (may be bloody) • Hypotension • Shock	• Stop the transfusion • Obtain cultures of the patient's blood and send with remaining blood to blood bank • Antibiotics as prescribed • Fluids or steroids as prescribed • Vasopressors may be needed
Graft versus host disease (GVHD)	Occurs in immunodeficient patients who receive lymphocytes; involves donor's lymphocytes mounting an attack against the recipient's tissues	Days to weeks after transfusion	• Fever • Rash • Stomatitis • Hepatitis • Severe diarrhea • Bone marrow suppression • Infection • Lymphadenopathy • Hepatosplenomegaly	• Steroids as prescribed • Methotrexate or azathioprine (Imuran) may be prescribed

8.5   Learning Activity

Identify the appropriate actions to take for suspected transfusion reaction in chronologic order.

1. _____
2. _____
3. _____
4. _____
5. _____
6. _____
7. _____
8. _____
9. _____

Answers to this activity can be found in the Answer Key.

Drugs Affecting Clotting

Drugs may affect clotting by interfering in multiple points in the intrinsic, extrinsic, or common pathways (Figure 8-4). The administration of more than one drug produces synergistic effects.

Platelet Aggregation Inhibitors

Many drugs inhibit platelet aggregation. Although this may be a desirable therapeutic effect for the specific purpose of impairing platelet aggregation to prevent the development of the platelet plug (i.e., white clot) and the intrinsic pathway (Box 8-7), this may also be an adverse effect (e.g., nonsteroidal antiinflammatory agents, quinidine).

Platelet aggregation inhibitors prevent platelet aggregation and platelet-mediated thrombosis. One mechanism of action is to impair the ability of the platelet to aggregate. The effect of this inhibition of platelet aggregation decreases after 24 hours. Another mechanism of action that occurs with these drugs is a decrease in the number of platelets called thrombotic thrombocytopenic purpura (TTP), though this is an undesirable effect. Treatment of TTP is discontinuance of the offending drug and may require administration of platelets. Monitor the patient on these medications for TTP and report petechiae, ecchymosis, or bleeding.

Cyclooxygenase (COX) inhibitors (e.g., aspirin) block synthesis of thromboxane A_2, inhibiting platelet aggregation. ADP pathway inhibitors (e.g., ticlopidine [Ticlid], clopidogrel [Plavix], and prasugrel [Effient]) block ADP from binding to its receptor, inhibiting platelet aggregation. Phosphodiesterase inhibitors (e.g., dipyridamole [Persantine] and cilostazol [Pletal]) increase cyclic adenosine monophosphate (cAMP) and lower levels of thromboxane A_2, inhibiting platelet aggregation.

Indications for oral antiplatelet agents include acute coronary syndrome, maintenance of coronary artery stent patency, and stroke prophylaxis for patients with carotid artery disease. The agents of choice for stent placement and stroke prophylaxis include clopidogrel (Plavix), aspirin, and the combination drug Aggrenox, which is dipyridamole and ASA. The agent used for a patient with peripheral arterial disease is cilostazol (Pletal). After vascular surgery, the patients are given dextran 40 as an antithrombotic to reduce blood viscosity, and as a volume expander in hypovolemia.

Intravenous platelet aggregation inhibitors are GP IIb/IIIa platelet receptor blockers (e.g., abciximab [ReoPro], eptifibatide [Integrilin], and tirofiban HCl [Aggrastat]). Each of these agents inhibits platelet aggregation, but there are differences between the agents (Table 8-13). Glycoprotein IIb/IIIa inhibitors block the glycoprotein IIb/IIIa platelet receptor. This interrupts the final common pathway for platelet aggregation by interfering with platelet aggregation via fibrinogen, vWF, and fibronectin. Indicated for acute coronary syndrome (ACS) with or without PCI, patients needing these agents require transfer to a higher level of care. Closely monitor the patient's bleeding time to determine the effectiveness of the agent. There is no specific reversal agent for these drugs, but treat bleeding with platelet transfusion.

Anticoagulants

Indirect thrombin inhibitors such as unfractionated heparin (UFH) or low-molecular-weight heparin (LMWH), and heparinoid (Orgaran) accelerate the formation of the antithrombin III-thrombin complex. The complex deactivates thrombin and prevents the conversion of fibrinogen to fibrin. The action of these drugs prevents new clot formation and extension of existing clots along with decreasing platelet aggregation. There is an unpredictable dose-response relationship with heparin, though the prediction of the response improves with weight dosing. There is a more predictable dose-response relationship with heparinoids. Clinical indications for these drugs include:

- Acute coronary syndrome (UFH or LMWH)
- Prevention or treatment of deep vein thrombosis (UFH, LMWH, or danaparoid)
- Pulmonary embolism (UFH or LMWH)
- Peripheral arterial emboli (UFH)
- Transient ischemic attack or ischemic stroke (UFH)
- Disseminated intravascular coagulation with clinical evidence of thromboembolism (UFH)

TABLE 8-12   Potential Adverse Effects of Blood Transfusion

Complication	Clinical Indications	Prevention/Treatment

Citrate intoxication and hypocalcemia caused by binding of citrate with calcium	• Paresthesia of fingertips and/or circumoral area
	• Chvostek sign
	• Trousseau sign
	• Muscle cramps, tremors
	• Increased deep tendon reflexes (DTRs) and carpopedal spasm
	• Abdominal cramps, biliary colic
	• Confusion or psychosis
	• Memory loss
	• Laryngospasm or stridor
	• Tetany (characterized by cramps, twitching of the muscles, sharp flexion of the wrist and ankle joints, and seizures)
	• ECG changes
	  • Prolonged QT interval
	  • Dysrhythmias
		• Monitor calcium in patients receiving multiple transfusions and/or patients with hepatic or renal disease
		• Administer 500 mg-1 g of calcium every 3-5 units of blood as prescribed

Hyperkalemia caused by hemolysis of stored blood and liberation of potassium
NOTE: The older the blood, the higher the potassium in the blood
	• Tachycardia progressing to bradycardia and cardiac arrest
	• Nausea, vomiting, intestinal colic, and diarrhea
	• Muscle weakness progressing to flaccid paralysis
	• Numbness and/or tingling of extremities
	• Increased DTRs
	• Fatigue
	• Lethargy, apathy, and/or mental confusion
	• Respiratory muscle weakness may cause hypopnea or dyspnea
	• Respiratory distress
	• Oliguria
	• Decreased contractility and cardiac output
	• ECG changes
	  • Tall, peaked T waves
	  • Wide QRS complex
	  • Prolonged PR interval
	  • Flattened to absent P wave
	  • Bradycardia
	  • Dysrhythmias
		• Monitor potassium closely in patients receiving stored blood (especially patients with renal insufficiency)
		• Dextrose and insulin may be prescribed acutely for patients with cardiac effects of hyperkalemia

Loss of 2,3-DPG (2,3-DPG is a byproduct of glucose metabolism on the hemoglobin molecule; banked [refrigerated] blood is low in 2,3-DPG; 2,3-DPG encourages unloading between hemoglobin and oxygen)	• Clinical indications of hypoxia (e.g., tachycardia, dysrhythmias, cyanosis, restlessness, and confusion)	• Especially a problem if massive amounts of banked blood are administered • Give fresh whole blood when possible for patients in need of multiple transfusions
Ammonia intoxication (occurs in older blood; especially a problem for patients with hepatic disease)	• Decreased cardiac output: hypotension • Confusion • Altered level of consciousness • Elevated serum ammonia	• Avoid use of older blood, especially for massive transfusion • Monitor for ammonia intoxication in patients with hepatic disease
Dilutional coagulopathy	• Prolonged PT and aPTT • Bleeding from needle site and/or wound	• Administer 2 units FFP and/or platelets for every 10 units of packed RBCs as prescribed
Hypothermia	• Decrease in body temperature • Decrease in tissue delivery of oxygen caused by shift of the oxyhemoglobin dissociation curve to the left resulting in increased affinity between hemoglobin and oxygen	• Warm blood to 35°-37° C if large quantities of blood are being administered

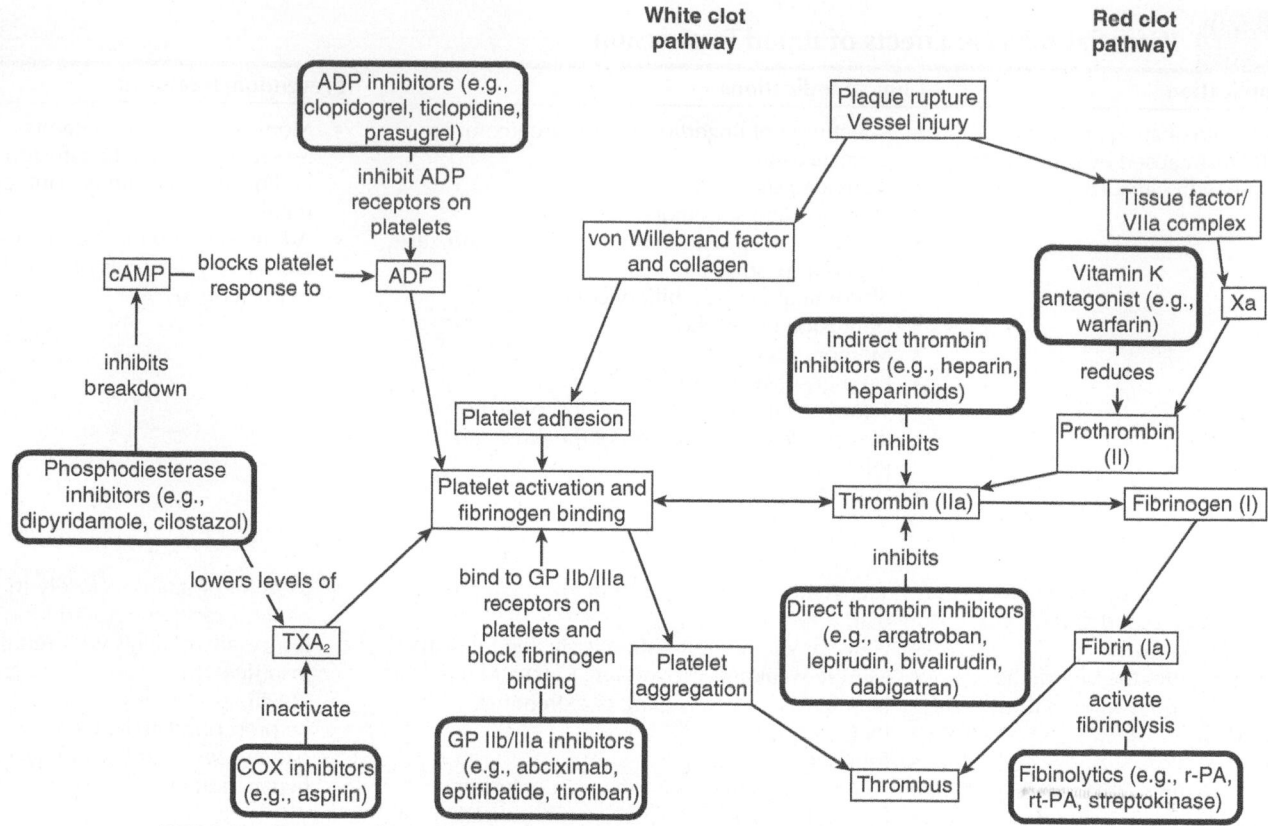

FIGURE 8-4 Drugs that affect clotting: Effects on pathways to thrombus formation. (From Dennison, R. D. [2013]. *Pass CCRN!* [4th ed.]. St. Louis, MO: Elsevier.)

BOX 8-7

Drugs Used to Decrease Platelet Aggregation

- COX inhibitors (e.g., aspirin)
- Phosphodiesterase inhibitors (e.g., dipyridamole [Persantine] and cilostazol [Pletal])
- ADP pathway inhibitors (e.g., ticlopidine [Ticlid], clopidogrel [Plavix], and prasugrel [Effient])
- GP IIb/IIIa platelet receptor blockers (e.g., abciximab [ReoPro], eptifibatide [Integrilin], and tirofiban HCl [Aggrastat])
- Combination agents (e.g., dipyridamole and aspirin [Aggrenox])
- Dextran 40 (LMD)

- Maintenance of arterial patency after PCI or fibrinolytic therapy (UFH or heparinoid)
- Maintenance of arterial line patency (UFH)
- Patients with or at risk of HIT having PCI

There are some important differences between UFH and LMWH to keep in mind. LMWH is more potent at inactivating factor Xa than inactivating thrombin. LMWH has a longer half-life than UFH. The half-life of LMWH is 4 to 6 hours compared with 1 to 2 hours for UFH. LMWH has 90% bioavailability, and UFH has only 30% bioavailability, which allows a more predictable anticoagulant response for LMWH. There is less risk of HIT with LMWH than UFH. The cost of LMWH is greater, but there is not a need for ongoing laboratory monitoring. The aPTT and the ACT laboratory parameter evaluate the therapeutic effect of UFH. With the use of

LMWH, monitoring of coagulation parameters is not required but may prolong the PT and aPTT. The reversal agent is protamine sulfate. A dose of 1 mg of protamine neutralizes approximately 100 units of heparin. Administer protamine slowly to avoid hypotension.

Direct thrombin inhibitors such as argatroban (Acova) and bivalirudin (Angiomax) inhibit thrombin activity. There is a predictable dose-response relationship. Administer argatroban for the treatment of HIT and associated thromboembolic complications. Administer bivalirudin for the treatment of acute coronary syndrome undergoing PCI. In addition, bivalirudin is being evaluated for use in ischemic stroke, DIC, and MI. There is no reversal agent for direct thrombin inhibitors and the aPTT or ACT evaluates the therapeutic effect. The oral anticoagulants, such as warfarin (Coumadin), limit the availability of vitamin K, which is necessary for the formation of factors II (prothrombin), VII, IX, and X, along with the anticoagulant proteins C and S. Warfarin prevents development of a clot and prevents extension of an existing clot and secondary thromboembolic complications. The indications for warfarin (Coumadin) include:

- Deep vein thrombosis
- Valvular heart disease
- Atrial dysrhythmias
- Postvalve replacement

The reversal agent for warfarin (Coumadin) is vitamin K, so it is important to note that a consistent intake of green leafy vegetables prevents a fluctuation in PT levels and allows for dose stabilization. The PT and INR evaluate the therapeutic effect of warfarin.

TABLE 8-13	Differences between the Intravenous Antiplatelet Agents		
Drug	**Half-Life**	**Duration of Inhibition**	**Renal Insufficiency Dosing**
Abciximab (Reopro)	10-30 minutes	Most significant, prolonged 18-36 hours to a week	No adjustment
Tirofiban (Aggrastat)	120 minutes	1-2 hours after cessation of infusion	Requires adjustment
Eptifibatide (Integrilin)	150 minutes	1-2 hours after cessation of infusion	Requires adjustment with a creatinine >2 mg/dL Contraindicated if serum creatinine is 4 mg/dL

Fibrinolytics

Fibrinolytics activate plasminogen to accelerate clot lysis. Recombinant plasminogen activators such as alteplase (Activase), reteplase (Retavase), and tenecteplase (TNKase) activate plasminogen to plasmin, which is the active agent that breaks and degrades the fibrin clot. In essence, these drugs speed up the normal process to allow early reperfusion. The need for fibrinolytics requires transfer of the patient to a higher level of care.

Fibrinolytic drugs are indicated for a number of conditions. These drugs are very effective in preventing heart damage to patients having a myocardial infarction if administered within 6 hours of infarct or the patient is still having ischemic chest pain. Fibrinolytics are also indicated for an ischemic stroke. Treatment should be initiated within 3 hours of symptoms. It is necessary to perform a CT to rule out hemorrhagic stroke and have that CT interpreted within the 3-hour window before administering the fibrinolytic. Drugs in this classification also treat patients with a massive pulmonary embolism.

Bleeding initiates a series of normal reactions that stop blood flow and maintains balance within the system. The reactions include reflex vasoconstriction, platelet aggregation, and blood coagulation, which cause blood to solidify, and clot resolution, which returns blood to the fluid state. In many clinical situations, drugs slow or stop this process, with the goal of preventing tissue damage from the decreased blood flow that occurs when the clotting process cuts off blood supply to an area. All drugs that alter coagulation interfere with the normal protective reflexes. The dangers of eliminating reflexes could include serious or even fatal bleeding episodes. Early identification of problems, transfer to and from higher levels of care, monitoring for adverse effects, and discharge planning require knowledge about the types of drugs and the administration, adverse effects, and nursing implications of drugs that affect clotting (Table 8-14).

ANEMIA

Anemia is a condition that develops when the blood lacks enough healthy RBCs or hemoglobin. Anemia is the most common blood condition in the United States. It affects about 3.5 million Americans. Women and people with chronic diseases are at increased risk of anemia. Certain forms of anemia are hereditary. Women in the childbearing years are particularly susceptible to iron-deficiency anemia because of the blood loss from menstruation and the increased blood supply demands during pregnancy. Older adults also may have a greater risk of

developing anemia because of poor diet and other medical conditions. Broad definitions of anemias include three groups:

- Anemia caused by blood loss
- Anemia caused by decreased or faulty RBC production
- Anemia caused by destruction of RBCs

Acute blood loss results in dramatic alterations in hemodynamic status and often needs emergent interventions. Chronic blood loss is more insidious and the body has time to compensate. Inadequate production of RBCs may be due to a number of disorders such as aplastic anemia, chronic inflammatory disease, end-stage renal disease, or malignancy, as well as chemotherapy and radiation treatments, dietary deficiencies, bone marrow transplantation, and certain drugs. An increase in the destruction of RBCs may be due to an immune-mediated response, hereditary spherocytosis, hemoglobin defects like sickle cell anemia, and mechanical trauma from replacement heart valves.

8.6 Learning Activity

Match the cause of the anemia to the pathophysiology.

_____ 1. Esophageal varices
_____ 2. Radiation or drugs
_____ 3. Hereditary
_____ 4. Malignancy
_____ 5. Lead poisoning
_____ 6. Crohn disease
_____ 7. Anorexia nervosa
_____ 8. Mismatched blood transfusion reaction
_____ 9. Trauma
_____10. Chronic kidney disease

a. Blood loss
b. Decreased or faulty red blood cell production
c. Destruction of red blood cells

Answers to this activity can be found in the Answer Key.

Hemoglobin is a main part of RBCs and binds oxygen. If there are too few or abnormal RBCs or the hemoglobin is abnormal or low, the cells in the body will not get enough oxygen. Symptoms of anemia occur because organs are not getting what they need to function properly. Because the main function of the RBC is oxygenation, anemia results in varying degrees of hypoxia.

TABLE 8-14   Selected Drugs That Affect Clotting

Drug	Administration	Adverse Effects	Nursing Implications
Indirect Thrombin Inhibitors			

Unfraction-ated heparin (UFH)	• Subcutaneous: Usually prophylactic, dose is 5000 units every 12 hours (also called *miniheparin*)
	• IV injection: Usually 80 units/kg (maximum 10,000 units) followed by infusion (only 60 units/kg recommended if patient is receiving fibrinolytics or GP IIb/IIIa inhibitors)
	• IV infusion: mix 25,000 units in 500 mL (50 units/mL) and infuse at 18 units/kg/hr (maximum 1000 units/hr) (only 12 units/kg recommended if patient is receiving fibrinolytics or GP IIb/IIIa inhibitors); dose is adjusted to achieve aPTT of 1.5-2.5 times the laboratory control
	• Note: The trend in IV weight-dosed heparin is to decrease the amount of heparin (60 units/kg for injection followed by 12 units/kg/hr for infusion) and desirable aPTT (45-60 seconds)
	• Maximum: 40,000 units/day
		• Hemorrhage with excessive aPTT
		• Hypertension or hypotension
		• Hypersensitivity reaction including bronchospasm
		• Fever
		• Hepatitis
		• Hyperkalemia especially in patients with renal failure
		• Thrombocytopenia (caused by HIT)
			• Monitor aPTT and platelet count, and for signs of hemorrhage
			  • Note petechiae and request platelet count if petechiae noted; heparin usually discontinued if platelet count is less than 100,000/mm^3
			  — Administer argatroban as prescribed for HIT
			• Note contraindications: known hypersensitivity, active bleeding, blood dyscrasias (except DIC), suspected intracranial hemorrhage, severe hypertension, peptic ulcer disease, open wounds, recent surgery, endocarditis, shock, and threatened abortion
			• Use cautiously in alcoholism, liver disease, renal disease, and in older adults
			• Monitor oral secretions, sputum, vomitus, NG aspirate, stool, and urine for blood
			• Ensure that protamine sulfate (antidote) is available
			• Avoid IM, arterial, or venous punctures if at all possible
			• Hold pressure for longer than usual if punctures are necessary
			• Do not discontinue suddenly: warfarin usually will have already been started and the PT within therapeutic range before heparin is discontinued
			• Do not aspirate before subcutaneous administration and do not massage after administration
			• Note that NTG interacts with heparin causing more heparin to be required to achieve a therapeutic aPTT; monitor aPTT closely with significant NTG dosage changes or discontinuance

Low-molecular-weight heparin (LMWH)	Enoxaparin (Lovenox) • SC: 30 mg bid Dalteparin sodium (Fragmin) • SC: 2500 units daily starting 1-2 hours before surgery and repeated qd for 5-10 days postoperatively Ardeparin (Normiflo) • SC: 50 antifactor Xa units/kg every 12 hours beginning the evening before surgery and continued until the patient is ambulatory Tinzaparin sodium (Innohep) • SC: 175 antifactor Xa units/kg daily for approximately 6 days or until adequate anticoagulation with warfarin	• Bleeding • Epidural or spinal hematoma (especially when used with patients with epidural or spinal anesthesia) • Fever • Elevation of liver enzymes • Thrombocytopenia • Chest pain	• Note that LMWH does not require routine laboratory monitoring because it does not usually alter PT or aPTT • Contraindications and cautions are as for heparin • Obtain baseline platelet count; monitor for petechiae • Monitor oral secretions, sputum, vomitus, NG aspirate, stool, and urine for blood • Ensure that protamine sulfate (antidote) is available • Avoid IM, arterial, or venous punctures if at all possible • Hold pressure for longer than usual if punctures are necessary • Administer deep subcutaneously but avoid IM injection

Rivaroxaban (Xarelto)	Oral tablet 15 mg and 20 mg with food; take 10-mg tablets with or without food • Nonvalvular atrial fibrillation: For patients with CrCl >50 mL/min: 20 mg orally once daily with the evening meal; for patients with CrCl 15 to 50 mL/min: 15 mg orally once daily with the evening meal • Treatment of DVT, PE, and reduction in the risk of recurrence of DVT and of PE: 15 mg orally twice daily with food for the first 21 days for the initial treatment of acute DVT or PE. After the initial treatment period, 20 mg orally once daily with food for the remaining treatment and the long-term reduction in the risk of recurrence of DVT and of PE • Prophylaxis of DVT following hip or knee replacement surgery: 10 mg orally once daily with or without food • Dosage form: tablets: 10 mg, 15 mg, and 20 mg	• Bleeding • Hypersensitivity reactions	• Risk of bleeding; can cause serious and fatal bleeding • Promptly evaluate signs and symptoms of blood loss • Use with caution in pregnant women due to the potential for obstetric hemorrhage and/or emergent delivery • Use not recommended with prosthetic heart valves • Avoid concomitant use with combined P-gp and strong CYP3A4 inhibitors (e.g., ketoconazole, itraconazole, lopinavir/ritonavir, ritonavir, indinavir, conivaptan) • Avoid concomitant use with drugs that are combined P-gp and strong CYP3A4 inducers (e.g., carbamazepine, phenytoin, rifampin, St. John's wort)
Fondaparinux (Arixtra)	• Prophylaxis of deep vein thrombosis: Arixtra 2.5 mg subcutaneously once daily after hemostasis has been established. The initial dose should be given no earlier than 6 to 8 hours after surgery and continued for 5 to 9 days. For patients undergoing hip fracture surgery, extended prophylaxis up to 24 additional days is recommended. Treatment of deep vein thrombosis and pulmonary embolism: Arixtra 5 mg (body weight <50 kg), 7.5 mg (50 to 100 kg), or 10 mg (>100 kg) subcutaneously once daily. Treatment should continue for at least 5 days until INR 2 to 3 achieved with warfarin sodium. • For subcutaneous use only; do not mix with other injections or infusions. • Single-dose, prefilled syringes containing 2.5 mg, 5 mg, 7.5 mg, or 10 mg of fondaparinux.	• Bleeding complications • Thrombocytopenia • Mild local irritation at injection site • Bleeding, rash, and pruritus may occur following subcutaneous injection • Anemia, insomnia, increased wound drainage, hypokalemia, dizziness, hypotension, confusion, bullous eruption, hematoma, postoperative hemorrhage, and purpura may occur	• Do not administer the initial dose earlier than 6 to 8 hours after surgery • Periodic routine complete blood counts (including platelet counts), serum creatinine level, and stool occult blood tests are recommended • The packaging (needle guard) contains dry natural rubber and may cause allergic reactions in latex-sensitive individuals • Risk of bleeding is increased with reduced renal or hepatic function • Spinal or epidural hematomas, which may result in long-term or permanent paralysis, can occur with the use of anticoagulants and neuraxial (spinal/epidural) anesthesia or spinal puncture; the risk of these events may be higher with postoperative use of indwelling epidural catheters or concomitant use of other drugs affecting hemostasis, such as NSAIDs

Direct Thrombin Inhibitors

Argatroban (Acova)	• IV infusion: mix 250 mg in 250 mL of normal saline (1 mg/mL); administer initially at 2 mcg/kg/min; no loading dose is given • Maximum: 10 mcg/kg/min • Reduce dosage in hepatic disease; start at 0.5 mcg/kg/min	• Bleeding: GI, genitourinary, or intracranial • Allergic reaction • Dyspnea • Hypotension • Fever • Diarrhea • Sepsis • Cardiac arrest	• Monitor PT, aPTT, CBC, and for signs of bleeding • Contraindications and cautions are as for heparin • Obtain baseline platelet count and aPTT; monitor aPTT every 4 hours • Anticoagulant effects are increased in patients receiving platelet aggregation inhibitors, fibrinolytics, or other anticoagulants • Monitor oral secretions, sputum, vomitus, NG aspirate, stool, and urine for blood • Avoid IM, arterial, or venous punctures if at all possible • Hold pressure for longer than usual if punctures are necessary • Protect infusion from direct sunlight

Continued

TABLE 8-14 Selected Drugs That Affect Clotting—cont'd

Drug	Administration	Adverse Effects	Nursing Implications
Bivalirudin (Angiomax)	• IV injection: 0.75-1 mg/kg followed by IV infusion • IV infusion: mix 250 mg in 250 mL of normal saline (1 mg/mL) and infuse at 1.75-2.5 mg/kg/hr for 4 hours then decrease infusion to 0.2 mg/kg/hr for an additional 14-20 hours if needed	• Bleeding • Back pain • Generalized pain • Headache • Nausea • Hypotension	• Monitor PT, aPTT, CBC, and for signs of bleeding • Contraindications and cautions are as for heparin • Obtain baseline platelet count and aPTT; ACT may also be used • Anticoagulant effects are increased in patients receiving platelet aggregation inhibitors, fibrinolytics, or other anticoagulants • Monitor oral secretions, sputum, vomitus, NG aspirate, stool, and urine for blood • Avoid IM, arterial, or venous punctures if at all possible • Hold pressure for longer than usual if punctures are necessary • Protect infusion from direct sunlight
Dabigatran (Pradaxa)	Nonvalvular atrial fibrillation: • For patients with CrCl >30 mL/min: 150 mg orally twice daily • For patients with CrCl 15-30 mL/min: 75 mg orally twice daily Treatment of DVT and PE: • For patients with CrCl >30 mL/min: 150 mg orally twice daily after 5-10 days of parenteral anticoagulation Reduction in the risk of recurrence of DVT and PE: • For patients with CrCl >30 mL/min: 150 mg orally twice daily after previous treatment • Dosage forms: Capsules: 75 mg and 150 mg	• Gastritis-like symptoms • Bleeding	• Instruct patients not to chew, break, or open capsules • Review recommendations for converting to or from other oral or parenteral anticoagulants • Temporarily discontinue Pradaxa before invasive or surgical procedures when possible, then restart promptly
Vitamin K Antagonists			

Warfarin (Coumadin, Panwarfin)	• PO: 2-10 mg daily depending on PT and international normalized ratio (INR)
	  • INR 2-3
	    • MI
	    • DVT prophylaxis or treatment
	    • Pulmonary embolus
	    • Valvular heart disease
	    • Atrial fibrillation
	    • Tissue heart valve
	  • INR 2.5-3.5
	    • Mechanical heart valve
		• Hemorrhage with excessive PT
		• Agranulocytosis, leukopenia
		• Hepatitis
		• Diarrhea
		• Fever
		• Rash
		• Skin necrosis: occurs during the first several days of warfarin therapy; lesions occur on extremities, breasts, trunk, and/or penis
		• Cholesterol microemboli causing purple toe syndrome
			• Monitor PT and for signs of hemorrhage
			• Note contraindications: known hypersensitivity, bleeding disorders, leukemia, peptic ulcer disease, liver disease, severe hypertension, endocarditis, acute nephritis, blood dyscrasias, eclampsia, suspected intracranial hemorrhage, open wounds, recent surgery, and threatened abortion
			• Use cautiously in alcoholism, pregnancy, lactation, during menses, during use of any drainage tube, in older adults, or in any patient in whom slight bleeding is dangerous
			• Ensure that vitamin K (AquaMephyton) is available
			• Avoid IM, arterial, or venous punctures if at all possible
			• Hold pressure for longer than usual if punctures are necessary
			• Monitor oral secretions, sputum, vomitus, NG aspirate, stool, and urine for blood
			• Do not discontinue suddenly
			• Teach patient to avoid trauma and increase amounts of vitamin K (green leafy vegetables), and how to monitor for bleeding
			• Teach the patient to report fever or rash; usually necessitates discontinuance

The body compensates for anemia by increasing cardiac output and respiratory rate, redistributing blood supply to the brain and heart, and increasing the kidney's production of erythropoietin.

All patients with anemia regardless of the type have tachycardia at rest from the patient's baseline. Keep in mind, the heart rate will increase in patients on beta-blockers, but may not go over the normal heart rate parameter of 80 to 100 bpm due to the medication. Tachycardia, hypotension, and orthostatic changes in vital signs may be present. Other predominant symptoms include fatigue, dyspnea, bone pain, altered mental status, dizziness, inability to concentrate, and confusion. The patient may appear with pallor or jaundice, and have tenderness with hepatosplenomegaly noted upon palpation and percussion.

In patients with anemia, urine and stool may test positive for blood. In severe anemia, the Hgb level is less than 7 g/dL and the Hct is less than 23%. Other findings vary with the cause of the anemia and include an increased reticulocyte count, decreased serum iron level, increased or decreased total iron-binding capacity, decreased ferritin levels, increased indirect bilirubin, and a positive Coombs test. Special types of radiographs detect the source of bleeding. A bone marrow biopsy evaluates the RBC production or detects malignancy.

The goals of care are focused on maintaining adequate gas exchange, avoiding dehydration due to bleeding, and controlling the level of fatigue. Patients with anemia have many basic nursing needs during the course of recovery. Maintain the patient in a high Fowler's position to alleviate shortness of breath and dyspnea. Provide adequate nutrition intake of iron, vitamin B_{12}, and folate. Provide education regarding the administration of iron. Administer oxygen as prescribed especially if the patient is dyspneic or having chest pain. Administer blood transfusion therapy if prescribed and monitor the patient for potential complications of the anemia itself along with the various treatments provided. Promote rest, assist the patient as needed, and protect from injury. Administer analgesics along with hydration as required in sickle cell crisis. The major complications of anemia are shortness of breath due to diminished oxygen-carrying capacity, and safety issues related to the patient's weakness and fatigue.

IMMUNOSUPPRESSION

Immunosuppression refers to a defect in the immunologic system that puts the patient at increased risk for infection. Although there are primary forms of immune dysfunction, the majority of cases of immunosuppression occur due to a complication of an underlying disease and/or treatments. Various drugs prescribed to suppress one part of the immune system may have untoward effects on other parts of the hematologic and immunologic systems. These drugs act primarily on the B cells and T cells and suppress not only the response to the allograft but also the patient's ability to fight bacteria, viruses, fungi, parasites, and neoplasms. The risk factors and etiology of immunosuppression include drugs, genetics, decreased neutrophil production, and HIV infection.

Neutropenia occurs when the total number of neutrophils is abnormally low. The greater the length of time neutropenia exists, the greater the risk for infection. Often, hospital admission is required when a patient is diagnosed with sepsis or acute leukemia complicated by neutropenia. The most common sites of infection are the lung, blood, skin, urinary tract, and GI tract.

Decreased neutrophil production occurs when the bone marrow infiltrates with malignant cells. In addition, recent history of high doses of antineoplastic chemotherapy, radiation therapy to the bone, and bone marrow transplantation may be the cause of a decrease in production of neutrophils. Neutropenia is also a factor in autoimmune disorders such as systemic lupus erythematosus (SLE) and rheumatoid arthritis (RA). Neutropenic patients do not have an adequate WBC to mount a response; therefore the classic indications of infection may be absent. Overwhelming sepsis causes increased use of the neutrophils. The clinical presentation of a patient with immunosuppression may include the following:

- Report of malaise, fever, chills, and night sweats
- Temperature exceeding 101° F (38.3° C)
- Tachycardia and hypotension
- Confusion
- Sore throat, pain with swallowing, and lymphadenopathy
- Dyspnea, shortness of breath, cough, crackles, and rhonchi
- Abdominal pain, diarrhea, and pain with urination and/or defecation
- Sinus pain and headache

The absolute neutrophil count (ANC) is the measure of the number of infection-fighting WBCs in the blood. The normal neutrophil count is 2500 to 6000. When there are 1000 or fewer neutrophils, the risk of infection is increased. When the ANC is lower than 500, neutropenia exists and the risk for getting a serious infection is present. Radiology procedures are noncontributory to the diagnosis of neutropenia, but may indicate the source of infection secondary to the neutropenia. A bone marrow biopsy would confirm the diagnosis.

The priority of collaborative care management is to anticipate the patient trajectory and support the patient until the WBCs are available to fight infection. Infection will result in febrile episodes. Protect the patient from sources of community or nosocomial infections and implement the following neutropenic precautions:

- Assess the daily ANC, WBC count, and differential
- Bathe to counteract infection by normal flora
- Inspect skin and mucous membranes every 4 hours
- Assess invasive sites every 4 hours for signs of portal infection
- Obtain cultures from any new sites with drainage
- Administer antibiotics as prescribed
- Monitor and supplement nutritional intake of vitamins, proteins, and fats
- Monitor, encourage, and supplement free water intake
- Anticipate a daily chest radiography for patients prone to pneumonia
- Encourage deep breathing and change of position every 2 to 4 hours
- Place gifts of fresh flowers and plants outside of the patient's area, yet try to keep them within the patient's vision
- Ensure that all patients' visitors are free of communicable disease
- Recommend private rooms for all patients at risk of infection

HIV INFECTION

HIV type 1 is a retrovirus that infects cells expressing CD4 on their cell membranes, primarily T_{11} lymphocytes. The HIV copies its RNA into the host cell's DNA and then remains quiet until activation of the host cell produces an immune response. Activation of the host CD4 cells also initiates replication and production of the HIV RNA when released into the circulation, infecting other cells expressing CD4.

Intimate sexual contact, contaminated needles, or contaminated blood products transmit HIV. A mother transmits HIV to the fetus and breast-feeding transmits the virus from mother to child.

Clinical manifestations of HIV infection (Box 8-8) vary depending on the disease stage. The initial stage of HIV infection lasts 4 to 8 weeks. High levels of the virus are in the blood and the patient experiences generalized flu-like symptoms. The virus then enters a latent stage. The virus remains inactive in the infected, resting CD4 cells, replicating only upon activation of the immune response. At this point, the level of the virus is high in the lymph nodes, but low in the blood. The T_c cells, which express CD8, are not infected by HIV. The B cells attempt to destroy the virus, but the T_c and the B cells are inadequate by themselves without T_{11} support. The duration of the asymptomatic latent stage ranges between 2 and 12 years. During this time, the number of CD4 cells declines. It is in the third stage that the patient begins to have opportunistic infections. The CD4 levels are usually below $500/mm^3$ and continue to decline while the level in the blood increases. This third stage lasts about 2 to 3 years. Once the CD4 count drops below $200/mm^3$,

Clinical Indications of HIV/AIDS

Initial Indications of HIV Infection
- Fever
- Headache
- Muscle aches
- Rash
- Chills
- Sore throat
- Mouth or genital ulcers
- Swollen lymph glands (mainly on the neck)
- Joint pain
- Night sweats
- Diarrhea

Indications of HIV Infection
- Fever
- Fatigue
- Swollen lymph nodes (often one of the first signs of HIV infection)
- Diarrhea
- Weight loss
- Cough
- Shortness of breath

Indications of Progression to AIDS
- Soaking night sweats
- Shaking chills or fever higher than 100° F (38° C) for several weeks
- Cough
- Shortness of breath
- Chronic diarrhea
- Persistent white spots or unusual lesions on tongue or in mouth
- Headaches
- Persistent, unexplained fatigue
- Blurred and distorted vision
- Weight loss
- Skin rashes or bumps

the disease has advanced to AIDS. Although HIV/AIDS infection was once considered a certain death sentence, early detection and treatment can now mean a normal life span for otherwise healthy Americans. People who begin taking antiretroviral drugs earlier live longer. By lowering the number of viral cells in the blood, antiretroviral therapy, or ART, also helps to prevent HIV transmission (Miller & Hodder, 2014). Assess for the presence of HIV when a patient presents with a known social history of IV drug abuse with shared needles, unprotected sexual conduct, and a history of blood transfusions in addition to general symptoms of fatigue, night sweats, sore throat, dyspnea, pain, and frequent occurrence of infections. Patients with HIV suffer from weight loss, diarrhea, elevated temperatures, skin and mucous membrane lesions, possible cachexia, and lymphadenopathy. Tachycardia, hypotension, and adventitious breath sounds are also usually present upon presentation.

A positive western blot test determines the diagnosis. The ELISA test is a less expensive screening for the HIV antibody. If the ELISA results in a false positive, a western blot confirms the diagnosis. In addition, if CD4 counts are less than $500/mm^3$, the HIV patient may demonstrate anergy with no reaction to a skin test panel. There may be infection present with unusual or opportunistic organisms (i.e., *Pneumocystis jiroveci*).

The goals of collaborative care for HIV patients are focused on education about prevention of the spread of HIV infection, maintenance of universal precautions, and containment of opportunistic infections. Address the patient's major psychosocial needs by helping the patient express fear and grief and deal with social isolation. The collaborative care team needs to understand the trajectory of the disease and provide for the needs of patients throughout the clinical course. Other aspects of care focus on nutrition, infection control, pharmacologic therapies, and ethical issues. In addition, the care team needs to monitor the patient frequently and implement treatment regimens as needed if the patient develops AIDS, dementia complex, and/or opportunistic infections. If dementia occurs, institute fall precautions and support for cognitive, motor, and behavioral dysfunction. Manage infections with antibiotics and antiretroviral therapy such as the following:

- Zidovudine
- Didanosine (ddI, Videx)
- Zalcitabine (ddC, Hivid)
- Stavudine (d4T, Zerit)
- Protease inhibitors: saquinavir (Invirase), indinavir (Crixivan), nelfinavir (Viracept), and/or ritonavir (Norvir)

ORGAN TRANSPLANT AND REJECTION

Transplantation is the act of transferring cells, tissues, or organs from one site to another. Transplantation of an organ (e.g., kidney, liver, heart, lung, pancreas) from a donor corrects a malfunction of an organ system. However, the immune system remains the most formidable barrier to transplantation as a routine medical treatment. The immune system has developed elaborate and effective mechanisms to combat foreign agents. These mechanisms are also involved in the rejection of transplanted organs, since the recipient's immune system recognizes the transplant as foreign.

Rejections occur through various mechanisms. A type III hypersensitivity reaction in the blood vessels of a graft occurs immediately after the transplant. A cytotoxic T lymphocyte can directly attack the allograft, which results in an acute rejection within days of the transplant. The B-lymphocytes can make antibodies against the allograft. The antibodies activate the complement pathways and attract platelets. Fibrin accumulates on the transplanted tissue, causing ischemia, which slowly rejects the transplant over months and years. In an attempt to prevent rejection, matching human leukocyte antigen (HLA) before transplantation and immunosuppressive therapy are the mainstays of the transplant regimen.

Allogeneic bone marrow transplant (BMT) is different from solid organ transplantation. In allogeneic BMT, the immune system itself is being transplanted into a new host; therefore, it may attack any tissue in the new host, resulting in graft versus host disease (GVHD). Because GVHD is usually a limited (although serious) problem, the majority of patients receiving allogeneic BMT can eventually discontinue immunosuppressive therapy. In patients receiving solid organs, the host's own immune system attacks the donated organ, necessitating life-long treatment with immunosuppressive agents.

The clinical indications of rejection include malaise, poor appetite, myalgia, and tenderness of the allograft. There may be swelling of the allograft and temperature exceeding 101° F (38.3° C).

Diagnostic tests for rejection are specific to the organ transplanted. The goal of collaborative care focuses on anticipating the patient trajectory with knowledge of when the various types of rejections occur and frequent monitoring for complications. Provide immunosuppression to halt the rejection if possible.

Understanding these mechanisms is important, as it aids in understanding the clinical features of rejection and, hence, in making an early diagnosis and delivering appropriate treatment. Knowledge of these mechanisms is also critical in developing strategies to minimize rejection and in developing new drugs and treatments that blunt the effects of the immune system on transplanted organs, thereby ensuring longer survival of these organs.

CANCER AND ONCOLOGIC EMERGENCIES

Cancer is a disease of cells characterized by abnormal cell growth, which begins with DNA damage. Either inherited mutations or acquired DNA damaging agents cause cancer (Figure 8-5). There is no single cause of cancer but rather there are many factors. Some predisposing factors to the development of cancer are genetic predisposition, tobacco, alcohol, hormones, immune deficiency, age, occupation, x-rays, sunlight, and a diet high in fat. While normal cell growth is regulated in response to need, malignant cells have disorderly division and uncontrolled growth pattern, are nonencapsulated, tend to metastasize, and often recur after treatment. Tumors are endogenous and classified by their tissue of origin. Malignant tumors (Box 8-9) draw nourishment from the body while contributing nothing to its functions. Grading of tumors involves categorizing tumors according to cell differentiation and the relationship to the tissue of order.

The stages of cancer are initiation, promotion, progression, and metastasis. The initial mutation occurs in the initiation

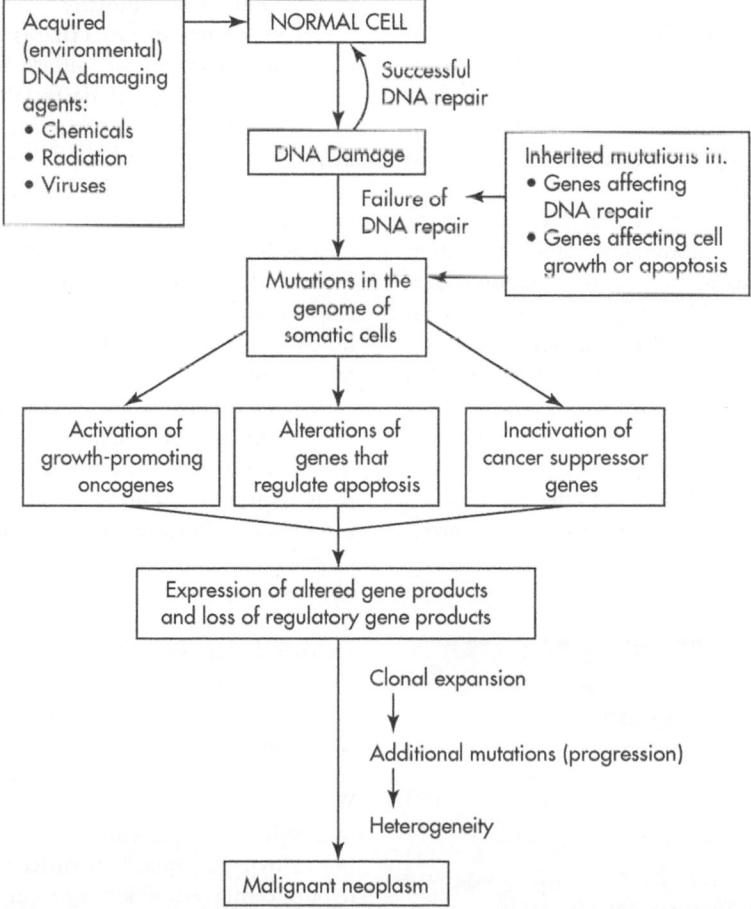

FIGURE 8-5 Pathophysiology of the development of malignancy. (From Price, S. A., & Wilson, L. M. [2003]. *Pathophysiology: Clinical concepts of disease processes* [6th ed.]. St. Louis, MO: Mosby.)

stage. The promotion stage occurs when the body's defenses fail to kill the mutations, but rather are stimulated to divide. In the progression stage, the tumor cells compete with one another and become more aggressive as they develop more mutations. Metastasis occurs through lymphatic or vascular circulation, direct extension, or seeding. The most common sites of metastasis are the lung, liver, bone, and brain. Prognostic factors include tumor size, nodal involvement, and metastasis. Staging involves categorizing the disease progression and includes the presence or absence of metastasis, and amount of organ involvement.

The patient with cancer may have a family history of cancer. He or she may present with changes in appetite, weight loss, energy level changes, or pain. Physical examination may include the presence of a mass and/or enlargement of lymph nodes. The seven warning signs of cancer include:

- Change in usual bowel and bladder function
- A sore that does not heal
- Unusual bleeding or discharge
- Thickening or a lump in the breast or elsewhere
- Indigestion or dysphagia
- Obvious change in wart or mole
- Nagging cough or hoarseness

Clinical manifestations of cancer are related to changes in organ function, the local effects of the tumor (e.g., compression of nerves or veins, or GI obstruction), ectopic hormones (i.e., paraneoplastic disorders), and nonspecific indications of tissue breakdown (e.g., weight loss or pathologic fractures). Diagnostic tests for cancer include serum studies such as CBC, platelet count, blood chemistries, and CEA. Biopsy and cytology studies are definitive tests used to identify presence of malignancy and cell type. Radiologic studies, such as x-rays, CT scans, MRI, radioisotope scanning, ultrasound, and thermography, are also important for screening and staging. Endoscopic examinations may also be important for screening and biopsy.

Collaborative management of cancer may include surgery, radiation, chemotherapy, and/or biotherapy. Cancer treatment may include a single type of treatment or a combination of surgery, radiation, chemotherapy, and biotherapy. Surgery includes excision of the tumor and a margin of healthy tissue. Surgical treatments can diagnose, cure, palliate, or ablate (e.g., removal of tumor-promoting hormones) the cancer. Radiation treatment can also cure, control, or palliate the cancer. Radiation may cause radiation syndrome (i.e., fatigue, malaise, headache, anorexia, nausea, and/or vomiting) or other effects specific to the irradiated site. Chemotherapy treatment can cure, control, or palliate the cancer. The goal of chemotherapy is to eliminate enough tumor cells so that the body's natural defenses can eradicate any remaining cells. These drugs are either antineoplastic agents or hormones and may be administered intravenously, intraarterially, regionally, or orally. Frequently, combination antineoplastic therapy is used to combat cancer. Common side effects of chemotherapy include nausea and vomiting, bone marrow depression, alopecia, fatigue, anorexia, stomatitis, menstrual irregularities, and aspermatogenesis. Biotherapy agents used in the treatment of cancer include interferons, interleukins, colony-stimulating factors, tumor necrosis factor, and monoclonal antibodies. These agents affect biologic responses. Patients with cancer also require nutritional support and attention to comfort with analgesics and sedatives.

An oncologic emergency and when care requirements are significant due to uncontrolled pain or complications are two of the main reasons cancer patients are admitted to a progressive care unit. Three oncologic emergencies to consider are superior vena cava syndrome, tumor lysis syndrome, and spinal cord compression.

Superior Vena Cava Syndrome

Superior vena cava syndrome is a progressive occlusion of the superior vena cava, which leads to venous distention of the head and upper extremities. It may be associated with cancer of the lung, non-Hodgkin's lymphoma, and metastatic breast cancer. Either the tumor or a thrombosis obstructs the superior vena cava, decreasing venous return to the heart, which decreases cardiac output and increases central venous pressure. The patient complains of clinical indications including headache, cough, dyspnea that is worse when lying down, dizziness, and a feeling of fullness in the head, face, and neck. Objective findings include facial rubor, conjunctival redness of the eye, swelling of the neck and face, and distended veins in the head, neck, and chest. Cyanosis on the trunk may be noted and the patient may be hypotensive. A mediastinal mass may be evident on chest x-ray; CT scan, bronchoscopy, and mediastinoscopy may be indicated. To manage a patient with superior vena cava syndrome, administer oxygen to maintain a SpO_2 of at least 90%. Increase oral fluids and administer IV fluids as prescribed. Administer anticoagulants as prescribed to prevent extension of the clot if that is the cause. Administer glucocorticoids and diuretics as prescribed. Glucocorticoids decrease the inflammation surrounding the tumor or the tumor itself if the tumor is steroid responsive, such as with lymphoma. Diuretics reduce venous return to reduce intracardiac pressure. Administer analgesics and antiemetics as indicated. Closely monitor the patient for sepsis, airway obstruction, and cardiopulmonary arrest.

Tumor Lysis Syndrome

Tumor lysis syndrome is the metabolic consequence of rapid tumor destruction by chemotherapy or, less commonly, radiation. This is more likely in rapidly growing tumors that are highly sensitive to chemotherapy, such as lymphomas and leukemias. When the chemotherapy or radiation kills the tumor cells, the intracellular components are released into the circulation, leading to hyperkalemia, hyperuricemia, hyperphosphatemia, and hypocalcemia. Acute kidney injury can occur. The patient may complain of anorexia, nausea, vomiting, or abdominal pain. He or she may have weakness, paralysis, spasms, palpitations, or

BOX 8-9	
Differences between Benign and Malignant Tumors	
Benign	**Malignant**
Grow slowly	Grow rapidly
Well-defined capsule	Not encapsulated
Not invasive	Invasive
Well differentiated	Poorly differentiated
Low mitotic index	High mitotic index
Do not metastasize	Can spread distantly (metastasis)

seizures. Hypocalcemia may occur, causing tetany along with evidence of positive Chvostek and Trousseau signs. Diagnostic studies will show the electrolyte imbalances and the hyperuricemia. BUN and creatinine may be elevated. To manage a patient with tumor lysis syndrome, administer oxygen to maintain a SpO_2 of at least 90%. Increase oral fluids and administer IV fluids as prescribed. Administer sodium bicarbonate if prescribed to help decrease uric acid moving into solution and thus eliminated in the urine. Note that this treatment is controversial. Administer allopurinol to decrease uric acid production and treat electrolyte imbalance. Assist in preparation of the patient for hemodialysis if necessary for acute kidney injury. Monitor the patient closely for dysrhythmias, renal calculi, and acute kidney injury.

Spinal Cord Compression

Spinal cord compression is the result of tumor invasion of the epidural space with compression of the spinal cord, potentially resulting in permanent paralysis. Myeloma, lymphoma, and breast, lung, prostate, or renal cancer patients are at highest risk. Back pain is the most significant early symptom of spinal cord compression; this pain usually increases when lying down. Urinary retention, constipation, impotence, and urinary or fecal incontinence may occur early, whereas motor or sensory impairments progressing to paralysis are late indications. Spinal x-ray, CT scans, bone scans, and myelograms diagnose spinal cord compression, though the MRI is likely to be most definitive. To relieve cord compression, administer corticosteroids (e.g., dexamethasone) as prescribed. Assist with additional therapies such as chemotherapy, radiation, or surgery to preserve neurologic function. Laxatives, stool softeners, and manual removal of fecal impaction may be necessary. In addition, an indwelling urinary catheter may be necessary for urinary retention.

COAGULOPATHY

Coagulopathy is a condition in which the blood's ability to clot (i.e., coagulate) is impaired. This condition can cause prolonged or excessive bleeding, which may occur spontaneously or following an injury or medical and dental procedures. Coagulopathy may cause uncontrolled internal or external bleeding.

The normal clotting process depends on the interplay of various proteins in the blood. Reduced levels or absence of blood-clotting proteins, known as clotting factors or coagulation factors, may cause coagulopathy. Genetic disorders, such as hemophilia and von Willebrand's disease, can cause a reduction in clotting factors. Vitamin K deficiency, liver disease, and anticoagulants such as warfarin will also cause coagulation problems. Coagulopathy may also occur because of dysfunction or reduced levels of platelets and immune thrombocytopenia (Table 8-15).

DISSEMINATED INTRAVASCULAR COAGULATION

Disseminated intravascular coagulation (DIC) is a syndrome characterized by thrombus formation and hemorrhage secondary to overstimulation of the normal coagulation process. This syndrome leads to massive intravascular clotting with resultant depletion in clotting factors and platelets and risk for bleeding. The etiology of DIC is always a secondary phenomenon and numerous risk factors have been identified (Table 8-16).

The pathophysiology of DIC (Figure 8-6) begins with damage to the vascular endothelium or damage to tissue. Thrombin generation causes thrombosis in the microcirculation (i.e., microclots), which causes ischemia distal to the clot. Thrombosis also causes consumption of clotting factors and platelets, which impairs the ability to make a stable clot and causes hemorrhage. Hemorrhage leads to the initiation of the fibrinolytic system causing production of FDPs, which perpetuate bleeding. Consider DIC as a consumptive coagulopathy that can be thought of as clotting (i.e., microclots), followed by bleeding (i.e., consumption of clotting factors and platelets), and more bleeding (i.e., effect of FDPs).

The clinical course of a patient with DIC will include history of a predisposing factor. Vigilance and knowledge of risk factors facilitate early recognition and initiation of treatment. Close monitoring for the clinical indications of DIC and early detection will facilitate a quick transfer to a higher level of care during the acute onset and supportive care during the recovery period. The patient with DIC will have the clinical indications of decreased perfusion, platelet dysfunction, and hemorrhage (Table 8-17).

8.7 Learning Activity

Match the coagulopathy with the associated pathology.

_____ 1. Hemophilia A
_____ 2. Hemophilia B
_____ 3. von Willebrand disease
_____ 4. Heparin-induced thrombocytopenia
_____ 5. Disseminated intravascular coagulation
_____ 6. Liver disease
_____ 7. Immune thrombocytopenic purpura
_____ 8. Thrombotic thrombocytopenic purpura

a. Activation of thrombin and consumption of platelets and clotting factors
b. Binding of immune complexes to platelets that are then destroyed by the spleen
c. Deficiency of von Willebrand factor
d. Deficiency of factor VIII
e. Deficiency of factor IX
f. Development of heparin-platelet factor 4 complex, which increases platelet activation and causes thrombocytopenia
g. Platelet aggregation and consumption
h. Inability to produce clotting factors

Answers to this activity can be found in the Answer Key.

TABLE 8-15 Inherited and Acquired Coagulopathies

Cause of Coagulopathy	Pathophysiology	Treatment
Hereditary Coagulopathies		
Hemophilia A	• X-linked recessive disorder; though considered a hereditary disorder, may occur as a new mutation in factor VIII gene • Deficiency of factor VIII • Inadequate factor VIII-von Willebrand factor (vWF) complex • Inadequate platelet adhesion	• Either highly purified factor VIII concentrate or recombinant factor VIII administration • DDAVP stimulates the endothelial cells to release vWF and plasminogen activator
Hemophilia B (Christmas disease)	• X-linked recessive disorder • Deficiency of factor IX	• Highly purified factor IX
von Willebrand disease	• Types 1 and 2 are inherited as autosomal dominant traits, and type 3 is inherited as autosomal recessive deficiency of vWF • Decreased platelet adhesion	• Usually mild and does not require treatment, though risk of bleeding is increased • Highly purified factor VIII concentrate that contains vWF • DDAVP stimulates the endothelial cells to release vWF and plasminogen activator
Acquired Coagulopathies		
Vitamin K deficiency	• Inadequate synthesis and regulation of prothrombin, procoagulant factors (VII, IX, and X), and anticoagulant regulators (proteins C and S)	• Parenteral administration of vitamin K • FFP in life-threatening hemorrhage or in preparation for emergency surgery
Liver disease	• Impaired clotting caused by diminished production of clotting factors, especially factor VII and less so factor IX • Impaired fibrinolysis caused by diminished production of plasminogen and alpha$_2$-antiplasmin • Decreased thrombopoietin results in decreased platelet production	• FFP • Platelets
Immune thrombocytopenic purpura (formerly known as *idiopathic thrombocytopenia purpura*)	Acute ITP • Secondary to infection, particularly viral, or other condition that results in large amounts of antigen in the blood, such as drug allergies or systemic lupus erythematosus • Antigen and antibodies form immune complexes that bind to receptors on platelets, which causes platelet destruction in the spleen Chronic ITP • Development of autoantibodies against platelet-specific antigens • Removal of the antibody-coated platelets removed by the spleen	• Glucocorticoids • IV immunoglobulins • Splenectomy may be considered • Immunosuppressive agents may be used
Thrombotic thrombocytopenic purpura	• Platelets aggregate and cause occlusion of arterioles and capillaries within the microcirculation • Platelet consumption • Organ ischemia	• Plasma exchange with fresh frozen plasma • Glucocorticoids • Splenectomy may be considered • Immunosuppressive agents may be used

One of the earliest findings in the DIC patient is that the platelet count is decreased (less than 150,000/mm^3). The PT and aPTT are prolonged, but these tests are less sensitive than other tests. The thrombin time is prolonged (>15 seconds) and the fibrinogen level is decreased by 50% or more, or less than 200 mg/dL. Use the fibrinogen level to evaluate patients who have contributing factors that do not permit monitoring platelet count. Because fibrinogen is elevated in pregnancy, sepsis, and neoplastic conditions, a decrease of 50% is a more accurate

indicator of DIC than an absolute value in these patients. The thrombin-antithrombin III (TAT) complex is decreased (usually less than 70% activity) and evaluates the activation of the coagulation system that occurs when thrombin is generated. Decreased antithrombin III indicates an accelerated coagulation process.

FDP measures the results of both fibrin and fibrinogen degradation. The FDPs are elevated (>40 mcg/mL) but may be reported as positive at a number of dilutions. The FDP diagnostic for DIC is positive at greater than 100 dilutions (reported positive at 1:100).

TABLE 8-16   **Etiology of Disseminated Intravascular Coagulation**

Etiology	Possible Risk Factors
Vascular injury or inflammation	• Shock • Vasculitis • Giant hemangioma • Dissecting aneurysm • Toxemia of pregnancy

Infection and sepsis	• Bacterial
	  • Gram negative (e.g., *Escherichia coli*, meningococcal)
	  • Gram positive (e.g., *Staphylococcus*, *Streptococcus*)
	• Viral (e.g., influenza, herpes, cytomegalovirus, adenovirus)
	• Rickettsial (e.g., Rocky Mountain spotted fever)
	• Protozoal (e.g., malaria)
	• Fungal (e.g., *Aspergillus, Candida, Histoplasma, Toxoplasma*)

Hematologic/immunologic	• Hemolytic blood transfusion reaction • Massive blood transfusion • Prolonged cardiopulmonary bypass • Sickle cell crisis • Thalassemia major • Polycythemia vera • Anaphylaxis • Systemic lupus erythematosus • Transplant rejection
Trauma	• Multiple traumas • Burns • Acute anoxia • Heat stroke • Crush injury • Head injury • Surgery

Neoplastic disorders	• Adenocarcinoma: produce the procoagulant mucin
	  • Pancreatic cancer
	  • Breast cancer
	  • Prostate cancer
	  • Ovarian cancer
	  • Lung cancer
	  • Colon cancer
	  • Stomach cancer
	• Cancer of the urinary tract
	• Sarcoma
	• Leukemia
	• Pheochromocytoma

Obstetric complications	• Abruptio placentae • Retained dead fetus • Retained placenta • Septic abortion • Hydatidiform mole • Amniotic fluid embolism • Acute fatty liver of pregnancy • Toxemia
Embolism	• Pulmonary embolism • Fat embolism • Amniotic fluid embolism
GI and GI accessory organs	• Necrotizing enterocolitis • Pancreatitis • Obstructive jaundice • Hepatitis • Cirrhosis • Acute hepatic failure

Continued

TABLE 8-16	Etiology of Disseminated Intravascular Coagulation—cont'd
Etiology	**Possible Risk Factors**
Pulmonary	• ARDS • Pulmonary embolism
Toxins	• Snake bites • Aspirin poisoning • Impure IV drugs
Prosthetic devices	• LeVeen or Denver shunt • Intraaortic balloon pump

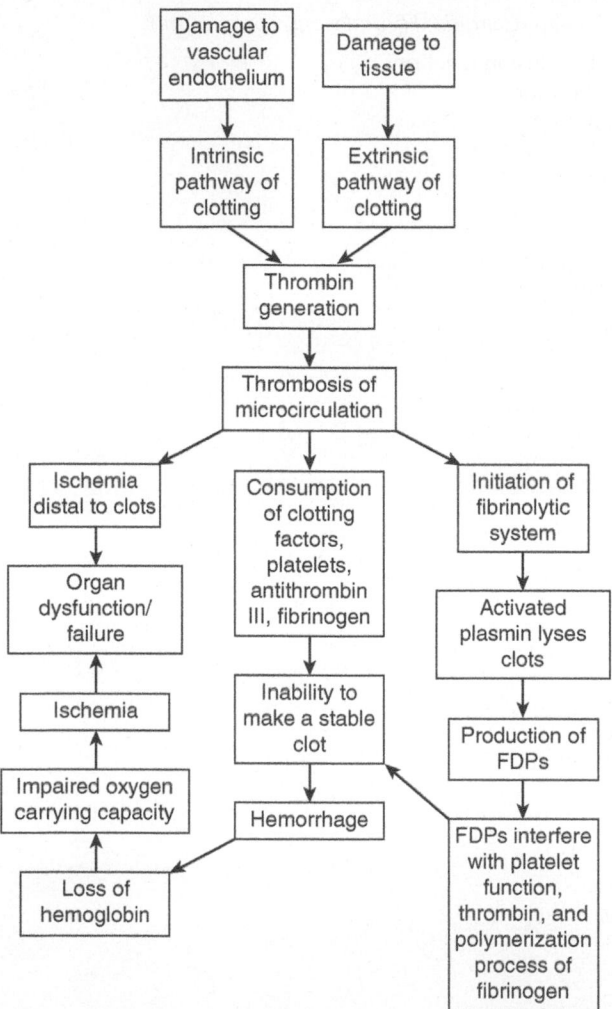

FIGURE 8-6 Pathophysiology of disseminated intravascular coagulation (DIC). *FDPs,* Fibrin degradation products. (From Dennison, R. D. [2013]. *Pass CCRN!* [4th ed.]. St. Louis, MO: Elsevier.)

The D-dimer is specific to the results of fibrin degradation and more specific for DIC than FDPs but less sensitive. The D-dimer is a product of fibrin degradation and is elevated (>250 ng/mL) or positive at greater than 1:8 dilutions. The D-dimer may be falsely positive postsurgically and in certain malignancies, deep vein thrombosis, and pulmonary embolism.

The protamine sulfate test is strongly positive in DIC. Add protamine sulfate to plasma to see if fibrin strands form. A positive test reflects the formation of excessive amounts of thrombin. In DIC, a clotting factor analysis will show a decrease in factors I, V, and VIII, and in fibrinogen.

A peripheral smear will show the presence of schistocytes, helmet cells, and red cell fragments. The Hgb and Hct decrease if blood loss is significant. The patient's arterial blood gas state is initially respiratory alkalosis, but it progresses to metabolic acidosis due to lactic acidosis. The patient's urine, stool, and sputum may be positive for blood. The collaborative health care team uses the results of diagnostic tests for a DIC scoring system (Table 8-18).

8.8   Learning Activity

Identify the direction of change of the following laboratory values in DIC, ↑ or ↓.

Platelets	
PT	
aPTT	
Fibrin split products	
Factors V, VIII	
Fibrinogen	

Answers to this activity can be found in the Answer Key.

The priority of collaborative management is to identify and closely assess high-risk groups for clinical indications of DIC. Monitor patients closely for thrombosis or bleeding by noting the presence of petechiae, ecchymosis, and acrocyanosis. Test all nasogastric aspirate or vomitus, stools, and urine for blood. Monitor the patient's oral secretions, pulmonary secretions, and gums for evidence of bleeding. Assess the patient's cardiovascular and perfusion status by monitoring level of consciousness, peripheral pulses, capillary refill, and urine output. Monitor laboratory studies for diagnostic indications of DIC.

Treatment begins with correction and control of the underlying causative factors. Surgical interventions such as debridement, abscess drainage, evacuation of the uterus, or removal of a tumor may be required. Administer antimicrobials for an infection, and antineoplastics are given for a malignancy. Early identification and elimination of the cause is always the first line of treatment along with facilitating the transfer of the patient to a higher level of care. The remaining focus of initial treatment is supportive measures to maintain airway, ventilation, and oxygenation until restoration of coagulation balance occurs. A priority in this stage is to administer oxygen to maintain a PaO_2 of 80 mm Hg and SpO_2 of 95%. Ensure patency of a peripheral intravenous catheter, and administer normal saline to replace volume until type and crossmatch are completed and blood is available to correct the hypovolemia, hypotension, hypoxia, and acidosis.

TABLE 8-17	Clinical Presentation of Disseminated Intravascular Coagulation
Category	Clinical Presentation
Decreased perfusion	• Brain: change in level of consciousness, focal neurologic signs, and/or seizures • Heart: chest pain, ST segment elevation or depression, and/or clinical indications of hypoperfusion • Lung: dyspnea, chest pain, and/or clinical indications of hypoxemia • Kidney: decreased urine output, occult or gross hematuria, proteinuria, and/or electrolyte imbalance • GI tract: abdominal pain, diarrhea, and/or occult or gross blood in stool • Skin: acral cyanosis of toes, fingers, lips, nose, or ears; mottling; coldness; and/or necrosis
Platelet dysfunction	• Petechiae: frequently the first indication of DIC • Ecchymoses • Purpura
Hemorrhage	• Tachycardia: Initially postural only, then profound tachycardia • Hypotension: Initially narrowed pulse pressure, then postural hypotension, then profound hypotension • Tachypnea • Overt bleeding in a patient with no previous bleeding history • Mucosal surfaces: gingival bleeding and/or epistaxis • GU: Hematuria • GI: Hematemesis, hematochezia, melena, and/or guaiac-positive stool • Pulmonary: hemoptysis • Gynecologic: vaginal bleeding • Skin: prolonged oozing from puncture points, IV sites, and wounds (referred to as surface bleeding), and/or bruising • Occult bleeding • Swollen joints and joint pain may indicate bleeding into the joint • Abdominal distention and rebound tenderness may indicate intraperitoneal bleeding • Back pain, leg numbness, and hypotension may indicate retroperitoneal bleeding • Headache, change in level of consciousness, and pupillary changes may indicate intracerebral hemorrhage • Visual changes: blurred vision; loss of visual fields may indicate retinal hemorrhage • Alterations in hemodynamic parameters: central venous pressure and cardiac output/cardiac index may be decreased

| TABLE 8-18 | DIC Scoring System |

Laboratory Test	0	1	2	3
Platelet count/nL	Greater than 100	Greater than 50	Less than 50	
D-dimer mcg/mL	Less than 1		1-5	Greater than 5
Fibrinogen g/L	Greater than 1	Less than 1		
Prothrombin index %	Greater than 70	40-70	Less than 40	

The DIC Scoring System requires the presence of a risk factor for DIC before the laboratory test results can be evaluated. If greater than or equal to 5, it is compatible with overt DIC. If less than 5, it is suggestive for nonovert DIC in a patient with an underlying disorder known to be associated with DIC. Adapted from Taylor, F. B., Toh, C. H., Hoots, W. K., Wada, H., & Levi, M. (2001). Towards definition, clinical and laboratory criteria, and a scoring system for disseminated intravascular coagulation. *Thromb Haemost, 86,* 1327-1330.

Administer IV heparin (usually 5 to 15 units/kg/hr) to stop the microclotting to maintain perfusion and protect vital organ function, A desirable aPTT is 1.5 to 2 times the control. Administer heparin as prescribed to patients with thrombosis who continue to bleed despite other rigorous treatment, which is often effective with underlying malignancy, acute promyelocytic leukemia, and purpura fulminans seen in sepsis. The heparin prevents further thrombosis in the microvasculature and prevents platelet aggregation. The heparin works with antithrombin III to neutralize circulating thrombin. The treatment with heparin continues to be controversial as it may potentiate or prolong bleeding, but it is thrombosis of small vessels, not hemorrhage, that has the greatest impact on morbidity and mortality in DIC. Heparin treatment is contraindicated in CNS or GI hemorrhage, DIC associated with hepatic failure, hemorrhagic obstetric causes (e.g., abruptio placentae), and recent surgical procedures. Administer antithrombin III to neutralize thrombin. Both of these agents may increase bleeding.

The desired outcome of efforts used to support coagulation is cessation of bleeding. Administer blood products as

TABLE 8-19 **Treatments for DIC**

Treatment	Rationale	Controversy
Heparin	• Prevents further microclots and prevents platelet aggregation • Works with antithrombin III to neutralize circulating thrombin	• May perpetuate bleeding
Antithrombin III	• Works with heparin to neutralize circulating thrombin	• May perpetuate bleeding
Clotting factors • Fresh frozen plasma • Cryoprecipitate • Platelets	• Reestablishes normal hemostatic potential	• "Fuel to the fire" theory attests that until the clotting process is stopped, clotting factors just increase the thrombosis and microclotting
Epsilon-aminocaproic acid (Amicar)	• Blocks the fibrinolytic system so that stable clots are not degraded • Decreases amount of FDPs that act as anticoagulant	• Clearance of microclots from occluded vessels may be delayed • Indicated only in primary fibrinolysis

TABLE 8-20 **Comparison of Nonimmune and Immune Heparin-Induced Thrombocytopenia**

Characteristic	HAT: Nonimmune (previously referred to as *HIT-I*)	HIT: Immune (previously referred to as *HIT-II*)
Onset	Days 1-4 of heparin administration	Day 5-10 of heparin administration
Route and dose	Primarily with high dose of IV heparin	Any route or dose
Effect on platelets	90,000-150,000/mm^3 for 1-5 days	Greater than 50% drop from baseline on days 7-10
Course	Platelet count may normalize No thrombosis	Thrombosis May be associated with life-threatening complications
Mechanism	Direct toxic effect	Immune-mediated
Antibodies	No	Yes
Treatment	Observation	Cessation of heparin and nonheparin anticoagulants

prescribed to replace missing clotting factors. Maintain platelet count above 50,000/mm^3. Platelet replenishment is a priority to assist in the reinitiation of effective clotting. Administer desmopressin acetate as prescribed to improve platelet function when platelet dysfunction is due to dextran, nonsteroidal anti-inflammatory agents, or aspirin; monitor for fluid overload, hyponatremia, and tachycardia. Administer fresh frozen plasma (FFP), which contains all clotting factors, to bleeding patients with markedly prolonged PT and aPTT. FFP also replenishes fibrinogen levels. Administer cryoprecipitate, which contains factors VIII and XIII and fibrinogen, to maintain fibrinogen levels above 125 mg/dL.

Many of the treatments just noted are initiated while the patient is being transitioned to a higher level of care. Patients with DIC require complex critical care nursing to stabilize and support them until adequate coagulation processes are restored. These patients may require intubation, mechanical ventilation, volume replacement, inotropes, vasopressors, select medications used only in a critical care setting such as hemostatic cofactors and antifibrinolytic agents, and hemodynamic monitoring. The care of the acute DIC patient is complex and controversy regarding selected treatment exists (Table 8-19).

8.9   Learning Activity

Discuss the controversy of the following therapies in the treatment of DIC.

a. Heparin	
b. Clotting factors	

Answers to this activity can be found in the Answer Key.

HEPARIN-INDUCED THROMBOCYTOPENIA

Heparin-induced thrombocytopenia (HIT) is a prothrombotic disorder caused by a subset of antibodies against platelet factor 4 (PF4)-heparin complexes with strong platelet-activating properties. There is a differentiation between heparin-associated thrombocytopenia (HAT) and HIT (Table 8-20).

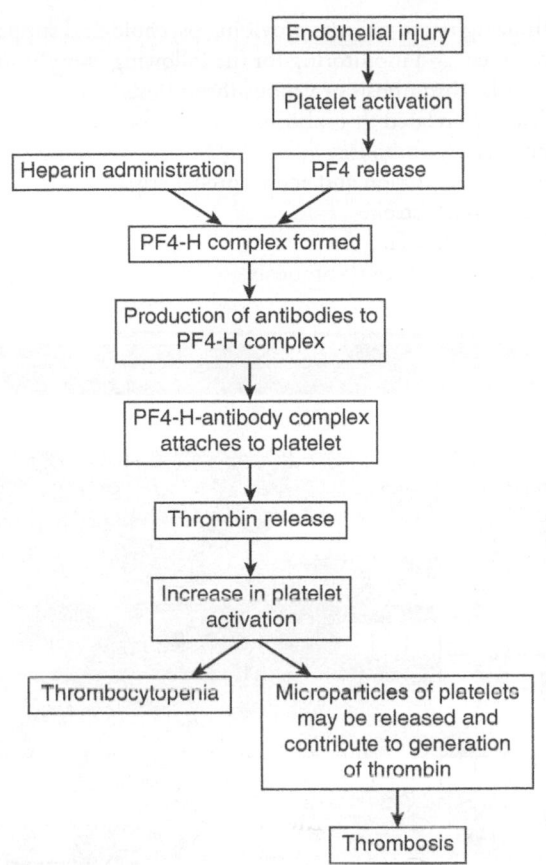

FIGURE 8-7 Pathophysiology of heparin-induced thrombocytopenia (HIT). *PF4-H,* Platelet factor 4-heparin. (From Dennison, R. D. [2013]. *Pass CCRN!* [4th ed.]. St. Louis, MO: Elsevier.)

The etiology of HIT is heparin administration or heparin-coated catheters. There is a greater risk with unfractionated heparin (3% to 5%) than with low-molecular-weight heparin (0.05%). The risk is higher with bovine heparin than with porcine heparin. Postoperative patients and those patients with underlying vascular endothelial cell injury or venous stasis are at a greater risk.

The pathophysiology (Figure 8-7) includes the development of PF4-heparin complex and production of antibodies to this complex. This complex then attaches to the platelet, causing thrombin release and activation of platelets; this results in thrombus formation and thrombocytopenia.

Subjective complaints are rare in the patient with HIT. The clinical presentation is usually a thrombotic event and a decreased platelet count. A venous clot is 4 times more likely than an arterial thrombus. Venous thrombosis may occur as a deep vein thrombosis, a pulmonary embolism, a cerebral venous thrombosis, or an adrenal infarction. An arterial thrombus may occur as a myocardial infarction, thrombotic stroke, limb arterial occlusion, renal or mesenteric arterial thrombosis, or aortic occlusion. The patient may present with skin lesions such as petechiae or with an acute systemic reaction. Bleeding rarely occurs.

The diagnosis of HIT is determined by a platelet count less than $100,000/mm^3$ or a 50% decrease from baseline platelet count. A platelet activation (functional) assay relies on the ability of the PF4-heparin antibody to activate platelets. This test is less sensitive but more specific. In addition, a serotonin release assay and platelet aggregation assay such as heparin-induced platelet aggregation may elicit further evidence. An enzyme-linked immunoassay (ELISA) for PF4-heparin antibodies is more sensitive but less specific. A 4T diagnostic scoring system has been established (Table 8-21).

TABLE 8-21 4T Scoring System for HIT

	2 Points	1 Point	0 Points
Thrombocytopenia	Platelet count fall greater than 50% from baseline AND platelet nadir greater than or equal to 20×10^9/L	Platelet count fall 30%-50% from baseline AND platelet nadir 10-19 $\times 10^9$/L	Platelet count fall less than 30% from baseline AND platelet nadir less than 10 $\times 10^9$/L
Timing of fall in platelet count	Clear onset between days 5 and 10 OR less than or equal to 1 day if heparin exposure within previous 30 days	Fall in platelet count consistent with onset between days 5 and 10 but timing is not clear due to missing platelet counts OR onset after day 10 of heparin exposure OR fall in platelet count less than or equal to 1 day if heparin exposure within previous 30-100 days	Fall in platelet count less than 4 days after recent heparin exposure
Thrombosis or related occurrence	New thrombosis, skin necrosis, or acute systemic reaction after UFH exposure	Progressive or recurrent thrombosis or unconfirmed but clinically suspected thrombosis	No thrombosis or thrombosis preceding heparin exposure
Thrombocytopenia: Possible other causes	None apparent	Possible other causes present	Probable other causes present

A score less than 4 = low probability of HIT, score of 4 to 5 = intermediate probability of HIT, and a score greater than 5 = high probability of HIT. From Crowther, M. A., Cook, D. J., Albert, M., Williamson, D., Meade, M., Granton, J., et al. (2010). The 4Ts scoring system for heparin-induced thrombocytopenia in medical-surgical intensive care unit patients. *J Crit Care, 25*(2), 287-293.

The focus of collaborative care management of HIT is to correct the coagulopathy. Discontinue the offending agent (i.e., heparin) and administer an alternative anticoagulant (e.g., argatroban or danaparoid) as prescribed. Warfarin decreases protein C activity and predisposes a patient to microvascular thrombosis and limb gangrene; therefore, until the platelet count normalizes, it is contraindicated. Plasmapheresis removes the pathogenic immunoglobulins. Priority nursing care focuses on the treatment of ischemic pain, maintaining skin integrity, minimizing tissue trauma, providing psychological support and reassurance, and monitoring for the following complications:

- Arterial thrombosis or venous thrombosis
- Catheter-related thrombosis
- Pulmonary embolism
- Adrenal infarction and acute adrenal crisis
- Thrombotic stroke
- Myocardial infarction
- Mesenteric artery thrombosis

8.10   Synthesis Learning Activity: Crossword Puzzle

Complete the following crossword puzzle related to cancer.

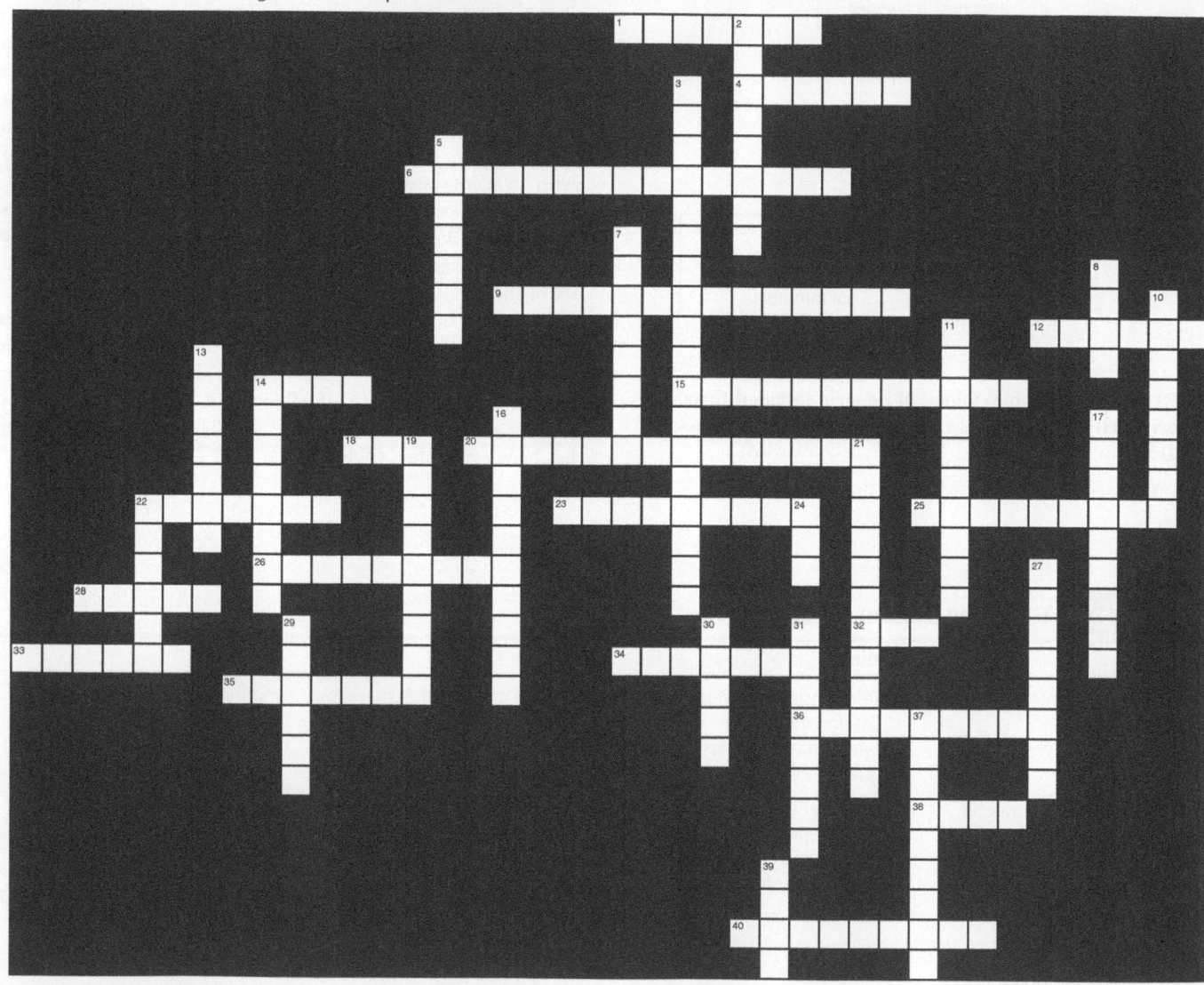

Answers to this activity can be found in the Answer Key.

ACROSS

1. Eating a healthy diet, exercising regularly, and not smoking are examples of _____ prevention
4. Used for definitive diagnosis and grading of a tumor
6. The orderly process in which proliferating cells are transformed into different and more specialized types
9. A malignant glandular neoplasm
12. 50% of us will develop _____ and 30% of us will die of _____
14. The word cancer is derived from the Greek word for _____
15. Benign tumors are usually _____ and well differentiated
18. Tumor staging system (abbrev.)
20. These syndromes are symptom complexes triggered by the malignancy but not directly related to the tumor
22. Exposure to _____ increases the risk of bladder cancer

23. Abnormal changes in the size, shape, and organization of mature cells; not cancer but may precede cancer

25. A malignant tumor of epithelial origin

26. This is a significant risk for patients receiving antineoplastic agents due to their effect on the bone marrow

28. This syndrome is frequently seen in small cell (oat cell) carcinoma of the lung (abbrev.)

32. This virus is associated with cervical cancer (abbrev.)

33. Carcinoma _____ is preinvasive

34. The most common symptoms of cancer

35. Tumor _____ are substances produced by malignant cells that can be tested for in the blood, urine, or cerebral spinal fluid; examples are CEA and PSA

36. Term for loss of cellular differentiation

38. A symptom of cancer late in the course that is controlled with increasing dosages of narcotics

40. This type of neoplasm metastasizes to other areas of the body

DOWN

2. Exposure to _____ increases the risk of lung cancer and mesothelioma

3. This bacterium is associated with stomach cancer (2 words)

5. Cells are most susceptible to injury during this phase of the cell cycle

7. The most common cancer in men

8. The most likely cancer to cause death in men and women

10. Cancer of blood-forming cells

11. The major cause of death related to cancer

13. The change in this unhealthy habit is the reason for the increase and now decreasing risk of lung cancer

14. Malnutrition that occurs with cancer that results in wasting and extensive loss of adipose tissue

16. An agent capable of causing cancer

17. Self-breast examination, blood pressure screening, and regular dental examinations are examples of _____ prevention

19. Cell _____ that cause cancer must be bad enough to change the cell so that when it divides, the new cells have the mutation but not bad enough to cause cell death

21. Because cancer cells are essentially body cells, normal cells are injured by this therapy

22. The most common cancer in women

24. Cancer is more likely as we _____ due to cancer taking a long time to develop, more exposure to carcinogens, and immunosenescence

27. Synonymous with tumor; not necessarily benign or malignant

29. Risk of cancer of the _____ is increased with alcohol intake and smoking

30. GI malignancies are most likely to metastasize to the _____

31. This serious skin cancer is related to skin exposure to ultraviolet radiation

37. Cancer of lymphatic tissue

39. Hair follicles here are affected most by antineoplastic agents

8.11   Synthesis Learning Activity: Crossword Puzzle

Complete the following crossword puzzle related to hematologic and immunologic conditions.

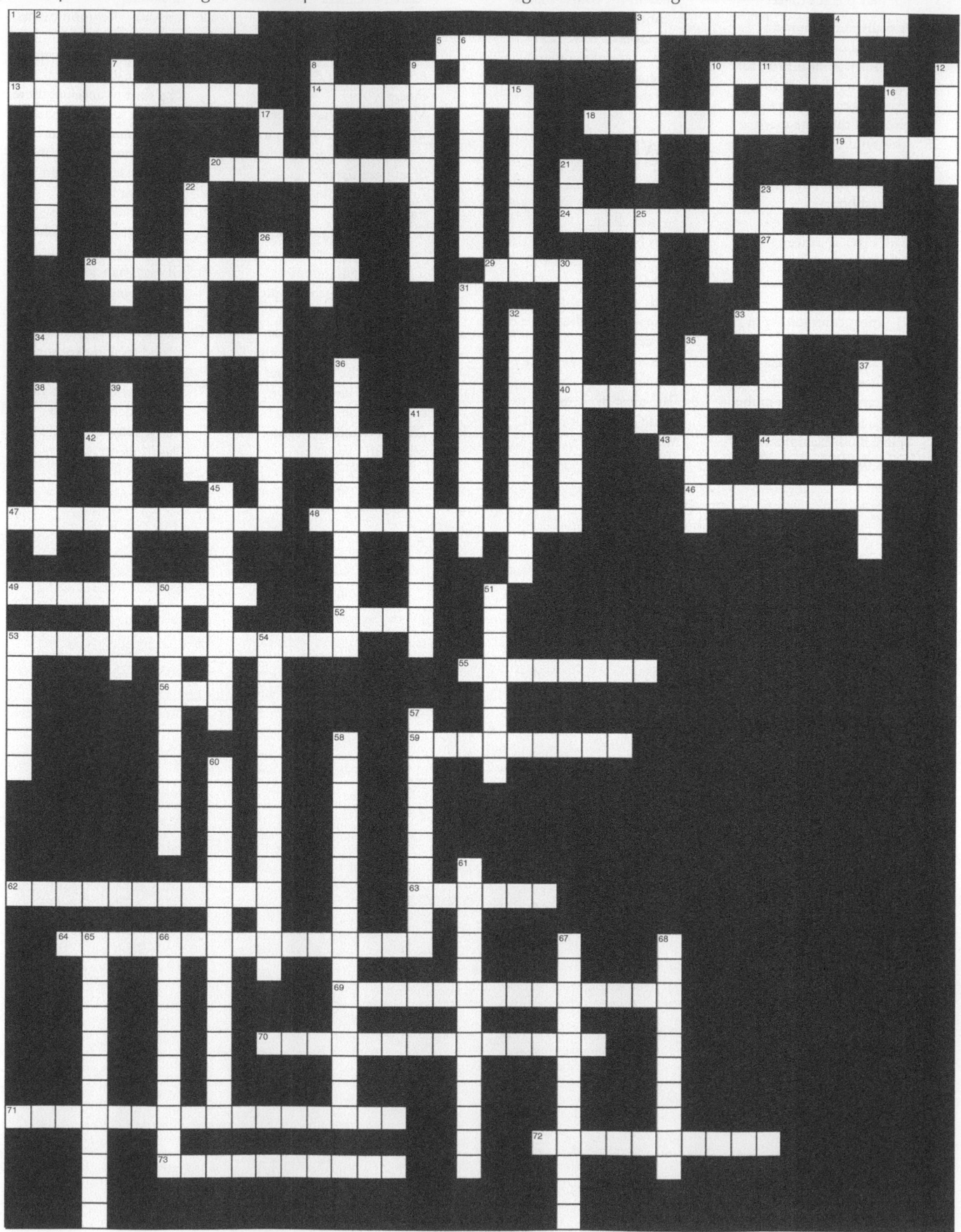

Answers to this activity can be found in the Answer Key.

ACROSS

1. The complex physiologic process for termination of bleeding
3. The major physiologic effect of anemia
4. This condition is characterized by widespread microclots, consumption of clotting factors and platelets, and impaired fibrinolysis (abbrev.)
5. This mediator is released by the mast cell in allergic reactions
10. Activated plasminogen; the active agent in the fibrinolytic process
13. The term for movement of neutrophils and phagocytes through pores of small blood vessels
14. This type of anemia is associated with increased RBC destruction, which causes jaundice
18. Factor X is sometimes referred to as _____ factor; deficient in hemophilia B
19. An increase in segmented neutrophils is referred to as a shift to the _____
20. This type of cell can engulf and digest microorganisms and cellular debris
23. The yellowish fluid that transports lymphocytes
24. The first sign of platelet dysfunction
27. The liquid portion of blood
28. The indirect thrombin inhibitor frequently used post-PCI (generic)
29. An increase in the number of immature neutrophils and other leukocytes in the blood is referred to as a shift to the _____
33. This type of immunity is mediated by B cells; involves the development of antigen-specific antibodies
34. A cascading system that can result in direct killing of invading organisms

40. The product of erythrocyte destruction
42. A leukocyte count that is higher than normal
43. The end result of fibrinolysis (abbrev.)
44. These cells are fixed macrophages in the liver
46. This type of immunity is mediated by the T cell
47. This type of platelet analysis determines the ability of platelets to aggregate
48. The term for a mature RBC
49. The blood parameter that indicates the percentage of RBCs in a given volume of blood
52. Anemia related to a deficiency of _____ causes nail changes and sores at the corners of the mouth
53. The primary regulator of the platelet circulating mass
55. The granulocyte that releases heparin and histamine
56. The immunoglobulin most important in allergic reactions
59. Glycoprotein IIb/IIIa inhibitor frequently used before and after PCI (generic)
62. This mediator causes vasoconstriction, pulmonary vasoconstriction, and platelet aggregation
63. The condition characterized by a reduction in the total number of circulating erythrocytes or a decrease in the quality or quantity of hemoglobin
64. This blood product is administered to replace factor VIII in patients with hemophilia
69. A synonym for antibody; made by B cells
70. The process of erythrocyte production
71. A decrease in the number of platelets
72. A type of agranular leukocyte; B cells and T cells are examples

73. This type of T cell serves to modulate the immune response; increased in AIDS

DOWN

2. This type of granulocyte is most significant in allergic reactions
3. The parenteral anticoagulant that acts as an indirect thrombin inhibitor (generic)
4. The most specific laboratory test for DIC
6. The clotting pathway that is initiated by endothelial injury
7. A leukocyte count that is lower than normal
8. The movement of neutrophils and monocytes toward an antigen
9. These cells are decreased in ITP, DIC, and HIT
10. This electrolyte may increase with administration of banked blood
11. A drug frequently administered to decrease platelet aggregation (abbrev.)
12. A platelet plug is sometimes referred to as a _____ clot
15. Chemical mediators of immunity and inflammation
16. The most abundant immunoglobulin
17. Normal adult hemoglobin (abbrev.)
21. An autoimmune disorder in which an IgG autoantibody is formed and binds to and destroys the platelets (abbrev.)
22. The sequential physiologic response that the body makes to injuries
23. A direct thrombin inhibitor that may be used for HIT (generic)
25. The clotting pathway that is initiated by tissue injury
26. This type of platelet analysis determines the number of platelets
30. A synonym for platelet

31. The adherence of phagocytes to the vessel wall
32. A leukocyte that releases granules when it ruptures
35. This objective finding may occur with hemolytic anemia
36. Heparin and _____ maintain the fluidity of the blood
37. A vitamin K antagonist; oral anticoagulant (generic)
38. This electrolyte may decrease with administration of banked blood
39. This coagulation study evaluates platelet function (2 words)
41. A cytokine synthesized by lymphocytes
45. This blood protein becomes fibrin when activated
50. An oral platelet aggregation inhibitor prescribed for several months after PCI with stents (generic)
51. This type of anemia is due to bone marrow suppression
53. The site of T cell distribution
54. This hormone is released from the kidney in response to low oxygen levels
57. This agranulocyte is the major phagocyte of the leukocytes
58. The first homeostatic mechanism
60. A common presenting symptom of leukemia and lymphoma
61. The process by which stem cells develop and differentiate into different types of blood cells
65. An immature erythrocyte
66. This type of anemia is caused by loss of intrinsic factor and malabsorption of vitamin B_{12}
67. The final stage of the clotting process
68. The reticulocyte count reflects activity of the _____ (2 words)

A 23-year-old female accountant complains of a rash on her ankles and shins, and easy bruising for 10 days. The rash is not itchy or painful. She denies recent contact with new soaps or detergents. The bruises occur on her arms and sides, unrelated to trauma. On further questioning, she reports nosebleeds, gum bleeding with flossing, and an unusually heavy menses 1 week ago. She had an upper respiratory infection 3 weeks ago, which has now resolved. On physical examination, she has no lymphadenopathy or hepatosplenomegaly. Her stool is guaiac positive.

a. Her signs and symptoms are most suggestive of what type of bleeding disorder? Select the most likely choice.
   ( ) Coagulation abnormality
   ( ) Abnormality of vascular integrity or platelet function

b. Select all the additional questions that you should ask.

Check or leave blank	Question
	Have you had bleeding problems in the past, particularly with procedures or trauma?
	Have you had your cholesterol checked?
	What medications and supplements—not prescribed by a physician—are you taking?
	Do you smoke?
	Do you drink alcohol? If so, how often?
	Do you use IV drugs?
	Do you have unprotected sex?
	Do you have exposure to any chemicals or radiation at work or at home?
	Does anyone in your family have a problem with bleeding?
	Have you had a recent unexpected loss of weight?
	Do you have any heartburn, dyspepsia, or chronic indigestion?

c. What laboratory tests would you expect to be ordered? Select all that would be indicated.

Check or leave blank	Laboratory Test
	Complete blood count (CBC)
	Peripheral smear
	Reticulocyte count
	Prothrombin time (PT) and activated partial thromboplastin time (aPTT)
	D-dimer
	Platelet function analyzer (or PFA-100 or platelet function screen)
	Bleeding time
	Lactic dehydrogenase (LDH)
	Viral titers for a chronic infection with HIV and hepatitis C
	Viral titers for an acute infection
	Thrombopoietin (TPO) levels
	Glucose level
	Chest x-ray
	Direct antiglobulin test
	Quantitative immunoglobulins
	Helicobacter pylori antigen assay

Answers to this activity can be found in the Answer Key.

The Neurologic System

ANATOMY AND PHYSIOLOGY

The neurologic system is composed of the central, peripheral, and autonomic nervous systems. The central nervous system (CNS) consists of the brain and spinal cord. The peripheral nervous system includes the cranial nerves, spinal nerves, and peripheral nerves. The autonomic nervous system (ANS) consists of the sympathetic nervous system (SNS) and the parasympathetic nervous system (PNS).

The neurologic system receives stimuli from the internal and external environment via sensory pathways and communicates that information between the body periphery and the CNS. It processes information received at reflex or conscious levels to determine appropriate responses and transmits information over motor pathways to organs responsible for responding to the stimuli.

Microscopic Anatomy and Physiology

Neuroglia, also called *glial cells*, make up 85% of the cells in the CNS. They provide support, nourishment, and protection to the neurons. Neuroglial cells are mitotic and can replicate themselves; therefore, most tumors of the CNS originate from these cells.

Microglia cells, oligodendroglia cells, astrocytes, and ependyma cells are the four types of neuroglial cells. Microglia cells are part of the reticuloendothelial system and are relatively rare in normal CNS tissue. The microglia cells can become mobile and travel to an area of neuron damage, enlarge and phagocytize tissue debris. Oligodendroglia cells are responsible for myelin formation in the CNS. Astrocytes may provide nutrients and regulate the chemical environment for neurons. Astrocytes also play a role in the blood-brain barrier along with the endothelium of the blood vessels. Astrocytes provide structure and support for nerve cells and may have an indirect role in synaptic transmission. Ependyma cells line the ventricles of the brain and the central canal of the spinal cord and aid in secretion of cerebrospinal fluid (CSF).

Neurons (Figure 9-1 and Table 9-1) are the unit of the nervous system that transmits nerve impulses. There are 10 billion neurons in the CNS with most of them in the cerebral cortex. Neurons cannot regenerate in the CNS, but they can regenerate in the peripheral nervous system by growing within the myelin if the cell body is intact.

Neurons are categorized by their direction, the number of processes, and their location. The direction of impulse formation may be afferent or efferent. Afferent sensory neurons transmit impulses to the spinal cord or brain. Efferent motor neurons transmit impulses away from the brain or spinal cord. Additionally, interneurons transmit impulses from sensory neurons to motor neurons.

Unipolar neurons have one process coming from the cell body and bifurcate into an axon and a dendrite. Bipolar neurons have two processes (one axon and one dendrite) coming from the cell body. Multipolar neurons have one axon and more than one dendrite. The location of the neuron is determined in relation to the brainstem. Upper motor neurons originate above the brainstem and lower motor neurons originate below the brainstem.

Neurophysiology

A chemical, electrical, mechanical, or thermal stimulus initiates impulse transmission. During an impulse transmission, a change in the permeability of the cell membrane to sodium occurs. An influx of sodium causes depolarization of the cell, which initiates an action potential. Repolarization and return to normal resting polarized (ready) state follows depolarization. Synaptic transmission is a unidirectional conduction of an impulse from one neuron to the next. As the impulse nears the end of the axon, there is a release of a neurotransmitter from the synaptic vesicles. The diffusion of the neurotransmitter across the synaptic gap changes the permeability of the cell membrane of the adjoining cell, thereby creating a continuation of the impulse to its end organ or cell. Three types of synapses exist:

- Axosomatic synapse: where the axon of one neuron synapses with the cell body of another neuron
- Axodendritic synapse: where the axon of one neuron synapses with the dendrite of another neuron
- Axoaxonic synapse: where the axon of one neuron synapses with the axon of another neuron

The absolute refractory period is the period of time when the nerve cannot be stimulated again regardless of the strength of the stimulus. The relative refractory period is the period of time when the nerve can only be stimulated by a strong impulse.

Presynaptic vesicles release cerebral neurotransmitters (Table 9-2), which act as a chemical bridge for the transmission of impulses from one neuron to another. After synaptic transmission,

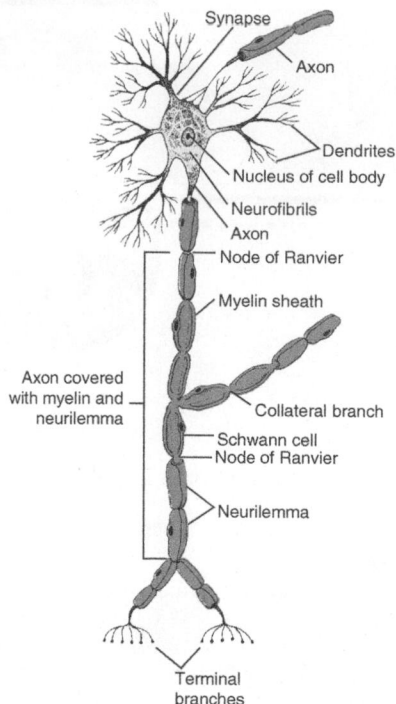

FIGURE 9-1 The neuron. (From Black, J. M., & Hawks, J. A. [2009]. *Medical-surgical nursing: Clinical management for positive outcomes* [8th ed.]. Philadelphia, PA: Saunders.)

TABLE 9-1	**Components of Neurons**
Component	**Function/Structure**
Cell body (soma)	• Contains nucleus
Nucleus	• Controls metabolic processes of cell
Cytoplasm	• Contains organelles to carry out metabolic functions
Axons	• Conduct impulses away from cell body to other neurons or to end organs • Only one axon per neuron • May be myelinated or unmyelinated
Dendrites	• Conduct impulses toward cell body, which receives nerve impulses from the axons of other neurons • May be more than one dendrite
Neurofibrils	• Consists of thin, threadlike fibers that form a network in the cytoplasm
Nissl bodies	• Structures that specialize in protein synthesis with RNA • Maintain and regenerate neuronal processes
Myelin sheath	• Consists of a white lipid substance between the nodes of Ranvier on the axon of some neurons • Acts as insulation to speed conduction of impulses down the axon sheath • Accounts for white color found in parts of brain and spinal cord • Formed by oligodendroglia in CNS and by Schwann cells in PNS
Nodes of Ranvier	• Constrictions occurring periodically along the axon where it is not covered by myelin • Allows rapid conduction of impulses by saltatory conduction (node to node)
Neurilemma	• Outer coating of the neurons in the peripheral nervous system • Provides for peripheral nerve regeneration
Synaptic knobs	• Contain vesicles that store neurotransmitter substances

an enzyme inactivates the neurotransmitter (e.g., cholinesterase deactivates acetylcholine). Neurotransmitters may be excitatory or inhibitory. Excitatory neurotransmitters promote conduction of the impulse from one cell to the next; inhibitory neurotransmitters increase the resistance to depolarization.

Cerebral Metabolism

Oxygen requirements of the brain are high in relation to its size. The brain has high metabolic energy requirements as well. The brain weight is 2% of the total body weight but receives 20% of the cardiac output and uses 20% of oxygen delivered. Cerebral oxygen consumption averages about 49 mL/min. The brain, especially the cerebral cortex, is very susceptible to a change in oxygen delivery, though the brainstem is the most resistant to hypoxic damage. Within seconds to minutes of anoxia, cytotoxic edema will occur, causing brain edema and neuron death.

Nutrient requirements of the brain are also high because of its high metabolic energy needs. Glucose is the main source of cellular energy (i.e., adenosine triphosphate [ATP]). The minimal storage of glucose in the brain necessitates a constant supply for normal brain function. At rest, the brain consumes 25% of body glucose. Triggered by the SNS, gluconeogenesis is a very important process because it causes the conversion of protein and fat to glucose, thereby protecting the brain. Also important in this protective mechanism is the fact that the brain does not require insulin to use glucose. Significant hypoglycemia is associated with neurologic symptoms. Confusion usually occurs if blood glucose is less than 50 to 70 mg/dL and loss of consciousness occurs if blood glucose is less than 20 mg/dL, and progresses to death. Although hyperglycemia does not cause direct neurologic effects, the osmotic effect may cause hyperosmolality and brain dehydration, such as is seen with hyperosmolar hyperglycemic state (HHS).

Vitamins required by the brain include thiamine (B_1), B_{12}, pyridoxine (B_6), and niacin (i.e., nicotinic acid). Thiamine is important in the Krebs cycle and deficiency of thiamine causes Wernicke encephalopathy. Vitamin B_{12} is important in the spinal cord and peripheral nervous system. Deficiency of B_{12} causes pernicious anemia and gradual deterioration of the CNS and peripheral nerves. Pyridoxine is a coenzyme that participates in many enzymatic reactions in the CNS. Neuropathy and seizures occur with pyridoxine deficiency. The synthesis of coenzymes requires niacin and a deficiency of niacin causes pellagra.

Blood-Brain Barrier

The blood-brain barrier is not a true structure but a special permeability characteristic of the brain capillaries and choroid plexus. It acts to limit transfer of certain substances into extracellular fluid (ECF) or CSF of the brain and prevents toxic substances from readily entering the extracellular space of the nervous system. Water, carbon dioxide, oxygen, glucose, and lipid-soluble substances cross the cerebral capillaries with ease. The uptake of other substances such as dyes and ions (e.g., Na^{++}, K^+) is much slower. The goal of

TABLE 9-2	Neurologic System Neurotransmitters		
Name	**Type**	**Region**	**Predominant Effect**
Acetylcholine	Cholinergic	• Basal ganglia • Pyramidal cells • Parasympathetic branch of ANS	Excitatory
Norepinephrine	Amine	• Hypothalamus • Brainstem • Sympathetic branch of ANS	Inhibitory/excitatory
Dopamine	Amine	• Basal ganglia • Brainstem	Inhibitory
Serotonin	Amine	• Hypothalamus • Brainstem	Inhibitory
Gamma-aminobutyric acid (GABA)	Amino acid	• Basal ganglia • Cerebellum • Spinal cord	Inhibitory
Glycine	Amino acid	• Spinal cord	Inhibitory
Beta-endorphins	Peptide	• Spinal cord	Inhibitory
Substance P	Peptide	• Pain fibers in spinal cord	Excitatory

the blood-brain barrier is to regulate the entry or removal of various substances to maintain homeostasis in the CNS environment. The blood-brain barrier has clinical significance in treating and diagnosing CNS disease. Unfortunately, the blood-brain barrier may hinder the effective use of certain drug therapies in the treatment of neurologic system problems. Trauma, induction of some toxic elements, intracranial tumor, and/or brain irradiation may alter the permeability of the blood-brain barrier.

Macroscopic Anatomy and Physiology
Scalp
The scalp is the five layers of skin covering the cranium. Use the mnemonic SCALP to remember the five layers.
- **S**kin: thicker than anywhere else in the body, and is hair-bearing.
- **C**onnective tissue: thin layer of fat and fibrous tissue that connects the skin to the underlying aponeurosis. Blood vessels are attached to this layer. The scalp is very vascular and the blood vessels here do not contract well when injured; as a result, a scalp laceration can result in significant blood loss.
- **A**poneurotica: tough layer of dense, fibrous tissue.
- **L**oose areolar tissue: loosely connects the epicranial aponeurosis to the pericranium and allows the superficial three layers of the scalp to move over the pericranium.
- **P**ericranium: the periosteum of the skull bones.

Skull
The skull (Figure 9-2) is the bony structure of the head, consisting of the cranium and the skeleton of the face. The skull is composed of an inner table and outer table separated by cancellous (spongy) bone. This structure allows for maximum strength and minimal weight. The cranium is a body vault that holds and protects the brain from external forces and has a volume capacity of approximately 1500 mL.

The cranium consists of eight bones: one frontal, occipital, ethmoid, and sphenoid bone and two parietal and temporal bones. The sphenoid bone divides the interior of the skull into three fossae (Figure 9-3). The anterior fossa contains the frontal lobes; the middle fossa contains the temporal, parietal, and occipital lobes; and the posterior fossa contains the cerebellum. The brain connects to the spinal cord via the foramen magnum, a large oval-shaped opening at the base of the skull.

Meninges
Meninges (Figure 9-4) are the protective coverings of the brain and the spinal cord. The pia mater is the delicate layer that adheres to the surface of the brain and spinal cord. This layer follows the sulci and gyri of brain and carries branches of cerebral arteries with it. Sulci are the shallow grooves or invaginations on the surface of the brain (deep sulci are referred to as *fissures*) and gyri are convolutions on the surface of the brain. The blood vessels of the pia mater form the choroid plexus, which produces CSF.

The arachnoid mater is the middle layer of the meninges. The subarachnoid space is between the arachnoid mater and the pia mater and contains the larger blood vessels of the brain, the CSF, and the arachnoid villi. Arachnoid villi are projections of arachnoid mater that serve as channels for absorption of CSF into the venous system. A subarachnoid hemorrhage is bleeding into the subarachnoid space between the arachnoid membrane and the pia mater surrounding the brain. The dura mater is the outermost layer of the meninges. The meningeal arteries and venous sinuses lie within clefts formed by separation of inner and outer layers of the dura mater. The epidural space is a potential space between the skull and the dura mater and is the site of an epidural hemorrhage or hematoma. The subdural space is a potential space between the dura mater and the arachnoid mater and is the site of a subdural hemorrhage or hematoma.

There are several folds of the dura mater (Figure 9-5). The falx cerebri separates the two cerebral hemispheres. It also separates the two cerebellar hemispheres. The tentorium cerebelli separate the cerebral hemispheres from the cerebellum. The diaphragma sella canopies the sella turcica, where the pituitary gland is located, and encloses the pituitary gland.

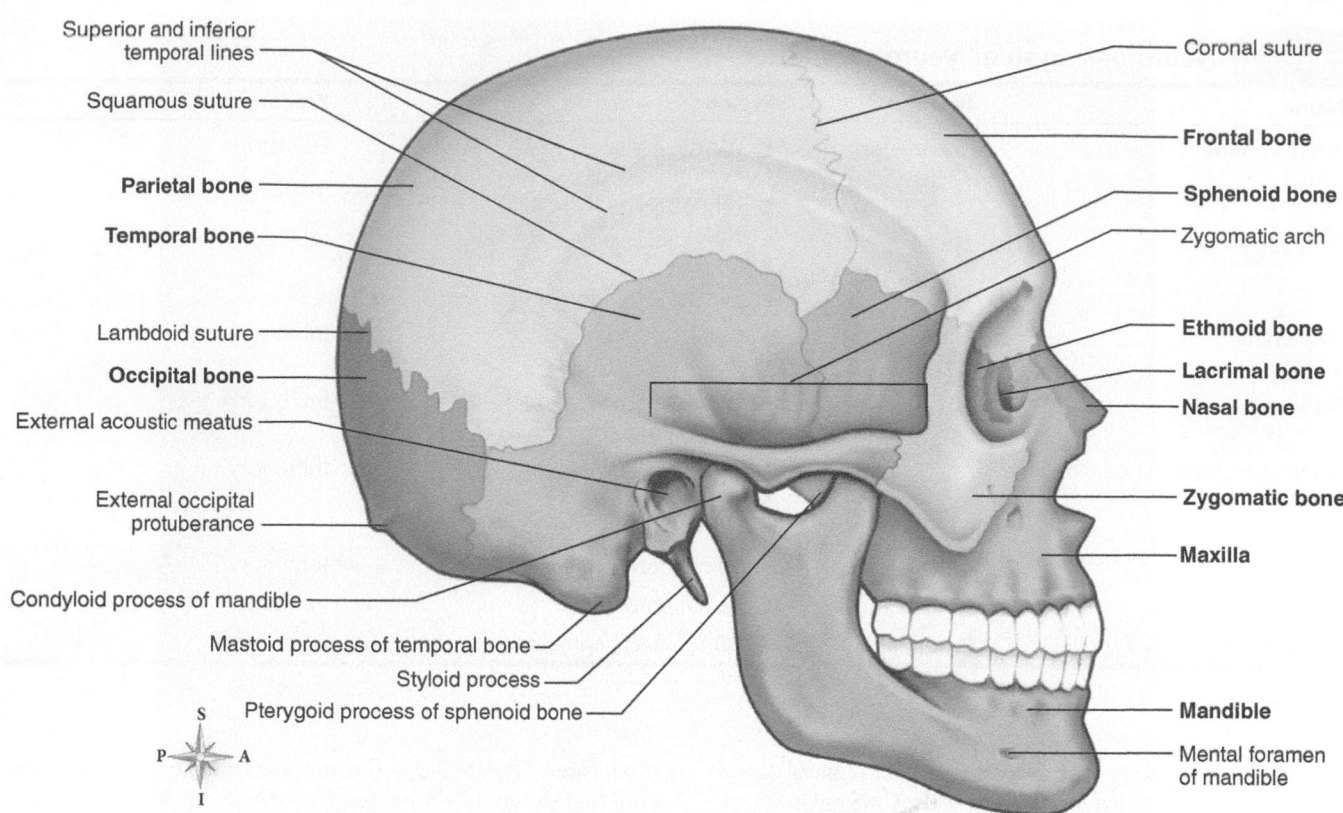

Superior and inferior temporal lines

Squamous suture

Parietal bone

Temporal bone

Lambdoid suture

Occipital bone

External acoustic meatus

External occipital protuberance

Condyloid process of mandible

Mastoid process of temporal bone

Styloid process

Pterygoid process of sphenoid bone

Coronal suture

Frontal bone

Sphenoid bone

Zygomatic arch

Ethmoid bone

Lacrimal bone

Nasal bone

Zygomatic bone

Maxilla

Mandible

Mental foramen of mandible

FIGURE 9-2 Lateral view of skull. (From Patton, K. T., & Thibodeau, G. F. [2016]. *Anatomy & physiology* [9th ed.]. St. Louis, MO: Mosby.)

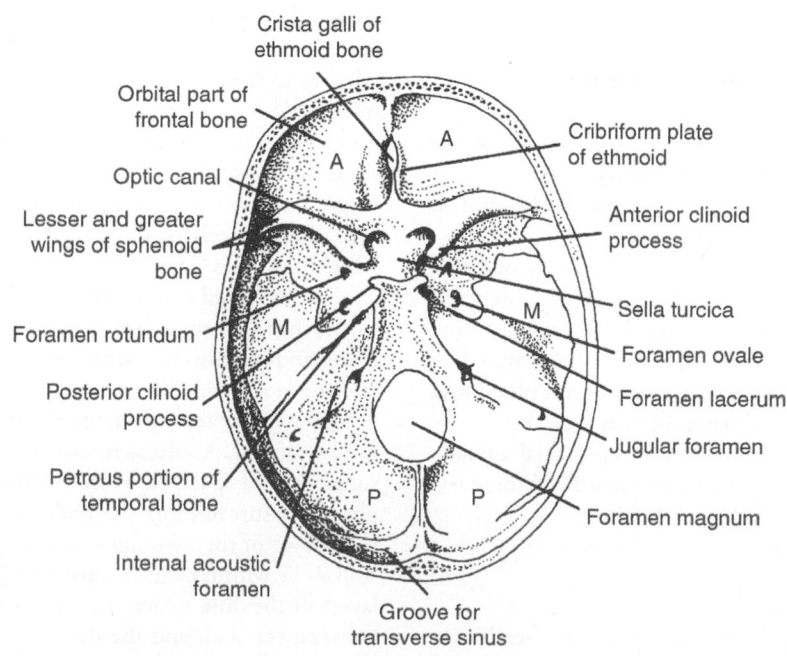

Crista galli of ethmoid bone

Orbital part of frontal bone

Optic canal

Lesser and greater wings of sphenoid bone

Foramen rotundum

Posterior clinoid process

Petrous portion of temporal bone

Internal acoustic foramen

Cribriform plate of ethmoid

Anterior clinoid process

Sella turcica

Foramen ovale

Foramen lacerum

Jugular foramen

Foramen magnum

Groove for transverse sinus

A = Anterior cranial fossa
M = Middle cranial fossa
P = Posterior cranial fossa

FIGURE 9-3 Bones that form the floor of the cranial cavity and the three fossae formed by these bones. (From Kinney, M., Dunbar, S., Brooks-Brunn, J. A., Molter, N., & Vitello-Cicciu, J. [1998]. *AACN clinical reference for critical care nursing* [4th ed.]. St. Louis, MO: Mosby.)

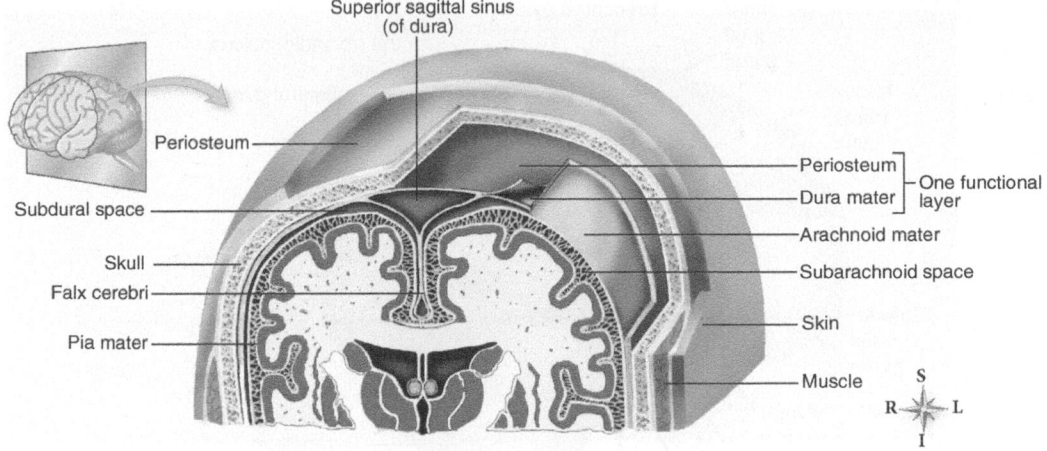

FIGURE 9-4 Coverings of the brain. (From Patton, K. T., & Thibodeau, G. F. [2016]. *Anatomy & physiology* [9th ed.]. St. Louis, MO: Mosby.)

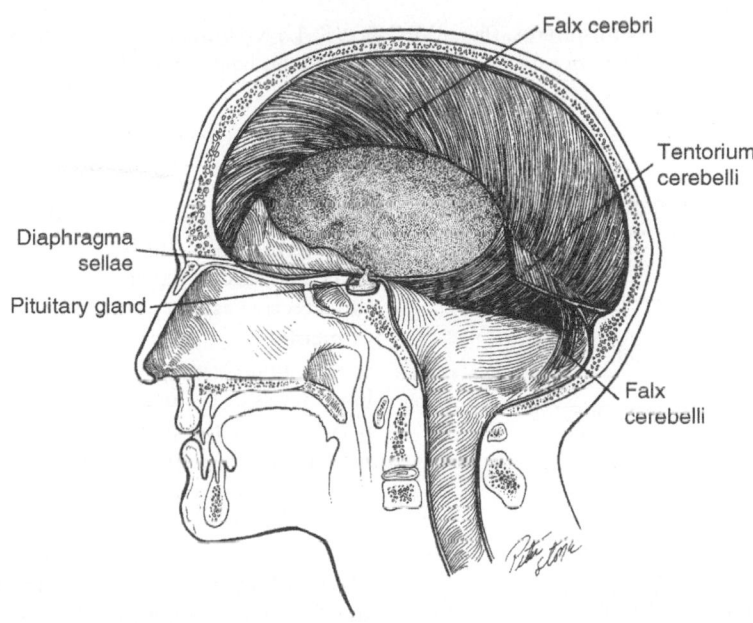

FIGURE 9-5 Folds of the dura. (From Kinney, M., Dunbar, S., Brooks-Brunn, J. A., Molter, N., & Vitello-Cicciu, J. [1998]. *AACN clinical reference for critical care nursing* [4th ed.]. St. Louis, MO: Mosby.)

Brain

The brain, divided into the cerebrum (i.e., telencephalon), brainstem, and cerebellum, weighs approximately 2 kg. The cerebrum consists of two cerebral hemispheres connected by the corpus callosum. Fissures are separations in the cerebral hemispheres and are similar to sulci except that they are deeper. The great longitudinal fissure divides the left and right cerebral hemispheres. The Fissure of Rolando (also referred to as *central sulcus*) divides the frontal lobe from the parietal lobes and separates the motor and sensory strips. The Fissure of Sylvius (also referred to as *lateral sulcus* or *Sylvian fissure*) divides the frontal lobe from the temporal lobes.

Cerebral cortical areas (Figure 9-6 and Table 9-3) include the frontal lobe, which contains the precentral gyrus (also referred to as the *motor strip*); the parietal lobe, which contains the postcentral gyrus (also referred to as the *sensory strip*); the temporal lobe; and the occipital lobe. Each of the two cerebral hemispheres of the brain receives sensory information from the opposite side of the body and controls skeletal muscles of the opposite side. Each hemisphere has specialization. The left cerebral hemisphere is specialized for analysis, problem solving, language, mathematics, abstract reasoning, and interpretation of symbols. The right cerebral hemisphere is specialized for visuospatial patterns, nonverbal communication, music, and artistic ability. Ninety percent of right-handed people are left hemisphere dominant. Sixty percent of left-handed people are right hemisphere dominant. Language centers are located in the dominant hemisphere; therefore, lesions occurring in the dominant hemisphere frequently cause aphasia.

The corpus callosum is a thick band of nerve fibers that connects the left and right sides of the brain. It transfers

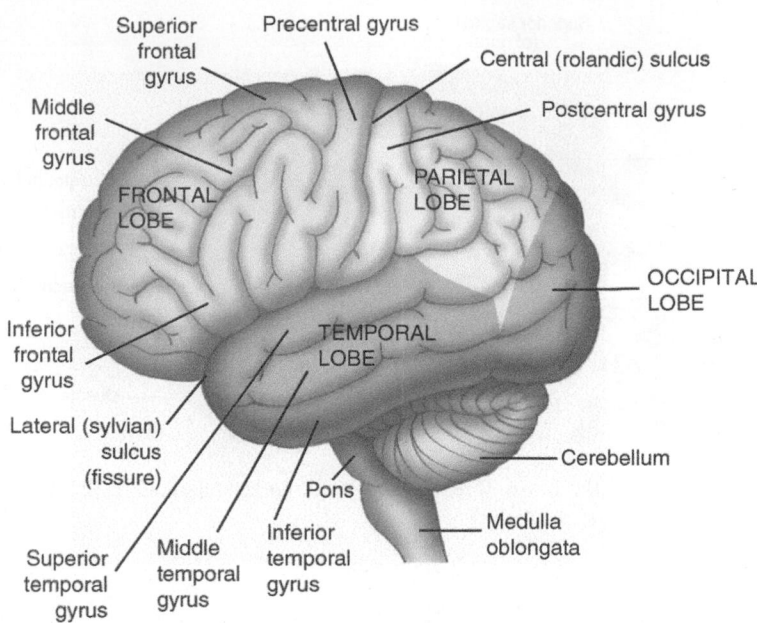

FIGURE 9-6 Cerebral hemispheres. (From McCance, K. L., & Huether, S. E. [2014]. *Pathophysiology: The biologic basis for disease in adults and children* [7th ed.]. St. Louis, MO: Mosby.)

TABLE 9-3	Cerebral Cortical Areas and Functions	

Cerebral Cortical Areas	Functions

Frontal lobe	• Personality
	• Behavior: ethical, moral, and social
	• Intellectual functions
	  ◦ Conscious thought
	  ◦ Abstract thinking
	  ◦ Judgment and foresight
	• Short-term memory
	• Voluntary motor function
	• Motor speech (Broca area in dominant hemisphere)

Parietal lobe	• Localization of sensory information to the body surface • Sensory integration and discrimination • Object recognition • Position sense • Body awareness • Body image
Temporal lobe	• Emotion • Long-term memory • Processing of olfactory, gustatory, and auditory input • Sensory speech (Wernicke area in dominant hemisphere)
Occipital lobe	• Processing of visual input

motor, sensory, and cognitive information between the brain hemispheres.

The diencephalon contains the thalamus, hypothalamus, and limbic system. The thalamus relays incoming messages to appropriate areas of the brain. The hypothalamus regulates temperature, food and water intake, sleep patterns, autonomic responses, and hormonal secretion of the pituitary gland. The limbic system regulates self-preservation behaviors, including aggression, basic drives (e.g., food, sex), the affective aspect of emotional behavior, and some aspects of memory.

The brainstem relays messages between the brain and the lower levels of the nervous system. It is the origin of all cranial nerves except the first and second. The brain stem has three sections: the mesencephalon (i.e., midbrain), the pons, and the medulla oblongata. The mesencephalon is the origin of the third and fourth cranial nerves. It contains both motor and sensory pathways and is the location of the reticular activating system (RAS), which is responsible for arousal from sleep, wakefulness, and focusing of attention. The pons is the origin of the fifth, sixth, and seventh cranial nerves and connects the cerebral cortex and the cerebellum. The pons contains both motor and sensory pathways and regulates respiratory rhythm. The medulla oblongata is the origin of the eighth, ninth, tenth, eleventh, and twelfth cranial nerves and connects the motor and sensory tracts of the spinal cord to the medulla. The medulla contains cardiac and respiratory centers.

The cerebellum is located in the posterior fossa. The cortex is the outer layer of the cerebellum and is made of gray matter consisting of neuron cell bodies that are six cell layers thick. The deeper layers of each hemisphere are white matter consisting of myelinated axons with four paired masses of gray matter known as *basal ganglia*. Basal ganglia are the major center of the extrapyramidal system. Their functions include regulation and control of motor integration, influencing posture, and allowing fine voluntary movements.

The cerebellum coordinates muscle movement with sensory input. It controls balance, influences muscle tone in relation to equilibrium, and affects locomotion and posture. The cerebellum also controls nonstereotyped movements and synchronizes muscle action.

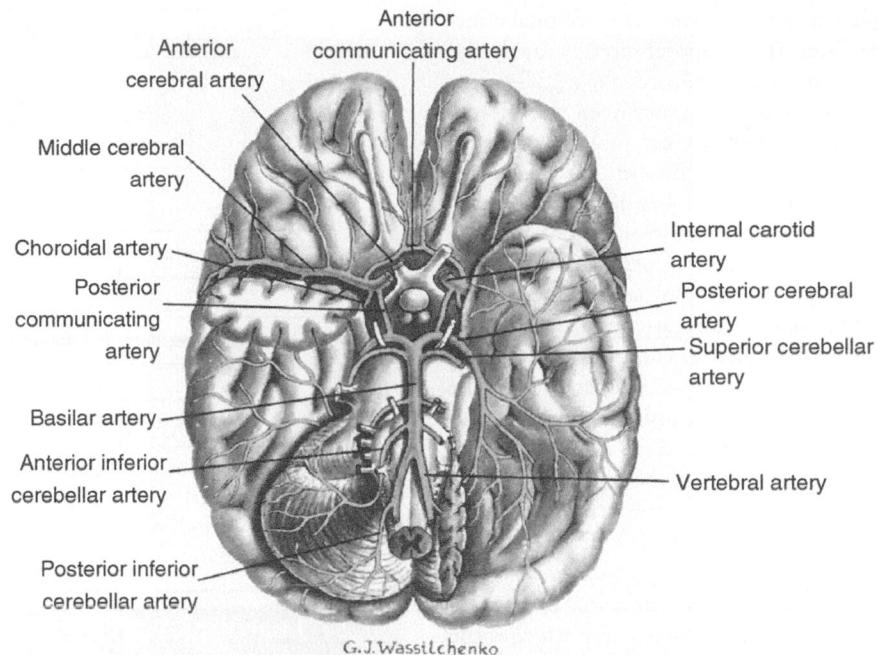

FIGURE 9-7 Arterial system of the brain. (From Urden, L., Stacy, K., & Lough, M. [2010]. *Critical care nursing: Diagnosis and management* [6th ed.]. St. Louis, MO: Mosby.)

9.1 Learning Activity

Match the area of the brain to the associated function.

_____ 1. Anterior frontal lobe
_____ 2. Posterior frontal lobe
3. Parietal lobe
_____ 4. Occipital lobe
_____ 5. Temporal lobe
_____ 6. Cerebellum
_____ 7. Medulla
_____ 8. Hypothalamus
_____ 9. Wernicke's area
_____ 10. Thalamus
_____ 11. Limbic system
_____ 12. Broca's area

a. Responsible for verbal expression
b. Regulates cardiac, vasomotor, and respiratory functions
c. Receives visual stimuli
d. Maintains equilibrium
e. Regulates endocrine and autonomic functions
f. Receives auditory stimuli
g. Receives sensory stimuli
h. Involved in emotional and sexual response
i. Responsible for language interpretation
j. Contains the motor strip which controls voluntary motor functions
k. Controls judgment, insight, and reasoning
l. Relays sensory and motor input to the cerebrum

Answers to this activity can be found in the Answer Key.

TABLE 9-4 Cerebral Artery Distribution

Artery	Areas
Anterior Circulation: Internal Carotid System	
Anterior cerebral arteries	• Superior surface of the frontal and parietal lobes • Medial surface of cerebral hemispheres • Basal ganglia • Corpus callosum • Hypothalamus
Middle cerebral arteries	• Lateral surfaces of frontal, parietal, and temporal lobes • Superior surface of temporal lobe • Subcortical structures (e.g., thalamus, hypothalamus, basal ganglia) • Precentral (motor) gyri • Postcentral (sensory) gyri
Posterior Circulation: Vertebrobasilar System	
Basilar artery	• Most of brainstem • Cerebellum
Posterior cerebral arteries	• Thalamus • Medial portion of occipital lobe • Inferior portion of temporal lobe • Vestibular organs • Cochlear apparatus

Cerebral Circulation
The Arterial System

The brain receives 20% of the cardiac output. The cerebral arterial circulation (Figure 9-7 and Table 9-4) consists of the anterior and the posterior circulation. The external carotid system arises from the common carotid arteries and makes up the occipital, temporal, and maxillary arteries. The occipital arteries supply the posterior fossa; the temporal arteries supply the temporal area; and the maxillary arteries form the middle meningeal arteries. The anterior circulation arises from the internal carotid artery and supplies most of the cerebral hemispheres. The vertebrobasilar arteries supply the cerebellum, brainstem, and areas of the occipital and temporal lobes of the cerebrum.

The internal carotid system feeds the anterior circulation of the brain, which accounts for 80% of cerebral perfusion. The anterior circulation includes the anterior cerebral arteries, the anterior communicating artery, the middle cerebral arteries, and the posterior communicating arteries. The anterior communicating artery connects the right and left anterior cerebral arteries to form the anterior section of the circle of Willis. The posterior communicating arteries connect the posterior cerebral arteries with the anterior circulation to form the posterior portion of the circle of Willis.

The posterior circulation makes up the vertebrobasilar system, and arises from the subclavian arteries. It joins at the lower border of the pons to form the basilar artery. It includes the posterior cerebral arteries, basilar artery, anterior spinal artery, and posterior spinal arteries. The anterior spinal artery supplies the anterior half of three quarters of the spinal cord and the medial aspect of the brainstem. The posterior spinal arteries traverse the spinal cord along the dorsal roots.

The internal carotids and vertebral arteries form the circle of Willis. If one of the carotid or vertebral arteries occludes, the circle of Willis permits collateral circulation. Unfortunately, many people have an incomplete circle of Willis, which prevents this collateral flow when injury or occlusion occurs. The circle of Willis is prone to aneurysmal formation due to multiple bifurcations.

The meningeal arteries are branches of the external carotid arteries that supply the dura mater. The internal carotid and vertebral arteries supply the pia mater and arachnoid mater. The anterior meningeal artery supplies the anterior portion of the dura; the middle meningeal artery supplies most of the dura; the posterior meningeal artery supplies the occipital area of the dura.

Cerebral Blood Flow

Cerebral blood flow (CBF) brings oxygen and nutrients to the brain tissue for cellular energy production and removal of waste products from the blood. CBF varies with changes in cerebral perfusion pressure (CPP) and the diameter of the cerebrovascular bed. Normal CBF is approximately 50 mL/100 g/min.

CPP is the net pressure gradient that causes cerebral blood flow to the brain. Mean arterial blood pressure (MAP) and intracranial pressure (ICP) affect the CPP. ICP is the pressure exerted by brain tissue, blood, and CSF against the inside of the skull.

SIDEBAR 9-2

Cerebral Perfusion Pressure

CPP is calculated as: MAP – ICP

Changes in MAP or ICP will affect CPP. MAP is calculated as: (SBP + [2 × DBP]) divided by 3. Normal MAP is 70 to 105 mm Hg; normal ICP is 5 to 15 mm Hg; so normal CPP is 60 to 100 mm Hg. CPP less than 50 mm Hg is associated with impaired neuronal functioning. Because ICP measurement requires intracranial pressure monitoring, transfer the patient to a higher level of care. ICP monitoring is not performed in the progressive care unit. Nurses on the progressive care unit need to rely on clinical indications of increased ICP.

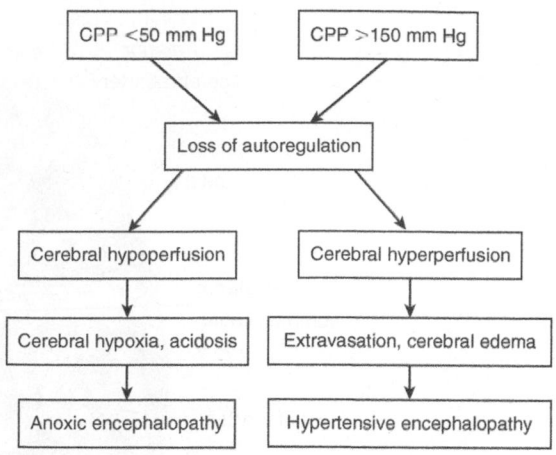

FIGURE 9-8 Effects of significant alterations in cerebral perfusion pressure. *CPP,* cerebral perfusion pressure. (From Dennison, R. D. [2013]. *Pass CCRN!* [4th ed]. St. Louis, MO: Elsevier.)

9.2   Learning Activity

Your patient has had a traumatic brain injury. His blood pressure is 80/50 mm Hg and his ICP is 20 mm Hg. Calculate his cerebral perfusion pressure. Should you be concerned? Why?

Answers to this activity can be found in the Answer Key.

Autoregulation is the ability of the brain to alter the diameter of the arterioles to maintain CBF at a constant level despite changes in CPP. When ICP approaches the MAP, CPP decreases to the point where autoregulation is impaired and CBF decreases (Figure 9-8). A low CPP caused by either a low MAP (e.g., cardiopulmonary arrest, shock) or a high ICP (e.g., cerebral edema, intracranial mass) causes hypoperfusion, resulting in anoxic encephalopathy. A high CPP caused by a high MAP (e.g., hypertensive crisis) causes hyperperfusion, resulting in brain edema and hypertensive encephalopathy.

Factors that increase CBF include hypercapnia, hypoxemia, decreased blood viscosity, hyperthermia, and vasodilating drugs. Factors that decrease CBF include hypocapnia, hyperoxemia, increased blood viscosity, hypothermia, intracranial hypertension, cerebral vasospasm, and drugs that increase blood pressure (e.g., vasopressors). Therapeutic drugs used to optimize cardiac output (CO), blood pressure (BP), and CPP and/or minimize oxygen consumption may result in decreased CO, BP, CPP, and CBF when used inappropriately or in excess. These include negative inotropes (e.g., beta-blockers, barbiturates), vasodilators (e.g., nitroprusside, nitroglycerin, nicardipine), and anesthetic agents. Therapies utilized to manage acute intracranial hypertension, which are aimed at lowering $Paco_2$ (i.e., hyperventilation), result in vasoconstriction, thereby reducing cerebral blood flow and oxygenation. Reserve hyperventilation therapy for situations that involve imminent herniation.

The Venous System

The cerebrum has external veins that lie in the subarachnoid space on surfaces of the hemispheres. There are also internal veins that drain the central core of the cerebrum and lie beneath the corpus callosum. Both external and internal venous systems empty into venous sinuses that lie between the dura layers. The superior

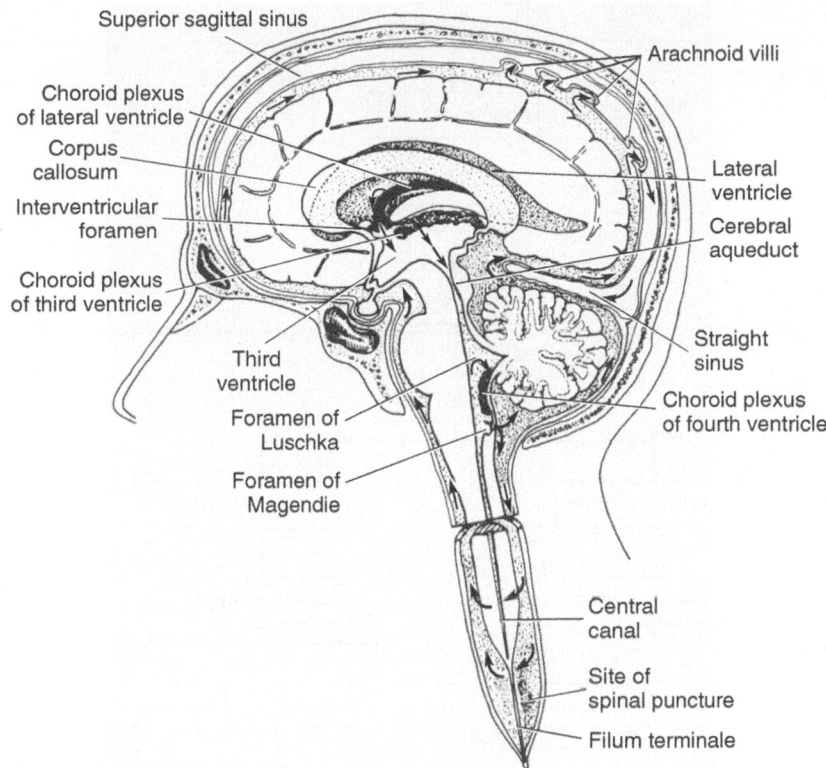

Superior sagittal sinus

Arachnoid villi

Choroid plexus
of lateral ventricle

Corpus
callosum

Lateral
ventricle

Interventricular
foramen

Cerebral
aqueduct

Choroid plexus
of third ventricle

Third
ventricle

Straight
sinus

Choroid plexus
of fourth ventricle

Foramen of
Luschka

Foramen of
Magendie

Central
canal

Site of
spinal puncture

Filum terminale

FIGURE 9-9 Lateral view of the ventricular system. Arrows show direction of CSF circulation. (From Kinney, M., Dunbar, S., Brooks-Brunn, J. A., Molter, N., & Vitello-Cicciu, J. [1998]. *AACN clinical reference for critical care nursing* [4th ed.]. St. Louis, MO: Mosby.)

sagittal sinus drains venous blood from the anterior portions of the brain. The cavernous sinus drains venous blood from the inferior portions of the brain. The transvenous sinus drains venous blood from the posterior portion of the brain, and the internal jugular veins collect blood from the venous sinuses in the dura.

Cerebrospinal Fluid

Cerebrospinal fluid (CSF) cushions the brain and spinal cord and allows compensation for changes in ICP. Displacement of CSF out of the cranial cavity compensates for increases in intracranial volume to prevent an increase in ICP. Of the approximately 120 to 150 mL of CSF, about 90 mL is distributed in the lumbar subarachnoid space, 25 mL is in the ventricles, and about 35 mL is distributed throughout the rest of the subarachnoid space. The brain synthesizes about 500 mL of CSF each day. The pressure exerted by the CSF is normally measured at less than 200 mm H_2O at the lumbar level with the patient in a side-lying position.

CSF is a transudate of plasma formed by the choroid plexus in the ventricles. The choroid plexus consists of sheets of epithelial cells that project into the lumen of the ventricular spaces. The lateral ventricles produce the majority (95%) of CSF. CSF is absorbed via the arachnoid villi, which return it to the systemic circulation by the internal jugular veins. The hydrostatic pressure gradient between the CSF and the venous sinus is one factor that determines CSF absorption.

CSF Communication System within the Brain

CSF circulates within the subarachnoid space and the ventricles (Figures 9-9 and 9-10). The ventricles are hollow spaces lined with ependyma and they contain specialized epithelium called the choroid plexus, which produces CSF. The lateral ventricles

are the largest of the ventricles. One lateral ventricle lies in each cerebral hemisphere. The third ventricle lies between the two lateral ventricles. The fourth ventricle lies in the posterior fossa.

Spine and Spinal Cord

The vertebral column is composed of 7 cervical, 12 thoracic, 5 lumbar, 5 sacral, and 4 coccygeal vertebrae. The spinal cord (Figure 9-11) is 42 to 45 cm in length, extending from the superior border of the atlas to the upper border of the second lumbar vertebrae (L2). It is continuous with the brainstem. As with the brain, the meninges include the pia mater, arachnoid mater, and dura mater. The central canal is the opening in the center of the spinal cord that contains CSF and communicates with the fourth ventricle. The central gray horns form an "H" and contain mostly cell bodies.

The anterior (or ventral) horn contains cell bodies of efferent, or motor, fibers. The posterior (or dorsal) horn contains cell bodies of afferent, or sensory, fibers. The lateral horns contain the preganglionic fibers of the autonomic system.

Columns of white matter are fiber tracts that surround the gray matter and contain mostly myelinated axons. Ascending tracts conduct sensory impulses from the spinal cord to the thalamus and cerebral cortex and include the posterior tracts (dorsal columns) and the anterior and lateral spinothalamic tracts. Descending tracts conduct motor impulses from the brain to motor neurons in the anterior horn and include the corticospinal lateral tract and the pyramidal lateral tract. Spinal tracts (Table 9-5) receive their name by column, origin, and termination. For example, the lateral corticospinal tract is located in the lateral column, originates in the cortex, and terminates in the spine; it is therefore a descending tract (cortex to spine).

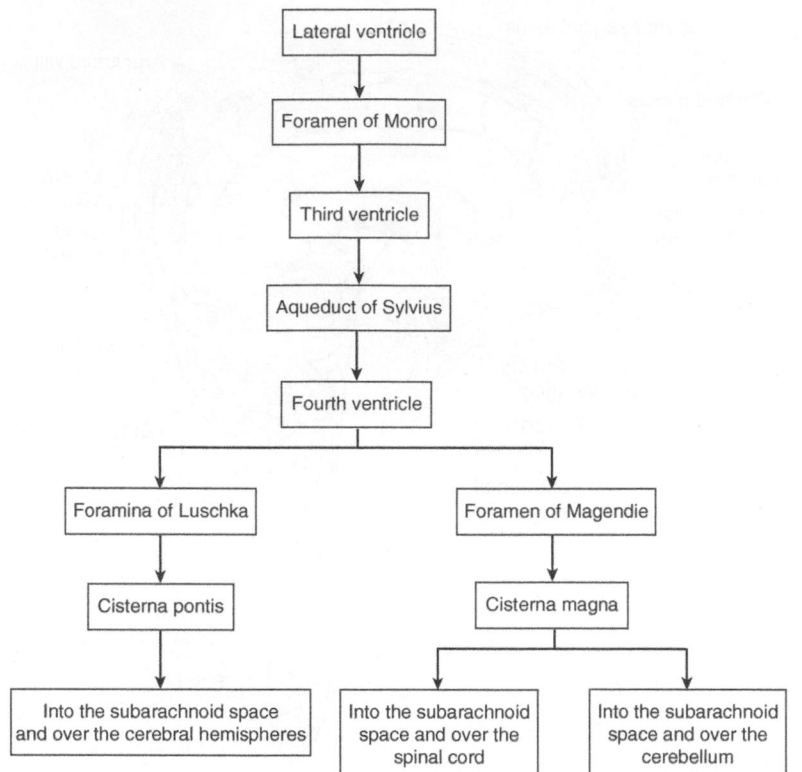

FIGURE 9-10 Circulation of CSF. (From Dennison, R. D. [2013] *Pass CCRN!* [4th ed.] St. Louis, MO: Elsevier.)

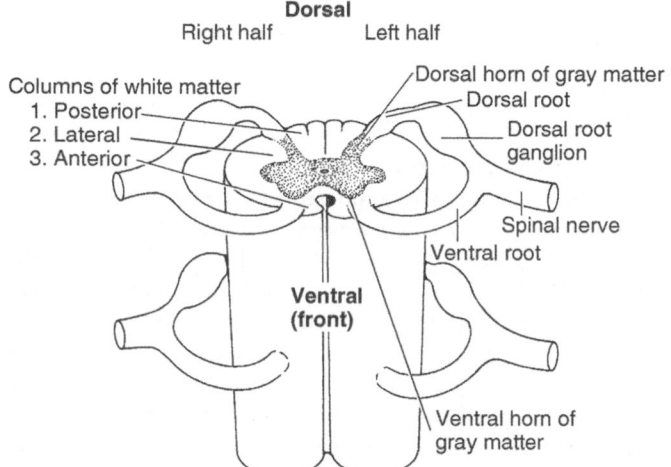

FIGURE 9-11 Segment of the thoracic spinal cord in cross section. (From Kinney, M., Dunbar, S., Brooks-Brunn, J. A., Molter, N., & Vitello-Cicciu, J. [1998]. *AACN clinical reference for critical care nursing* [4th ed.]. St. Louis, MO: Mosby.)

Upper motor neurons (UMNs) are located in the cerebral cortex and brainstem. Cell bodies lie in the motor area of the cerebral cortex. Axons pass through the spinal cord to synapse with the lower motor neurons. Damage to UMNs causes spastic paralysis and hyperactive reflexes.

Lower motor neurons (LMNs) are located in the spinal cord. Cell bodies lie in the anterior horn of gray matter in the spinal cord. Axons directly innervate striated muscle fibers. Damage to LMNs causes flaccid paralysis and areflexia.

The spinal cord mediates the reflex arc (Figure 9-12) by causing an involuntary response to a stimulus (e.g., touching a hot stove causes reflex withdrawal of hand). It serves as the communicating pathway between the brain and the peripheral nervous system. The stimulus does not go beyond the spinal cord to the brain, and it does not require cerebral interpretation. The receptor organ (sensory receptor) contains sensory fibers that are sensitive to the stimulus. The afferent neuron (sensory neuron) sends the impulse to the spinal cord. The interneuron passes the impulse from the sensory neuron to the motor neuron. The effector neuron (motor neuron) sends the impulse to the effector organ and responds to the impulse. The effector organ also serves as the communicating pathway between the brain and the peripheral nervous system. In our example, it sends the message of pain to the brain.

Peripheral Nervous System

The spinal segments consist of 31 pairs of spinal nerves: 8 cervical (C1-C8), 12 thoracic (T1-T12), 5 lumbar (L1-L5), 5 sacral (S1-S5), and 1 coccygeal. The fibers of spinal nerves include both motor fibers and sensory fibers. Motor fibers originate in the anterior gray column of the spinal cord, form the ventral root of the spinal nerve, and pass to the skeletal muscles. Sensory fibers originate in the spinal ganglia of dorsal roots. Peripheral branches distribute to the visceral and somatic structures as mediators of sensory impulses to the CNS. Each spinal nerve innervates a specific portion of the skin, identified as the dermatome for that spinal nerve (Figure 9-13 and Table 9-6). Spinal nerves form various nerve plexuses that innervate the skin and muscles throughout the body.

- The cervical plexus innervates C1-C4.
- The brachial plexus innervates C5-C8 and T1.
- The lumbar plexus innervates L1-L4.
- The sacral plexus innervates L4-L5 and S1-S4.

TABLE 9-5	**Spinal Cord Tracts and Functions**				
Tract	**Column**	**Direction**	**Functions**		**Sidedness**
Spinothalamic					
Lateral spinothalamic	Lateral	Ascending	• Pain • Temperature		Contralateral
Anterior spinothalamic	Anterior	Ascending	• Light touch • Pressure • Pain • Temperature		Contralateral
Spinotectal	Lateral	Ascending	• Tactile stimulation arousing consciousness		Contralateral
Spinocerebellar					
Dorsal spinocerebellar	Lateral	Ascending	• Reflex proprioception • Muscle tone and synergy		Ipsilateral
Ventral spinocerebellar	Lateral	Ascending	• Reflex proprioception • Muscle tone and synergy		Contralateral
Medial Lemniscal System					
Fasciculus gracilis	Posterior	Ascending	• Position sense • Vibratory sense • Pressure • Tactile localization • Two-point discrimination		Ipsilateral
Fasciculus cuneatus	Posterior	Ascending	• Position sense • Vibratory sense • Pressure • Tactile localization • Two-point discrimination		Ipsilateral
Pyramidal					
Lateral corticospinal	Lateral	Descending	• Voluntary movement		Contralateral
Ventral corticospinal	Lateral	Descending	• Voluntary movement		Ipsilateral
Extrapyramidal					
Rubrospinal	Lateral	Descending	• Synergy and muscle tone		Contralateral
Lateral vestibulospinal	Anterior	Descending	• Posture and equilibrium		Ipsilateral
Medial vestibulospinal	Anterior	Descending	• Posture and equilibrium		Contralateral
Lateral reticulospinal	Lateral	Descending	• Muscle tone		Ipsilateral
Medial reticulospinal	Anterior	Descending	• Muscle tone		Ipsilateral
Tectospinal	Anterior	Descending	• Vision and hearing		Contralateral

Cranial Nerves

Twelve pairs of cranial nerves (Table 9-7) carry impulses to and from the brain. The cranial nerves may have motor or sensory functions or both.

Autonomic Nervous System

The autonomic nervous system (ANS) consists of two neuron chains that carry information from the CNS to peripheral effector organs. A preganglionic neuron is the cell body outside

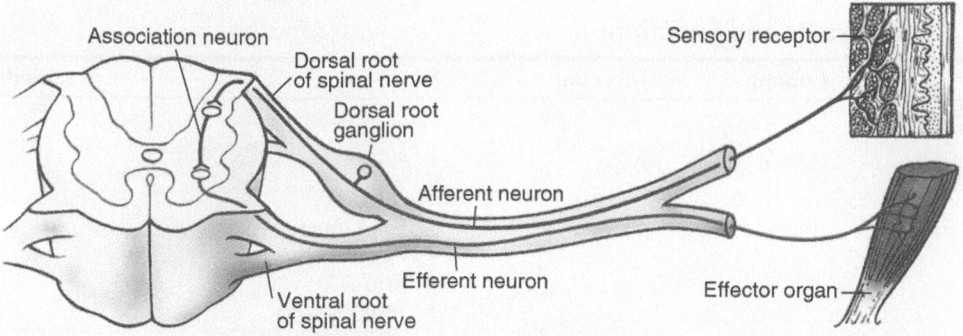

FIGURE 9-12 Basic diagram of a reflex arc, including the sensory receptor, afferent neuron, association neuron, efferent neuron, and effector organ. (From Lewis, S. M., Heitkemper, M. M., & Dirksen, S. R. [2000]. *Medical-surgical nursing* [5th ed.]. St Louis, MO: Mosby.)

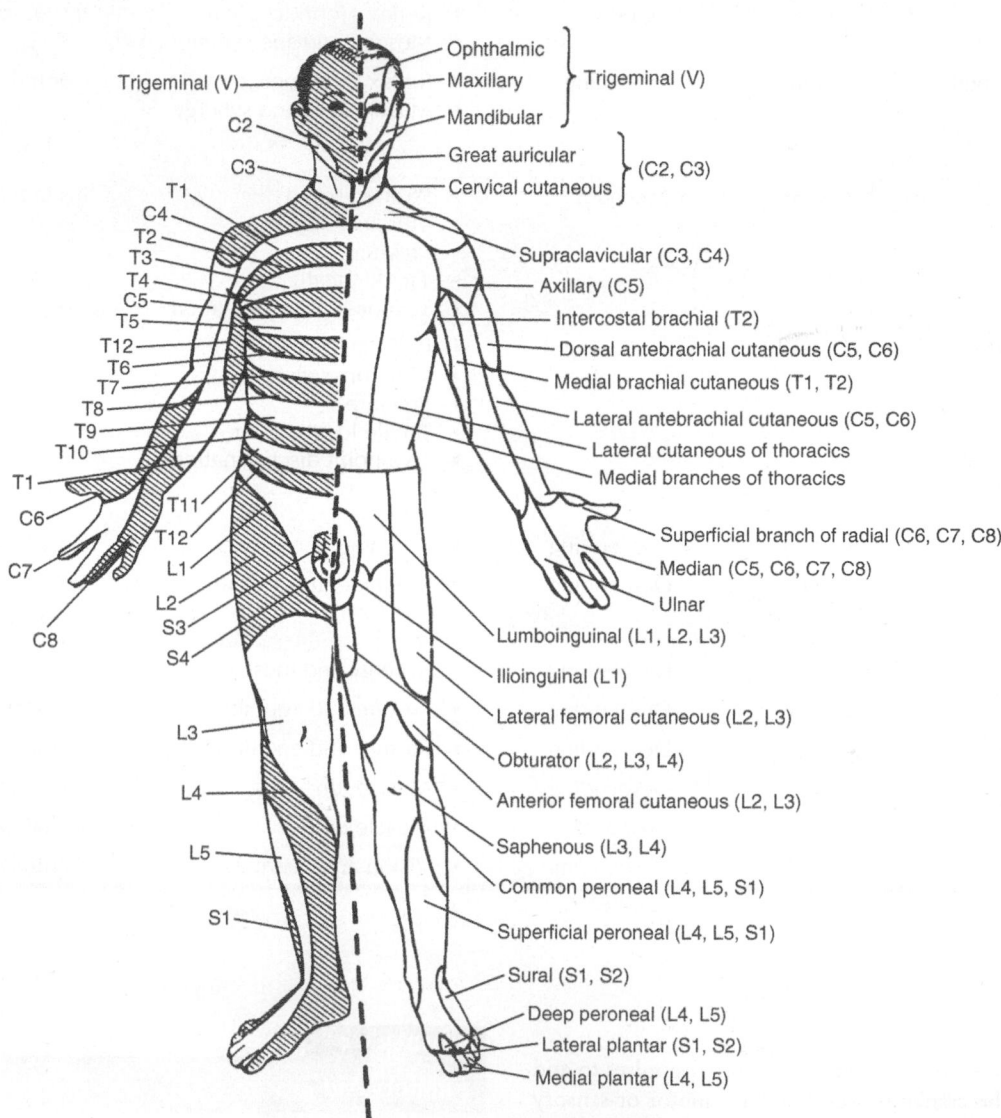

FIGURE 9-13 *Left,* Dermatome distribution. *Right,* Peripheral distribution of cutaneous nerves. (From Long, B. C., Phipps, W. J., & Cassmeyer, V. L. [1993]. *Medical-surgical nursing: A nursing process approach* [3rd ed.]. St Louis, MO: Mosby.)

the CNS. The postganglionic neuron is the cell body inside the CNS. The preganglionic neuron axon terminates on the postganglionic neuron cell bodies that are located throughout the body in autonomic ganglia. In the sympathetic branch, cell bodies are located in the spinal cord from T1 to L2. In the parasympathetic branch, cell bodies are located in the nuclei of cranial nerves III, VII, IX, or X or in the spinal cord from

S2 to S4. The postganglionic neuron axon terminates and innervates the specific effector organs of the ANS.

Neurotransmitters form a chemical bridge in transmission of a nerve impulse. The sympathetic branch neurotransmitters are epinephrine and norepinephrine; the parasympathetic branch neurotransmitter is acetylcholine. The ANS controls activities of the viscera at an unconscious level. It consists of

TABLE 9-6 Relationship of Spinal Cord Segments to Peripheral Nerves, Muscles, and Functional Ability

Spinal Cord Segment	Peripheral Nerves	Muscles	Functional Ability
C3-5	Phrenic nerve	Diaphragm	Diaphragmatic chest excursion
C5	Spinal accessory nerve	Trapezius	Shoulder shrug
C5-6	Axillary nerve Musculocutaneous nerve Radial nerve	Deltoid Biceps Brachioradialis	Arm elevation Forearm flexion
C6-8	Radial nerve	Triceps Extensor carpi radialis and ulnaris Flexor carpi radialis and ulnaris	Forearm extension Wrist extension Wrist flexion
C8, T1	Median nerve Ulnar nerve	Adductor pollicis Dorsal interossei	Handgrip Finger spreading
T1-T12	Thoracic and lumbosacral branches	Intercostals Rectus abdominis and obliques	Intercostal chest excursion Rotation at waist
L1-L3	Femoral nerve	Iliopsoas Quadriceps	Hip flexion Knee extension
L2-4	Deep peroneal nerve Sciatic nerve	Extensor hallucis and digitorum Biceps femoris and hamstrings	Foot dorsiflexion Knee flexion

two parallel systems that regulate visceral organs by acting in opposing manners (Table 9-8).

The sympathetic branch (also called *adrenergic*) dominates in crises and is frequently referred to as the *fight or flight system*. Physiologic or psychologic stressors innervate the SNS and promote activities that prepare the body for the crises. The parasympathetic branch (also called *cholinergic*) dominates in moments of calm or "steady state" and promotes activities that restore the body's energy sources.

9.3 Learning Activity

Identify the following physiologic alterations as being associated with either the sympathetic or parasympathetic branch.

	Sympathetic	Parasympathetic
Bronchodilation		
Coronary artery dilation		
Hypersalivation		
Increased serum glucose		
Increased perspiration		
Increased intestinal motility		
Pupil constriction		
Tachycardia		

Answers to this activity can be found in the Answer Key.

PHYSIOLOGY OF PAIN

The progressive care nurse focuses primarily on acute (nociceptive or physiologic) pain. Chronic pain may result from unrelieved acute pain. Acute pain occurs when mechanisms such as surgery, trauma, or disease cause inflammation and cellular damage. Pain is a signal or warning of the extent of tissue damage. This warning enables a patient to initiate protective behaviors to minimize the damage and promote tissue repair.

Acute pain activates the SNS responses such as increased heart rate, blood pressure, and respiratory rate. This response is proportional to the intensity and extent of the stimuli; however, wide variations exist among patients. The response is time-limited with resolution or healing of the underlying problem. If inadequately managed, pain can persist after repair of injured tissue. Somatic or visceral describes the origin and type of acute pain. Somatic pain arises from the tissues (e.g., skin, muscle, and bone). Patients describe this type of pain as sharp, dull, aching, or cramping. The pain may be localized or diffuse and may radiate. Visceral pain arises from the organs (e.g., liver, pancreas, and bowel) and may be well or poorly localized or referred. Patients describe this type of pain as sharp, stabbing, and a deep ache.

Nociceptors are peripheral neurons, primarily afferent peripheral fibers, which sense unpleasant or potentially damaging noxious stimuli. Two examples of these fibers are delta and C fibers. A delta nociceptor is a large, thinly myelinated fiber that rapidly conducts impulses generated in response to mechanical or thermal stimuli, which results in sharp, well-localized pain. The C fibers are smaller and unmyelinated. The C fibers slowly conduct impulses generated in response to all noxious stimuli, which results in poorly localized, dull and aching pain. More than 75% of nociceptors are C fibers. Repeated exposure to chemical mediators or repeated noxious stimuli, known as peripheral sensitization, may result in the lowering of nociceptor activation.

Nociception is the neurochemical process of transmitting pain response to a peripheral noxious (e.g., thermal, mechanical, or chemical) stimulus to an intact spinal cord and brain. There

TABLE 9-7   Cranial Nerve Summary

Number	Name	Functions
I	Olfactory	Sensory • Smell
II	Optic	Sensory • Vision acuity • Peripheral visual fields
III	Oculomotor	Motor • Upward, lateral eye movement • Pupillary constriction • Eyelid elevation
IV	Trochlear	Motor • Downward, medial eye movement
V	Trigeminal	Sensory • Sensation of scalp and face • Sensation of cornea of eye Motor • Temporal and masseter muscles
VI	Abducens	Motor • Outward lateral eye movement
VII	Facial	Sensory • Sweet and salty taste on anterior two thirds of tongue Motor • Muscles of facial expression • Eyelid closure • Lacrimal and salivary glands
VIII	Vestibulo-cochlear (acoustic)	Sensory • Hearing • Equilibrium and balance
IX	Glossopha-ryngeal	Sensory • Sour and bitter taste on posterior one third of tongue • Pharynx Motor • Parotid gland
X	Vagus	Sensory • Pharynx, larynx, neck Motor • Palate, larynx, pharynx • Swallowing • Cardiac muscle • Secretory glands of pancreas and GI tract
XI	Spinal accessory	Motor • Shoulder and neck movement • Sternocleidomastoid and trapezius muscles
XII	Hypoglossal	Motor • Tongue strength and movement

TABLE 9-8   Autonomic Nervous System: Sympathetic and Parasympathetic Branch Function

	Sympathetic (Adrenergic)	Parasympathetic (Cholinergic)
Eyes	• Pupils dilate	• Pupils constrict
Heart	• Heart rate increases • Contractility increases • Coronary arteries dilate	• Heart rate decreases • Contractility decreases • No effect on coronary arteries
Lungs	• Bronchodilation	• Bronchoconstriction
Liver	• Glycogenolysis and lipolysis	• Glycogenesis
GI	• Salivary flow decreases • Gastric mobility and secretion decrease • Intestinal motility decreases	• Salivary flow increases • Gastric mobility and secretion increase • Intestinal motility increases
Urinary bladder	• Bladder relaxes • Sphincter closes	• Bladder contracts • Sphincter opens
Adrenal glands	• Secrete epinephrine, norepinephrine	• No effect
Skin	• Piloerection (goose pimples) • Increased perspiration	• No effect

are four basic stages of nociception: transduction, transmission, perception, and modulation (Table 9-9). The perception of pain requires integration of many factors (e.g., physiologic factors, psychosocial factors, and past experience) and often leads to emotional responses such as anger and anxiety. Nociception does not always lead to pain. Endogenous endorphin release may blunt the perception of pain. Pain can also occur without nociception (e.g., phantom limb pain).

Chronic pain has no arbitrarily fixed duration. Chronic pain extends beyond the expected period of healing. Chronic pain serves no useful purpose and the SNS is unresponsive. Chronic pain often has a disproportionate response to the stimulus and/or physical findings. Neuropathic pain, which involves abnormal processing of sensory input in the PNS or CNS due to injury or impairment, is often involved. A patient describes chronic pain as either continuous or intermittent sensations of burning, shooting, shock-like, tingling, and/or jabbing pain. Chronic pain can result from conditions such as nerve root compression, diabetic neuropathy, Guillain-Barré syndrome, phantom limb pain, and complex regional pain syndrome.

The key physiologic concepts of neuroplasticity and central sensitization provide an explanation of chronic pain. Neuroplasticity is the ability of neurons to change their response to stimuli following sustained exposure to noxious stimuli. Central sensitization is a heightened excitability that results in an exaggerated response to stimuli, an expansion of the pain distribution, and a lower threshold

TABLE 9-9	Nociception Stages	
Stage	**Steps**	**Interventions**
Transduction	• Noxious stimuli damage cells, release substances (e.g., prostaglandins, serotonin, substance P, histamine) causing inflammation and sensitivity • An action potential generates an electrical impulse in response to stimuli	• NSAIDs target inflammation • Anticonvulsants and local anesthetics block ion exchanges involved in the action potential
Transmission	• Neurotransmitter (e.g., glutamate, substance P) are released to bind to NMDA receptors and facilitates transmission to dorsal horn in spinal cord • Impulses travel to brainstem, thalamus, and cortex via ascending tracts	• Opioids reduce release of substance P • NMDA receptor antagonists (e.g., ketamine, dextromethorphan) inhibit glutamate binding
Perception	• Reticular activating system: Automatic response alerts individual to respond to pain • Somatosensory cortex: Localization, characterization, and preservation of pain information • Limbic system: Site of emotional-behavioral response to pain	• Opioids binding to their receptors in the brain alter the perception of pain • Distraction and relaxation may modify pain perception by limiting signals to process
Modulation	• Neurons release inhibitory amino acids (GABA, glycine), neuropeptides (endogenous opioids), serotonin, and norepinephrine to bind with receptors to raise the threshold for nociceptor activation and prevent the release of other neurotransmitters (e.g., substance P) • Emotions (e.g., fear, anxiety, anticipation, stress) can increase pain	• Baclofen binds to GABA receptors and mimics its inhibitory effects • Opioids activate descending inhibitory pathways • Tricyclic antidepressants prevent the reuptake and storage of serotonin and norepinephrine, which makes them more available

(i.e., hyperalgesia) for noxious stimuli. In addition, the patient perceives normally benign stimuli as painful (i.e., allodynia).

NEUROLOGIC ASSESSMENT

Chief Complaint

The chief complaint is a statement from the patient on why he or she is seeking help and includes the duration of the problem. Many possible neurologic symptoms might prompt the patient and/or family to seek help. The patient or family may report a change in consciousness (e.g., difficulty staying awake). There may be a complaint of a headache, which can be focal or generalized, and unilateral or bilateral. Headaches may occur with or without a fever. If associated with a fever, the headache may be from an infectious process, such as meningitis or encephalitis. Headache without a fever may be due to a subarachnoid hemorrhage (SAH), intracerebral hemorrhage, or tumor. If the patient states the chief complaint is "the worst headache of my life," this is strongly suggestive of an SAH. It is important to determine the time of day of the headache because, for example, an early morning headache is suggestive of a tumor. The patient or family may report a seizure, which may be either a new onset or, if the patient has a history of epilepsy, an increase in frequency.

Complaints of visual changes may be present. Visual changes may be described as a loss of a portion of the visual field, diplopia (i.e., double vision), nystagmus (i.e., fast, uncontrollable movements of the eyes), or photophobia. Photophobia (i.e., eye discomfort in bright light) may occur in patients with an increased ICP or meningitis.

The patient or family members may report impaired speech. The impaired speech may include dysarthria (i.e., difficulty with articulation due to a motor disorder of the muscles controlling the mouth, tongue, and larynx) or aphasia (i.e., impaired understanding or expression of verbal and/or written language). Along with this, the patient may also note dysphagia (i.e., difficulty with swallowing).

The family may describe changes in the patient's mood, such as depression, euphoria, or emotional lability. Changes in thought processes, such as hallucinations, delusions, illusions, or paranoia, or changes in cognition may also be a complaint. Family may note and report changes in behavior such as hygiene habits, inappropriate laughter, or frequent crying. The patient may have noted a change in motor function, such as a tremor, paresis (i.e., weakness of voluntary muscles), or paralysis. There may also be complaints of a change in gait, dizziness, syncope, or vertigo, or a change in sensory function. Examples of sensory function changes are pain, paresthesia (i.e., a burning or prickling sensation), or anesthesia (i.e., loss of sensation). The patient often describes these changes as decreased sensation, numbness, or tingling. Memory changes or difficulties with activities of daily living (ADLs) are often a concern. There is a wide range of potential symptoms associated with neurologic assessment to evaluate.

History of Present Illness

Query the patient about the onset of his or her symptoms or complaint. Ask whether the onset was sudden or gradual. Use terms easily understood by the patient and family. Ask about associated symptoms, such as pain, headache, nausea and/or vomiting, vertigo, numbness or weakness, and seizures. Define pain using a pain description tool, such as *OPQRST*.

O: Onset. Did your pain start suddenly or gradually get worse and worse? What were you doing when the pain started?

P: Provocation and Palliation. What provokes or worsens the pain? What relieves the pain? What was used but did not relieve pain? Is there a pattern to the pain?

Q: Quality. What does the pain feel like? The patient may describe it in terms such as stabbing, stinging, lightning-like, or pounding.

R: Region and Radiation. Where is the pain located? Does the pain radiate and to where? Dermatomal relationships should be noted.

S: Severity. How severe is the pain on a 0 to 10 scale with 0 being no pain and 10 being the most severe pain?

T: Timing. Is the pain intermittent or continuous? How does the occurrence of pain relate to other events or activities?

Past Medical History

Inquire from the patient and family the relevant past medical history. Ask about congenital disorders, childhood diseases, infectious neurologic conditions, or a previous diagnosis of a neuromuscular disease. Congenital disorders include spina bifida, cerebral palsy, and Down syndrome. Childhood diseases or conditions related to neurologic disorders include poliomyelitis and epilepsy. Infectious neurologic conditions that are rare in adults and children include encephalitis and meningitis. Ask about any history of neuromuscular disease, such as multiple sclerosis, myasthenia gravis, amyotrophic lateral sclerosis (ALS), Parkinson disease, or Alzheimer disease. Also, inquire about any history of head trauma or spinal cord injury. Query the patient about a history of cancer, including specifics, such as type, stage, and therapy. Cardiovascular disease can also cause neurologic complications. Ask about coronary artery diseases such as angina and myocardial infarction, valvular heart disease, endocarditis, dysrhythmia (especially atrial fibrillation), hypertension, hyperlipidemia, and ventricular aneurysm. Ask about a history of cerebrovascular disease, especially ischemic or hemorrhagic stroke, and carotid artery disease, including the presence of a bruit or a prior carotid endarterectomy. Explore the patient's history of diabetes mellitus, chronic kidney disease, and/or a past occurrence of pulmonary embolism because these conditions increase a patient's risk for neurologic problems. To determine a patient's sensory impairment, ask about the use of eyeglasses, contact lenses, hearing aids, or prostheses.

Family History

A family history of cardiac disease, hypertension, diabetes mellitus, cancer, and cerebrovascular disease, especially ischemic or hemorrhagic stroke, increases the risk for neurologic problems and complications. Also ask about any neurologic disorders in the family, such as epilepsy, ALS, Huntington's disease, muscular dystrophy, neurofibromatosis, Tay-Sachs disease, myasthenia gravis, multiple sclerosis, or Alzheimer disease. Explore any family history of tremor, dementia, and psychiatric disorders.

Social History

Obtain information regarding the patient's relationship with his or her spouse or significant other, and the family structure. Ask about educational level and occupation, focusing on possible exposure to toxins such as solvents, pesticides, arsenic, and lead. Also, explore the patient's stress level and usual coping mechanisms, dietary habits and caffeine intake, and recreational and exercise habits. If the patient smokes, record tobacco use as pack-years. Calculate pack-years as the number of packs per day times the number of years the patient has been smoking. Record alcohol consumption as number of beverages per month, week, or day. Determine drug use or abuse and toxin exposure. Inquire about recent travel, especially international travel. Determine the patient's hand dominance and record this valuable information.

Medication History

Determine the dose, frequency, and time of the last dose of any prescribed medication. Ask the patient about nonprescribed drugs including over-the-counter remedies, herbs, and drugs of abuse. Determine the patient's current understanding of actions and side effects of any drugs taken. Drugs frequently used for neurologic problems include:
- Tranquilizers
- Sedatives
- Aspirin
- Anticonvulsants
- Antihypertensives
- Platelet aggregation inhibitors

In addition, drugs taken for other reasons may cause neurologic problems. The drugs that can cause neurologic symptoms include:
- Tranquilizers
- Sedatives
- Aspirin
- Anticoagulants
- Alcohol

Vital Signs

Cushing Triad

Cushing triad is an increased systolic BP with a decreased diastolic BP (widened pulse pressure), bradycardia, and an abnormal respiratory pattern. It is a *late* sign of increased ICP and impending herniation. Although this triad is of great concern, changes in level of consciousness (LOC), pupil changes, or motor changes precede these triad signs.

Blood Pressure

Because the cranium is an inexpansible vault, intracranial hemorrhage cannot result in hypotension because herniation would result before significant hypotension would occur. Consider other sources of bleeding, such as peptic ulcer or trauma, when hypotension occurs. Hypotension has significant physiologic implications because it decreases CPP and general neurologic deterioration occurs due to inadequate perfusion to the brain.

Systolic hypertension may occur as a component of Cushing triad; it represents compensation for the increase in ICP. It may also indicate a change in arterial resistance and be associated with vessel occlusion as seen in stroke. Hypertensive crisis may result in cerebral encephalopathy when the limits of autoregulation are exceeded (i.e., CPP >150 mm Hg).

Pulse pressure is the difference between systolic and diastolic pressure. The normal pulse pressure is 30 to 40 mm Hg. An increased (i.e., widening) pulse pressure is a component of Cushing's triad.

Heart Rate

Sinus bradycardia may be a manifestation of intracranial hypertension and is a component of Cushing's triad. Hypoxia, hemorrhage, and general neurologic deterioration may result in sinus tachycardia and ventricular dysrhythmias. Atrial dysrhythmias such as premature atrial contractions, atrial fibrillation, or atrial flutter may be an etiologic factor in ischemic stroke.

Ventilatory Rate and Rhythm

Several ventilatory patterns are indicative of neurologic dysfunction. Ventilatory patterns correlate to the level of CNS activity (Figure 9-14).

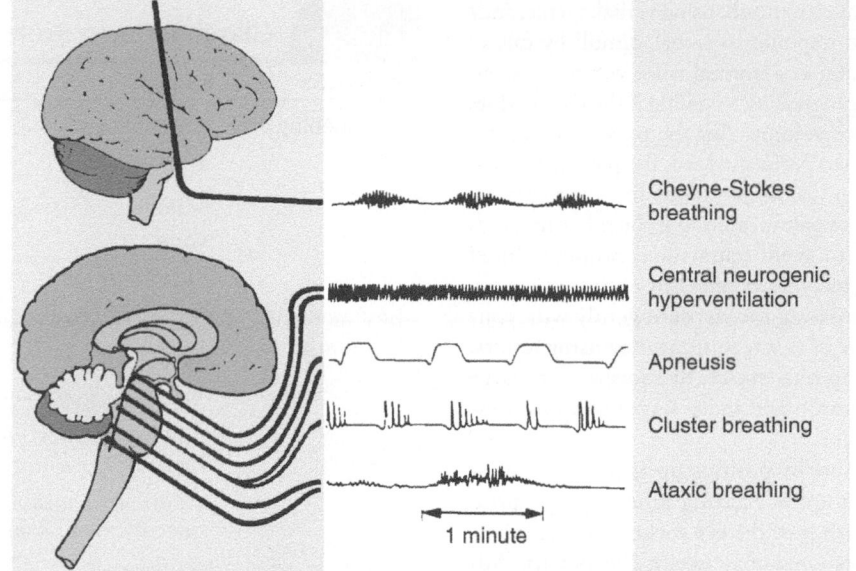

FIGURE 9-14 Abnormal ventilatory patterns with corresponding level of central nervous system activity. (From McCance, K. L., & Huether, S. E. [2014]. *Pathophysiology: The biologic basis for disease in adults and children* [7th ed.]. St. Louis, MO: Mosby.)

CNS depression from injury, disease, or drugs can cause bradypnea, a regular ventilatory rhythm with a rate of less than 12 breaths/min. Cheyne-Stokes breathing is an increasing rate and depth of ventilation followed by decreasing rate and depth of ventilation and then apnea. Bilateral lesions of the cerebral hemispheres, a lesion of the basal ganglia, a cerebellar or upper brainstem lesion, or a metabolic condition are causes of Cheyne-Stokes breathing. CNS hyperventilation is a sustained increased rate and depth of ventilation. Lesions of the lower midbrain and upper pons or secondary to a transtentorial herniation may be cause for CNS hyperventilation. Apneustic breathing is apnea with inspiration followed by exhalation; it is associated with lesions of the mid- to lower pons. Cluster (or Biot) breathing is 3 to 4 breaths of identical rate and depth followed by apnea, which is then repeated; it is caused by lesions of the lower pons or upper medulla. Ataxic breathing has no pattern to ventilation; it is completely irregular, with mostly apnea and associated with a lesion of the medulla.

9.4 Learning Activity

Think about the following ventilation patterns and identify the site of lesion that would cause them.

Pattern	Site of Lesion
CNS hyperventilation	
Cheyne-Stokes breathing	
Cluster (or Biot)	
Ataxic	
Apneustic	

Answers to this activity can be found in the Answer Key.

Temperature

In shock states, drug overdose, metabolic coma, diabetic coma, or terminal stages of neurologic disease, subnormal temperature may occur. Elevated temperatures occur with systemic infection, CNS infection, subarachnoid hemorrhage (SAH), seizures, or hyperactivity. Extremely elevated temperature may be associated with injury to the hypothalamus. It is important to differentiate central neurogenic fever from infectious fever. In central fevers, the body does not generally respond to antipyretics. Treat central neurogenic fevers with external cooling methods.

General Appearance

Upon assessment, it is important to note the patient's general appearance. Attire should be appropriate to the patient's age and the environment. Assess grooming including the hair, teeth, nails, and general hygiene. Evaluate the patient's general behavior, including demeanor and affect. Note the patient's facial expressions and body language. Describe a patient's mood, such as euphoric, angry, or depressed. Take notice of the patient's posture, particularly any gestures, fidgeting, restlessness, or rigidity. Evaluate the patient's gait by looking for uncoordinated movements of the body known as ataxia. Physical defects that may be present include:

- Hemiparesis (i.e., weakness on one side)
- Hemiplegia (i.e., paralysis of one side)
- Facial asymmetry
- Ptosis (i.e., drooping of the eyelid)
- Tremor
- Amputations

Mental Status and Cognition
Level of Consciousness

The patient's level of consciousness (LOC) is the most sensitive clinical indicator of a change in neurologic status. Consciousness refers to the state of awareness of self, environment, and responses to environment and arousal is a measure of being awake. Arousal is a function of the RAS in the midbrain. Awareness involves interpreting sensory input and giving an appropriate response and requires both an intact RAS and intact cerebral hemispheres.

Evaluate the patient's response to stimuli, using verbal, tactile, and/or painful stimuli. Evaluate response to verbal stimuli by calling the patient by name, speaking at a normal voice volume. Use an increased loudness of voice progressing to yelling if the patient does not respond to normal voice volume. Ask the patient to make a fist with his or her hand; when performed, ask the patient to open the fist. Perform evaluation of tactile stimuli by touching or shaking the patient. Only evaluate painful stimuli if the other methods are unsuccessful. Take care to avoid trauma and bruising caused by pinching. The following techniques can elicit response to pain:

- Perform a sternal rub, rubbing the sternum gently with your knuckle; discontinue use of this technique if bruising results.
- Apply pressure to the trapezius muscle by squeezing the large muscle mass between thumb and index finger or apply pressure to the Achilles tendon.
- Apply supraorbital pressure by pushing up against the supraorbital ridge with your thumb, exerting gentle upward pressure; take care not to push into the eye socket because injury to the eye or a vagal response may occur. Do not use this technique in patients with a facial or cranial fracture.
- Apply pressure to the nail bed using the flat surface of a pen or pencil. This method does not evaluate central pain but rather evaluates peripheral pain, which is useful in determining sensory and motor function. This method to assess pain is performed in concert with other pain assessment techniques. Document this assessment technique because the resulting movement from the patient is likely reflexive rather than an accurate response.

The patient's LOC is normal when the patient arouses easily, maintains wakefulness, speaks coherently, and responds appropriately to stimuli. The many labels used to describe levels of consciousness create confusion. The best practice is to describe the patient's response to stimuli and behavior rather than use labels. Some common labels used include the following:

- Hypersomnia refers to prolonged sleeping time with a normal sleep pattern.
- Lethargy, obtundation, and stupor all indicate diminishing LOC.
- Coma refers to the absence of awareness and responsiveness caused by a structural lesion or metabolic condition.
- Persistent vegetative state refers to the situation when the patient is unaware of self and surroundings while maintaining sleep-wake patterns along with eye opening but without response to stimuli; brainstem and hypothalamic functions are intact.
- Locked-in syndrome refers to consciousness with near-complete paralysis with the patient able to answer questions with eye blinking; vision and hearing are preserved. This state is due to a lesion of the midbrain or pons.
- Brain death refers to the absence of all cortical and brainstem functions.

Glasgow Coma Scale

The Glasgow Coma Scale (GCS) (Table 9-10) is a standardized observation method to evaluate the responsiveness in patients with traumatic brain injury. Record the best or highest response for E (eye), M (motor), and V (verbal) responses. Record the responses separately, along with a quantitative score. Note whether certain responses cannot be evaluated because of endotracheal intubation or tracheostomy or aphasia or if the eyes are swollen shut. Parameters of the GCS are a minimum of three and a maximum (normal) of 15. Consider a change of two points or more clinically significant.

TABLE 9-10 Glasgow Coma Scale

Parameter	Response	Score
Eye opening	Spontaneous	4
	To speech	3
	To pain	2
	None	1
	Untestable	U
Best motor response	Obeys commands	6
	Localizes pain	5
	Withdraws from pain	4
	Abnormal flexion (decorticate posturing)	3
	Abnormal extension (decerebrate posturing)	2
	None	1
	Untestable	U
Best verbal response	Oriented	5
	Confused	4
	Inappropriate	3
	Incomprehensible	2
	None	1
	Untestable	U

9.5 Learning Activity

A patient is admitted to your unit after a craniotomy. Since the last neuro check an hour ago, his clinical presentation has changed. He now opens his eyes only when you ask him to do so, and he answers questions but is confused about where he is and the date. He is moving all four extremities and will briefly squeeze your hand when you ask him to do so. What is his Glasgow Coma Scale (GCS)? Should you notify the physician?

Answers to this activity can be found in the Answer Key.

National Institutes of Health Stroke Scale

The National Institutes of Health Stroke Scale (NIHSS) (Table 9-11) scores the severity of presenting clinical presentation in patients with suspected stroke. A score of more than 25 indicates severe neurologic deficit. Complete an NIHSS score to determine a baseline assessment upon admission. Repeat NIHSS scores every 2 hours after treatment, 24 hours post onset of symptoms, 7 to 10 days post onset of symptoms, and 3 months post onset of symptoms.

Cognitive Function

To evaluate the patient's orientation, ask specific questions of the patient and observe his or her behavior. The patient may be alert but confused. Assess the patient's orientation to time by asking the patient to give today's date or to state the year. Assess orientation to place by determining the patient's ability

TABLE 9-11   **National Institutes of Health Stroke Scale**

Item/Domain	Response	Score
1A. Level of consciousness	Alert, keenly responsive	0
	Not alert but arousable by minor stimulation to obey, answer, or respond	1
	Not alert and requires repeated stimulation to attend, or is obtunded and requires strong or painful stimulation to make movements (not stereotyped)	2
	Responds only with reflex motor or autonomic effects or totally unresponsive, flaccid, and areflexic	3
1B. LOC questions Ask the month and patient age; must be exactly right	Answers both correctly	0
	Answers one correctly or patient unable to speak due to any reason other than aphasia or coma	1
	Answers neither correctly, or too stuporous or aphasic	2
1C. LOC commands Ask patient to open and close eyes and then grip and release nonparetic hand	Performs both tasks correctly	0
	Performs one task correctly	1
	Performs neither task correctly	2
2. Best gaze Only horizontal movements tested	Normal	0
	Partial gaze palsy	1
	Forced deviation or total gaze paresis not overcome by oculocephalic maneuver	2
3. Visual Tested by confrontation	No visual loss	0
	Partial hemianopia	1
	Complete hemianopia	2
	Bilateral hemianopia (blind from any cause including cortical blindness)	3
4. Facial palsy Encourage the patient to show teeth or raise eyebrows and close eyes; score symmetry of grimace in response to noxious stimuli in the poorly responsive or noncomprehending patient	Normal symmetric movement	0
	Minor paralysis (flattened nasolabial fold, asymmetry on smiling)	1
	Partial paralysis (total or near-total lower face paralysis)	2
	Complete paralysis (absence of facial movement upper/lower face)	3
5. Motor arm Extend left arm palm down at 90 degrees (sitting) or 45 degrees (supine) 5a Left arm 5b Right arm	No drift—holds for full 10 seconds	0
	Drifts down before 10 seconds but does not hit bed/support	1
	Some effort against gravity, but cannot get up to 90 (or 45 if supine) degrees	2
	No effort against gravity; limb falls	3
	No movement	4
6. Motor leg Extend leg and flex at hip to 30 degrees 6a Left leg 6b Right leg	No drift—holds for full 5 seconds	0
	Drifts down before 5 seconds but does not hit bed/support	1
	Some effort against gravity	2
	No effort against gravity; limb falls	3
	No movement	4
7. Limb ataxia Finger/nose and heel/shin done on both sides; not ataxia if hemiplegic or unable to comprehend; ataxia must be out of proportion to any weakness present	Absent	0
	Present in one limb	1
	Present in two limbs	2
8. Sensory	Normal	0
	Mild-to-moderate sensory loss; pinprick less sharp or dull on affected side	1
	Severe-to-total sensory loss; patient unaware of being touched	2

Continued

TABLE 9-11	National Institutes of Health Stroke Scale—cont'd	
Item/Domain	**Response**	**Score**
9. Best language Name items; read short sentences	No aphasia; normal	0
	Mild-to-moderate aphasia; some loss of fluency or comprehension	1
	Severe aphasia—fragmentary communication; listener carries burden of communication	2
	Mute, global aphasia; no usable speech or auditory comprehension	3
10. Dysarthria If not obviously present, have patient read	Normal	0
	Mild-to-moderate dysarthria; slurs some words	1
	Severe dysarthria; so slurred as to be unintelligible, or mute	2
11. Extinction/inattention	No abnormality	0
	Inattention to any sensory modality or extinction to bilateral simultaneous stimulation in one sensory modality	1
	Profound hemi-inattention or extinction to more than one modality; does not recognize own hand	2

From National Institutes of Health. (n.d.). NIH stroke scale. Retrieved from www.ninds.nih.gov/doctors/NIH_Stroke_Scale_Booklet.pdf.

to identify surroundings (e.g., where are you now?) or the ability to state their address (e.g., where do you live?). Assess orientation to person by determining the ability of the patient to identify himself or herself by name (e.g., who are you? what is your name?) or the recognition of friends and family (e.g., who is this?). Assess orientation to situation by determining the ability of the patient to identify why he or she is in the hospital (e.g., why are you here?).

Test memory by asking the patient questions or performing tests. Ask the patient to state his or her birthday or birthplace to test remote memory. Test recent memory by asking the patient what he or she ate for breakfast. Test short-term recall by asking the patient to repeat three or four objects 3 to 5 minutes after informing him or her to remember the objects. Ask a question about a current event to test a patient's general knowledge. To evaluate attention span, determine whether the patient is able to stay on a subject and perform calculations. Illusions, hallucinations, delusions, or paranoia are all indicative of alterations in thought content. Test calculation skills by asking the patient to count backward from 100 by 7s (i.e., 100, 93, 86, 79, etc.) or spell the word "world" backward if unable to count backward. Evaluate judgment by asking the patient why he or she is in the hospital or by providing a hypothetical situation such as "what would you do if there was a fire in the wastebasket?" Test abstraction by asking the patient what the phrase "a rolling stone gathers no moss" or "people in a glass house should not throw stones" means. Evaluate speech and language by noting punctuation, rhythm, stream of talk, sentence structure, and appropriate use of words. Speech should be fluent with expression of connected thoughts. If the patient cannot utilize or understand verbal communication, determine whether he or she can understand or utilize gestures, or if the patient can understand written language or write messages. Identify the presence of speech disorders. The following are types of speech disorders:
- Dysphonia: difficulty producing sound.
- Dysarthria: difficulty with articulation.
- Dysprosody: a lack of inflection while talking.

TABLE 9-12	Muscle Strength Grading Scale
Grade	**Description**
0/5	No movement or muscle contraction
1/5	Trace; no movement but evidence of muscle contraction
2/5	Not greater than gravity; movement with gravity eliminated
3/5	Greater than gravity; movement against gravity
4/5	Slight weakness; movement against some resistance
5/5	Normal; movement against full resistance

- Aphasia: impaired understanding or expression of verbal and/or written language.
- Receptive (sensory) aphasia is caused by a lesion in Wernicke's area in the temporal lobe.
- Expressive (motor) aphasia is caused by a lesion in Broca's area in the frontal area.
- Global aphasia occurs if both receptive and expressive aphasia are present; the person is also unable to read or write.

Motor Function

When assessing muscle size, look for symmetry. The presence of atrophy or hypertrophy is abnormal. Movement and strength of extremities (Table 9-12) should be spontaneous and symmetric. The patient should be able to assume a position of comfort.

Test arm strength by evaluating the strength of the flexor and extensor muscle groups against resistance; ask the patient to push or pull while you hold his or her arm. Test for pronator drift by having the patient hold his or her arms out in front of the body with palms up and eyes closed. Normally the patient should be able to hold the arms even for at least 20 seconds. When there is unilateral weakness, the weak arm begins to drift and pronate (i.e., turn palm downward). Test leg strength by

TABLE 9-13 Locating Site of Motor Problems

	Lower Motor Neuron	Upper Motor Neuron	
		Pyramidal Tract	Extrapyramidal Tract
Effect	• Flaccid paralysis • Areflexia	• Spastic paralysis with hyperactive reflexes • Positive Babinski reflex	• No paralysis • Altered muscle tone and abnormal movements
Muscle appearance	• Atrophy • Small muscular contractions (fasciculation)	• Mild atrophy from disuse	• Tremor when at rest
Muscle tone	• Decreased	• Increased	• Increased
Muscle strength	• Decreased or absent	• Decreased or absent	• Normal
Coordination	• Absent or poor	• Absent or poor	• Slowed

evaluating the strength of the flexor and extensor muscle groups against resistance; ask the patient to push or pull while you hold his or her leg. Ask the patient to raise one leg at a time to 30 degrees off the bed from a supine position and hold in place for a count to 5 while you observe for drift.

Hypotonicity is present when there is little resistance to passive movement; flaccidity is present when there is no resistance to passive movement. Flaccid paralysis is generally associated with lower motor neuron lesions though it does occur during spinal shock seen early in spinal cord injury. Hypertonia is increased muscle resistance to passive movement; rigidity is increased muscle resistance to passive movement of a rigid limb that is uniform through both flexion and extension. For example, paratonic rigidity may occur in coma and is a sign of diffuse cerebral dysfunction. Clinically, spasticity results from the loss of inhibition of motor neurons, causing excessive muscle contraction. This ultimately leads to hyperreflexia, an exaggerated deep tendon reflex. Spastic paralysis is associated with upper motor neuron lesions and emerges after resolution of the early flaccidity stage. Clonus is the continued rhythmic contraction of a muscle after applying a stimulus. Clonus is associated with tetany and hyperreflexia such as with hypocalcemia.

Upper motor neurons involve the brain or the spinal cord. Lower motor neurons involve the cranial nerves, spinal nerves, or peripheral nerves. The differences between upper motor neuron versus lower motor neuron lesions are summarized in Table 9-13.

Coordination

Test coordination by evaluating point-to-point movements and rapid, rhythmic alternating movements. The following are examples of tests to evaluate point-to-point movements:
• Perform the finger-nose test by asking the patient to touch his or her nose with a finger with the eyes open and then closed.
• Perform the finger-finger test by asking the patient to touch your finger with his or her finger with the eyes open and then closed; you should not move your finger between the open eyes test and the closed eyes test.
• Perform the heel-shin test by asking the patient to run the heel of one foot down the opposite leg from the knee to the foot.

The following are examples of tests that evaluate rapid, rhythmic alternating movements:
• Perform the pronation-supination test by asking the patient to rapidly pronate and supinate his or her hand.

• Perform the patting test by asking the patient to rapidly pronate and supinate his or her hand against a leg.
• Perform the figure-of-eight test by asking the patient to draw a figure of eight in the air with his or her great toe.

Evaluate gait using the tandem gait test. Ask the patient to walk heel-to-toe in a straight line. Normally, the patient should have the ability to walk heel-to-toe without difficulty. A loss of balance indicates cerebellar dysfunction. The following are examples of abnormal gaits:
• Spastic gait is when the patient's leg is stiff and moved slowly, and the toes and lateral aspect of the foot scrape the floor as the leg is moved; it indicates a corticospinal tract lesion.
• Steppage gait occurs when each step lifts the foot very high with a distinctive slapping sound as it hits the floor; it indicates a peripheral nerve injury.
• Ataxic gait occurs when feet are broad-based and steps are unsteady and staggering; it indicates a cerebellar or dorsal column lesion.
• Propulsive gait occurs when the body leans forward, steps are short, momentum is increased, and falls are common; it indicates a basal ganglia dysfunction, such as Parkinson disease.
• Waddling gait occurs when the pelvis opposite the weight-bearing hip drops and the trunk inclines, causing a waddle; it indicates proximal muscle weakness, such as in muscular dystrophy.
• Scissors gait occurs when the thighs are held together and each foot is alternately brought forward; it indicates an upper motor neuron lesion.

Test a patient's stationary balance by using the Romberg test. Ask the patient to stand with feet together and arms extended in front with eyes closed while you stand close enough to catch the patient if he or she should start to fall. Normally, the patient is able to stand erect and steady. Consider slight swaying as normal. If the patient loses his or her balance, it indicates a loss of position sense and/or cerebellar dysfunction.

Involuntary Movements

Involuntary movements include posturing and tremors. Posturing may occur spontaneously or in response to pain in comatose patients. Posturing may be abnormal flexion or extension, opisthotonos, or flaccidity. In abnormal flexion (Figure 9-15), also called decorticate posturing, the arms are flexed toward the body and the legs are extended; this posturing indicates a cerebral lesion. In abnormal extension (see Figure 9-15), also called decerebrate posturing, the arms are extended, and the wrists are

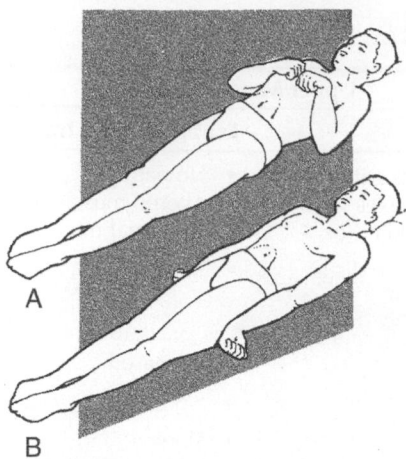

FIGURE 9-15 A, Abnormal flexion (decorticate) posturing. **B,** Abnormal extension (decerebrate) posturing. (From Urden, L., Stacy, K., & Lough, M. [2014]. *Critical care nursing: Diagnosis and management* [7th ed.]. St. Louis, MO: Mosby.)

TABLE 9-14	Dermatomal Levels for Bedside Assessment	
Anatomic Location	**Spinal Level**
Front of neck	C3
Thumb	C6
Ring and little fingers	C8
Nipple line	T4
Umbilicus	T10
Groin crease	L1
Knee	L3
Anterior ankle and foot	L5

externally rotated and the legs are extended; this posturing indicates a midbrain or brainstem lesion.

Opisthotonos, also referred to as arching, is an extension of arms and legs, with arching of the back and neck. It may indicate a brainstem injury. Flaccid posture occurs when the entire body is flaccid even with painful stimulation.

Tremors are classified as either nonintentional or intentional. A nonintentional tremor occurs at rest, such as in Parkinson disease. An intentional tremor occurs with movement and indicates cerebellar disease. Asterixis is a flapping tremor of the wrist and associated with metabolic encephalopathy such as hepatic or renal failure. Stress or age may induce tremors.

Sensory Function
Ability to Perceive Sensation
Sensory testing involves evaluating superficial touch, superficial pain, skin temperature, vibration, deep sensation, and position sense. Test superficial sensation by lightly touching the patient's skin with a wisp of cotton. Test superficial pain with a light pinprick on the skin with a sterile needle. Although rarely performed, test skin temperature by placing hot and cold test tubes on the skin. Temperature is only tested when the patient is unable to distinguish sensation. Test deep sensation and vibratory sense using a tuning fork on the joints of the thumbs and great toes. Test position sense by positioning the great toe or thumb upward or downward with eyes closed and asking the patient to identify the position. Test for deep pain by putting pressure on the Achilles tendon, calf muscles, and upper arm muscles.

Evaluate cortical/discriminatory sensation by using one- and two-point touch. For two-point discrimination, touch the patient with two points at varying degrees of separation to see if the patient feels only one point or two points. Evaluate double simultaneous stimulation (i.e., tactile inattention testing) by asking the patient to differentiate between one point and two points when being touched by one or two points on opposite sides of the body in corresponding locations. Test stereognosis by placing common objects in the patient's hand with his or her eyes closed and asking the patient to identify the object. Test topognosis by asking the patient to identify which finger is being touched with his or her eyes closed. Finally, test graphesthesia by tracing numbers or letters on the patient's skin with his or her eyes closed and ask him or her to identify the number or letter.

Agnosia is the inability to recognize objects through the special senses. There are five types of agnosia; each correlates to lesions in specific areas of the brain:
- Visual agnosia indicates a lesion in the occipital lobe.
- Auditory agnosia indicates a lesion in the temporal lobe.
- Tactile agnosia indicates a lesion in the parietal lobe.
- Body parts and relationships agnosia indicates a lesion in the parietal lobe.
- Autotopagnosia is the inability to orient parts of the body, and is due to a parietal or thalamic lesion.

There are various degrees of sensory loss including the following:
- Anesthesia: complete loss of sensation.
- Dysesthesia: impaired sensation.
- Hyperesthesia: increased sensation.
- Hypoesthesia: decreased sensation.
- Paresthesia: a burning, tingling sensation.

A dermatome (Table 9-14 and Figure 9-13) is the skin area supplied by sensory fibers of a single spinal nerve. Sensory loss below a dermatomal level is due to a spinal cord lesion. Sensory loss along a dermatome is associated with a spinal nerve lesion. Distribution of sensory loss may also be along the peripheral nerve distribution (see Figure 9-13).

Cranial Nerve Function
Olfactory (I)
Test the patient's ability to identify familiar odors (e.g., coffee, cloves, tobacco, and alcohol). Test each nostril separately with the patient's eyes closed. Normal olfactory function is the ability to identify familiar odors. Abnormal function, anosmia is the inability to identify familiar odors, but this test is rarely performed in acute care.

Optic (II)
There are several aspects to testing the optic nerve, including vision and funduscopic evaluation. If indicated, test the patient's visual acuity using a Snellen chart. Ask the patient to read lines of the Snellen chart from a distance of 20 feet. Record the number on the lowest line that the patient can read with 50% accuracy. Perform the test with the patient wearing glasses or contact lenses if he or she requires them. If the patient cannot see well enough to read the Snellen chart, ask how many fingers you are holding up. If the patient cannot see well enough to tell you how many fingers you are holding up, assess whether he or she blinks to visual threat. To test near-vision, ask the patient to read newsprint at a distance

of 12 inches or by using a Rosenbaum pocket screener held 14 inches from the patient. The normal response is the ability to read print at 12-14 inches. Test visual fields by confrontation. Compare the patient's visual field to the examiner's visual field with the eye on the same side covered. Loss of vision can be total or a portion of the visual field. The following are types of visual field losses:

- Unilateral blindness caused by a lesion of the eye, retina, or optic nerve.
- Bitemporal hemianopsia is a partial blindness in which vision is missing in the outer half of both the right and left visual field; it indicates a lesion of the optic chiasm or a lesion causing pressure on the optic chiasm (e.g., pituitary tumor).
- Homonymous hemianopsia is a visual field defect involving either the two right halves or the two left halves of the visual field of both eyes caused by a lesion of the right or left optic tract.
- Right or left homonymous hemianopsia with macular sparing is due to a lesion of the right or left geniculocalcarine tract.
- Quadrantanopsia is the loss in the same quadrant of vision in each eye.

Assess for papilledema with a funduscopic examination. If papilledema is present, the optic disk protrudes forward and the disk margins are blurry. It may be an indication of intracranial hypertension.

Oculomotor (III), Trochlear (IV), Abducens (VI)

Test these cranial nerves together. They control many motor aspects related to the function of the eye. Always ask if the patient experiences any double vision, and if so, when it is worse. Observe the position of the patient's eyelids. Ptosis is a drooping of the upper eyelid. The lid may droop only slightly, or it may cover the pupil entirely. Ptosis may indicate injury to the oculomotor (III) nerve.

Pupil size is normally 2 to 6 mm; a change of more than 1 mm is clinically significant. Note any of the following abnormal states:

- Pinpoint (and nonreactive) is indicative of a pontine lesion or an effect of medication, such as opiates (e.g., morphine) or miotics (e.g., pilocarpine).
- Midsize (2-6 mm) but nonreactive indicates a midbrain lesion. Unilateral large (greater than 6 mm) and nonreactive (may be referred to as *blown* or *Hutchinsonian pupil*) is a result of pressure on the oculomotor nerve on the same side.
- Bilateral large (greater than 6 mm) and nonreactive indicates a brainstem lesion or an effect of medication, such as parasympatholytics (e.g., atropine) or sympathomimetics (e.g., epinephrine).

Pupils should be equal. Unequal pupils are referred to as *anisocoria.* There is a normal variation in 15% to 20% of the population, who have slightly unequal pupils (1 mm or less difference). A difference of more than 1 mm or a change from baseline is abnormal. Ipsilateral (i.e., same side) pupil dilation is caused by an injury to the parasympathetic fibers of the oculomotor nerve. The cause of ipsilateral pupil constriction is an injury to the sympathetic fibers of the oculomotor nerves (e.g., Horner syndrome). Pupils are often large during or after a seizure, but persistent mydriasis may reflect anticholinergic or sympathomimetic toxicity.

The shape of pupils is normally round. An oval pupil may precede a dilated pupil as a sign of pressure on the oculomotor nerve. It is associated with intracranial pressure of 18 to 35 mm Hg. An irregularly shaped pupil, such as one that is keyhole

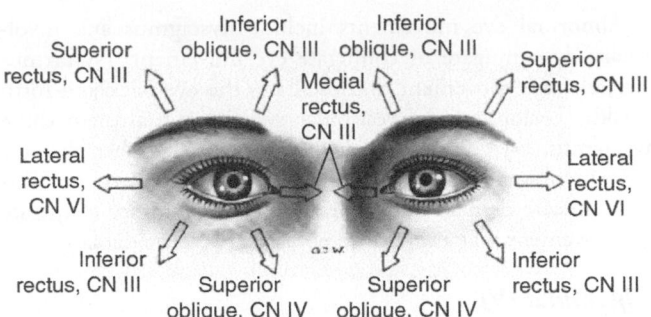

FIGURE 9-16 The six cardinal positions of gaze. (From Seidel, H. M., et al. [1991]. *Mosby's guide to physical examination* [2nd ed.]. St Louis, MO: Mosby.)

shaped, may occur in patients after cataract removal due to concurrent iridectomy.

Normally, pupils are in the midposition. Both eyes deviated toward one side is an abnormal finding; it is indicative of a unilateral pontine lesion. A fixed lesion such as a tumor, stroke, or hemorrhage would cause pupils to move toward the lesion and away from the hemiparesis. A downward deviation of both eyes, frequently with inward convergence, indicates a thalamic lesion. In cranial nerve III palsy, a downward deviation of one eye occurs. A medial deviation of one eye occurs in cranial nerve IV palsy. When a patient is having a seizure, pay close attention to which direction the eyes are deviated. The eyes will deviate to the side contralateral to the seizure focus area.

Test reactivity to light by first darkening the room. Shine a small, bright penlight in front of each eye. Note pupil constriction as the direct reaction and pupil constriction of the opposite pupil as a consensual reaction. Normal findings are a brisk bilateral direct and consensual reaction to light. Sluggish or absent reaction is abnormal and may indicate cranial nerve III pressure or injury, hypothermia, or barbiturate intoxication. Hippus, also known as pupillary arhetosis, is a spasmodic, rhythmic, but irregular, dilating, and contracting pupillary movement between the sphincter and dilator muscles. The rhythm of the contractions represents a galloping horse. Hippus is particularly noticeable when testing pupil function with a light, but it is independent of eye movements or changes in illumination. The occurrence of hippus is usually normal; however, pathologic hippus can occur. Pathologic hippus, the phenomenon of increased oscillation or amplitude, is associated with aconite poisoning, altered mental status, trauma, cirrhosis, and renal disease, and suggests a common pathway of frontal lobe dysfunction.

Test accommodation ability by asking the patient to focus on a distant object and continue to focus on the object as it moves closer. Pupils should dilate when focusing on a far object and constrict and converge inward when focusing on a near object.

Test for the ciliospinal reflex by squeezing the trapezius muscle and observing the reaction of the pupil on the same side. Normally, there is ipsilateral pupil dilation with the trapezius squeeze. It is an abnormal reaction if there is no response, and is indicative of an interruption of the sympathetic fibers of cranial nerve III.

Test extraocular movements (EOMs) by asking the patient to keep the head straight and follow your finger with the eyes. Move your finger in the direction of the six cardinal positions of gaze (Figure 9-16). A normal response occurs when both eyes move conjugately in the direction of your finger. If one or both eyes do not move to follow your finger, it is indicative of cranial nerve injury or an isolated muscular dysfunction.

Abnormal eye movements include nystagmus and involuntary dysconjugate or conjugate eye movement. Nystagmus is a jerky eye movement that oscillates the eye back and forth quickly. Lesions of the vestibular system or brainstem cause nystagmus. Dysconjugate eye movement occurs when the eyes move involuntarily and do not move in the same direction. This may indicate damage to the brainstem. Involuntary conjugate eye movement may indicate cerebral hemispheric damage.

Trigeminal (V)

The trigeminal nerve has both a sensory branch and a motor branch. The sensory branch is tested using the superficial sensation and superficial pain tests as described in the Sensory Function section in this chapter. Test the three branches (i.e., ophthalmic, maxillary, and mandibular) on both sides. It is abnormal if there is no detection of touch or pain. Test the corneal blink reflex by touching the cornea with drops of sterile normal saline. The expected response, a bilateral blink, indicates intact trigeminal (V) and facial (VII) nerves. A decreased or absent blink may indicate injury to the trigeminal nerve. Contact lens wearers often have a diminished corneal blink reflex.

Test the motor branch of the trigeminal nerve by inspecting the face for muscle atrophy and tremor. Palpate the masseter muscle while the patient clenches his or her teeth. Palpate the temporal muscles as the patient squeezes his or her eyes closed. Asymmetry of muscle strength may indicate injury to the trigeminal nerve.

Facial (VII)

The facial nerve also has both a motor branch and a sensory branch. Test the motor branch by evaluating the symmetry of facial expressions while the patient raises the eyebrows, frowns, smiles, and closes the eyelids tightly. Asymmetry of facial expression, the loss of the nasolabial fold, or the eyelid remaining open manifests a facial nerve injury (i.e., Bell palsy). Test the sensory branch by evaluating the patient's ability to taste sweet and salty on the anterior two-thirds of the tongue; however, in acute care testing the ability to taste is rare. The inability to taste indicates an injury to the facial nerve (VII).

Acoustic (VIII)

The acoustic nerve is associated with hearing and balance. Testing hearing acuity evaluates the cochlear branch of the acoustic nerve. Perform the whisper test by having the patient's face turned away from you, then whisper to see if the patient can hear the whispered word phrase and differentiate between hearing and lip reading. Test each ear separately.

To perform the Weber test, place a tuning fork at the midline vertex of the skull. A normal response is one in which the patient hears equally on both sides. An abnormal response occurs when a patient indicates a difference between the two ears. A positive Weber test may indicate a conductive or sensorineural loss. Further testing is necessary to determine the type of hearing loss.

To perform the Rinne test, place a tuning fork on the mastoid; when the patient can no longer hear the sound by bone, move the tuning fork to in front of the ear. Air conduction is usually twice that of bone conduction so the patient should still be able to hear the sound in front of the ear. The inability to hear the sound by air after the cessation of Sythe sound by bone indicates a conductive hearing loss as is associated with middle ear infection or a foreign body in the ear canal.

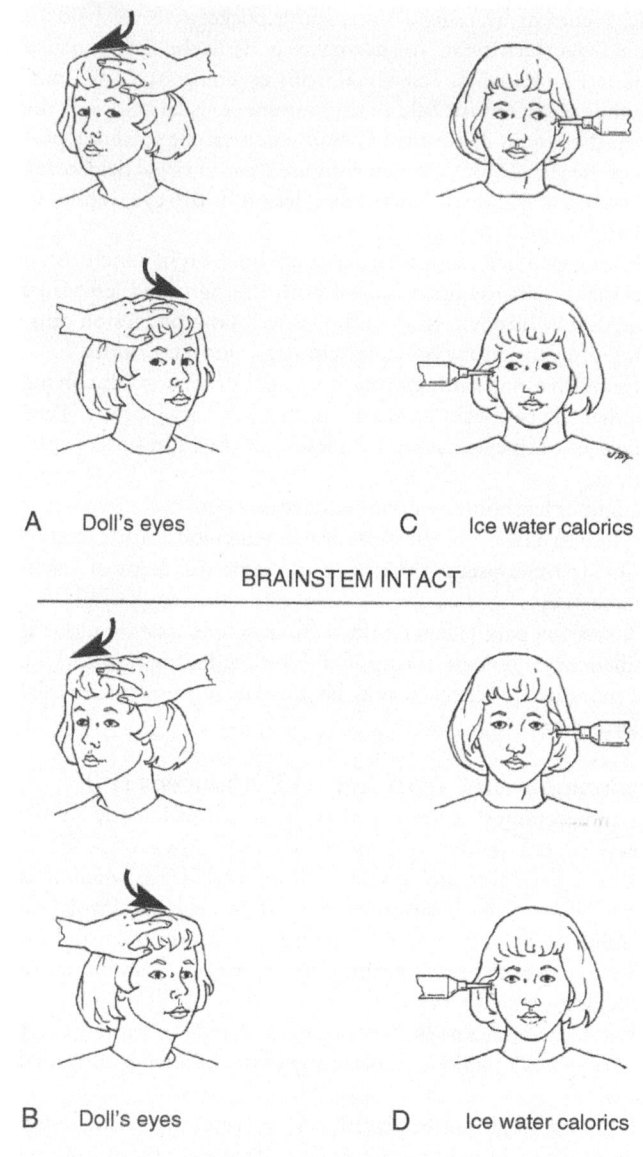

A   Doll's eyes   C   Ice water calorics

BRAINSTEM INTACT

B   Doll's eyes   D   Ice water calorics

BRAINSTEM NOT INTACT

FIGURE 9-17 A, Oculocephalic (doll eyes) reflex with normal response: eyes move in the direction opposite the direction that the head is turned. **B,** Oculocephalic (doll eyes) reflex with abnormal response: eyes either move in the same direction as the head is being turned or stay midline. **C,** Oculovestibular (caloric) reflex with normal response: nystagmus is present, and there may be conjugate movement toward the irrigated ear. **D,** Oculovestibular (caloric) reflex with abnormal response: no nystagmus or dysconjugate movement of the eyes. (From Beare, P. G., & Myers, J. L. [1994]. *Principles and practice of adult health nursing* [2nd ed.]. St Louis, MO: Mosby.)

Although there is no direct test for the vestibular branch, symptoms such as nystagmus, vertigo, nausea, vomiting, pallor, sweating, and hypotension indicate problems in this area. The reflexes involving the vestibular system include the oculocephalic reflex and the oculovestibular reflex. Reflexes of the vestibular branch of the acoustic nerve and connections with the oculomotor (III) nerve and acoustic (VIII) nerve provide information regarding integrity of the brainstem.

Ensure radiologically clearance of the cervical spine, and then test for the oculocephalic reflex, also called doll eyes reflex (Figure 9-17), on unconscious patients. Due to the unconscious state, you will need to hold the eyes open. Rotate the head side to side and observe eye movement. A normal response is that the eyes move in the opposite direction of the head. If the eyes stay midline or turn to the same direction as the head (i.e., absence of doll eyes), it indicates compression in the midbrain-pontine area.

Before testing the oculovestibular reflex (also called *caloric testing*) (see Figure 9-17), ensure that the tympanic membrane is intact and there is no basal skull fracture. Elevate the head of the bed 30 degrees. The examiner, usually a physician, injects 30 to 50 mL of iced water over 30 seconds into the ear canal and against the tympanic membrane. A normal response of nystagmus with deviation toward the irrigated ear indicates that the pons and midbrain are intact. Keep in mind that this test may be painful to the patient. No eye movement or dysconjugate eye movement is one criterion used for determining brain death.

Glossopharyngeal (IX), Vagus (X)

Test the glossopharyngeal and vagus nerves together. Test phonation by asking the patient to say "Ah" and observe for bilateral elevation of the soft palate. An abnormal response is no elevation of the palate on one side. Test speech by listening to the patient's speech and ask that the patient change the volume and pitch of his or her voice. Note any hoarseness, which may indicate damage to the laryngeal branch of the vagus (X) nerve.

Test taste by evaluating the ability to taste sour and bitter on the posterior one-third of the tongue. Test swallowing by holding the tongue down with a tongue blade and touching each side of the pharynx with a cotton swab. Palpate the elevation of the larynx with the swallow. If the patient is conscious, give a sip of water. A normal response is an involuntary swallow or gag when the palate is stroked, an elevation of the larynx with the swallow, and an effective swallow. These responses indicate intactness of the glossopharyngeal (IX) and vagus (X) nerves. Test the cough reflex by touching the hypopharynx with a suction catheter. An involuntary cough indicates intactness of glossopharyngeal (IX) and vagus (X) nerves.

Spinal Accessory (XI)

Test the spinal accessory nerve by inspecting the sternocleidomastoid and trapezius muscles for size and symmetry. Ask the patient to shrug the shoulders as you push down on the shoulders with your hands and to turn his or her head to each side against resistance. Injury to the spinal accessory (XI) causes asymmetry and poor muscle strength.

Hypoglossal (XII)

Test the hypoglossal nerve by inspecting the tongue for atrophy, fasciculations and alignment and evaluating tongue strength. Use your index finger to test tongue strength when the patient pushes his or her tongue against the cheek. Presence of atrophy or fasciculations, deviation from midline, or a decrease in tongue strength is associated with injury to the hypoglossal (XII) nerve. In addition, ask the patient to say "light, tight, and dynamite" to assess the patient's ability to speak the letters L, T, D, and N clearly. The speech should be clear.

9.6 Learning Activity

For each cranial nerve, identify the name; whether it's motor, sensory, or both; and the method of assessment.

Cranial Nerve Number	Name	M (motor), S (sensory), or B (both)	Method of Assessment
I			
II			
III			
IV			
V			
VI			
VII			
VIII			
IX			
X			
XI			
XII			

Answers to this activity can be found in the Answer Key.

TABLE 9-15	Grading Scale for Deep Tendon Reflexes
Grade	Description
0	Absent
1+	Diminished
2+	Normal
3+	More brisk than average but may be normal
4+	Hyperactive with clonus

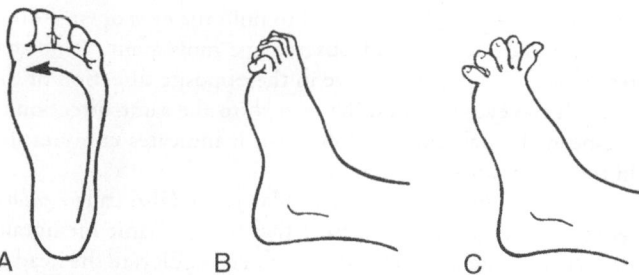

FIGURE 9-18 Babinski reflex. A, Method of stroking sole of foot. **B,** Normal response (absence of Babinski reflex). **C,** Abnormal response (presence of Babinski reflex).

TABLE 9-16	Deep Tendon Reflexes	
Reflex	Response	Spinal Nerves
Biceps	Elbow flexion	C5-6
Brachioradialis	Wrist extension	C5-6
Triceps	Elbow extension	C7-8
Patellar	Knee extension	L2-4
Achilles	Foot extension	S1-2

Reflexes
Deep Tendon (Also Called Muscle-stretch) Reflexes
Test deep tendon reflexes (DTRs) by tapping the tendon with a reflex hammer. A normal response is contraction of the muscle and a jerk of the affected limb. Hyporeflexia is a less than a normal contraction. Hypocalcemia, hyperphosphatemia, hypomagnesemia, and an LMN lesion may cause of hyporeflexia. Hyperreflexia is a greater than normal contraction and may include the presence of clonus. Hypercalcemia, hypophosphatemia, hypermagnesemia, and a UMN lesion may cause hyperreflexia. Grade DTRs using a grading scale (Table 9-15). The DTRs' location can be correlated to a spinal level (Table 9-16).

Superficial Reflexes
Test for abdominal reflexes by stroking the abdomen toward the umbilicus with the blunt end of a cotton-tipped applicator. A normal response is that the umbilicus moves toward the quadrant stroked; an abnormal response is no response to the stroke. Absence of superficial abdominal reflexes indicates a lesion at T7 to T9 for the upper abdomen and T11 to T12 for the lower abdomen.

To evaluate the plantar reflex, stroke the sole of the foot with a blunt instrument (Figure 9-18). In adults, a normal response occurs when the toes curl downward. An abnormal response (i.e., Babinski reflex) is an extension of the great toe and fanning of the other toes. The presence of a Babinski reflex is an indication of a UMN lesion.

Pathologic Reflexes
The Babinski reflex, described previously, is a pathologic reflex, as are the grasp, sucking, and glabellar reflexes. The grasp and sucking reflexes are infantile reflexes and indicate diffuse cerebral dysfunction. Test for the grasp reflex by placing something, such as a finger, in the patient's hand. The grasp reflex is when the patient grasps your finger and will not release the grasp on command. Test for the sucking reflex by touching the corner of the patient's mouth. The sucking reflex is when the patient

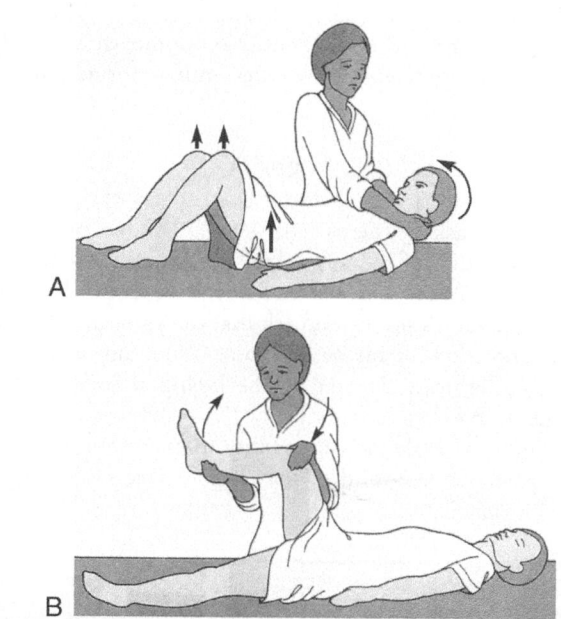

FIGURE 9-19 Brudzinski **(A)** and Kernig **(B)** signs. (From Barker, E. [2008]. *Neuroscience nursing: A spectrum of care* [3rd ed.]. St. Louis, MO: Mosby.)

purses his or her lips and starts to suck. Test for the glabellar reflex test by tapping the patient's forehead. The glabellar reflex is when the patient repeatedly blinks. This reflex indicates diffuse cerebral dysfunction.

Miscellaneous Clinical Findings
Clinical Indications of Meningeal Irritation
Nuchal rigidity is indicative of meningeal irritation caused by infection or hemorrhage. Brudzinski sign and Kernig sign (Figure 9-19) are also indications of meningeal irritation.

Before performing the test for the Brudzinski sign, obtain radiologic clearance of the cervical spine. To test for the Brudzinski sign, ask the patient to bring his or her chin toward the chest and move the head forward. A Brudzinski sign is the presence of neck pain and involuntary adduction and flexion of the legs when the head moves forward; this indicates irritation of the meninges by infection or blood, such as in SAH. Test for the Kernig sign by placing the patient on his or her back, assisting the patient to flex the thigh toward the chest until the hip is at a 90-degree angle, and then extend the leg at the knee. Kernig sign is the inability to extend the leg fully when flexing the thigh toward the abdomen and neck pain may occur; this indicates irritation of the meninges by infection or blood, as from an SAH.

DIAGNOSTIC STUDIES

To determine and monitor patients with neurologic disorders, several common diagnostic studies are used. These tests include a complete blood cell count and differential, serum glucose, chemistry tests including osmolality and electrolyte levels, clotting profiles, arterial blood gas levels, toxicology screens, urinalysis, and CSF analysis. With the CSF analysis, compare the patient's values against normal CSF values (Table 9-17) and request a culture and sensitivity test. When conducting a CSF analysis, number the test tubes to differentiate between traumatic puncture and hemorrhage. If the first test tube is bloody but others are clear, consider trauma; an SAH would cause all test tubes to be equally bloody.

Several radiologic examinations assess neurologic problems. A skull series may be useful in detecting skull abnormalities (e.g., fractures, erosion), noting shifts in the pineal gland, or noting the presence of intracranial air or abnormal calcifications. A spine series elicits vertebral integrity and alignment of the spine along with diagnosis of fractures, dislocations, bony defects, or degenerative processes. To delineate further abnormalities, more invasive diagnostic studies (Table 9-18), such as angiography, CT scans, MRIs, perfusion studies, and myelography, are performed.

TABLE 9-17	Normal Characteristics of Cerebrospinal Fluid
Characteristic	**Normal Value**
Appearance	Clear colorless
Specific gravity	1.007
Glucose level	50-75 mg/dL or approximately 60% serum level
Protein	Lumbar: 15-45 mg/dL (increases when blood present)
Lactate	10-20 mg/dL
Cells	White blood cells: 0-5/mm³
	Red blood cells: 0/mm³
pH	7.35
Pressure	70-180 mm H_2O, measured in lumbar level with patient in the lateral decubitus position
Volume	Ventricular system and subarachnoid space contain approximately 125-150 mL of CSF

9.7 Learning Activity

Applying the Synergy Model, select the appropriate level in the following case scenarios

A. A 60-year-old woman is admitted with left-sided hemorrhagic stroke resulting from hypertension. She is experiencing right-sided weakness. Resilience level _____

B. An 80-year-old man is transferred from the critical care unit. He is still comatose after a massive intracranial hemorrhage several days ago. Vulnerability level _____

C. A 75-year-old woman is admitted after falling at home and hitting her forehead. She has been on warfarin due to chronic atrial fibrillation. She is presently awake and neurologically intact. Stability level _____

Answers to this activity can be found in the Answer Key.

TABLE 9-18	Neurologic Diagnostic Studies	
Study	**Purposes**	**Comments**

Angiography	• Visualizes extracranial and intracranial vasculature
	• Identifies aneurysm, AVM, vasospasm, vascular tumors
	• Detects arterial occlusion and allows delivery of intraarterial therapy to restore blood flow
		• May cause local hematoma, vasospasm, vessel occlusion, allergic reaction to contrast media, transient or permanent neurologic dysfunction
		• Before test:
		  • Keep patient NPO for 4 hours and provide sedation before the study
		  • Check for allergy to iodine
		  • Evaluate renal function
		• After the test:
		  • Ensure hydration postprocedure (contrast medium used)
		  • Maintain bed rest for 8-12 hours depending on method used for stasis at the puncture site
		  • Monitor arterial puncture point for hemorrhage or hematoma
		  • Monitor neurovascular status of affected limb
		  • Monitor for indications of systemic emboli
		  • Reevaluate renal function

Continued

TABLE 9-18   Neurologic Diagnostic Studies—cont'd

Study	Purposes	Comments
Cisternogram	• Views CSF flow • Identifies hydrocephalus • Evaluates CSF leakage through a dural tear • Evaluates abnormality of structures at the base of the brain and upper cervical cord region	• Contraindicated in intracranial hypertension
Computerized tomography (CT); computerized axial tomography (CAT)	• Views intracranial structures: size, shape, location, shifts • Differentiates between tumors, hemorrhage, and infarction • Identifies hydrocephalus, brain edema, infectious processes, trauma, aneurysm, hematoma, AVM, brain atrophy, and subacute and old brain infarction • Evaluates arterial system if CT angiography studies performed	• Patient must be cooperative • Contrast media may be used; contrast media may be used after a noncontrast CT. For a patient scheduled for a head CT with contrast, the patient must have a 20-gauge or higher IV placed above the patient's wrist • Check for allergy to iodine or seafood before study if contrast will be given • Sedation may be given • Monitor for signs of allergic reaction • Encourage fluids • Evaluate renal function when contrast media used

Digital subtraction angiography (DSA): brain; spine	• Visualizes the vasculature, especially carotid and larger cerebral arteries
	• Evaluates occlusive vascular disease
	• Identifies tumors, aneurysms, AVM, and vascular abnormalities
		• May be done intravenously or intraarterially
		• If IV: less invasive with fewer complications than cerebral angiography
		• If intraarterial, care as for angiogram
		• Contrast media are used
		   • Check for allergy to iodine or seafood before study
		   • Patient will be NPO for 4-8 hours before the study
		   • Monitor for signs of allergic reaction
		   • Encourage fluids

Electroencephalography (EEG)	• Differentiates epilepsy from mass lesion • Detects focus of seizure activity • Evaluates drug intoxication • Evaluates electrical function of the brain, which may be abnormal in the presence of cerebrovascular alterations • Localizes tumor, abscess, and other mass lesions • May be used in designation of brain death	• Stimulants, anticonvulsants, tranquilizers, and antidepressants may be withheld for 24-48 hours before the study • Hair shampooed before and after study
Electromyography (EMG); nerve conduction velocity studies	• Detects muscle disease • Identifies peripheral neuropathies, nerve compression • Identifies nerve regeneration and muscle recovery	• Patient must be cooperative • Contraindicated in patients taking anticoagulants, with bleeding disorders, or with skin infection • May be uncomfortable for patient
Electronystagmography (ENG)	• Detects nystagmus, which may aid in identification of cerebellar or vestibular problem	
Evoked potential studies	• Evaluate brain's electrical potentials (responses) to external stimuli; evaluate sensory and somatosensory neurologic pathways • Identify neuromuscular disease, cerebrovascular disease, spinal cord injury, traumatic brain injury, peripheral nerve disease, and tumors • Determine prognosis in traumatic brain injury • Contribute to diagnosis of multiple sclerosis and brainstem injury	• Hair is shampooed before and after study

TABLE 9-18	Neurologic Diagnostic Studies—cont'd	
Study	**Purposes**	**Comments**
Isotope ventriculography	• Visualizes CSF circulation system	• No CSF withdrawn • May cause meningeal irritation and aseptic meningitis
LP or cisternal puncture	• Obtains CSF for analysis • Measures CSF opening pressure (roughly equivalent to intracranial pressure for most patients if done recumbent and no blockage is present)	• Cisternal puncture is higher risk but may be used if scar tissue prevents lumbar puncture • Patient must be cooperative • Contraindicated in patients with intracranial hypertension because herniation may occur • Contraindicated in bleeding disorders and in patients receiving anticoagulants • Patient kept flat for 4-8 hours afterward to prevent headache • May cause headache, low back pain, meningitis, abscess, CSF leak, or puncture of spinal cord
Magnetic resonance angiography (MRA)/magnetic resonance imaging (MRI)	• As for CT • Visualizes tissue state (diffusion and perfusion) so that early ischemic changes are apparent (CT cannot visualize most early changes) • Identifies vascular lesions, tissue abnormalities, hemorrhage, infarction, epileptic foci, and multiple sclerosis • Identifies patency of large veins and venous sinuses • Identifies brainstem abnormalities • Identifies type, location, and extent of brain injury	• Patient must be cooperative • Contraindicated in patients with any implanted metallic device, including pacemakers • Tends to overestimate degree of stenosis • Sedation is often required for patients who are claustrophobic or who have neurologic injury
Magnetic resonance spectroscopy (also known as *nuclear magnetic resonance [NMR] spectroscopy*)	• Measures biochemical changes in the brain tissue • Detects abnormal changes as in brain tumors, epilepsy, stroke, and traumatic brain injury	• Patient must be cooperative • Contraindicated in patients with any implanted metallic device, including pacemakers
Myelography	• Visualizes spinal subarachnoid space • Detects spinal cord lesions and cord or nerve root compression • Detects pressure on spinal nerve roots	• If done with oil-based iophendylate (Pantopaque), patient must lie flat for 4-8 hours after study • May cause headache, nerve root irritation, allergic reaction, or adhesive arachnoiditis • If done with water-soluble metrizamide (Amipaque), patient should have head of bed elevated • May cause headache, nausea, vomiting, back and neck ache, chest pain, seizures, hallucinations, speech disorders, dysrhythmias, or allergic reaction • Encourage fluid intake with either type of dye
Nerve conduction velocity studies	• Identify peripheral neuropathies and nerve compression	• Needle electrodes are used
Oculoplethysmography (OPG)	• Indirectly measures ocular artery pressure • Reflects adequacy of cerebrovascular blood flow in the carotid artery	• Contraindicated in patients who have undergone eye surgery within the last 6 months, who have had lens implants or cataracts, or who have had retinal detachment • May cause conjunctival hemorrhage, corneal abrasions, or transient photophobia
Pneumoencephalography	• Visualizes ventricular system and subarachnoid space • Identifies intracranial tumors • Identifies brain atrophy	• Care as for LP • Contraindicated in patients with intracranial hypertension • May cause headache, nausea, vomiting, autonomic dysfunction, herniation, subdural hematoma, air embolus, or seizures • Patient kept flat for 12-24 hours after the study

Continued

TABLE 9-18   Neurologic Diagnostic Studies—cont'd

Study	Purposes	Comments
Positron emission tomography (PET) or single photon emission-computerized tomography (SPECT)	• Evaluates oxygen and glucose metabolism • Measures cerebral blood flow, which may be altered by traumatic brain injury, seizure, ischemia, stroke, or neoplasm • Also used to evaluate dementia, depression, schizophrenia, and Alzheimer's disease	• Patient must be cooperative • Contraindicated in pregnant and breastfeeding patients
Radioisotope brain scan	• Identifies tumors, cerebrovascular disease, infarction, trauma, infectious processes, seizures	• Generally replaced by CT scan • Reassure patient that amount of radioactive material is minimal • Patient must be cooperative • Contraindicated in pregnant and breast-feeding patients
Regional cerebral blood flow (xenon [^{133}Xe] inhalation)	• Evaluates blood flow to the cerebral cortex • Identifies cerebrovascular disease • Detects regions of increased or decreased perfusion • Determines presence of collateral blood flow • Evaluates the effect of vasospasm on tissue perfusion	• Assure patient that amount of radioactive material is minimal • Contraindicated in pregnant and breastfeeding patients
Skull x-rays	• Detects skull fracture, facial fracture, tumor, bone erosion, cranial anomalies, air-fluid level in sinuses, abnormal intracranial calcification, and radiopaque foreign bodies	• Linear and basal fractures frequently missed by routine x-rays • Contraindicated in pregnant patients
Somatosensory evoked potential (SSEP)	• Evaluates neural pathways involving the spinal cord, brainstem, thalamus, and cerebral cortex • Useful in diagnosis of multiple sclerosis, brain tumor, and spinal cord injury • Useful in determination of brain death	
Somnography	• Records EEG during sleep • Evaluates sleep and sleep disorders	
Spinal cord angiography	• Differentiates between spinal AVM, angioma, tumor, and ischemia	• As for angiogram • May cause thrombosis of spinal vessels and allergy to contrast agent
Spine x-rays	• Detects vertebral dislocation or fracture, degenerative disease, tumor, bone erosion, or calcification • Identifies structural spinal deficits and rules out associated cervical spine injuries	• Care must be taken to prevent fracture displacement and spinal cord injury • C1-C2 view best obtained via open mouth; C6-C7 best obtained with arms pulled down
Suboccipital puncture	• Obtains CSF for analysis • Measures CSF pressure • Rarely performed but may be useful when LP is contraindicated	• May cause trauma to the medulla
Transcranial Doppler	• Measures blood flow velocity through the cerebral arteries • Identifies vasospasm, emboli, vascular stenosis, and brain death	• Quality of findings and interpretation varies with user • Transtemporal window required (lacking in 14% of general population)
Ventriculography	• Obtains CSF for analysis • Measures CSF pressure • Is used especially when intracranial hypertension contraindicates LP	• May cause meningeal irritation, seizures, herniation, intracerebral or intraventricular hemorrhage

9.8   Synthesis Learning Activity: Crossword Puzzle

Complete the following crossword puzzle related to neurologic anatomy, physiology, and assessment.

Answers to this activity can be found in the Answer Key.

ACROSS

2. The term for the opening at the base of the skull where the brain connects to the spinal cord (2 words)

4. The term for difficulty with swallowing

14. CSF is produced in capillary networks called ___ plexuses

15. This type of aphasia is also referred to as motor aphasia

17. The term for the intrinsic ability of the cranium's contents to change to prevent increase in ICP

21. The part of the brain that coordinates muscle movement with sensory input

22. This branch of the autonomic nervous system is frequently referred to as "fight or flight"

23. This type of cell forms the blood-brain barrier

24. The term for the protective coverings of the brain and spinal cord

26. The middle layer of the meninges is the _____ mater; blood vessels and CSF are located here

29. A diagnostic study to evaluate the brain's electrical activity (abbrev.)

30. A primary neurotransmitter for the sympathetic nervous system

31. The term for an unpleasant sensation

33. The vascular structure that is invaluable for collateral circulation (3 words)

35. The term for an unsteady or staggering gait

36. Another term for sympathetic

40. The term for double vision

41. MAP − ICP; normally 60 to 100 mm Hg (abbrev.)

48. During this refractory period, the nerve cannot be stimulated again
50. A pathologic reflex of grasping whatever is placed in the hand with failure to release on command
51. The term for an abnormal sensitivity to light
52. The enzyme that breaks down acetylcholine
53. This cranial nerve controls lateral eye movement
54. The term for the brain's ability to tolerate increases in volume without a corresponding increase in pressure
56. The term for the intrinsic ability of the cerebral blood vessels to dilate or constrict to stabilize cerebral blood flow
59. This lobe controls vision
60. The cranial nerve that controls visual acuity
61. The nodes of _____ allow rapid conduction of impulses by saltatory conduction
62. SBP + (2 x DBP) divided by 3; normally 70 to 105 mm Hg (abbrev.)
63. The type of paralysis seen with LMN lesion
64. The sympathetic and parasympathetic nervous systems constitute the _____ nervous system
66. This cranial nerve controls swallowing
67. A check for arm weakness is to ask the patient to hold his or her arms even and observe for _____
68. The term for difficulty with articulation
70. The outermost layer of the meninges is the _____ mater
72. A chemical that acts as a bridge for transmission of impulses
76. These neurons are responsible for myelin formation in the CNS
78. _____ sign is pain in the neck when the leg is extended; indicates meningeal irritation
79. The term for the inability to understand or express verbal communication
83. These lobes control sensory function

84. The term for loss of half of the visual field
87. These nerve cells provide support, nourishment, and protection of the neurons
88. The term for the loss of motor function
89. The type of paralysis seen with UMN lesion
93. This area of the midbrain is responsible for wakefulness (3 words)
95. The unidirectional conduction of an impulse from one neuron to the next
97. These cells are responsible for the transmission of nerve impulses
99. The brain must have a continuous supply of oxygen and _____

DOWN

1. The cranial nerve that controls sensation on the face
3. This is the predominant neurotransmitter for the parasympathetic nervous system
5. The respiratory centers are located in the _____
6. The term for a loss of sensation
7. This pressure is the pressure exerted from the intracranial contents (abbrev.)
8. In chronic _____ state, the patient is unaware of self and surroundings
9. This test should never be performed if the patient has clinical indications of intracranial hypertension (abbrev.)
10. This acts as a cushion for the brain and the spinal cord (abbrev.)
11. _____ triad is a late indication of intracranial hypertension
12. The scoring system used to standardize observation of responsiveness in neurologic patients
13. The term for the inability to recognize objects through the special senses
14. Another term for parasympathetic
16. These neurons transmit impulses away from the spinal cord or brain

18. The cranial nerves, spinal nerves, and peripheral nerves constitute the _____ nervous system
19. The spinal _____ extends from the brainstem to L2
20. The component of the neuron that conducts impulses toward the cell body
25. This posturing is also referred to as abnormal extension
27. The term for slow movement
28. This type of aphasia is also referred to as sensory aphasia
32. This type of nerve cell is part of the reticuloendothelial system and is responsible for phagocytosis
34. This band of brain tissue connects the left and right cerebral hemispheres (2 words)
35. The component of the neuron that conducts impulses away from the cell body to other neurons or to end organs
37. The contraction of a muscle and a jerk of the affected limb, which is tested by tapping the tendon with a hammer (abbrev.)
38. The cranial nerve that controls pupillary constriction
39. A synapse between the axon of one neuron and the cell body of another neuron would be referred to as _____
42. The normal response to stroking the sole of the foot is the _____ reflex
43. The fold of the dura that separates the cerebral hemispheres from the cerebellum
44. This portion of the brainstem controls cardiac and respiratory centers
45. Another term for body
46. This branch of the autonomic nervous system may be described as "steady state"
47. The term for CSF leak from the nose
49. This bone divides the interior of the skull into 3 fossae: anterior, middle, and posterior

50. Four paired masses of gray matter in the deeper layers of each hemisphere are called the basal _____
55. This portion of the skull has 8 bones
57. Peripheral pain may be tested with pressure to the _____ (2 words)
58. The posterior portion of these lobes controls voluntary motor function
61. This is a test of balance to check for cerebellar dysfunction
65. The term for arching associated with brainstem injury
69. This spinal tract carries pain, temperature, light touch, pressure, and pain
71. This posturing is also referred to as abnormal flexion
73. This type of hydrocephalus is most likely to occur from trauma, including surgical trauma
74. The term for CSF leak from the ears
75. The cranial nerve that allows you to smile
77. This area of the diencephalon is responsible for temperature regulation
80. The term for the skin covering the cranium
81. This type of neuron has one axon and more than one dendrite
82. These nerve cells line the ventricles of the brain and aid in secretion of CSF
85. Neurons that transmit impulses to the spinal cord or brain
86. The term for a lack of inflection while talking
90. The innermost layer of the meninges is the _____ mater
91. These may be partial or generalized
92. The coating or sheath that speeds transmission along the axon
94. This lobe controls long-term memory
96. This nerve originates at C3, C4, C5 and innervates the diaphragm
98. The most important assessment parameter in a patient with a neurologic condition (abbrev.)

SPECIFIC PATIENT HEALTH PROBLEMS

Intracranial Hypertension

The cranium is an inexpansible vault. Brain tissue, CSF, and intravascular blood fill the intracranial cavity to its capacity. Increased ICP correlates to an increase in intracranial volume. Possible causes included brain edema, mass lesions, cerebrovascular alterations, and hydrocephalus. Cerebral edema, either cytotoxic or vasogenic, is the most common cause of intracranial hypertension and may be localized or generalized. Intracellular swelling of neurons and glial cells causes cytotoxic edema. Conditions that cause the swelling include hypoosmolality, hypoxia, and cardiac arrest. With hypoosmolality, the serum osmolality and sodium are low. Water will enter the neurons and glial cells in an attempt at equalizing intracellular and extracellular osmolality. The result is cytotoxic edema. Hypoxia decreases ATP production, impairing the sodium-potassium pump, allowing sodium and water to enter the cells. Cardiac arrest, a cause of anoxic encephalopathy, is one cause of cytotoxic edema.

An increase in extracellular fluid causes vasogenic edema. In vasogenic edema, there is a breakdown of the blood-brain barrier and an increase in vascular permeability with leakage of plasma proteins. Vasogenic edema begins locally, and then becomes generalized. The conditions that cause vasogenic edema include trauma, such as from contusion, tumors, hemorrhage, abscesses, and surgical trauma, such as craniotomy.

A hematoma, neoplasm, abscess, or trauma may cause a mass lesion in the intracranial cavity. Hematomas may be located in the epidural space or subdural space or may be intracerebral (i.e., within the brain matter). Neoplasms may be from a primary brain tumor or metastatic tumor, where the original site is other than the brain. A bacterial or fungal infection may cause an abscess. Trauma may cause intracranial hypertension due to local edema; the contusion may act as a mass lesion.

Arterial vascular occlusions may cause cerebrovascular alteration. Venous outflow obstruction causes alterations by decreasing venous return from the head. Neck rotation, hyperextension, hyperflexion, tracheostomies, and a cervical collar are examples of causes of venous outflow obstructions. Increased intrathoracic pressure may decrease venous return to the heart, resulting in decreased blood flow to the brain, and therefore, decreased venous return. Intrathoracic pressure increases during the Valsalva maneuver from coughing, vomiting, or straining at stool. Positive pressure mechanical ventilation and positive end-expiratory pressure also increase intrathoracic pressure with potential resultant increase in ICP. A hypertensive crisis will cause an increase in CPP, which may in turn cause intracranial hypertension. Causes of vasodilation, which will increase the volume of blood inside the cranium and increase ICP, include hypercapnia, hypoxia, and vasoactive drugs.

Hydrocephalus is a medical condition in which there is an abnormal accumulation of CSF in the ventricles, or cavities, of the brain. Causes of hydrocephalus include an increase in production of CSF or a decrease in reabsorption of CSF. Choroid plexus papilloma may cause an increase in the production of CSF. The conditions of SAH or meningitis cause a communicating hydrocephalus. A tumor, hemorrhage, surgical or traumatic edema, or obstructing outflow of CSF due to infarction may cause noncommunicating hydrocephalus.

Intracranial volume is composed of brain tissue, circulating blood, and CSF. Brain tissue is normally approximately 80%

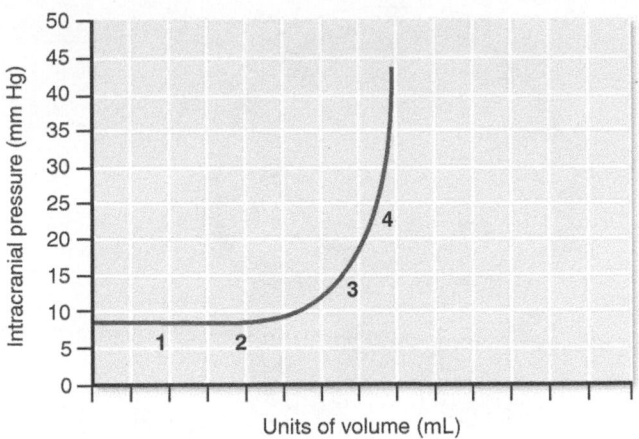

FIGURE 9-20 Intracranial pressure-volume curve. *1,* High compliance and low elastance. *2,* Lower compliance and higher elastance. *3,* High elastance and low compliance. *4,* Herniation. (See text for more complete description.) (From Carlson, K. K. [Ed.]. [2009]. *Advanced critical care nursing.* St. Louis, MO: Saunders.)

to 88% of intracranial volume. Circulating blood volume is normally approximately 2% to 10% of intracranial volume and CSF is normally approximately 10%. Significant cerebral atrophy occurs in the elderly, people affected by Alzheimer dementia, and alcohol or drug abusers. Atrophy results in less than 80% of intracranial volume being brain tissue, creating traction on the bridging vessels, which increases the risk of intracranial bleeding. In these instances, hemorrhage or hematoma may be substantial before visible symptoms.

The cranium is an inexpansible vault, and inside the cranium is a closed system with the three fluctuating volumes discussed in the previous paragraph. Compensation is the ability of the cranium's contents to change or rearrange to maintain stable intracranial volume. Compensation is more effective when the volume increase is slower. If the volume of one of the three constituents of the intracranial cavity increases, a reciprocal decrease in volume of one or both of the others will occur to prevent an increase in intracranial volume and resultant pressure. Initially, displacement from the cranium to the lumbar cistern as well as a decrease in production and increase in reabsorption of CSF decreases the CSF. Compression of the low-pressure venous system decreases blood volume by shunting blood to the venous sinuses. A relationship between volume and pressure exists (Figure 9-20). As successive units of any of the three volumes are added to the cranium, a critical point is reached. Each additional unit of volume added increases ICP dramatically and herniation results (Figure 9-21 and Table 9-19).

The pathophysiologic sequence of intracranial hypertension (Figure 9-22) begins with an increase in the brain volume, CSF volume, or blood volume. Compliance is the brain's ability to tolerate increases in volume without a corresponding increase in pressure. Compliance is poor if a small increase in volume causes a large increase in pressure. Decompensation occurs when the brain loses its ability to compensate. Pressure on the cerebral vessels slows blood flow to the brain. Diminished circulation produces ischemia and an accumulation of carbon dioxide and lactic acid. Hypoxia and hypercapnia trigger vasodilation, which increases blood volume and brain edema. Brain edema increases ICP further. Compression of cerebral vessels occurs and causes further ischemia. Eventually cerebral circulation stops and brain death occurs.

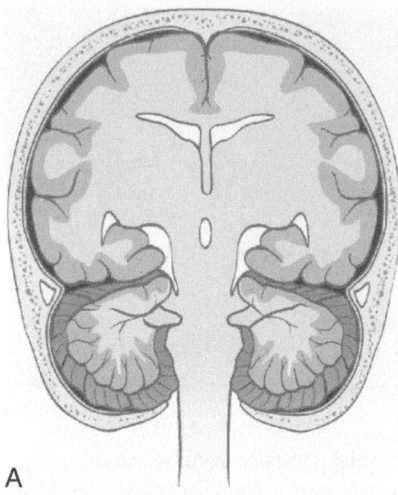

A

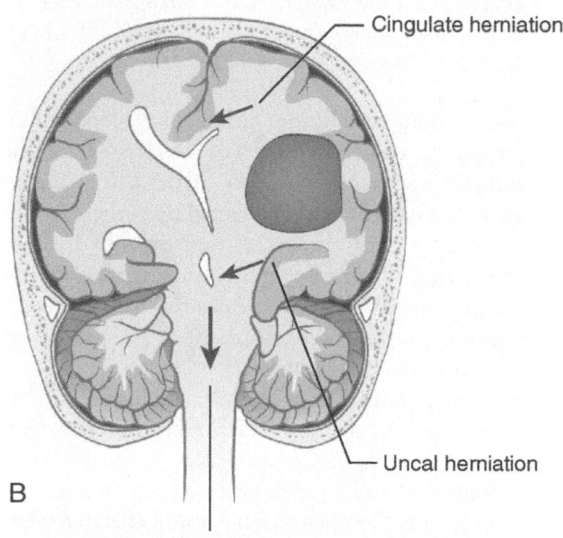

Cingulate herniation

Uncal herniation

B

Central herniation

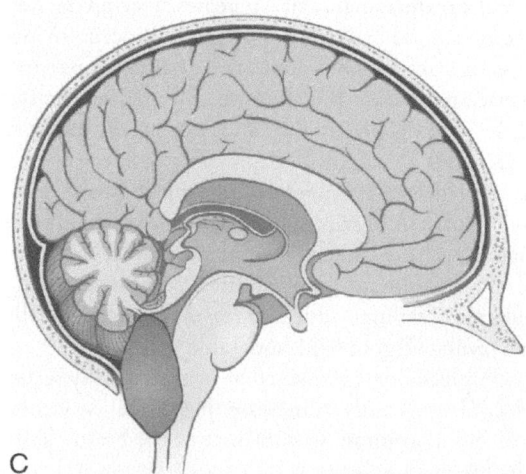

C

FIGURE 9-21 Herniation syndromes. A, Normal intracranial structures. **B,** Supratentorial herniation syndromes. **C,** Cerebellar tonsil herniation. (From McCance, K. L., & Huether, S. E. [2014]. *Pathophysiology: The biologic basis for disease in adults and children* [7th ed.]. St. Louis, MO: Mosby.)

The compensatory and decompensatory changes indicative of intracranial hypertension occur in a sequential process (Figure 9-23). With intracranial hypertension, changes in the patient's LOC, cranial nerve function, motor function, and vital signs occur.

Yawning, restlessness, and confusion manifest changes in LOC in the early stage. Confusion is the earliest and most sensitive clinical finding in a patient with deteriorating loss of consciousness. Late changes include a diminishing LOC and posturing.

Cranial nerve changes involve cranial nerves II, III, V, IX, and X. Ipsilateral pupil changes, including change in size and shape (oval), conjugate eye deviation, and a sluggish reaction to light, manifest early changes in the oculomotor (III) nerve. Late changes are ipsilateral pupil changes of one or both pupils. The pupils may be dilated and nonreactive to light. Ptosis and, with brainstem lesions, dysconjugate eye movement may be present. Optic (II) visual changes include diplopia. Papilledema is more likely to occur when ICP rises slowly rather than quickly. Trigeminal (V) nerve changes manifest as an impaired corneal reflex. Glossopharyngeal (IX) and vagus (X) changes result in impaired gag reflex and swallowing.

Motor changes are contralateral to the actual area affected by the neurologic problem; therefore, they are manifested on the opposite side as the lesion. They are due to compression or pressure in the corticospinal tracts. Early motor signs are paresis and plegia. A late motor sign is posturing.

Vomiting may occur especially with lesions below the tentorium. Pressure on the vomiting center in the brainstem causes projectile vomiting without nausea. Headache with increasing severity may occur. Normal protective reflexes such as cough, gag, and corneal reflexes may be decreased or absent and seizures may occur.

Vital sign changes include Cushing triad, which is due to pressure on, or ischemia of, the vasomotor center in the brainstem. Components of Cushing triad are an increased systolic BP, a widening pulse pressure (due to the diastolic BP being normal or decreased along with an increased systolic BP), bradycardia, and respiratory pattern changes. Changes in respiratory patterns are dependent on the location of the injury. Central hyperthermia may occur late in intracranial hypertension due to pressure on the thermoregulatory center in the hypothalamus.

Diagnostic studies performed to determine the cause of the intracranial hypertension include CT scan, cerebral angiography, skull x-ray, EEG, evoked potentials, and ECG. A diagnostic test that is contraindicated is a lumbar puncture if intracranial hypertension is suspected. The procedure may cause a downward cerebellar herniation with medullary herniation and death. A CT scan may show the cause of intracranial hemorrhage (ICH) or intracerebral shifts. Cerebral angiography may show the cause of intracranial hypertension. An EEG evaluates brain wave activity and evoked potentials assess brainstem integrity. An ECG may show a prolonged QT interval or dysrhythmias, especially with SAH.

The first and most important interventions in caring for patients with neurologic illness or injury are to prevent causes of intracranial hypertension when possible and monitor closely for clinical indications of intracranial hypertension. Recognize the factors that increase ICP (Box 9-1) and prevent as many of these factors as possible. Monitor for neurologic changes during nursing care activities, such as turning, suctioning, oral care, and bathing. Some of these factors that increase ICP are necessary and required aspects of nursing care. Continually assess the patient during these activities and space the activities to allow the ICP to return to normal before performing another activity that may increase the ICP.

Proper positioning is required to promote and maintain adequate venous drainage from the head. Maintain the patient's head and neck in a straight alignment to prevent compression of the jugular veins. Prevent compression of jugular veins by

TABLE 9-19 Herniation Syndromes

Type of Herniation	Description	Symptomatology	Comments
Supratentorial			
Cingulate (or subfalcine) herniation	Expanding lesion of one hemisphere shifts laterally and forces the cingulate gyrus under the falx cerebri; compression of vessels causes brain edema, ischemia, and intracranial hypertension	• No specific clinical manifestations • May have altered LOC or plegia • Cheyne-Stokes breathing pattern may be seen	• Not life-threatening but a sign of brain decompensation • If condition not controlled, uncal or central herniation will occur
Uncal herniation	Expanding lesion in middle fossa or temporal lobe causes a lateral displacement, which pushes the uncus of the temporal lobe over the edge of the tentorium; uncus may be lacerated by sharp edge of tentorium	• First symptom is unilateral (ipsilateral) pupil dilation with sluggish reaction to light → fixed, dilated pupils • Decreased LOC • Ventilatory pattern change • Contralateral hemiplegia progressing to posturing	• Most common herniation syndrome • Life-threatening when hemorrhage or brainstem compression occurs
Central (or transtentorial) herniation	Expanding lesions of the frontal, parietal, or occipital lobes or severe generalized edema causes downward displacement of the basal ganglia and diencephalon through the tentorial notch, causing pressure on the midbrain	• First symptom is change in level of consciousness • Small, reactive pupils → fixed, dilated pupils • Ventilatory pattern changes → apnea • Decorticate posturing → flaccidity	• May be preceded by cingulate or uncal herniation • Life-threatening
Transcalvarial herniation	Extrusion of brain tissue through the cranium	• No specific clinical manifestations	• May occur through an opening from a skull fracture, craniotomy site, or burr hole • Risk of infection
Infratentorial			
Upward transtentorial herniation	Expanding mass lesion of cerebellum, brainstem, or fourth ventricle causes protrusion of the central area of the cerebellum and the midbrain upward through the tentorial notch	• First symptom is unilateral (ipsilateral) pupil dilation • Obstructive hydrocephalus occurs with rapid deterioration of neurologic status	• May be life-threatening
Downward cerebellar (or tonsillar) herniation	Expanding lesion of the cerebellum exerts downward pressure, sending cerebellar tonsils through the foramen magnum; compression and displacement of the medulla oblongata occur	• Coma • Flaccid paralysis • Respiratory and cardiac arrest occur	• May be a complication of lumbar puncture when LP is performed in presence of high ICP • Causes death

tracheostomy ties or a cervical collar. Frequently assess the tracheostomy ties or cervical collar to ascertain that they are secure but not too tight and loosen if necessary.

To prevent an increase in ICP caused by a Valsalva maneuver, instruct the patient to exhale when turning in bed and to cough with the mouth open if coughing is necessary. Teach the patient to avoid straining, bending, or sneezing. Administer stool softeners as indicated to prevent constipation and straining at stool. Treat nausea with antiemetics to prevent vomiting. When positioning the patient, avoid hip flexion greater than 90 degrees. Discourage isometric exercise and do not use the footboard to prevent foot drop. Use high-top tennis shoes to prevent foot drop in place of a footboard.

Administer analgesics and/or sedatives before activities that may increase ICP. Closely assess the patient's response to head of bed (HOB) elevation by evaluating changes in ICP, clinical indications, and vital signs. Although elevation of the HOB to 30 degrees promotes venous drainage from the brain, it may decrease cerebral blood flow by decreasing BP.

Suctioning can cause a significant increase in ICP. To prevent an increase in ICP associated with suctioning, suction only if necessary and limit suctioning to 10 seconds with a negative pressure of less than 120 mm Hg.

Oxygen and carbon dioxide levels affect cerebral vessels, which affects vascular tone and cerebral oxygenation. Monitor the respiratory effort and ventilation pattern. Hypercapnia and/or

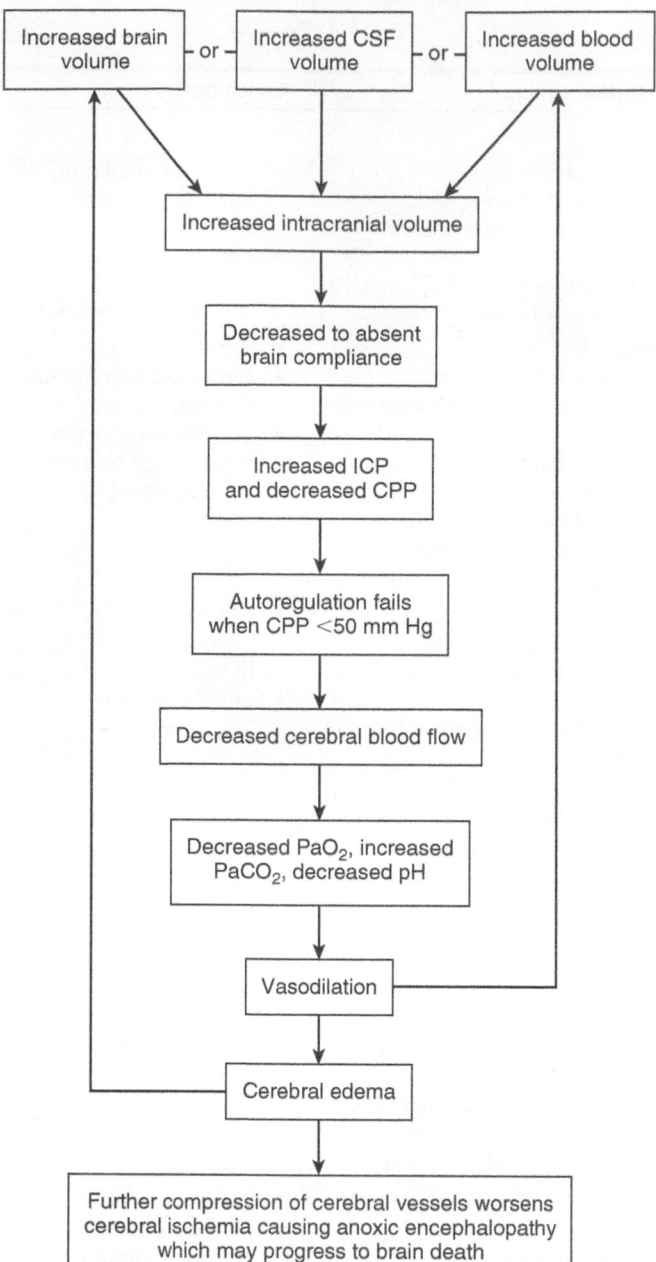

FIGURE 9-22 Summary of pathophysiology of intracranial hypertension. (From Dennison, R. D. [2013]. *Pass CCRN!* [4th ed.]. St. Louis, MO: Elsevier.)

hypoxemia may cause vasodilation and increase ICP. Obtain arterial blood gases and monitor pulse oximetry (SpO_2).

Attempt to maintain the patient's euvolemic state. Monitor the patient's fluid balance and administer IV fluids to the patient as prescribed. Avoid hypotonic fluids such as D_5W, which may contribute to brain edema.

If CSF leakage is noted, do not pack the nose or ears. Apply a mustache dressing under the nose or a 4 × 4 inch gauze over the ear. Confirm that the fluid draining from the nose or ears is CSF by testing it for glucose; CSF will test positive for glucose but mucus will not.

Reduce the patient's anxiety by frequently reorienting the patient to person, place, date, and time. Explain all procedures thoroughly to the patient and family. Maintain a calm, quiet environment for the patient. Prevent loud noises and disturbing conversations. Be careful to not conduct or allow emotionally disturbing conversations to occur at the bedside. Encourage the family to touch the patient and speak to him or her encouragingly. Let them know that many patients report awareness even during altered LOC.

Maintain the patient in a normothermic state (less than 38° C or 100.5 F). Treat hyperthermia aggressively in patients with neurologic illness or injury because temperature elevations are associated with significant increase in metabolic rate and oxygen consumption. Brain injury causes central neurogenic fever and reflects hypothalamic dysfunction. Characterized by a lack of sweating and absence of tachycardia, the condition may persist for days. Central neurogenic fever is best controlled by external cooling such as a hyperthermia blanket, applying ice packs, and/or using a fan to cool the skin. Avoid the complication of shivering when using a hypothermia blanket by implementation of a shivering protocol. Shivering is both an anticipated consequence and, potentially, a major adverse effect of therapeutic hypothermia. Even mild hypothermia can elicit a vigorous thermoregulatory defense to maintain body temperature at the hypothalamic set point. In healthy humans, peripheral vasoconstriction is triggered at 36.5° C and shivering at 35.5° C. Temperature thresholds for vasoconstriction and shivering are often higher than normal in brain-injured patients; therefore, these thermoregulatory defenses may occur more vigorously and at higher temperatures in these individuals. Control of shivering is essential for effective cooling, as shivering fights the cooling process, makes attaining target temperature difficult, is extremely uncomfortable, and can trigger massive increases in systemic and cerebral energy consumption and metabolic demand. Turn the hypothermia blanket off when the temperature reaches 38° C (100.5° F) because the temperature of a neurologic patient will tend to drift downward after removal of the hypothermia blanket. Small doses of promethazine HCl (Phenergan) decrease shivering. Sedation with opioids, α2-receptor agonists, or propofol may be necessary to prevent shivering.

Peripheral fever is associated with infection and characterized by sweating and tachycardia. Control peripheral fever with antipyretics such as acetaminophen (Tylenol).

Treat intracranial hypertension by decreasing metabolic requirements of the brain. Administer prophylactic anticonvulsants that are for no longer than 7 days as prescribed. Administer mannitol or hypertonic saline (2% or 3% solution) as prescribed. Because mannitol administration may cause a rebound effect with increased ICP, hypertonic saline solution is preferred. Surgical intervention may be required for removal of a mass lesion or hematoma. A hemicraniectomy, in which a portion of the skull is removed to allow for the brain to swell, may be performed. In severe ICP, a bilateral craniectomy may be performed. Hyperventilation therapy is only used for impending herniation because cerebral ischemia results.

Monitor the patient for complications such as emboli, infection, atelectasis, pressure ulcers, and contractures. Implement nursing measures to prevent the complications. Turn and position the patient, encourage deep breathing, utilize pneumatic compression devices, avoid dehydration, maintain infection control measures, and perform range-of-motion exercises for the patient. Continually assess the patient for permanent neurologic residual deficits, herniation, and brain death.

Encephalopathy

Encephalopathy is defined as a global mental status dysfunction as a manifestation of a systemic or brain disorder. Encephalopathy is a general term describing a disease that affects the function

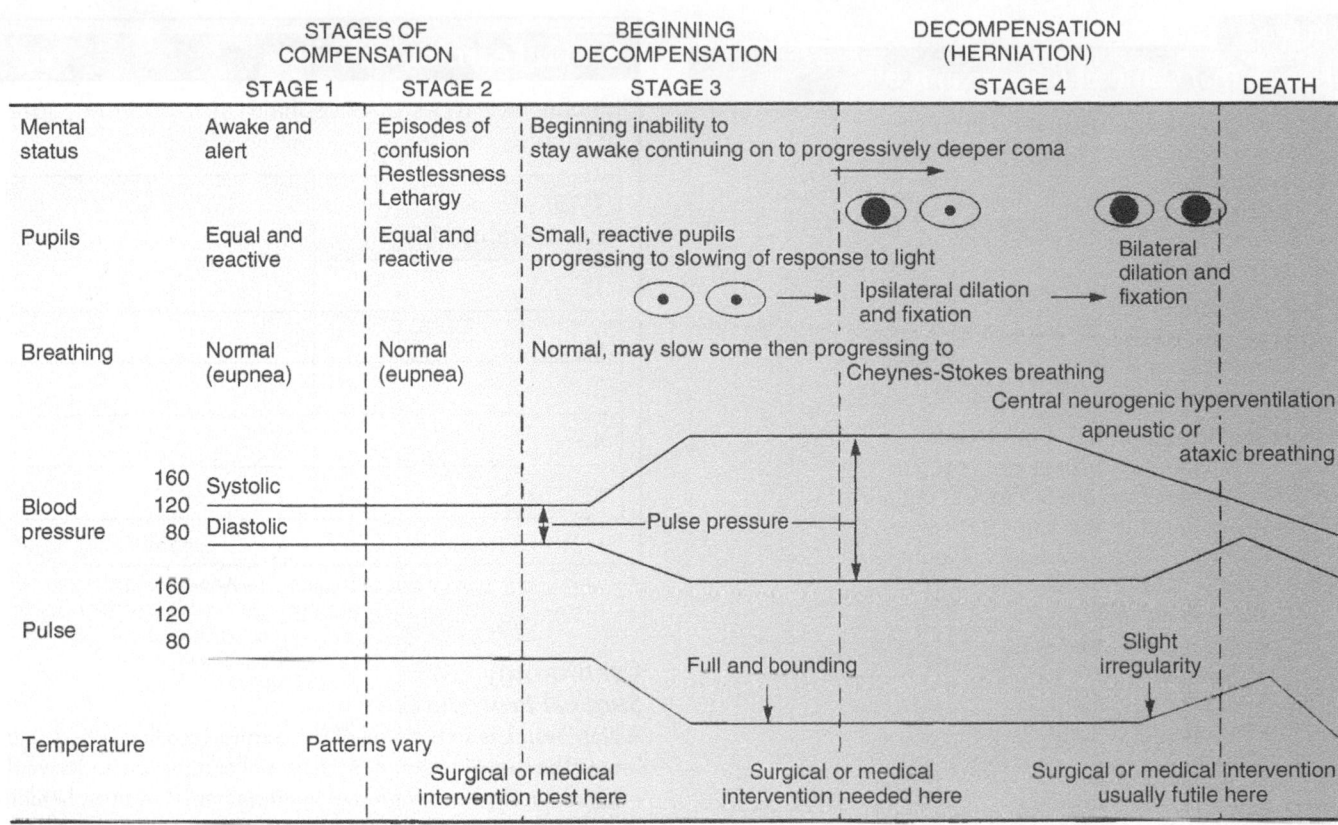

FIGURE 9-23 Clinical correlates of compensated and decompensated phases of intracranial hypertension. (From Beare, P. G., & Myers, J. L. [1994]. *Principles and practice of adult health nursing* [2nd ed.]. St Louis, MO: Mosby.)

9.9 Learning Activity

List 10 factors that can increase Intracranial pressure that can and should be eliminated.

1. _____
2. _____
3. _____
4. _____
5. _____
6. _____
7. _____
8. _____
9. _____
10. _____

Answers to this activity can be found in the Answer Key.

9.10 Learning Activity

Identify five interventions that can help prevent increased intracranial pressure.

1. _____
2. _____
3. _____
4. _____
5. _____

Answers to this activity can be found in the Answer Key.

or structure of your brain. There are many types of encephalopathy and brain disease. Some types are permanent and some are temporary. Some types are present from birth and never change; others are acquired after birth and may get progressively worse.

Alterations in cerebral perfusion pressure (CPP) (see Figure 9-8) may cause encephalopathy. Anoxic encephalopathy occurs when CPP is less than <50 mm Hg and is most likely caused by an event such as cardiac arrest or severe hypotension, in which the brain received an inadequate oxygen supply for a period. Hypertensive encephalopathy occurs when CPP is more than 150 mm Hg and the extremely elevated hydrostatic pressure in cerebral arteries causes fluid to be pushed into brain tissue, causing cerebral edema. Uremic or hepatic encephalopathy occurs due to a buildup of toxins normally removed by functioning kidneys or liver. Water, electrolyte (especially sodium), glucose, or vitamin abnormalities and toxins cause metabolic encephalopathy. Thiamine (vitamin B_1) deficiency commonly associated with alcoholism triggers Wernicke encephalopathy especially with the administration of glucose without adequate thiamine replacement. Carbon monoxide and cyanide poisoning also cause a metabolic encephalopathy because they prevent hemoglobin from transporting oxygen to tissues, causing cerebral anoxia. Infection from bacteria, viruses, and fungus may also cause encephalopathy.

The clinical presentation of encephalopathy varies with the cause. Objective findings vary, but in mild encephalopathy, memory loss and subtle personality changes occur. Severe encephalopathy may present as dementia, loss of consciousness, or seizures. Diagnostic testing may aid in clarification of the cause.

Factors That Cause an Increase in ICP

Ventilation and/or Oxygenation Problems
- Airway obstruction
- Hypercapnia
- Hypoxia
- Suctioning without hyperoxygenation
- Deep breathing

Position Changes
- Prone position
- Trendelenburg position
- Extreme hip flexion (greater than 90 degrees)

Decreased Venous Return from Head
- Neck flexion, hyperextension, or rotation
- Tight tracheostomy ties or cervical collar
- Increased intrathoracic pressure
  - Positive pressure mechanical ventilation
  - Positive end-expiratory pressure
  - Valsalva maneuver
    - Straining at stool
    - Vomiting
    - Coughing
    - Isometric exercise
  - Suctioning

Increased Metabolic Rate
- Hyperthermia
- Seizure activity
- Rapid eye movement (REM) sleep

Stress
- Disturbing conversation
- Noise
- Bright lights
- Pain or noxious stimuli

9.11   Learning Activity

Identify five types of encephalopathy and the cause of each.

Type of Encephalopathy	Cause
1.	
2.	
3.	
4.	
5.	

Answers to this activity can be found in the Answer Key.

Craniotomy
Surgical Procedures

A craniotomy is an opening of the cranium to allow access to the brain. The surgeon uses a supratentorial craniotomy to access the cerebral hemispheres for removing intracranial tumors, hematomas, abscesses, or epileptic foci. A craniotomy is also used to clip or ligate aneurysm or arteriovenous (AV) malformations in the anterior circulation. Additional reasons to perform a craniotomy include to place a ventriculovenous, ventriculopleural, or ventriculoperitoneal shunt; debride fragments and necrotic tissue; or elevate and realign bone fragments. To access the brainstem and cerebellum to allow removal of cerebellar tumors and hemorrhages, acoustic neuromas, or tumors of the brainstem or cranial nerves, the surgeons performs an infratentorial craniotomy.

A transsphenoidal approach, referred to as a transsphenoidal hypophysectomy, is frequently used to remove the pituitary gland. With a transsphenoidal hypophysectomy, the surgeon generally goes through the nose to the floor of the brain through the sphenoid bone. The surgeon enters the sella turcica through the floor of the nose and the sphenoid sinus. Indications for a transsphenoidal hypophysectomy include a pituitary tumor or to control pain associated with metastatic cancer.

A craniectomy is the removal of a portion of the cranium. Cranioplasty is the repair of the cranium, with a synthetic material used in most instances. Burr holes are small holes drilled through the cranium to allow access to underlying structures. Burr holes provide an access to evacuate an epidural or subdural hematoma and/or insert an intraventricular catheter for CSF drainage. In addition, burr holes provide the access for insertion of another form of ICP monitoring device such as a subarachnoid screw.

Preoperatively, a priority in the collaborative care management of neurosurgical patients is to control the patient's pain and discomfort and complete the preparations required for each type of surgical procedure. Administer small doses of fentanyl or morphine as prescribed, but avoid oversedation. Oversedation impairs the patient's LOC, the most important assessment parameter. The preoperative anticonvulsant drug of choice is levetiracetam (Keppra). The patient's hair and body are washed with an antimicrobial shampoo and soap the night before surgery and

---

The priorities of care for a patient with encephalopathy are to maintain the airway, oxygenation, and ventilation. Administer oxygen to maintain SpO_2 of greater than or equal to 92% unless contraindicated. If the patient is conscious and can follow instructions, encourage the patient to deep breathe. In the presence of audible rhonchi, instruct the patient to cough with the mouth open to decrease sustained elevations of ICP. Assess the patient's swallow competency and have suction equipment available. Resolve any impairment in neurologic function, if possible, through treatment of the cause. Maintain adequate hydration and electrolyte balance by administering isotonic fluids as prescribed. Monitor closely for indications of overhydration or dehydration by evaluation of urine output and urine specific gravity hourly. Maintain the patient's nutritional status. Enteral nutritional support is preferred. Prevent patient injury by assessing the potential risks and initiating appropriate interventions. Administer prophylactic anticonvulsants as prescribed and use protective measures if seizure occurs. Perform passive ROM and reposition the patient every 2 hours. Perform frequent skin assessment and skin care. Instill artificial tears every 2 hours to prevent corneal abrasions in patients who do not blink. Reorient the patient to time and place often and encourage the family's participation in reality orientation.

the operative area is usually clipped in the operating room (OR) or the OR holding area. Record a baseline neurologic status. This baseline status includes the patient's LOC and Glasgow Coma Score. In addition, document the deficits in communication and cognitive, motor, sensory, and cranial nerves. Inform the patient and family what to expect after surgery. Prepare the patient and family that equipment such as IV catheter(s), oxygen therapy, an indwelling bladder catheter, and sequential compression stockings may be present postoperatively. Inform the patient and family that if mechanical ventilation or an intraventricular catheter and ICP monitor are required postoperatively to expect a transfer to a higher acuity unit.

Teach the patient and family that the patient may experience a mild to moderate headache after surgery. Other discomforts that the patient may experience are photophobia, periorbital edema, and bruising. Instruct the patient to notify the nurse if he or she develops a headache or other symptoms. There may also be a head dressing and drain present. Administer medications or other interventions to relieve symptoms.

Postoperatively, the priority in collaborative care management is to prevent, monitor for, and treat clinical indications of intracranial hypertension. Perform frequent neurologic assessments and compare the results with the patient's preoperative status. Check visual acuity on patients who have undergone a hypophysectomy. Teach the patient to avoid the causes of intracranial hypertension (see Box 9-1). To promote jugular vein drainage, advise the patient to avoid twisting of the head or neck or flexion of the neck, and support the head, neck, and shoulders when turning the patient in bed. Control conditions that may increase the cerebral metabolic rate. To decrease environmental stimuli, avoid excessive noise, upsetting conversations, bright lights, and extremes of room temperature. Plan nursing activities so that there is spacing in between and do not perform activities in clusters. Assess the patient's tolerance to nursing care activity before implementation of any activity.

Position the patient appropriately to prevent complications, promote venous drainage, and avoid restriction of blood flow. Supratentorial craniotomy patients should have the HOB elevated 30 degrees. If removal of a large mass or bone flap occurred, do not allow the patient to lie on the operative side. Position the patients who have had an infratentorial craniotomy supine, with a small pillow under the nape of the neck. Do not allow the patient to lie completely supine for 48 hours. Patients who have undergone a transsphenoidal craniotomy, such as those who have had a hypophysectomy, should have the HOB elevated to 30 degrees. Position patients who received the placement of an interventricular shunt flat on the nonoperative side. The surgeon may prescribe other specific positioning restrictions.

Monitor the patient's vital signs, airway, breathing, and circulatory status and implement measures to maintain airway, oxygenation, and ventilation. Encourage the patient to deep breathe but avoid coughing. When audible rhonchi are present, coughing is necessary; therefore, instruct the patient to cough with the mouth open. Administer oxygen to maintain SpO_2 of greater than or equal to 92% unless contraindicated. Assess the patient's gag reflex and swallowing competency and have suction equipment available.

Monitor the patient for hypertension or hypotension and administer fluids and/or medication to maintain adequate cerebral perfusion. Maintain adequate hydration and electrolyte balance and monitor closely for indications of fluid overload or deficit. Fluid overload can predispose the patient to brain edema. A fluid deficit can decrease CPP and cause cerebral ischemia. Evaluate the patient's urine output and urine specific gravity hourly. Administer isotonic fluids as prescribed and avoid D_5W and other hypotonic solutions.

Administer anticonvulsants for seizures, antipyretics and cooling blankets for hyperthermia, and sedation as indicated for shivering and restlessness. Administer treatments for intracranial hypertension as prescribed. These are most likely to include mannitol or hypertonic saline infusions but may include return to surgery.

Assess the head dressing hourly and notify the surgeon if large amounts of drainage are noted. Assess the patient for the presence of rhinorrhea, otorrhea, and excessive swallowing. Apply a mustache dressing for rhinorrhea. Apply a 2 × 2 inch dressing over the ear for otorrhea or a sterile URI bag. Apply cool compresses to decrease periorbital edema.

Assess the patient for the presence of a headache and provide interventions and medications for relief. Inform the patient and family to notify the nurse at the onset of a headache. Severe pain is not normal, and if it occurs, notify the physician. Administer small doses of morphine or fentanyl, but avoid oversedation. When the patient can take oral medications, acetaminophen with oxycodone (Percocet) or hydrocodone (Lorcet) is usually used.

Prevent injury and promote safety for the patient. Institute seizure precautions, and if seizures do occur, administer anticonvulsants as prescribed. Perform passive ROM, reposition the patient every 2 hours, and perform frequent skin assessment. Instill artificial tears every 2 hours to prevent corneal abrasions in patients who do not blink. Create a moisture chamber using plastic wrap. Do not put tubes, such as a suction catheter or nasogastric tube, into the nose if the patient has had a transsphenoidal approach procedure and warn the patient not to blow or pick the nose. Orient the patient to time and place often and encourage family participation in reality orientation.

Monitor for and prevent patient from infection. Administer prophylactic and/or therapeutic antibiotics as prescribed. Monitor the head dressing and drains for any purulent drainage. Assess the wound during aseptic dressing changes for redness, swelling, induration, and drainage, and drainage of CSF. A CSF leak increases the risk of intracranial infection. Be aware that a CSF leak is normal for up to 72 hours after a transsphenoidal hypophysectomy. A CNS infection can cause encephalitis or meningitis. Clinical indications of CNS infection include headache, photophobia, nuchal rigidity, fever, and positive Kernig and Brudzinski signs. The treatment for a CNS infection is antibiotics and monitoring for complications. Intracranial hypertension from brain edema usually peaks in about 48 to 72 hours. Monitor the patient for brain ischemia, infarction, cerebral hemorrhage, and CSF leak. Hydrocephalus may occur but it is frequently transient due to swelling.

Prevent deep vein thrombosis (DVT) with the use sequential compression devices rather than graduated elastic stockings because these patients are at high risk for DVT. Apply the sequential compression devices before surgery and use whenever the patient is in bed. Administer low-dose heparin or low-molecular-weight heparin as prescribed.

Prevent a stress ulcer, frequently referred to as *Cushing ulcer*, with administration of histamine$_2$ receptor antagonists or proton pump inhibitors prophylactically. Monitor the patient for clinical indications of occult and overt GI bleeding.

Hemorrhagic Stroke

A hemorrhagic stroke is a neurologic deficit caused by interruption of blood flow to the brain due to vessel rupture. The hemorrhage results from a weakened vessel that ruptures and bleeds into the surrounding brain. The blood accumulates and compresses the surrounding brain tissue.

The etiology of hemorrhagic stroke includes intraparenchymal brain hemorrhage (IPBH), also called intracerebral hemorrhage (ICH), intraventricular hemorrhage (IVH), and subarachnoid hemorrhage (SAH). The causes of IPBH include trauma or hypertensive rupture of a cerebral vessel, vascular intracerebral tumor, anticoagulants, bleeding disorders, spontaneous hemorrhagic conversion of a cerebral infarct, fibrinolytic use in ischemic stroke, and arteriovenous malformation (AVM) rupture. An AVM is a tangle of abnormal arteries and veins where the arteries feed directly into veins without a capillary bed. AVMs are always congenital and may occur in other circulatory systems, including the spinal cord. Although AVM rupture usually causes IPBH, it can also result in IVH and SAH.

The patient with a hemorrhagic stroke may complain of headache. Seizure, focal neurologic deficit, hypertension, decreased LOC, and other signs of elevated ICP occur in IPBH. Clinical presentation of AVM may include headache, seizure, and focal deficits. An AVM can be symptomatic without hemorrhage.

A noncontrast head CT scan within 45 minutes of arrival to the ED can immediately show IPBH. Another radiology procedure used to diagnose IPBH is an MRI. MRI can also be used to diagnose IPBH. Contrast-enhanced CT and MRI, CT angiography and venography, and MRA and venography can be used to diagnose structural lesions that cause IPBH. CT angiography and contrast CT are also used to identify patients who may develop enlargement of a hemorrhage.

Collaborative management priorities include protecting and maintaining the patient's airway, ventilation, and oxygenation. Administer oxygen as needed to maintain SpO$_2$ greater than or equal to 92% unless contraindicated. Prevent aspiration by positioning the patient on the lateral side. Provide safety by ensuring suction equipment is available at the bedside. When suctioning the patient, endotracheal administration of lidocaine may reduce the risk of increased ICP. A patient without airway protective reflexes due to decreased LOC or with a focal deficit requires endotracheal intubation. Sedation is necessary before intubation. Monitor the patient's vital signs and if the SBP is >180 mm Hg or MAP is >130 mm Hg and ICP is stable with no signs and symptoms of increased ICP, maintain the MAP at 110 mm Hg or BP 160/90 mm Hg. The American Heart Association (AHA) does not have specific recommendations for medications for this condition, but the focus of care is to correct any bleeding diatheses and hold oral anticoagulants regardless of surgical intervention.

Surgical or endovascular treatment may be required. There are no definitive recommendations on the timing or type of surgery used. Surgery can be craniotomy or stereotactic radiosurgery to evacuate the clot. Surgery should be considered when it is a complicated hemorrhage of the cerebellum, the

hemorrhage is supratentorial and >30 mL, or the hemorrhage is within 1 cm of the brain surface. If the AVM may not be safely excised to control hemorrhage, a stereotactic radiosurgery procedure is performed. In addition, an endovascular treatment with glue embolization may treat the AVM. This involves the injection of glue into the arterial pedicle to cause thrombosis and block blood flow into the malformation. Endovascular treatment may also include embolization of the AVM with Silastic beads and/or preoperative embolization followed by a surgical excision.

Posthemorrhage care includes monitoring vital signs and performing neurologic assessments. Strict glycemic control and management of hyperthermia are important to prevent complications, morbidity, and mortality. DVT prophylaxis, infection prevention, and wound care (in the event of craniotomy) prevent complications. It is not recommended to administer prophylactic seizure medication unless the patient has demonstrated seizure activity due to IPBH.

IVH typically is the result of an aneurysmal or AVM rupture, or extension of IPBH. Clinical presentation, diagnosis, and treatment are specific to those disease states.

SAH is hemorrhage into the subarachnoid space most commonly caused by cerebral aneurysms, weakened, bulging areas on an intracranial artery. The most common site for cerebral aneurysms to develop is on the circle of Willis or an area of bifurcation. Large aneurysms can act as space-occupying lesions. The etiology of aneurysm comes from degenerative states such as hypertension and diabetes mellitus, as well as induced damage from smoking. The major cause for cerebral aneurysms is smoking. Connective tissue disorders such as lupus can also contribute to aneurysm formation and genetics may be a factor. The familial incidence of cerebral aneurysm is 2% to 3%.

Risk factors for SAH can be dependent on the size and location of the aneurysm, as well as patient sex and race. Stress and inflammation may have a role in SAH. SAH risk is greater in patients who are hypertensive and who smoke. Formation, growth, and rupture of aneurysm is difficult to predict and dependent on many factors. Aneurysm types include:

- Saccular or berry aneurysm has a distinct sac and stem shape; it is the most common type of aneurysm.
- Fusiform aneurysm has an amorphous shape and lacks a stem.
- Traumatic aneurysm is due to external cerebral trauma.
- Mycotic aneurysm is caused by septic emboli originating from a different, infected site in the body and is very rare.

The pathophysiologic sequence that occurs with hemorrhagic stroke has similarities and differences depending on the cause (Figure 9-24). Two common risks to note are rebleeding and vasospasm.

The majority of patients with hemorrhagic stroke experience a sudden, severe headache, frequently described as "the worst headache of my life." Patients also describe it as a "thunder clap" or "like being hit in the head." The headache is localized, progressing to generalized, and may radiate to the neck and back. Because blood is irritating to meninges, meningeal symptoms (nuchal rigidity, photophobia, decreased LOC, Brudzinski and Kernig signs) and nausea and vomiting are common. Patients with SAH frequently state they had a less severe headache in the 2 to 8 weeks before their hemorrhage. This is due to a warning, or sentinel, leak. Sentinel leaks are associated with an increased risk of rebleeding (i.e., ruptured aneurysm rupturing again)

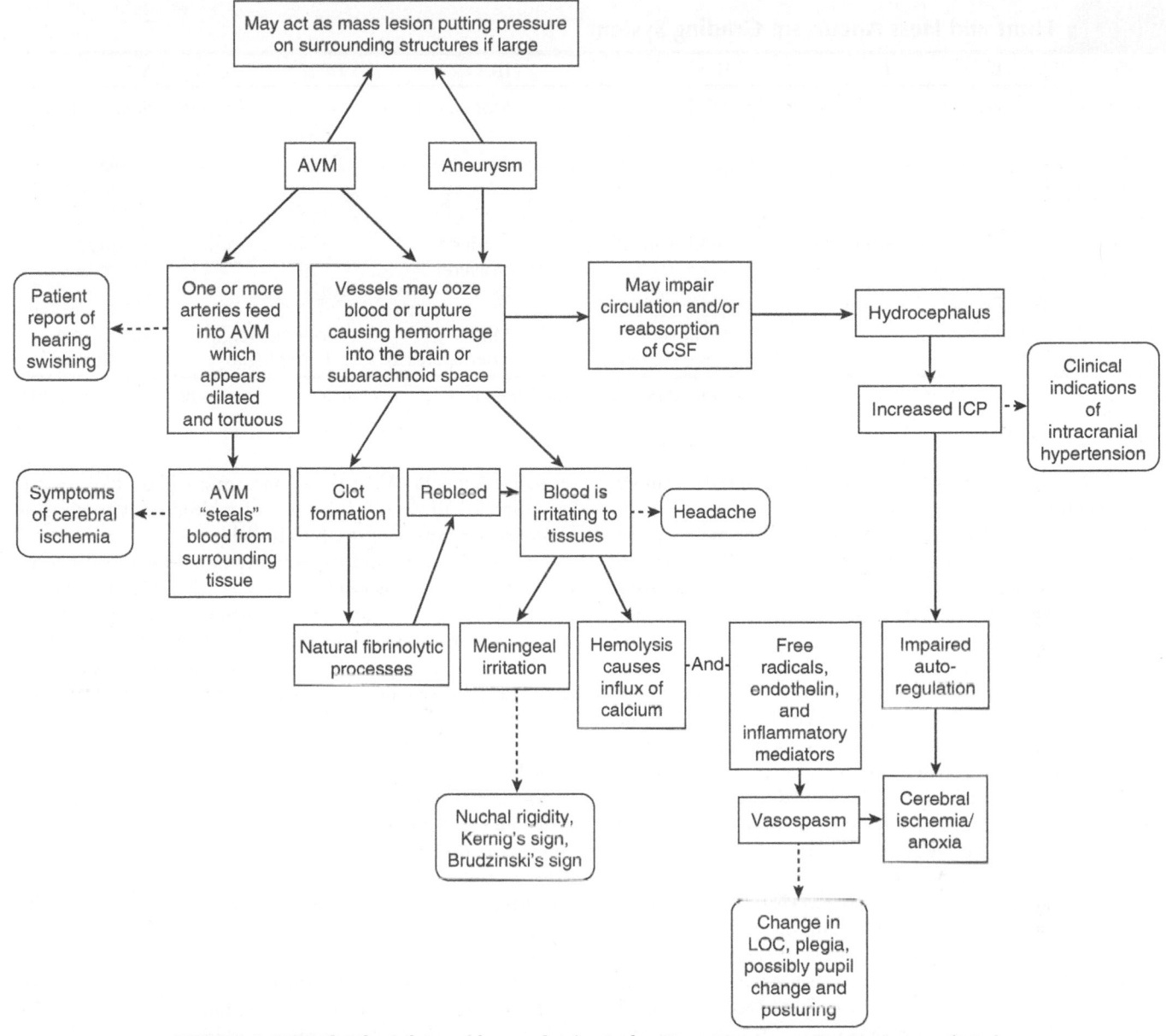

FIGURE 9-24 Pathophysiology of hemorrhagic stroke. Dotted lines connect pathology to clinical presentation. *AVM,* Arteriovenous malformation; *CSF,* cerebrospinal fluid; *ICP,* intracranial pressure; *LOC,* level of consciousness. (From Dennison, R. D. [2013]. *Pass CCRN!* [4th ed.]. St. Louis, MO: Elsevier.)

unless surgical treatment is performed. Sentinel headaches may be associated with nausea and vomiting, diplopia, and/or blurred vision.

Patients with hemorrhagic stroke commonly present with severe hypertension, as this is the most frequent cause of ICH. Focal neurologic deficits such as hemiplegia or ptosis may be present. The patient may demonstrate restlessness progressing to an altered LOC, positive Kernig and Brudzinski signs, hyperthermia, and seizures. The site and size of the hemorrhage determine the specific clinical presentation. The Hunt and Hess scale grade the severity of SAH (Table 9-20).

Laboratory findings may show a coagulation problem evident by an abnormal PT/aPTT. Hyponatremia may be present due to syndrome of inappropriate antidiuretic hormone (SIADH) or cerebral salt wasting. ECG changes that occur with SAH include flattened, peaked, or inverted T wave; presence of U wave; and/or QT prolongation. Torsades de pointes

dysrhythmia has been associated with SAH and other dysrhythmias are common. An echocardiography may show a decreased ejection fraction due to a "stunned" myocardium, but the mechanism is unknown.

A radiologic test that may be done is a noncontrast head CT, which can aid in diagnosing SAH, IPBH, IVH, and hydrocephalus. A CT is the initial imaging of choice. Perform an MRI to diagnose SAH if CT fails to show SAH but suspicion remains high. CT angiography locates the aneurysm, but the gold standard remains angiography. Three-dimensional angiography is optimal for identifying the size, location, and anatomy of the aneurysm. If the CT is nondiagnostic and there are no clinical indications of intracranial hypertension, a lumbar puncture may be performed. It is important to number the tubes. If only test tube number 1 is bloody, it is a traumatic tap. If all the test tubes are bloody, it is likely that the patient has an SAH. Elevation in protein will also be present in the CSF tapped.

TABLE 9-20	Hunt and Hess Aneurysm Grading System					
Grade	**0**	**I**	**II**	**III**	**IV**	**V**
Description	No bleed	Minimal bleed	Mild bleed	Moderate bleed	Moderate → severe bleed	Severe bleed
LOC	Alert	Alert	Awake	Drowsy	Stupor	Coma; moribund appearance
Headache	None	Minimal	Mild → moderate	Moderate → severe	Moderate → severe	Moderate → severe
Nuchal rigidity	None	Slight	Yes	Yes	Yes	Yes
Neurologic deficit	None	No	Minimal (e.g., cranial nerve palsy)	Mild (e.g., hemiparesis)	Moderate (e.g., hemiplegia)	Severe (e.g., posturing)

From Hunt, W. E., & Hess, R. M. (1968). Surgical risk as related to time of intervention in the repair of intracranial aneurysms. *J Neurosurg, 28*(1), 14-20. http://dx.doi.org/10.3171/jns.1968.28.1.0014.

An SAH of more than 5 days will yield a CSF that is dark amber or xanthochromatic.

The priority of collaborative management is to maintain the patient's airway, ventilation, and oxygenation. Administer oxygen as needed to maintain SpO_2 greater than or equal to 92% unless contraindicated. Prevent the occurrence of aspiration by positioning the patient on the side and provide for patient safety by maintaining suction equipment at the bedside. Patients without airway protective reflexes due to decreased LOC or focal deficits require endotracheal intubation. Sedation is necessary before intubation.

Monitor and treat the patient for clinical indications of increased ICP and elevated blood pressure. Control blood pressure, but the AHA does not recommend a specific level and drug choice. A desirable SBP is below 160 mm Hg. To achieve this level, administer labetalol (Normodyne) as prescribed as long as the patient's heart rate is above 60. Perform neurologic examinations frequently to assess for neurologic deterioration and report changes immediately.

Minimize the potential for rebleeding by instituting aneurysm precautions and assisting in patient preparation for surgical or interventional neuroradiology procedures. When the aneurysm ruptures again, rebleeding occurs. About half of all aneurysms that rebleed do so within the first 6 hours after the initial hemorrhage. Rebleeding is associated with a poor prognosis. The risk factors for rebleeding include:

- Large aneurysms
- High Hunt and Hess scale score
- Decreased LOC
- History of a sentinel headache
- SBP >160 mm Hg
- Long delay in surgical treatment

Aneurysm precautions are implemented to prevent bleeding episodes. Nursing care includes efforts to decrease environmental stimuli and providing a quiet, dimly lit private room. Enforce bed rest with the HOB elevated 15 to 30 degrees. Instruct visitors that the patient should not be upset in any way and limit the number of visitors and duration of visits. Patients demonstrating restlessness or extreme pain may require intubation to control the ICP. When providing nursing care, instruct the patient to avoid the Valsalva maneuver. Advise him or her to cough with the mouth open and exhale when turning in bed. Administer stool softeners as ordered and do not perform any rectal procedures (e.g., rectal temperature, enemas). Treat the presence of fever with acetaminophen. Administer antifibrinolytics, such as aminocaproic acid (Amicar) or tranexamic acid (Cyklokapron), as prescribed to decrease the risk of rebleeding if surgical or endovascular treatment needs to be delayed.

SAH due to aneurysm requires surgery or endovascular treatment to secure the aneurysm and prevent rebleeding. Prepare the patient for surgery or interventional neuroradiology procedures. The treatment options are surgical clipping or endovascular coiling. Research has failed to demonstrate which procedure, clipping or coiling, is better at definitively treating ruptured aneurysms. The effectiveness depends on the patient's acuity; comorbidities; age; treating facility; and location, size, and morphology of the aneurysm, but it is recommended to treat as early as possible after SAH.

Surgical clipping requires a craniotomy to access the aneurysm. An occlusion of the neck of the aneurysm with a surgical clip blocks the aneurysm from the healthy circulation. Endovascular coiling employs an angiographic technique to treat the aneurysm. Detachable coils are made of soft platinum. The device molds itself into the inner diameter of the aneurysmal dilation to cause thrombosis, forming a clot. Eventually the base of the aneurysm endothelializes and cuts itself off from the healthy circulation. Coils are placed in the aneurysm under fluoroscopy until the aneurysm is occluded and no coil mass protrudes into the healthy artery. Three-dimensional angiography is best suited for endovascular aneurysm treatment.

Provide postoperative care as described in the craniotomy section. Postoperative and postprocedural interventions include monitoring for clinical indications of intracranial hypertension or rebleeding. Prevent and monitor for clinical indications, and treat intracranial hypertension (see Intracranial Hypertension section). Monitor the patient for ischemia related to vasospasm following SAH due to aneurysm. Vasospasm is a pathologic narrowing of arteries after SAH. The result of vasospasm is delayed cerebral ischemia (DCI) and cerebral infarction. Recognize the factors that increase the risk of the occurrence and severity of vasospasm. Vasospasm is a risk until approximately 21 days after SAH. The peak incidence is at 7 to 10 days. Monitor for the following clinical indications of vasospasm:

- Presence or worsening of a headache
- Change in LOC or confusion
- Visual changes and/or pupil change
- Seizure
- New or worsening of focal neurologic deficit such as hemiparesis, aphasia

Evaluate and report the results of radiologic studies performed. Perform transcranial Doppler studies daily after SAH or more often if indicated. Note flow velocity trends. Intracranial blood flow velocities that are greater than 100 to 120 cm/second suggest a vasospasm. Velocities greater than 200 cm/second suggest severe vasospasm. Correlate the study results with the patient's clinical assessment. Perfusion CT or MRI can be used to diagnose ischemia associated with vasospasm. Angiography is the definitive study for diagnosis of a cerebral vasospasm. An angiography will show a narrowing of arterial vessels before clinical indications of vasospasm are noted.

Administer medication for vasospasm as ordered. Nimodipine (Nimotop) is a calcium channel blocker that is most commonly used to prevent vasospasm and reduce resultant ischemia and poor outcomes. The dosage is 60 mg orally every 4 hours for 21 days post-SAH. Adverse effects include hypotension, and if that occurs, reduce the dose to 30 mg every 2 hours.

Maintain euvolemia and monitor serial hemoglobin and hematocrit results. Administer transfusions to anemic patients as prescribed. Induce hypertension for SAH patients with vasospasm-induced DCI, unless the patient is already hypertensive or his or her cardiac status precludes it. Achieve induced hypertension with maintenance of euvolemia and medically induced hypertension. The AHA does not recommend specific therapies to induce hypertension.

If medical management fails, as evidenced by continued symptoms and arterial narrowing on imaging, the physician may perform transluminal cerebral balloon angioplasty via angiography to open the segment of the artery in vasospasm. In accessible arteries, the physician inserts a balloon-tipped catheter, but vessel rupture may occur, and once the balloon is deflated, vasospasms may return. An intraarterial injection of a vasodilating agent, such as verapamil or nicardipine, to relieve vasospasm of vessels too distal for the use of angioplasty is an option, but complications of this treatment include intracranial hypertension and brain ischemia.

Monitor the patient closely for complications. In addition to vasospasm and rebleeding, brain edema resulting in intracranial hypertension, hydrocephalus, fluid and electrolyte imbalance, hyperthermia, seizures, dysrhythmias, deep vein thrombosis, pulmonary embolism, and hyperglycemia are major complications. Monitor for and treat intracranial hypertension as previously discussed. Hydrocephalus may require a temporary diversion with an intraventricular catheter or lumbar drain and more long-term management through placement of a ventriculoperitoneal shunt. Diabetes insipidus (DI), syndrome of inappropriate antidiuretic hormone (SIADH), and cerebral salt wasting syndrome (CSW) cause fluid and electrolyte imbalance. Seizures may develop early or late. Administer prophylactic anticonvulsants prescribed. The increase in BP, increase in metabolic rate and oxygen demand, and compromised ventilation and oxygenation during seizure activity could be devastating. Monitor for dysrhythmias such as prolonged QT interval and torsades de pointes. Prevent deep vein thrombosis and pulmonary embolism with sequential compression devices on the lower extremities and ambulate the patient as soon as possible. Strictly control glycemic levels and patient temperature.

As with any health issue, patient education is a priority nursing intervention. Provide the patient and family education on nonpharmacologic therapies recommended. Discuss the importance of weight normalization and cessation of tobacco use and provide referrals to appropriate health care resources. Advise the patient to limit alcohol consumption to 1 to 2 alcoholic beverages daily. If alcohol is a problem for the patient, refer him or her to Alcoholics Anonymous or another appropriate resource. Stress the importance of regular aerobic exercise in moderation and provide information on stress reduction using complementary therapies such as relaxation, imagery, and biofeedback.

Advise the patient to be current with a pneumococcal vaccination and to get an annual flu vaccination. Teach the patient to recognize symptoms of recurrence and when to call the physician. Patient teaching on pharmacologic agents include those that control hypertension, hyperlipidemia, and diabetes mellitus.

9.12 Learning Activity

Your patient has had a hemorrhagic stroke. She has nuchal rigidity and decerebrate posturing. She does not vocalize at all and will not open her eyes even to pain. What is her Glasgow Coma Score? What grade bleed is this on the Hunt and Hess aneurysm grading scale?

GCS_____ Hunt and Hess _____

Answers to this activity can be found in the Answer Key.

9.13 Learning Activity

Identify the following factors as being associated with which complication of subarachnoid hemorrhage: vasospasm or rebleed.

	Vasospasm	Rebleed
Occurs either immediately after the bleed or between 7 and 10 days after the bleed		
Caused by calcium influx into the vessel		
Occurs any time after 3 days		
Treated by hyper-volemic hemodilu-tion and calcium channel blockers		
Caused by lysis of the protective clot		
Prevented by early clipping if the patient is stable enough		

Answers to this activity can be found in the Answer Key.

Symptoms Occurring during Transient Ischemic Attacks

Anterior Circulation	Posterior Circulation
• Ipsilateral monocular visual defect (amaurosis fugax) or homonymous hemianopsia	• Bilateral visual defect; diplopia
• Contralateral sensory or motor defects	• Bilateral sensory or motor defects
• Aphasia (if dominant hemisphere affected)	• Dysphagia
• Ipsilateral headache	• Occipital headache
• Seizure activity	• Vertigo, syncope (drop attack), dizziness, ataxia

Ischemic Stroke

Transient ischemic attack (TIA) is an episode of neurologic impairment attributed to focal cerebral ischemia (Box 9-2) that resolves within 24 hours (usually less than 1 to 2 hours) without lasting deficits. It may be described as injury to the zone of penumbra without central infarction.

Ischemic stroke is a sudden, severe disruption of the cerebral circulation caused by thrombus or embolus with a subsequent loss of neurologic function. Lacunar stroke is a special subset of thrombotic stroke seen almost exclusively in hypertensive patients and affects the deep white matter. A lacunar stroke is a small, perforating vessel thrombosis.

Thrombosis may be caused by:

• Intracranial arteriosclerosis
• Carotid artery atherosclerosis
• Hypertension
• Hypercoagulability (e.g., polycythemia)
• Mural thrombi from dysrhythmia (e.g., atrial fibrillation) or ventricular aneurysm
• Bacterial endocarditis
• Valvular heart disease
• Prosthetic cardiac valves
• Deep vein thrombosis with patent foramen ovale
• Air or fat embolism

Risk factors for ischemic stroke are similar to those for myocardial infarction, and include a family history of stroke; hypertension; smoking; diabetes mellitus; valvular heart disease; coronary artery disease; heart failure; hyperlipidemia; dysrhythmias, especially atrial fibrillation; hypercoagulability, such as is seen with polycythemia; obesity; and a sedentary lifestyle. Drugs, including alcohol, especially heavy episodic consumption; stimulants (e.g., cocaine, phenylpropanolamine); and oral contraceptives have been implicated.

The pathophysiology of ischemic stroke (Figure 9-25) is the result of vascular occlusion with resultant ischemia and infarction. The neurologic deficits correlate to the vessel or vessels occluded and the area or areas of the brain affected by the ischemia and infarction.

The patient may have history of TIA, hypertension, cardiovascular disease, arteriosclerosis, and/or diabetes mellitus. The onset of clinical manifestations is sudden. Thrombotic stroke frequently occurs during periods of rest. A decrease in cardiac output and blood pressure with less flow through an area of

critical stenosis is the most likely cause of the stroke. Embolic stroke is more likely to occur when the patient is active. The objective findings will vary, depending on the location of the vessel involved and the extent of injury (Box 9-3).

Laboratory findings may show elevated lipid levels. The serum glucose may be low or high. Although diabetes mellitus is a risk factor for ischemic stroke, physiologic stress makes hyperglycemia more likely in stroke even in nondiabetics. In addition, hypoglycemia may mimic stroke. A baseline clotting profile is desirable before administering fibrinolytics, but the only laboratory value required by the AHA before fibrinolytic therapy is glucose. An ECG may show dysrhythmias as a possible cause of cerebral emboli. A Holter monitor may identify a transient dysrhythmia. Echocardiography may show an intracardiac source for cerebral emboli, such as ventricular aneurysm or bacterial endocarditis.

Radiologic studies can provide important diagnostic information and guide treatment regimens. Doppler carotid studies may show carotid artery stenosis. A noncontrast CT may be normal early in ischemic stroke. A CT identifies the location and characteristics of subacute and old infarcts, the presence or absence of gross hemorrhage, and the presence or absence of a mass lesion. The CT may also show a distortion or shift of the ventricles. A CT is also performed 24 hours postfibrinolytic therapy to rule out ICH. Noncontrast CT is the only imaging needed before fibrinolysis, and should be completed within 45 minutes of arrival to the ED. The presence of early ischemic changes may be seen on an MRI when a CT still looks normal. A cerebral angiography identifies occlusion, stenosis, aneurysms, and hemorrhage of the arterial system. CT angiography and CT perfusion can demonstrate areas of arterial occlusion, penumbra, and infarct.

The priority of collaborative management for a patient with an ischemic stroke is to maintain airway, ventilation, and oxygenation. Administer oxygen as needed to maintain SpO_2 greater than or equal to 92% unless contraindicated. Prevent aspiration by positioning the patient on the side and have suctioning equipment available at the bedside. Patients without airway protective reflexes due to decreased LOC or focal deficit require endotracheal intubation. Sedation is necessary before intubation.

Utilize the NIHSS (see Table 9-11) to determine baseline neurologic assessment and to assess changes in neurologic status. Immediately report any changes in neurologic status. Correct the possible causes and contributing factors of ischemia. Assist in electrical or pharmacologic conversion of atrial fibrillation or administer anticoagulants to prevent mural thrombi. Management of ischemic stroke includes prompt assessment including CT scan to rule out hemorrhagic stroke and initiation of fibrinolytics if indicated (Figure 9-26).

Decrease the patient's BP s as indicated in acute ischemic stroke to maintain perfusion to the penumbra. If intravenous or intraarterial fibrinolysis or mechanical fibrinolysis is going to be used, BP should be treated if the SBP is >185 mm Hg or DBP is >110 mm Hg. During therapy, BP should be ≤180/105 mm Hg and monitored every 15 minutes during treatment and for 2 hours after. Then, monitor the BP every 30 minutes for 6 hours, and every 1 hour for 24 hours. If none of these therapies are being applied, treat the BP only if the SBP is >220 mm Hg or DBP is >120 mm Hg. Agents should be short acting and easily titratable. Administer IV infusions of labetalol (Normodyne), nicardipine (Cardene), nitroprusside

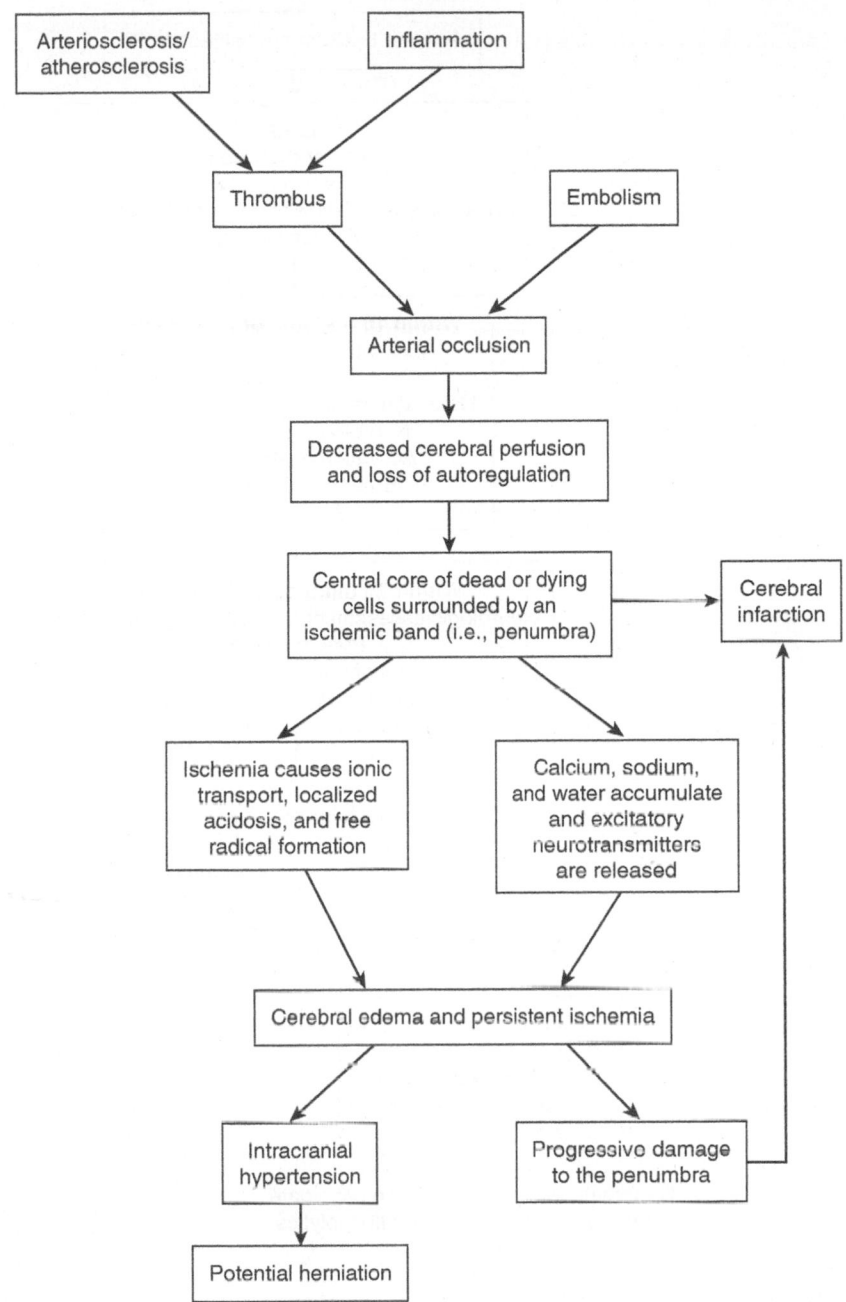

FIGURE 9-25 Pathophysiology of ischemic stroke. (From Dennison, R. D. [2013]. *Pass CCRN!* [4th ed.]. St. Louis, MO: Elsevier.)

Focal Neurologic Deficits Related to Location of Vascular Occlusion

Anterior Cerebral Artery
- Impaired gait
- Contralateral paralysis of leg and foot
- Personality changes: flat affect; inappropriate emotional responses
- Mental impairment

Middle Cerebral Artery
- Hemiplegia of face and arm on contralateral side
- Contralateral sensory deficit
- Aphasia if dominant hemisphere affected
- Homonymous hemianopsia
- Apraxia, agnosia, neglect if nondominant hemisphere affected
- Dysarthria
- Dysphagia

Posterior Cerebral Artery
- Cortical blindness
- Perseveration (abnormal persistence of a response)
- Homonymous hemianopsia

Vertebral or Basilar Artery
- Weakness of tongue
- Ipsilateral facial numbness and weakness
- Dizziness
- Nystagmus
- Dysarthria
- Dysphagia
- Ataxia
- "Locked-in" syndrome (quadriplegia and mutism with intact consciousness)

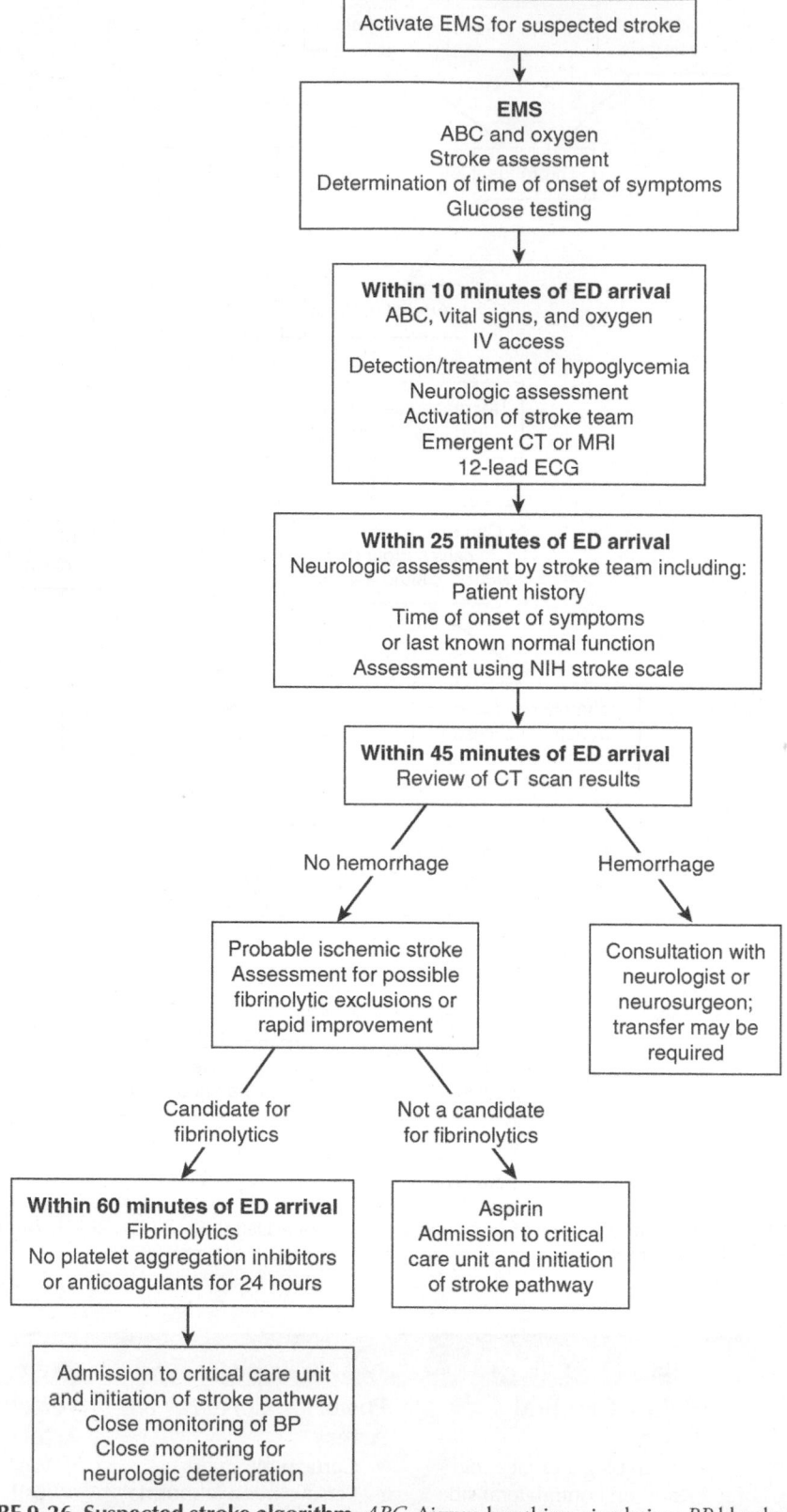

FIGURE 9-26 Suspected stroke algorithm. *ABC,* Airway, breathing, circulation; *BP,* blood pressure; *CT,* computed tomography; *ECG,* electrocardiogram; *EMS,* emergency management system; *IV,* intravenous; *MRI,* magnetic resonance imaging; *NIH,* National Institutes of Health. (From Dennison, R. D. [2013]. *Pass CCRN!* [4th ed.]. St. Louis, MO: Elsevier. Data from Jauch, E. C., Cucchiara, B., Adeoye, O., Meurer, W., Brice, J., Chan, Y. Y., et al. [2010]. Part 11: Adult stroke: 2010 American Heart Association guidelines for cardiopulmonary resuscitation and emergency cardiovascular care. *Circulation, 122* [18 suppl 3], S818-828.).

(Nipride), hydralazine (Apresoline), or enalaprilat (Vasotec) as prescribed.

The goal of fibrinolytic administration is the lysis of an occluding clot to restore blood flow to the compromised but viable penumbra. Administer IV fibrinolysis within 60 to 90 minutes of arrival in ED. There are seven "Ds" of stroke care:

- Detection of early indications and determination of time of onset. Time of onset is either witnessed or the time that last known normal neurologic function was noted.
- Dispatch of emergency medical care.
- Delivery of the patient to the nearest facility capable of implementing the most current stroke guidelines.
- Door and rapid triage in the emergency department.
- Data collected to aid in decision making: Baseline CT and/ or MRI to exclude intracranial hemorrhage and other risk factors for intracranial hemorrhage. Obtain history, complete physical examination, and evaluate laboratory values. The only data needed for fibrinolytics are time of onset, non-contrast head CT, and glucose.
- Decision to administer fibrinolytics is made by determining whether the patient meets the criteria for fibrinolytics and does not have contraindications (Box 9-4).
- Drug should be administered within 3 to 4.5 hours of the onset of symptoms depending on the patient.

Administer fibrinolytics (Table 3-23) via intravenous or intraarterial routes or by mechanical thrombectomy. Intravenous recombinant tissue plasminogen activator (rtPA)/alteplase (Activase) administration dosage is a total of 0.9 mg/kg, with a maximum dose of 90 mg. Of this total dose, give 10% over 1 minute. Administer the remaining 90% over 60 minutes. Alteplase is the only drug FDA approved for such use.

Administer intraarterial fibrinolysis via a catheter placed into the cerebral circulation under fluoroscopy. Alteplase is the most likely drug used in this method. The AHA guidelines recommend that if no improvement occurs in the patient after IV fibrinolytics, it is reasonable to attempt intraarterial fibrinolysis. Intraarterial fibrinolysis has a 6-hour window for initiating treatment after the patient last had normal neurologic function.

Mechanical thrombectomy is a procedure used alone or in conjunction with IV/IA alteplase. The physician places a clot retriever arterially via angiography to the site of the thrombus. There are two types of retrievers: a coil and a stent. The stent type has shown better outcomes. During the procedure, a suction type device removes debris.

Management of the patient after IV/IA fibrinolysis or mechanical thrombectomy includes the monitoring of vital signs and neurologic status. BP management is as previously described and depending on treatment. The patient should have a repeat CT at 24 hours postfibrinolytic therapy to evaluate for any hemorrhage.

Medications administered in addition to fibrinolytics include a 325-mg oral aspirin beginning 24 to 48 hours after presentation. Other antiplatelet agents in later stages of ischemic stroke (i.e., 24 hours and later) have not demonstrated any benefit. Do not administer anticoagulants or platelet aggregation inhibitors during the acute phase or for 24 hours after fibrinolytic.

Prepare the patient for surgical procedures as requested. The need for surgery is dependent on size and location of the clot and the patient's neurologic status and indicated for patients with signs of cerebrovascular insufficiency who have not had

---

BOX 9-4

Inclusion and Exclusion Criteria for the Use of Fibrinolytics in Ischemic Stroke

Inclusion
- Diagnosis of ischemic stroke causing measurable neurologic deficit
- Onset of symptoms less than 3-4.5 hours before initiation of infusion
- Age greater than or equal to 18 years

Exclusions if within 3 Hours of Onset of Symptoms
- Head trauma or previous stroke within previous 3 months
- Suspicion of intracerebral hemorrhage by symptoms or CT or history of previous hemorrhagic stroke
- Puncture of a noncompressible artery within the previous 7 days
- Uncontrolled hypertension (i.e., systolic BP greater than 185 mm Hg or diastolic BP greater than 110 mm Hg)
- Evidence of active bleeding on physical examination
- Significant risk of bleeding (e.g., platelet count 100,000/mm^3, use of anticoagulants with aPTT greater than upper limit of normal, INR greater than 1.7, or PT greater than 15 seconds)
- Serum glucose less than 50 mg/dL
- CT evidence of multilobar infarction (i.e., hypodensity greater than one-third of cerebral hemisphere)

Relative Exclusions if within 3 Hours of Onset of Symptoms
- Only minor neurologic deficit or rapidly resolving neurologic deficit
- Seizure at onset with postictal neurologic deficit
- Major surgery or serious trauma within 14 days
- Recent (i.e., within 21 days) gastrointestinal or genitourinary hemorrhage
- Recent (i.e., within 3 months) acute myocardial infarction

Additional Exclusions if Not within 3 Hours but within 4.5 Hours of Onset of Symptoms
- Age greater than 80 years
- Severe stroke (i.e., NIHSS greater than 25)
- On anticoagulant therapy regardless of INR
- History of both diabetes and prior ischemic stroke

---

a completed stroke. Surgeries accompanied by angiography include an endarterectomy or carotid artery angioplasty with or without stenting and/or an intraarterial mechanical embolectomy with or without fibrinolytic administration. Craniotomy may be required for evacuation of a clot in cases of subsequent hemorrhage. A decompressive hemicraniectomy is indicated in cases of severe cerebral edema, hemispheric shifting, and potential herniation.

Collaborative management after ischemic stroke includes preventing, monitoring for, and treating if needed clinical indications of intracranial hypertension (see Intracranial Hypertension section). This is particularly important during the first 72 hours. The patient should be in a specialized stroke unit with standardized order sets. A priority care focus is to maintain fluid and electrolyte balance and nutritional status. Administer IV fluids as prescribed and initiate early enteral feedings within 24 to 48 hours if the patient is unable to take food by mouth.

Assess the patient's gag and swallow reflexes before giving PO fluids. Use a bedside dysphagia screening tool routinely. Strict glycemic control is vital to improving patient outcome.

Initially, place the patient on bed rest to decrease metabolic requirements. Administer stool softeners to prevent constipation and straining as prescribed. Treat any episodes of hyperthermia with antipyretics, passive cooling (i.e., fans), and cooling blankets.

Assess the patient's ability to communicate and establish a means of communication. Consult a speech therapist as soon as possible in patients with aphasia. Protect the patient from injury by providing assistance during ambulation and be aware that the patient may have postural imbalance related to hemiparesis or hemiplegia. Orient the patient often and provide explanations of care. Confusion and disorientation as well as memory deficits may occur concomitantly with aphasia. Encourage family members to visit and teach them how to reorient the patient. Administer anticonvulsants as prescribed.

Prevent the hazards of immobility. Reposition the patient every 2 hours and perform passive ROM exercises every 2 hours. Teach the family to perform ROM exercises and have them demonstrate to ensure understanding. Assist with active ROM exercises when the patient is able to assist. Maximize the patient's independence in ADLs and allow the patient to do whatever he or she can. Provide emotional support and encourage participation in support groups. Provide instruction and counseling regarding lifestyle modification and need for pharmacologic therapy.

Monitor the patient for complications including persistent neurologic trauma, brain edema, and fluid and electrolyte imbalance. Monitor the patient for seizures, but only administer anticonvulsants with evidence of seizure activity, not prophylactically. Spastic paralysis may cause contractures; therefore, ROM, splints, and ongoing physical therapy can prevent this complication. Prevent deep vein thrombosis and pulmonary embolism with prophylactic subcutaneous low-molecular-weight heparin (LMWH) or unfractionated heparin and sequential compression devices. Other complications include pneumonia, urinary tract infection, urosepsis, and pressure ulcers.

Teach the patient about nonpharmacologic therapies that will be helpful in recovery. Instruct the patient regarding weight normalization and dietary modifications. Consult the dietician and provide information on a low-saturated- fat, 2- to 3-g sodium diet. If the patient has diabetes mellitus, consult the diabetes educator to discuss an ADA diet for control of blood glucose and reinforce teaching. Instruct the patient to limit alcohol consumption to 1 to 2 alcoholic beverages daily. If alcohol is a problem for the patient, refer him or her to Alcoholics Anonymous or another appropriate resource. Stress the importance of regular aerobic exercise in moderation and provide information on stress reduction using complementary therapies such as relaxation, imagery, and biofeedback.

Explain to the patient and family how to recognize symptoms of TIA or stroke and when to call the physician. Teach the patient and family about pharmacologic agents given in the hospital and that will continue at home. These include medications that control hypertension, hyperlipidemia, and diabetes mellitus. Instruct the patient and family on other medications prescribed for the patient, such as platelet aggregation inhibitors and/or anticoagulants. Recommend a yearly flu vaccine and ask if the patient has ever received a pneumococcal vaccination. If he or she has not, or if it has been longer than 5 years, recommend that he or she receive it, preferably before leaving the hospital.

9.14   Learning Activity

List five ways that the use of fibrinolytics for ischemic stroke is different from the use of fibrinolytics for myocardial infarction.

1. _____
2. _____
3. _____
4. _____
5. _____

Answers to this activity can be found in the Answer Key.

Status Epilepticus

A seizure is a sudden, paroxysmal episode of exaggerated activity or abnormal behavior caused by excessive discharge of cerebral neurons. Seizures are classified (Table 9-21) according to clinical presentation features and duration.

Status epilepticus is seizure activity of 30 minutes or more in duration. This condition results from a single seizure or a series of seizures in which there is no return of consciousness between seizures. A more current definition is seizure activity lasting at least 10 minutes because treatment for status epilepticus is initiated within 10 minutes, preventing the continuation of seizure activity for 30 minutes.

Seizures may occur in patients with a preexisting history of seizure disorder due to withdrawal from anticonvulsant medications. Acute alcohol withdrawal and acute withdrawal from chronically used drugs that have sedative or depressant effects, such as barbiturates, place a patient at risk for seizure. Any acute condition that lowers the seizure threshold can induce a seizure in patients with a history of seizure.

Patients with no prior history of seizure disorder may develop seizures from brain trauma and brain tumors, and ischemic or hemorrhagic stroke. CNS infections, such as meningitis, encephalitis, and abscess, and all types of encephalopathy can cause seizure. Seizure can occur from hypoglycemia and electrolyte imbalances, including hyponatremia, hypocalcemia, and hypomagnesemia. Drug or alcohol withdrawal can cause a seizure in a patient with no prior history of seizure. Drug toxicity, including lidocaine, meperidine, theophylline, salicylates, cyclic antidepressants, and cocaine, places a patient at risk for seizure. Lastly, sepsis may also cause seizure.

The pathophysiology of prolonged generalized seizures (Figure 9-27) relates to increased cerebral blood flow, SNS stimulation, compromise of the patient's airway and ventilation, and clonic-tonic activity. The results of these pathophysiologic events have neurologic, cardiac, respiratory, and renal consequences.

The patient's history may include a precipitating event or condition. The patient or family may report a history of seizure. They may also report a history of noncompliance in taking anticonvulsant drugs. There may also be a history of chronic drug or alcohol use. Seizure activity produces an alteration in LOC, as well as tonic and/or clonic body movements. The patient may be incontinent of urine or stool. There may be involuntary motor activities such as lip smacking, swallowing, or chewing.

Several laboratory findings may be abnormal. Serum chemistry analysis may show an increase in blood urea nitrogen (BUN) if the patient's seizure was a result of uremia or hyperosmolality, and electrolytes may show hyperkalemia. Increased liver function studies occur in patients with hepatic failure. Toxicology

TABLE 9-21 Types of Seizures

Type	Features	Duration
Generalized: Loss of Consciousness		
Absence (petit mal)	• Momentary loss of consciousness • Blank stare, cessation of activity • Eye blinking, lip smacking may occur • May lose muscle tone	Seconds
Tonic-clonic (grand mal)	• May be preceded by an aura and a cry from forced expiration • Loss of consciousness • Symmetric tonic-clonic extremity movements • May experience apnea with cyanosis until tonic phase ends • May bite tongue, may be incontinent • Postictal fatigue, muscle soreness, confusion, lethargy, and/or headache	3-5 minutes
Myoclonic	• Short, abrupt muscle contractions of arms, legs, and torso • Contractions may be symmetric or asymmetric	Seconds
Clonic	• Muscle contraction and relaxation but slower than with myoclonic seizure	Several minutes
Tonic	• Abrupt increase in muscle tone of torso and face • Flexion of arms; extension of legs	Seconds
Atonic	• Abrupt loss of muscle tone • May cause falling and injuries related to fall	Seconds
Partial: Focal at Onset but May Evolve into a Generalized Seizure		
Simple partial	• Consciousness not impaired • Abnormal unilateral movement of arm, leg, or both • Patient may sense abnormal smell, sound, or sensation, such as numbness, tingling, or burning • Tachycardia or bradycardia, tachypnea, skin flushing, epigastric discomfort	Seconds to minutes
Complex partial	• Loss of consciousness but eyes may be open • Lip smacking, chewing, picking at clothing • Mumbling, speaking in repetitive phrases • Posturing or jerking movements • Postictal confusion, amnesia common	Minutes

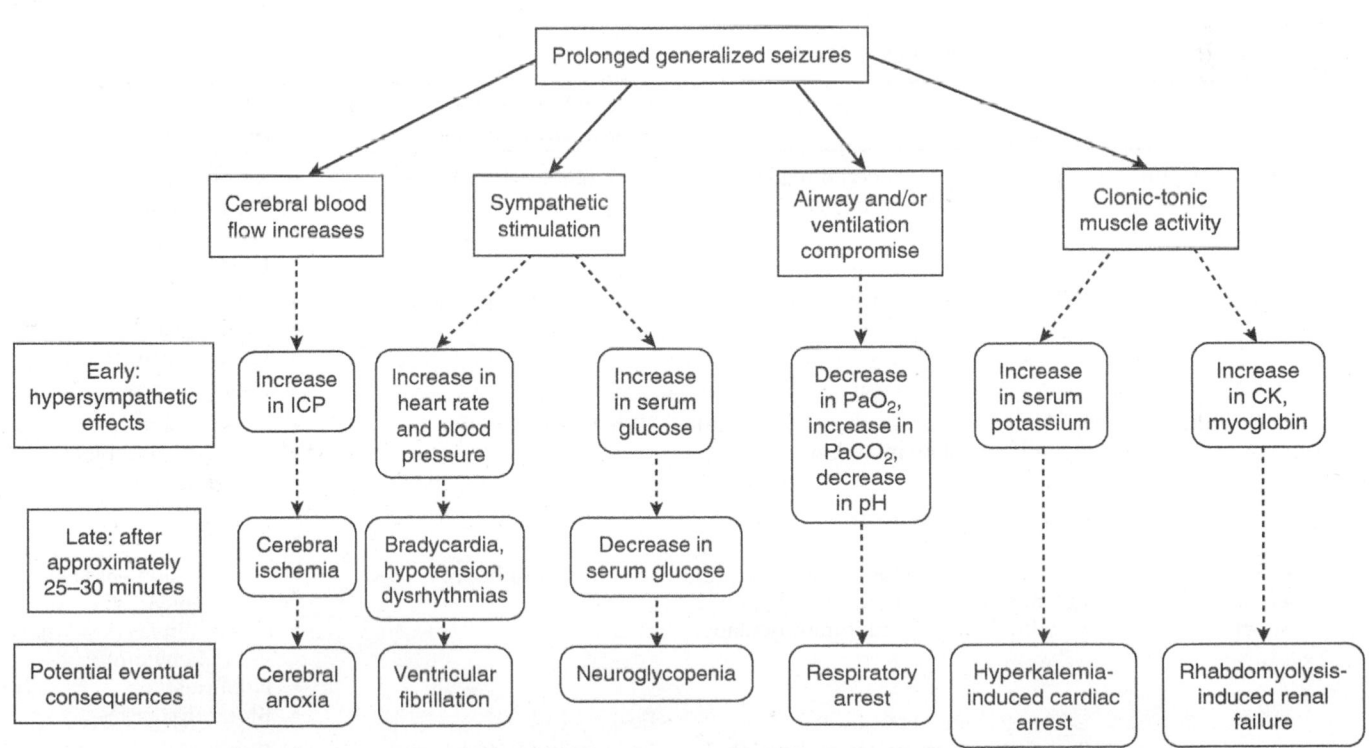

FIGURE 9-27 Pathophysiology of status epilepticus. Dotted lines connect pathology to clinical presentation. *CK,* Creatine kinase; *ICP,* intracranial pressure; *PaCO$_2$,* partial pressure of carbon dioxide in arterial blood; *PaO$_2$,* partial pressure of oxygen in arterial blood. (From Dennison, R. D. [2013]. *Pass CCRN!* [4th ed.]. St. Louis, MO: Elsevier.)

screens for drug and alcohol levels may indicate an intake at a level that places the patient at risk for seizure. Anticonvulsant drug levels may be subtherapeutic, which may indicate an issue of noncompliance. Serum glucose increases early in the seizure, but it may also decrease late in the seizure. Lactic acid and creatinine kinase (CK) levels may be increased. Arterial blood gases may show hypercapnia and hypoxemia. The urinalysis may indicate that myoglobinuria is present. Results of a lumbar puncture may show an infection such as meningitis to be the cause.

Radiologic findings in a skull x-ray may show the cause of the seizure. CT, MRI, or MRA may indicate the presence of pathologic conditions, such as mass lesions. An EEG will show the seizure activity. An EEG at rests may detect seizure activity, but the patient may also need a provocation EEG to detect abnormalities. In a provocation EEG, the patient is sleep deprived and stimulated with lights and noise to induce seizure activity.

The priority care focus for a patient having a seizure is to establish and maintain the airway and adequate ventilation. Insert an artificial airway if ventilation and oxygenation are inadequate. Utilize a nasopharyngeal airway or nasotracheal intubation if the mouth is not accessible. Do not try to force the mouth open. Monitor the patient's ABGs and pulse oximetry. Maintain oxygenation with the administration of oxygen as needed to maintain SpO_2 greater than or equal to 92% unless contraindicated. Prevent aspiration by positioning the patient on his or her side. Do not just turn the head to the side. Have suction equipment available at the bedside and suction as indicated. The patient may require mechanical ventilation for prolonged hypoventilation.

Protect the patient from injury and prevent complications during seizure. Call for help and do not leave the patient. Loosen constrictive clothing and remove the pillow from under the head. Do not restrain the patient, but gentle guiding of extremities is acceptable. Pad the side rails with blankets or pillows and assess the patient for injury. Remain aware of the surroundings and maintain the patient's privacy.

Assess for and eliminate causes or contributing factors for seizures. Analyze the serum for glucose, sodium, potassium, calcium, phosphorus, magnesium, and BUN. Screen for drugs, such as barbiturates, tricyclic antidepressants, and alcohol. Obtain anticonvulsant drug levels. Obtain blood cultures if the patient has hyperthermia. Correct the contributing factors that lower seizure threshold, such as hypoxemia, acid-base imbalance, electrolyte imbalance, hyperthermia, or hypermetabolism.

Stop seizure activity with medication. Initiate an IV and administer 100 mg thiamine and 50 mL of $D_{50}W$ if alcohol ingestion or hypoglycemia is suspected. Administer thiamine with dextrose to prevent Wernicke encephalopathy, especially if the patient has chronic malnutrition. Administer benzodiazepine or other drugs (Table 9-22) if seizures persist after dextrose and thiamine administration.

Administer benzodiazepines to stop a seizure already in progress. Lorazepam (Ativan) is usually the drug of choice; however, diazepam (Valium) may also be given. Other anticonvulsant medications (Table 9-23) can be administered after benzodiazepine to prevent recurrence. The newer maintenance medications have fewer side effects and are prescribed based on the drugs' narrow- or broad-spectrum effects. Some of the more commonly used newer agents include levetiracetam (Keppra), clonazepam (Klonopin), valproic acid (Depakene), and divalproex sodium (Depakote). Older drugs such as phenytoin (Dilantin), fosphenytoin (Cerebyx), or phenobarbital may also be prescribed. Agents given for refractory status epilepticus include pentobarbital (Nembutal), midazolam (Versed), and propofol (Diprivan). Reduce the IV medication infusion rate as prescribed after at least 12 hours without seizures. Monitor patients receiving anticonvulsant medications closely for

TABLE 9-22 **Intravenous Anticonvulsant Drugs**

Drug	IV Dosage	Time to Stop Seizure/Duration of Anticonvulsant Effect	Adverse Effects
Lorazepam (Ativan)	0.1 mg/kg (not to exceed 8 mg/kg) at a rate no faster than 2 mg/min	6-10 minutes/12-24 hours	• Respiratory depression • Tachycardia • Hypotension • Dysrhythmias
Diazepam (Valium)	0.15-0.25 mg/kg at a rate of no faster than 5 mg/min	1-3 minutes/30 minutes	• Respiratory depression • Tachycardia • Hypotension • Dysrhythmias
Phenytoin sodium (Dilantin)	10-20 mg/kg at a rate no faster than 50 mg/min; must be mixed in saline	30 minutes/24 hours	• Hypotension • Dysrhythmias; blocks • Hepatitis • Nephritis • Blood dyscrasias
Fosphenytoin (Cerebyx)	15-20 mg/kg phenytoin equivalent (PE) at a rate no faster than 150 mg/min; may be administered intramuscularly	15 minutes/24 hours	• Hypotension (less risk than phenytoin) • Dysrhythmias (less risk than phenytoin) • Nephritis • Blood dyscrasias
Phenobarbital (Phenobarbital sodium, Luminal)	20 mg/kg at a rate no faster than 50 mg/min (not actively seizing) or 100 mg/min (actively seizing)	20-30 minutes/48 hours	• Respiratory depression • Hypotension • Angioedema • Thrombophlebitis

complications related to medications. Assess the patient for hypotension, which is an adverse reaction of many of the anticonvulsant drugs. Administer fluids as prescribed and assess effectiveness. Monitor for respiratory depression, particularly if the patient has received benzodiazepines. Ensure that emergency equipment is nearby. If respiratory depression occurs, ventilation with a manual resuscitation bag and mask may be required. Endotracheal intubation may also be required.

Monitor and document the duration of the seizure activity, the patient's LOC, any medications given, and the response. Document the presence or absence of an aura. If an aura was present, the nature of the aura, such as visual, auditory, smell, or taste, should be described. Also, document the presence or absence of a cry. Document the onset of the seizure, noting the site of initial body movements, deviation of the head and/or eyes, chewing and salivation, posture of the body, and sensory changes. During the tonic and clonic phases, note the movement of the body during the progression. Also, note skin color, airway patency, pupillary eye direction, incontinence, and duration of each phase. Document the duration and behavior of the relaxation phase. During the postictal phase, note its duration, the patient's general behavior and memory of events, orientation, pupillary changes, headache, aphasia, and any injuries. Document the duration from aura to relaxation, and the drugs administered. Clear and concise documentation of the seizure event is a major advantage in the differentiation of a seizure disorder.

Postseizure collaborative management includes assessing the patient's condition closely and monitoring to prevent complications. The HOB should be elevated to 30 degrees to prevent aspiration. If indicated, insert a nasogastric tube to prevent vomiting and aspiration. Monitor the cardiac rate and rhythm and BP. Make sure that cardiovascular emergent drugs are available. Assess the patient's neurologic status frequently. Provide reassurance and comfort during the postictal period. Reassure and reorient the patient as he or she awakens and provide privacy and a calm environment. Discretely clean the patient if he or she was incontinent and allow the patient to sleep. Monitor serum drug concentrations and adjust drug dosages as prescribed to maintain optimal levels. Maintain fluid and electrolyte balance. Assess laboratory findings such as electrolytes, including calcium and magnesium, serum CK to detect rhabdomyolysis, and renal and hepatic function. Document the diagnostic findings, which may include serum electrolytes and diagnostic imaging such as CT, MRI, and EEG. Prepare the patient for surgical procedures that may be required for removal of tumor, hematoma, or abscess that may have caused the seizure.

Monitor the patient for complications and assess for injury that may have occurred during the seizure. Also, assess for aspiration or signs and symptoms of acute respiratory failure. Analyze acid-base imbalance, which can be either respiratory or metabolic acidosis. Monitor the patient's serum glucose, as hypoglycemia is common after a seizure because of the energy expended. If the patient is hypoglycemic, administer parenteral dextrose as required. The hypermetabolic state caused by seizure may damage cells; therefore, monitor for hyperkalemia and elevated CK and note any change in urine color. Cola-colored urine, in conjunction with elevated potassium and CK, may indicate myoglobinuria. Myoglobinuria can lead to rhabdomyolysis and renal failure. Administer fluids, mannitol, and sodium bicarbonate as prescribed. Monitor the patient for hyperthermia and treat with antipyretics and/or a hypothermia blanket for elevated temperatures. Continually monitor and assess the patient for residual neurologic deficits.

TABLE 9-23 Medications Used for Seizures

Classification	Medication
AMPA receptor antagonist	Perampanel (Fycompa)
Calcium channel modulator	Levetiracetam (Keppra, Keppra XL)
Carbonic anhydrase inhibitor	Acetazolamide (Diamox)
Carboxamide	Carbamazepine (Tegretol) Eslicarbazepine (Aptiom) Oxcarbazepine (Trileptal) Rufinamide (Banzel)
GABA analog	Gabapentin (Neurontin) Pregabalin (Lyrica) Progabide (Gabrene) Vigabatrin (Sabril)
GABA reuptake inhibitor	Tiagabine (Gabitril)
K-channel opener	Ezogabine/Retigabine (Potiga)
NMDA receptor blocker	Felbamate (Felbatol) Sodium Channel Modulators Lacosamide (Vimpat) Lamotrigine (Lamictal) Phenytoin (Dilantin)
Succinimide	Ethosuximide (Zarontin) Methsuximide (Celontin)
Sulfamate-substitute monosaccharide	Topiramate (Topamax, Topamax ER, Qudexy XR)
Sulfonamide	Zonisamide (Zonegran)
Valproic acid	Divalproex Sodium (Depakote) Valproic Acid (Depakene)
Barbiturate	Phenobarbital Primidone (Mysoline)
Benzodiazepine	Clobazam (Onfi) Clonazepam (Klonopin, Epitril, Rivotril) Diazepam (Valium, Diastat) Lorazepam (Ativan)

9.15 Learning Activity

List five observations to make and five interventions to perform during a seizure.

Observations to Make	Interventions

Answers to this activity can be found in the Answer Key.

9.16   Learning Activity

List two adverse effects of each of the following anticonvulsive medications that the nurse should monitor.

Drug	Adverse Effects
Lorazepam (Ativan)	
Diazepam (Valium)	
Phenytoin sodium (Dilantin)	
Fosphenytoin (Cerebyx)	
Phenobarbital (Phenobarbital sodium, Luminal)	

Answers to this activity can be found in the Answer Key.

9.17   Synthesis Learning Activity: Clinical Vignette

A 68-year-old man arrives in the ED with new onset of right-sided weakness and aphasia. He has a history of hypertension, hyperlipidemia, and type 2 diabetes mellitus. His medications include lisinopril (Prinivil) 30 mg PO daily in the AM, metformin hydrochloride extended release (Glucophage XR) 1500 mg PO daily in the AM, and atorvastatin (Lipitor) 80 mg daily in the PM. His wife reports that the patient's father died of a stroke when he was 63 years of age, and that there is a family history of hypertension and diabetes. A Stroke Alert is called.

1. Which is the correct order for treatment of stroke?
   a. Determination of time of onset of symptoms, neurologic assessment, emergent CT scan, fibrinolytics if indicated
   b. Determination of time of onset of symptoms, emergent CT scan, neurologic assessment, fibrinolytics if indicated
   c. Glucose testing, activation of stroke team, neurology consult, fibrinolytics if indicated
   d. Glucose testing; activation of stroke team; emergent CT scan; 325 mg aspirin, chewed

CT scan indicates an ischemic stroke. Fibrinolytic therapy is initiated intravenously. Within 60 minutes of initiation, the patient's symptoms improve. He is admitted to the progressive care unit. Prescriptions include:
   • Neurologic assessment with vital signs every 2 hours and as indicated
   • Speech and language consult to evaluate swallowing
   • NPO until speech therapist clears patient for swallowing, then PO medications may be administered
   • Lisinopril (Prinivil) 30 mg PO daily in the AM
   • Metformin hydrochloride extended release (Glucophage XR) 1500 mg PO daily in the AM
   • Pantoprazole sodium (Protonix) 40 mg PO in the AM
   • Atorvastatin (Lipitor) 80 mg PO daily in the PM
   • Point-of-care glucose testing three times/day before meals
   • Consult physical therapy for rehabilitation assessment
   • Out of bed with assistance after rehab consult
   • Sequential compression device applied to lower legs when in bed
   • Notify the physician of worsening of signs/symptoms

2. During the first assessment, the nurse notes that there is mild drift of the right arm and leg, and mild aphasia. The nurse should:
   a. Document the assessment
   b. Notify the physician of worsening signs/symptoms
   c. Cancel the rehabilitation consult
   d. Repeat the assessment in 15 minutes

3. Four hours after the initial neurologic assessment, the patient demonstrates improved strength in the right arm and leg, although he is still weaker on the right. Aphasia appears to be resolved. The speech and language consultant arrives and performs a dysphagia test. The patient is cleared to take medication and have a soft diet. That evening, the nurse begins teaching with the patient and his wife. Which of the following should the nurse teach first?
   a. Information about fibrinolytics
   b. Information on new drugs he is receiving
   c. Importance of monitoring glucose
   d. Signs and symptoms of stroke

Answers to this activity can be found in the Answer Key.

9.18   Learning Activity

Match the following sign or symptom associated with the neurologic condition.

_____ 1. Brainstem lesion
_____ 2. Subarachnoid hemorrhage
_____ 3. Status epilepticus
_____ 4. Dural tear
_____ 5. Postcraniotomy
_____ 6. Upper motor neuron lesion
_____ 7. Meningeal irritation
_____ 8. Intracranial hypertension
_____ 9. Hydrocephalus

a. Kernig sign
b. Change in LOC, pupillary changes, respiratory pattern changes, Cushing triad
c. Periorbital edema
d. Increased lumbar pressure (LP), vomiting
e. Rhinorrhea
f. "Worst headache of my life"
g. Myoglobinuria
h. Absence of doll eyes (i.e., oculocephalic reflex)
i. Babinski reflex

Answers to this activity can be found in the Answer Key.

9.19   Synthesis Learning Activity: Crossword Puzzle

Complete the following crossword puzzle dealing with neurologic conditions and treatment.

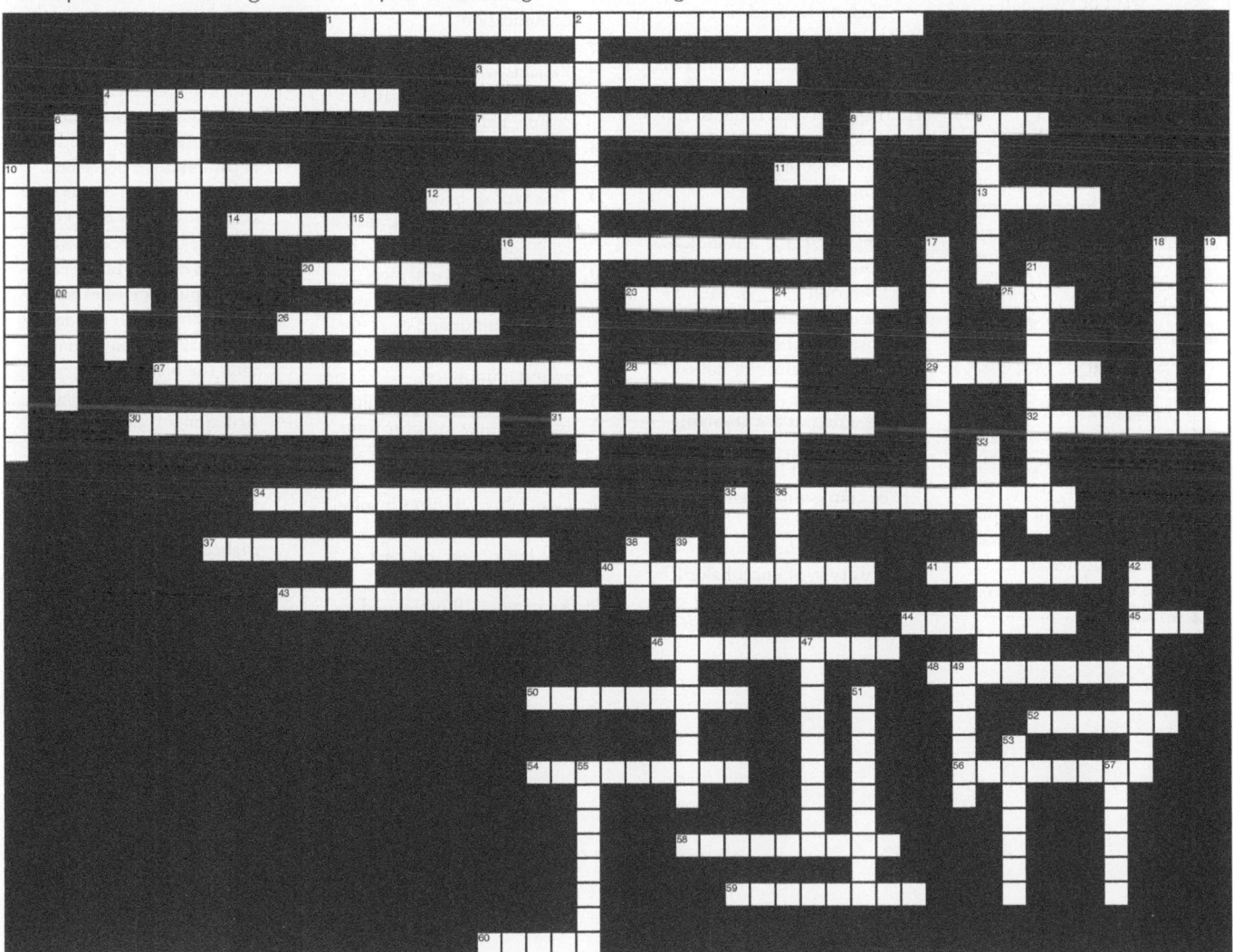

Answers to this activity can be found in the Answer Key.

ACROSS

1. Common cause of secondary brain injury (2 words)
3. Stroke causes _____ paresis or plegia
4. Brainstem lesions may cause this type of eye movement
7. Head of bed should be flat after this type of craniotomy
8. The primary symptom of hemorrhage from a cerebral aneurysm is sudden, severe _____
10. A major risk factor for stroke
11. A _____ hole is drilled into the cranium to allow access for aspiration of a clot or to place an intracranial catheter for monitoring ICP
12. Used to reduce peripheral fever
13. The first sign of uncal herniation is a dilated, sluggish, or nonreactive _____
14. _____ triad of vital sign changes is a late sign of intracranial hypertension
16. This complication may occur after craniotomy, traumatic brain injury, hemorrhagic stroke, or meningitis
20. This type of skull fracture of the temporal bone may tear the middle meningeal artery and cause epidural hematoma
22. State of unconsciousness in which the patient cannot be awakened
23. This type of stroke is caused by aneurysm or arteriovenous malformation
25. The first sign of tentorial herniation is a change in _____ (abbrev.)
26. This type of cerebral edema is caused by hyponatremia, ischemia, or hypoxia
27. Used to reduce central fever (2 words)

28. The _____ in the CSF is reduced in bacterial meningitis
29. CSF is produced in capillary networks called _____ plexuses
30. This type of craniotomy is often used for removal of the pituitary gland
31. This type of hydrocephalus may be caused by SAH or meningitis
32. This type of hematoma is caused by an arterial bleed and causes rapid deterioration
34. HOB should be elevated after this type of craniotomy
36. Rupture of a cerebral aneurysm is sometimes referred to as a _____ hemorrhage because the blood vessels are located in this space
37. This type of drug is most likely to be used first to control seizures
40. Uncal herniation causes dilation of the _____ pupil
41. Tight cervical collar or tracheostomy ties may increase ICP by compressing these veins
43. Monitor patients with status epilepticus for this indication of rhabdomyolysis
44. Elevation _____ in the CSF occurs in meningitis
45. Focal cerebral ischemia that resolves within 24 hours (abbrev.)
46. Opening of the cranium
48. Diabetes _____ is a complication of head trauma or craniotomy that causes polyuria
50. Bruise on the brain
52. This type of encephalopathy is caused most often by out-of-hospital cardiac arrest

54. This type of cerebral edema is caused by breakdown of the blood-brain barrier from trauma, tumor, abscess, or hemorrhage
56. An abnormal weakness of an artery; most commonly occurs in the circle of Willis
58. Herniation with a downward shift of the brain causing the brainstem to be pushed through the foramen magnum
59. This type of stroke is caused by thrombus or embolism
60. A side-to-side herniation

DOWN

2. This dysrhythmia is a common cause of ischemic stroke (2 words)
4. Prolonged QT interval frequently seen in SAH may cause this serious cardiac complication
5. Repair of the cranium
6. Patients with status epilepticus may have _____ and require parenteral dextrose
8. Shifting of the brain within or out of the cranium
9. This type of partial seizure is associated with loss of consciousness
10. Central _____ is associated with injury to the hypothalamus and does not respond to antipyretics such as acetaminophen
15. This type of hydrocephalus is most likely to occur from trauma, including surgical trauma
17. Generalized seizures involve these phases (2 words)
18. The most common type of cerebral aneurysm
19. An osmotic diuretic used for increased ICP

21. This hypothesis states that the cranium is an inexpansible vault and if one of the three intracranial volumes increases, one of the other components must decrease or there will be a resultant increase in ICP
24. This type of encephalopathy is caused by severe elevation of BP
33. Inflammation of the meninges
35. A subjective sensation that often precedes a seizure
38. Autoregulation fails if the _____ is <50 mm Hg or >150 mm Hg (abbrev.)
39. This drug is frequently used to prevent/treat vasospasm (generic)
42. Patients with status epilepticus have elevated CK and _____
47. This type of herniation occurs with bilateral processes such as cerebral edema; also called central herniation
49. This type of rigidity occurs with meningeal irritation from infection or blood
51. A complication of cerebral aneurysm, which occurs most commonly about 3 to 5 days after the bleed; treated with calcium channel blockers
53. A complication of cerebral aneurysm, which frequently occurs about 7 to 10 days after the bleed
55. This type of intracranial hematoma is caused by a venous bleed and causes symptoms that develop over several days
57. This electrolyte is affected by diabetes insipidus, syndrome of inappropriate ADH, and cerebral salt wasting syndrome

Multisystem

SHOCK

Shock is a life-threatening clinical syndrome of insufficient perfusion of cells and vital organs that results in tissue hypoxia. In the shock state, perfusion is inadequate to sustain life, and this inadequate perfusion results in cellular, metabolic, and hemodynamic derangements. It is important to note that shock is not determined by the BP level, and the patient may not be significantly hypotensive, especially early in a shock state. Failure to detect and treat shock promptly can lead to multiple organ dysfunction syndrome (MODS) and death. Early detection and treatment can dramatically affect mortality.

Shock is categorized as hypovolemic, cardiogenic, or distributive. Hypovolemic shock is due to inadequate intravascular volume. Cardiogenic shock is due to pump failure. Obstructive shock is a type of cardiogenic shock caused by physical obstruction of blood circulation and inadequate blood oxygenation. The mechanical impediment prevents diastolic filling of the ventricles, leading to a significant fall in cardiac index. Causes of obstructive shock are tension pneumothorax, cardiac tamponade, massive pulmonary thromboembolism, heart valve stenosis, cardiac tumor, pulmonary hypertension, and coarctation of the aorta. Distributive shock, also called vasogenic shock, results from excessive vasodilation, relative hypovolemia, and the impaired distribution of blood flow. Septic shock, which carries significant mortality, is the most common form of distributive shock. Septic shock results from massive vasodilation caused by the release of mediators of the inflammatory process in response to overwhelming infection. Anaphylactic shock is another common form of distributive shock and results from massive vasodilation caused by release of histamine in response to a severe allergic reaction from drugs or toxins, including insect bites, transfusion reactions, and heavy metal poisoning. Distributive neurogenic shock due to neurologic injury is the result of massive vasodilation caused by suppression of the sympathetic nervous system.

Systemic inflammatory response syndrome (SIRS) is the systemic response to a variety of insults that begin as local inflammation. The scope of SIRS is more global than local inflammation. Consider the vasodilation and increased capillary permeability of local inflammation as a normal healing process and the more global vasodilation and increased capillary permeability of SIRS as being life threatening. The clinical suspicion and established criteria (Table 10-1) of SIRS, sepsis, shock, and multisystem organ dysfunction syndrome

(MODS) by an experienced clinician is also important. MODS is a clinical syndrome (Box 10-1) in which progressive and potentially irreversible physiologic dysfunction of two or more organs or organ systems is induced by a primary or secondary injury.

Shock is initiated by a decreased tissue oxygenation caused by a decrease in circulating blood volume (i.e., hypovolemic), decrease in ability of the heart to pump blood (i.e., cardiogenic), and/or a decrease in vascular tone (i.e., distributive). There are four stages of shock: initial, compensatory, progressive, and refractory. In the initial stage, subclinical hypoperfusion caused by inadequate delivery and/or inadequate extraction of oxygen is present. Although the progressive care unit nurse does not perform hemodynamic monitoring and measurement, astute physical assessment can detect early subtle changes in patient condition and an understanding of the hemodynamic principles of cardiac output (CO) and cardiac index (CI) is required to provide quality, safe care. In early shock, CO/CI are decreased but there are no clinical indications of hypoperfusion; however, this decrease in CO/CI is detectable with good assessment skills to note changes in patient condition and/or non invasive hemodynamic monitoring. In the compensatory stage (Figure 10-1), the neuroendocrine systems attempt to

TABLE 10-1	Differentiation Criteria of SIRS, Early Sepsis, Late/Severe Sepsis, Shock, and MODS
Condition	**Criteria**
SIRS	Temperature >38° C (100.4° F) or < 36° C (96.8° F) Heart rate >90 Respiratory rate >20 or $Paco_2$ <32 mm Hg WBC >12,000/mm^3, <4000/mm^3, or >10% bands
Sepsis	Suspected or present source of infection with SIRS
Severe sepsis	Lactic acidosis, SBP <90 mm Hg or SBP drop ≥40 mm Hg of normal
Septic shock	Severe sepsis with hypotension, despite adequate fluid resuscitation
MODS	Evidence of dysfuntion of two or more organ systems

Clinical Findings in MODS

Heart
- Myocardial depression and hypotension
- Life-threatening dysrhythmias
- Myocardial ischemia/infarction
- Chest pain
- ECG indicators of myocardial infarction
- Positive CK-MB and troponin
- Heart failure: S_3, crackles, dyspnea, JVD, hepatomegaly, edema
- Increased intracardiac pressures (i.e., CVP, PAP, PAOP)
- Cardiac arrest

Brain
- Restlessness, confusion, altered level of consciousness
- Decrease in Glasgow Coma Score of 1 or more
- Focal signs (e.g., hemiparesis or hemiplegia, aphasia) may be present

Lungs
- Hypoxemia with PaO_2/FiO_2 ratio of less than 250 mm Hg
- Decreased static compliance
  - Increased work of breathing
  - Increased peak and plateau pressure if patient on mechanical ventilation
- Diffuse pulmonary infiltrates on chest x-ray
- Necessity of mechanical ventilation with PEEP 7.5 cm H_2O or greater

Kidney
- Urine output less than 0.5 mL/kg/hr
- Elevated BUN and creatinine
- Decreased urine creatinine clearance

Gastrointestinal
- Diminished bowel sounds
- Poor tolerance of enteral feedings
- Occult or overt GI bleeding

Liver
- Hypoglycemia
- Elevated bilirubin and jaundice
- Elevated AST, ALT, and LDH
- Decreased albumin

Hematologic
- Decreased platelets
- Elevated aPTT/PT
- Decreased fibrinogen
- Positive D-dimer
- Bleeding in a patient without a prior history of bleeding; petechiae; blood in sputum, vomitus, nasogastric aspirate, urine, or stool

Metabolic
- Metabolic acidosis
- Serum lactate greater than 4 mmol/L

Cardiac Output/Index

Cardiac output (CO) is the volume of blood pumped by the heart per minute and is the product of the amount of blood per heart beat (called the stroke volume) times the number of heart beats in a minute (heart rate). For an average size adult (70 kg) at rest, this flow of blood from the heart into the circulation would be about 5 liters per minute.

Cardiac index (CI) is a parameter that relates the cardiac output (CO) from the left ventricle in a minute to body surface area (BSA), thus relating heart performance to the size of the individual. Normal CI is 2.5 to 4.0 liters/minute/m².

Clinical indications suggestive of decreased CO/CI include tachycardia, hypotension, cool and clammy skin, and decreased urine output.

10.1   Learning Activity

Match the pathophysiology with the type of shock.

_____ 1. Anaphylactic
_____ 2. Cardiogenic
_____ 3. Hypovolemic
_____ 4. Neurogenic
_____ 5. Septic

a. Massive vasodilation caused by the release of inflammatory mediators in response to overwhelming infection
b. Inability of the heart to effectively pump
c. Inadequate intravascular volume
d. Vasodilation caused by the release of histamine from mast cells
e. Vasodilation resulting from suppression or loss of the sympathetic nervous system

Answers to this activity can be found in the Answer Key.

The clinical presentation of shock demonstrates a progression through states of subclinical hypoperfusion, SNS innervation, hypoperfusion, and profound hypoperfusion (Table 10-2). The patient's cardiac index decreases and distinct clinical findings emerge in each stage.

In the initial stage, there are no clinical indications, but an expert nurse may detect that "something is different." The SNS stimulation in the compensatory stage produces clinical signs and symptoms. The patient may voice feelings of anxiety, fear, impending doom, and thirst. Objective findings include tachycardia and blood pressure changes. The systolic BP increases or stays the same while the diastolic BP increases, resulting in a decrease in pulse pressure. Because diastolic BP is a reflection of arterial elasticity, the vasoconstriction caused by the SNS causes an elevation in diastolic BP and a narrowing of the pulse pressure earlier than a decrease in systolic BP or MAP. When repositioning the patient from a lying to sitting position, orthostatic effects occur, decreasing the BP. Other findings present in this stage include tachypnea and cool, pale, and clammy skin. In addition, bowel sounds are decreased as well as urine output (<0.5 mL/kg/hr).

compensate and restore tissue perfusion to vital organs. During the progressive stage of shock (Figure 10-2), there is an inability of the compensatory mechanisms to maintain tissue perfusion. In the refractory stage (Figure 10-3), the shock state is irreversible and refractory to conventional therapy with manifestations of progressive organ dysfunction and/or failure.

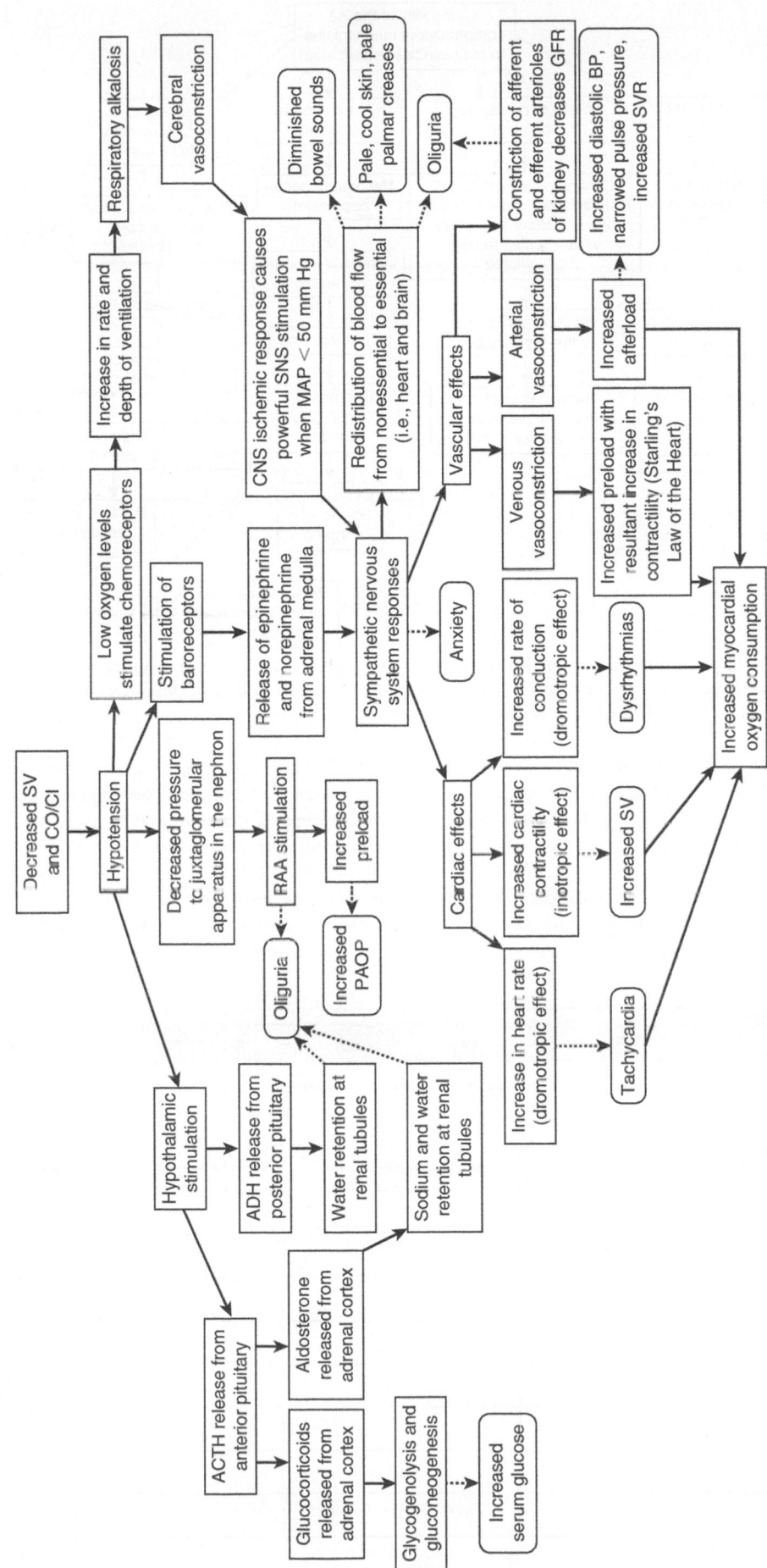

FIGURE 10-1 Pathophysiology of shock: compensatory stage. Dotted lines connect pathology to clinical presentation. *ACTH,* Adrenocorticotropic hormone; *ADH,* antidiuretic hormone; *BP,* blood pressure; *CO/CI,* cardiac output/cardiac index; *CNS,* central nervous system; *GFR,* glomerular filtration rate; *PAOP,* pulmonary artery occlusive pressure; *RAA,* renin-angiotensin-aldosterone; *SV,* stroke volume; *SVR,* systemic vascular resistance. (From Dennison, R. D. [2013]. *Pass CCRN!* [4th ed.]. St. Louis, MO: Elsevier.)

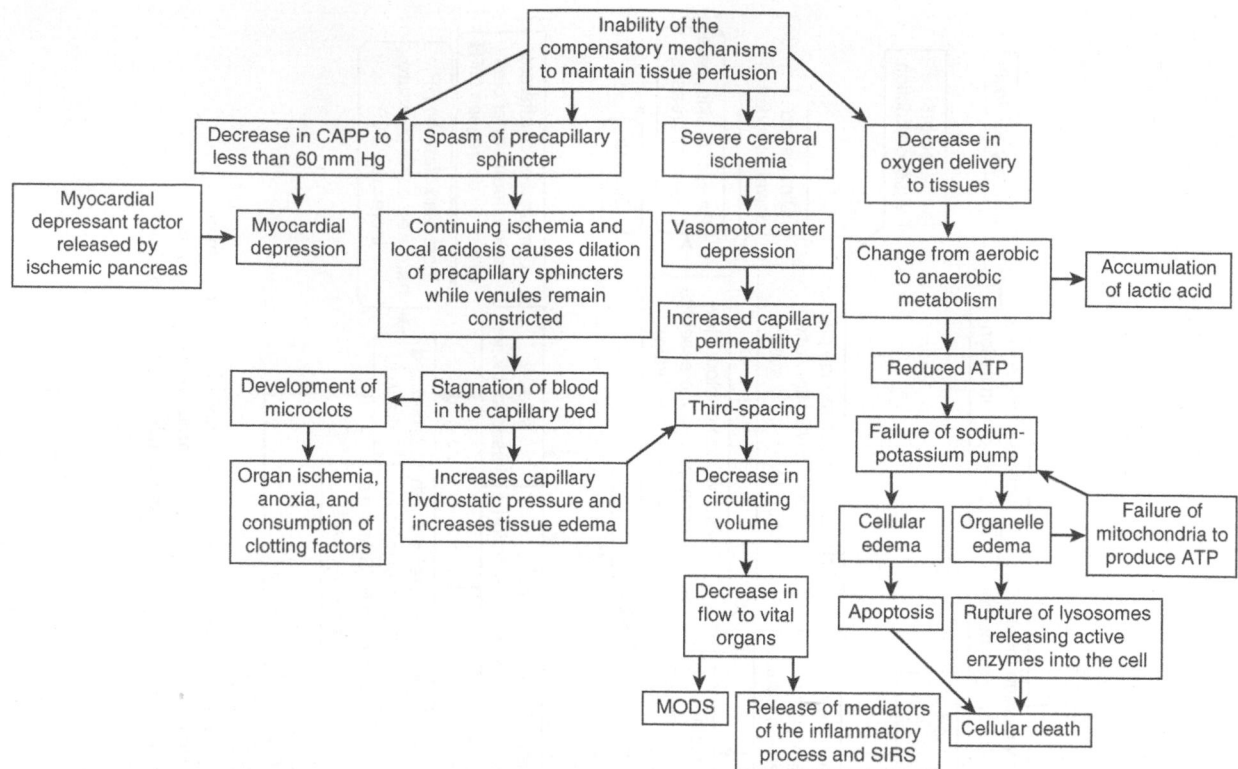

FIGURE 10-2 Pathophysiology of shock: progressive stage. *ATP,* Adenosine triphosphate; *CAPP,* coronary artery perfusion pressure; *MODS,* multiple organ dysfunction syndrome. (From Dennison, R. D. [2013]. *Pass CCRN!* [4th ed.]. St. Louis, MO: Elsevier.)

Even though the SNS shunts blood to the central nervous system (CNS) during this state, neurologic findings such as irritability, restlessness, and confusion occur early because the CNS is very sensitive to changes in oxygen and glucose.

Hypoperfusion findings are evident in the progressive stage. Subjectively, the patient may complain of anorexia, nausea, chest pain, palpitations, and dyspnea. Objective indications of hypoperfusion include tachycardia, dysrhythmias, hypotension (MAP <70 mm Hg), hypothermia, tachypnea, bluish and mottled appearance of skin, and peripheral cyanosis. The patient's gastrointestinal (GI) system, renal system, and CNS are affected as evidenced by vomiting and absent bowel sounds, anuria (i.e., negligible or <100 mL/24 hr), and lethargy or coma. With progression to the refractory stage, there is profound hypoperfusion, altered hemodynamic changes (Table 10-3), organ failure, and clinical evidence of MODS.

10.2   Learning Activity

Identify the following findings of shock as occurring during the compensatory, progressive, and/or refractory stages of shock.

	Compensatory	Progressive	Refractory
Tachycardia			
Dysrhythmias			
Cool, pale skin			
Disseminated intravascular coagulation			
Mottling of extremities			
Neurologic changes: lethargy, coma			
Oliguria			
Anuria			

10.2 Learning Activity—cont'd

	Compensatory	Progressive	Refractory
Acute respiratory distress syndrome			
Narrow pulse pressure			
Profound hypotension despite vasopressors			
Dysrhythmias			
Hypotension			
Decreased bowel sounds			
Thirst			
Neurologic changes: irritability, confusion			
Nausea			
Neurologic changes: focal signs			

Answers to this activity can be found in the Answer Key.

Decreased oxygen delivery to the tissues (DO$_2$) is common to all forms of shock except the early stage of septic shock. Early in septic shock, the CO/CI and the DO$_2$ are increased, but the extraction and utilization of oxygen by the tissues are impaired. Calculations can determine oxygen delivery and oxygen delivery indices. Normal oxygen delivery is approximately 1000 mL/min and normal oxygen delivery index is approximately 600 mL/min/m^2.

SIDEBAR 10-2

Calculation of Oxygen Delivery

Oxygen delivery (DO$_2$) = CO × (Hgb × 1.34 × SaO$_2$) × 10; normal approximately 1000 mL/min

Oxygen delivery (DO$_2$I) = CI × (Hgb × 1.34 × SaO$_2$) × 10; normal approximately 600 mL/min/m^2

Why is this important to me? The three factors that affect the delivery of oxygen to the tissues are (1) SaO$_2$, (2) hemoglobin (Hgb), and (3) cardiac index. A reduction in any of these three factors impairs oxygen delivery to the tissues. Another concern is that even with normal oxygen delivery, when oxygen consumption is increased (e.g., with fever, anxiety, seizures, or restlessness), there may still be an oxygen deficit at the tissue level.

Mixed venous oxygen saturation (SvO$_2$) is the percentage of oxygen bound to Hgb in blood returning to the right side of the heart. This value reflects the amount of oxygen "left over" after the tissues remove what they need. A decrease in SvO$_2$ indicates a decrease in the delivery of oxygen (i.e., SaO$_2$, Hgb, or cardiac index) or the consumption of oxygen is increased; therefore, a reduced oxygen reserve exists. Obtain a mixed venous oxygen saturation with an oximeter at the distal end of a pulmonary artery catheter as it is positioned in a pulmonary arteriole and includes all of the venous blood returning from the superior vena cava, inferior vena cava, and the coronary veins. Once the blood reaches the pulmonary artery and arteriole, all of the venous blood has "mixed" to reflect the average amount of oxygen remaining. The measurement reflects the amount of oxygen remaining after all tissues in the body have removed oxygen from the Hgb. In addition, the mixed venous sample captures the blood before it is reoxygenated in the pulmonary capillary on the way back to the pulmonary vein.

Because monitoring a pulmonary artery catheter requires a critical care admission and the use of this catheter has declined dramatically, measurements from a central venous catheter in the superior vena cava (ScvO$_2$) replaces the SvO$_2$ and are interpreted in the same manner. The ScvO$_2$ replaces the SvO$_2$ and identifies changes in a patient's tissue oxygen extraction in the progressive care unit. Although the value may be incorrect at times, a blood gas sample obtained from the superior vena cava (which reflects venous return from only the head and upper extremities) will have the same meaning as a SvO$_2$. The SvO$_2$ or ScvO$_2$ can help to determine whether the cardiac index and oxygen delivery are high enough to meet a patient's needs. The monitoring of mixed venous samples is valuable in the assessment of shock and can be very useful if measured before and after treatment changes. The normal SvO$_2$ value is 60% to 80%. Decreased SvO$_2$ to less than 60% indicates a decrease in oxygen reserve caused by either a decrease in tissue oxygen delivery (DO$_2$) or an increase in tissue oxygen consumption (VO$_2$). A decrease in the DO$_2$ occurs with a decrease in SaO$_2$, CO, or Hgb. An increase in the VO$_2$ resultant decrease in SvO$_2$ and occurs from fever, agitation, and/or seizures.

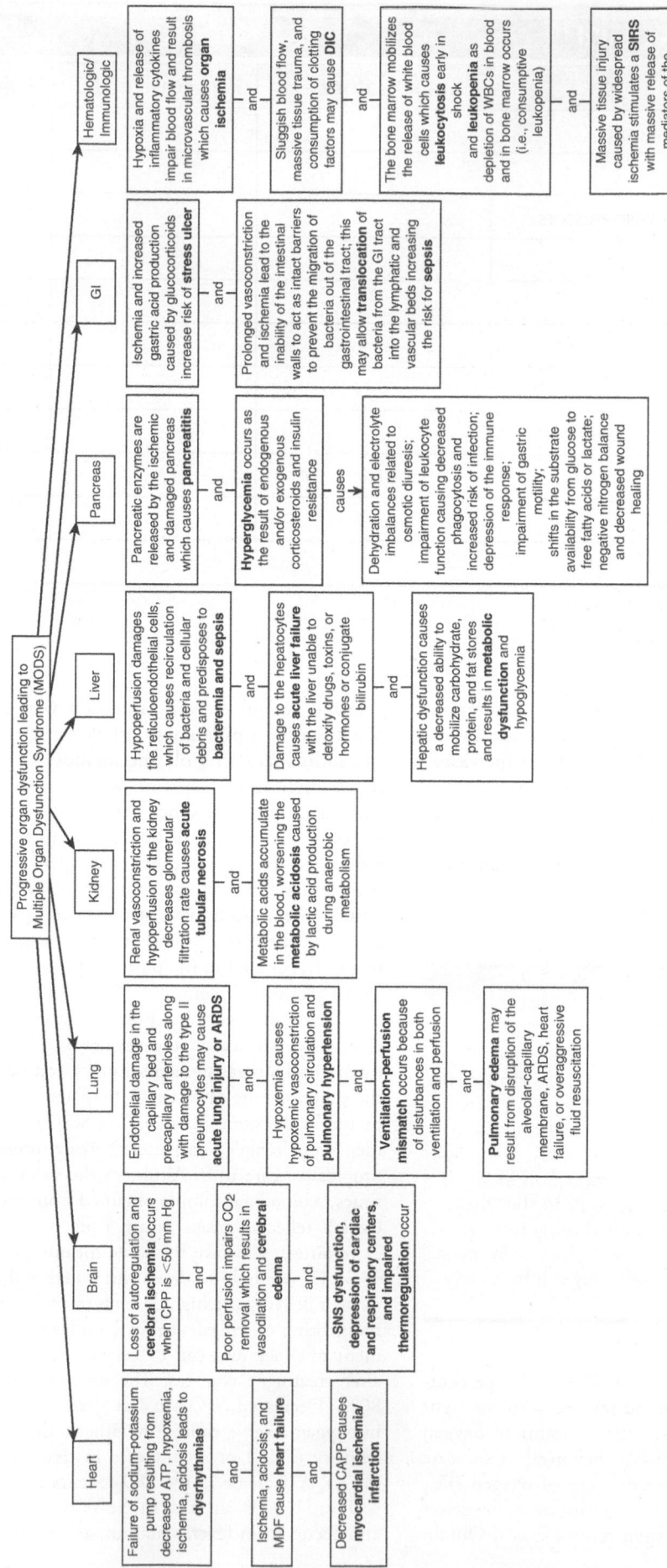

FIGURE 10-3 **Pathophysiology of shock: refractory stage.** *ARDS,* Acute respiratory distress syndrome; *ATP,* adenosine triphosphate; *CAPP,* coronary artery perfusion pressure; *CPP,* cerebral perfusion pressure; *DIC,* disseminated intravascular coagulation; *GI,* gastrointestinal; *MDF,* myocardial depressant factor; *MODS,* multiple organ dysfunction syndrome; *SIRS,* systemic inflammatory response syndrome; *SNS,* sympathetic nervous system; *WBC,* white blood cell. (From Dennison, R. D. [2013]. *Pass CCRN!* [4th ed.]. St. Louis, MO: Elsevier.)

TABLE 10-2 Clinical Presentation of the Stages of Shock

	Initial: Subclinical Hypoperfusion	Compensatory: SNS Innervation	Progressive: Hypoperfusion	Refractory: Profound Hypoperfusion
Cardiac index	2.2-2.5 L/min/m²	2-2.2 L/min/m²	Less than 2 L/min/m²	Less than 1.8 L/min/m²
Clinical indications	• No clinical indications of hypoperfusion but "something is different" • Detected by invasive hemodynamic monitoring	• Tachycardia • Narrowed pulse pressure • Tachypnea • Cool skin • Oliguria • Diminished bowel sounds • Restlessness → confusion	• Dysrhythmias • Hypotension • Tachypnea • Cold, clammy skin • Anuria • Absent bowel sounds • Lethargy → coma	• Life-threatening dysrhythmias • Hypotension despite potent vasopressors • ARDS • DIC • Hepatic dysfunction/failure • ATN • Mesenteric ischemia/infarction • Myocardial ischemia/infarction • Failure • Cerebral ischemia/infarction

TABLE 10-3 Hemodynamic Alterations in Shock

	Hypovolemic	Cardiogenic	Septic	Anaphylactic	Neurogenic
HR	High	High	High	High	Normal or low
BP	Normal → Low	Normal → Low	Low	Normal → Low	Normal → Low
CO/CI	Low	Low	High → Low	Normal → Low	Normal → Low
CVP	Low	High	Low	Low	Low
SVR/SVRI	High	High	Low	Low	Low
SvO_2	Low	Low	High → Low	Low	Low

HR, Heart rate; BP, blood pressure; CO, cardiac output; CI, cardiac index; CVP, central venous pressure; SVR, systemic vascular resistance; SVRI, systemic vascular resistance index; SvO_2, mixed venous oxygen saturation.

10.3 Learning Activity

Complete this table by putting ↑, ↓, or normal in the empty cells.

Type of Shock	CO/CI	RAP/PAP/PAOP	SVR	SvO_2/$ScvO_2$
Hypovolemic				
Cardiogenic				
Septic				
Anaphylactic				
Neurologic				

Answers to this activity can be found in the Answer Key.

10.4 Learning Activity

Match these general treatments of shock with the factor of oxygen delivery or consumption that they are intended to affect.

_____ 1. Isotonic crystalloids
_____ 2. Red blood cells
_____ 3. Oxygen
_____ 4. Mechanical ventilation
_____ 5. Inotropic agents
_____ 6. Sedation
_____ 7. PEEP
_____ 8. Surgical intervention to stop bleeding
_____ 9. Treatment of metabolic acidosis
_____ 10. Hypothermia

a. Improved DO_2 by improving SaO_2
b. Improved DO_2 by improving Hgb
c. Improved DO_2 by improving cardiac index
d. Diminished VO_2

Answers to this activity can be found in the Answer Key.

A variety of diagnostic serums, arterial blood gases, cultures, and urine test abnormalities (Table 10-4) indicate shock in varying stages. Other diagnostic tests isolate the cause or stage of shock. One important serum level to obtain is lactate. The serum lactate level rises early in the shock state and correlates closely with the degree of hypoperfusion. Levels above 2 mmol/L are associated with increased mortality. It is important to remember when drawing a serum lactate level that an arterial or central venous line should be used. The need to apply a tourniquet for a peripheral venous draw causes a false-positive value.

The priority of collaborative management of patients with all forms of shock is to maximize oxygen delivery to the tissues. First, maintain optimal Hgb and vascular volume. Monitor central venous pressure (CVP) or pulmonary artery occlusive pressure (PAOP) measurements when available to assess venous return to the heart (i.e., preload). Insert two intravenous (IV) catheters immediately, especially in cases of hemorrhage. These catheters should be short and large-gauge to allow rapid administration of fluids or blood if required. When an IV access is not available, administer fluid and blood products via an intraosseous route. To access the intraosseous site, place a rigid needle through the bone cortex into the medullary cavity, preferably in the anterior aspect of the tibia 1 to 3 cm below the proximal tibial tuberosity. The most frequently used site is the anteromedial aspect of the upper tibia as it lies just under the skin and can easily be palpated and located. The anterior aspect of the femur, the superior iliac crest, and the head of the humerus are other sites that are used. Access to and use of the intraosseous route requires immobilization of the limb.

Volume replacement is a priority for hypovolemic and vasogenic shock and may be necessary even in cardiogenic shock to achieve optimal volume and preload. Fluid resuscitation uses several types of fluids (Box 10-2). Crystalloids (Table 10-5) are solutions with dextrose or electrolytes. Crystalloids are safe, effective, inexpensive, and usually the initial fluid type used.

Hypertonic crystalloids (e.g., 3% saline) have been advocated for trauma resuscitation, but there is no evidence of the benefit of hypertonic crystalloid over isotonic crystalloid solutions (Patanwala, Amini, & Erstad, 2010). Colloids are large molecule (i.e., protein or starch) solutions considered when the patient's response to initial efforts is insufficient. Colloids not only stay in the vascular space better than crystalloids, but also may contribute to intravascular colloidal oncotic pressure to pull more fluid into the vascular space.

Colloids may be used in neurogenic shock or hypovolemic shock, except in the case of early burns. Septic and anaphylactic shock are both associated with increased capillary permeability, so avoid colloids in the initial stage. The following are examples of colloids used in shock:

- Albumin: plasma protein component; most costly but least likely to cause complications
- Dextran: contains polymers of high-molecular-weight polysaccharides; may cause coagulopathy by decreasing platelet aggregation; causes allergic reactions; may cause acute tubular necrosis and renal failure, but this is rare
- Hetastarch: contains polymers of hydroxyethyl starch; may cause coagulopathy by decreasing platelet aggregation; may elevate serum amylase levels, but they return to normal 5 to 7 days after hetastarch

Use blood and blood products to achieve a specific physiologic goal, such as to increase oxygen delivery or clotting

---

TABLE 10-4 Diagnostic Abnormalities in the Stages of Shock

Diagnostic Test	Abnormality
Serum Chemistry	
Sodium	Increased early; increased or decreased late
Potassium	Decreased early; increased late
Chloride	Decreased early; increased late
Bicarbonate	Normal early; decreased late
CO_2	Normal early; decreased late
Glucose	Increased early; decreased late
BUN	Increased
Creatinine	Increased
Total protein, albumin	Decreased
Bilirubin	Increased late
Amylase, lipase	Increased late
Ammonia	Increased late
CK	Increased
Liver enzymes (AST, ALT, LDH)	Increased
Lactate	Increased; correlates with degree of hypoperfusion
CBC	
Hemoglobin, hematocrit	Decreased if due to hemorrhage
Hematocrit	Increased if due to cause other than hemorrhage
WBC	Increased early, decreased late
Clotting Studies	
PT, aPTT	May be prolonged
Platelets	Decreased
Arterial Blood Gases	Respiratory alkalosis progresses to metabolic acidosis; there may also be decreased PaO_2 and SaO_2
Blood Cultures	May identify organism if septic shock
Urine	
Urine creatinine clearance	Decreased
Urine specific gravity	Increased early, decreased late
Urine osmolality	Increased early, decreased late
Urine sodium	Decreased
Heavy pigments	Present
Myoglobinuria	May be present due to muscle tissue destruction (e.g., crush injuries, muscle ischemia/necrosis, electrical burns, and seizures)
Hemoglobinuria	May be present due to a mismatched blood transfusion reaction and/or fresh water near-drowning

BOX 10-2

Types of Fluids Used for Fluid Resuscitation

Crystalloids	Colloids	Blood and Blood Products
Isotonic: NS; LR (D$_5$NS, D$_5$LR)	Albumin	Whole blood
Hypotonic: ½NS (D$_5$½NS, D$_5$W)	Dextran 70/75	Packed RBCs
Hypertonic: 3% saline; D$_{10}$W; TPN	Hetastarch (Hespan)	Fresh frozen plasma

D$_5$LR, 5% dextrose in lactated Ringer's; D$_5$NS, 5% dextrose in normal saline; D$_5$½NS, 5% dextrose in 0.45% saline; D$_5$W, 5% dextrose in water; D$_{10}$W, 10% dextrose in water; NS, normal (0.9%) saline; ½NS, 0.45% saline; LR, lactated Ringer's; TPN, total parenteral nutrition (usually 25% dextrose).

NOTE: Dextrose solutions are in parentheses because even though 5% dextrose adds to osmolality in the bottle or bag, this small amount of dextrose is metabolized so quickly when in the body that it should not be considered in the osmolality of the solution. So consider D$_5$NS as NS, D$_5$½NS as ½NS, and D$_5$W as water. This last example is why D$_5$W is avoided except in extreme hyperosmolar conditions. In significant volumes, D$_5$W will dilute electrolytes, particularly sodium, and potentially causes neurologic changes, including seizures.

TABLE 10-5   Crystalloids

	Isotonic	Hypotonic	Hypertonic
Osmolality	250-350 mOsm/L (which is similar to blood osmolality of 280-295 mOsm/L)	Less than 250 mOsm/L	Greater than 350 mOsm/L
Uses	• Tend to stay in the vascular space better than other crystalloids • Require replacement with 3 mL for every 1 mL lost because they do equilibrate across fluid compartments	• Tend to leave the vascular space and replace the interstitial space better than the vascular space	• Pull fluid from the interstitial space into the intravascular space • Expands intravascular volume over isotonic crystalloids without the adverse effects of colloids • Monitor closely for clinical indications of fluid overload when these solutions are administered

Examples	0.9% saline
	• Composition
	  • 154 mEq of sodium
	  • 154 mEq of chloride
	  • Water
	• Osmolality is 289 mOsm/L
	• pH is 5.7
	• Large volumes may cause metabolic (hyperchloremic) acidosis
	Lactated Ringer's
	• Composition
	  • 130 mEq/L
	  • 109 mEq/L chloride
	  • 4 mEq/L potassium
	  • 3 mEq/L of calcium
	  • 28 mEq/L of lactate
	  • Water
	• Osmolality is 273 mOsm/L
	• pH 6.7
	• Lactate is added as a buffer to make the solution less acidic (than without the lactate)
	• Lactate is converted to bicarbonate by the liver so large volumes may cause metabolic alkalosis and this solution should be avoided in patients who have liver disease
		Half normal (0.45%) saline
		• Composition
		  • 77 mEq of sodium
		  • 77 mEq of chloride
		  • water
		D$_5$W
		• Composition
		  • 50 g of dextrose
		  • Water
		• Note that though D$_5$W is isotonic in the bottle, the body quickly metabolizes the dextrose and free water is left; avoid this solution except in extremely hyperosmolar patients (e.g., HHS, DI)
			Hypertonic (3% saline)
			• 513 mEq of sodium
			• 513 mEq of chloride
			D$_{10}$W (10% dextrose in water)
			• Composition
			  • 100 g of dextrose/L
			  • Water
			D$_{50}$W (50% dextrose in water)
			• Composition
			  • 25 g of dextrose/50 mL ampule
			  • Water
			Total parenteral nutrition solution
			• Central
			  • 250 g of dextrose/L
			  • Protein, electrolytes, vitamins vary
			  • Water
			• Peripheral
			  • 100 g of dextrose/L
			  • Protein, electrolytes, vitamins vary
			  • Water

capability. These products contain plasma proteins to add to intravascular colloidal oncotic pressure. The red blood cell (RBC) is the only solution that increases the CaO$_2$ (content of oxygen in arterial blood) because the Hgb molecule carries 97% of all oxygen. Blood is indicated when the patient has lost blood and there are clinical indications of hypoperfusion. Use blood as prescribed for patients with evidence of acute hemorrhage and

hemodynamic instability or inadequate oxygen delivery (Kaur, Basu, & Kaur, 2011).

Consider blood transfusion if the Hgb is less than 7 g/dL in patients requiring mechanical ventilation, in resuscitated trauma patients, and in patients with stable cardiac disease (Kaur, Basu, & Kaur, 2011; Napolitano et al., 2009). The major disadvantages of blood and blood products are the cost and risk of blood transfusion reactions or blood-transmitted disease, such as HIV, hepatitis, or cytomegalovirus.

Several factors affect the selection process for replacement solutions. Do not use colloids in situations with increased capillary permeability. In other situations, there is no difference in effectiveness between crystalloids and colloids (Perel & Roberts, 2011), and because colloids are considerably more costly, the first choice in most situations is crystalloids. Use blood only when specifically indicated because blood administration is associated with an increased risk of SIRS and mortality.

Consider the volume of fluid replacement. A typical fluid challenge is 250 to 500 mL of normal saline over 5 minutes. Monitor the BP, CVP if available, and clinical indicators of fluid overload (e.g., dyspnea, jugular venous distention, S_3, systolic flow murmur, crackles). If the patient is hemorrhaging, immediately complete a type and crossmatch. Type-specific blood or O negative may be given in severe hemorrhage but because the use of O negative may make future crossmatching more difficult, avoid unless absolutely necessary. Take care during fluid resuscitation to prevent the occurrence of hypothermia. Hypothermia impairs tissue oxygen delivery by shifting the oxyhemoglobin dissociation curve to the left and impairs coagulation. Warm fluids as prescribed if the patient has cold agglutinins, the body temperature is low (35° C or less) at the initiation of fluid resuscitation, or multiple units of blood or multiple liters of IV fluids are needed. Avoid overheating the patient, which may cause vasodilation and precipitate a decrease in preload.

10.5 Learning Activity

List two fluids in each category.

Isotonic crystalloids		
Hypotonic crystalloids		
Hypertonic crystalloids		
Colloids		
Blood or blood products		

Answers to this activity can be found in the Answer Key.

Take care to avoid excess fluid resuscitation, which is associated with increased incidence of bleeding, abdominal hypertension and abdominal compartment syndrome, acute respiratory distress syndrome (ARDS), MODS, and death. In trauma patients, return of the MAP between 70 and 80 mm Hg may cause clot disruption and increased bleeding. Permissive hypotension with a MAP of 60 mm Hg is an approach that may be used until surgical intervention is available (Morrison et al., 2011). Most patients in shock require fluid replacement, administration of venous vasodilators, and/or diuretics as prescribed to decrease the preload in patients in cardiogenic shock.

Maintain optimal cardiac contractility and cardiac index. Monitor the patient's ECG, MAP, CVP if available, and neurologic status while facilitating transfer to a higher level of care. The patient in cardiogenic shock will typically require the administration of inotropes (e.g., dobutamine) to increase contractility and venous vasodilators (e.g., nitroglycerin [NTG]) to decrease preload. Although arterial vasodilators (e.g., nitroprusside) decrease afterload, the patient in cardiogenic shock may be too hypotensive for their use and an intraaortic balloon pump would be used instead to decrease afterload and increase coronary artery perfusion pressure. Correct metabolic acidosis because it affects cardiac contractility. Although this is usually accomplished by treatment of the cause of the tissue hypoxia that is causing the lactic acidosis, sodium bicarbonate may be given in severe metabolic acidosis (i.e., pH <7.0).

Although generally contraindicated in patients with cardiogenic shock, because they increase afterload and myocardial oxygen consumption, vasopressors (Table 10-6) are useful in the distributive forms of shock to maintain vascular tone. In an effort to maintain MAP above 60 mm Hg to maintain perfusion pressure, vasopressors are used, but by constricting the vessels, they may actually decrease blood flow to organs, even though the MAP is higher. Although the patient will not receive vasopressors while on the progressive care unit, treatment may be initiated before transfer and these are important concepts to understand.

To improve the patient's oxygenation and perfusion status, implement strategies to improve the Hgb and oxygen saturation (SpO_2). Maintain optimal oxygen saturation and monitor the SpO_2 and arterial blood gases. Ensure an adequate patient airway. Initially, administer oxygen at 5 to 6 L/min. High oxygen concentrations may be necessary depending on the SpO_2 and arterial blood gas values. CPAP may be of help before transfer, intubation, and the initiation of mechanical ventilation. The patient may require PEEP, and/or extracorporeal membrane oxygenation (ECMO) for respiratory muscle fatigue, respiratory acidosis, and/or refractory hypoxemia. Monitor the patient's SpO_2, arterial blood gases, or chest x-ray. Observe for indications of decreased lung compliance indicative of ARDS (e.g., increased work of breathing).

Although improving SaO_2, Hgb, and cardiac index is crucial to improve oxygen delivery to tissues, it is also important to minimize oxygen consumption of the tissues. Maintain patient comfort and bed rest. Provide adequate rest periods from nursing care and treat pain and anxiety with the administration of analgesics and anxiolytics as required, but be cautious to avoid cumulative effect. Control the patient's body temperature. Treat hyperthermia with cooling blankets and set at 1° below the patient's temperature to avoid drift and resultant shivering. Avoid overheating the patient, which may increase myocardial oxygen consumption and cause vasodilation, reducing preload and cardiac output. Provide patient and family support and keep the patient and family informed. Encourage the patient and family to discuss fears and concerns.

Prevent injury caused by decreased perfusion. Limit sedatives and other CNS depressants. Administer drugs only by the IV route because peripheral perfusion and drug absorption are impaired. A central venous catheter with a multiple-lumen catheter is preferred for drug administration.

Maintain or improve the patient's nutritional status. Provide enteral feedings unless absolutely contraindicated (e.g., paralytic ileus or structural obstruction). Use of the GI tract is important to prevent bacterial translocation, which is the movement of bacteria from the GI tract into the lymphatics or vascular beds. Glutamine, arginine, and omega-3 fatty acids may be important in the prevention of sepsis, septic shock,

TABLE 10-6 **Selected Vasopressors**

Drug	Administration	Adverse Effects	Nursing Implications
Norepineph-rine bitartrate (Levophed)	• IV infusion: mix 4 mg in 250 mL (16 mcg/mL) and infuse at 0.1-0.3 mcg/kg/min; titrate to BP response • Administer through central venous catheter if possible; if administered peripherally, use a large vein • Do not administer with alkaline solutions	• Bradycardia • Ventricular dysrhythmias • Hypertension • Anxiety • Headache • Tremor • Dizziness • Chest pain • Metabolic (lactic) acidosis • Severe vasoconstriction may cause renal or mesenteric necrosis • Local necrosis with high dosages or if infusion infiltrates	• Monitor BP, HR, ECG, urine output, neurologic status • Note contraindications: known hypersensitivity, ventricular fibrillation, tachydysrhythmias, pheochromocytoma, narrow-angle glaucoma • Use cautiously in peripheral vascular disease, hyperthyroidism, CAD, hypertension, psychoneurosis, diabetes, patient receiving MAO inhibitors or tricyclic antidepressant, and in older adults • Note that this drug may cause a fluid shift from intravascular to interstitial space, causing depletion of intravascular volume • Do not use discolored solution • Prevent extravasation as necrosis may occur; treat with phentolamine (Regitine)
Dopamine hydro-chloride (Intropin)	• IV infusion: mix 400 mg in 250 mL (1600 mcg/mL) and infuse at 0.5-20 mcg/kg/min depending on desired effect • Maximum: 20 mcg/kg/min • Administer through central venous catheter if possible; if administered peripherally, use a large vein • Do not administer with alkaline solutions	• Tachycardia • Ventricular ectopy • Hypertension or hypotension • Nausea, vomiting • Dyspnea • Headache • Palpitations • Chest pain in patients with CAD • Tissue necrosis with high dosages or extravasation	• Monitor BP, HR, ECG, PA, PAOP, SVR, CI, urine output • Note contraindications: known hypersensitivity, uncorrected tachydysrhythmias, ventricular fibrillation, pheochromocytoma, hypertrophic cardiomyopathy, and in patients receiving MAO inhibitors • Use cautiously in peripheral vascular disease • Consider the cause of hypotension instead of automatically initiating dopamine to increase the blood pressure; *improve perfusion* by treating the cause of hypotension (e.g., volume replacement, inotropes, preload, or afterload reduction) • Provide volume expansion during weaning; taper gradually to wean • Do not administer if discolored • Prevent extravasation as necrosis may occur; treat extravasation with phentolamine (Regitine)
Phenylephrine (Neo-Synephrine)	• IV infusion: mix 30 mg in 500 mL (60 mcg/mL); usual dose is 0.5-10 mcg/kg/min • Rapid onset and short duration • Preferred agent in patients with tachycardia	• Reflex bradycardia • Ventricular dysrhythmias • Hypertension • Nausea, vomiting • Paresthesia • Palpitations • Anxiety • Restlessness • Headache • Tremor • Chest pain	• Monitor BP, HR, ECG • Note contraindications: known hypersensitivity, ventricular fibrillation, tachydysrhythmias, pheochromocytoma, narrow-angle glaucoma • Use cautiously in older adults and those with hyperthyroidism, CAD, hypertension, psychoneurosis, diabetes mellitus, peripheral vascular disease • Prevent extravasation as necrosis may occur; treat with phentolamine (Regitine) • Treat reflex bradycardia with atropine • Discard if discolored or precipitate present

continued

TABLE 10-6   **Selected Vasopressors—cont'd**

Drug	Administration	Adverse Effects	Nursing Implications
Epinephrine hydro-chloride (Adrenalin)	• IV infusion: mix 1 mg in 250 mL (4 mcg/mL) and infuse at 1-10 mcg/min (0.05-1 mcg/kg/min); titrate to desired effect • Administer through central venous catheter if possible; if administered peripherally, use a large vein • Do not administer with alkaline solutions	• Tachycardia • Dysrhythmias • Palpitations • Anxiety • Restlessness • Headache • Dizziness • Tremor • Cerebral hemorrhage • Chest pain • Hyperglycemia	• Monitor BP, HR, ECG • Note contraindications: glaucoma, organic brain damage, cardiomegaly • Use cautiously in older adults and those with hyperthyroidism, chest pain, hypertension, psychoneurosis, diabetes mellitus • Prevent extravasation as necrosis may occur; treat with phentolamine (Regitine) • Discard if discolored or precipitate present
Vasopressin (Pitressin)	• IV infusion: 0.01-0.04 units/min	• Bradycardia • Hypertension • Fever • Water intoxication (SIADH), hyponatremia • Nausea, abdominal cramps • Tremor • Headache • Seizures • Coma • Constriction of cardiac arteries, resulting in chest pain and myocardial ischemia	• Monitor BP, HR, daily weight, serum sodium • Note contraindications: known hypersensitivity, nephritis • Use cautiously in coronary artery disease

SIRS, and MODS. The use of arginine in the presence of sepsis is controversial and safety is still questionable. Provide parenteral feeding, trace elements, and vitamins as prescribed if enteral feedings are contraindicated or if parenteral supplementation of enteral feedings is required to meet calorie and protein requirements. Closely monitor serum potassium, magnesium, and phosphate levels and replace or restrict as indicated.

Maintain renal perfusion and the glomerular filtration rate (GFR). Insert an indwelling urinary catheter to monitor hourly urine output. Monitor the BUN, creatinine, urine creatinine clearance, and urine sodium. Replace volume as indicated by CVP, urine output, insensible fluid loss, or clinical indications of dehydration. Monitor the patient closely for change in the color of urine, which may indicate the presence of myoglobinuria or hemoglobinuria, which are both associated with increased risk of acute tubular necrosis.

Maintain glycemic control and recognize that hyperglycemia is related to stress and insulin resistance and occurs in patients without a diagnosis of diabetes mellitus. Maintain serum glucose between 140 and 180 mg/dL. Although there has been considerable debate on the desirable serum glucose level over the last decade, the body of evidence related to this question indicates that there is no mortality benefit but there is an increased hypoglycemia risk associated with glucose control maintained within the 80 to 110 mg/dL range (Sandrock & Albertson, 2010). Measure serum glucose by point-of-care testing every hour until serum glucose is less than 180 mg/dL, and then every 4 hours. Capillary glucose measurements may be inaccurate in edematous, vasoconstricted, or poorly perfused patients; therefore, an arterial or venous catheter should be placed for sampling. Administer insulin as prescribed. Insulin is usually administered subcutaneously at meals and bedtime and adjusted according to serum glucose level in the progressive care unit. If the patient is taking nothing by mouth, do glucose checks every 6 hours and treat hypoglycemia with parenteral dextrose.

Monitor the patient for the complications of dysrhythmias, GI ulceration, deep vein thrombus (DVT), and mesenteric ischemia and/or infarction. Conduct continuous monitoring and administer the appropriate antidysrhythmic agents depending on the rhythm displayed. Observe for bleeding and administer stress ulcer prophylaxis with H_2 receptor antagonists or proton pump inhibitors as prescribed. Administer DVT prophylaxis with low-molecular-weight heparin subcutaneously and the use of an antithrombic sequential pump device as prescribed. To detect mesenteric ischemia and/or infarction, monitor the patient for abdominal pain and bloody diarrhea, and prep the patient for surgery if intestinal perforation occurs.

Monitor the patient for indications of organ failure and MODS. ARDS, disseminated intravascular coagulation (DIC), hepatic failure, acute tubular necrosis (ATN), myocardial infarction (MI), and cerebral infarction occur often with shock. Provide emotional support to the patient and family. Keep the patient informed regarding what is going to occur and why. Provide the family with accurate information and maintain hope but do not give false reassurance.

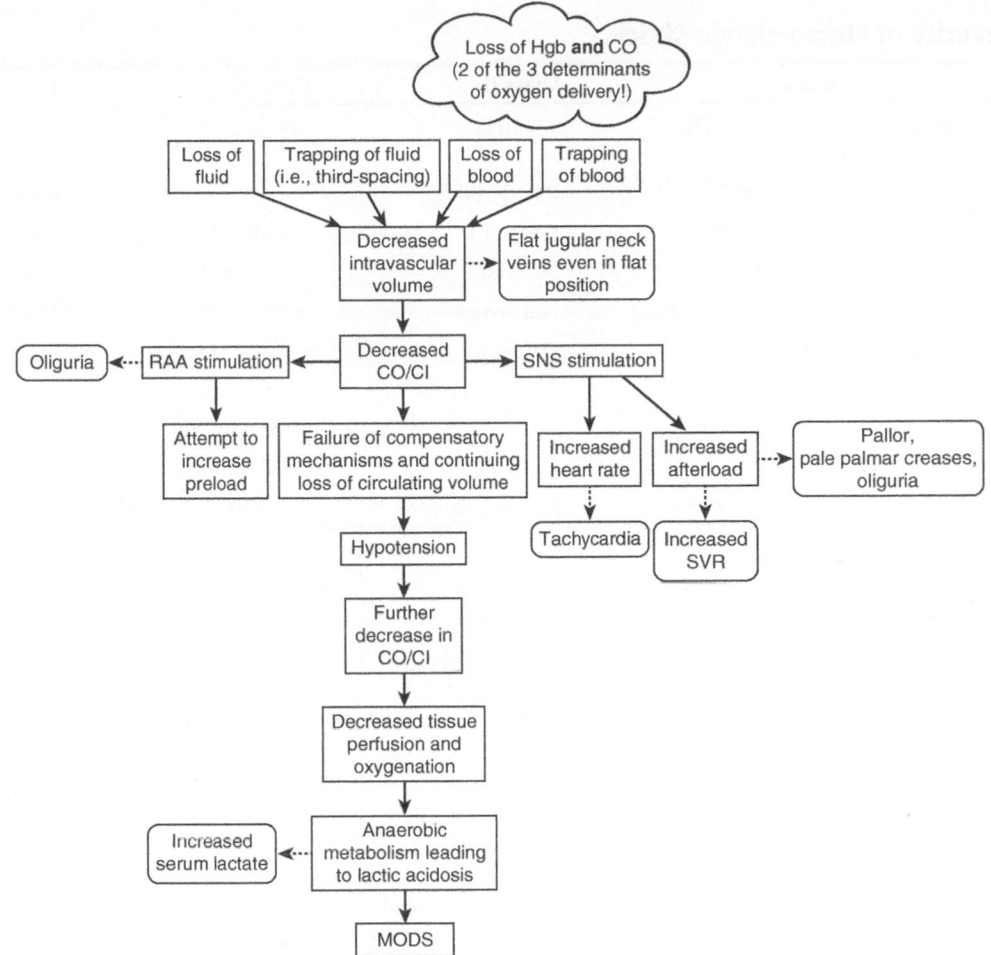

FIGURE 10-4 **Pathophysiology of hypovolemic shock.** Dotted lines connect pathology to clinical presentation. *CI*, Cardiac index; *CO*, cardiac output; *Hgb*, hemoglobin; *MODS*, multiple organ dysfunction syndrome; *RAA*, renin-angiotensin-aldosterone; *SNS*, sympathetic nervous system; *SVR*, systemic vascular resistance. (From Dennison, R. D. [2013]. *Pass CCRN!* [4th ed.]. St. Louis, MO: Elsevier.)

Hypovolemic Shock

An inadequate intravascular volume causes hypovolemic shock. The inadequate intravascular volume may occur from external blood loss, fluid loss, and internal sequestration of either blood or fluid. External losses of blood stem from bleeding due to GI issues (e.g., esophageal varices, peptic ulcers, hemorrhoids); genitourinary issues (e.g., antepartal or post-partum bleeding, hematuria); amputation; major blood vessel disruption, which may be overt or occult; and coagulopathy. Coagulopathy may be congenital (e.g., hemophilia) or acquired (e.g., DIC, excessive anticoagulation). Fluid loss may occur by GI, renal, and cutaneous routes. GI loss occurs in patients with vomiting, diarrhea, or nasogastric suction. Renal fluid loss is due to conditions such as DKA, HHS, diabetes insipidus, hypoaldosteronism (i.e., Addison disease), diuretics, or osmotic dyes. Causes of fluid loss from the cutaneous route are burns, exudative wounds, and excessive perspiration (e.g., heat exhaustion).

Fluids, sequestered internally in various spaces within the body, prevent fluid from being available in the intravascular space. Internal fluid sequestration may result in the development of ascites (e.g., peritonitis, pancreatitis, cirrhosis, and intraabdominal malignancies), pleural effusion, pericardial effusion, or intestinal lumen (e.g., intestinal obstruction).

Third spacing is the trapping of fluid into spaces that are neither intravascular nor intracellular. Blood may also be trapped into the hemoperitoneum or retroperitoneal cavity (e.g., hemorrhagic pancreatitis, ruptured spleen, lacerated liver), into the thorax (i.e., hemothorax) or mediastinum (i.e., hemomediastinum), into the false lumen of a dissecting aortic aneurysm, and/or into soft tissue with pelvic or long bone fractures.

The pathophysiology of hemorrhagic shock (Figure 10-4) stems from a decrease in intravascular volume and inadequate perfusion. Remember that while the loss of fluid decreases cardiac index, loss of blood causes a decrease in cardiac index and Hgb, two of the three components of oxygen delivery, accentuating the negative impact on oxygen delivery to the tissues and accentuating tissue hypoxia.

The clinical presentation for hypovolemic shock is the same as for most other types of shock but with some specific findings. Subjectively, the recent history will likely reveal a precipitating factor. Objective findings include flat neck veins, decreased CVP, and decreased urine output. Classification parameters (Table 10-7) delineate the severity of hemorrhagic shock.

Evaluation of fluid status and estimation of losses is important in the ongoing assessment of a patient with hypovolemia and hypovolemic shock. Along with oral and IV intake and

TABLE 10-7	Severity of Hemorrhagic Shock			
Indicator	Class I	Class II	Class III	Class IV
Blood loss (% of blood volume)	Less than 15%	15-30%	30-40%	Greater than 40%
Blood loss (mL)	Less than 750 mL	750-1500 mL	1500-2000 mL	Greater than 2000 mL
Heart rate/min	Less than 100	Greater than 100	Greater than 120	140 or greater
Blood pressure	Normal	Normal	Decreased	Decreased
Pulse pressure	Widened or normal	Narrowed	Narrowed	Narrowed
Capillary refill	Normal	Delayed	Delayed	Delayed or absent
Ventilatory rate/min	14-20	20-30	30-40	Greater than 35
Urine output (mL/hr)	30 or greater	20-30	Less than 20	Negligible
Skin appearance	Cool, pink	Cool, pale	Cold, moist, pale	Cold, clammy, cyanotic
Neurologic status	Slightly anxious	Mildly anxious	Anxious, confused	Confused, lethargy

Adapted from American College of Surgeons (2008). *ATLS: Advanced trauma life support for doctors* (8th ed.). Chicago, American College of Surgeons.

urine output, the measurement of intake and output includes estimation of insensible losses, tube drainage, and soiled dressings. Weigh dressings and convert to a volume, using 1 kg being equal to 1000 mL.

Specific diagnostic tests for a patient in hypovolemic shock include serum hematology, peritoneal lavage, and computed tomography (CT scan). The hematocrit (Hct) will be elevated if the shock is due to dehydration but decreased if due to blood loss. A diagnostic peritoneal lavage detects intraabdominal bleeding. A CT scan of the chest or abdomen is useful to detect the source of bleeding.

The collaborative management of a patient with hypovolemic shock is the same as for shock in general, but with a focus on replacement of lost fluid or blood. Identify the high-risk patient and monitor for clinical indications of hypoperfusion. The first priority is always to support ventilation and circulation and treat the cause. Compress any compressible vessels and prepare the patient for surgery if it is necessary to control bleeding. Other interventions may include the administration of medications as appropriate, such as antidiarrheals for diarrhea or insulin for hyperglycemia. Administer appropriate volume replacement via two large-gauge IV catheters. Initially, administer normal saline at a rapid rate. Give a blood transfusion for class III and IV when the fluid lost is blood. Monitor for fluid overload during replacement therapies. Utilize the autotransfusion technique to decrease the risk of transfusion-transmitted disease, if appropriate.

Cardiogenic Shock

An impaired ability of the heart to pump blood effectively causes cardiogenic shock. The most common cause of cardiogenic shock is decreased contractility due to acute MI with a loss of 40% of the left ventricular myocardium. This occurs with large anterior MI or acute MI in patients with history of previous MI or MIs and preexisting left ventricular dysfunction. Cardiogenic shock may also stem from myocardial ischemia with preexisting left ventricular dysfunction, myocardial contusion, cardiac surgery, dilated cardiomyopathy, myocarditis, severe heart failure (HF), and a ventricular aneurysm. In addition, an overdosage of myocardial depressant drugs (e.g., beta-blockers, calcium

channel blockers, or barbiturates) and acute rejection of cardiac transplant can also cause cardiogenic shock. A stunned or hibernating myocardium (transient cardiogenic shock) results from the following:

- Cardiac surgery: related to hypothermia, cardioplegic arrest
- Reperfusion injury
- Post-CPR
- Hypoxemia
- Acidosis
- Hypoglycemia
- Electrolyte imbalance

Dysrhythmias, cardiac tamponade, and/or a noncompliant ventricle (e.g., left ventricular hypertrophy, right ventricular hypertrophy) cause impaired filling of the heart chambers. Impaired emptying, which may be referred to as obstructive shock, is caused by valve dysfunction such as chronic stenosis or regurgitation, acute papillary muscle rupture, ventricular septal rupture, rupture of the ventricular free wall, intracardiac tumor, massive pulmonary embolism, tension pneumothorax, dissecting thoracic aortic aneurysm, coarctation of the aorta, and restrictive or hypertrophic cardiomyopathy.

The pathophysiology of cardiogenic shock (Figure 10-5) begins with an inability of the heart to pump blood effectively. Coronary artery perfusion pressure (CAPP) is significantly affected by a decrease in cardiac index and an increase in PAOP, both of which occur with the pump failure that occurs in cardiogenic shock. This decrease in CAPP causes worsening myocardial ischemia and worsening contractility and cardiac index, which further worsens CAPP, often referred to as the vicious cycle of cardiogenic shock.

The clinical presentation for cardiogenic shock is the same as for shock in general, but with some specific findings. The recent history may include a history of precipitating factors such as chest pain, dyspnea, and thirst along with anxiety, fear, and a feeling of impending doom. The objective findings of cardiogenic shock include the symptoms of left and right ventricular failure with shock. Classic left ventricular failure (LVF) findings include tachycardia, dysrhythmias, pulsus alternans, S_3, dyspnea, tachypnea, and crackles. Note that tachycardia may not be evident if the patient is receiving beta-blockers. Classic findings of right

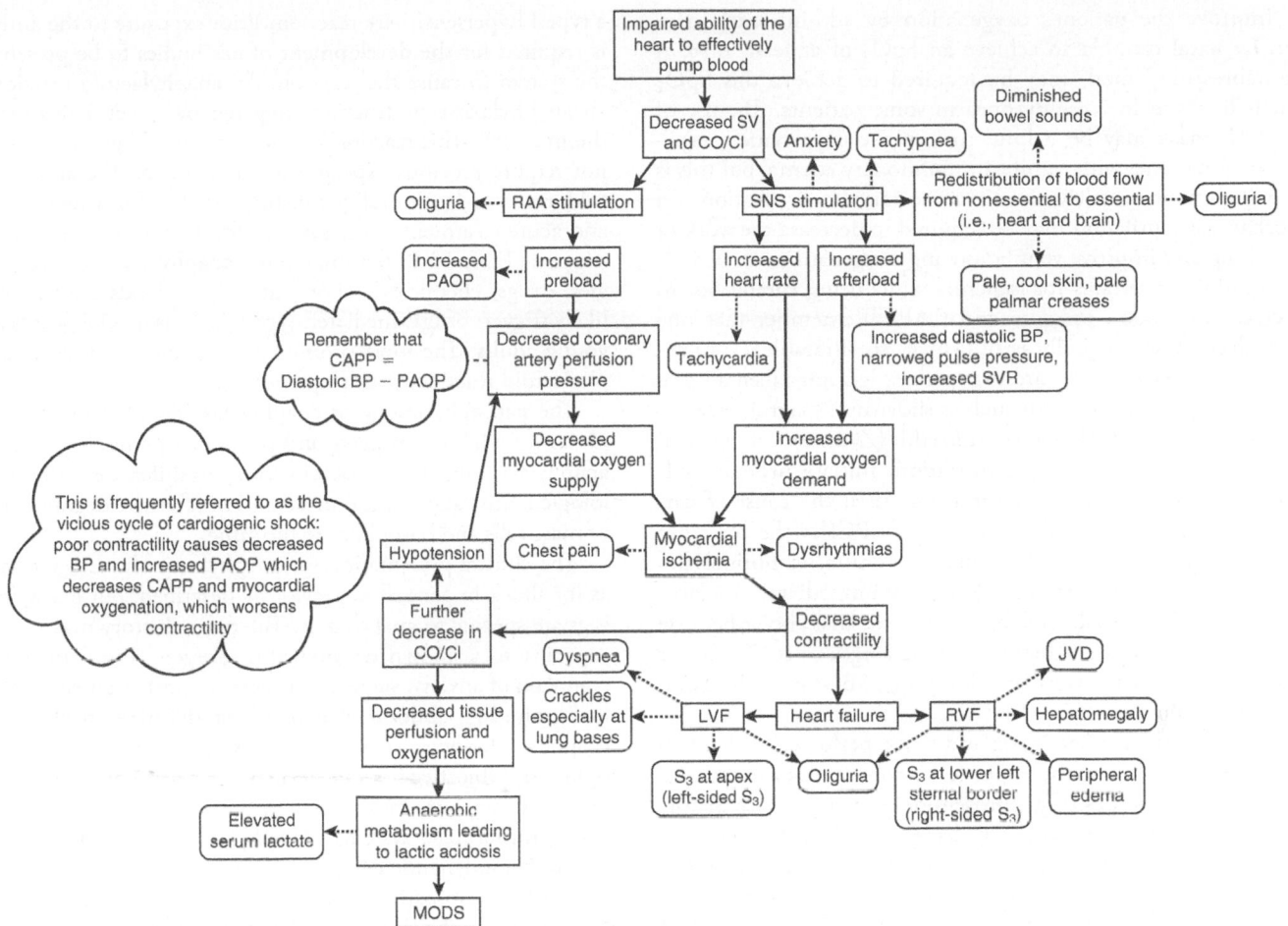

FIGURE 10-5 Pathophysiology of cardiogenic shock. Dotted lines connect pathology to clinical presentation. *BP,* Blood pressure; *CAPP,* coronary artery perfusion pressure; *CI,* cardiac index; *CO,* cardiac output; *LVF,* left ventricular failure; *MODS,* multiple organ dysfunction syndrome; *PAOP,* pulmonary artery occlusive pressure; *RAA,* renin-angiotensin-aldosterone; *RVF,* right ventricular failure; *SNS,* sympathetic nervous system; *SV,* stroke volume; *SVR,* systemic vascular resistance. (From Dennison, R. D. [2013]. *Pass CCRN!* [4th ed.]. St. Louis, MO: Elsevier.)

ventricular failure (RVF) are jugular venous distention, hepatosplenomegaly, and peripheral edema. Hemodynamic alterations (see Table 10-3) demonstrate a decreased CO/CI, elevated CVP and PAOP, and increased systemic vascular resistance.

Serum diagnostic test results in cardiogenic shock will show elevations in the cardiac enzymes and troponin levels if the cause of the cardiogenic shock is acute MI or myocardial contusion. The patient's arterial blood gases may reveal significant hypoxemia caused by the pulmonary edema and then respiratory acidosis as the patient fatigues and acute respiratory failure occurs. Eventually, metabolic acidosis with tissue hypoxia occurs, causing lactic acidosis.

An electrocardiogram (ECG) may reveal acute (i.e., ST segment elevation, pathologic Q waves) or old MI (pathologic Q waves without ST segment elevation) changes. Dysrhythmias may be present. Persistent ST segment elevations in anterior leads suggest a ventricular aneurysm.

Diagnostic radiology examinations used in cardiogenic shock include the chest x-ray (CXR) and echocardiography. The CXR may show pulmonary vascular congestion. Echocardiography may reveal the cause of cardiogenic shock. This test determines ventricular wall motion abnormalities seen in myocardial

ischemia or infarction. Global wall motion abnormality is present in cases of cardiomyopathy or myocarditis. Echocardiograms detect cardiac tamponade and valve abnormalities (e.g., ruptured ventricular septum, and ruptured papillary muscle with acute mitral regurgitation). A cardiac catheterization may be performed and this procedure may reveal the cause of the cardiogenic shock and abnormal intracardiac pressures.

Collaborative management for cardiogenic shock is the same as for shock in general with some specific differences. Closely monitor high-risk patients for clinical indications of hypoperfusion and transfer to a higher level of care for continuous invasive hemodynamic monitoring to be able to detect early changes in cardiac index. Prevent and treat the shock by implementation of the following:

- Early reperfusion for acute MI using percutaneous coronary intervention (PCI) or fibrinolytics
- Pericardiocentesis for cardiac tamponade
- Fibrinolytics and anticoagulants for pulmonary embolus
- Surgery for removal of intracardiac tumors, valve replacement, septal repair, etc.
- Emergency decompression followed by chest tube for tension pneumothorax

Improve the patient's oxygenation by administering oxygen by nasal cannula to achieve an SpO_2 of at least 92%. A nonrebreathing mask may be required to achieve this SpO_2 but is likely to increase dyspnea in some patients. The use of a CPAP mask may be helpful to improve oxygenation, especially for patients with significant pulmonary edema, but this is also likely to increase dyspnea in some patients. Intubation and mechanical ventilation may be required to decrease the work of breathing and improve ventilation and oxygenation.

Administer nitrates for ischemia while being careful not to decrease the blood pressure and CAPP. Remember that one nitroglycerin sublingually is 400 mcg, so titratable IV nitroglycerin is preferred. Ensure that patient has not taken an oral phosphodiesterase inhibitor such as sildenafil (Viagra), tadalafil (Cialis), vardenafil (Levitra), udenafil (Zydena), or avanafil (Stendra) before nitrate administration. Initiate prompt evaluation for emergency reperfusion options if the cause of cardiogenic shock is an acute MI. Primary PCI is the preferred treatment if the facilities are available. Administer fibrinolytics to open the coronary vessels if PCI is not immediately available within 90 minutes. Fibrinolytics are not the first choice because the complication rate is higher and the length of stay is longer than PCI. Coronary artery bypass graft (CABG) may also be an option in some cases.

Optimize the cardiac index and tissue perfusion with pharmacologic agents. Use inotropes (e.g., dobutamine) to increase *contractility*. Diuretics (e.g., furosemide) or venous vasodilators (e.g., nitroglycerin [NTG]) will decrease *preload*. Give arterial vasodilators (e.g., nitroprusside [NTP]) to decrease *afterload*, but their use in cardiogenic shock is limited by hypotension and contraindicated in acute myocardial ischemia due to the risk of coronary artery steal. When coronary artery steal occurs, blood shunts from ischemic areas to the nonischemic areas. Exercise caution with giving all arterial vasodilators in acute myocardial ischemia because they are likely to decrease aortic root pressure and CAPP. Careful titration of all vasodilators is required to maintain the MAP above the 60 mm Hg required to perfuse the vital organs. To control tachycardia, give antidysrhythmics or the physician may perform a cardioversion procedure. Pacemakers control bradycardias. Anxiolytics (e.g., lorazepam [Ativan]) may be helpful to decrease the heart rate by decreasing anxiety. Since beta-blockers decrease contractility, they are contraindicated during cardiogenic shock.

The use of an intraaortic balloon pump (IABP) or ventricular assist device (VAD) achieves afterload reduction without pharmacologic agents. IABP is especially helpful in patients who have very high afterload that is refractory to arterial vasodilators or who are too hypotensive to utilize arterial vasodilators to reduce afterload. IABP or VADs may also serve as a bridge to transplant if the patient is a candidate for cardiac transplantation. The physician inserts a left ventricular assist device or biventricular assist device percutaneously (i.e., Impella). Register the patient for cardiac transplantation if appropriate.

Anaphylactic Shock

Anaphylactic shock results from massive vasodilation caused by the release of histamine in response to a severe allergic reaction. Anaphylaxis is a systemic response to a specific antigen, usually occurring within 1 hour of exposure. Anaphylaxis is an immunoglobulin E (IgE)-mediated response, which is an example of a type I hypersensitivity reaction. Prior exposure to the antigen is required for the development of antibodies to be present in the system to cause the reaction. An anaphylactoid reaction is an anaphylaxis-type reaction triggered by direct activation of the mast cell. This reaction is a nonimmune response and does not require previous exposure to the antigen. The anaphylactoid reaction is clinically indistinguishable from anaphylaxis and acute treatment is the same as for anaphylaxis. The major triggers (Table 10-8) that may cause anaphylaxis are food allergies, drugs, chemicals, venom, and dyes. Foods are the most likely triggers of IgE-mediated-type reactions in adolescents and young adults. The most prominent substances that cause anaphylactoid reactions are drugs and dyes.

The pathophysiology of anaphylaxis (Figure 10-6) is complex. Although the triggers and the initial pathophysiology of anaphylactic and anaphylactoid reactions differ, the pathophysiologic events and clinical presentation after the degranulation of mast cells and basophils are the same.

The clinical presentation for anaphylactic shock is the same as for shock in general as previously described, but many findings are specific to anaphylaxis. The recent history may include exposure to a known or unknown allergen. The patient may complain of anxiety, vague uneasiness, warmth, nausea, abdominal cramping, abdominal pain, chest tightness, palpitations, dyspnea, dizziness, vertigo, pruritus, and a feeling of throat tightness. Objective findings of anaphylactic shock (Table 10-9) involve cutaneous, cardiovascular, pulmonary, neurologic, GI, and genitourinary systems. Anaphylactic shock may quickly lead to hemodynamic compromise and death.

Specific diagnostic serum laboratory and arterial blood gas analyses aid in the differential diagnosis of anaphylactic shock. Serum IgE levels may be used to confirm an allergic origin of the shock. Eosinophils will be elevated in anaphylactic shock. Initially, arterial blood gases show a respiratory alkalosis with hypoxemia. Eventually, respiratory and metabolic acidosis results as hypoventilation and tissue hypoxia occur.

Collaborative management of anaphylactic shock is as for shock in general, but there are several treatments specific to anaphylactic shock. Prevention aims to identify a high-risk patient, avoid exposure to allergens, and monitor closely for clinical indications of allergic reaction and hypoperfusion.

Maintain the patient's airway, oxygenation, and ventilation. Assess the airway for clinical indications of angioedema (i.e., edema of uvula, respiratory distress, stridor, hypoxemia). If angioedema is present, assist with endotracheal tube insertion early to prevent complete airway obstruction. If edema is too severe to allow endotracheal intubation, a cricothyrotomy may be necessary. Administer oxygen at 5 to 6 L initially and adjust to maintain SpO_2 at 95% unless contraindicated. A 100% nonrebreathing mask may be required, but keep in mind that the mask may increase the sensation of dyspnea. Mechanical ventilation may be required.

Remove the offending agent and slow the absorption of antigen. If the anaphylaxis is due to a sting, remove the stinger if possible to do without squeezing. Apply ice to the site of the sting or bite. Discontinue any infusion of dye, drug, or blood if that is the precipitating factor. Perform dermal decontamination with soap and water if the allergen is exposed to skin. Do not initiate gastric lavage to remove ingested antigens due to the risk of aspiration.

Modify or block the effects of biochemical mediators with pharmacologic agents and fluids. Administer the sympathomimetic

TABLE 10-8 **Triggers of IgE-Mediated and Non-IgE Reactions**

	IgE-Mediated Reactions	Non-IgE Anaphylactoid Reactions
Food	• Fish • Shellfish (e.g., shrimp, lobster, crab, scallops) • Eggs • Milk products • Soy • Wheat • Strawberries • Legumes (e.g., peanuts, soybeans) • Nuts (e.g., walnuts, pecans, cashews, almonds) • Chocolate • Food additives (e.g., sulfites, MSG) • Meat tenderizer	

Drugs	• ACE inhibitors (e.g., captopril, enalapril)
	• Acetylcysteine (Mucomyst)
	• Allergic extracts in hyposensitization therapy
	• Allopurinol (Zyloprim)
	• Anesthetics
	  • Local anesthetics: lidocaine, procaine, cocaine
	  • General anesthetics: thiopental, etomidate, ketamine
	• Animal serums: antitoxins, antivenins
	• Antibiotics
	  • Beta-lactam antibiotics
	  • Penicillin
	  • Cephalosporins
	  • Tetracycline
	  • Macrolides
	• Barbiturates
	• Blood and blood products: blood transfusion incompatibilities, albumin
	• Enzymes
	  • Pancreatic
	  • Papaya enzyme
	   — Meat tenderizer
	   — Chymopapain (used in chemical discectomy)
	• Insulin: pork or beef
	• Iodine-containing solutions (e.g., Betadine)
	• Narcotics: morphine, meperidine, codeine
	• Neuromuscular blockers
	• Protamine sulfate
	• Thiazide diuretics (e.g., hydrochlorothiazide)
	• Vaccines
		• Aspirin
		• Nonsteroidal antiinflammatory agents (NSAIDs: ibuprofen, indomethacin)
		• Opiates (morphine, Demerol, codeine)
		• Thiamine
		• Dextran
		• Gamma globulin

Dyes	• Iodine-containing contrast media (e.g., Renografin)	• Radiopaque contrast media • Fluorescein
Venoms	• Snakes • Hymenoptera (e.g., wasps, hornets, bees, yellow jackets, fire ants) • Spiders • Jellyfish • Stingrays • Deer flies • Scorpions	
Chemicals and biologics	• Materials (e.g., latex) • Hand lotions • Soap • Perfume • Animal dander	

agent epinephrine (0.1 mg [100 mcg]) intravenously over 5 to 10 minutes initially as prescribed when clinical indications of cardiovascular compromise are present. Note the difference in dosage from the treatment of 1 mg (1:10,000) epinephrine given for pulseless ventricular tachycardia and ventricular fibrillation. Stop the administration of the epinephrine injection if dysrhythmias or chest pain occurs. Start an IV infusion of epinephrine at 1 to 4 mcg/min if there is an inadequate response to the IV injection. Administer intramuscular epinephrine (0.3-0.5 mg) every 5 to 10 minutes for patients with less severe symptoms; the thigh

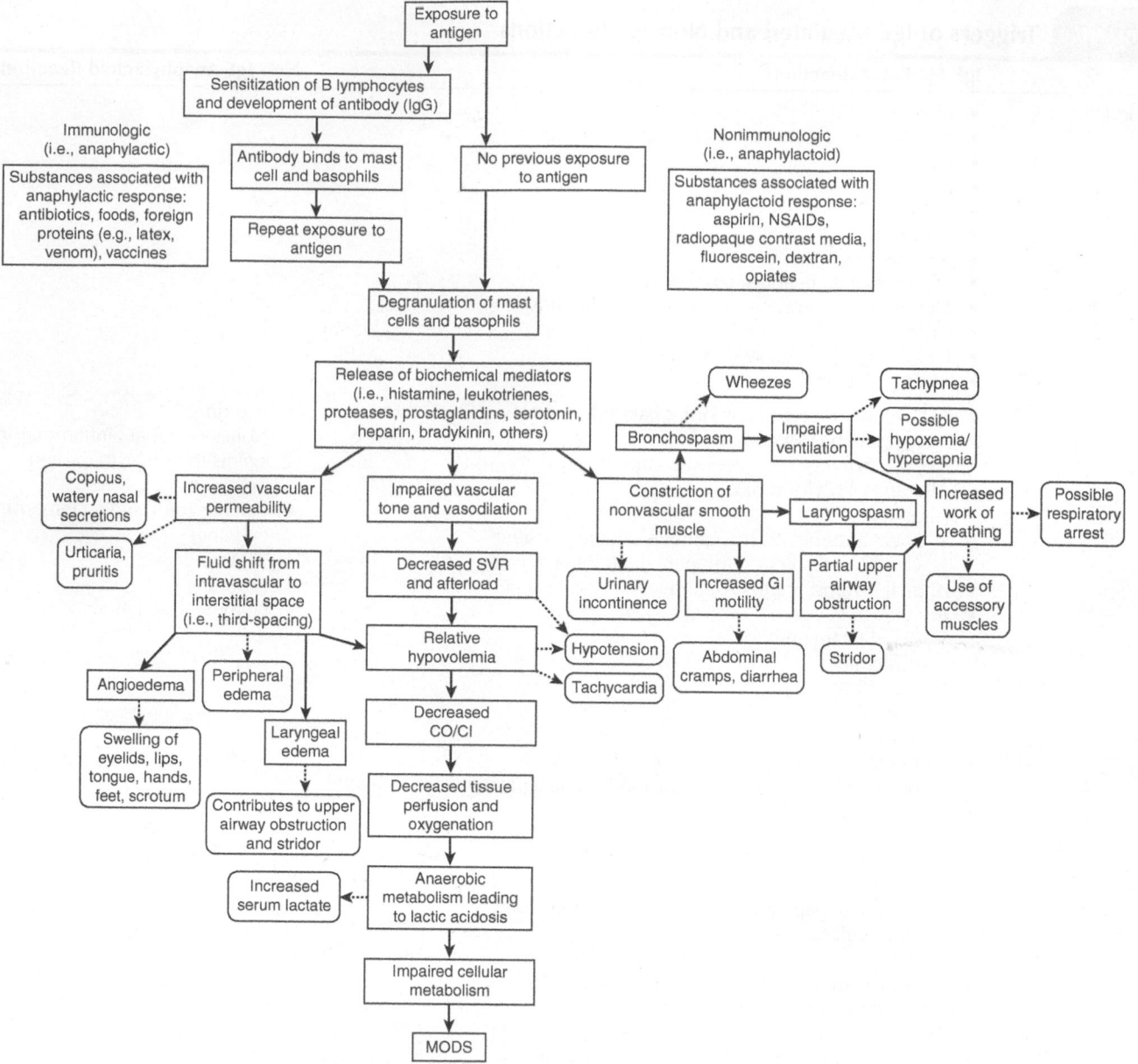

FIGURE 10-6 Pathophysiology of anaphylactic shock. Dotted lines connect pathology to clinical presentation. *CI,* Cardiac index; *CO,* cardiac output; *GI,* gastrointestinal; *NSAID,* nonsteroidal antiinflammatory drug; *SVR,* systemic vascular resistance. (From Dennison, R. D. [2013]. *Pass CCRN!* [4th ed.]. St. Louis, MO: Elsevier.)

is the preferred injection site over the upper arm. Administer IV glucagon (3.5-5 mg) as prescribed for patients taking beta-blockers with hypotension refractory to epinephrine and fluids because glucagon can stimulate an increase in heart rate and contractility even with beta-blockade. Repeat the glucagon if there is no BP response in 10 minutes. Monitor the patient who receives glucagon for nausea, vomiting, hypokalemia, and hyperglycemia.

Administer drugs to block histamine receptors as prescribed. Diphenhydramine (Benadryl) 25 to 50 mg IV, IM, or PO blocks H1 receptors and ranitidine (Zantac) 50 mg IV or famotidine (Pepcid) 20 mg IV blocks H2 receptors. Administer steroids as prescribed to stabilize mast cells, decrease capillary permeability, and prevent any delayed reactions. IV methylprednisolone sodium succinate (Solu-Medrol) 100 mg or hydrocortisone sodium succinate (Solu-Cortef) 100 to 200 or 500 mg is given. Oral prednisone 40 to 60 mg daily may also be used.

Administer bronchodilators as prescribed to reverse the bronchoconstriction caused by histamine, SRS-A, and bradykinin bronchodilators. Albuterol and/or ipratropium bromide (Atrovent) is given via intermittent or a continuous nebulizer for wheezing refractory to epinephrine.

Replace fluids with 1 to 2 L of normal saline as prescribed. To maintain MAP and tissue perfusion, fluids, inotropes, and/or vasopressors may also be necessary.

Neurogenic Shock

Neurogenic shock results from massive vasodilation caused by suppression of the sympathetic nervous system. A cervical or high thoracic (i.e., T6 or above) spinal cord injury is the most common cause. However, note that neurogenic shock is not the same as spinal shock; spinal shock results from a loss of neurologic function below the level of the injury but is not necessarily

TABLE 10-9	Objective Findings Present in Anaphylactic Shock
System	**Objective Findings**
Cutaneous	Local: an identifiable site of allergen exposure, bite, sting, or envenomation may be evident as localized redness, swelling, and pruritus Generalized: • Angioedema (edema of membranous tissues): swelling of eyes, lips, tongue, hands, feet, and genitalia • Flushing • Warm to hot skin • Urticaria • Conjunctival injection, tearing • Watery rhinorrhea, sneezing • Erythema more in upper extremities
Cardiovascular	• Tachycardia • Hypotension • Dysrhythmias • ST and T wave changes consistent with ischemia • Shock • Cardiac arrest may occur
Pulmonary	• Hoarseness • Cough • Prolonged expiration • Breath sound changes: stridor, wheezing, crackles, rhonchi • Respiratory arrest may occur
Neurologic	• Restlessness • Headache • Paresthesia • Change in level of consciousness • Seizures
Gastrointestinal	• Dysphagia • Vomiting • Hyperactive bowel sounds • Diarrhea
Genitourinary	• Urinary incontinence • Urine output: may be decreased • Vaginal bleeding

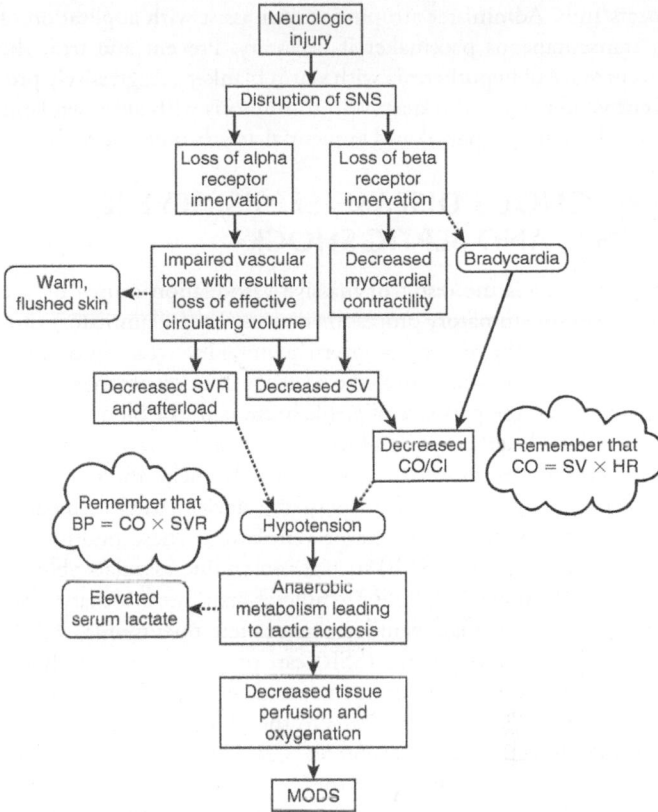

FIGURE 10-7 Pathophysiology of neurogenic shock. Dotted lines connect pathology to clinical presentation. *BP,* blood pressure; *CI,* cardiac index; *CO,* cardiac output; *HR,* heart rate; *MODS,* multiple organ dysfunction syndrome; *SNS,* sympathetic nervous system; *SV,* stroke volume; *SVR,* systemic vascular resistance. (From Dennison, R. D. [2013]. *Pass CCRN!* [4th ed.]. St. Louis, MO: Elsevier.)

associated with inadequate tissue perfusion. Other causes of neurogenic shock include head injury, insulin shock, general anesthesia, spinal anesthesia, epidural block, and drugs such as barbiturates, phenothiazines, and sympathetic blocking agents (e.g., antihypertensives). In addition, exposure to unpleasant circumstances (e.g., fright, pain) may be an etiology of neurogenic shock.

The pathophysiology of neurogenic shock (Figure 10-7) occurs from a disruption of the sympathetic nervous system. Consider that loss of alpha innervation causes vasodilation and loss of beta innervation causes bradycardia and myocardial depression.

The clinical presentation of neurogenic shock is the same as shock in general but with some differences. The recent history may include an identifiable cause of the neurogenic shock. Specific objective findings for neurogenic shock include

bradydysrhythmias that may progress to asystole; hypotension; hypothermia; warm, dry, flushed skin; hemodynamic instability; and neurologic deficit. The neurologic deficits include paralysis below the level of spinal cord injury and neurologic changes related to head injury.

The collaborative management of neurogenic shock is the same as for shock in general as previously discussed with some specific differences. Identify high-risk patients and monitor them closely for clinical indications of hypoperfusion. Prevent further neurologic injury and treat the cause of the neurogenic shock. For instance, implement early immobilization of the spine with suspected spinal injury along with the elevation of the head of the bed to 30 degrees to decrease spinal cord edema. In the case of anesthesia-induced shock, reverse the anesthesia and rewarm the patient. To prevent and treat insulin-related shock, monitor patients for the clinical indications of hypoglycemia and measure serum glucose as required. Administer 10 to 15 g of carbohydrate if the patient is conscious or 50 mL of $D_{50}W$ if unconscious.

Attempt to maintain MAP and tissue perfusion is another major focus of care. Maintain the MAP greater than 70 mm Hg. Administer crystalloids and colloids as prescribed. Hypertonic saline may be used. The colloid albumin has traditionally been advocated, but recent studies and a meta-analysis show no benefit to the use of colloids. Monitor the patient closely for pulmonary or cerebral edema. Administer inotropes and/or vasopressors as prescribed; these may be necessary for hypotension. Maintain the patient's heart rate at 60 to 100 beats/min. Administer atropine and/or assist with application of a transcutaneous pacemaker if necessary. Prevent and treat the occurrence of hypothermia with warm blankets. Aggressively prevent venous stasis and deep vein thrombosis with anticoagulants (e.g., low-dose heparin) and sequential antithrombotic devices.

INFECTIOUS DISEASE, SEPSIS, SEVERE SEPSIS, AND SEPTIC SHOCK

Septic shock is the result of massive vasodilation caused by the release of inflammatory process mediators. The inflammatory process occurs in the response to overwhelming infection. Infection is an inflammatory response to the presence of microorganisms, and bacteremia is the presence of viable bacteria in the blood.

Modern health care employs many types of invasive devices and procedures to treat patients and to help them recover. Infections may be associated with the devices used in medical procedures, such as catheters or ventilators. These health care–associated infections (HAIs) such as central line–associated blood-stream infections (CLABSIs), catheter-associated urinary tract infections (CAUTIs), ventilator-associated pneumonia (VAP), and surgical site infections (SSIs) can progress to sepsis, shock, and death. CLABSIs result in thousands of deaths each year and billions of dollars in added costs to the U.S. health care system, yet these infections are preventable. CAUTIs involve any part of the urinary system, including the urethra, bladder, ureters, and kidneys. CAUTIs are the most common type of HAI reported. Among CAUTIs acquired in the hospital, the majority are associated with an indwelling urinary catheter. The most important risk factor for developing a CAUTI is prolonged use of the urinary catheter; therefore, catheters should only be used for appropriate indications and should be removed as soon as they are no longer needed. An SSI is an infection that occurs after surgery in the surgical area. SSIs can sometimes be superficial infections involving the skin only, but other SSIs are more serious and can involve subcutaneous or deeper tissues under the skin, organs, or implanted material. VAP is a lung infection that develops in a person who is on a ventilator. The infection may occur if microorganisms enter the patient's lungs through the endotracheal tube. The Centers for Disease Control (CDC) provides guidelines and tools to the health care community to prevent and treat these HAIs. All these conditions are frequently a precursor to sepsis, and can lead to septic shock and death. Research has shown that a significant portion of these infections can be prevented.

Sepsis is the systemic inflammatory response syndrome (SIRS) caused by infection. Severe sepsis is associated with organ dysfunction. In septic shock, sepsis is present with hypotension despite adequate fluid resuscitation along with the presence of perfusion abnormalities. Several factors (Table 10-10) influence the development of septic shock. Immunosuppression and factors that cause bacteremia and septicemia, and microorganisms influence the development of septic shock. The gram-negative bacteria *Escherichia coli, Enterobacter,* and *Pseudomonas aeruginosa* are the most likely microorganisms to cause the problem. Other gram-negative bacteria, gram-positive bacteria, viruses, fungi, and parasites can cause septic shock but are less likely. However, drug-resistant gram-positive bacteria are increasingly the cause of sepsis.

The pathophysiology of septic shock (Figure 10-8) is complex involving a multitude of mediators and mechanisms. Endothelial cell dysfunction causes pathologic changes in all organ systems.

TABLE 10-10	Factors Influencing the Development of Septic Shock
Factors	**Etiology**
Immunosuppression	• Extremes of age • Malnutrition • Alcoholism or drug abuse • Debilitation • Malignancy • AIDS • History of splenectomy • Chronic health problems (diabetes mellitus, liver disease, heart disease [e.g., coronary artery disease or heart failure], renal failure) • Bone marrow suppression • Immunosuppressive therapies (e.g., immunosuppressive drugs, antineoplastic drugs, antibiotic therapy, corticosteroids)
Mechanisms of exposure to microorganisms	• Invasive procedures and devices • Pulmonary procedures • Diagnostic procedures • Surgical procedures or wounds • Traumatic wounds or burns • Genitourinary infection • Untreated GI disease (cholelithiasis, intestinal obstruction, appendicitis, diverticulitis) • Peritonitis • Food poisoning • Prolonged hospitalization • Translocation of GI bacteria (NPO status, decreased peristalsis, and GI ischemia contribute to proliferation of GI bacteria and translocation of these bacteria into blood or lymph)
Microorganisms	Gram-negative bacteria • *Escherichia coli* • *Klebsiella* • *Enterobacter* • *Pseudomonas aeruginosa* • *Proteus mirabilis* • *Enterococcus* • *Serratia marcescens* • *Bacteroides* organisms • *Haemophilus influenzae* Gram-positive organisms • *Staphylococcus aureus* • *Staphylococcus epidermidis* • *Streptococcus pneumoniae* • *Clostridium* organisms • *Pneumococcus* Other organisms • Viruses • Fungi • *Rickettsia* • *Spirochaeta* • Protozoa • Parasites

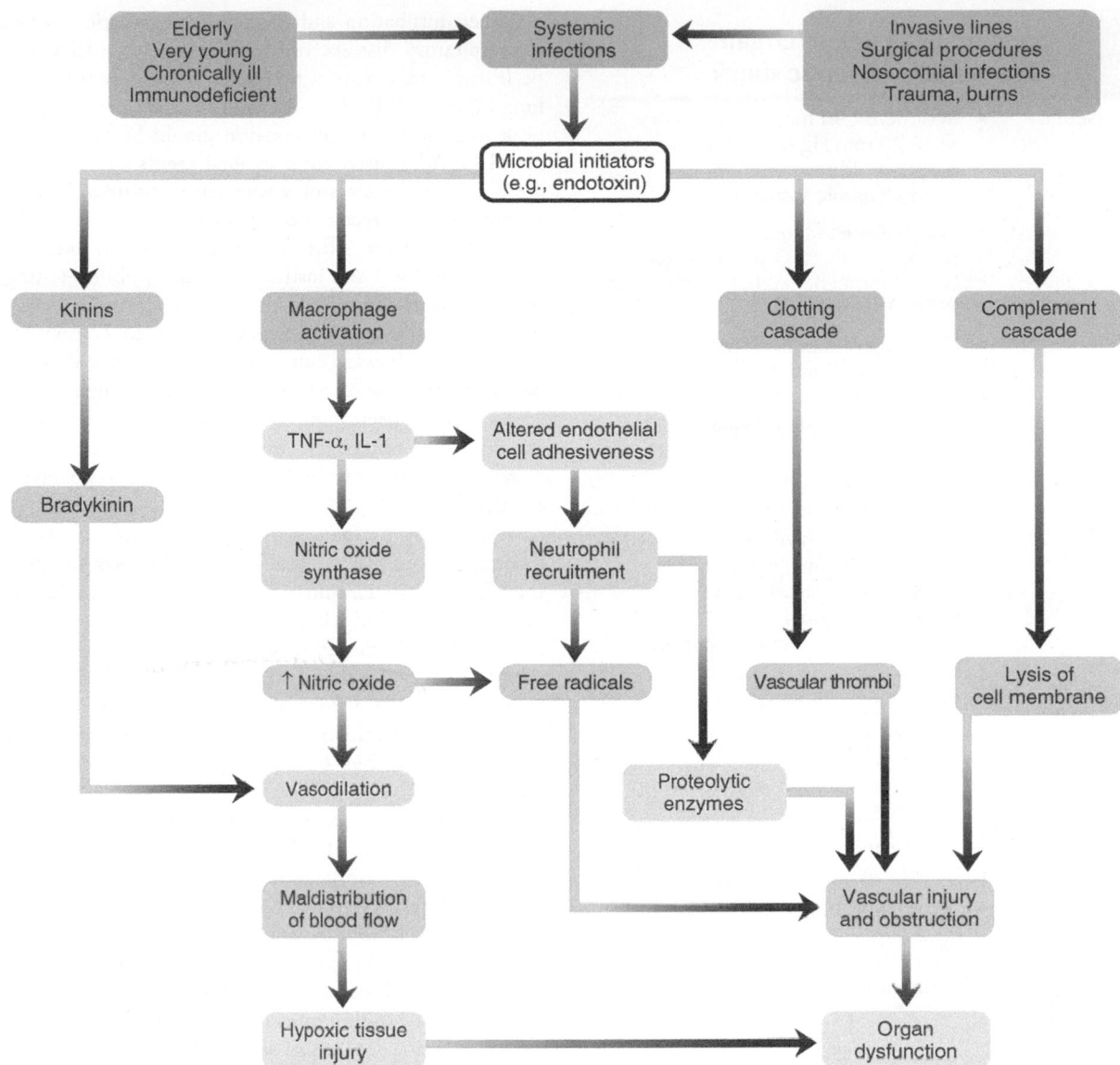

FIGURE 10-8 Pathophysiology of septic shock. (From Copstead, L., & Banasik, J. [2013]. *Pathophysiology* [5th ed.]. St. Louis, MO: Saunders.)

The recent history of a patient with septic shock includes documented or suspected infection. In addition to the manifestations of infection, such as fever and altered mental status, the patient will also exhibit evidence of two or more of the SIRS criteria (see Table 10-1). In the case of severe sepsis, there is evidence of organ dysfunction (Table 10-11) along with the sepsis criteria. Clinical indications of global hypoxia including a systolic BP of 90 mm Hg or less or MAP of 65 mm Hg or less and a serum lactate of at least 4 mmol/L are present in septic shock.

Although the collaborative management for septic shock is the same as for shock as previously discussed, there are significant additions. Identify a high-risk patient and monitor closely for clinical indications of infection and sepsis. Assess patients for hyperthermia, increased respiratory rate, elevated glucose caused by insulin resistance, poor gastric motility and retention of enteral feedings, and elevated serum lactate despite a clinical picture of increased cardiac index. Employ prevention measures to prevent infection and sepsis. Use good hand washing techniques, prevent cross-contamination, and avoid intrusive procedures if possible. Implement patient care measures to facilitate early identification of infection. Monitor color and characteristics of sputum, urine, stools, wounds, etc. Culture secretions and wounds as indicated. Prepare the patient for surgery for any of the following:

- Removal of all necrotic tissue
- Drainage of abscess
- Early debridement of burn eschar
- Prompt stabilization of fractures to minimize soft tissue damage, inflammation, and infection

Perform meticulous oral and airway care. Implement measures to prevent VAP. Provide IV, intraarterial, pulmonary artery, and urinary catheter care according to CDC guidelines or hospital policy. Render meticulous wound care based on the appearance of wounds. If possible, avoid NPO status on patients to prevent translocation of enteric bacteria into the lymphatics and vascular bed. Give enteral feedings if possible. Prophylactic antibiotic therapy is controversial today as more and more microorganisms become resistant to available antibiotic therapy.

TABLE 10-11	Specific Evidence of Organ Dysfunction in Septic shock
Cardiovascular	• Systolic BP 90 mm Hg or less or MAP 70 mm Hg or less for 1 hour despite fluid resuscitation • Hemodynamic instability
Respiratory	• PaO_2/FiO_2 less than 250 • Bilateral infiltrates on chest x-ray • Need for mechanical ventilation and PEEP greater than 7.5 cm H_2O
Renal	• Doubling of baseline creatinine or 2 times upper limit of normal • Urine output less than 0.5 mL/kg/hr for 1 hour despite adequate fluid resuscitation
Hematologic	• Platelet reduction • Thrombocytopenia less than 100,000 platelets/mm^3 • Decrease of platelets by 50% from highest value in last 3 days • INR greater than 1.2 • PTT/aPTT greater than upper limit of normal • Increased D-dimer
Metabolic	• pH less than 7.3 (or base deficit greater than 5) • Serum lactate more than upper limit of normal
Central nervous system	• Altered LOC • Confusion
Hepatic	• Serum bilirubin greater than 2 mg/dL for 2 days • Liver enzymes greater than 2 times upper limit of normal

Many physicians prefer to have clinical indications of infection before prescribing antibiotic therapy.

The focus of collaborative management is on restoration of tissue perfusion, normalization of cellular metabolism, and provision of early goal-directed therapy during the first 6 hours after severe sepsis or septic shock is recognized. The use of evidence-based guidelines (Figure 10-9) is crucial in reducing mortality.

When an infection is suspected or confirmed, two or more indications of SIRS (see Table 10-1) are present, the MAP is less than 65 mm Hg after 20 mL/kg fluid bolus, and/or serum lactate is at least 4 mmol/L, initiate the treatment guidelines to achieve the following:

• CVP of 8-12 mm Hg
• MAP of 65 mm Hg or greater
• SvO_2 of 70% or greater
• Urine output greater than 0.5 mL/kg/hr

Recommendations for resuscitation and management also include intubation and mechanical ventilation, cultures, antimicrobials, fluid replacement, pharmacologic agents, removal of toxins, correction of hypothermia, and the monitoring complications of shock and clinical indications of organ failure (Marik, 2011)

When intubation and mechanical ventilation are required for respiratory distress, use low settings of tidal volume and peak inspiratory plateau pressures to avoid ventilator-induced lung injury (VILI). The tidal volume is set at 6 mL/kg and the peak inspiratory plateau pressure should be no more than 30 cm H_2O. Administer antimicrobial agents after blood cultures are obtained. In cases of severe sepsis, initiate antimicrobials within 1 hour of recognition of severe sepsis; it is not necessary to wait for cultures. The clinical presentation, likely microorganism, and local and institutional susceptibility testing guide the administration of broad-spectrum antimicrobials with a planned reassessment of efficacy after 48 to 72 hours (Levins, 2010). When drawing cultures, one blood draw should be percutaneous and one blood draw should be through each vascular access that has been in place for more than 48 hours. Cultures should also be obtained from other sites (e.g., CSF, pulmonary secretions, urine, or wound) when indicated as possible sources of infection.

Implement preload correction measures if the CVP is less than 8 mm Hg. Crystalloid fluid boluses are given until the CVP is 8 to 12 mm Hg. Colloids are not indicated and may be harmful and hypertonic crystalloids are not recommended at this time. If the CVP is more than 15 mm Hg and the MAP is greater than 110 mm Hg, nitroglycerin is administered until the CVP is less than 12 or the MAP is less than 90 mm Hg. Afterload correction measures are instituted if the MAP is less than 65 mm Hg after 2 L of crystalloids are given.

Administer vasopressors as necessary to maintain a MAP of at least 65 mm Hg. If the diastolic BP is less than 40 mm Hg, start vasopressors immediately and concurrently with fluid resuscitation (Marik, 2011). The initial agent advocated is norepinephrine (2-20 mcg/min), but dopamine (5-20 mcg/kg/min) may also be used. A recent large, prospective multicenter randomized controlled trial (SOAP trial) indicated higher mortality with use of dopamine versus norepinephrine. This same study also found a higher mortality in patients with shock receiving steroids and dopamine (DeBacker et al., 2010). Previously, low-dose dopamine (less than 5 mcg/kg/min) was thought to provide renal protection and is currently not advocated. Phenylephrine is preferred if the heart rate is greater than 120 beats/min. Vasopressin at 0.03 units/min should be added if the patient remains hypotensive despite a reasonable dose of norepinephrine. Very low doses (0.01-0.04 units/min) of vasopressin improve MAP in septic shock. Terlipressin, a longer-acting synthetic analog of vasopressin, has a longer half-life and has similar hemodynamic effects to vasopressin. The use of these agents requires an arterial catheter for continuous monitoring of blood pressure. In addition, consider corticosteroids if the patient is vasopressor dependent. A cosyntropin stimulation test is recommended. To perform this test, a baseline cortisol level is drawn, and then ACTH 250 mcg is given intravenously with a remeasurement of cortisol at 30 and 60 minutes. A change in the cortisol level of less than 9 mcg/dL suggests adrenal insufficiency. If the cosyntropin stimulation test is negative, hydrocortisone 50 mg IV every 6 hours along with fludrocortisone 50 mcg PO daily is recommended for the adrenal insufficiency in severe sepsis. If the MAP is greater than 110 mm Hg, nitrates such as nitroglycerin or hydralazine may be used.

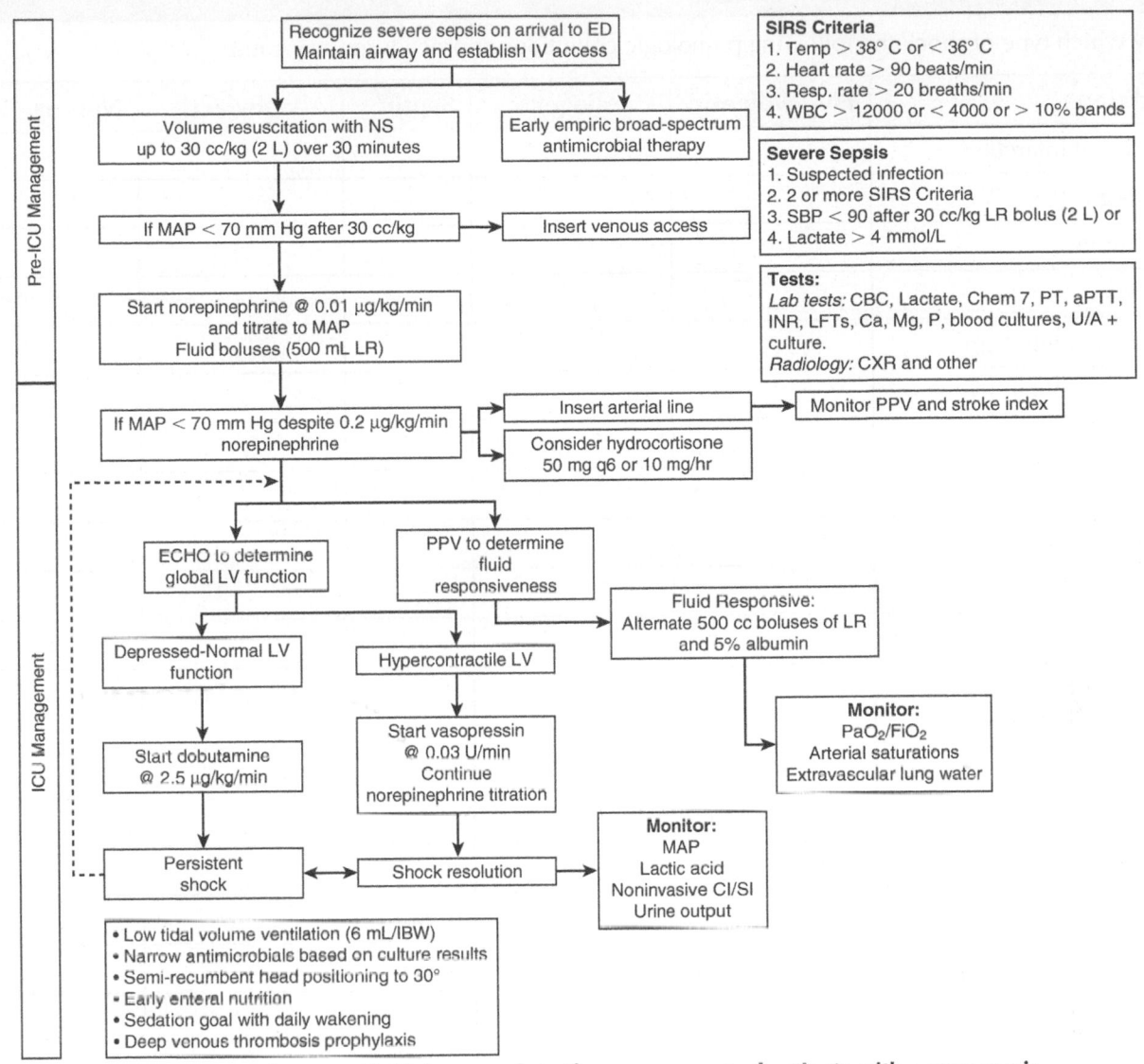

FIGURE 10-9 Suggested initial approach to the management of patients with severe sepsis and septic shock. *Ca,* Calcium; *CI,* cardiac index; *ED,* emergency department; *IBW,* ideal body weight; *ICU,* intensive care unit; *INR,* international normalized ratio; *LFT,* liver function test; *LR,* lactated Ringer's; *LV,* left ventricular; *MAP,* mean arterial pressure; *Mg,* magnesium; *NS,* normal saline; *P,* phosphate; *PPV,* pulse pressure variation; *PT,* prothrombin time; *aPTT,* activated partial prothrombin time; *SBP,* systolic blood pressure; *SI,* stroke index; *SIRS,* systemic inflammatory response syndrome; *U/A,* urinalysis; *WBC,* white blood cell. (Adapted from Marik, P. E. [2011]. Surviving sepsis: Going beyond the guidelines. *Ann Intensive Care, 1*[1], 17.)

Provide several measures to optimize oxygen delivery. If the ScvO₂ is less than 70% after the earlier-listed therapies and the hemoglobin is less than 10 g/dL, administer red blood cells. Platelets are indicated if the platelet counts are less than 5000/mm³ or when less than 30,000/mm³ if there is significant risk for bleeding. If the ScvO₂ is less than 70% after earlier-listed therapies and hemoglobin is greater than 10 g/dL, administer dobutamine (Dobutrex) or dopamine (Intropin). If the heart rate is more than 120 beats/min, digoxin may be considered. Administer prescribed corticosteroids in an effort to decrease inflammation and antithrombotic aspects of sepsis. Control of serum glucose as described in the general discussion of shock is a priority.

Administer antimicrobials to treat infection and neutralize toxins. Prepare the patient for surgical procedures such as the

drainage of an abscess, debridement of a wound, and reduction of a fracture. Use of experimental therapies may be implemented, but these may only be available for compassionate use. Employ efforts to control hyperthermia. Monitor the patient's core body temperature. Administer antipyretics as indicated with recognition that fever is an important defense mechanism (Cunha, 2012). The indications for treatment of fever include severe cardiopulmonary disease with body temperatures greater than 38.8° C (102° F), brain injury, and extreme hyperpyrexia (i.e., body temperature greater than 41.1° C [106° F]). The treatment guidelines recommend reducing temperatures slowly to 38.8° C (102° F) to prevent chills, shivering, and a rebound increase in body temperature. Treatment includes the use of antipyretics (e.g., acetaminophen) and environmental cooling methods such as fans, cooling blankets, and tepid soaks.

10.6 Learning Activity

Identify which type of shock the following pathologic conditions or procedures may cause.

Condition	Hypovolemic	Cardiogenic	Septic	Anaphylactic	Neurogenic
Myocardial infarction					
Bee sting					
Head injury					
Diarrhea					
Pulmonary embolism					
Ruptured gallbladder					
Esophageal varices					
Ruptured papillary muscle					
Insulin shock					
Ascites					
IVP dye					
Cervical or high thoracic spinal cord injury					
Invasive procedures					
Burns					
Blood transfusion reaction					
Spinal anesthesia					
Trauma					
Malnutrition					
Chemotherapy					

Answers to this activity can be found in the Answer Key.

10.7 Learning Activity

Match the specific therapies with the type of shock for which they may be used. You may list more than one therapy for each form of shock, and the therapies may be used more than once.

_____ 1. Anaphylactic
_____ 2. Cardiogenic
_____ 3. Hypovolemic
_____ 4. Neurogenic
_____ 5. Septic

a. Intravenous fluids
b. Corticosteroids
c. Blood
d. Vasopressors
e. Inotropes
f. Intraaortic balloon pump (IABP)
g. Pacemaker
h. Epinephrine
i. Antihistamines
j. Antimicrobials
k. Treatment of cause
l. Oxygen
m. Vasodilators

Answers to this activity can be found in the Answer Key.

SYSTEMIC INFLAMMATORY RESPONSE SYNDROME AND MULTIPLE ORGAN DYSFUNCTION SYNDROME

Systemic inflammatory response syndrome (SIRS) is the extensive inflammation or the clinical response to that inflammation that can occur in patients with disorders such as infection, pancreatitis, ischemia, multiple traumas, shock, or immunologically mediated organ injury. Multiple organ dysfunction syndrome (MODS) is the presence of progressive impairment of function in two or more organ systems in an acutely ill patient such that maintenance of homeostasis is lost without intervention. MODS may be either primary or secondary. Primary MODS occurs when there is a direct injury to the specific dysfunctional organ. Secondary MODS occurs as a sequel to trauma or infection that results in the systemic inflammatory response and dysfunction of organs elsewhere in the body.

There are several etiologies for the development of SIRS. SIRS can develop from mechanical tissue damage from trauma, burns, crush injuries, and surgical procedures. Intraabdominal and intracranial abscesses, ischemic/necrotic tissue due to prolonged shock, MI, pancreatitis, and DIC may also lead to SIRS

development. Microbial invasion, especially in patients with immunosuppressed states during surgery/trauma, community exposure, and/or nosocomial exposure, is a common cause of SIRS. Endotoxin release from gram-negative sepsis and translocation of bacteria from the gut are other causes of SIRS. Sepsis is the most common single etiologic factor, but 40% to 50% of MODS patients do not have positive blood cultures. Patients with global perfusion deficits from shock and cardiopulmonary arrest and regional perfusion deficits such as vascular injury, vascular repair procedures, and thromboembolic events are also at risk for the development of SIRS. Acute direct injury to an organ or organs, or a secondary response due to SIRS causes MODS.

The pathophysiology of MODS (Figure 10-10) is similar to sepsis and involves the action of multiple mediators and endothelial injury. The result is hypoxia, tissue ischemia, and damage to multiple organs. The patient with MODS may have some or all of the clinical findings in Box 10-1.

SIRS clinical presentation demonstrates two or more of the established criteria related to heart rate, respiratory rate, temperature, and white blood cell count (see Table 10-1). There are risk factors, potential inflammatory/immune effects, and complications (Table 10-12) for each body system.

10.8 Learning Activity

Complete the following table that describes the four physiologic alterations that are likely to be seen in systemic inflammatory response syndrome (SIRS). The criteria for SIRS are two of these four parameters.

Heart rate	Greater than _____			
Respiratory rate	Greater than _____	OR	Paco$_2$	Less than _____
Temperature	Greater than _____	OR	Less than _____	
WBC	Greater than _____	OR	Less than _____	

Answers to this activity can be found in the Answer Key.

In MODS, the defined parameters and degree of organ dysfunction (Table 10-13) range from normal to severe. Each organ system demonstrates specific dysfunction (Table 10-14) parameters reflective of MODS.

Collaborative management of a patient with SIRS and MODS focuses on the prevention and treatment of any infection and improvement of oxygen delivery to the tissues. Prevent and treat infection the same as discussed in the previous septic shock discussion. To maximize oxygen delivery, maintain the patient's cardiac index, Hct, and SaO$_2$. Maintain the cardiac index within normal limits because increasing the cardiac index to 4.5 L/min/m^2 or greater is effective in reducing mortality. Administer crystalloid fluids only because of increased capillary permeability in these conditions. Administer inotropes (e.g., dobutamine) as prescribed. Administer vasopressors (e.g., dopamine, norepinephrine) as prescribed when SVR is

very low and adequate filling volume established. Maintain Hct at approximately 30% to 32% and administer blood and blood products as prescribed. Correct coagulopathies with the administration of fresh frozen plasma, platelets, and vitamin K as prescribed. Maintain SaO$_2$ greater than 95%. Ensure adequate airway, administer oxygen, and initiate mechanical ventilation with PEEP as needed. Monitor the patient's SvO$_2$ for decreased SvO$_2$ to less than 60%, which indicates that oxygen delivery is impaired or oxygen consumption is increased. Assess the patient's SaO$_2$, cardiac index, and Hgb levels along with causes of increased consumption (e.g., shivering, fever, seizures). Increased SvO$_2$ to greater than 80% indicates that oxygen extraction is impaired. Continue to minimize oxygen consumption of the tissues, maintain or improve nutritional status, and monitor for complications such as shock, organ failure, and death as discussed in the previous shock section.

10.9 Learning Activity

Match the sign/symptom of dysfunction with the organ that is dysfunctional.

_____ 1. Brain
_____ 2. Heart
_____ 3. Blood
_____ 4. Kidneys
_____ 5. Liver
_____ 6. Lungs

a. Decreased PaO_2/FiO_2 ratio
b. Oliguria
c. Hypoglycemia
d. Decrease in Glasgow Coma Scale score
e. Prolonged PT, aPTT, decreased platelets
f. Increased CVP/PAOP

Answers to this activity can be found in the Answer Key.

10.10 Synthesis Learning Activity: Crossword Puzzle

Complete the following crossword puzzle related to shock, SIRS, and MODS.

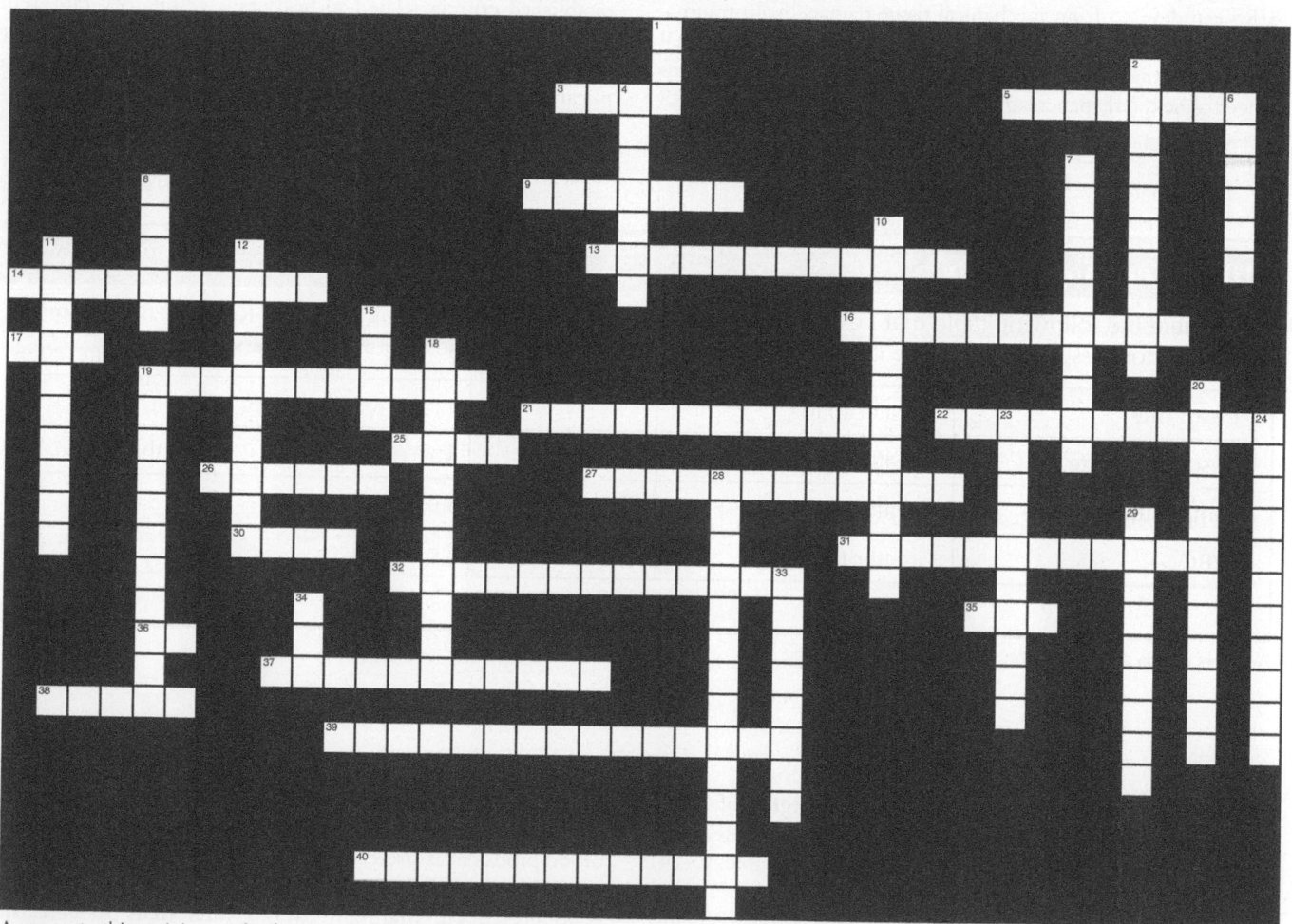

Answers to this activity can be found in the Answer Key.

ACROSS

3. The frequently fatal result of SIRS; previously referred to as multisystem organ failure (abbrev.)
5. Type of IV fluids that are used to increase intravascular colloidal oncotic pressure

9. This stage of shock is associated with a decrease in tissue oxygenation but no clinical indications of hypoperfusion
13. This type of drug may be used in vasogenic shock to restore normal vascular tone (plural)

14. The type of shock caused by suppression of the sympathetic nervous system
16. The first-line drug for anaphylactic shock (generic)
17. The type of coagulopathy seen in MODS (abbrev.)

19. A complication of administering large volumes of IV fluid and blood that may cause shifting of the oxyhemoglobin dissociation curve to the left
21. This type of drug may be used to decrease preload or afterload in cardiogenic shock (plural)

22. The type of shock caused by the inability of the heart to pump effectively
25. A mechanical therapy used in cardiogenic shock to increase CAPP and decrease afterload (abbrev.)
26. Infection with SIRS
27. This type of shock is caused by antigen-antibody response, IgE, and the release of histamine and other mediators
30. The type of acute respiratory failure seen in MODS (abbrev.)
31. This type of IV fluid contains solutes and may be categorized as hypotonic, isotonic, or hypertonic
32. An anaphylactic-like reaction that does not require previous exposure; not mediated by IgE, and probably triggered by the complement system
35. The type of acute kidney injury seen in MODS (abbrev.)

36. The most common cause of cardiogenic shock (abbrev.)
37. The stage of shock when compensatory mechanisms are no longer effective in maintaining tissue perfusion
38. The condition of insufficient perfusion of cells and vital organs
39. H1 receptor antagonist (generic)
40. The consequence of muscle destruction; may cause renal failure

DOWN

1. The branch of the autonomic nervous system responsible for the early compensatory response to hypoperfusion in shock (abbrev.)
2. The inotropic agent used most often in cardiogenic shock (generic)

4. A colloid solution that contains large starch molecules; affects platelet aggregation
6. This type of shock is associated with mediator release in response to overwhelming infection
7. The presence of viable bacteria in the blood
8. This type of IV infusion is required for hemorrhage to the point of hypoperfusion
10. The stage of shock dominated by neuroendocrine responses to hypoperfusion
11. The drug most commonly associated with anaphylactic shock (generic)
12. The term for the edema of the mucous membranes seen in anaphylactic shock
15. A systemic response of the immune system to microorganisms, tissue trauma, toxins, burns, etc. (abbrev.)

18. An alkaline buffer used for severe metabolic acidosis
19. Type of shock caused by loss of intravascular volume
20. Third-spacing is the shift of fluid from the intravascular space to the _____ space, pleural space, pericardial space, and peritoneal space
23. The stage of shock associated with irreversible organ damage
24. VO_2 is oxygen _____
28. A consequence of hemolytic blood transfusion reaction; may cause renal failure
29. The mediator seen in anaphylactic shock that causes vasodilation and increased capillary permeability
33. DO_2 is oxygen _____
34. The hemodynamic parameter that is increased in hypovolemic and cardiogenic shock (abbrev.)

COMPLEX WOUNDS

Complex wound is the term used recently to group those well-known difficult wounds, either chronic or acute, that challenge medical and nursing teams. The major groups of complex wounds (Table 10-15) include diabetic wounds, pressure sores, chronic venous ulcers, postinfection soft tissue gangrene, and ulcers resulting from vasculitis. These wounds defy cure using conventional and simple dressing therapy and currently have a major socioeconomic impact. Often, patients receive treatment of these complex wounds in the progressive care unit by multidisciplinary teams.

In most cases, surgical treatment of these types of wounds is unavoidable, because the extent of skin and subcutaneous tissue loss requires reconstruction with grafts and flaps. New technologies, such as the negative pressure device (i.e., wound vac), have been used on these wounds with some success. Wound care may be broadly divided into nonoperative and operative methods. For stage I and II pressure ulcers, wound care is usually conservative (i.e., nonoperative). For stage III and IV lesions, surgical intervention (e.g., flap reconstruction) may be required, though conservative treatment occurs on some of these lesions because of coexisting medical problems. Approximately 70% to 90% of pressure ulcers are superficial and heal by secondary intention. Successful medical management of complex pressure ulcers and other types of complex wounds relies on the following key principles:

- Reduction of pressure
- Adequate debridement of necrotic and devitalized tissue
- Control of infection
- Meticulous wound care

Immediately after wounding, tissue repair begins with hemostasis. Healing then involves a complex chain of events coordinated by key cells, principally macrophages, which use an array of polypeptide growth factors. These newly identified factors act to induce migration and multiplication of cells, as well as the production of other growth factors. The interrelated processes of epithelialization, angiogenesis, fibroplasia, and collagen synthesis occur only when appropriate cells receive growth factor–encoded signals.

Comprehensive wound management includes prevention. Patients at risk of developing chronic wounds such as pressure sores or venous ulcers should be watched and receive appropriate preventive measures. The use of a grading scale, such as the Braden scale, estimates the risk, and surveillance of inpatients at risk has reduced the incidence of pressure sores. The assessment of existing wounds includes consideration of factors that can affect healing, such as nutrition, hydration, diabetes, or ischemia. Management consists of debridement, the control of infection, and the promotion of natural healing.

The modern view of wound care considers a wound to be a temporary structure established to effect healing. Following this view, the design of modern dressings nurtures the cellular environment of the wound. A myriad of dressing materials are available. Ultimately, dressing design may resemble the technology of tissue culture. Previously, there were prolonged hospital stays for chronic wound treatment with multiple and frequently painful dressing changes. Currently, there are insufficient resources to allow chronic inpatient treatment of all wounds and patients are less prepared to accept prolonged morbidity. New parameters for dressings have emerged. A dressing is no longer a passive adjunct to healing, but is an active element of wound management designed to debride the wound, control infection, and promote

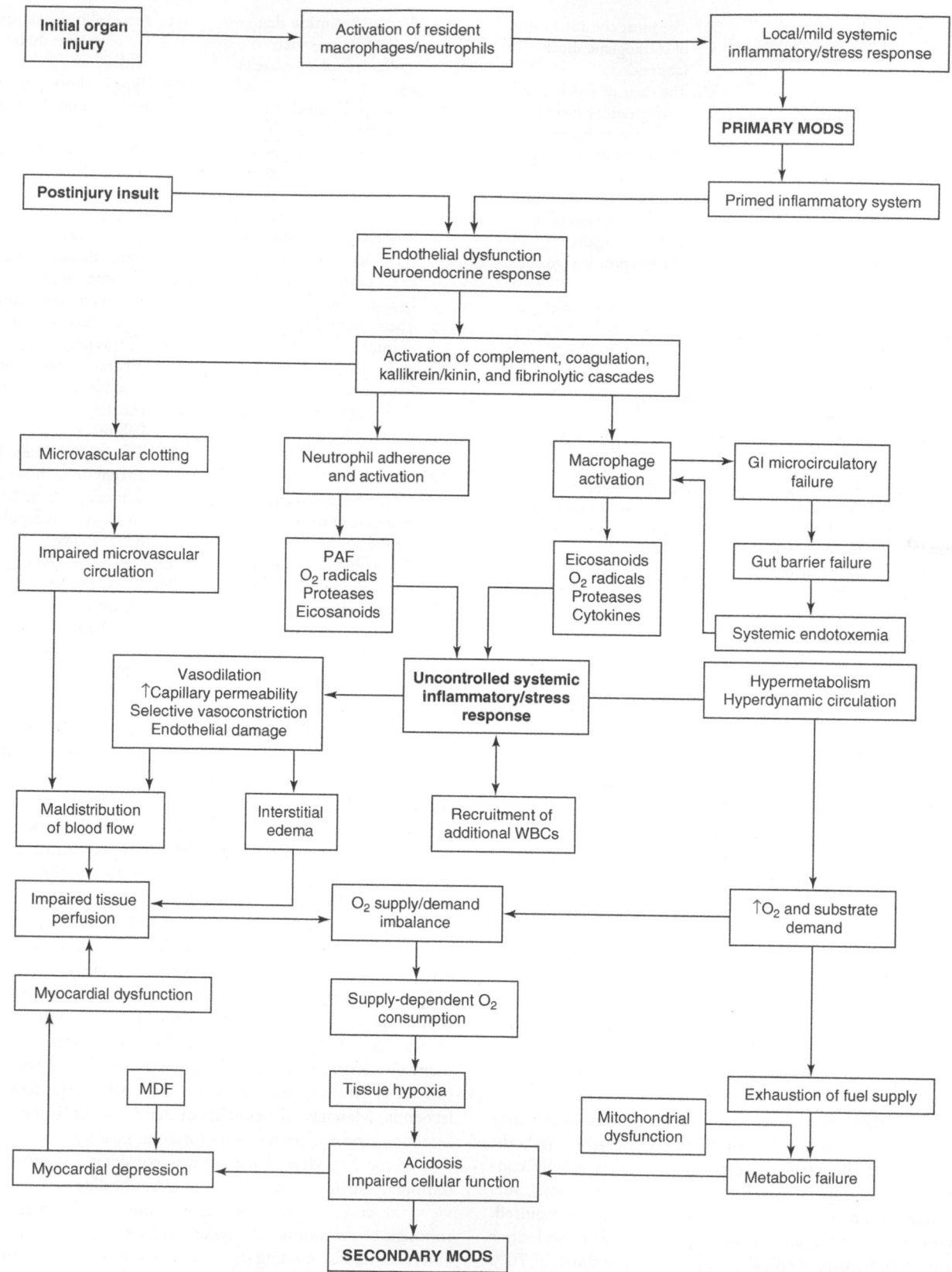

FIGURE 10-10 **Pathophysiology of multiple organ dysfunction syndrome (MODS).** *GI,* Gastrointestinal; *MDF,* myocardial depressant factor; *PAF,* platelet-activating factor; *WBC,* white blood cell. (From McCance, K. L., & Huether, S. E. [2014]. *Pathophysiology: The biologic basis for disease in adults and children* [7th ed.]. St. Louis, MO: Mosby.)

TABLE 10-12 Systems Assessment with Potential Inflammatory/Immune Effect and Complications

System	Risk Factors	Effect on IIR	Assessment	Potential Complications
CNS	• Invasive drains • ICP monitoring • Surgical incision • Cranial nerve involvement • Spinal cord injury	• Increased microbial access • IIR activation • Impaired natural defenses	• LOC, GCS • CCP • Inflammation at wound • Respiratory depression • Skin breakdown	• CNS infection • Aspiration • Corneal abrasions • Skin breakdown
Pulmonary	• Artificial airway • Mechanical ventilation • Barotrauma • High FiO_2 levels	• Bypass of natural airway defenses • Increased microbial access • Activation of alveolar macrophages with toxic mediator release • Altered surfactant production	• Dyspnea • Use of accessory muscles • Thick, discolored sputum • Wheezes, crackles, rhonchi • Decreased compliance • Increased V/Q mismatching • Increased intrapulmonary shunt infiltrates on chest x-ray • Respiratory acidosis ($\downarrow$ pH, $\uparrow$ $PaCO_2$) • Hypoxemia ($\downarrow$ PaO_2, $\downarrow$ SaO_2, SpO_2) • Hypoxia ($\downarrow$ SvO_2, $\uparrow$ lactate)	• Aspiration • Atelectasis • Pneumonia • ARDS • Oxygen toxicity
CV	• Invasive monitoring • Poor perfusion	• Increased microbial access • Tissue ischemia → IIR activation with third spacing and edema • Cellular activation and mediator release	• Changes in HR, BP, CO/CI, PAP, PAOP, CVP/RAP, SVR • Cold, pale skin • Inflammation at access sites • Diminished pulses • Narrowed pulse pressure • Urine output • Dysrhythmias • Myocardial ischemia or infarction • Positive cardiac isoenzymes, troponin • $\uparrow$ lactate	• Reperfusion injury • Cellulitis • Bacteremia/sepsis • Endothelial damage and clotting abnormalities
GI	• Nasogastric tube • Antacid therapy • H_2-blocker therapy • Stress ulceration • Antibiotics • Ileus	• Gastric pH → bacterial colonization • IIR activation • Inhibition of normal flora's protective function • Inability to clear bacterial load	• Bowel sounds • Upper or lower GI bleeding • Abdominal distention • Diarrhea • Constipation, impaction • Ileus • Stress ulceration/erosion • Guaiac + stool • Enteric organisms on blood culture • Jaundice • Ascites • Drug clearance • Abnormal bleeding • Liver enzymes • Hypoglycemia • Ammonia • Plasma proteins • Clotting factors • Hepatomegaly/splenomegaly	• Colonization of esophagus and tracheobronchial tree • Pneumonia • Overgrowth of pathogenic organisms in the GI tract (e.g., *C. difficile*) • Translocation of bacteria to the lymph and blood

TABLE 10-12	Systems Assessment with Potential Inflammatory/Immune Effect and Complications—cont'd

System	Risk Factors	Effect on IIR	Assessment	Potential Complications
GU	• Bladder catheter • Antibiotics • Hyperglycemia	• Increased microbial access • Altered normal flora in vagina • Promotion of yeast growth	• Changes in urine output • Malodorous urine or vaginal discharge • Peripheral edema • CVP/RAP, PAP, PAOP • BUN and creatinine • Metabolic acidosis (↓ pH, ↓ HCO_3)	• Urinary tract infection • Septicemia • *Candida* infections

ARDS, Acute respiratory distress syndrome; *BP,* blood pressure; *BUN,* blood urea nitrogen; *CCP,* cerebral perfusion pressure; *CNS,* central nervous system; *CO/CI,* cardiac output/cardiac index; *CV,* cardiovascular; *CVP/RAP,* central venous pressure/right atrial pressure; *FiO₂,* fraction of inspired oxygen; *GCS,* Glasgow Coma Score; *GI,* gastrointestinal; *GU,* genitourinary; *H₂,* histamine type 2 receptor; *HCO₃,* bicarbonate; *HR,* heart rate; *ICP,* intracranial pressure; *IIR,* inflammatory/immune response; *LOC,* level of consciousness; *Paco₂,* partial pressure of carbon dioxide in arterial blood; *PaO₂,* partial pressure of oxygen in arterial blood; *PAOP,* pulmonary artery occlusive pressure; *PAP,* pulmonary artery pressure; *SaO₂,* oxygen saturation of hemoglobin in arterial blood; *SpO₂,* oxygen saturation of hemoglobin by pulse oximetry; *SvO₂,* oxygen saturation of hemoglobin in venous blood; *SVR,* systemic vascular resistance.
Adapted from Huddleston Secor, V. (1996). *Multiple organ dysfunction & failure: Pathophysiology and clinical implications* (2nd ed.). St Louis, MO: Mosby.

TABLE 10-13	Definitions of Degrees of Organ Dysfunction

Organ System	Parameter	Normal	Organ Dysfunction			
			Mild	Moderate	Severe	Extreme
CV	Systolic BP (mm Hg)	Greater than 90	Less than 90 but fluid responsive	Less than 90, not fluid responsive	Less than 90, not fluid responsive	Less than 90, not fluid responsive
	Arterial pH	At least 7.3	At least 7.3	At least 7.3	Less than 7.3	Less than 7.2
Pulmonary	PaO₂/FiO₂ (mm Hg)	Greater than 400	301-400	201-300	101-200	Less than 100
CNS	GCS	15	13-14	10-12	7-9	At least 6
Coagulation	Platelet count (1000/mL)	Greater than 120	81-102	51-80	21-50	Less than or equal to 20
Renal	Creatinine (mg/dL)	Less than 1.5	1.5-1.9	2-3.4	3.5-4.9	Less than or equal to 5
Hepatic	Bilirubin (mg/dL)	Less than 1.2	1.2-3.5	3.6-7	7.1-14	Greater than 14

Data from Bone, R. C. (1997). Managing sepsis: What treatments can we use today? *J Crit Illn, 12*(1), 15.

healing. The ideal dressing must be easy to apply and painless to remove, and require fewer changes and fewer human resources. It must be robust enough for outpatients to use.

Not all wounds require surgical debridement, but removal of necrotic tissue from the wound edges and cavity is required for healing. Traditionally, wounds were debrided with "wet to dry" dressings: layered wet gauze inserted into the wound, allowed to dry, and then removed with necrotic material attached. These dressings required frequent changes that were often painful. Recent developments in dressing technology have introduced hydrogels and other occlusive dressings. These allow in situ degradation of necrotic material, which is then absorbed into the fluid phase of the dressing.

Great confusion arises in clinical practice between the significance of a positive wound swab and the risk of invasive infection. Wound healing is only significantly retarded when a sufficient bacterial load (>105 bacteria/g of tissue) is present. In practical terms, an open draining wound without necrotic tissue colonizes,

but the bacteria present are usually insufficient in number to affect healing. In contrast to colonization, invasive infection retards healing and leads to wound breakdown. For most wounds, all that is required to reduce bacterial counts to tolerable levels is to clean away accumulated debris. Use topical antiseptics to irrigate, cleanse, and debride wounds. In general, they do not promote the development of drug resistance, but they vary in antibacterial effect, and some species, especially pseudomonas, are resistant.

Cleansing noninfected "clean" wounds is best carried out with saline. For purulent wounds, a range of antiseptics is available, but delayed healing occurs with some. Chlorhexidine 0.05% is the most widely used antiseptic. It has a lower incidence of contact dermatitis and less tissue toxicity. Cetrimide 1% has a marked detergent action. It is often used for soiled traumatic wounds; however, the agent's in vitro cytotoxicity makes it unpopular for routine use. Povidone-iodine is particularly useful against staphylococci, but is less effective against pseudomonas species. It is also associated with contact hypersensitivity as well

TABLE 10-14 Clinical Presentation of Specific Organ Dysfunction

System Dysfunction	Clinical Parameter
Pulmonary system: acute respiratory distress syndrome (ARDS) in the absence of pulmonary embolism or bilateral pneumonia	• Predisposing factor such as sepsis • Unexplained hypoxemia • Bilateral pulmonary infiltrates consistent with pulmonary edema • PaO_2/FiO_2 ratio less than 300 • PAOP less than 18 mm Hg (to rule out cardiac pulmonary edema)
Hematologic (DIC): absence of liver failure, major hematoma, or anticoagulation therapy	• Fibrin degradation products (FDPs) greater than 1:40 or D-dimer greater than 2 mg/L • Thrombocytopenia or a 25% drop from a previous value • Prolonged aPTT • INR greater than 1.2 • May have clinical evidence of bleeding
Renal: absence of diuretic within 2 hours of urine analysis	• Urine output less than 0.5 mL/kg/min • Serum creatinine abnormal and urinary sodium greater than 40 mmol/L • If previous renal insufficiency, an increase in creatinine by 2 mg/dL not due to myoglobinuria
Hepatobiliary: absence of preexisting liver disease	• Serum bilirubin greater than 2 mg/dL for 2 days • Alkaline phosphatase, ALT, AST, gamma-glutamyl transferase (GGT) over twice laboratory normal
Central nervous system: absence of sedation or paralyzing agents that would alter the patient's ability to respond	• Decrease in Glasgow Coma Score by 1 point
Metabolic	• Serum lactate level increased

TABLE 10-15 Complex Wounds

Surgical wounds	• Open nonhealing postsurgical wounds • Localized incisions • Infected and/or draining wounds • Complicated surgical wounds
Pressure ulcers with complication	• Multiple stage II • Stage III or IV
Other wounds	• Infections requiring IV antibiotics • Wounds requiring frequent dressing changes • Amputations • Diabetic ulcers • Necrotizing fasciitis • Osteomyelitis • Peripheral vascular disease • Venous stasis • Post trauma • Burns • Fistulas

as toxicity from systemic absorption, which limits its use as an irrigant in large, deep cavities. The use of hypochlorite solutions (i.e., bleach) has declined due to concerns about tissue toxicity.

Systemic antibiotics do not penetrate necrotic tissue and have little to offer in the management of chronic wounds. Avoid topical antibiotic applications because they are ineffective and foster multiple drug-resistant strains of bacteria. Antibiotics are only appropriate when there is invasive infection, such as cellulitis.

An active dressing aims to establish an optimum microenvironment for healing the wound. It must maintain the wound temperature and moisture level, permit respiration, and allow epithelial migration. Optimal wound temperature is required for the function of cells such as macrophages, neutrophils, and fibroblasts. The respiration of these cells also requires adequate transfer of oxygen and carbon dioxide across the wound surface. The most favorable environment for the mobility and respiration of cells is a moist wound. Studies of the moist wound environment have shown enhanced epithelial migration, fibroblast function, and collagen production. These findings supported the development of occlusive dressings.

Semipermeable adhesive films such as Opsite and Tegaderm are permeable to gas and water vapor, but are a barrier to bacteria and water. They are generally reserved for the definitive closure of superficial, partial thickness wounds where comfort and ease of management are important. Apply the dressings and leave in place for several days, but remove if exudate builds up and leaks occur. Stretch the film to facilitate easier removal.

Hydrocolloid dressings such as Comfeel and Duoderm are adhesive, water- and gas-impermeable membranes. When the inner layer contacts the exudate, it forms a gel. They provide an excellent seal around the edges of the wound and can protect pressure areas. The hydrocolloids absorb exudate and help to debride the wound. Warn the patients that the wound may, at first, become smelly and appear to enlarge. The dressing needs changing when the gel leaks out. To avoid frequent changes, the dressing should have a diameter at least 2 cm bigger than the wound. The hydrocolloids can be used in the presence of necrotic material, but tend to have problems with overwhelming exudate buildup in large wounds or those where there is anaerobic colonization.

Alginate dressings such as Kaltostat and other alginates are derivatives of seaweed. The wound exudate activates the alginate dressing to produce a hydrophilic gel. Like hydrocolloids, alginates absorb the noncellular components of the exudate. Alginates provide a satisfactory dressing for lightly contaminated wounds and cavities. They are generally unsatisfactory in the presence of dry, necrotic tissue as there is no exudate to activate them. Removal of the dressing is easy because the alginates are not adhesive and removed by lavage, but held in place by another dressing. Depending on the amount of exudate, change alginates dressings twice a week.

Highly absorbent synthetic foams, Lyofoam and Allevyn, absorb large volumes of exudate from discharging wounds, reducing the need for dressing changes. These dressings combined with a hydrogel treat necrotic wounds that require debriding.

Hydrogel dressings include Intrasite, based on starch polymers. They provide moisture to the wound and encourage debridement. Hydrogels are best suited to dry necrotic wounds, but they also absorb exudate while maintaining the products of tissue repair and degradation, including growth factors and lysosomes, in contact with the wound. If the wound is clean, replace the gel once or twice a week. Infected wounds require daily dressings.

The wound assessment determines the suitable dressing. An adhesive film dressing is adequate for superficial partial thickness wounds. Wounds with mild to moderate exudate indicate the use of hydrocolloid dressings. Contaminated, moderate to heavy exudated wounds indicate the use of an alginate dressing. Heavy exudate wounds can use foam dressing and dry necrotic wounds require a hydrogel dressing. Definitive protocols for these dressings are yet to be established. Currently, adhesive films are used for a superficial wound, hydrocolloids are used for shallow ulcers, and alginates are used for the deep cavities. Foams are used as an adjunct for heavily exudative wounds. Hydrogels are used increasingly in the debridement of dry or necrotic ulcers, particularly when used with an adhesive film to retain the gel at the wound surface. Straightforward surgical and traumatic wounds require simple, low-cost dressings because healing is likely to be rapid and uncomplicated. Dressing choices for complicated wounds reflect a growing understanding of wound healing physiology. However, comparison of dressings continues to be largely anecdotal and management protocols are still evolving. Choices of dressings increasingly represent a cost/benefit analysis where the high cost of the latest dressing is balanced against savings in time and labor involved in dressing changes.

PALLIATIVE CARE

Palliative care means patient and family-centered care that optimizes quality of life by anticipating, preventing, and treating suffering. Palliative care throughout the continuum of illness involves addressing physical, intellectual, emotional, social, and spiritual needs and facilitating patient autonomy, access to information, and choice. The Synergy Model that guides progressive care nursing correlates with the philosophy and concepts of palliative care.

Hospitals are ethically obligated to offer such programs because the principles of beneficence and nonmaleficence require that hospitals, in addition to clinicians, seek to improve the quality of life and relieve the pain and suffering of all patients to the best of their ability. The National Consensus Project for Palliative Care (2013) updated the Clinical Practice Guidelines for Quality Palliative Care, which provides an educational framework and blueprint for the structure and provision of palliative care. Patients deserve the best quality of health care hospitals can provide at all stages of illness. Meet the complex needs of dying patients most effectively through the use of dedicated palliative care program. These palliative programs should include appropriate patient populations, patient and family-centered care, initiation of palliative care, continuity of care across settings, equitable access to care, comprehensive care, use of an interdisciplinary team, attention to relief of suffering, emphasis on communication, and skill in attending to the dying patient and bereaved survivors, as well as addressing regulatory issues.

The mission of the National Consensus Project for Quality Palliative Care is to create clinical practice guidelines that improve the quality of palliative care in the United States. Specifically, the Clinical Practice Guidelines for Quality Palliative Care promote quality palliative care, foster consistent and high standards in palliative care, and encourage continuity of care across settings. Since there is shared responsibility for palliative care across health care settings, the emphasis is on collaborative partnerships within and between hospitals, community centers, hospices, and home health agencies to ensure quality, continuity, and access to palliative care. The progressive care nurse requires education on palliative care nursing, specifically addressing the following eight domains of care:

Domain 1: Structure and Processes of Care
Domain 2: Physical Aspects of Care
Domain 3: Psychological and Psychiatric Aspects
Domain 4: Social Aspects of Care
Domain 5: Spiritual, Religious, and Existential Aspects of Care
Domain 6: Cultural Aspects of Care
Domain 7: Care of the Patient at the End of Life
Domain 8: Ethical and Legal Aspects of Care

10.11 Learning Activity

Identify whether the following statements are True (T) or False (F).

T F 1. Patients with chronic contaminated wounds containing necrotic tissue should be treated with systemic antibiotics.

T F 2. Hydrogels can be used to absorb exudate and debride necrotic tissues.

Answers to this activity can be found in the Answer Key.

10.12   Synthesis Learning Activity: Clinical Vignette

The patient is a 73-year-old male, retired postman. He was a heavy smoker of 2 packs/day until 5 years ago. The patient presented with increased shortness of breath, yellowish sputum production over the last week, and slight fever at 38.3° C 2 days before admission. He has a history of chronic bronchitis and is on Ventolin and Atrovent inhalers. His last FEV_1 in 1999 was 0.8 L/min. In 1996, the patient was admitted to the ICU and on mechanical ventilation with pneumococcal pneumonia with severe sepsis. He has had a pneumococcal vaccination and yearly influenza vaccinations.

The patient complains of dark urine and hasn't voided in the last 8 hours. He has used the Ventolin inhaler 4 times in the last couple of hours without relief.

The patient is admitted at 2300. He weighs 80 kg. He had labored breathing at 35/min, with a prolonged expiratory time and accessory muscle use. Temperature is 38.2° C; heart rate: 110/min; blood pressure: 90/50 mm Hg. He has jugular venous distension, peripheral edema, and fine crackles at both lung bases. A bruit is noted over the right carotid artery. Chest x-ray shows hyperinflation and possible bronchiectasis in both lung bases. There is also a possible left lower lobe infiltrate. ECG shows right axis deviation and inverted T waves in V_1-V_4.

Laboratory results include:

Sodium	148 mEq/L
Potassium	3.5 mEq/L
BUN	15 mg/dL
Lactate	1 mmol/L
Hgb	15.6 g/dL
Hct	47%
WBC	12,500 mm^3
Platelets	175,000 mm^3
aPTT	35 seconds
INR	1.3
ABGs on room air:	
pH	7.27
PaO_2	56 mm Hg
HCO_3	26 mEq/L
$Paco_2$	55 mm Hg

At 2340, BiPAP was initiated in the ED with 40% oxygen. Methylprednisolone (Solu-Medrol) 40 mg IV q 6 hours and cefuroxime (Ceftin) 1 gm IV q 8 hours are also initiated.

Normal saline 500 mL was administered over 1 hour after bladder catheter revealed only 20 mL of dark yellow urine with absence of blood on the strip reagent. D_5NaCl 0.9% + KCl 40 mg/L was initiated at 80 mL/hour after a saline infusion was completed.

Does the patient described in this case study meet criteria for SIRS, sepsis, severe sepsis, or septic shock?

_____

_____

Answers to this activity can be found in the Answer Key.

10.13   Learning Activity

Applying the Synergy Model to practice, what level would a 91-year-old male without family support who had a postoperative infection and requires complex dressing changes on discharge be given?

_____ a. Level 1

_____ b. Level 2

_____ c. Level 3

_____ d. Level 4

Answers to this activity can be found in the Answer Key.

10.14   Synthesis Learning Activity: Clinical Vignette

A 26-year-old female is admitted with fever, chills and lower abdominal pain. She denies dysuria and cough. She has a history of a seizure disorder and has been taking phenytoin (Dilantin) for many years. She has no costovertebral tenderness and there is no obvious source of infection.

Temperature: 39.4° C

HR: 125 bpm, BP 75/40→90/50 mm Hg after 2 L NS

A. Is the patient in SIRS, sepsis, or shock? What criteria determine this?

_____

_____

_____

Diagnostics:

Urinalysis

5-20 WBC/hpf

Bacteria seen

Serum

WBC 11,000 mcL, 22% bands, Hgb normal, platelets normal

LFTs normal, electrolytes, amylase normal

Creatinine 139 mg/dl

Radiology

CXR clear

CT (with contrast) chest & abdomen: free fluid pelvis, edematous left kidney

B. Is the patient in SIRS, sepsis, or shock at this point? What is/are the differentiating factor(s)?

_____

_____

_____

Treatment:

Started on emperic antibotics (Cefotaxime [Claforan], ciprofloxacin [Cipro], ampicillin [Omnipen, Principen], metronidazole [Flagyl]) after cultures

12 hours later:

HR increased to 180 bpm, BP 65/P mm Hg by palpation despite fluids

RR 40+breaths/minute with significant dyspnea

Chest x-ray shows bilateral pulmonary infiltrates

ABGs: pH 7.23; PaO_2 100 mm Hg on 80% oxygen; $Paco_2$ 33 mm Hg; HCO_3 14 mEq/L

Serum lactate 2.6 mmol/L

Increased transaminases, decreased urine output

Increased INR to 2.4

The rapid response team is called and she is intubated, mechanical ventilation is initiated, and a central venous catheter is inserted. A norepinephrine (Levophed) infusion is initiated for BP support.

Intubated, mechanical ventilation, central venous catheter, arterial catheter, vasopressor

Blood cultures: Gram-negative bacillus 2/2 bottles

C. Is the patient in SIRS, sepsis, or shock at this point? What is/are the differentiating factor(s)?

_____

_____

Answers to this activity can be found in the Answer Key.

Behavioral/Psychosocial

HISTORY AND PHYSICAL EXAMINATION

In patients presenting with behavioral or psychosocial problems, the first step to treatment is to assess the patient's history. Identify preexisting psychiatric, psychologic, and social problems. Evaluate pre-illness coping mechanisms and identify sources of support from family, friends, pets, and spirituality.

Determine the patient's family history. Investigate if the patient has a health care proxy, living will, or durable power of attorney. Obtain contact information, such as home and cell phone numbers for family members. Determine the current family structure and identify who the family caregivers are. Determine the current and available support system. Ask about any family concerns and the best visiting time, and the preferred method of meeting and communicating with the health care team.

Attempt to determine the patient's chief complaint. Ask the patient and family about the history of the present illness, especially current symptoms and medications. Determine the type of medication ordered, dosage, when it was ordered, and the last dose taken. Note any changes related to medication use. Identify current use/abuse of substances including alcohol and prescribed, over-the-counter medications and other drugs. Investigate the patient's past medical history. Elicit information about previous illnesses or injuries, previous hospitalizations, review of body systems, and allergies. Learning about the social history of the patient is also an important part of the assessment process. Determine whether there is any history of substance abuse. Ask if there has been any major family trauma or stress. Determine the patient's educational level and current responsibilities such as a job, financial obligations, spouse, parents, children, and pets. Inquire about family structure and identify who makes or influences health care decisions. Identify the individuals who are in regular contact with the patient; this may include immediate or extended family or friends who the patient identifies as his or her support system.

Perform a physical, cognitive, and behavioral oral examination on the patient. Assess the patient's ability to concentrate and level of judgment, and identify any confusion. Note sleep patterns, level of agitation, and interaction with family and staff. Review the findings from other diagnostic studies such as serum laboratory analysis, urinalysis, and other diagnostic tests such as an angiography, computed tomography (CT) scan, and electroencephalogram (EEG). Assess and reassess each episode of delirium/disorientation and coping along the acute care environment continuum.

Mental Status Examination

Conduct a mental status assessment. Examine the patient's general appearance by assessing hygiene and grooming. Note whether the patient's clothing is clean and is age, fit, and weather appropriate. Note whether the patient's eye contact is consistent, intermittent, or poor. Note whether the patient is cooperative and if the patient's motor activity reveals purposeful movement. Note any restlessness or tremor. Evaluate the patient's speech. Look for changes in speech patterns and/ or idiosyncrasies and whether the speech is slurred, loud, or soft. Note if the patient's speech is rapid or forced, which may indicate he or she feels pressured. A patient suffering from a behavior or psychosocial problem reports or demonstrates varied emotions (Box 11-1); therefore, assess affect and mood.

In addition to changes in affect, mood, and speech, a patient with behavioral problems may also have alterations in thought, perception, and cognition. Thought can refer to the ideas or arrangements of ideas that result from thinking. Thought process is the use of the mind to consider something carefully, but the following alterations that impede the process are often present in behavioral or psychosocial disturbances:

- Blocking: cessation in the flow of thought or speech
- Flight of ideas: leap from one idea to another, distracted from thoughts and speech by things in the environment
- Looseness of association: no logical connection between sentences
- Circumstantial: thoughts or speech that contains excessive details about the topic but finally reaches the intended point
- Tangential: thoughts that are logical and directed that may be related to the topic but take off in a different direction and do not address the question or specific topic

Thought content is a description of what the patient is thinking. Patients may be phobic, suspicious, or paranoid. They may have feelings of hopelessness or guilt. Determine whether the patient is delusional (i.e., a persistent belief or perception held despite evidence to the contrary). Examples of delusion include being controlled, grandeur, persecution, nihilistic, and somatic. Ask the patient if he or she sees or hears things that others do not. Determine whether the patient is fixated on a single idea and if so, what idea. Determine whether the thought content presented is consistent with the patient's affect. Assess for any ideation or distortion of thought in addition to thoughts or plan of suicide or homicide. If there is any concern regarding possible interest in committing suicide or homicide, ask this directly, including a search for details (e.g., specific plan, time, etc.). Bringing up the topic will not trigger suicidal thoughts.

BOX 11-1	
Affect and Mood Alterations in Behavioral and Psychosocial Disturbance	
Affect: Emotion That the Patient Demonstrates	**Mood: Emotion That the Patient Reports**
Normal: emotions consistent with the situation and conversation	Calm and cooperative
Anxious, worried	Hostile
Flat: demonstrates no emotion	Depressed
Inappropriate: Emotions demonstrated are not consistent with the situation or maturity level	Elated
	Anxious
Labile: Emotions demonstrated fluctuate high to low rapidly and inconsistently without respect to the situation	Agitated
Guarded: appears wary or overly cautious in conversation	

Adapted from Mackenzie, M. J., Carlson, L. E., Ekkekakis, P., Paskevich, D. M., & Culos-Reed, S. N. (2013). Affect and mindfulness as predictors of change in mood disturbance, stress symptoms, and quality of life in a community-based yoga program for cancer survivors. Retrieved from *www.hindawi.com/journals/ecam/2013/419496/*

TABLE 11-1 Types of Abnormal Hallucinations

Type	Perception of
Auditory	Voices or other sounds
Visual	Images
Gustatory	Taste
Tactile	Touch
Olfactory	Odors
Kinesthetic	Bodily movement
Somatic	Something occurring within one's own body

These questions have never been shown to plant the seeds for an otherwise unplanned event and may provide critical information, so they should be asked!

Perceptual disturbances include hallucinations and illusions. Hallucinations are sensory perceptions that do not result from an external stimulus and occur in an awake state. An illusion is a false interpretation of an external sensory stimulus such as a coat hanging over a chair perceived as a person sitting there. Consider hypnagogic and hypnopompic hallucinations normal. Hypnagogic hallucinations are associated with the semiconsciousness state immediately preceding sleep. Hypnopompic hallucinations are associated with the semiconsciousness preceding waking. Consider auditory, visual, gustatory, tactile, olfactory, kinesthetic, and somatic hallucinations (Table 11-1) abnormal.

Cognition is the set of all mental abilities and processes related to knowledge. These abilities include knowledge, attention, memory, judgment, evaluation, reasoning, computation, problem solving, decision making, comprehension, and language. Cognition is conscious and unconscious, concrete or abstract, as well as intuitive (e.g., knowledge of a language) and conceptual (e.g., model of a language). Cognitive processes use existing knowledge and generate new knowledge. To assess cognition, observe the patient's orientation to person, place, time, and situation. Immediate recall, short-term memory, and long-term memory are assessed. Evaluate intelligence, concentration, judgment, and insight. Determine whether the patient is able to understand information relayed. Determine the ability of the patient to focus and pay attention, make sound decisions, and understand the current situation intact.

Diagnostics

Initially, the purpose of several diagnostic studies completed is to rule out medical conditions and/or substance abuse. Indicated serum laboratory studies evaluate CBC, hemoglobin, hematocrit, thyroid panel, liver studies, and renal function. Perform a urinalysis and urine toxicology screen. In addition, perform a serum toxicology screen. For all women from 10 to 50 years old, ensure that a pregnancy examination is performed. In addition, perform specific diagnostic tests such as CT scans, electroencephalography (EEG), and cerebral blood flow studies as prescribed.

11.1 Learning Activity
Match the following hallucinations with the correct definition.

_____ 1. Auditory
_____ 2. Visual
_____ 3. Gustatory
_____ 4. Hypnopompic
_____ 5. Tactile
_____ 6. Olfactory
_____ 7. Kinesthetic
_____ 8. Somatic

a. Feeling sensations when not being touched
b. Seeing images that are not present
c. Smelling odors that are not present
d. Perceiving a taste without an identifiable cause
e. Hearing voices or sounds that are not there
f. Vivid dreamlike hallucination upon awakening
g. Perceiving movement of the body without cause
h. Feeling that something is occurring within one's own body

Answers to this activity can be found in the Answer Key.

BOX 11-2

Erikson's Stages of Psychosocial Development (Adulthood Only)

Young Adulthood (18-40 Years of Age)
Conflicts: intimacy versus self-isolation or self-absorption
Developmental tasks
- Accepts self
- Establishes independence
- Establishes a vocation to make worthwhile contributions
- Learns to appraise and express love responsibly
- Establishes intimate bond with another
- Establishes and manages residence
- Finds congenial social group
- Decides on option of a family
- Formulates philosophy of life
- Establishes role in community

Middle Adulthood (40-60 Years of Age)
Conflicts: generativity versus self-absorption and stagnation
Developmental tasks
- Develops new satisfaction as a mate
- Supportive to mate
- Develops sense of unity with mate
- Assists offspring to become happy, responsible adults
- Takes pride in accomplishments of self and mate
- Balances work with other roles; assists aging parents
- Achieves social and civic responsibility
- Maintains active organizational membership
- Accepts physical changes of middle age
- Makes an art of friendship
- Balances leisure with service pursuits
- Develops more depth of personal philosophy by reevaluating values and examining assets

Older Adulthood (60 Years of Age to Death)
Conflicts: Integrity versus despair
Developmental tasks
- Continued self-development
- Adapts to family responsibilities
- Maintains self-worth, pride, and usefulness
- Deals with loss of spouse, friends, and upcoming end to life

PSYCHOSOCIAL LIFE CYCLE

Patients and family members come to the progressive care unit at all phases of the life cycle. Growth and development of the patient and family members influence psychosocial needs, response to illness, and behaviors. Illness and changes in body image may present serious psychological stress. The patient and family need an assessment of psychosocial illness impact on current growth and development needs. Erikson (1968) described eight stages of the life cycle with four being before adulthood. The adult stages are significant in progressive care (Box 11-2).

MASLOW'S HIERARCHY OF NEEDS

The manner in which the fulfillment of basic human needs occurs depends on personal abilities, environment, and life experience. According to Maslow's Hierarchy of Needs

TABLE 11-2 **Maslow's Hierarchy of Needs**

Physiologic	Oxygen, food, water, and sleep
Safety and security	Protection and freedom from anxiety
Love and belonging	Freedom from loneliness and alienation
Esteem and recognition	Freedom from a sense of worthlessness, inferiority, and helplessness
Self-actualization	Aesthetic needs, self-fulfillment, creativity, and spirituality

(Table 11-2), the needs are progressive, but primary needs must be met before dealing with higher-level needs. Needs change throughout the life cycle. Human needs of the acutely ill patient (Figure 11-1) include physical, social, and psychological components. Illness may require a refocusing on the achievement of basic needs.

11.2 Learning Activity

Match the level of Maslow's Hierarchy of Needs to the example.

_____ 1. Physiologic   a. Creativity
_____ 2. Safety and   b. Water
         security   c. Promotion at work
_____ 3. Love and   d. Marriage
         belonging   e. Home security
_____ 4. Esteem and
         recognition
_____ 5. Self-actualization

Answers to this activity can be found in the Answer Key.

PATIENT- AND FAMILY-CENTERED CARE

The family systems theory suggests that individuals do not exist in isolation, but rather as a part of an emotional family unit. Families are systems of interconnected and interdependent individuals and are composed of related parts that interact together as a whole. Understanding patients and families does not occur in isolation. Patient- and family-centered care recognizes that the quality, safety, and delivery of health care improve when the expertise of health care professionals partner with the experience of patients and families. The use of patient- and family-centered care provides professional insight into dysfunctional family relationships along with learning their effective coping mechanisms and available support. Patient- and family-centered care facilitates an understanding of family cultural patterns and dynamics, including communication, power, economics, and interaction. In the progressive care unit, nurses use patient- and family-centered care to design policies, programs, and individual care plans for the best possible outcomes for patients, their families, and health care providers.

A family system is a group of individuals bonded together by their interests. It is usually a community whose members nurture and support one another. Members have set rules, roles,

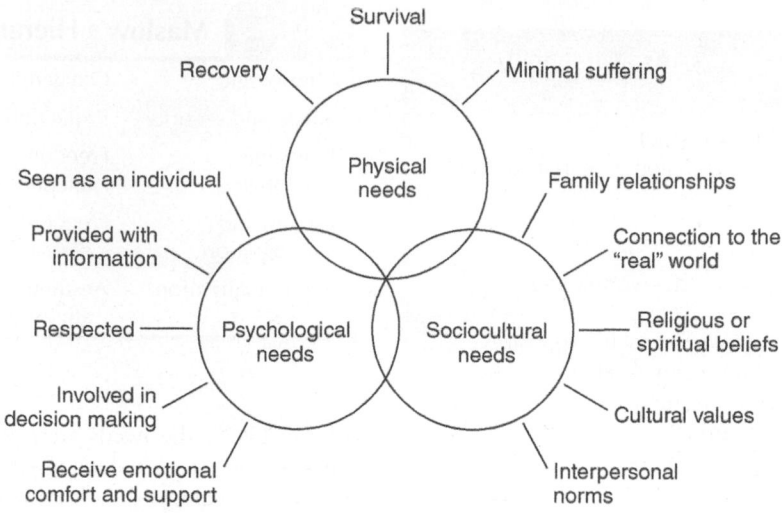

FIGURE 11-1 Human needs of the critically ill patient. (From Kinney, M. et al. [1998]. *AACN's clinical reference for critical care nursing* [4th ed.]. St. Louis, MO: Mosby.)

power structure, communication style, and problem-solving techniques influenced by cultural factors and spiritual support that allow them to accomplish tasks. Illness often alters the rules, roles, power, etc., in the family, which creates stress and the need for adaptation to the new environment and situation. Family caregivers exposed to environmental stressors develop role strain, which if not recognized and effectively managed can lead to exhaustion.

PROGRESSIVE CARE ENVIRONMENT

The patient care environment can directly affect the ability to meet a patient's needs. The patient has a need for rest and sleep; therefore, the doors on patient rooms should be closed and the bright fluorescent lighting dimmed. Staff awareness and behavior can have a profound effect on modifying the environment. The progressive care unit is often a transitional environment because patients more often than not transfer in and out of the unit depending on their clinical status and acuity level. The progressive care nurse needs to understand the stress experienced by the patient as he or she moves from one care environment to another along with the patient's ability to cope. The progressive care environment needs to provide for additional privacy and be conducive to the patient's normal rest patterns. Patients received on the progressive care unit from the critical care unit may have experienced some form of delirium. Progressive care nurses need to employ strategies to create a healing environment.

STRESS

Stress, defined as a mental, emotional, or physical tension or strain, occurs when an individual encounters various types of stimuli. Illness is a stressful situation. Directed interventions by the nurse can lessen stress and/or the impact of stress on the patient and family. Nursing presence and the anticipation of patient needs are associated with less stressful experiences. There are many stressors (Box 11-3) in a progressive care unit setting. Psychological stressors for acutely ill patients

and their families are powerlessness, sleep deprivation, grief and loss, sensory overload or deprivation, pain, and post-traumatic stress disorder. Selye (1976) identified two types of stress: distress and eustress. Distress can occur from noxious stimuli. Eustress results from nonthreatening stimuli. Noxious psychosocial stimuli can overwhelm the body's compensatory ability to maintain homeostasis and can elicit a stress response. The major neural response to a stressful stimulus is activation of the sympathetic nervous system. Psychoneuroimmunologic research has identified a relationship between stress and immune function. Crisis is the state that occurs when one's usual ways of coping are inadequate to deal with the stress. Patient and family coping mechanisms (Table 11-3 and Table 11-4) need to be identified and developed. Interventions to decrease or eliminate stress include:

- Maintain a calm, restful environment.
- Provide for as much independence of the patient as possible.
- Provide contact with reality and the outside world.
- Encourage use of coping mechanisms.

TABLE 11-3	Coping Mechanisms for Stress
Type	**Example**
Action	Taking walks, cleaning house, gardening, or singing
Cognitive	Problem solving or reading about the issue
Spiritual	Prayer
Interpersonal	Talking with support person
Emotional	Use of psychological defense mechanisms (see Table 11-4)

TABLE 11-4	Psychological Defense Mechanisms
Defense Mechanism	**Description**
Suppression	Conscious, deliberate forgetting of unacceptable or painful thoughts, impulses, feelings, or acts
Repression	Unconscious, involuntary forgetting of unacceptable or painful thoughts, impulses, feelings, or acts
Denial	Treating obvious reality factors as though they do not exist because they are consciously intolerable
Rationalization	Attempting to justify feelings, behaviors, and motives that would otherwise be intolerable by offering a socially acceptable, intellectual, and apparently logical explanation for an act or decision
Compensation	Making extra effort to achieve in one area to offset real or imagined deficiencies in another area
Sublimation	Directing energy from unacceptable drives into socially acceptable behavior
Projection	Unconsciously attributing one's own unacceptable qualities and emotions to others
Regression	Going back to an earlier level of emotional development and organization
Withdrawal	Separating oneself from interpersonal relationships in order to avoid emotional expression or responsiveness

PSYCHOSOCIAL CARE ISSUES

Several common psychosocial care issues occur in progressive care patients and families. Many of these psychosocial issues and concerns are interdependent. For example, inadequately managed pain may lead to feelings of powerlessness, anxiety, and depression, which in turn will heighten the perception of pain. Powerlessness, sleep deprivation, and grief and loss are the most common psychosocial issues patients and families deal with in the progressive care unit.

Powerlessness

Powerlessness is a perceived lack of control over the outcome of a specific situation or problem, and the patient's perception that any action he or she takes will not affect the outcome. Symptoms that manifest powerlessness include apathy, withdrawal, resignation, lack of decision making, aggression, anger, and fatalism. An individual's self-esteem and self-concept along with where the individual is in the life cycle influence the ability of an event to engender a sense of powerlessness. Progressive care patients may experience loss of their ability to control even the most basic of functions, including the ability to communicate, breathe on their own, and control bladder and bowel function. In addition, depending on the institution's philosophy, participation in decision making may be limited. Patients being transferred from a higher-acuity level of care may be skeptical, fearful of being cared for improperly, and afraid to be alone. Interventions to decrease feelings of powerlessness include:

- Recognize the potential for feelings of powerlessness; particularly at risk are individuals who usually are in a position of power or control in their daily life.
- Support the patient's sense of control by offering alternatives related to activity times, treatment times, diet, routine hygiene, diversionary activities, and visitation.
- Assist the patient in identifying activities that he or she can perform independently.
- Keep the patient informed about his or her treatment.
- Encourage the patient's involvement in decision making related to treatment.
- Increase the patient's control as his or her condition improves.

Sensory Overload/Deprivation

Sensory overload occurs on an acute care unit due to the increased frequency and intensity of stimulation of the senses with nonmeaningful stimuli. Contributing factors include constant noise and lights, alarms, and chatter of unfamiliar voices. The primary intervention for sensory overload is to eliminate or limit nonmeaningful sensory stimulation. Monitor only those patients with clinical indications for monitoring and collaborate with the interprofessional team to determine those patients in the progressive care unit who should be monitored (i.e., ECG, pulse oximetry) and what parameters to use. Use the American Heart Association's Practice Standards for ECG Monitoring in Hospital Settings (Drew & Funk, 2006).

Pulse oximeters typically measure oxygen saturation best in patients who have adequate peripheral perfusion and are not moving. The newest pulse oximetry technology improves accuracy in states of low perfusion and increased motion. Delaying a setting (e.g., from the time the event initially occurs to when an alarm is triggered) on the SpO_2 alarm to 15 seconds or 19 seconds can reduce the frequency of alarms by 50% and 70%, respectively; most desaturations recover within a short period. Setting the alarm threshold based on each patient's condition also can reduce the frequency of alarms. Reducing the SpO_2 alarm threshold from 90% to 88% results in a 45% decrease in the number of alarms. When both a 15-second delay and an alarm threshold of 88% were applied, a "six-fold reduction" was demonstrated in the number of SpO_2 alarms. The combination of both customized alarm delay and threshold settings optimizes the SpO_2 (Welch, 2011).

Customize the alarms to meet the needs of individual patients. Set customized alarms within 1 hour of assuming care of a patient and as the patient's condition changes. Consider updating pulse oximetry equipment to decrease false alarms (Gross, Dahl, & Nielson, 2011). Develop a culture of suspending alarms when nurses perform patient care that may produce false alarms.

Sensory deprivation occurs on an acute unit due to the decreased frequency, intensity, or variety of stimulation of the senses with meaningful stimuli. Contributing factors include an absence of windows, clocks, and calendars along with constant noise, lights, technical language, lack of familiar faces, and deprivation of familiar touches, sounds, smells, and tastes of the usual environment. Encourage family visitation and ask the family to bring familiar objects to the hospital. Put a calendar and clock where the patient can see them. Patients who have transitioned from a higher-acuity level of care may have experienced a decrease in the amount, consistency, and/or quality of sleep that occurs in a 24-hour period. Sleep fragmentation occurs when a patient fails to complete a full sleep cycle that includes both rapid eye movement and non-rapid eye movement sleep. Circadian rhythm, the 24-hour cycle that is linked to light and dark phases of the day, can be disturbed. Biologic functions affected by circadian rhythms include the heart rate, metabolic rate, breathing rate, and temperature. Imbalance in the secretion of melatonin can result in a wide range of sleep disorders. The goal of interventions to combat sleep deprivation is to restore normal sleeping patterns. Prepare the environment to optimize sleep and rest by shutting off lights, limiting noise, and providing adequate pain relief. There may be a need to use short-term pharmacologic agents to treat sleep deprivation, but long-term use should be discouraged.

Grief and Loss

The grief reaction is the emotional response to a loss in which something valued is changed or altered so that it no longer has its previously valued traits. The acute illness experience can precipitate a grief reaction by both the patient and family. Grief may result from loss or potential loss of health, body image, role, and financial security. The degree of grief experienced correlates to the meaning of the loss, adequacy of coping, and availability of support. It is important to recognize and appreciate the cultural variation in the expression of grief. Allow the patient and family members to express grief in their own way. Provide ongoing, honest information to the patient and family regarding the patient's illness and expected recovery. Teach the patient and family about the normal grief response and always offer privacy.

Each individual may grieve differently due to age, gender, and personal, religious, and cultural differences. Ask the patient and family about cultural and individual preferences. Consider using the distress screening tool to ascertain the degree of psychosocial, spiritual, and physical distress. To address the needs of adult patients, as well as the needs of their caregivers or family, including children, the progressive care nurse provides information and tools to improve their comfort and skills in dealing with this type of loss. Assess the patient and family for the following:

- Assessment of suicide risk
- Assessment of coping mechanisms and patient resiliency
- Assessment of risk of complicated grief
- Timing of assessments
- Management/treatment

Provide nonpharmacologic management by acknowledging the loss, educate the patient and family, and assist with lifestyle management (e.g., rest, exercise, social connections, spiritual support, home support, compassionate care benefits program). In some situations, administer pharmacologic management (e.g., benzodiazepines). Provide information on other types of support such as patient and caregiver support groups, online support groups, spiritual care and/or faith-based communities, and hospice and palliative care programs. Refer to a bereavement counselor, psychologist, or psychiatrist as appropriate or if requested (AHRQ, 2011).

SPECIFIC PATIENT HEALTH PROBLEMS

Anxiety Disorders

Anxiety is a state of uneasiness, apprehension, and worry. The subjective experience differs from one individual to another and has both physiologic and psychological components. Often, the person does not know the cause of the unpleasant emotional state with increased feelings of tension and helplessness. There are several different types of anxiety. A panic disorder is a sudden-onset anxiety in the form of fear and panic (i.e., panic attack). A phobia is an irrational or illogical fear of an object, situation, or event. An obsessive-compulsive disorder (OCD) is recurrent, persistent, intrusive thoughts and feelings (i.e., obsessions), coupled with behaviors that are ritualistic and repetitive (i.e., compulsions). Posttraumatic stress disorder (PTSD) is persistent or repeated reexperiences of a traumatic event that has occurred in the past through thoughts and memories that induce an anxiety response. Substance-induced anxiety disorder refers to the development of anxiety symptoms with substance withdrawal or within a month of substance-abuse cessation.

Predisposing factors for anxiety include genetic predisposition, preexisting diseases, and developmental causes. Preexisting diseases that may cause anxiety include hyperthyroidism, hyperparathyroidism, pheochromocytoma, vestibular disorders, seizure disorders, dysrhythmias, and other cardiac disorders. A major depressive disorder is a psychological illness that can trigger anxiety. In addition, the development of anxiety may stem from age, stress, sleep deprivation, changes in health status, central nervous system (CNS) stimulant substance abuse, CNS depressant withdrawal, and/or trauma. In adolescents, triggers of anxiety include peer pressure related to appearance, substance abuse, pressure to achieve, and puberty. Life changes such as marriage, divorce, childbirth, menopause, career pressures, and the loss of parents may trigger anxiety in adults. Anxiety in older adults stems from the loss of a spouse, significant other, or friends along with diminished independence and health.

Although not well understood, the pathophysiologic process of anxiety is a disruption of modulators within the CNS. The autonomic nervous system mediates the majority of the symptoms. Studies suggest that an imbalance of certain neurotransmitters (i.e., chemical messengers in the brain) may contribute to anxiety disorders. The neurotransmitters targeted in anxiety disorders are gamma-aminobutyric acid (GABA), serotonin, dopamine, and epinephrine. Serotonin appears to be specifically important in feelings of well-being, and deficiencies are highly related to anxiety and depression. Stress hormones such as cortisol also play a role.

Objective indicators of anxiety include tachycardia, tachypnea, elevated BP, pallor, tremors, dilated pupils, and nystagmus. Subjectively, patients with anxiety often report a history of excessive anxiety or worry for more than 6 months. They also report an inability to control feelings and have three or more of the following symptoms:

- Restlessness, feeling keyed up
- Fatigue
- Difficulty concentrating
- Irritability
- Muscle tension
- Sleep disturbances: difficulty falling or staying asleep, not feeling rested
- Sexual problems
- Apprehensive, fearfulness, and/or helplessness
- Tightness in chest and/or shortness of breath
- Dizziness
- Choking feeling

Collaborative management of patients with anxiety focuses first on the treatment of the cause. Pulse oximetry is helpful to rule out hypoxemia as a cause of anxiety. Administer oxygen by nasal cannula at 2 to 6 L/min if indicated to maintain SpO_2 of 95% unless contraindicated. In patients with COPD, use pulse oximetry to guide the oxygen administration to keep the SpO_2 of ~90%. Start an IV access for fluid and medication administration if indicated. Always consider a physiologic cause of anxiety and treat any identified cause. To rule out medical conditions, diagnostic tests performed on patients with anxiety include basic CBC, chemistry profile, along with serum and urine drug screens, as indicated. An ECG may show dysrhythmias, particularly sinus tachycardia, PACs, and PVCs.

Provide a safe, quiet environment and decrease stimulation by darkening the room. Assess the patient's psychiatric status, especially suicidal ideation and agitation level. Ensure continuous observation of the patient and establish a trusting relationship with the patient by using the following nursing interventions:

- Maintain a calm manner when approaching the patient.
- Acknowledge the patient's feelings and fears.
- Use a calm tone, and speak clearly and distinctly.
- Maintain eye contact when speaking with the patient.
- Communicate honestly.
- Assist in problem solving.

The standard approach to treating most anxiety disorders is a combination of talk therapy, such as cognitive-behavioral therapy (CBT), and an antidepressant medication (Table 11-5). A selective serotonin reuptake inhibitor (SSRI) is typically the first choice, with a serotonin-norepinephrine reuptake inhibitor (SNRI) being an alternative. If patients do not respond to these drugs, tricyclic antidepressants may be helpful. For patients who are not helped by antidepressants or who need help rapidly because antidepressants take several weeks to be effective, consider short-term benzodiazepine therapy. Benzodiazepines (e.g., diazepam [Valium], lorazepam [Ativan], chlordiazepoxide [Librium]) are effective medications for most anxiety disorders and have been the standard of treatment for years. However, their long-term daily use is associated with a risk for dependency and abuse. Therefore, in most cases, the SSRIs and other newer antidepressants are now frontline agents.

Dementia

Dementia is the term used to describe the symptoms of a large group of illnesses that cause a progressive decline in functioning. It is a broad term to describe a loss of memory, intellect, rationality, social skills, and normal emotional reactions. Dementia causes significant impairment in a person's daily functioning.

TABLE 11-5 Psychopharmacologic Agents Used in Treatment of Anxiety Disorders

Classification	Adverse Effects	Nursing Implications
SSRIs • Fluoxetine (Prozac) • Sertraline (Zoloft) • Paroxetine (Paxil) • Fluvoxamine (Luvox) • Citalopram (Celexa) • Escitalopram (Lexapro)	• Sexual dysfunction, including lowered sex drive • Weight gain • Agitation, nausea, and diarrhea • Increased risk for suicidal thoughts and behavior in young people ages 18-24 • Heart-related birth defects	• Use lowest effective dose possible in the elderly. • Monitor patients with cardiovascular conditions closely. • Monitor for any worsening of depressive symptoms or changes in behavior, especially during the first few months of treatment. • Discuss the potential risks of these drugs during pregnancy and breastfeeding.
SNRIs • Venlafaxine (Effexor) • Duloxetine (Cymbalta)	• Impaired sexual function • Increased blood pressure and heart rate • Severe withdrawal symptoms, including dizziness and nausea • Risk of overdose • Complications in newborns • Generally mild, including dry mouth, nausea, and sleepiness • Liver damage	• Approved for adults only. • Monitor patients with heart problems closely. • Educate patients on risk of overdose and avoid acute withdrawal. • Avoid last semester of pregnancy. • Avoid in patients with narrow-angle glaucoma, liver or kidney diseases, or ETOH abuse.
Tricyclic antidepressants • Imipramine (Tofranil) • Nortriptyline (Pamelor) • Desipramine (Norpramin) • Clomipramine (Anafranil)	• Sleep disturbance • Orthostatic hypotension • Weight gain • Sexual dysfunction • Mental disturbance	• Closely monitor elderly patients and those with a history of seizures, cardiovascular conditions, closed-angle glaucoma, and urinary retention or obstruction.

Continued

TABLE 11-5   Psychopharmacologic Agents Used in Treatment of Anxiety Disorders—cont'd

Classification	Adverse Effects	Nursing Implications

Benzodiazepines
• Alprazolam (Xanax)
• Clonazepam (Klonopin)
• Lorazepam (Ativan)
	• Daytime drowsiness
	• Hung-over feeling
	• Paradoxical confusion or delirium
	• Intellectual impairment
	• Agitation
	• Worsen respiratory problems
	• Ataxia and reduced motor coordination
	• Increased risk of falling and accidents
	• Birth defects
	• IV administration can cause phlebitis
	• Withdrawal symptoms, such as sleep disturbance and anxiety, stomach distress, sweating, and insomnia
		• Use short term.
		• Teach patient to avoid use with alcohol.
		• Monitor elderly patients closely because they are more susceptible to side effects and should be started at half the dose prescribed for younger people.
		• Warn the patient to be cautious performing tasks that require mental alertness (e.g., driving, using machinery).
		• Do not use in pregnant women or nursing mothers because of associated birth defects.
		• Monitor IV sites closely and change site if redness or swelling occur.
		• Monitor for tolerance that develops; drugs lose their effectiveness with continued use at the same dosage and dependency can occur within 3 weeks.
		• Monitor for withdrawal symptoms within hours or days after stopping the medication, which can last 1-3 weeks.
		  • The longer the duration of therapy and/or the higher the dose, the more severe these symptoms can become.
		  • Tapering off gradually is the best approach to stop taking these drugs. Certain medications (such as antiseizure drugs, antidepressants, and buspirone) may also help with withdrawal.
		• Monitor for paradoxical reaction; the most common paradoxical reactions are increased anxiety, irritability, and agitation; however, more severe effects can also occur, including mania, hostility and rage, aggressive or impulsive behavior, and hallucinations.

Nonbenzodiazepines • Buspirone (Buspar)	• Dizziness • Nausea • Drowsiness • Excitement • Headache	• Note that this drug does not have any sedative, muscle relaxant, or anticonvulsant effects. • Lasts only 2-3 hours and takes 2-3 weeks for symptom relief to occur. • Teach the patient to take with food, which facilitates achieving a steady state concentration. • Increases the risk of digitalis toxicity because it is highly protein bound and displaces digoxin.
Beta-blockers • Propranolol (Inderal) • Atenolol (Tenormin)	• Light-headedness • Sleepiness • Nausea • Unusually slow pulse	• Monitor the patient for complications, such as dysrhythmias.

Dementia is a chronic global deterioration of cognitive functioning that results from a disorder of the brain or an organic disease. Dementia is chronic and progressive in nature and the clinical presentation includes personality, behavioral, emotional, and functional changes in the patient. Predisposing factors for the development of dementia include aging, cerebrovascular disease, brain tumors, and Alzheimer disease. Other conditions such as hypothyroidism, hypercalcemia, neurosyphilis, HIV infection, substance abuse, normal-pressure hydrocephalus, and trauma such as a chronic subdural hematoma can cause dementia. Vitamin deficiencies, such as deficiencies of folic acid, vitamin B_{12}, and niacin, may also cause dementia.

The pathophysiology of dementia is dependent on the etiology. There is a chronic global deterioration of cognition. Cognitive malfunctioning occurs preceded by deterioration in emotional control, social behavior, and motivation. Cognitive malfunctioning interferes with memory, intellect, learning, orientation, comprehension, calculation, language, and judgment.

TABLE 11-6	Medications Used in Treatment of Dementia		
Classification	**Mechanism of Action**	**Indications**	**Adverse Effects**
Cholinesterase inhibitors • Donepezil (Aricept) • Rivastigmine (Exelon) • Galantamine (Razadyne)	• Prevent the breakdown of acetylcholine and support communication among nerve cells by keeping acetylcholine levels high, which is important for learning and memory. • Delay worsening of symptoms for 6 to 12 months on average for about half the people who take them.	All stages (Aricept) Mild to moderate: • Alzheimer disease • Vascular dementia (Razadyne) • Parkinson disease dementia (Aricept) • Lewy body dementia	• Nausea, vomiting • Loss of appetite • Diarrhea • Loses effect over time
N-methyl-D-aspartate blockers • Memantine (Namenda)	• Regulate the activity of glutamate, a chemical messenger involved in the brain functions of learning and memory. • Some research has shown that combining memantine with a cholinesterase inhibitor may have beneficial results.	Moderate to severe: • Alzheimer disease • Vascular dementia • Parkinson disease dementia • Lewy body dementia	• Dizziness • Loses effect over time

Subjective complaints of a patient with dementia include memory loss, confusion, and a decline in cognitive functioning and judgment. The objective signs and symptom of dementia range from a general lack of orientation to focal neurologic signs. The patient lacks orientation to situation, time, place, and person. The patient may suffer from aphasia, apraxia, and agnosia along with demonstrated behavioral disturbances and a shallow, flat affect. Focal neurologic signs present include exaggeration of deep tendon reflexes, Babinski reflex, pseudobulbar palsy, gait abnormalities, and weakness of extremities. Diagnostic examinations include the mini-mental status examination (www.healthandwelfare.idaho.gov/Portals/0/Medical/Medicaid CHIP/MiniMental.pdf). To rule out other medical causes, obtain a basic CBC, serum chemistry, and urinalysis. A priority focus in collaborative management for a patient suffering from dementia is to provide treatment of the cause, supportive care, and a safe environment. Assess the patient's psychiatric status, especially suicidal ideation, and sensory status, such as hearing and visual deficits. Optimally, place the patient in a quiet, private room with minimal stimulation that permits continuous observation. Use the patient's name during conversation, keep the conversations simple and short, and frequently reorient the patient to person and place.

One challenge in caring for patients with dementia is the assessment of pain. A tool that may be used is the Pain Assessment in Advanced Dementia (PAINAD) (Warden, Hurley & Volicer, 2003). This tool uses five behavioral indicators of pain including (1) breathing, (2) vocalization, (3) facial expression, (4) body language, and (5) consolability (Horgas & Miller, 2008). Retrieve this tool from www.healthcare.uiowa.edu/igec/tools/pain/PAINAD.pdf and use to determine when the patient with dementia requires analgesics and to evaluate response to analgesics.

There is no cure for most types of dementia; however, there are drug treatments (Table 11-6) available to slow or minimize the disease progression and alleviate symptoms. Administer

drugs as prescribed for dementia. Interview the family members to determine current safety issues. Utilize the information provided by families to guide the plan of care. Evaluate patient risk for making unsafe decisions and the potential for wandering and falling. Avoid physical restraints, but continuous companions may be necessary to ensure safety. Monitor the patient for complications such as violence, falls, decreased awareness of environment, and decreased self-care.

Dementia often causes a number of behavioral and psychological symptoms, which can be very distressing. These may include depression, anxiety, sleeplessness, hallucinations, ideas of persecution, misidentification of relatives or places, agitation, and aggressive behavior. These symptoms may respond to reassurance, a change in the environment, or removal of the source of any distress such as pain. However, sometimes medication may be required for relief.

Major tranquilizers control agitation, aggression, delusions, and hallucinations. Haloperidol (Haldol) is one commonly used drug. In modest doses, this drug tends to cause symptoms similar to Parkinson disease such as stiffness, shuffling gait, and shakiness, and older people are very prone to these side effects. Some are unable to tolerate even low doses of haloperidol.

Newer tranquilizers such as risperidone (Risperdal) have fewer Parkinson-like side effects. Risperidone appears to be helpful for the treatment of aggression and psychosis, but may be associated with a slight increase in risk of stroke. Olanzapine (Zyprexa) and quetiapine (Seroquel) are also used, but there is some evidence that olanzapine may also be associated with increased risk of stroke.

Symptoms of depression are extremely common in people with dementia. Treat depression with antidepressant agents, but take care to minimize side effects.

Anxiety states, accompanied by panic attacks and unreasonable fearfulness, can be very distressing for a person with dementia and place considerable stress on family and caregivers. While benzodiazepines are very effective for reducing anxiety in the short term, most individuals rapidly become tolerant to

TABLE 11-7	**Delirium versus Dementia**	
	Delirium	**Dementia**
Onset	Rapid: hours to days	Gradual: months to years
Orientation	Impaired	Impaired
Memory	Impaired: short-term and remote	Predominantly short-term memory impaired; remote memory stays intact
Level of consciousness	Disturbed, often fluctuates over 24-hour period	Alert, steady
Sleep-wake cycle	Erratic, disturbed over the course of the day, no patterns	No acute change; however, day-night reversal is common over time
Etiology	Evidence of general medical condition, trauma, substance use or withdrawal, or toxin	No evidence of medical illness, trauma, substance use or withdrawal, or toxin to account for changes
EEG	Diffuse slowing	Slowing may occur
Duration	Brief (if effectively treated)	Chronic
Symptoms	Fluctuate over 24 hours	Consistent pattern
Sensory/perception	Hallucinations common	Misidentification and delusions

their effects so they become less beneficial with time. In addition, withdrawal of benzodiazepines is often associated with a rebound of anxiety symptoms.

Persistent waking at night and nighttime wandering can cause difficulty for the patient and caregiver. Many drugs commonly prescribed for dementia can cause excessive sedation during the day, leading to an inability to sleep at night. Increased stimulation during the day can reduce the need for sleep-inducing medications at night. Medication to treat sleep disturbances should be a last resort, as people may become dependent on these and withdrawal of the medication results in rebound sleeplessness and anxiety.

Delirium

Delirium is an acute change (i.e., hours to days) in consciousness, cognition, and disturbance in attention not due to dementia. Accompanied by personality, behavioral, emotional, and functional changes, delirium is transient in nature but usually reversible. There are significant differences between delirium and dementia (Table 11-7). Delirium may result from or be related to a general medical condition, such as trauma or infection; the use/abuse of or withdrawal from a prescribed, illegal, or over-the-counter substance; exposure to a toxin; and/or a combination of these. In fact, causes of delirium include almost any disorder or drug. Treatment is correction of the cause and supportive measures.

Delirium may occur at any age but is more common among the elderly. At least 10% of elderly patients admitted to the hospital have delirium, and 15% to 50% experience delirium at some time during hospitalization (Juang, 2015). Delirium is also common after surgery and among nursing home residents and ICU patients. When delirium occurs in younger people, it is usually due to drug use or a life-threatening systemic disorder.

Patients who experience delirium during hospitalization are more likely to develop dysrhythmias, posttraumatic stress disorder, and cognitive decline. They are also more likely to be discharged to a place other than home. Evidence shows a correlation between development of ICU delirium and an increased number of days on mechanical ventilation, ICU length of stay,

and hospital length of stay, along with a higher 6-month mortality rate (Slooter, 2013).

Delirium due to certain conditions (e.g., hypoglycemia, drug or alcohol intoxication, infection, iatrogenic factors, drug toxicity, electrolyte imbalance) typically resolves rapidly with treatment. However, recovery may be slow (days to even weeks or months), especially in the elderly, resulting in longer hospital stays, increased risk and severity of complications, increased costs, and long-term disability. Some patients never fully recover from delirium. For up to 2 years after delirium occurs, risk of cognitive and functional decline, institutionalization, and death is increased. Morbidity and mortality rates are higher in patients who have delirium when admitted to the hospital or who develop delirium during hospitalization; 35% to 40% of hospitalized patients with delirium die within 1 year (Girard et al., 2010). There are many predisposing risks for delirium. Men are more likely than women to develop delirium and the elderly are at high risk. Other predisposing factors can be categorized as history or clinical course, environmental factors, and pharmacologic agents (Box 11-4).

The pathophysiology of delirium is dependent on the etiology. There is always an acute (i.e., hours to days) deterioration of cognition with fluctuating level of awareness.

Emotional, behavioral, cognitive, and sleep/wake cycle prodromal symptoms may be present and include anxiety, irritability, restlessness, disorientation, and an inability to sleep or stay asleep. Cognitive malfunction occurs in memory, intellect, learning, orientation, calculations, language, and judgment.

Subjective complaints of the patient with delirium include difficulty concentrating, memory loss, confusion, and a decline in cognitive function and judgment. Objective findings seen in delirium are a lack of orientation to situation, time, place, and person. Behavioral disturbances and functional decline are present and may progress to stupor, coma, seizures, and death if underlying etiology is not effectively treated. The patient may say things that do not make sense and report seeing, hearing, and feeling things that are not there. The patient may have paranoid delusions. The family will report that the patient is acting differently from normal.

BOX 11-4

Predisposing Risks for Delirium

History or Clinical Course

- History of delirium
- History of dementia
- History of mental illness or psychological problems
- History of alcohol or substance abuse
- History of falls
- Severe illness
- Cardiac surgery
- Cardiopulmonary bypass
- Prolonged surgery
- Electrolyte imbalance: sodium and potassium
- Hypoxia
- Infection
- Severe pain
- Impaired eyesight or hearing
- Malnutrition
- Renal or hepatic disease
- Fracture or trauma

Environmental Factors

- Critical care
- Sleep deprivation
- Sensory overload/sensory deprivation
- Noise
- Hypothermia or hyperthermia
- Physical restraints

Pharmacologic Agents

- Anticholinergics, including anti-histamines (e.g., diphenhydramine [Benadryl] and disopyramide [Norpace])
- Opioids
- Benzodiazepines
- Tricyclic antidepressants
- Corticosteroids
- General anesthetics
- H_2 receptor blockers
- Diuretics
- Withdrawal from alcohol, nicotine, or drugs

Delirium states include hyperactive, hypoactive, or mixed forms. Patients with the hyperactive form are agitated, pulling at tubes and picking at sheets and clothing, and exhibit combative behavior and progressive sedation. Often, providers fail to recognize the hypoactive form because the patient is calm with inattentiveness and decreased mobility. The mixed form may have both presentations.

A common tool used to diagnose delirium is the Confusion Assessment Method (CAM). The four components of CAM are (1) acute change or fluctuating course of mental status, (2) inattention, (3) altered level of consciousness, and (4) disorganized thinking (Ely, 2001; Inouye et al., 1990). If features 1 and 2 and either feature 3 or 4 are present, delirium is present. Each feature relies on standard components of a neurologic assessment. Diagnostic tests performed include the diagnostic studies to determine the cause of the delirium and the mini-mental status examination (Folstein, Folstein, & McHugh, 1975). The patient with delirium due to being in the critical care unit may present with altered consciousness, decreased attention span, disorientation, confusion, memory loss, labile emotions, and perceptual distortions, such as hallucinations, paranoia, and combativeness.

The first priority of collaborative care is the prevention of predisposing factors for delirium. Get the patient out of bed into a chair or ambulate as soon as possible. Initiate efforts to facilitate communication with an intubated patient or one who has a tracheostomy; contact speech therapy as soon as possible. Ensure use of eye glasses and hearing aids if required. Treat pain and promote rest and sleep. Avoid the use of drugs known to predispose the patient to delirium.

When delirium does occur, eliminate causes of delirium if possible. Encourage the family to visit and reorient the patient. The presence of familiar persons may be calming and helpful.

Also, attempt to provide continuity of nursing staff to lessen the number of adjustments required by the patient and family. Place personal belongings at the bedside. Place a clock and calendar in the room. Ask the patient to bring in familiar pictures and music.

Use the patient's name during conversation. Keep conversations simple and short. Frequently reorient the patient to person, place, time, and situation. Encourage family and staff not to argue with the patient about his or her hallucinations, if present. Do not use physical restraints but rather use a family member or a companion to talk to the patient, talk about current events, and alert the nurse to the patient's attempts to remove tubes, etc. Remove all unnecessary tubes, catheters, and drains as soon as possible. Assist the patient to ambulate and sit in a chair.

Adjust the lighting to simulate night and day, and maintain the sleep-wake cycles while allowing for short naps throughout the day. During the day, ensure good lighting and open the curtains. Plan uninterrupted nighttime sleep and do not awaken the patient unless truly necessary. Provide a safe environment with a quiet room with minimal stimulation, which will also allow continuous observation. Decrease the noise level on alarms and decrease extraneous conversation and other noise. Earplugs may also be an option. The Environmental Protection Agency (EPA) (1974) recommends that daytime noise levels in a hospital not exceed 45 dB and that nighttime levels not exceed 35 dB.

Evaluate the risk for making unsafe decisions and the potential for falling. Monitor for complications of violence, falls, decreased awareness of environment, and decreased self-care (e.g., feeding, toileting, hygiene).

Administer drugs to calm and sedate the patient as prescribed. The drug used most often is haloperidol. The usual IV or intramuscular (IM) dose is 1 mg. Haldol may also be given orally if the patient is cooperative and able to take and swallow the medication. Monitor the patient's ECG because prolonged QT interval and resultant torsades de pointes may occur. Chlorpromazine (Thorazine) may also be used; the dose is 25 mg IV or IM initially followed by 25 to 50 mg every 1 to 4 hours.

Depression

Depression is a disturbance of mood associated with anhedonia (i.e., loss of interest and/or pleasure in usual activities) or an increase in sadness or negative thinking not associated with medication withdrawal, bereavement, or another medical condition. The feeling of sadness and hopelessness may be manifested by loss of interest in people, dissatisfaction, difficulty in making decisions, and crying. The patient may say that he or she is a failure, being punished, or is considering hurting himself or herself.

There are several predisposing factors for the development of depression. Genetic predisposition, severe psychosocial stressors, hormonal imbalance, and sudden changes in substance use are factors that predispose a patient to depression. Medical conditions such as diabetes, myocardial infarction, cardiac surgery, cancer, or stroke along with medication side effects can also predispose a patient to depression.

The pathophysiology of depression is not well defined, but it is associated with a disturbance in CNS serotonin activity. Current evidence points to a complex interaction between neurotransmitter availability and receptor regulation and sensitivity underlying the affective symptoms. Clinical and preclinical trials suggest a disturbance in central nervous system serotonin (5-HT) activity as an important factor. Other neurotransmitters implicated include norepinephrine (NE), dopamine (DA), glutamate, and brain-derived neurotrophic factor (BDNF) (Hasler, 2010).

The patient with depression will subjectively complain of a depressed mood or anhedonia for a period of 2 months or more. He or she may express feelings of guilt, worthlessness, hopelessness, and recurrent thoughts of death and/or suicide. The patient may have a history of attempted suicide, thoughts or plans of suicide, or recurrent thoughts of death. In addition, he or she may report the occurrence of sleep disturbances such as insomnia, hypersomnia, and feeling unrested, as well as an inability to concentrate. Physical symptoms such as low energy and fatigue, changes in appetite, weight loss or gain, decreased libido, amenorrhea, and constipation may be a problem. Psychomotor symptoms of agitation, restlessness, the need to keep moving or psychomotor retardation with a generalized slowing down of movements, physical reactions, and speech may be present in depressed patients. Objective signs and symptoms present in a patient with depression may be an appearance indicative of poor hygiene and a lack of concern regarding appearance. The patient may be tearful and have a flat affect, along with quiet speech, little eye contact, psychomotor retardation, or evidence of psychotic symptoms such as hallucinations or delusions.

To rule out a medical cause for depression, perform serum and urine drug screens and a serum alcohol level. Thyroid function studies rule out hypothyroidism, and a CBC with differential eliminates the condition of anemia. A CT scan and MRI of the head may detect masses or structural abnormalities as the cause of the depression.

Collaborative management focuses on inspiring hope and facilitating coping. Provide information necessary to identify the patient's needs and to visualize the future realistically. Provide a safe environment and complete an assessment of psychiatric status especially for suicidal ideation. Provide a quiet room with minimal stimulation that allows for continuous observation. Use a nonjudgmental approach with the patient and provide frequent contacts to assure the patient of the staff's concern. If suicide is a concern, someone is to stay with the patient at all times.

Assist with treatment of depression by administering and monitoring the patient's response to antidepressant therapy. Categories of antidepressants include selective serotonin reuptake inhibitors (SSRIs) (e.g., citalopram [Celexa], escitalopram [Lexapro], fluoxetine [Prozac], paroxetine [Paxil], sertraline [Zoloft]), monoamine oxidase inhibitors (MAOIs) (e.g., isocarboxazid [Marplan], nialamide [Niamid], phenelzine [Nardil]), and tricyclic antidepressants (TCAs) (e.g., imipramine [Tofranil], amitriptyline [Elavil], clomipramine [Anafranil], imipramine [Tofranil], nortriptyline [Pamelor]). Assist the physician with electroconvulsant (ECT) therapy, light therapy, and transcranial magnetic stimulation if indicated. Monitor for complications of violent behavior and/or suicide. Provide patient education and counseling related to treatment methods and changes to report to the primary care provider.

Substance Use Disorders

Substance dependence is a maladaptive pattern of substance use, leading to clinically significant impairment or distress. Three or more of the following conditions, occurring at any time in the same 12-month period, manifest substance dependence:

- Tolerance
- Substance is taken in larger amounts or over a longer period than was intended
- Persistent desire or unsuccessful efforts to cut down or control use
- Much time spent in activities necessary to obtain the substance
- Important social, occupational, or recreational activities are given up or reduced because of usage
- Use is continued despite knowledge of physical or psychological problems caused by usage

Substance abuse is a pattern of continued substance use causing clinically significant impairment once or more in a 12-month period (APA, 2000). Substance abuse leads to a failure to fulfill role obligations at work, home, or school. Substance use in physically hazardous situations is a danger to the abuser and society. Legal problems and/or social or interpersonal problems related to the substance use may occur.

Several factors may predispose a patient to substance abuse. Substance abuse occurs more frequently when a family history of substance abuse or dependence exists. There is evidence of a genetic predisposition, but environmental exposure also influences the problem. Patients are more prone to the problem when they suffer from an inability to cope effectively. Peer pressure and group modeling, especially in adolescence, can lead to a substance abuse problem. Patients with substance abuse problems report a related history of usage and requests for help with addictions. A pattern of drug-seeking behavior of a particular medication (e.g., narcotic pain medication or tranquilizers) without an organic basis may be evident and the patient may demonstrate abusive or threatening behavior when denied drugs. In any type of addiction, relapse is common even with treatment.

Subjectively, the patient may self-report or family/friends may report the substance abuse. Patients may request help with addiction and be emotionally distressed and crying. Objective indications of substance abuse range from inappropriate behavior to stupor or coma. The patient may exhibit intoxication or erratic behavior including impaired judgment, aggression, and a labile mood. Speech may be slurred or rambling and the gait unsteady. Other findings may include the presence of nystagmus and impaired memory or attention. Diagnostic serum and urine drug screens will identify the agent(s) ingested. Collaborative management focuses on providing a safe environment and assessing the patient's psychiatric status, especially for suicidal ideation. Provide close monitoring for progression of symptoms. The Clinical Institute Withdrawal Assessment of Alcohol Scale (CIWA-Ar) is a widely accepted tool to facilitate assessment and treatment of alcohol withdrawal (see Chapter 6) (Sullivan et al., 1989). Provide a quiet room with minimal stimulation that allows for continuous observation. Determine whether the patient has suicidal ideation and/or plans for suicide. Avoid restraints, but the patient may be secluded and/or 1:1 observation required to ensure patient safety. Prevent withdrawal seizures by administering benzodiazepines as prescribed and monitor for the following complications:

- Cardiac dysrhythmias
- Hypertension or hypotension
- Respiratory depression
- Seizures
- Coma

Substance Abuse Withdrawal

Withdrawal from a substance may cause a specific syndrome due to the cessation of (or reduction in) substance use that has been heavy and prolonged. Withdrawal causes clinically significant distress or impairment that is unrelated to a general medical condition or another mental disorder. A patient who intentionally or unintentionally ceases to take a dependent substance will develop symptoms within hours to a few days following the cessation. Multiple objective signs and symptoms may be evident. Two or more of the following develop within hours to a few days after cessation:

- Autonomic hyperactivity
- Hand tremors
- Insomnia
- Nausea or vomiting
- Visual, tactile, or auditory hallucinations
- Psychomotor agitation
- Anxiety
- Seizures

The priority focus of collaborative management for a withdrawal syndrome is to maintain airway, breathing, ventilation, and circulation. Obtain vital signs (blood pressure, pulse, respiratory rate, and temperature) every 15 to 30 minutes until the patient is stable. Continually assess the cardiac rate and rhythm. Administer oxygen by nasal cannula at 2 to 6 L/min if indicated to maintain SpO_2 of 95% unless contraindicated. In patients with COPD, use pulse oximetry to guide oxygen administration to maintain a SpO_2 of ~90%. Obtain IV access for fluid and medication administration. Provide a safe environment and complete an assessment of the patient's psychiatric status,

especially for suicidal ideation. Provide a quiet room with minimal stimulation that allows for continuous observation. Use a nonjudgmental attitude when caring for the patient. Keep conversations simple and short. Frequently reorient the patient to person and place. Avoid restraints, but 1:1 observation of patient may be required to ensure patient safety. Administer and monitor the response of benzodiazepines prescribed to prevent seizures. Monitor the patient for complication of delirium tremens (DTs), which can progress to coma and death quickly.

Alcohol Withdrawal Syndrome

Alcohol withdrawal syndrome (AWS) consists of a spectrum of clinical manifestations that vary in severity and duration upon cessation of alcohol intake in the alcohol-dependent patient. Clinical presentations of AWS are part of a clinical continuum, but the sequence of events may be inconsistent, and is dependent on the degree of alcohol abuse. There are four stages of alcohol withdrawal (refer to Chapter 6).

To assess objectively the severity of AWS, a scale called the Clinical Institute Withdrawal Assessment for Alcohol Scale was developed (https://umem.org/files/uploads/1104212257_CIWA-Ar.pdf) (Sullivan et al., 1989). This scale is a 10-step assessment (scored from 0 to 67 points) of signs and symptoms of AWS. The initial score can be administered upon admission to the hospital and repeated hourly thereafter for signs of progression. A patient with a score of greater than 20 should be transferred to a higher-acuity level of care immediately, with the goal of reducing his or her score to less than 10 within the first 24 hours.

Aggression and Violence

Aggression is forceful physical or verbal behavior that may or may not cause harm to others. Violence is the ultimate maladaptive coping response and is the acting out of aggression that results in injury to others or destruction of property. The accumulation of stress in patients and family members who have feelings of desperation and lack the coping skills to resolve a situation by other means may trigger violence. Predisposing factors to violence include substance abuse, stress reactions, inability to cope, direct intent to injure (i.e., assault), and history of trauma, violence, or abuse. Aggression and violence can be present with personality disorders, organic illness, psychiatric illness, and/or substance abuse or withdrawal. Neglect, the failure to care for oneself or another person properly, can also be a form of abuse.

Elder abuse is the infliction of physical, emotional/psychologic, sexual, or financial harm on an older adult. Elder abuse can also take the form of intentional or unintentional neglect of an older adult by the caregiver. If medical conditions, medications, or treatments cannot explain symptoms, investigate to determine if cues signal elder abuse or neglect. Symptoms of elder abuse and neglect range from outward clinical signs of physical abuse (e.g., bruises) to neglect (e.g., lack of clothing, food, shelter, and health care). Report suspected abuse to social services.

A patient with aggression and violent tendencies demonstrates cognitive, behavioral, and physiologic findings. The patient may act paranoid and lack the ability to think clearly and rationally. Behavioral signs may include anger, yelling, and the use of profanity. The patient may be agitated and pacing about. Verbal threats and physical violence such as striking, pushing, and kicking staff may occur. Physiologic findings include tachycardia, tachypnea, elevated blood pressure, and increased muscle tension.

The priority focus of the collaborative management for the aggressive or violent patient is to ensure your personal safety and the safety of other staff members, as well as the safety of the patient, family, and other visitors. At the first indication of physical threat, call security and/or the police for assistance. Conduct frequent assessments of psychiatric status, especially suicidal ideation. Provide the patient and family members support and information. Attempt to determine what the patient wishes if able to comprehend the situation. Monitor for complications of assault, homicide, and/or suicide.

Suicide

Suicide is the willful taking of one's own life. Suicide may be premeditated or impulsive. Predisposing factors to suicide include family history, prior attempts at suicide, substance abuse, depression, physical illnesses, violent environmental factors, and an anniversary of the suicide/death of a loved one. If a patient admits to suicidal ideation, determine if he or she has developed a plan.

Provide a safe environment and assess the patient's psychiatric status. Provide a quiet room with minimal stimulation that allows for continuous observation. Do not leave the patient alone. Clear the environment of any potential harmful items, which the patient could use for self-harm or harm to others. Use a nonjudgmental approach with the patient. Avoid physical restraint, but one-on-one observation is required to ensure patient safety. Resolve immediate medical crisis needs before dealing with mental health issues. Also, provide support to family members.

Bipolar Disorders

The primary symptoms of bipolar disorder are dramatic and unpredictable mood swings. The condition varies from a depressive state to a manic state. Mania symptoms may include excessive happiness, excitement, irritability, restlessness, increased energy, less need for sleep, racing thoughts, high sex drive, and a tendency to make grand and unattainable plans. Depression symptoms may include sadness, anxiety, irritability, loss of energy, uncontrollable crying, change in appetite causing weight loss or gain, increased need for sleep, difficulty making decisions, and thoughts of death or suicide. Self-injury, often referred to as cutting, self-mutilation, or self-harm, is an injurious attempt to cope with overpowering negative emotions, such as extreme anger, anxiety, and frustration. It is usually repetitive, not a one-time act. Suicide is a very real risk for people with bipolar disorder, but treatment greatly lowers the risk. There are several types of bipolar disorder (Table 11-8); all involve episodes of depression and mania to a degree. They include bipolar I, bipolar II, cyclothymic disorder, mixed bipolar, and rapid-cycling bipolar disorder.

Mania

Mania is a condition in which the patient has an episode of elevated, irritable, or expansive mood lasting at least 1 week. There is a marked impairment in functioning. Findings are not due to any substance or general medical condition. Bipolar mania is a combination of mood swings from mania to depression.

There is a genetic predisposition to the condition of mania. Other factors that predispose the condition include severe psychosocial stressors, hormonal imbalance, and a sudden decrease

TABLE 11-8	Types of Bipolar States
Type	**Symptoms**
Bipolar I	At least one manic episode in his or her life; a manic episode is a period of abnormally elevated mood, accompanied by abnormal behavior that disrupts life
Bipolar II	Moods cycling between high and low over time, but the "up" moods never reach full-on mania
Rapid cycling	Four or more episodes of mania or depression in 1 year
Mixed bipolar	Both mania and depression simultaneously or in rapid sequence
Cyclothymia	Milder symptoms than in bipolar disorder

in substance use. The pathophysiology of mania is thought to involve the dysregulation of neurotransmitters.

A patient with mania will likely have a history of manic or hypomanic episodes. He or she is likely to complain of racing thoughts and has little need for sleep. Often, there is an increase in use of prescribed or illegal drugs to calm the patient. Mania leads to risky behaviors, such as abuse of credit cards and reckless spending and multiple sex partners. Mania causes interference with job performance. The mania often causes the development of unrealistic future plans. The patient may have an arrest history and previous or current plans for suicide.

Observation of the patient will likely reveal fidgeting and pacing. The patient will have difficulty staying on topic and will have flight of ideas. Inappropriate elation, euphoria, and laughing may occur along with grandiosity. Assess any injuries the patient may have suffered during the manic state.

Diagnostic studies include serum alcohol levels and urine drug screens. An ECG may show tachycardia, atrial dysrhythmias, PACs, and PVCs. Other diagnostic laboratory and radiology studies are done to rule out medical causes of the mania and/or identify current injury.

A priority focus during an episode of mania is to provide a safe environment and the conduction of a psychiatric assessment, especially suicidal ideation. Provide a quiet room with minimal stimulation that allows for continuous observation. Use a nonjudgmental approach with the patient. Avoid restraints, but 1:1 observations may be required to ensure patient safety.

Use prevention strategies to manage aggressive behavior in all clinical settings. Identify behaviors or actions that escalate and deescalate violent behavior. Nursing interventions focus on communication and development of the nurse-patient relationship, cognitive interventions, patient education, creating a calm and therapeutic environment, and violence prevention. Observe every 15 minutes for behaviors and physical conditions and document. The Joint Commission (2015) defines two types of restraints based on the purpose for the restraints. Behavioral restraints are used most frequently in the emergency department for the control of aggressive/violent behavior or behavior that is dangerous to self or others. When using behavioral restraints, offer liquid, nutrition, comfort, and bathroom every 2 hours. Remove the restraints every 2 hours for no less than 5 minutes for range of motion and skin care. Medical/surgical restraints are used for care management of a patient on a medical/surgical or progressive care unit who is exhibiting behavior that is interfering with treatment (e.g., pulling on IV, indwelling urinary catheter, or dressings). Observe every 2 hours for behaviors and physical conditions and document. Offer liquid, nutrition, comfort, and bathroom every 2 hours. Remove restraints every 2 hours for no less than 10 minutes for range of motion and skin care.

Control the mania with administration of antipsychotics for psychosis, if present, until the mood stabilizers take effect. Mood stabilizers, such as lithium, anticonvulsants (e.g., divalproex sodium [Depakote], lamotrigine [Lamictal], and carbamazepine [Tegretol]), antipsychotics (e.g., aripiprazole [Abilify], risperidone [Risperdal], and olanzapine [Zyprexa]), and benzodiazepines (e.g., lorazepam [Ativan], clonazepam [Klonopin], and alprazolam [Xanax]) are used to control the mania and antidepressants are used the control the depression. Administer beta-blockers to block effects of excess catecholamines. Provide counseling to deal with the cycling of moods, behavior, and interpersonal relationships. Monitor the patient for complications of self-injury or suicide.

Psychosis

Psychosis is a severe psychiatric disorder characterized by personality disorganization, loss of contact with reality, and deterioration of normal social functioning. The condition can be acute or chronic lasting from a few days to several months. The condition may be functional or organic.

Factors that lead to the functional type of psychosis are severe depression, mania, schizophrenic disorder, or a brief psychotic episode. The predisposing factors for the organic type of psychosis are the ingestion of a toxic substance, shock or trauma, slow onset dementia, and rapid onset delirium, but the pathophysiology of the condition is poorly understood.

During mania, the patient or family may report a previous history of psychotic episodes, confusion, or amnesia. The patient may report paranoid ideation, fears about safety, loss of energy, and self-medication. Delusions and hallucinations, usually auditory, may be present. Other findings that may be present in mania are avolition (i.e., inability to initiate activities including self-care), alogia (i.e., absence of speech), anhedonia, and a flat affect. The patient may have disorganized speech or incoherence. Conversation may indicate confusion, loss of touch with reality, and loss of orientation to time, place, and person. In mania, there may be increased agitation or bizarre behavior, grossly exaggerated behaviors, and/or psychomotor retardation (i.e., visible generalized slowing down of movements, physical reactions, and speech). Diagnostic tests include a urinalysis, especially if the person is an elderly female. Perform serum and urine drug screens. CT scans reveal if any masses or structural changes have occurred in the cranium. Perform other diagnostic laboratory and radiology studies as indicated to rule out other medical causes.

The priority of collaborative management is to provide a safe environment and the conduction of a psychiatric assessment, especially for the presence of suicidal ideation. Provide a quiet room with minimal stimulation that allows continuous observation. Use a nonjudgmental approach with the patient. Keep conversations simple, short, reality based, and concrete. Acknowledge the patient's delusion and/or hallucinations while maintaining reality (e.g., "I believe that you are hearing voices, but I do not hear them."). Avoid arguing with the patient about his or her experience. Provide support for the feelings that the symptoms may be generated (e.g., "It must be frightening to hear those voices."). Frequently reorient the patient to person, place, time, and situation. Avoid restraints, but 1:1 observation of the patient may be required to ensure patient safety.

Assist with management of psychosis by administration of antipsychotic medications to reduce psychosis. Administer anxiolytic medications adjunctively with antipsychotic medications to reduce anxiety and/or induce sleep. Consult with the patient's current psychiatrist or refer to a psychiatrist if previously not treated for psychosis. Monitor for complications of extrapyramidal symptoms (EPSs), neuroleptic malignant syndrome, incontinence, and coma.

11.3 Learning Activity

Identify the assessment findings in each of the following conditions that would help you distinguish it from the others.

Condition	Subjective Assessment	Objective Assessment
Anxiety disorder		
Depression		
Mania		
Hallucinations		
Psychosis		
Dementia		
Delirium		

Answers to this activity can be found in the Answer Key.

11.4   Synthesis Learning Activity: Crossword Puzzle

Complete the following crossword puzzle related to psychosocial conditions.

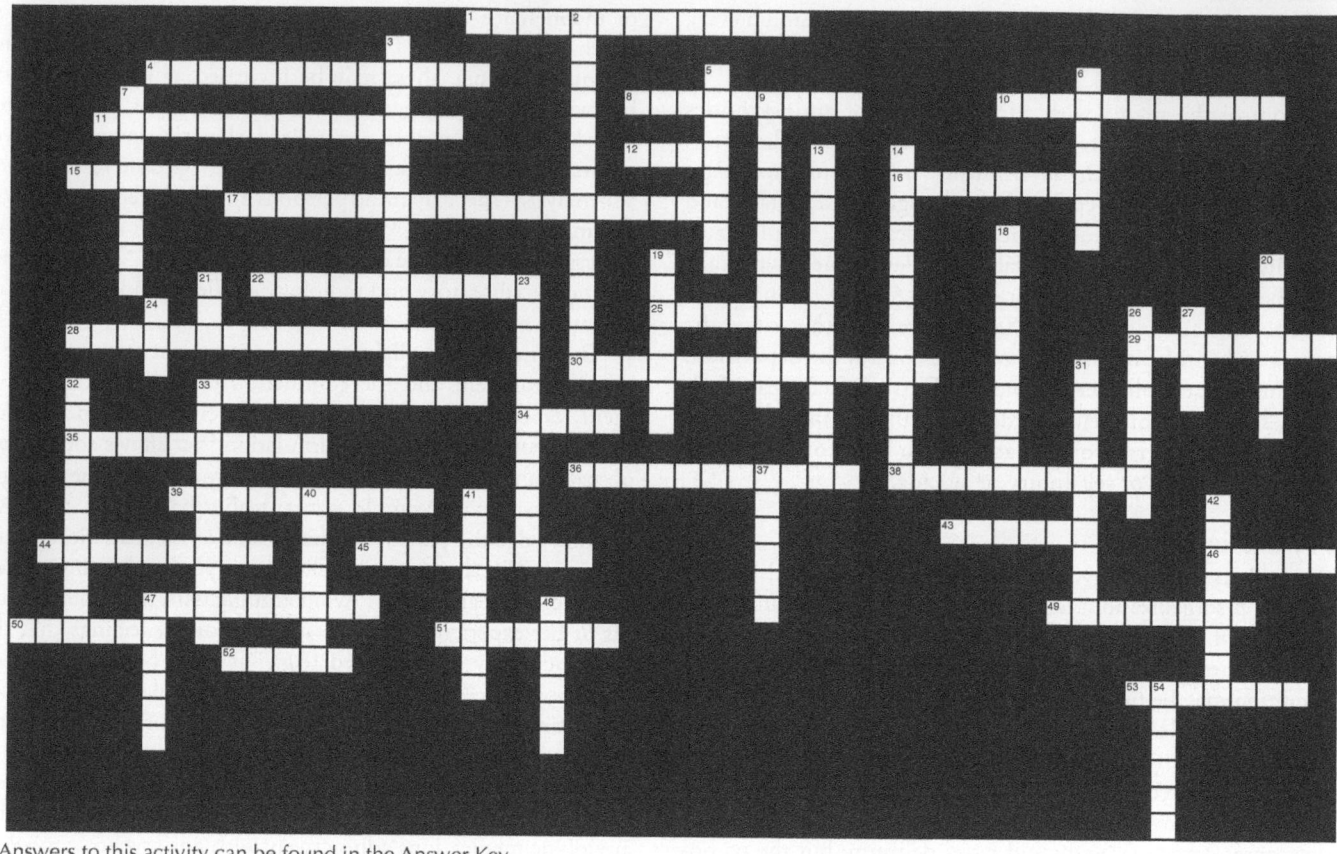

Answers to this activity can be found in the Answer Key.

ACROSS

1. A non-goal–directed speech that leaps from one idea to another (3 words)
4. A perceived lack of control over the outcome of a specific situation or problem
8. These are fixed false beliefs
10. The type of hallucination that occurs upon awakening
11. This chemical type of drug is administered to decrease anxiety and is also used to decrease the risk of seizures during substance withdrawal
12. Affect is said to be _____ if it demonstrates no emotion
15. The state that occurs when one's usual ways of coping are inadequate to deal with stress
16. There is an increase in this type of thinking in depression
17. The term for tolerance to a substance and inability to stop use (2 words)

22. These medications are used to decrease anxiety
25. The term for not attending to the emotional, physical, or mental care needs of another who cannot care for himself or herself
28. Thoughts or speech that contain excessive details about the topic but finally reach the intended point
29. According to Erikson, young adulthood is focused on _____ versus self-isolation
30. The term for recurrent substance use resulting in a failure to fulfill major role obligations at work, home, or school (2 words)
33. Sensory _____ is a decreased frequency, intensity, or variety of stimulation of the senses with meaningful stimuli
34. The emotion that the patient reports
35. Hallucinations are this type of disturbance

36. A state of sorrow over the loss of a loved one
38. The term for discomfort caused by separation from significant relationships, places, events, and objects
39. The term for going back to an earlier level of emotional development
43. The term for demonstrated emotion
44. This mental disorder is characterized by hallucinations and delusions
45. The lack of pleasure
46. An elevated or irritable mood of at least 1 week duration
47. The inability to initiate activities that is seen in psychosis
49. The involuntary cessation in the flow of thought or speech
50. The term for treating obvious reality factors as though they do not exist because they are consciously intolerable

51. According to Erikson, older adulthood is focused on integrity versus _____
52. The emotional response to a loss in which something valued is changed or altered
53. A language disturbance seen in dementia

DOWN

2. The term for sensory perceptions when there are no sensory stimuli
3. This functional type of drug is used for mood stabilization
5. This is the type of stress that occurs in response to nonthreatening stimuli
6. This disorder is characterized by feelings of helplessness and tension
7. An acute change (hours to days) in consciousness and cognition not due to dementia
9. The term for cognitive ability

13. The ability to focus and pay attention

14. Talking with a support person would be this type of coping mechanism

18. A brief test of specific aspects of cognitive function

19. The inability to recognize or identify objects despite intact sensory function

20. The inability to perform motor activities despite intact motor function

21. A tool commonly used to diagnose dementia (abbrev.)

23. The term for directing energy from unacceptable drives into socially acceptable behaviors

24. The term for recurrent, persistent, intrusive thoughts and feelings coupled with ritualistic and repetitive behaviors (abbrev.)

26. This is the type of stress that occurs in response to noxious stimuli

27. The term for persistent or repeated reexperiencing of a traumatic event that has occurred in the past, which induces an anxiety response (abbrev.)

31. The term for the logical, directed thought that may "circle the topic" but does not make a point or answer the intended question

32. The term for unconscious, involuntary forgetting of unacceptable or painful thoughts, impulses, feelings, or acts

33. An alteration in mood characterized by sadness and negative self-concept

37. This hierarchy of needs contends that physiologic needs for oxygen and nutrients take priority over love and belonging

40. The term for willful taking of one's own life

41. The ability to make sound decisions

42. A chronic global deterioration of cognition

47. The absence of speech

48. Emotions are said to be ____ when they fluctuate high to low rapidly and inconsistently without respect to the situation

54. A spiritual form of coping mechanism

11.5   Synthesis Learning Activity: Clinical Vignette

Mr. D is a 67-year-old widower of 2 years who retired 3 months ago from his position as a mechanical engineer. He lives alone in his home of 30 years. His son has accompanied him to the ED. He presents to the ED unshaven and disheveled with poor eye contact. He mumbles in response to questions in soft, low tones and is difficult to understand. He keeps stating that he is in awful shape, he has no memory, he is of no good use to himself or anyone else, and they should just let him die. When pressed to do so, he reluctantly identifies the correct year, date, and day. He is aware he has been brought to a hospital. His sleep is erratic, his appetite is poor, he has generalized weakness, and his gait is unsteady. His son reports that his father typically is meticulous about his appearance and is very articulate. He states that he last saw his father 2 weeks ago when they had gone out to dinner and had done some grocery shopping. At that time, Mr. D was well-groomed, walking steadily and independently, and actively involved in their conversation, his son said. He is concerned that his father has had a stroke.

a. What additional information might you need about Mr. D?	
b. What laboratory tests might be helpful?	
c. What would be a preliminary diagnosis for Mr. D and what are the data that support that diagnosis?	
d. What would be priority care issues for Mr. D?	

Answers to this activity can be found in the Answer Key.

11.6   Synthesis Learning Activity: Synergy Model

Using the Synergy Model in practice, determine the resource level of a homeless woman admitted to the hospital for observation following an attempted suicide. The patient cut her wrists, has no identification, and refuses to talk with the staff.

a. Level 1

b. Level 2

c. Level 3

d. Level 4

e. Level 5

Answers to this activity can be found in the Answer Key.

Learning Activities Answers

CHAPTER 2

2.1

1. Information collection and problem identification
2. Identification of possible solutions or actions
3. Analysis of the possible consequences of each solution or action
4. Selection of the best possible solution or action for implementation
5. Implementation of the solution or action
6. Evaluation of the results

2.2

a	1. Utilitarianism
d	2. Egoism
f	3. Deontology
c	4. Paternalism
g	5. Social contract
e	6. Natural law
b	7. Teleology

2.3

b	1. Veracity
e	2. Confidentiality
c	3. Autonomy
g	4. Nonmaleficence
f	5. Fidelity
d	6. Justice
a	7. Advocacy

2.4

Any eight of the following:
Progressive muscle relaxation (PMR)
Breathing
Meditation
Comeditation
Guided imagery
Massage
Hypnosis
Biofeedback
Therapeutic (or healing) touch
Purposeful touch
Music therapy
Aromatherapy
Pet therapy
Humor
Acupuncture

2.5

Any five of the following:
To have questions answered honestly
To be assured the best care possible is being given to the patient
To know the prognosis
To feel there is hope
To know specific facts about the patient's progress
To be called at home about changes in the patient's condition
To know how the patient is being treated medically
To feel hospital personnel care about the patient
To receive information about the patient daily
To have understandable explanations
To know exactly what is being done for the patient
To know why things were done for the patient
To see the patient frequently
To talk to the doctor every day
To be told about transfer plans

2.6

Any five of the following:
Communication
Trust
Respect
Understanding and acceptance of team members' roles
Competence
Shared responsibility and accountability
Shared goal setting
Flexibility
Administrative support

2.7

Choose any of the change models in Table 2-10 and describe how you would implement each aspect of the model to change practice.

Model	Planned Change
Lewin (1951) Model of Change	Status quo (diagnosis of problem) Unfreezing (develop the solution) Disequilibrium (overcome resistance) Moving (implement change) Refreezing (reestablishing balance) Equilibrium
Lippitt, Watson, and Westley (1958) Seven Phases of Planned Change	Aware of need for change Development of relationship between client system and change agent Definition of the change problem Establishment of change goals and exploration of options for achievement Implementation of the plan for change Acceptance and stabilization of the change Redefinition of the relationships of the change entities
Havelock (1973) Six Phases of Planned Change	Building a relationship Diagnosing the problem Acquiring relevant resources Choosing a solution Gaining acceptance Stabilizing the innovation and generating self-renewal
Rogers (1995) Diffusion of Innovation Model	Knowledge Persuasion Decision Implementation Confirmation
Prochaska (2000) Prochaska et al. (2001) Transtheoretical Model	Pre-contemplation: the individual is not thinking of change Contemplation: the individual is thinking of but not committed to change in the near future Preparation: the individual intends to change in the near future Action: the individual actively attempts to change Maintenance: the individual sustains the change over time
Kotter (1995) Process for Leading Change	Establish a sense of urgency Form a powerful guiding coalition Create a vision Communicate a vision Empower others to act on the vision Plan for and create short-term wins Consolidate improvements and produce still more change Institutionalize new approaches
Berwick (2003) From Description to Prescription	Find sound innovations Find and support innovators Invest in early adopters Make early adopter activity observable Trust and enable reinvention Create slack for change Lead by change

2.8

a. False
b. True
c. False
d. False
e. False

2.9

g	1. Islam (Muslim)
e	2. Catholicism
a	3. Judaism
c	4. Hinduism
d	5. Christian Scientist
f	6. Seventh-Day Adventist
b	7. Jehovah's Witnesses

2.10

c	1. Developing a clinical practice guideline for a common clinical condition or procedure
a	2. Designing and conducting a research study when the available evidence base is inadequate
b	3. Conducting a systematic review of available evidence related to a clinical issue
d	4. Initiation of an evidence-based clinical change
e	5. Appraisal of the effect of an evidence-based clinical change
a	6. Conducting a literature search for available evidence related to a clinical question

2.11

a. Bulletin boards for current articles
b. Journal clubs
c. Patient care conferences
d. Protocol and procedure development
e. Care paths

2.12

Any five of the following:
    Goal-oriented
    Less flexible
    Requires longer time in the performance of learning tasks
    Impatient in the pursuit of objectives
    Finds little use for isolated facts
    Strives for recognition and success
    Has multiple responsibilities, all of which draw upon his or her time
    Experienced in the "school of life"
    Requires a more constant and ideal learning environment
    Usually comes to the teaching program on a voluntary basis
    Wishes to be involved in mutual planning of learning experiences
    Likes to participate in diagnosing needs for learning, formulating learning objectives, and evaluating learning
    Expects a climate of mutual respect, trust, and collaboration that supports learning

2.13

A. Patient's Characteristics

Resiliency Level: (5) Able to mount response, strong coping mechanisms, endurance.

Vulnerability Level: (3) Somewhat susceptible, somewhat protected; in hospital high-acuity unit.

Stability Level: (3) Able to maintain steady state for limited time, medically treated with close observation. Scheduled for Monday, but with signs or symptoms of instability will be brought immediately.

Complexity Level: (3) complex surgical procedure, routine family dynamics, typical presentations.

Predictability Level: (5) Highly predictable, usual and expected course; follows pathway.

Resource Availability Level: (5) Extensive knowledge and skills available, good insurance and adequate finances, personal and psychological support, strong social system available.

Participation in Care Level: (3) Patient needs some assistance in care due to denial. Family had full capability and willingness for participation of patient/family in care. Wife or one daughter will rotate and someone will remain in hospital with patient.

Participation in Decision Making Level: (5) Full participation

B. Nurse Dimensions

Clinical Judgment Level: (3) Stable at present, needs a competent nurse that recognizes patterns and trends, and reacts to unexpected outcomes.

Advocacy/Moral Agency Level: (1) Aware of patient rights, works on behalf of patient/family, and aware of ethical conflicts and issues that may surface.

Caring Practices Level: (1) Maintains a safe environment, focuses on basic and routine needs of patient based on standards and protocols.

Collaboration level: (3) Initiates and participates in team meetings and discussions regarding patient care and/or practice issues. Recognizes and critiques multidisciplinary participation in care decisions.

Systems Thinking level: (1) Utilizes standardized processes, sees patient and family within the isolated environment of the unit, sees self as key resource for patient/family.

Response to Diversity level: (1) Assesses diversity. Recognizes practices based on diversity that may have negative impact, recognizes barriers.

Clinical Inquiry level: (3) Utilizes policies, procedures, standards, and guidelines adapting to patient needs.

Recognizes subtle changes in patient condition and begins to compare and contrast possible care alternatives.

Facilitator of Learning level: (3) Adapts planned educational programs to meet individual patient's need. Sees the patient/family as having input into educational goals and incorporates patient/family perspective into individualized education plan.

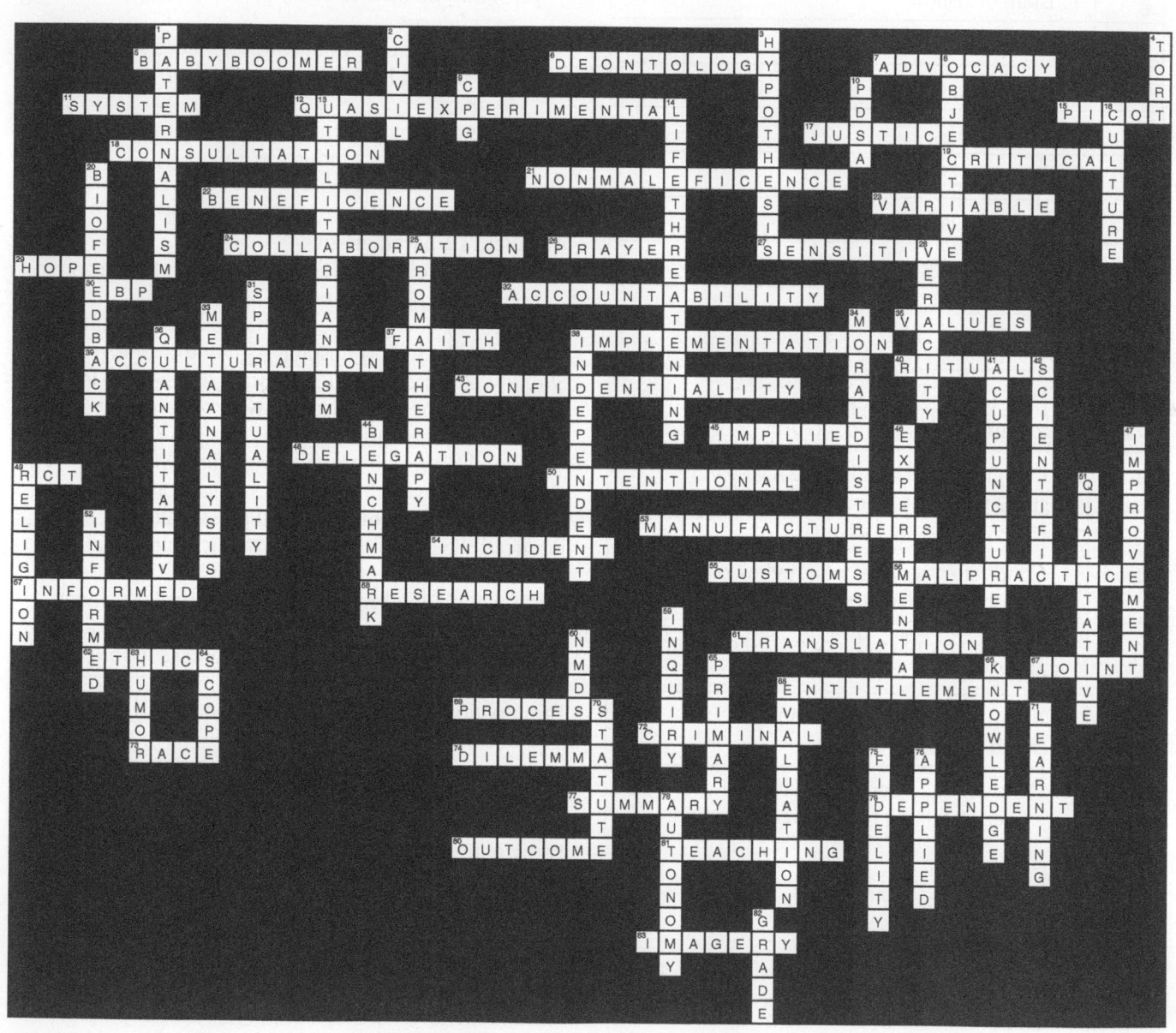

CHAPTER 3

3.1

Myocardial Oxygen Supply	Myocardial Oxygen Demand
Coronary artery patency	Heart rate
Diastolic pressure	Preload
Diastolic time	Afterload
Oxygen extraction: hemoglobin; SaO_2	Contractility

3.2

Structure	Coronary Artery
Anterior left ventricle	LAD
AV node	Most commonly RCA; less commonly LCA
Bundle branches	LAD
Inferior left ventricle	RCA
Lateral left ventricle	LCA
Left atrium	LCA
Posterior left ventricle	Most commonly RCA; less commonly LCA
Right atrium	RCA
Right ventricle	RCA
SA node	Most commonly RCA; less commonly LCA
Septum	LAD

3.3

Remember that you were asked to identify primary effects. If you gave answers other than these, perhaps you were thinking of the secondary effects, especially those mediated by the SNS or the resultant effect of a decrease in preload on contractility.

Conditions				
Aortic stenosis	___Heart Rate	___Preload	↑ LV Afterload	___Contractility
Bradydysrhythmias	↓ Heart Rate	↑ Preload	___Afterload	___Contractility
Cardiac tamponade	___Heart Rate	↓ Preload	___Afterload	___Contractility
Cardiogenic shock	___Heart Rate	↑ Preload	↑ Afterload	↓ Contractility
Cardiomyopathy	___Heart Rate	___Preload	___Afterload	↓ Contractility
HF	___Heart Rate	↑ Preload	↑ Afterload	↓ Contractility
Hypertension	___Heart Rate	___Preload	↑ LV Afterload	___Contractility
Hypovolemia	___Heart Rate	↓ Preload	___Afterload	___Contractility
Left ventricular myocardial infarction	___Heart Rate	___Preload	___Afterload	↓ Contractility

Conditions				
Neurogenic shock	↓ Heart Rate	↓ Preload	↓ Afterload	___Contractility
Pulmonary hypertension	___Heart Rate	___Preload	↑ RV Afterload	___Contractility
Right ventricular myocardial infarction	___Heart Rate	↑ RV Preload ↓ LV Preload	___Afterload	↓ Contractility
Septic shock - early	___Heart Rate	↓ Preload	↓ Afterload	↑ Contractility
Septic shock - late	___Heart Rate	↓ Preload	↓ Afterload	↓ Contractility
Tachydysrhythmias	↑ Heart Rate	↓ Preload	___Afterload	___Contractility
Treatments				
Aminophylline	___Heart Rate	___Preload	↓ RV Afterload	___Contractility
Digoxin (Lanoxin)	↓ Heart Rate	___Preload	___Afterload	↑ Contractility
Dobutamine (Dobutrex)	___Heart Rate	↓ Preload	↓ Afterload	↑ Contractility
Dopamine (3-5 mcg/kg/min)	↑ Heart Rate	___Preload	___Afterload	↑ Contractility
Dopamine (5-10 mcg/kg/min)	↑ Heart Rate	___Preload	↑ Afterload	↑ Contractility
Dopamine (>10 mcg/kg/min)	↑ Heart Rate	___Preload	↑ Afterload	___Contractility
Fluid challenge	___Heart Rate	↑ Preload	___Afterload	___Contractility
Furosemide (Lasix)	___Heart Rate	↓ Preload	↓ RV Afterload	___Contractility
Intraaortic balloon pump	___Heart Rate	___Preload	↓ Afterload	___Contractility
Isoproterenol (Isuprel)	↑ Heart Rate	↓ Preload	↓ Afterload	↑ Contractility
Milrinone (Primacor)	___Heart Rate	↓ Preload	↓ Afterload	↑ Contractility
Nesiritide (Natrecor)	___Heart Rate	↓ Preload	↓ Afterload	___Contractility
Nitroglycerin	___Heart Rate	↓ Preload	* Afterload	___Contractility
Nitroprusside (Nipride)	___Heart Rate	↓ Preload	↓ Afterload	___Contractility
Phenylephrine (Neo-Synephrine)	___Heart Rate	___Preload	↑ Afterload	___Contractility
Propranolol (Inderal)	↓ Heart Rate	___Preload	___Afterload	↓ Contractility
Vasopressin (Pitressin)	___Heart Rate	___Preload	↑ Afterload	___Contractility

*Nitroglycerin will decrease afterload if dosage is greater than 1 mcg/kg/min or approximately 70 mcg/min in a 70-kg patient.

3.4

b	1. Increase in heart rate, contractility, conductivity
d	2. Dilation of the renal and mesenteric arteries
a	3. Vasoconstriction
c	4. Vasodilation and bronchodilation

3.5

c	1. Alpha$_1$
d	2. Beta$_1$
a	3. Beta$_2$
b	4. Dopaminergic

3.6

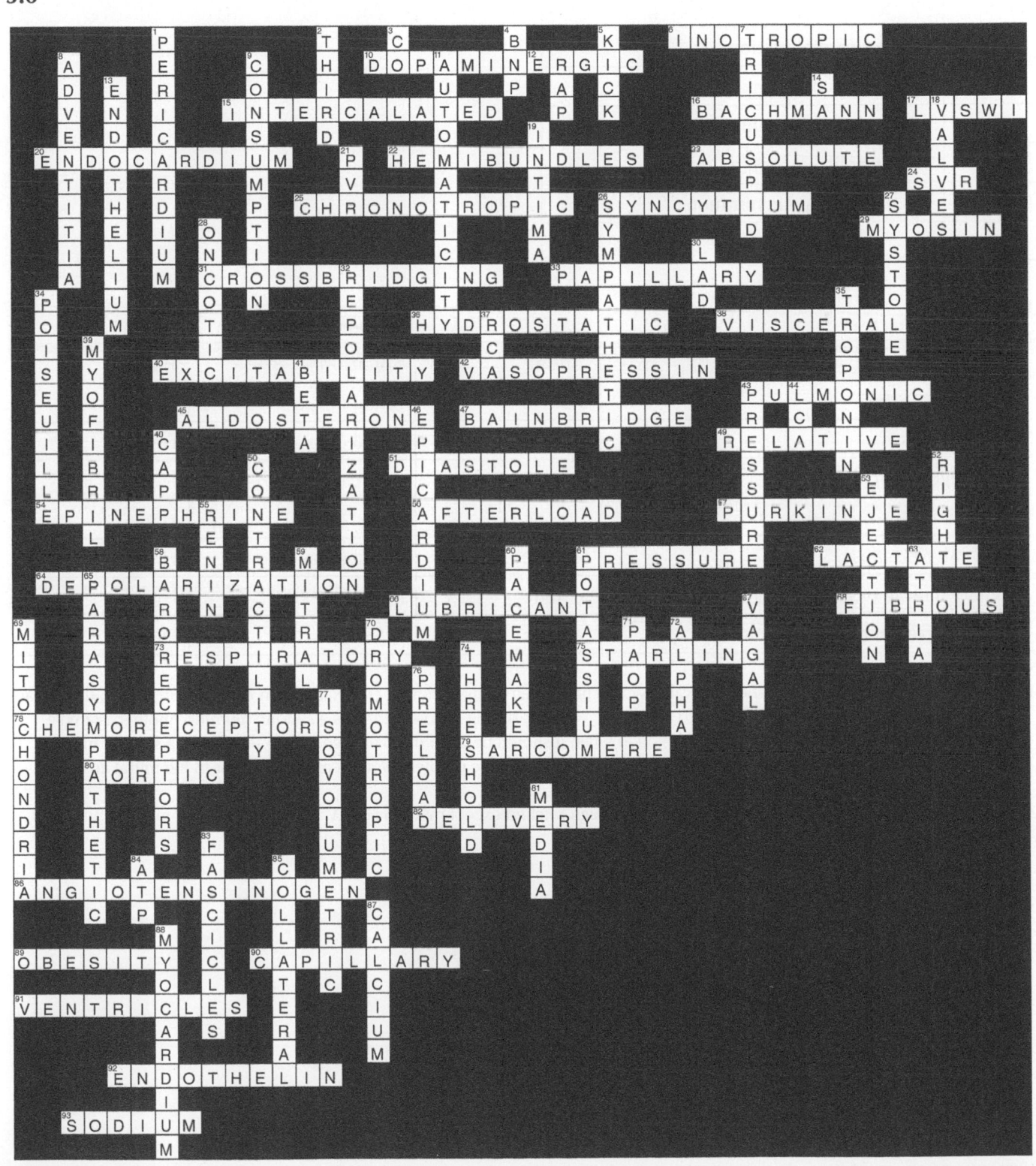

3.7

k	1. S_1
i	2. S_2
a	3. Physiologic split of S_2
f	4. Paradoxical split of S_2
b	5. Fixed, wide split of S_2
h	6. S_3
m	7. S_4
c	8. Pericardial friction rub
j	9. Midsystolic click
g	10. Holosystolic murmur
d	11. Systolic ejection murmur
l	12. Early diastolic murmur
e	13. Mid- to late-diastolic murmur

3.8

Condition	Timing	Location	Pitch
Mitral regurgitation	Systolic	Mitral (apex)	High
Mitral stenosis	Diastolic	Mitral (apex)	Low
Aortic regurgitation	Diastolic	Aortic (base)	High
Aortic stenosis	Systolic	Aortic (base)	High
Mitral valve prolapse	Systolic	Mitral (apex)	High
Papillary muscle dysfunction or rupture	Systolic	Mitral (apex)	High
Ventricular septal defect or rupture	Systolic	LLSB	High

Notes:

(1) To figure out timing, consider when the valve would have been open or closed. For example, in mitral regurgitation, the mitral valve would not be closed when it should be closed, which is during systole, so this is a systolic murmur. Another example would be that the aortic valve would not be open when it should be open in aortic stenosis, so this is also a systolic murmur.

(2) To figure out location, consider the auscultatory areas; a mitral valve problem would cause a murmur in the mitral auscultatory area, which is at the apex.

(3) To figure out pitch, remember that all murmurs are high-pitched except murmurs of AV valve stenosis (i.e., mitral or tricuspid stenosis).

3.9

k	1. Normal sinus rhythm
e	2. Sinus bradycardia
j	3. Sinus tachycardia
b	4. Premature atrial contraction
f	5. Atrial fibrillation
c	6. Atrial flutter
p	7. Supraventricular tachycardia
g	8. Premature junctional contraction
h	9. Junctional escape rhythm
m	10. Accelerated junctional rhythm
o	11. Junctional tachycardia
d	12. Premature ventricular complex
n	13. Accelerated idioventricular rhythm
t	14. Ventricular tachycardia
s	15. Ventricular fibrillation
i	16. Asystole
a	17. First-degree AV block
l	18. Second-degree AV block, type I
q	19. Second-degree AV block, type II
r	20. Third-degree AV block

3.10

a. Ventricular fibrillation
b. Sinus bradycardia with wide QRS (BBB should be assessed for on 12-lead ECG)
c. Supraventricular tachycardia; this is a regular narrow QRS tachycardia with no discernible P waves; the P waves could be hidden in the QRS or T wave, so there is no way to identify where above the ventricle the rhythm originates, but the rate of 180 beats/min suggests an atrial origin.
d. Idioventricular (escape) rhythm
e. Underlying sinus rhythm (atrial rate is 90 beats/min); there is a third-degree AV block with a ventricular escape rhythm (ventricular rate is 35 beats/min)
f. Underlying rhythm is sinus rhythm (atrial rate is 80 beats/min); there is a second-degree type I (i.e., Wenckebach) AV block present; conduction ratio is 3:2 and ventricular rate is 40-50 beats/min
g. Ventricular tachycardia (monomorphic)
h. Underlying rhythm is sinus tachycardia (atrial rate is 145 beats/min); there is a second-degree type II block present; conduction ratio is variable but the PR interval of the conducted P wave is consistent
i. Sinus rhythm with two unifocal PVCs

3.11

g	1. II, III, aVF
e	2. V_{4R}
b	3. I, aVL
f	4. V_1, V_2
a	5. V_3, V_4
c	6. V_5, V_6
d	7. V_8, V_9

3.12

a. LBBB: Note indicative changes of BBB in V_6 (LV lead) and the wide QRS is totally below the isoelectric line in V_1.
b. RBBB: Note indicative changes of BBB in V_1 (RV lead) and the wide QRS is totally above the isoelectric line in V_1.

3.13

a. Right axis deviation: Note negative QRS in I and positive QRS in aVF. Right atrial enlargement: Note tall, peaked P wave in lead II and dominant initial component of the P wave in V_1. Right ventricular hypertrophy: Note dominant R in V_1 along with RAD, RAE, and strain pattern (i.e., asymmetric T-wave inversion in V_1 and V_2).
b. Normal axis: Note positive QRS in I and isoelectric QRS in aVF. Left atrial enlargement: Note wide, notched P wave in lead II. Left ventricular hypertrophy: Note deep S wave (must be doubled since voltage was halved when the ECG was recorded) in V_1 and tall R wave in V_5. To check for voltage criteria, add the S in V_1 or V_2 and the R in V_5 or V_6. Since the sum is greater than 35 mm (40 in this case), voltage criteria for LVH is met.

3.14

a. Normal axis: Note positive QRS in I and positive QRS in aVL. ST segment elevation is noted from V_1-V_6. Pathologic Q waves are noted in V_2 and V_3. There is a small R wave in V_1, so the negative wave in that lead is an S wave. This ECG shows evidence of hyperacute anterior MI with injury extending to the septal and lateral walls.
b. Left axis deviation: Note positive QRS in I and negative QRS in aVF. ST segment elevation and pathologic Q waves are noted in II, III, and aVF indicative of acute inferior MI. Reciprocal changes in the V leads (ST segment depression from V_1-V_5) suggests posterior wall involvement also. Posterior wall leads are indicated.

3.15

g	1. Acute myocardial infarction
k	2. Hypercalcemia
n	3. Hyperkalemia
b	4. Hypocalcemia
l	5. Hypokalemia
e	6. Left atrial enlargement
f	7. Left bundle branch block
h	8. Left ventricular hypertrophy
d	9. Pericarditis
m	10. Variant angina
j	11. Right atrial enlargement
i	12. Right bundle branch block
c	13. Right ventricular hypertrophy
a	14. Wellens syndrome

3.16

f	1. Ventricular fibrillation
g	2. Stable monomorphic ventricular tachycardia
a	3. Asystole
h	4. Symptomatic bradycardia
i	5. Pulseless electrical activity
d	6. Stable SVT
c	7. Acute-onset atrial fibrillation
f	8. Pulseless ventricular tachycardia
j	9. Junctional tachycardia
h	10. Complete AV block with ventricular escape rhythm
b	11. Sinus tachycardia
e	12. Torsades de pointes

3.17

Adenosine (Adenocard)	Unclassified
Amiodarone (Cordarone)	III
Atropine	Unclassified
Digoxin	Unclassified
Diltiazem (Cardizem)	IV
Dofetilide (Tikosyn)	III
Esmolol (Brevibloc)	II
Flecainide (Tambocor)	IC
Ibutilide (Corvert)	III
Lidocaine (Xylocaine)	IB
Metoprolol (Lopressor)	II
Procainamide (Pronestyl)	IA
Propranolol (Inderal)	II
Quinidine	IA
Sotalol (Betapace)	II & III
Verapamil (Calan)	IV

3.18

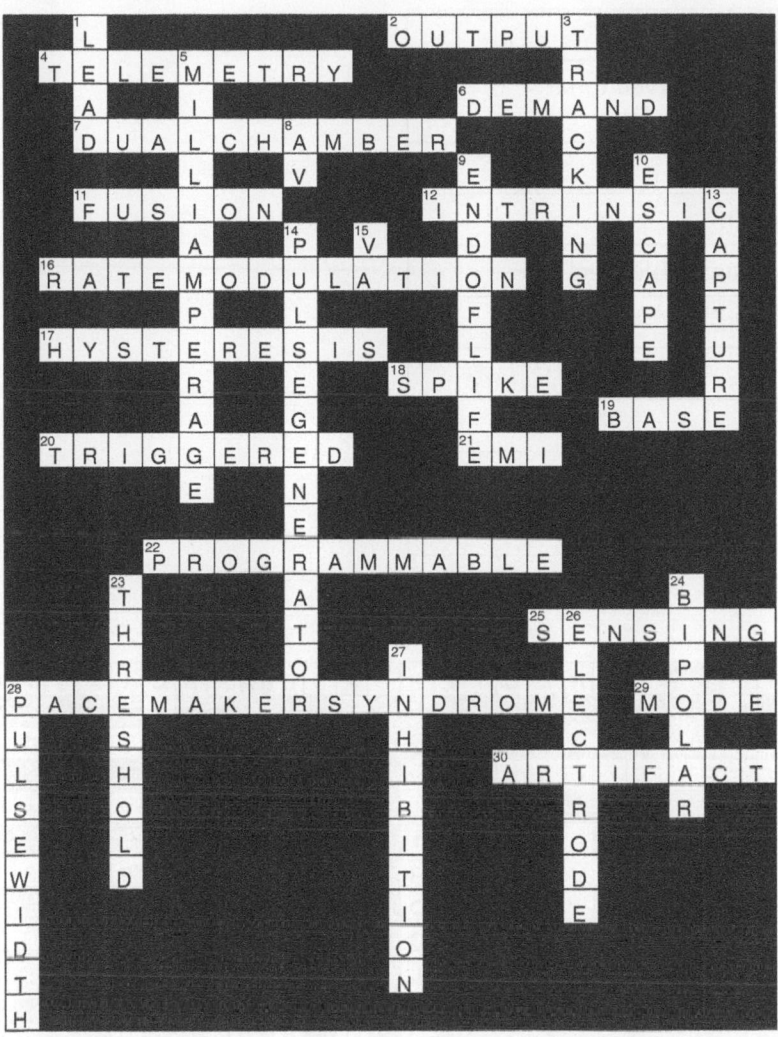

3.19

a. Interpretation: VVI with normal function; complex #4 is a PVC and it is sensed appropriately

b. Interpretation: DVI function with failure to sense; complex #5 shows atrial pacing with an intrinsic ventricular complex that is not sensed

c. Interpretation: VVI with intermittent failure to capture; after the third paced complex, there is a nonconducted pacing spike; after the fourth paced complex, there is a nonconducted pacing spike

3.20

Nonmodifiable	Modifiable
Heredity	Hypertension
Advancing age	Diabetes mellitus or glucose intolerance
Male gender	Hyperlipidemia
	Hyperhomocysteinemia
	Sedentary lifestyle
	Stress
	Obesity
	Cigarette smoking
	Oral contraceptives (especially in smokers)

3.21

a	1. Fibrinolytics
a	2. Percutaneous interventional procedures (PCI)
g	3. ACE inhibitors
c, d	4. Nitroglycerin
c	5. Calcium channel blockers
b, h	6. Beta-blockers
e, h	7. ASA
e, f	8. Heparin
e	9. Glycoprotein IIb/IIIa inhibitors
i, j	10. Intraaortic balloon pump (IABP)

3.22

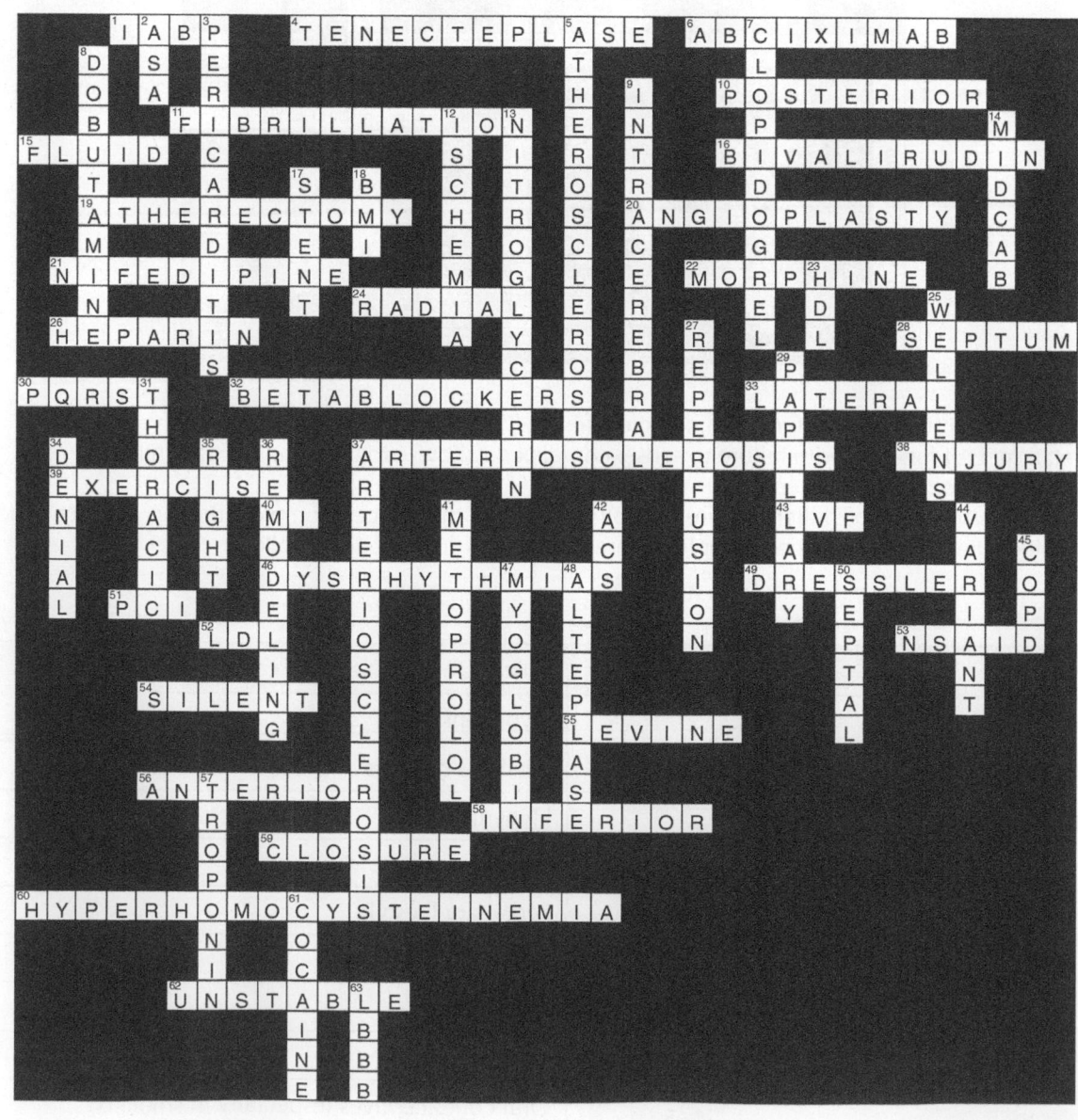

3.23

Causes	Left	Right
Aortic stenosis	✓	
Cardiac tamponade	✓	✓
Cardiomyopathy	✓	✓
Mitral stenosis	✓ (Forward failure)	✓ (Backward failure)
Myocardial infarction (left)	✓	
Myocardial infarction (right)		✓
Pulmonary embolism	✓ (Forward failure)	✓ (Backward failure)
Pulmonary hypertension		✓
Systemic hypertension	✓	

Sign/Symptom	Left	Right
Abnormal liver function studies		✓
Ascites		✓
Atrial dysrhythmias	✓	✓
Crackles audible over lungs	✓	
Dyspnea	✓	
Elevated CVP		✓
Hepatomegaly		✓
Jugular venous distention		✓
Mental confusion	✓	
Murmur of mitral regurgitation	✓	
Murmur of tricuspid regurgitation		✓
Orthopnea	✓	
Peripheral edema		✓
S_3, S_4 at apex	✓	
S_3, S_4 at sternum		✓
Weight gain	✓	✓

3.24

a. Yes. EF less than 40%.

b. Systolic. This is pump failure as evidenced by S_3.

c. Because she has acute decompensated heart failure, IV diuretics would be warranted. Aldactone, an aldosterone antagonist, would likely be helpful. She is already receiving an ACE inhibitor. Inotropic agents may be used.

d. Continuous renal replacement therapy, such as continuous venous-venous hemofiltration, might be used. Cardiac resynchronization therapy with a biventricular pacemaker may be indicated. Also, a frank discussion of end-of-life care with the patient and family is indicated.

e. D

3.25

Drug	Arterial Dilator	Venous Dilator
Clevidipine (Cleviprex)	✓	
Dobutamine (Dobutrex)	✓	✓
Fenoldopam (Corlopam)	✓	
Hydralazine (Apresoline)	✓	
Milrinone (Primacor)	✓	✓
Minoxidil (Loniten)	✓	
Morphine sulfate		✓
Nifedipine (Procardia)	✓	✓
Nitroglycerin (less than 1 mcg/kg/min)		✓
Nitroglycerin (greater than 1 mcg/kg/min)	✓	✓
Nitroprusside (Nipride)	✓	✓
Phentolamine (Regitine)	✓	✓
Prazosin (Minipress)	✓	✓

3.26

a, b, d, g, j, m	1. Right ventricular failure
b, c, g, l	2. Left ventricular failure
e	3. Left ventricular MI
a, f	4. Right ventricular MI
a, e, h, n	5. Cardiac tamponade
g	6. Valvular dysfunction
i, k	7. Chronic arterial insufficiency

3.27

a.
- BP 220/140 mm Hg
- Left ventricular failure (dyspnea, tachypnea, S₃, crackles, hypoxemia, pulmonary edema on chest x-ray) (NOTE: You would expect tachycardia, but remember that the beta-blocker has prevented this SNS compensatory mechanism.)
- Left ventricular hypertrophy (displaced PMI, cardiomegaly on chest x-ray, ventricular strain and large R waves in left ventricular leads)
- Renal insufficiency (decreased urine output, elevated BUN and creatinine maintaining the normal 10:1 ratio)
- Occipital headache

b. Indomethacin (Indocin) and other NSAIDs inhibit the synthesis of prostaglandins (which are vasodilators) so they increase BP and cause sodium and fluid retention
c. Heart, brain, kidney, retina
d. Yes. Hypertensive emergency warrants an admission to a critical care unit, once stabilized would be transferred to progressive care unit
e. Reduction of MAP by 25%
f.

Vasodilator	• Nitroprusside (Nipride) • Nitroglycerin (Tridil) • Hydralazine (Apresoline) • Nicardipine (Cardene)
ACE inhibitor	• Enalapril (Vasotec)
Alpha-blocker	• Phentolamine (Regitine)
Beta-blocker	• Esmolol (Brevibloc)
Alpha- and beta-blocker	• Labetalol (Normodyne)

g. 24 mL/hr
h.
- Nausea, vomiting, abdominal pain: patient report
- Headache, tinnitus: patient report
- Coronary artery steal: evidence of myocardial ischemia such as chest pain, ST segment elevation
- Nitroprusside-induced intrapulmonary shunt: decrease in SpO₂, decrease in SaO₂ and PaO₂ on ABGs
- Methemoglobinemia: decrease in SpO₂, decrease in SaO₂ on ABGs, increase in methemoglobin levels
- Thiocyanate toxicity: metabolic acidosis, confusion, hyperreflexia, seizures, elevated thiocyanate levels
i. No. Nifedipine has never been FDA approved for sublingual (or bite and swallow) use and should not be used because of the precipitous drops in BP that may occur.
j. Labetalol would have been preferable because nitroprusside's effect of causing direct vasodilation may increase intracranial pressure.
k.
- Murmur of aortic regurgitation (high-pitched diastolic murmur) heard best in aortic (second right intercostal space at the right sternal border) area
- BP differences from left arm to right arm or left leg to right leg
- "Ripping" or "tearing" chest pain
- Chest pain that radiates to the back
- Hypotension or shock
- Widening of mediastinum on chest x-ray

3.28

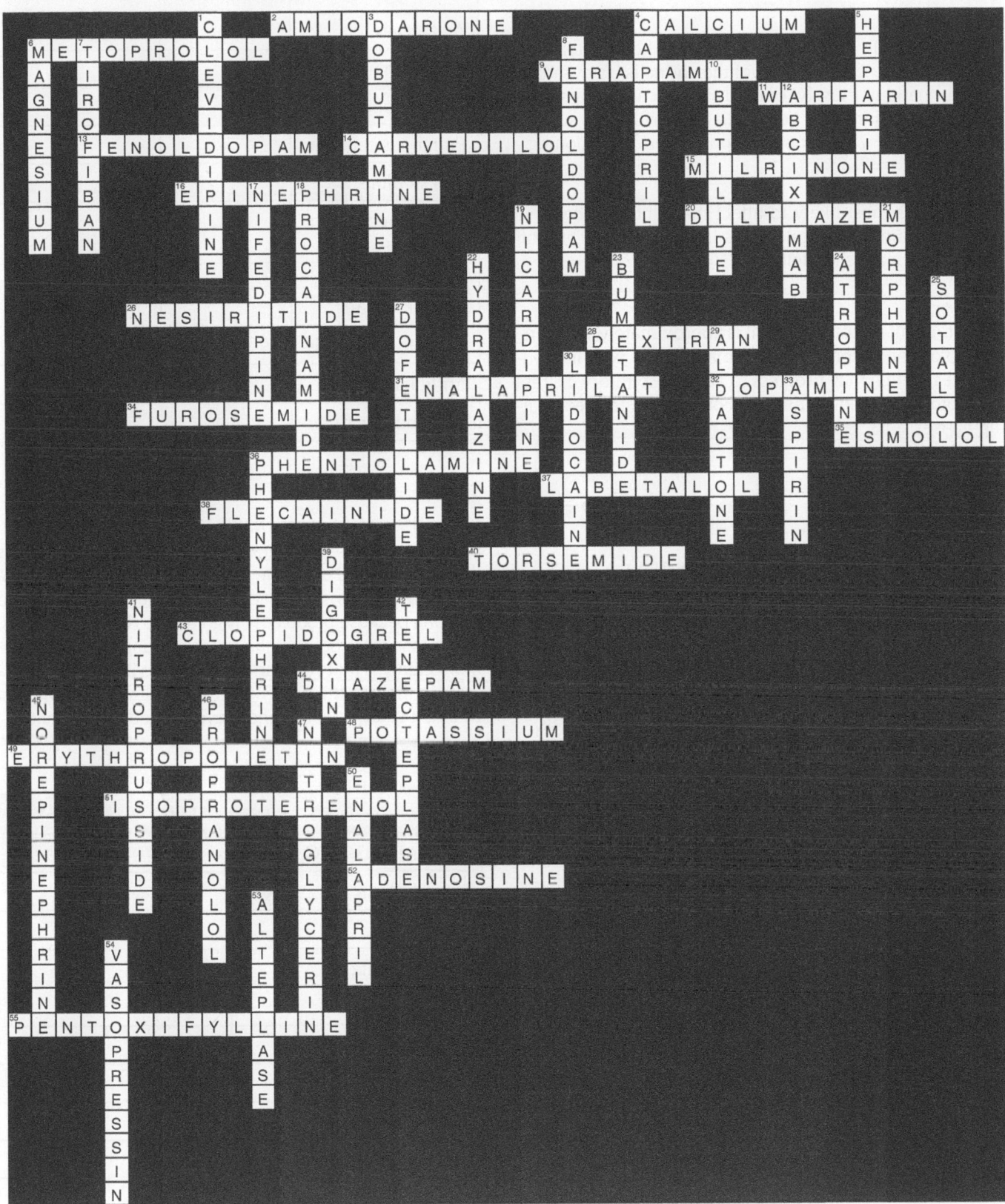

CHAPTER 4

4.1

Parasympathetic stimulation decreases heart rate, so a significant risk of stimulation of the carina is bradycardia. Monitor patients closely for bradycardia caused by stimulation of the carina and ventricular dysrhythmias, such as PVCs, caused by hypoxemia/hypoxia during suctioning.

4.2

Aspiration is most likely to affect the right lung because the right main stem bronchus is larger and straighter off the trachea than is the left.

4.3

Since the half-life of surfactant is approximately 14 hours, a hypoxic injury that causes damage to the type II pneumocytes, which may progress to acute respiratory distress syndrome between 12 and 18 hours after the precipitating cause.

4.4

	Primary	Accessory
Inspiration	Diaphragm External intercostals	Scalene Sternocleidomastoid
Expiration	None; expiration is normally passive	Internal oblique External oblique Rectus abdominis Internal intercostals Transverse abdominis

4.5

b	1. V_T
d	2. TLC
e	3. FVC
f	4. RV
a	5. FEV_1
c	6. VC
g	7. FRC

4.6

	Restrictive	Obstructive
Obesity hypoventilation syndrome	x	
Asthma		x
Pneumothorax	x	

	Restrictive	Obstructive
Atelectasis	x	
Pneumonia	x	
Kyphoscoliosis	x	
Pulmonary edema	x	
Mucus plugs		x
Lung cancer (bronchial)		x
Lung cancer (parenchymal)	x	
Chronic bronchitis		x
Artificial airway		x
Bronchospasm		x

4.7

Remember: good lung down, no lung down. The reason that you want the nonoperative lung down in lobectomy is that you want the operative lung up to encourage reexpansion because air rises and to optimize the V/Q matching to the lung because blood flow is greater to dependent areas. The reason that you want the operative lung down in pneumonectomy is that you want secretions to pool and consolidate in the hemithorax where the lung has been removed so that it takes up space and prevents mediastinal shift.

4.8

	Left	Right
Increased 2,3-DPG		x
Hypothermia	x	
Hypercapnia		x
Hyperthermia		x
Acidosis		x
Decreased 2,3-DPG	x	
Hypocapnia	x	
Alkalosis	x	
Hypophosphatemia	x	
Massive blood transfusion	x	

4.9

SaO_2
Hemoglobin
Cardiac output/index

4.10

Condition	Breath Sound Change or Changes
Emphysema	Diminished breath sounds
Atelectasis	Diminished breath sounds Bronchial or bronchovesicular breath sounds Crackles
Pneumonia	Diminished breath sounds Bronchial or bronchovesicular breath sounds
Chronic bronchitis	Rhonchi Wheezes may also be present
Pneumothorax	Diminished or absent breath sounds
Pulmonary fibrosis	Diminished breath sounds Crackles
Asthma	Wheezes Rhonchi
Pulmonary edema	Crackles Wheezes (referred to as *cardiac asthma*) may be present
Pleurisy	Pleural friction rub
Hemothorax	Diminished or absent breath sounds
Pleural effusion	Diminished breath sounds
Pulmonary embolism	Crackles Pleural friction rub if pulmonary infarction develops

4.11

	Answer
1.	Respiratory acidosis with hypoxemia
2.	Respiratory alkalosis
3.	Metabolic acidosis
4.	Metabolic alkalosis
5.	Compensated respiratory acidosis with significant hypoxemia
6.	Mixed disorder: Respiratory and metabolic acidosis with significant hypoxemia
7.	Mixed disorder: Respiratory alkalosis and metabolic alkalosis
8.	Mixed disorder: Respiratory acidosis and metabolic alkalosis*

	Answer
9.	Mixed disorder: Respiratory alkalosis and metabolic acidosis*
10.	Normal
11.	Metabolic acidosis with hypoxemia
12.	Respiratory acidosis with partial compensation and hypoxemia
13.	Metabolic acidosis with partial compensation
14.	Respiratory alkalosis with partial compensation
15.	Metabolic alkalosis with partial compensation and hypoxemia

*Without history and previous gases, what looks like a mixed disorder could be compensation and vice-versa. Remember that a midline pH makes a mixed disorder with both an acidosis and an alkalosis more likely, whereas a leaning pH makes compensation more likely.

4.12

a.	Respiratory acidosis
b.	Metabolic alkalosis
c.	Respiratory acidosis (but with elevated bicarbonate; chronic compensated respiratory acidosis with decompensation)
d.	Metabolic alkalosis
e.	Respiratory alkalosis
f.	Metabolic acidosis

4.13

TURBINATES
CRICOTHYROID   COMPLIANCE   EPIGLOTTIS
MAST   ALKALOSIS   SPIROMETRY
SHUNT   TACHYPNEA
PERFUSION   MITOCHONDRIA
WOB   AFFINITY   MACROPHAGE
COMPENSATION   VESICULAR   GLOTTIS
LEFT   CARBONDIOXIDE   OROPHARYNX   LINGULA
VENTILATION   CLUBBING   AGING
RUB   RESISTANCE
NASOPHARYNX   TONSIL   OXIMETRY
LARYNGOPHARYNX
CAPNOGRAPHY   RESTRICTIVE   ALVEOLAR
ELASTASE
CENTRAL   HYPOXEMIA
BRONCHOVESICULAR   LARYNX   TRACHEA
HYPOVENTILATION
PROPRIOCEPTORS   MIXED
CARINA   RHONCHI
BRONCHIAL
PNEUMOCYTE   HYPOXIA
FLAT   ANEMIA
DYSPNEA   ACIDOSIS   ACINUS
PULMONARYHYPERTENSION   EUPNEA

4.14

a. The term *hypoxemia* indicates that there is decreased oxygen in the blood, whereas *hypoxia* indicates that there is decreased oxygen in the tissue.

b. Because hypoxemia indicates a decrease in blood oxygen, blood parameters are used, such as PaO_2 (<80 mm Hg) or SaO_2 or SpO_2 (<95%).

c. Clinical indications of oxygen deficit are not evident until the tissues are deficient. The brain is a very sensitive indicator of low oxygen, so restlessness and confusion are indications that brain oxygen levels are low. The adrenal glands are also sensitive to low oxygen levels, and they release catecholamines to cause tachycardia and tachypnea. Central cyanosis may also occur. Serum arterial lactate levels would increase due to the shift to anaerobic from aerobic metabolism.

d. Absolutely. Since hypoxemia is present when PaO_2 is <80 mm Hg and SaO_2 is <95%, the tissues are still able to maintain normal oxygen levels by increasing the amount of oxygen that they extract. This would be reflected by a decrease in SvO_2. Generally, consider a PaO_2 of <60 mm Hg and SaO_2 of <90% as consistent with both hypoxemia AND hypoxia. You can also relate this to the oxyhemoglobin dissociation curve because a PaO_2 of 60 mm Hg and an SaO_2 of 90% is when the curve changes from horizontal to vertical, so any decrease in PaO_2 results in a more significant decrease in SaO_2.

e. Absolutely. Even with a normal PaO_2 and SaO_2, if the hemoglobin or cardiac output/index is reduced, oxygen delivery to the tissues is deficient and hypoxia occurs. Some other factors to consider are shift of the oxyhemoglobin dissociation curve to the left, decreased extraction by the tissues such as occurs in sepsis, and local perfusion issues such as peripheral vascular disease.

4.15

d	1. Nonrebreathing mask
e	2. Venturi mask
a	3. Nasal cannula
b.	4. Tracheostomy collar
c	5. Partial rebreathing mask

4.16

Any 10 of the following:
Acute respiratory distress syndrome (early)
Aminoglycosides
Amyotrophic lateral sclerosis
Anesthesia
Aspiration pneumonitis
Asthma
Atelectasis
Chest trauma
CNS depressant drugs
COPD with acute exacerbation
Cystic fibrosis
Epiglottis
Fat embolism
Guillain-Barré syndrome
Head trauma
Kyphoscoliosis
Morbid obesity
Multiple sclerosis
Muscle paralytics
Muscular dystrophy
Myasthenia gravis
Near-drowning
Neuromuscular blocking drugs

Organophosphate poisoning
Pleural effusion
Pneumonia
Pneumothorax
Poliomyelitis
Pulmonary edema
Pulmonary embolism
Pulmonary fibrosis
Sleep apnea
Smoke inhalation
Spinal cord injury
Status asthmaticus
Surgery: especially thoracic, abdominal, flank incision
Tracheal obstruction

4.17

Classification	Example
1. Beta$_2$-adrenergic agonists	• Salmeterol (Serevent) • Metaproterenol (Alupent, Metaprel) • Albuterol (Proventil, Ventolin) • Pirbuterol (Maxair) • Bitolterol (Tornalate) • Terbutaline (Brethine, Brethaire)
2. Anticholinergic agents	• Ipratropium bromide (Atrovent)
3. Methyxanthines	• Aminophylline • Theophylline (Theobid, Quibron) • Oxtriphylline (Choledyl SA)
4. Electrolyte	• Magnesium

4.18

d	1. Upper airway obstruction
f	2. Airway secretions
i	3. Overdosage of narcotics
h	4. Bronchospasm
b, c	5. Pneumothorax
a, b	6. Pneumonia
j	7. Postoperative pain
g	8. ARDS
e	9. Myasthenic crisis
b	10. Atelectasis

4.19

Any five in each column.

Pulmonary	Nonpulmonary
Chest trauma: Pulmonary contusion	Sepsis (number one cause)
Near-drowning	Shock or prolonged hypotension
Hypervolemia, pulmonary edema	Septic shock
Inhalation of toxic gases and vapors	Hypovolemic shock
Smoke	Anaphylactic shock
Chemicals	Cardiogenic shock
Oxygen toxicity	Neurogenic shock
Pneumonia	Multisystem trauma
Aspiration pneumonitis	Burns
Radiation pneumonitis	Cardiopulmonary bypass
Pulmonary embolism	Disseminated intravascular coagulation (DIC)
Radiation	Toxemia of pregnancy
Drugs: Bleomycin	Acute pancreatitis
	Diabetic coma
	Head injury
	Drug overdosage
	Multiple blood transfusions

4.20

1. Elevate the head of the bed 45 degrees.
2. Ensure appropriate positioning of feeding tube.
3. Check for gastric residuals and initiate measures to facilitate peristalsis or hold feedings if indicated.
4. Keep the cuff of the endotracheal tube or tracheostomy tube inflated to 20-30 cm H_2O.

4.21

PaO$_2$ (mm Hg)	Paco$_2$ (mm Hg)	pH	Stage
68	30	7.48	II
88	25	7.52	I
45	55	7.28	IV
52	40	7.40	III

4.22

Any three in each column.

Hyper-coagulability	Alteration In Blood Vessel	Venous Stasis
Malignancy	Trauma	Prolonged bed rest or immobilization
Oral contraceptives high in estrogen, especially in smokers	IV drug use	Obesity
Dehydration and hemoconcentration	Aging	Advanced age
Fever	Vasculitis	Burns
Sickle cell anemia	Varicose veins	Pregnancy
Pregnancy	Diabetes mellitus	Postpartum period
Polycythemia vera	Atherosclerosis	Congestive heart failure
Thrombocytopenia	Inflammatory process	Myocardial infarction
Abrupt discontinuance of anticoagulants		Bacterial endocarditis
Sepsis		Recent surgery especially legs, pelvis, or abdomen
		Thrombus formation in heart (AF)
		Cardioversion

4.23

b	1. Pulmonary contusion
c	2. Closed pneumothorax
d	3. Hemothorax
a	4. Tension pneumothorax

4.24

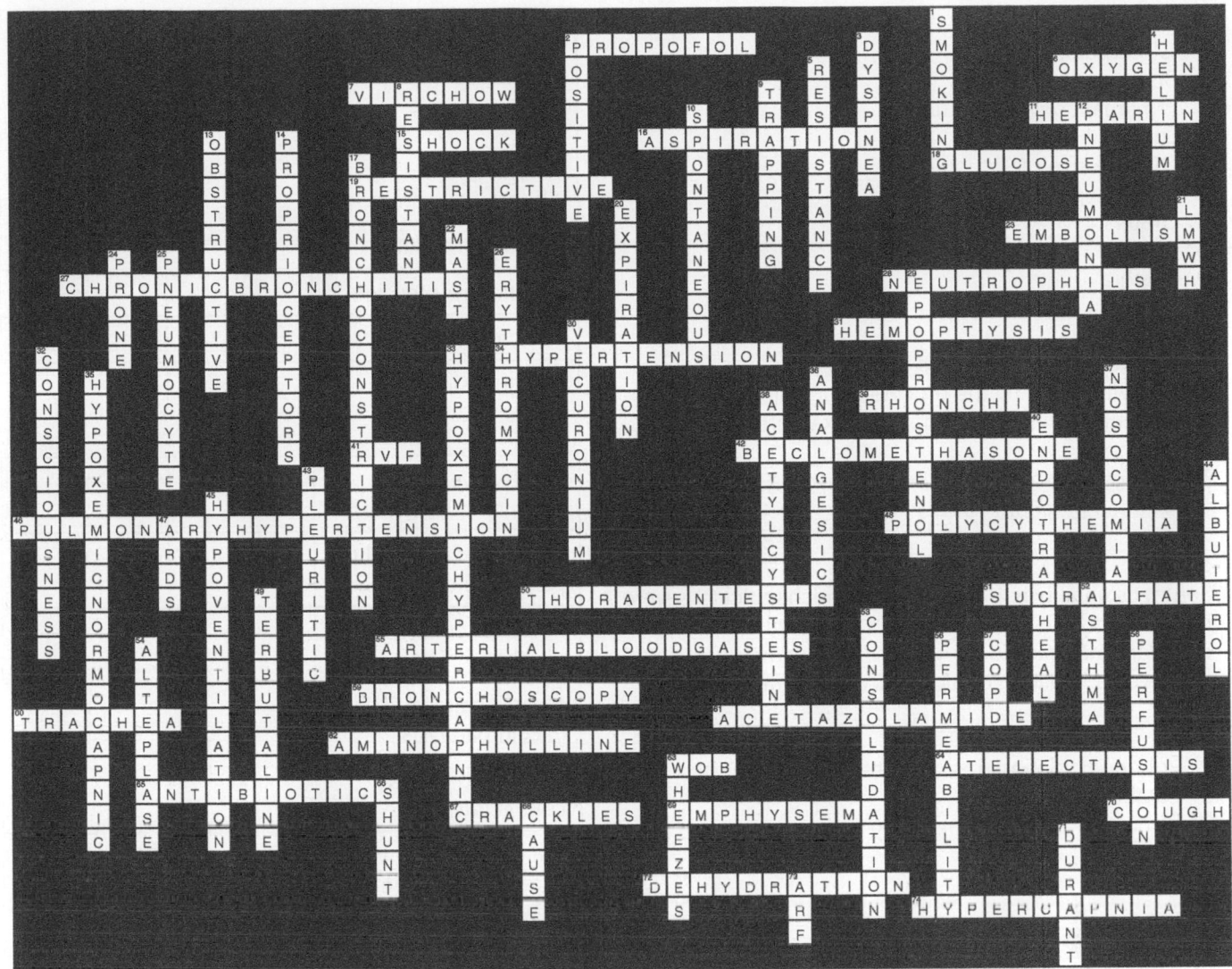

4.25

h	1. Resiliency—level 5
g	2. Vulnerability—level 1
f	3. Stability—level 5
a	4. Complexity—level 3
e	5. Resource availability—level 1
d	6. Participation in care—level 3
b	7. Participation in decision making—level 1
c	8. Predictability—level 5

4.26

1. High
2. a, b, d; V/Q scan is modified to include decreased amount of dye and increased time of scan. The spiral CT is now the treatment of choice for PE, but safety has not been determined in pregnant states.
3. Initially unfractionated heparin, then low–molecular-weight heparin, which is stopped immediately prior to delivery
4. alteplase (tPa) and warfarin (Coumadin)

CHAPTER 5

5.1

1 Glomerulus
2 Bowman's capsule
3 Proximal convoluted tubule
4 Loop of Henle
5 Distal convoluted tubule
6 Collecting ducts
7 Ureters
8 Bladder
9 Urethra

5.2

Water moves by the process of <u>osmosis.</u>
Electrolytes move by the process of <u>diffusion.</u>
The sodium-potassium pump is an example of <u>active transport.</u>
The use of a pushing force, such as hydrostatic pressure, is called <u>filtration.</u>

5.3

Serum osmolality is 433 mOsm/kg, which indicates severe dehydration. This is an example of a hyperglycemic hyperosmolar state caused by glucose intolerance associated with recent initiation of high-glucose enteral feedings.

5.4

1. Volume depletion (i.e., prerenal)
2. Catabolism
3. GI hemorrhage

5.5

Condition	Normal Anion Gap	Increased Anion Gap
Shock		×
Renal failure		×
Diarrhea	×	
Diabetic ketoacidosis		×
Salicylate overdose		×
Renal tubular acidosis	×	
Rhabdomyolysis		×
Carbonic anhydrase inhibitors	×	
Ethylene glycol poisoning		×

5.6

a. Hypercalcemia
b. Hypokalemia
c. Hypomagnesemia

5.7

Sign/Symptom	Excess (Hyper)	Deficit (Hypo)
Sodium		
Weight gain	×	
Abdominal cramps		×
Flushed, dry skin	×	
Postural hypotension		×
Headache		×
Hypertension	×	
Potassium		
Flat T waves, prominent U waves		×
Decreased GI motility, paralytic ileus		×
Intestinal colic, diarrhea	×	
Muscle cramps → flaccid paralysis		×
Decreased cardiac contractility	×	
Tall, peaked T waves, widened QRS complex	×	
Calcium		
Tetany		×
Decreased deep tendon reflexes	×	
Neuromuscular weakness, flaccidity	×	
Seizures		×
Bone or flank pain	×	
Laryngospasm		×
Phosphorus		
Tetany	×	
Fatigue		×
Chest pain		×
Dyspnea		×
Increased deep tendon reflexes	×	
Abdominal cramps	×	

Sign/Symptom	Excess (Hyper)	Deficit (Hypo)
Magnesium		
Decreased deep tendon reflexes	×	
Anorexia, nausea, vomiting		×
Cardiopulmonary arrest	×	
Lethargy	×	
Dysrhythmias, especially torsades de pointe		×
Facial flushing	×	

5.8

a. Potassium
b. Potassium, calcium, magnesium
c. Calcium
d. Calcium, phosphorus
e. Magnesium, phosphorus
f. Potassium, chloride

5.9

a. A patient receiving regular doses of furosemide.
1. Hypovolemia
2. Hyponatremia
3. Hypokalemia
4. Hypocalcemia
5. Hypomagnesemia
6. Metabolic alkalosis (due to hypochloremia and hypokalemia)
b. A patient with persistent vomiting.
1. Hypovolemia
2. Hyponatremia
3. Hypokalemia
4. Metabolic alkalosis (due to hypochloremia and hypokalemia)
c. A patient with acute kidney injury (oliguric phase).
1. Hypervolemia
2. Hyponatremia
3. Hyperkalemia
4. Hypocalcemia
5. Hyperphosphatemia
6. Hypermagnesemia
7. Metabolic acidosis
d. A patient with diabetic ketoacidosis (before treatment).
1. Hyperkalemia
2. Hypophosphatemia
3. Hypermagnesemia
4. Metabolic acidosis

e. A patient receiving multiple units of banked blood.
1. Hyperkalemia
2. Hypocalcemia
3. Hypomagnesemia

5.10

Condition	Prerenal	Intrinsic	Postrenal
Acute pyelonephritis		×	
Aminoglycosides		×	
Benign prostatic hypertrophy			×
Contrast dyes		×	
Diuretics	×	×	
Glomerulonephritis		×	
Goodpasture's syndrome		×	
Hemorrhage	×		
Hepatorenal syndrome	×		
Hypersensitivity reactions		×	
Intraabdominal tumor			×
Malignant hypertension		×	
Neurogenic bladder			×
Prolonged hypotension		×	
Renal calculi			×
Rhabdomyolysis with myoglobinuria		×	
Septic shock	×		

5.11

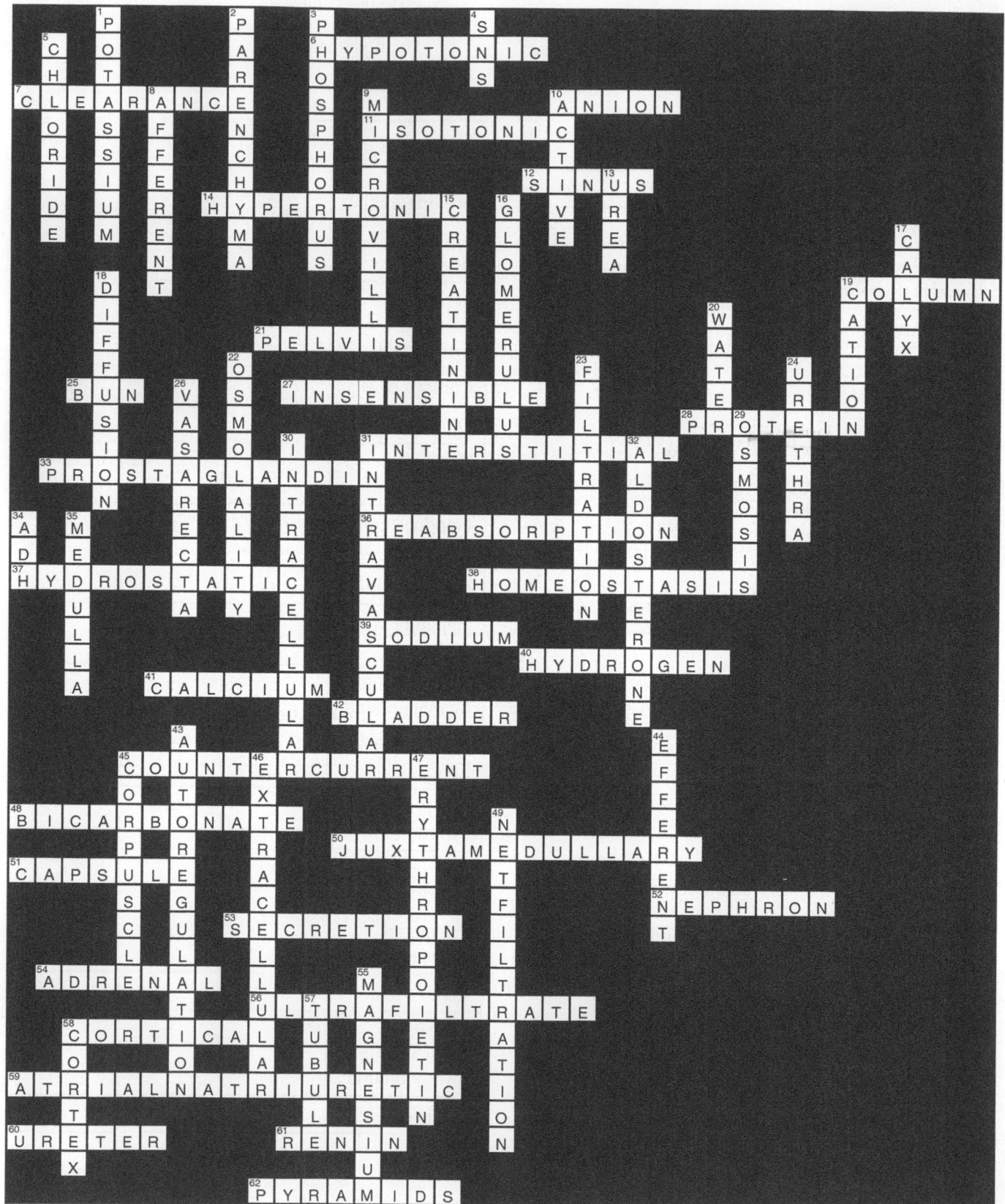

5.12

A. No, the patient needs an isotonic solution, such as NS, as the initial fluid replacement to stay in the vascular space. Decisions about the next liter(s) will be determined primarily by the patient's serum sodium and osmolality.

B. No, hypotonic solution, such as 0.45% NS, is needed to move fluid into the cells.

C. No, the patient is already alkalotic and lactate is converted to bicarbonate by the liver; the patient lost sodium, so hanging D_5NS is more appropriate.

5.13

A. b
B. c
C. a
D. b

CHAPTER 6

6.1

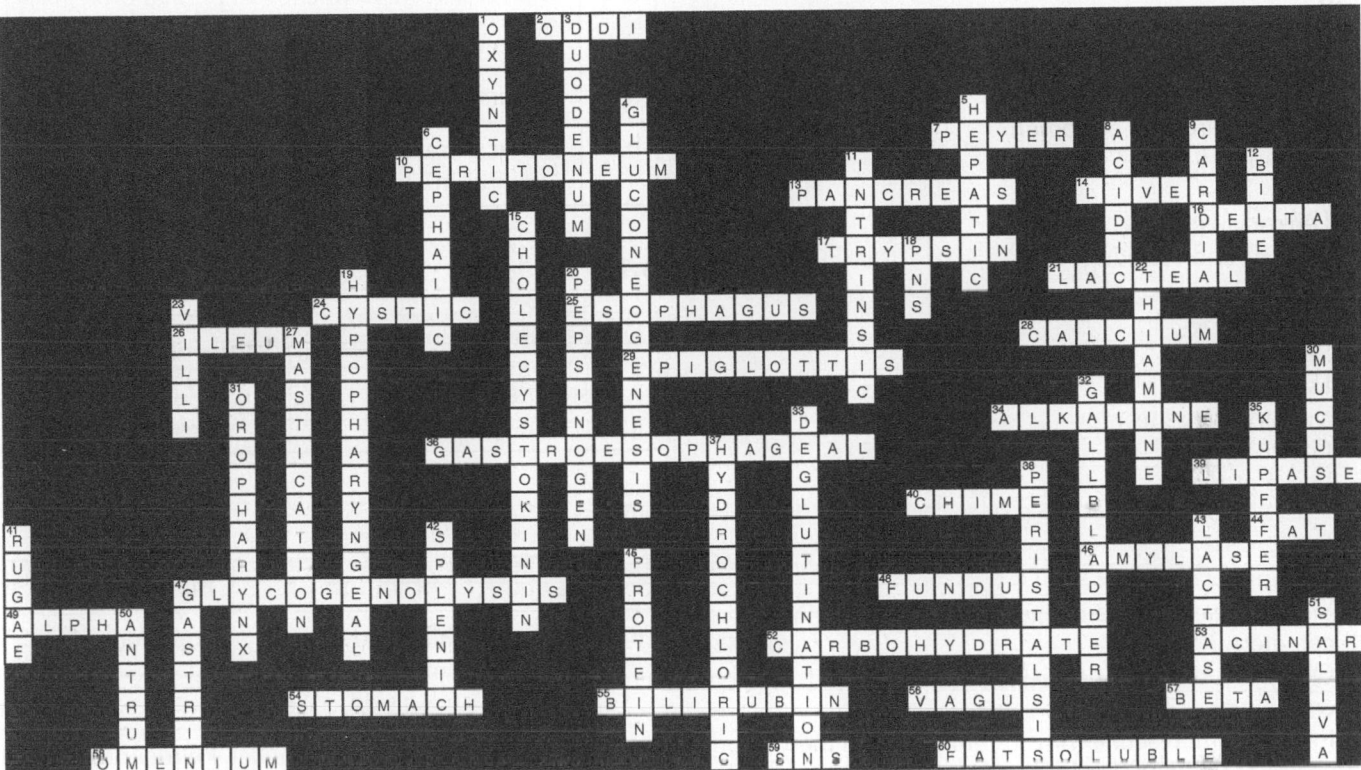

6.2

1. Liver disease (e.g., cirrhosis, hepatitis)
2. Biliary obstruction (e.g., cholelithiasis)
3. Excessive hemolysis (e.g., hemolytic blood transfusion reaction)

6.3

Type	Example
1. Antacids	Aluminum hydroxide and magnesium hydroxide (Maalox) Aluminum hydroxide, magnesium hydroxide, and simethicone (Mylanta) Aluminum hydroxide and magnesium trisilicate (Gaviscon)
2. Histamine (H$_2$) receptor antagonists	Cimetidine (Tagamet) Ranitidine (Zantac) Famotidine (Pepcid) Nizatidine (Axid)
3. Proton pump inhibitors	Omeprazole (Prilosec) Lansoprazole (Prevacid) Esomeprazole (Nexium)
4. Mucosal barrier	Sucralfate (Carafate)

6.4
The half-life of serum prealbumin is 2 to 3 days versus albumin with a half-life of 19 to 20 days. Therefore, serum transferrin will show improvement or decline more quickly.

6.5
2428 calories

6.6
- Abdominal pain
- Rebound tenderness
- Abdominal distention
- Rigid "boardlike" abdomen
- Diminished bowel sounds
- Fever
- Leukocytosis
- Nausea and vomiting

6.7
1. Peptic ulcer
2. Esophageal varices
3. Mallory-Weiss tear
4. Gastritis
5. Vascular tumor

6.8
1. Administer oxygen
2. Insert at least 2 large-gauge (16 or 18) intravenous catheters
3. Obtain blood samples for H&H and type and crossmatch
4. Initiate normal saline infusion initially and then blood products when prescribed and available

6.9
1. Sclerotherapy of varices
2. Ligation of varices
3. Intrahepatic (e.g., TIPS) or portosystemic shunt
4. Pharmacologic agents: octreotide acetate (Sandostatin) or vasopressin (Pitressin)

6.10

a, f	1. Splenic engorgement
g	2. Stretching of the liver capsule
d	3. Decrease in the metabolism of testosterone
c	4. Decrease in metabolism of aldosterone
a, c	5. Decrease in production of plasma proteins
e	6. Decrease in metabolism of estrogen
a	7. Decrease in production of clotting factors
b	8. Decrease in conjugation and excretion of bilirubin

6.11

Indicated	Contraindicated
Aldosterone antagonist (potassium-sparing)	Thiazide

6.12

Sign	Description	Indicates
Ballance	Dullness over right flank with patient on left side	Ruptured spleen
Grey-Turner	Ecchymosis to flank	Retroperitoneal bleeding
Cullen	Ecchymosis around umbilicus	Intraperitoneal bleeding
Coopernail	Ecchymosis of scrotum or labia	Pelvic fracture
Kehr	Left shoulder pain	Splenic rupture
Chvostek	Spasm of the facial muscles elicited by tapping on the facial nerve	Hypocalcemia
Trousseau	Carpal spasm induced by inflating a BP cuff on the upper arm to a pressure exceeding systolic blood pressure	Hypocalcemia

6.13

Clinical Finding	Condition(s)
Elevated lipase, amylase	Acute pancreatitis
Sudden, painless hematemesis	Esophageal varices
Decreased protein	Acute pancreatitis, liver disease, malnutrition
Rebound tenderness	Peritonitis
Jaundice	Liver disease, biliary obstruction, hemolysis
Hypocalcemia	Acute pancreatitis
Bleeding tendencies	Liver disease
Elevated ammonia	Hepatic failure, hepatic encephalopathy
Bloody diarrhea	Intestinal infarction
Hyperbilirubinemia	Liver disease, biliary obstruction, hemolysis
Fetor hepaticus	Hepatic failure
High-pitched rushing bowel sounds	Small bowel obstruction
Succussion splash	Pyloric obstruction
Management	**Condition**
Irrigate NG tube until clear	Upper GI bleed
Neomycin and lactulose	Hepatic failure; hepatic encephalopathy
Sclerosis during endoscopy	Esophageal varices
Aldosterone antagonist diuretics	Hepatic failure; hepatic encephalopathy
NPO status	Pancreatitis
Sengstaken-Blakemore tube	Esophageal varices
Volume and blood replacement	GI bleed
Billroth I or II	Gastric ulcer

6.14

Situation	Level I Minimally Stable	Level III Moderately Stable	Level V Highly Stable
34-year-old married businessman who has had a small bowel resection for Crohn's disease.	×		
36-year-old mechanic with cirrhosis and newly diagnosed liver cancer who is on the transplant list. He is separated from his wife and lives with his parents.		×	
18-year-old man with abdominal trauma due to MVA in which his girlfriend was killed.			×

6.15

1. b, c, d. Naproxen, history of smoking, age
2. c. Omeprazole (Prilosec)

6.16

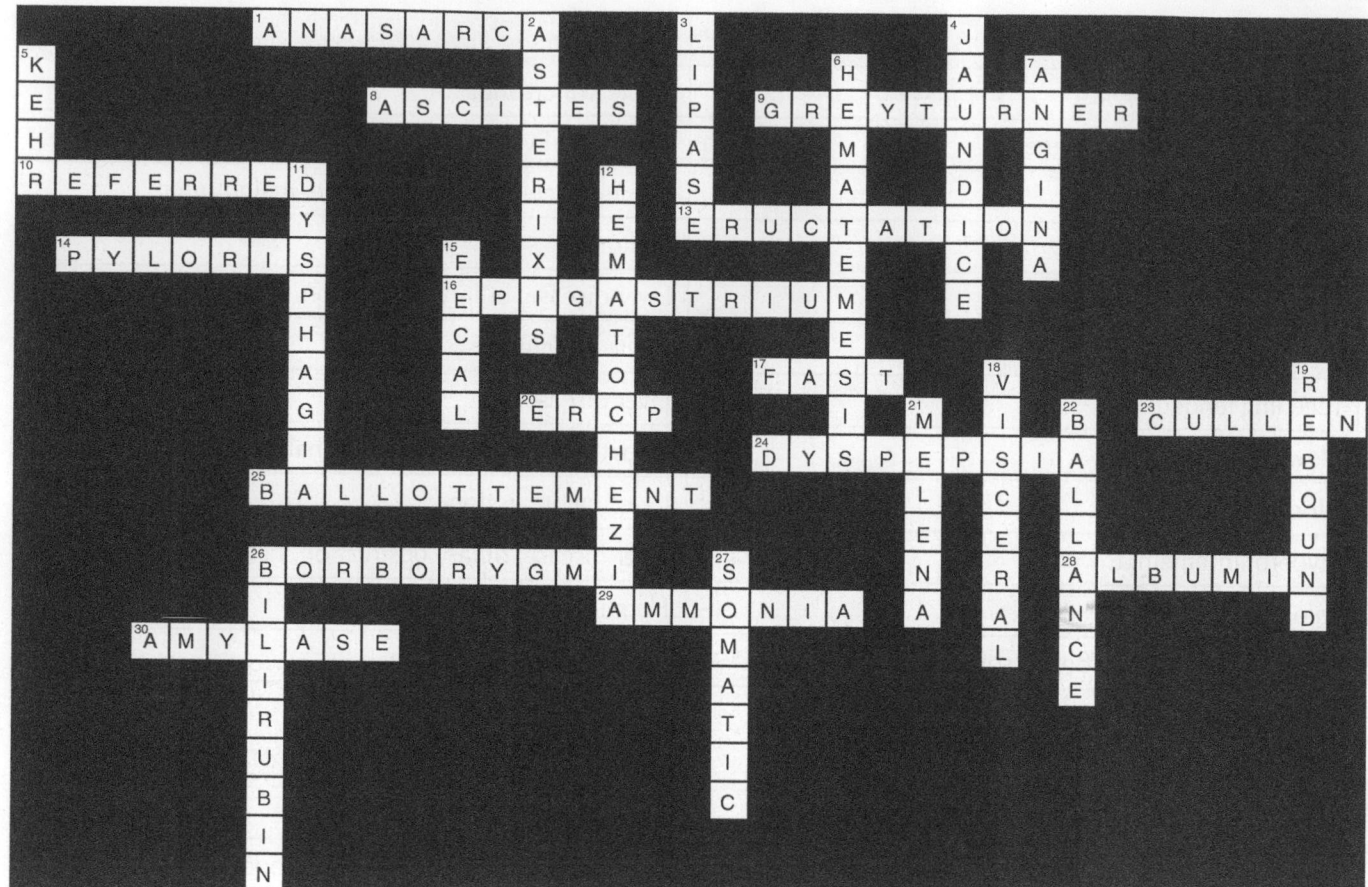

6.17

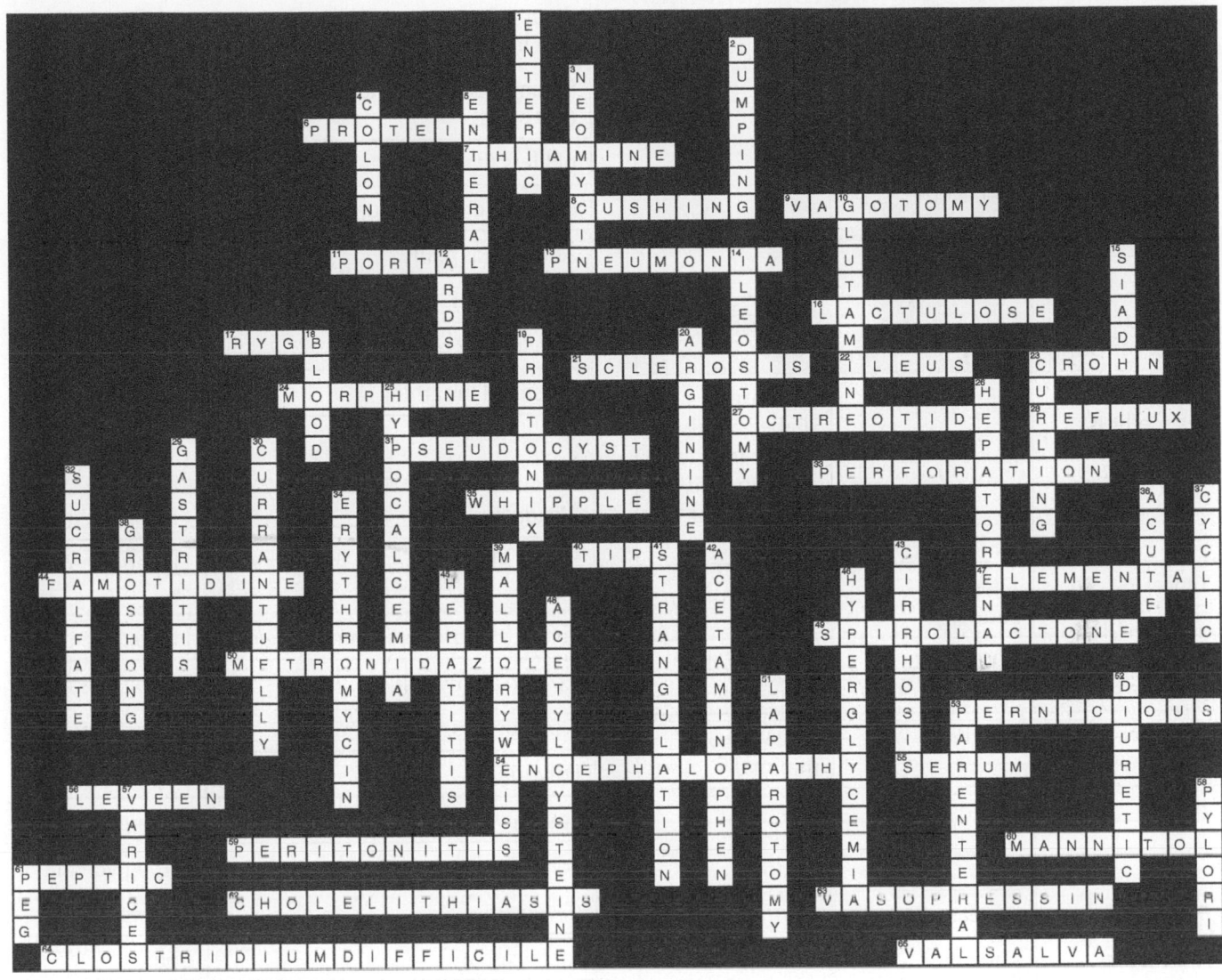

CHAPTER 7

7.1
Predictability—Level 1
Participation in decision making—Level 5
Resource availability—Level 3
Complexity—Level 1
Resiliency—Level 1
Participation in care—Level 1

7.2

Clinical Presentation	DKA	HHS
Type of diabetes mellitus	1	2 or non-diabetic with intolerance to glucose load (e.g., enteral feeding)
Onset	Gradual or sudden	Gradual
Typical serum glucose range	600 mg/dL	1100 mg/dL
Presence of ketosis	Positive	Negative or minimal
pH	Acidosis	Normal or minimally acidotic
Anion gap	Increased	Normal
Respiratory pattern	Kussmaul breathing (rapid and deep)	Normal or tachypneic (rapid and shallow)
Breath odor	Acetone (fruity)	Normal
Serum osmolality	295-330 mOsm/kg	330-450 mOsm/kg
Serum sodium	Decreased, normal, or increased	Normal or increased
Serum potassium	Increased initially; drops with rehydration and correction of acidosis	Decreased
BUN	Mildly increased	Severely increased
Average fluid deficit	4-8 L	8-15 L

7.3

Serum glucose greater than 300 mg/dL	Both
Serum glucose greater than 600 mg/dL	HHS
pH less than 7.3	DKA
Positive serum and urine ketones	DKA
Abdominal pain	DKA
Dehydration	Both
Lethargy → coma	Both
Kussmaul breathing	DKA

7.4

Headache	Hypoglycemia
Serum glucose greater than 300 mg/dL	Hyperglycemia
Serum glucose less than 50 mg/dL	Hypoglycemia
Cold, clammy skin	Hypoglycemia
Nervousness, tremors	Hypoglycemia
Polyuria	Hyperglycemia
Lethargy → coma	Hyperglycemia
Seizures → coma	Hypoglycemia
Glycosuria	Hyperglycemia
Tachycardia	Both
Agitation, difficulty with concentration	Hypoglycemia
Weakness, fatigue	Hyperglycemia
Fruity breath	Hyperglycemia
Abdominal pain	Hyperglycemia

7.5

b, c, d	1. DKA
b, c, d	2. HHS
a	3. Hypoglycemia

7.6

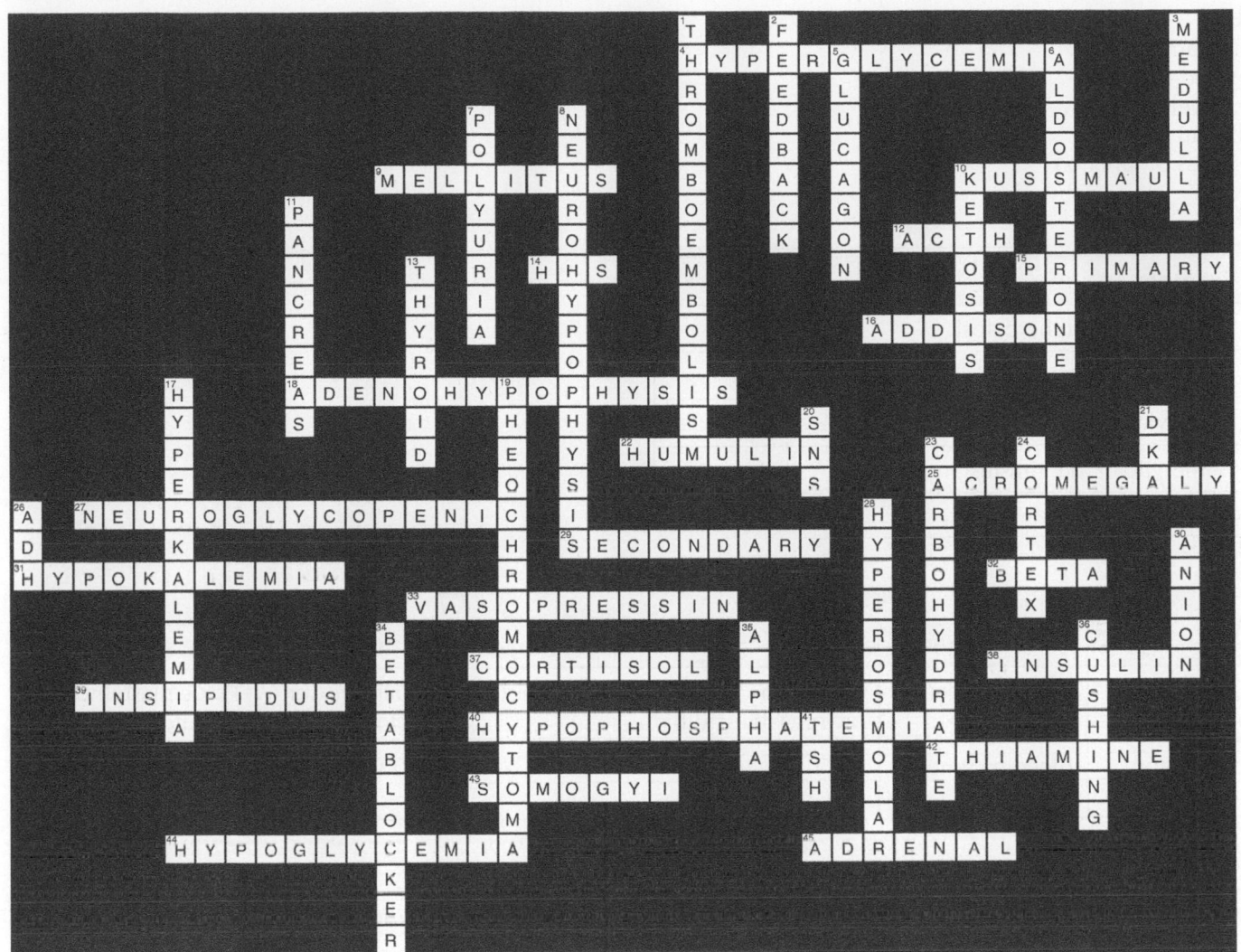

CHAPTER 8

8.1
a. Warmth
b. Redness
c. Swelling
d. Pain
e. Loss of function

8.2

Example	Type
Skin testing for tuberculosis	IV
Poststreptococcal glomerulonephritis	III
Anaphylaxis to penicillin	I
Hemolytic blood transfusion reaction	II

8.3

	Platelet Plug	Intrinsic Pathway	Extrinsic Pathway	Common Pathway	Fibrinolytic System
Activation	Intimal defect	Hageman factor (XII)	Tissue thromboplastin (III)	Stuart-Prower factor (X)	Tissue plasminogen activator
Laboratory test	Bleeding time	aPTT	PT	aPTT, PT	Fibrin split products

8.4

a	1. Aspirin
c	2. Heparin
b, f	3. Warfarin
e	4. rt-PA
d, e	5. Streptokinase
a	6. Clopidogrel

8.5
1. Stop transfusion.
2. Maintain IV access with normal saline and new administration set.
3. Reassure the patient; stay at the bedside.
4. Notify physician and blood bank.
5. Recheck blood numbers and type.
6. Treat symptoms appropriately.
7. Return unused portion of blood in blood bag and administration set to the blood bank.
8. Collect and send blood and urine samples to the laboratory; send another urine specimen 24 hours after transfusion reaction.
9. Document the transfusion reaction and treatment administered.

8.6

a	1. Esophageal varices
b	2. Radiation or drugs
b	3. Hereditary
b	4. Malignancy
b	5. Lead-poisoning
b	6. Crohn disease
b	7. Anorexia nervosa
c	8. Mismatch blood transfusion reaction
a	9. Trauma
b	10. Chronic kidney disease

8.7

d	1. Hemophilia A
e	2. Hemophilia B
c	3. von Willebrand disease
f	4. Heparin-induced thrombocytopenia
a	5. Disseminated intravascular coagulation
h	6. Liver disease
b	7. Immune thrombocytopenic purpura
g	8. Thrombotic thrombocytopenic purpura

8.8

Platelets	↓
PT	↑
aPTT	↑
Fibrin split products	↑
Factors V, VIII	↓
Fibrinogen	↓

8.9

a. Heparin	May perpetuate bleeding
b. Clotting factors	May perpetuate clotting

8.10

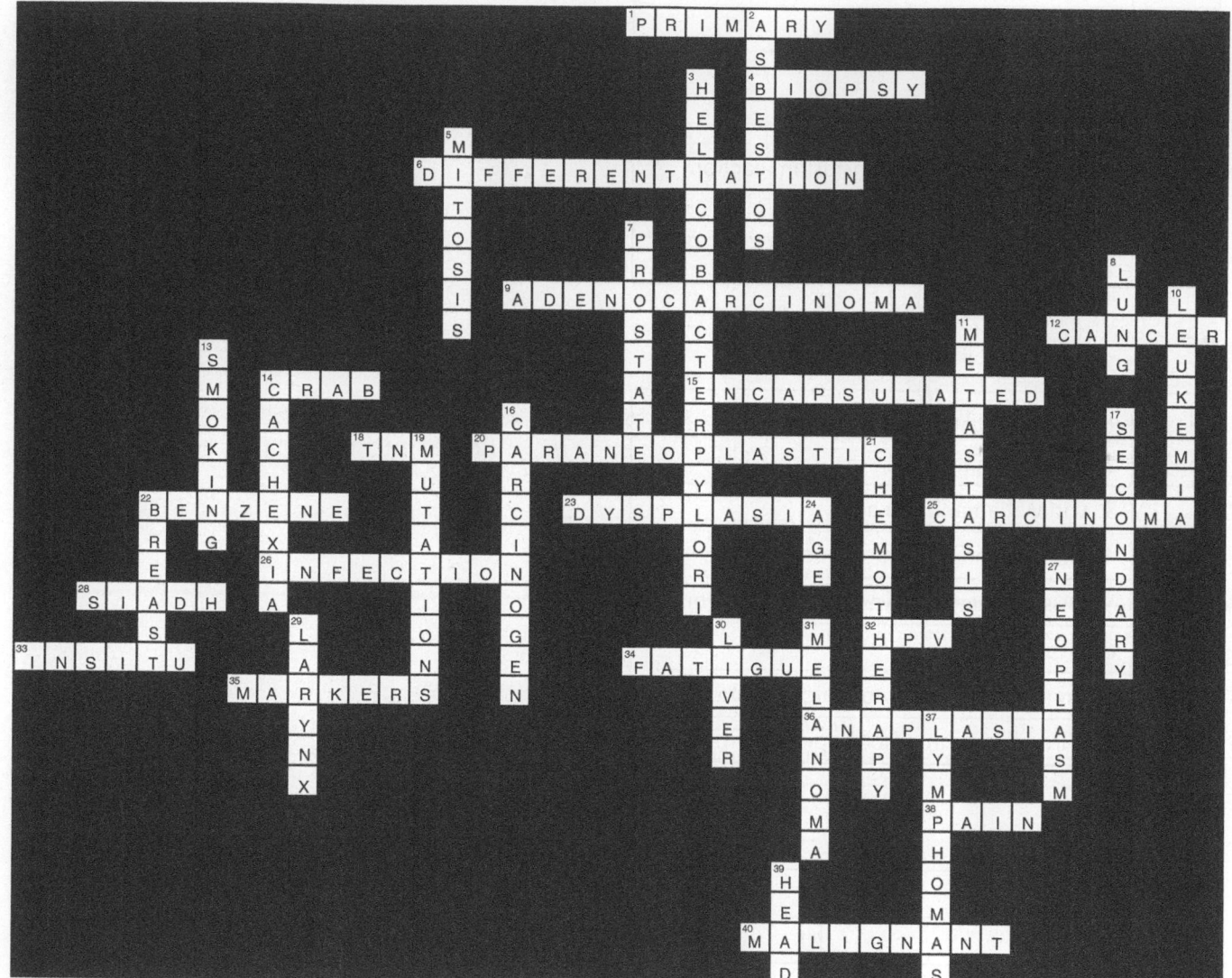

8.11

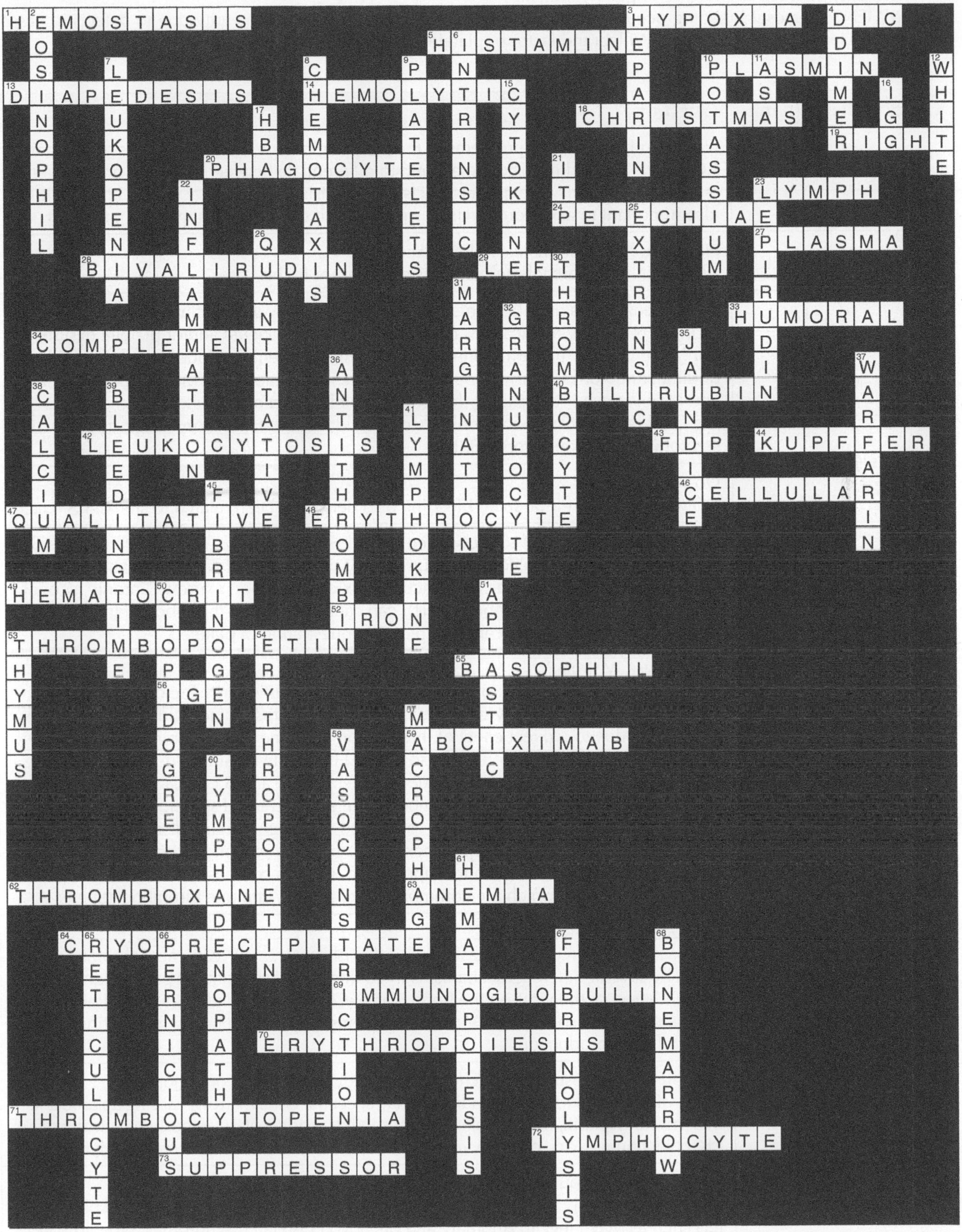
1 HEMOSTASIS
3 HYPOXIA
4 DIC
5 HISTAMINE
10 PLASMIN
13 DIAPEDESIS
14 HEMOLYTIC
18 CHRISTMAS
19 RIGHT
20 PHAGOCYTE
23 LYMPH
24 PETECHIAE
27 PLASMA
28 BIVALIRUDIN
29 LEFT
33 HUMORAL
34 COMPLEMENT
40 BILIRUBIN
42 LEUKOCYTOSIS
43 FDP
44 KUPFFER
46 CELLULAR
47 QUALITATIVE
48 ERYTHROCYTE
49 HEMATOCRIT
52 IRON
53 THROMBOPOIETIN
55 BASOPHIL
56 IGE
59 ABCIXIMAB
62 THROMBOXANE
63 ANEMIA
64 CRYOPRECIPITATE
69 IMMUNOGLOBULIN
70 ERYTHROPOIESIS
71 THROMBOCYTOPENIA
72 LYMPHOCYTE
73 SUPPRESSOR
2 EOSINOPHIL
3 HEPARIN
4 DDIMER
6 INTRINSIC
7 LEUKOPENIA
8 CHEMOTAXIS
9 PLATELETS
10 POTASSIUM
12 WHITE
15 CYTOKINE
22 INFLAMMATION
25 EXTRINSIC
26 QUANTITATIVE
30 THROMBOCYTE
31 MARGINATION
32 GRANULOCYTE
35 JAUNDICE
36 ANTITHROMBIN
37 WARFARIN
38 CALCIUM
39 BLEEDINGTIME
41 LYMPHOKINE
45 FIBRINOGEN
50 CLOPIDOGREL
51 APLASTIC
53 THYMUS
54 ERYTHROPOIETIN
57 MACROPHAGE
58 VASOCONSTRICTION
60 LYMPHADENOPATHY
61 HEMATOPOIESIS
65 RETICULOCYTE
66 PERNICIOUS
67 FIBRINOLYSIS
68 BONEMARROW

8.12

a. Abnormality of vascular integrity or platelet function

    COMMENT: Mucosal bleeding occurs when there is an abnormality in vascular integrity due to defects in vessel wall, or deficiency or defects in von Willebrand factor or platelets.

b.

Check or leave blank	Question
✓	Have you had bleeding problems in the past, particularly with procedures or trauma? COMMENT: Bleeding history may help to differentiate between acquired and congenital disorders. In this case, her history is more consistent with an acquired process. It is also important to ask about menses, specifically if they have changed from the past.
	Have you had your cholesterol checked? COMMENT: Hypercholesterolemia is not relevant in this case.
✓	What medications and supplements—not prescribed by a physician—are you taking? COMMENT: Many medications can cause thrombocytopenia and/or platelet dysfunction. Medications that commonly cause thrombocytopenia include heparin, quinidine, quinine, antibiotics, many immunosuppressive medications, chemotherapeutic agents, and H2-blockers. Medications that impair platelet function include aspirin, clopidogrel, and related P2Y12 antagonists, nonsteroidal antiinflammatory drugs, and selective serotonin release inhibitors (SSRIs).
	Do you smoke? COMMENT: Not relevant. No bleeding disorders have been related to smoking.
✓	Do you drink alcohol? If so, how often? COMMENT: Excessive alcohol consumption is a frequent cause of acute and chronic thrombocytopenia. Alcohol can be acutely toxic to the bone marrow. Chronic alcohol abuse can lead to liver cirrhosis, which can cause decreased thrombopoietin levels and hypersplenism, which can cause increased sequestration of platelets.
✓	Do you use IV drugs? COMMENT: It is important to ask about HIV and hepatitis C risk factors. HIV can cause thrombocytopenia by several different mechanisms including decreased platelet production due to a direct effect of the virus on the bone marrow. Immune-mediated increased platelet destruction can also occur. HIV-positive patients may also be taking medications that affect platelet production. Hepatitis C and B can cause liver cirrhosis with a resultant decrease in thrombopoietin and increased splenic sequestration of platelets. Hepatitis C may also be associated with autoimmune disorders such as immune thrombocytopenia. It is important to know if a patient has hepatitis B because it can be reactivated with immunosuppression, such as corticosteroids or azathioprine, and with rituximab, which are commonly used to treat immune thrombocytopenia.
✓	Do you have unprotected sex? COMMENT: It is important to ask about HIV risk factors. HIV can cause thrombocytopenia by several different mechanisms including decreased platelet production due to a direct effect of the virus on the bone marrow. Immune-mediated increased platelet destruction can also occur. HIV-positive patients may also be taking medications that affect platelet production.
✓	Do you have exposure to any chemicals or radiation at work or at home? COMMENT: Some toxins and radiation may affect the bone marrow, causing aplastic anemia, myelodysplasia, or leukemia. Patients should be asked about exposure to cleaning fluids, paint thinners, and other chemicals that they may use at work, home, or with hobbies.
✓	Does anyone in your family have a problem with bleeding? COMMENT: Family history is useful when considering inherited disorders of platelets such as May-Hegglin Anomaly and other MYH9-related syndromes, type IIb von Willebrand disease, Wiskott-Aldrich Syndrome, and others associated with decreased platelet number or function.

Check or leave blank	Question
✓	Have you had a recent unexpected loss of weight? COMMENT: It is important to inquire about systemic symptoms such as weight loss, fevers, night sweats, and fatigue when evaluating a hematologic disorder because various malignancies and infections can cause cytopenias.
✓	Do you have any heartburn, dyspepsia, or chronic indigestion? COMMENT: *H. pylori* may be associated with ITP. Many patients are symptomatic with this infection. Approximately 50% of treated patients' corrected platelet count with *H. pylori* treatment is >40,000/mm^3 at the start of the therapy.

c.

Check or leave blank	Laboratory Test
✓	Complete blood count (CBC) COMMENT: When you suspect thrombocytopenia, it is important to check for anemia and leukopenia as well. The patient should be asked whether any abnormalities have been noted on previous blood tests. Results of any prior tests should be obtained for comparison. This information will help to establish whether the thrombocytopenia is an acute or chronic problem.
✓	Peripheral smear COMMENT: It is always important to review the morphology of WBCs, RBCs, and platelets when evaluating for any type of cytopenia. The presence of schistocytes may indicate disseminated intravascular coagulation (DIC) or thrombotic thrombocytopenic purpura (TTP). The presence of immature cells may suggest an intrinsic bone marrow disorder. Very large platelets may suggest an inherited thrombocytopenia. It is important to rule out pseudothrombocytopenia due to platelet clumping. Clumping on the slide is purely artifact and can be avoided by redrawing the sample in a citrate or heparinized tube. It is also important to exclude any concurrent red blood cell disorders that would take you away from the diagnosis of immune thrombocytopenia such as spherocytes or a microangiopathic hemolytic anemia.
✓	Reticulocyte count COMMENT: The reticulocyte count is important to ascertain if the low platelet count is associated with RBC loss, which could be due to bleeding or a more general hematologic process associated with the thrombocytopenia, such as a warm antibody hemolytic anemia or microangiopathic hemolytic anemia.
✓	Prothrombin time (PT) and activated partial thromboplastin time (aPTT) COMMENT: The PT and aPTT are important to obtain for several reasons. First, if normal, they exclude a blood coagulation defect that can give thrombocytopenia (e.g., DIC). Second, they should be normal in a patient with immune thrombocytopenia only.
✓	D-dimer COMMENT: The D-dimer should be normal in a patient with immune thrombocytopenia. An abnormal D-dimer should prompt one to think of another reason for the thrombocytopenia (e.g., disseminated intravascular coagulation [DIC]).
	Platelet function analyzer (or PFA-100 or platelet function screen) COMMENT: A platelet count of greater than 100,000 mm^3 is required to perform a platelet function screen accurately. Therefore, this assay should not be performed.

Check or leave blank	Laboratory Test
	Bleeding time COMMENT: A bleeding time should be done only when the platelet count is known. In ITP, a patient may have a normal bleeding time even at a lower platelet count. The bleeding time screens for abnormal platelet function, and would be helpful in a patient with mucosal bleeding but with a normal platelet count. The bleeding time should be done only by technicians who are experts in the technique. In practice, this assay is no longer commonly performed. The platelet function analyzer (PFA) has been accepted by many as a substitute for the bleeding time. It is not clear if it is an adequate substitute. Neither assay should be performed on anemic or thrombocytopenic samples. Neither the bleeding time nor PFA assays predict bleeding risk.
✓	Lactic dehydrogenase (LDH) COMMENT: LDH is released from cytosol from lysed RBCs or platelets. A normal LDH supports the diagnosis of immune thrombocytopenia. An elevated LDH makes one think of consumptive disorders such as thrombotic thrombocytopenia purpura or hemolytic uremic syndrome.
✓	Viral titers for a chronic infection with HIV and hepatitis C COMMENT: HIV and hepatitis C are associated with chronic immune thrombocytopenia. Assaying for disease positivity is important to ascertain an etiology of chronic immune thrombocytopenia.
	Viral titers for an acute infection COMMENT: A recent viral respiratory infection may have triggered this patient's thrombocytopenia, but identifying the virus will not be helpful in diagnosing or treating this patient.
	Thrombopoietin (TPO) levels COMMENT: Thrombopoietin is a hormone that promotes platelet production. Thrombopoietin levels are currently measured for research purposes only.
	Glucose level COMMENT: The blood glucose is irrelevant to any of the bleeding disorders you may be considering.
	Chest x-ray COMMENT: This is not necessary for diagnosis or treatment.
✓	Direct antiglobulin test COMMENT: Patients with immune thrombocytopenia can also have an antibody-mediated autoimmune hemolytic anemia. This concurrence of these two disorders is called Evan syndrome.
✓	Quantitative immunoglobulins COMMENT: This assay can recognize common variable hypogammaglobulinemia, which is frequently associated with immune thrombocytopenia. It also is useful to detect hypergammaglobulinemic states, as seen in HIV and hepatitis, and it excludes myeloma as an etiology for thrombocytopenia. Additionally, if a patient is found to be IgA deficient, further testing is required. Some people with IgA deficiencies may develop anti-IgA antibodies. When those with anti-IgA are given blood component transfusions that contain IgA (such as plasma or immunoglobulin treatments), they may experience a severe anaphylactic transfusion reaction.
✓	*Helicobacter pylori* antigen assay COMMENT: As mentioned above, this infection may be associated with immune thrombocytopenia. Treatment for this condition can ameliorate the disorder in some patients. Please note that measurement of *H. pylori* antibodies should not be done when the patient is getting IV immunoglobulin.

CHAPTER 9

9.1

k	1. Anterior frontal lobe
j	2. Posterior frontal lobe
g	3. Parietal lobe
c	4. Occipital lobe
f	5. Temporal lobe
d	6. Cerebellum
b	7. Medulla
e	8. Hypothalamus
i	9. Wernicke's area
l	10. Thalamus
h	11. Limbic system
a	12. Broca's area

9.2

To calculate mean arterial pressure: $[SBP + (DBP \times 2)] \div 3$: $80 + (2 \times 50) = 180$, then divide by $3 = 60$.

To calculate cerebral perfusion pressure: MAP − ICP: $60 - 20 = 40$ mm Hg.

Should you be concerned? YES! CPP <50 is associated with loss of autoregulation, hypoperfusion of the brain, and anoxic encephalopathy.

9.3

	Sympathetic	Parasympathetic
Bronchodilation	×	
Coronary artery dilation	×	
Hypersalivation		×
Increased serum glucose	×	
Increased perspiration	×	
Increased intestinal motility		×
Pupil constriction		×
Tachycardia	×	

9.4

Pattern	Site of Lesion
CNS hyperventilation	Lower midbrain or upper pons
Cheyne-Stokes breathing	Cerebral hemispheres, basal ganglia, cerebellar lesion, or upper brain stem
Cluster (or Biot)	Lower pons or upper medulla
Ataxic	Medulla
Apneustic	Mid to lower pons

9.5

GCS: 13. You should notify the physician because this is a change in his neurologic status.

9.6

Cranial Nerve Number	Name	M (motor), S (sensory), or B (both)	Method of Assessment
I	Olfactory	S	• Evaluate the patient's ability to identify familiar odors
II	Optic	S	• Evaluate visual acuity using Snellen chart or newsprint • Evaluate the optic disc during funduscopic examination
III	Oculomotor	M	• Evaluate the ability to open eyes widely • Check size, shape, position, and reactivity of the pupils • Have the patient follow your finger with his or her eyes through the six cardinal positions of gaze • Look for abnormal eye movement
IV	Trochlear	M	• Have the patient follow your finger with his or her eyes through the six cardinal positions of gaze
V	Trigeminal	B	• Evaluate ability of the patient to detect light touch, superficial pain, and temperature on the forehead, cheeks, and jaw • Touch the cornea with a wisp of cotton and check for bilateral blink • Palpate the strength of the masseter muscles with the patient clinching his or her teeth and the strength of the temporal muscles with the patient squeezing his or her eyes shut
VI	Abducens	M	• Have the patient follow your finger with his or her eyes through the six cardinal positions of gaze
VII	Facial	B	• Ask the patient to smile and assess symmetry • Test the patient's ability to taste salt and sugar on the anterior tongue
VIII	Acoustic	S	• Evaluate ability of the patient to hear when speaking at normal voice volumes • Note any vertigo, nystagmus, nausea, vomiting, pallor, sweating, or hypotension
IX	Glossopharyngeal	B	• Evaluate the patient's ability to speak; note any hoarseness • Look for bilateral elevation of the palate with phonation • Test the patient's ability to taste sour and bitter on the posterior tongue • Evaluate the patient's ability to swallow • Test the gag reflex by stroking the palate with a tongue blade and looking for gag reflex • Evaluate cough reflex by touching the hypopharynx with a suction catheter
X	Vagus	B	• Tested with glossopharyngeal
XI	Spinal accessory	M	• Ask the patient to shrug his or her shoulders as you push down on them with your hands • Palpate the sternocleidomastoid and trapezius muscles for size and symmetry
XII	Hypoglossal	M	• Look for midline alignment when the patient protrudes his or her tongue • Look for fasciculations of the tongue

9.7

A. Level 3—Moderately resilient
B. Level 1—Highly vulnerable
C. Level 5—Highly stable

9.8

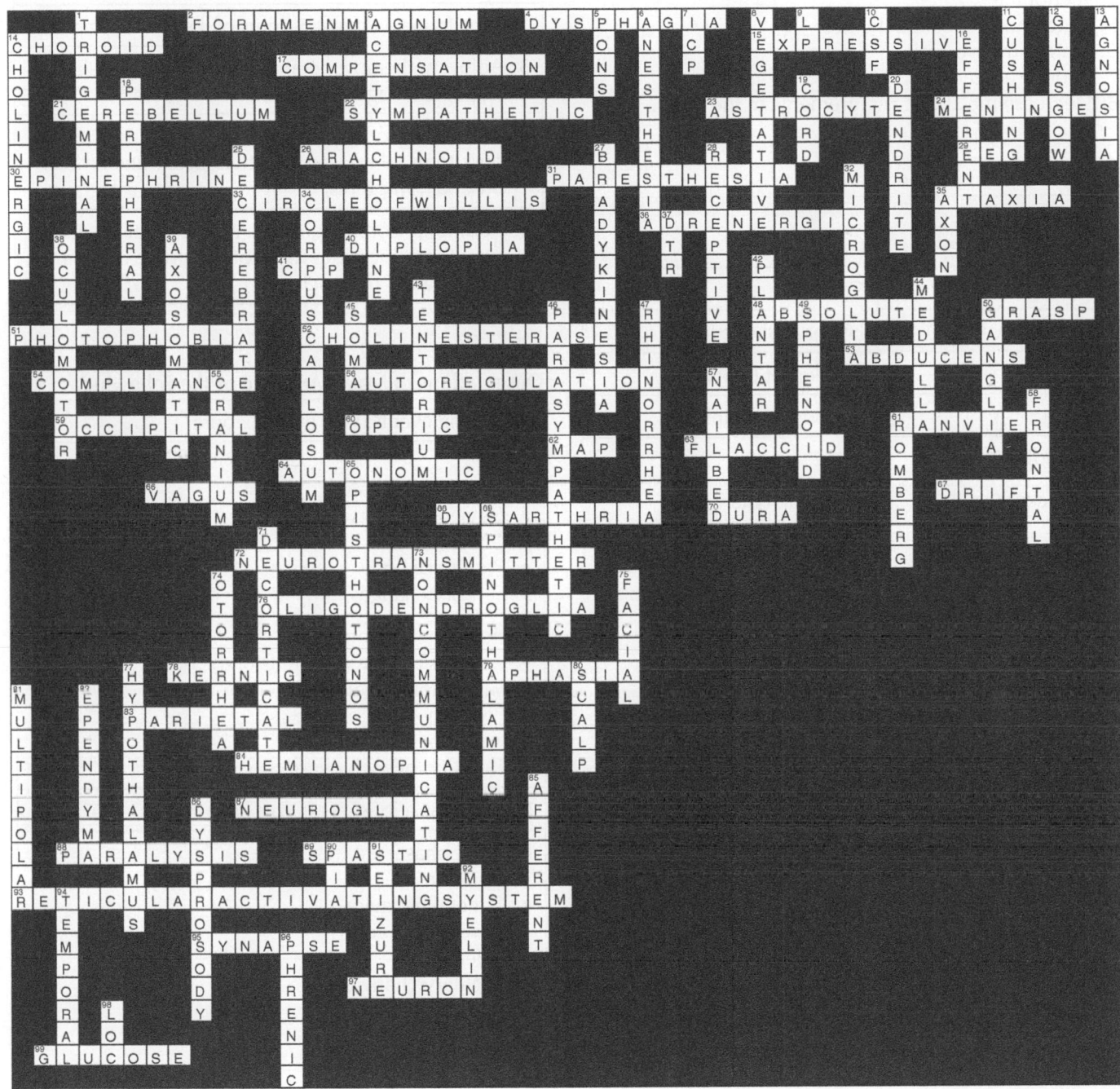

9.9

1. Neck twisting or flexion
2. Valsalva maneuver
3. Airway obstruction
4. Pain or noxious stimuli
5. Disturbing conversation
6. Noise
7. Bright lights
8. Tight tracheostomy ties or cervical collar
9. Seizure activity
10. Hyperthermia

9.10

Any five of the following:
1. Assess neurologic status frequently.
2. Maintain adequate venous drainage from head.
3. Prevent Valsalva maneuver.
4. Prevent increase in ICP associated with oral suctioning.
5. Space nursing care activities.
6. Maintain euvolemia.
7. Reduce anxiety.
8. Decrease metabolic requirements of the brain.

9.11

Any five of the following:

Type of Encephalopathy	Cause
Anoxic	Cardiac arrest
Hypertensive	Hypertensive crisis
Uremic	Buildup of toxins
Hepatic	Buildup of toxins
Metabolic	Diabetes
Wernicke	Thiamine (vitamin B_1) deficiency
Infection	Bacteria, virus, fungus

9.12

GCS: 4
Hunt and Hess: Grade V

9.13

	Vasospasm	Rebleed
Occurs either immediately after the bleed or between 7 and 10 days after the bleed		×
Caused by calcium influx into the vessel	×	
Occurs any time after 3 days	×	
Treated by hypervolemic hemodilution and calcium channel blockers	×	
Caused by lysis of the protective clot		×
Prevented by early clipping if the patient is stable enough		×

9.14

1. Dose: 0.9 mg/kg with maximum dose of ≤90 mg with the initial bolus being 10% of this total dose over 1 minute and the remaining 90% of this total dose infused over 60 minutes
2. Time frame: within 4.5 hours of the initial symptoms
3. Adjuvant therapy: no anticoagulants or platelet aggregation agents for the first 24 hours
4. Additional contraindication of awakening with symptoms (eliminates ability to determine time of onset of symptoms)
5. Additional contraindication of seizure at onset of symptoms (increases risk that the stroke is hemorrhagic rather than ischemic)

9.15

Observations to Make (Any Five of the Following)

Preceding events: Was there an aura?
Onset: • Body movements • Deviation of head and eyes • Chewing and salivation • Posture of body • Sensory changes
Tonic and clonic phases: • Progression of movements of the body • Skin color and airway • Pupillary changes • Incontinence • Duration of each phase
Level of consciousness during seizure
Postictal phase: • Duration • General behavior • Memory of events • Orientation • Pupillary changes • Headache • Aphasia • Injuries
Duration of entire seizure
Medications given and response

Interventions (Any Five of the Following)

Do not leave patient; provide privacy from other patients and visitors
Loosen clothing

Open airway, but do not try to pry mouth open; nasopharyngeal or nasotracheal airways may be used if necessary
Turn patient to side
Administer oxygen
Do not restrain; gentle guiding of extremities is acceptable
Pad side rails with blankets or pillows
Administer anticonvulsants (e.g. diazepam, phenytoin)
Reorient patient after seizure
Clean patient if incontinence has occurred
Allow patient to sleep

9.16

Drug	Adverse Effects (Any Two of the Following)
Lorazepam (Ativan)	• Respiratory depression • Tachycardia • Hypotension • Dysrhythmias
Diazepam (Valium)	• Tachycardia • Hypotension • Dysrhythmias
Phenytoin sodium (Dilantin)	• Hypotension • Dysrhythmias; blocks • Hepatitis • Nephritis • Blood dyscrasias
Fosphenytoin (Cerebyx)	• Hypotension • Dysrhythmias • Nephritis • Blood dyscrasias
Phenobarbital (Phenobarbital sodium, Luminal)	• Hypotension • Angioedema • Thrombophlebitis

9.17

1. b. Review the algorithm for Treatment of Ischemic Stroke. The most important information is determination of the time of onset of symptom. Fibrinolytics cannot be administered after 3 to 4.5 hours. Since (c) and (d) do not include determination of time of onset, they are not correct. It is important that the CT scan be completed within 10 minutes of ED arrival; the neurologic assessment (a) is performed after the CT scan.

2. a. The scenario only states that the patient is improved, not that the symptoms are completely gone. This is the nurse's baseline assessment. She should notify the physician (b) if the next assessment shows deterioration. There is no need to cancel the rehabilitation consult (c). The next assessment should be done as ordered (d); there is no indication that the patient is worsening. If the nurse notices a worsening of condition during routine nursing care, it would be appropriate to repeat the assessment at that time.

3. d. The patient should have received information about fibrinolytics (a) prior to receiving them. If the patient has any additional questions, the nurse should answer them, but this is not the priority. The only new drug (c) the patient is receiving is pantoprazole (Protonix). The nurse should explain this drug prior to administering it, but, again, it is not the priority. Patient teaching on the importance of regular glucose monitoring (c) should be done; however, given that the patient just had treatment for stroke, information on signs and symptoms (d) should be the priority.

9.18

h	1. Brainstem lesion
a, f	2. Subarachnoid hemorrhage
g	3. Status epilepticus
e	4. Dural tear
c	5. Postcraniotomy
i	6. Upper motor neuron lesion
a	7. Meningeal irritation
b	8. Intracranial hypertension
d	9. Hydrocephalus

9.19

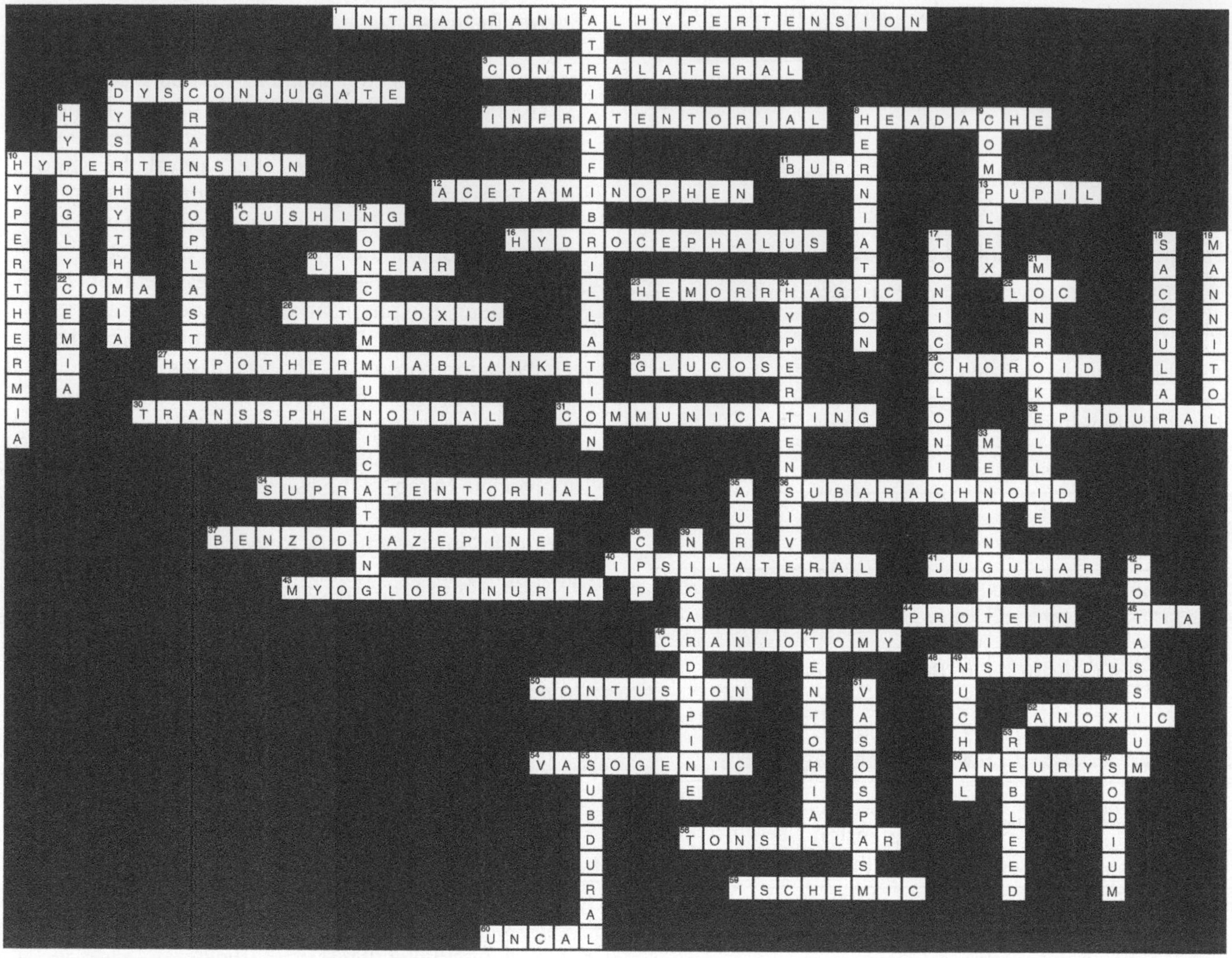

Crossword answer grid containing the following filled-in answers:

INTRACRANIAL HYPERTENSION, CONTRALATERAL, DYSCONJUGATE, INFRATENTORIAL, HEADACHE, HYPERTENSION, BURR, ACETAMINOPHEN, PUPIL, CUSHING, HYDROCEPHALUS, LINEAR, COMA, HEMORRHAGIC, CYTOTOXIC, HYPOTHERMIA BLANKET, GLUCOSE, CHOROID, TRANSSPHENOIDAL, COMMUNICATING, EPIDURAL, SUPRATENTORIAL, SUBARACHNOID, BENZODIAZEPINE, IPSILATERAL, JUGULAR, MYOGLOBINURIA, PROTEIN, CRANIOTOMY, INSIPIDUS, CONTUSION, ANOXIC, VASOGENIC, ANEURYSM, TONSILLAR, ISCHEMIC, UNCAL

CHAPTER 10

10.1

d	1. Anaphylactic
b	2. Cardiogenic
c	3. Hypovolemic
e	4. Neurogenic
a	5. Septic

10.2

	Compensatory	Progressive	Refractory
Tachycardia	✓	✓	
Dysrhythmias		✓	✓
Cool, pale skin	✓		
Disseminated intravascular coagulation			✓
Mottling of extremities		✓	✓

	Compensatory	Progressive	Refractory
Neurologic changes: lethargy, coma		✓	✓
Oliguria	✓		
Anuria		✓	✓
Acute respiratory distress syndrome			✓
Narrow pulse pressure	✓		
Profound hypotension despite vasopressors			✓
Hypotension		✓	✓
Decreased bowel sounds	✓	✓	
Thirst	✓	✓	
Neurologic changes: irritability, confusion	✓		
Nausea		✓	
Neurologic changes: focal signs			✓

10.3

Type of Shock	CO/CI	RAP/PAP/PAOP	SVR	SvO₂/ScvO₂
Hypovolemic	↓	↓	↑	↓
Cardiogenic	↓	↑	↑	↓
Septic	↑	↓	↓	↑
Anaphylactic	↓	↓	↓	↓
Neurologic	↓	↓	↓	↓

10.4

c	1. Isotonic crystalloids
b, c	2. Red blood cells
a	3. Oxygen
a	4. Mechanical ventilation
c	5. Inotropic agents
d	6. Sedation
a	7. PEEP
b	8. Surgical intervention to stop bleeding
c	9. Treatment of metabolic acidosis
d	10. Hypothermia

10.5

Isotonic crystalloids	Normal (0.9%) saline	Lactated Ringer's
Hypotonic crystalloids	Half-normal (0.45%) saline	5% dextrose in water
Hypertonic crystalloids	3% saline	10% dextrose in water
Colloids	Albumin	Dextran 70
Blood or blood products	Whole blood	Red blood cells

10.6

Condition	Hypovolemic	Cardiogenic	Septic	Anaphylactic	Neurogenic
Myocardial infarction		✓			
Bee sting				✓	
Head injury					✓
Diarrhea	✓				
Pulmonary embolism		✓			
Ruptured gallbladder			✓		
Esophageal varices	✓				
Ruptured papillary muscle		✓			
Insulin shock					✓
Ascites	✓				
IVP dye				✓	
Cervical or high thoracic spinal cord injury					✓
Invasive procedures	✓		✓		
Burns	✓		✓		
Blood transfusion reaction				✓	
Spinal anesthesia					✓
Trauma	✓		✓		
Malnutrition			✓		
Chemotherapy			✓		

10.7

a, b, d, h, i, k, l	1. Anaphylactic
e, f, k, l, m, and possibly g	2. Cardiogenic
a, k, l, and possibly c	3. Hypovolemic
a, d, k, l and possibly g	4. Neurogenic
a, d, j, k, l, and possibly b and e	5. Septic

10.8

Heart rate	Greater than **90 beats/min**			
Respiratory rate	Greater than **20 beats/min**	OR	Paco$_2$	Less than **32 mm Hg**
Temperature	Greater than **38° C (100.4° F)**	OR	Less than **36° C (96.8° F)**	
WBC	Greater than **12,000 cells/mm^3**	OR	Less than **4000 cells/ mm^3**	

10.9

d	1. Brain
f	2. Heart
e	3. Blood
b	4. Kidneys
c	5. Liver
a	6. Lungs

10.10

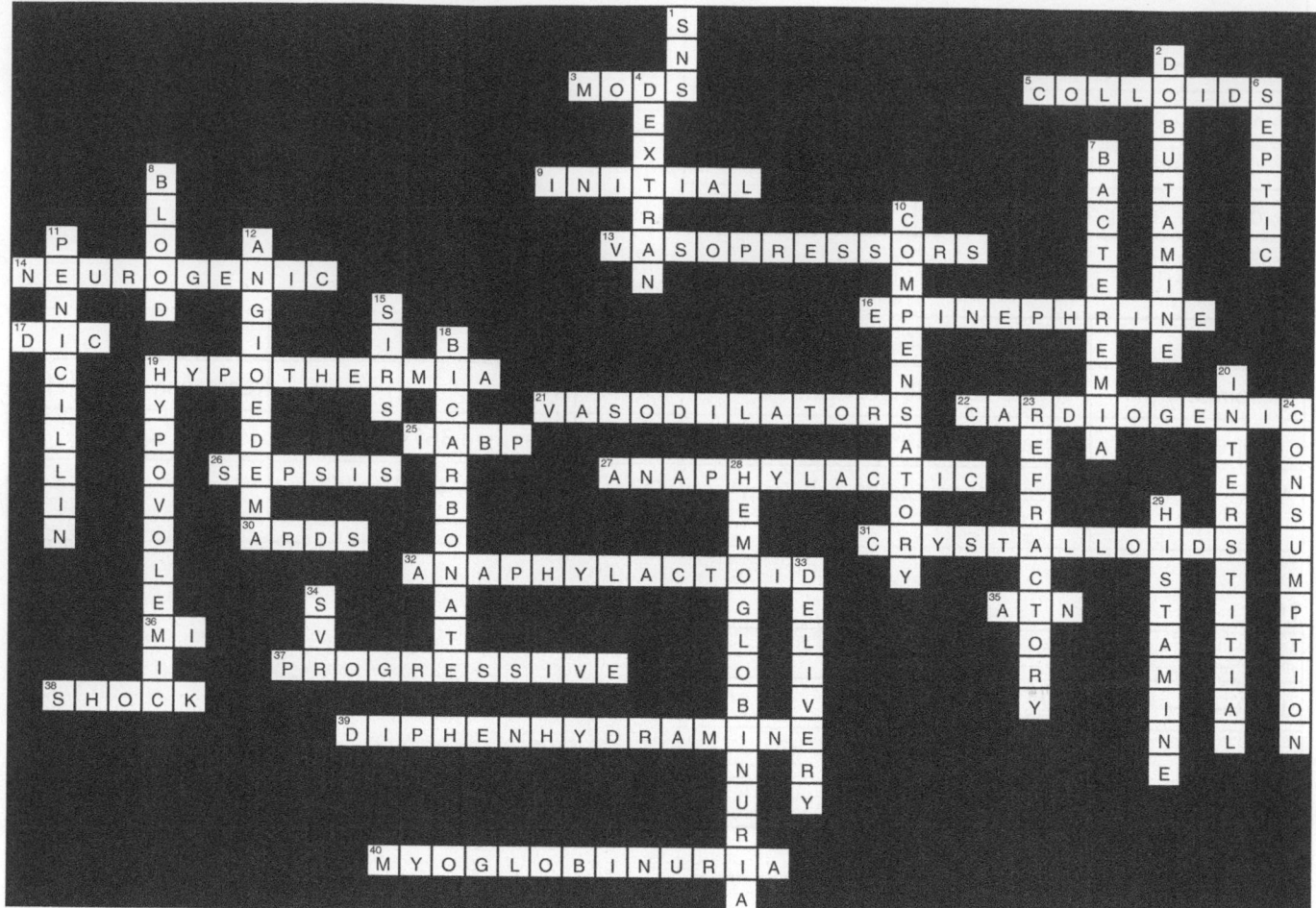

10.11

1. False
2. True

10.12

The patient does meet criteria for SIRS with a temperature of 38.2° C, respiratory rate of 35/minute, and heart rate of 110/minute. The patient does not meet criteria for sepsis at this point because there is no definitive infection though pneumonia is suspected. There is a need for investigation of possible sources of infection. There is no evidence of organ dysfunction (i.e., severe sepsis) at this point. Even though the BP is borderline low, there is no identified infectious cause and the serum lactate is normal, so there is no septic shock at this point. Other causes for the BP should be investigated.

10.13

a. Level 1

10.14

A. SIRS; meets criteria for SIRS, but no identified infection
B. Sepsis; meets criteria for SIRS and now has an identified source of infection
C. Shock; meets criteria for SIRS and sepsis and is now hypotensive despite fluids; acidotic; has an elevated serum lactate and an elevated INR

CHAPTER 11

11.1

e	1. Auditory
b	2. Visual
d	3. Gustatory
f	4. Hypnopompic
a	5. Tactile
c	6. Olfactory
g	7. Kinesthetic
h	8. Somatic

11.2

b	1. Physiologic
e	2. Safety and security
d	3. Love and belonging
c	4. Esteem and recognition
a	5. Self-actualization

11.3

Condition	Subjective Assessment	Objective Assessment
Anxiety disorder	• Apprehension and nervousness • Tremors • Tightness in chest • Dizziness	• Tachycardia, elevated BP, and tachypnea • Dilated pupils
Depression	• Hopeless feeling • Inability to concentrate • Low energy, fatigue, and loss of appetite • Depressed mood • Decreased libido • Recurrent thought of death	• Appearance sloppy • Flat affect • Tearful • Little eye contact • Slowness of movement • Quiet
Mania	• Racing thoughts • Risky or reckless behaviors • Little need for sleep	• Increased activity • Flight of ideas • Distractibility • Elation • Grandiosity
Hallucinations	• Patient reports having visions or hearing voices	• Patient is talking or responding to voices or other perceptual disturbances
Psychosis	• Paranoid ideas • Confusion or amnesia • Fears about safety	• Delusions and/or hallucinations • Agitation or bizarre behavior • Appears out of touch with reality • Inability to initiate activities • Lack of pleasure

Condition	Subjective Assessment	Objective Assessment
Dementia	• Memory loss • Speech impairment • Decline in cognitive function • Gradual onset	• Decrease in orientation and judgment • Aphasia • Apraxia • Agnosia • Shallow affect
Delirium	• Disorientation • Hallucinations • Acute onset	• Etiology identified; may include medical condition, trauma, substance use or withdrawal, and toxins • Fluctuating level of consciousness

11.4

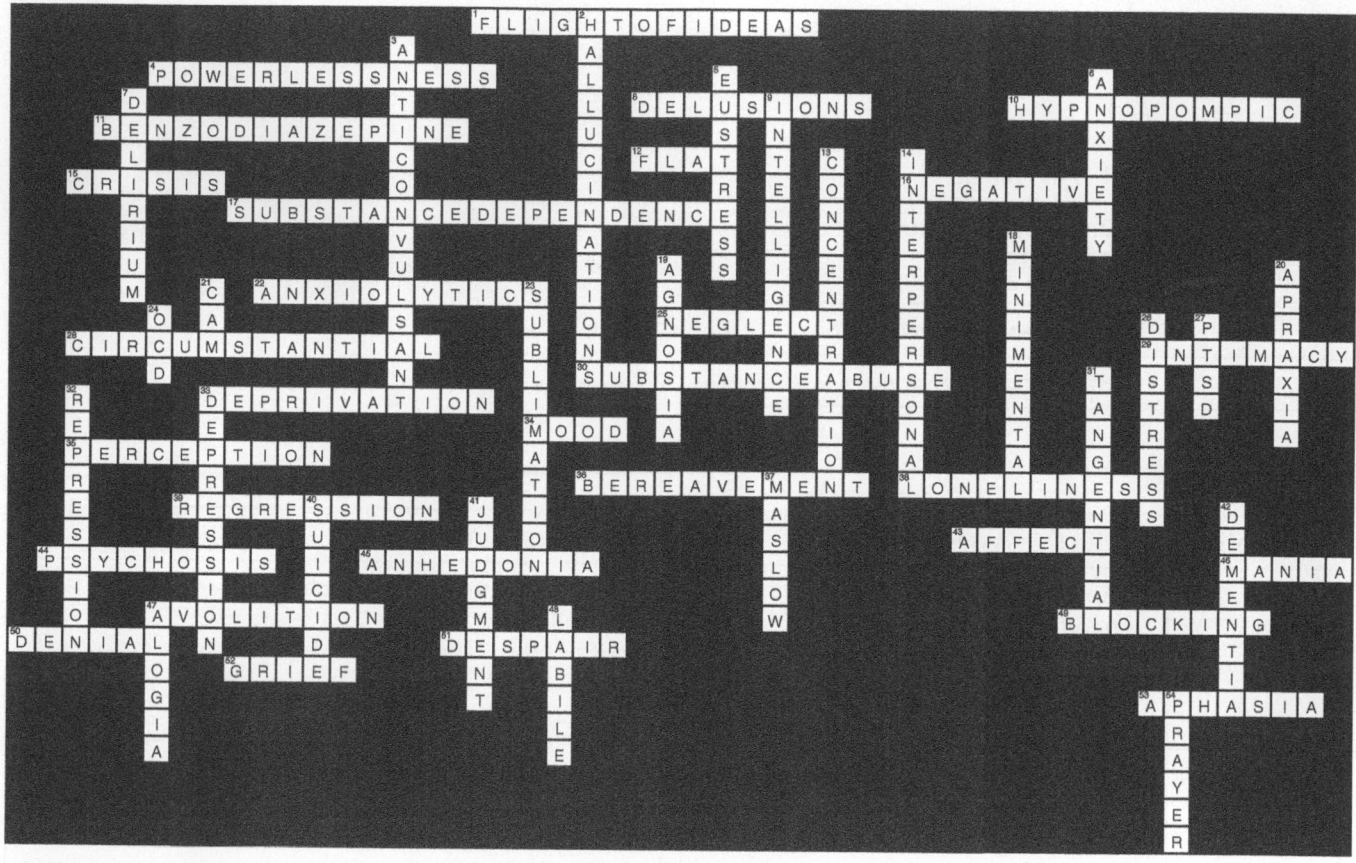

11.5

a. Does he have a history of medical or emotional issues?
   Is he currently taking any medication?
   Completion of neurologic exam.
b. CBC/electrolyte panel
   Toxicology screen
   Urinalysis
c. Delirium as evidenced by acute mental status change.
   Rule out depression: No reported medical cause for the change. He is oriented to person, place, and time.
   Rule out sepsis, stroke, and substance use: There is no evidence for this, but given the rapid change, these and other causes of delirium should be ruled out.
   Most likely not dementia due to acute onset.
d. Safety.
   Physical stabilization: Assess vital signs and labs, and intervene as indicated. If no abnormality is identified, consider a mental health issue such as depression.
   Emotional stabilization: Consider initiating treatment for depression if no physical problems are identified.

11.6

a. Level 1

References and Selected Readings

Chapter 1

American Association of Critical-Care Nurses. (2013a). *Certification exam handbook*. Retrieved from www.aacn.org/wd/certifications/docs/certexamhandbook.pdf.

American Association of Critical-Care Nurses. (2013b). *Exam statistics*. Retrieved from www.aacn.org/wd/certifications/content/statistical.pcms?menu=certification.

American Association of Critical-Care Nurses. (2013c). *Exam passing scores*. Retrieved from www.aacn.org/wd/certifications/content/exampassing-scores.pcms?menu=certification.

Altman, M. (2011). Let's get certified: Best practices for nurse leaders to create a culture of certification. *AACN Advanced Critical Care, 22*(1), 68–75.

Cary, A. H. (2001). Certified registered nurses: Results of the study of the certified workforce. *American Journal of Nursing, 101*(1), 44–52.

Fitzpatrick, J. C., Campo, T. M., Graham, G., & Lavandero, R. (2010). Certification, empowerment, and intent to leave current position and the profession among critical care nurses. *American Journal of Critical Care, 19*(3), 218–229.

Kendall-Gallagher, D., & Blegen, M. A. (2009). Competency and certification of registered nurses and safety of patients in intensive care units. *American Journal of Critical Care, 18*(2), 106–116.

Stromborg, M., Niebuhr, B., Prevost, S., Fabrey, L., Muenzen, P., Spence, C., & Valentine, W. (2005). Specialty certification: More than a title. *Nursing Management, 36*(5), 36–46.

Teal, J. (2011). Certifiably excellent. *AACN Adv Crit Care, 22*(1), 83–88.

Wade, C. H. (2010). Perceived effects of specialty nurse certification: a review of the literature. *Journal of Nursing Administration, 40*(10 Suppl), S5–13.

Chapter 2

Alfare-LeFevre, R. (2013). *Critical thinking, clinical reasoning, and clinical judgment: A practical approach* (5th ed.). St. Louis, MO: Saunders.

Armola, R. R., Bourgault, A. M., Halm, M. A., Board, R. M., Bucher, L., Harrington, L., & Medina, J. (2009). Upgrading the American Association of Critical-Care Nurses' evidence-leveling hierarchy. *American Journal of Critical-Care, 18*(5), 405–409.

Armola, R. R., Bourgault, A. M., Halm, M. A., Board, R. M., Bucher, L., Harrington, L., & Medina, J. (2009). AACN levels of evidence: What's new? *Critical Care Nurse, 29*(4), 70–73.

American Association of Critical-Care Nurses. (2005). *AACN standards for establishing and sustaining healthy work environments*. Retrieved from www.aacn.org/WD/HWE/Docs/HWEStandards.pdf.

American Association of Critical-Care Nurses. (2008). *Mission, vision and values*. Retrieved from www.aacn.org/wd/aacninfo/content/mission-vision-values-ethics.pcms?menu=aboutus.

American Association of Critical-Care Nurses. (2010). *Core curriculum for progressive care nursing* (1st ed.). St. Louis, MO: Saunders Elsevier.

American Association of Critical-Care Nurses. (2011). *AACN Practice Alert. Family presence: visitation in the adult ICU*. Retrieved from www.aacn.org/WD/practice/docs/practicealerts/family-visitation-adult-icu-practicealert.pdf.

American Association of Critical-Care Nurses. (2012a). *About critical care nursing*. Retrieved from www.aacn.org/wd/publishing/content/pressroom/aboutcriticalcarenursing.pcms?menu=publications.

American Association of Critical-Care Nurses. (2012b). *Certification exam handbook*. Retrieved from www.aacn.org/dm/mainpages/certificationhome.aspx.

American Association of Critical-Care Nurses. (2012c). *Moral distress*. Retrieved from www.aacn.org/wd/practice/content/ethic-moral.pcms?menu=practice.

American Association of Critical-Care Nurses. (2003). *The AACN Synergy Model for Patient Care*. Retrieved from www.aacn.org/wd/certifications/content/synmodel.pcms.

American Association of Critical-Care Nurses Certification Corporation. (2013). *PCCN test plan*. Retrieved from www.aacn.org/WD/Certification/content/pccnexamblueprint.pcms?menu=Certification.

American Nurses Association. (2001). *Code of ethics for nurses with interpretative statements*. Washington, DC: American Nurses Publishing.

American Nurses Association. (2012a). *What is nursing?* Retrieved from www.nursingworld.org/EspeciallyForYou/What-is-Nursing.

American Nurses Association. (2012b). *The nursing process*. Retrieved from www.nursingworld.org/Especially ForYou/What-is-Nursing/Tools-you-need/Thenursingprocess.htm.

American Nurses Association. (2012d). *Nursing-sensitive indicators*. Retrieved from www.nursingworld.org/MainMenuCategories/ThePracticeof-ProfessionalNursing/PatientSafetyQuality/Research-Measurement/The-National-Database/Nursing-Sensitive-Indicators_1.

APRN Consensus Work Group and the National Council of State Boards of Nursing APRN Advisory Committee. (2008). *Consensus model for APRN regulations: Licensure, accreditation, certification & education*. Retrieved from www.aacn.nchc.edu/Education/pdf/APRNreport.pdf.

Barden, L. (Ed.). (2005). *AACN standards for establishing and sustaining healthy work environments: A journey to excellence*. Aliso Viejo, CA: American Association of Critical-Care Nurses.

Bell, L. (Ed.). (2015). *AACN scope and standards for acute and critical care nursing practice* (2nd ed.) Aliso Viejo, CA: American Association of Critical-Care Nurses.

Benner, P. (2002). Living organ donors: Respecting the risks involved in the "gift of life." *American Journal of Critical Care, 11*, 266–268.

Braude, H. D. (2012). Conciliating cognition and consciousness: The perceptual foundations of clinical reasoning. *Journal of Evaluation in Clinical Practice, 18*(5), 945–950.

Burke, W., Evans, B. J., & Jarvik, G. P. (2014). Return of results: Ethical and legal distinctions between research and clinical care. *American Journal of Medical Genetics Part C: Seminars in Medical Genetics, 166C*(1), 105–111. Retrieved from www.ncbi.nlm.nih.gov/pubmed/24616381. *doi:10.1002/ajmg.c.31393*.

Centers for Medicare and Medicaid Services. (2004). *Interpretative guidelines-responsibilities of Medicare participating hospitals in emergency cases*. Retrieved from www.cms.hhs.gov/manuals/Downloads/som107ap_v_emerg.pdf.

Choiniere, D. B. (2010). The effects of hospital noise. *Nurse Administration Quarterly, 34*(4), 327–333.

Ciliska, D. K., Pinelli, J., DiCenso, A., & Cullum, N. (2001). Resources to enhance evidence-based nursing practice. *AACN Clinical Issues, 12*(4), 520–528.

Chuly, M., & Burns, S. M. (2010). *AACN essentials of progressive care nursing* (2nd ed.). New York: McGraw-Hill, Inc.

Curley, M. (2012, November 2). *Reflections on 15 years of synergy: Transcending practice and education to clinical research*. Seventh Annual Nursing Research Conference. Retrieved from www.udel.edu/nrc/archive/nrc-2012/downloads/presentations/Reflection_10_24-12_handout.pdf.

Curley, M. A. Q. (2007). *Synergy: The unique relationship between nurses and patients*. Indianapolis, IN: Sigma Theta Tau International.

Curley, M. A. Q. (1998). Patient-nurse synergy: Optimizing patients' outcomes. *American Journal Critical Care, 7*(1), 64–72.

Curtin, L., & Flaherty, M. J. (1982). *Nursing ethics: Theories and pragmatics*. Bowie, MD: Robert J. Grady Company.

Dennison, R. D. (2005). Creating an organizational culture for medication safety. *Nursing Clinics North America, 40*(1), 1–23.

Dennison, R. D. (2013). *Pass CCRN* (4th ed.). St. Louis, MO: Elsevier.

Dracup, K., & Bryan-Brown, C. W. (1999). Empathy: A challenge for critical care. *American Journal of Critical Care, 8*(4), 204–205.

Ecklund, M. M., & Stamps, D. C. (2002). The Synergy Model in practice: Promoting synergy in progressive care. *Critical Care Nurse, 22*(4), 60–67.

Elinson, J. (1987). Advances in health assessment discussion panel. *Journal Chronic Disease, 40*(Suppl 1), 83S–91S.

Environmental Protection Agency. (1974). *Information on levels of environmental noise requisite to protect public health and welfare with an adequate margin of safety.* Retrieved from www.nonoise.org/library/levels74/levels74.htm.

Epstein, E. G., & Delgado, S. (2010, September 30). Understanding and addressing moral distress. *Online Journal of Issues in Nursing, 15*(3), manuscript 1.

Exley, M., White, N., & Martin, J. H. (2002). Transplantation: Why families say no to organ donation. *Critical Care Nurse, 6*, 44–51.

Frank, G. (2001). EMTALA: An expert tells us what it's all about. *Journal of Emergency Nursing, 27*, 65–67.

Giger, J. N. (2013). *Transcultural nursing: Assessment and intervention.* St. Louis, MO: Elsevier.

Gray, J. A. M. (1997). *Evidence-based healthcare: How to make health policy and management decisions.* London: Churchill Livingstone.

Guido, G. W. (2010). *Legal and ethical issues in nursing* (5th ed.). Upper Saddle River, NJ: Prentice Hall.

Haig, K. M., Sutton, S., & Whittington, J. (2006). SBAR: A shared mental model for improving communication between clinicians. *Joint Commission Journal on Quality and Patient Safety, 32*(3), 167–175.

Health Resources and Services Administration. (2001). *Cultural competence works. Using cultural competence to improve the quality of health care for diverse populations and add value to managed care arrangements.* Retrieved from www.hrsa.gov/financeMC/ftp/cultural-competence.pdf.

Holley, A. B. (2010). *Sleep in the ICU.* Retrieved from www.medscape.com/viewarticle/723907.

Institute for Healthcare Advancement. (2012). *What is health literacy?* Retrieved from www.iha4health.org.

Institute for Healthcare Improvement. (2011). *Science of improvement: How to improve.* Retrieved from www.ihi.org/knowledge/Pages/HowtoImprove/ScienceofImprovementHowtoImprove.aspx.

Institute of Medicine. (2006). *Keeping patients safe: Transforming the work environment for nurses.* Washington, DC: The National Academies Press.

Joint Commission on Accreditation of Healthcare Organizations (JCAHO). (2014). *National Patient Safety Goals.* Retrieved from www.jointcommission.org/standards_information/npsgs.aspx.

Johnson, S. A., & Romanello, M. L. (2005). Generational diversity. Teaching and learning approaches. *Nurse Educator, 30*(5), 212–216.

Jonsen, A. R., Siegler, M., & Winslade, W. J. (2010). *Clinical ethics: A practical approach to ethical decisions in clinical medicine* (7th ed.). New York, NY: McGraw-Hill.

Kinney, M., Dunbar, S., Brooks-Brunn, J. A., Molter, N., & Vitello-Cicciu, J. (1998). *AACN clinical reference for critical care nursing* (4th ed.). St. Louis, MO: Mosby.

Kotter, J. P. (1995). Leading change: Why transformation efforts fail. *Harvard Business Review, 73*(1), 59–68.

Kübler-Ross, E. (1969). *On death and dying.* New York, NY: Macmillan.

Leske, J. (1991). Overview of family needs after critical illness: from assessment to intervention. *AACN Clinical Issues in Critical-Care Nursing, 2*(2), 220–229.

Leonard, M., Graham, S., & Bonacum, D. (2004). The human factor: The critical importance of effective teamwork and communication in providing safe care. *Qual Saf Health Care, 13*(1 Suppl), i85–i90.

Lewis, L., & Vickers, A. (2008). Unit based shared governance leads the journey of creating a healthy work environment. *Critical Care Nurse, 28*(2), 53–54.

McCaffery, M. (1968). *Nursing practice theories related to cognition, bodily pain and main environment interactions.* Los Angeles, CA: University of California, Los Angeles.

McCaffery, M. (2002). Teaching your patient to use a pain rating scale. *Nursing 2002, 32*(8), 17.

Melnyk, B., & Fineout-Overholt, E. (2015). *Evidence-based practice in nursing and healthcare: A guide to best practice* (3rd ed.). Philadelphia: Wolters Kluwer.

Matthews, E. E. (2011). Sleep disturbances and fatigue in critically ill patients. *AACN Advanced Critical Care, 22*(3), 204–224.

National Council of State Boards of Nursing. (1996). *Assuring competence.* Retrieved from www.ncsbn.org/public/resources/ncsbn_competence_two.htm.

National Council of State Boards of Nursing. (2015). *Joint Statement on Delegation American Nurses Association (ANA) and the National Council of State Boards of Nursing (NCSBN).* Retrieved from www.ncsbn.org/Delegation_joint_statement_NCSBN-ANA.pdf.

O'Grady, P., & Malloch, K. (2011). Quantum Leadership: Advancing Innovation, Transforming Health Care. Jones & Bartlett Learning: Sudbury MA.

Payen, J.-F., Bru, O., Bosson, J. L., Lagrasta, A., Novel, E., Deschaux, I., et al. (2001). Assessing pain in critically ill sedated patients using a behavioral pain scale. *Critical Care Medicine, 29*(12), 2258–2263.

Quality and Safety Education for Nurses. (2012). *Quality and safety competencies.* Retrieved from www.qsen.org/competencies.php.

Schmalenberg, C., & Kramer, M. (2008). Clinical units with the healthiest work environments. *Critical Care Nurse, 28*(3), 65–77.

Stevens, K. R. (2012). ACE Star Model of EBP: Knowledge transformation. Academic Center for Evidence-Based Practice, The University of Texas Health Science Center at San Antonio. Retrieved from www.acestar.uthscsa.edu.

Straus, S. E., Glasziou, P., Richardson, W. S., & Haynes, R. B. (2011). *Evidence-based medicine: How to practice and teach it* (4th ed.). Edinburgh: Churchill Livingstone.

U.S. Census Bureau. (2011). *Projection of the population by sex, race, and Hispanic origin for the United States: 2010-2050.* Retrieved from www.census.gov/population/www/projections/reports.html.

Yoder-Wise, P. (2011). *Leading and managing in nursing* (5th ed.). St. Louis, MO: Mosby.

Chapter 3

Aehlert, B. (2012). *ECGs made easy* (5th ed.). St. Louis, MO: Mosby.

Ahrens, T. (2010). Stroke volume optimization versus central venous pressure in fluid management. *Critical Care Nurse, 30*(2), 71–73.

American Heart Association. (2012). *Advanced cardiac life support (ACLS). Provider manual supplementary material.* Retrievd from www.hearttraining.com/media/documents/ACLS%20Renewal%20Folder/ACLS%20Supplementary%20Material.pdf.

Baird, M. S., & Bethel, S. (2010). *Manual of critical care nursing. Nursing interventions and collaborative management* (6th ed.). St. Louis, MO: Mosby Elsevier.

Barill, T. P. (2012). *The six second ECG: A practical guide to basic and 12 lead ECG interpretation.* Palm Springs, CA: Skillstat Learning, Inc. Retrieved from http://skillstat.com/wp-content/uploads/2014/10/SixSecondECG-Chapters-1-3.pdf.

Burns, S. (2014). *Core curriculum for progressive nursing* (3rd ed.). Palo Vista, CA: AACN.

Burns, S. (2014). *AACN essentials of progressive nursing* (3rd ed.). Palo Vista, CA: AACN.

Chuly, M., & Burns, S. M. (2010). *AACN essentials of progressive care nursing* (2nd ed.). New York, NY: McGraw-Hill.

Deutschman, C. S., & Neligan, P. J. (2010). *Evidence-based practice of critical care.* Philadelphia, PA: Saunders Elsevier.

Evenson, L., & Farnsworth, M. (2010). Skilled cardiac monitoring at the bedside: An algorithm for success. *Critical Care Nurse, 30*(5), 14–22.

Farwell, A. L. (2010). Saving muscle: Evidence-based strategies for reducing door-to-balloon times for ST-segment elevation myocardial infarction patients. *Journal of Emergency Nursing, 36*(3), 231–237.

Field, J. M., Hazinski, M. F., Sayre, M. R., et al. (2010). Part 1: Executive summary: 2010 American Heart Association guidelines for cardiopulmonary resuscitation and emergency cardiovascular care. *Circulation, 122*(18 Suppl 3), S640–S656.

Fletcher, B., & Thalinger, K. K. (2010). Prasugrel as antiplatelet therapy in patients with acute coronary syndromes or undergoing percutaneous coronary intervention. *Critical Care Nurse, 30*(5), 45–54.

Fox, L., Kirkendall, C., & Craney, M. (2010). Continuous ST-segment monitoring in the intensive care unit. *Critical Care Nurse, 30*(5), 33–44.

Gheorghiade, M., Vaduganathan, M., Fonarow, G. C., & Bonow, R. O. (2013). Rehospitalization for heart failure: Problems and perspectives. *Journal of the American College of Cardiology, 61*(4), 391–403. Retrieved from http://dx.doi.org/10.1016/j.jacc.2012.09.038.

Grannito, M. H., Norton, C. K., Sher, R., & Baldia, C. (2010). Takotsubo cardiomyopathy. Implications for nursing practice. *Advanced Emergency Nursing Journal, 32*(1), 83–91.

Guyton, A. C., & Hall, J. T. (2011). *Textbook of medical physiology* (12th ed.). Philadelphia, PA: Saunders.

Hays, A. J., & Wilkerson, T. D. (2010). Management of hypertensive emergencies: A drug therapy perspective for nurses. *AACN Advanced Critical Care, 21*(1), 5–14.

Hazinski, M. F., Nolan, J. P., Billi, J. E., et al. (2010). Part 1: Executive summary: 2010 international consensus on cardiopulmonary resuscitation and emergency cardiovascular care science with treatment recommendations. *Circulation, 122*(16 Suppl 2), S250–S275.

Herlihy, B. (2011). *The human body in health and illness* (4th ed.). Philadelphia, PA: Saunders Elsevier.

James, P. A., Oparil, S., Carter, B. L., et al. (2014). Evidence-Based Guideline for the Management of High Blood Pressure in Adults: Report From the Panel Members Appointed to the Eighth Joint National Committee (JNC 8). *JAMA, 311*(5), 507–520. http://dx.doi.org/10.1001/jama.2013.284427.

Jones, B., Higginson, R., & Santos, A. (2010). Critical care: Assessing blood pressure, circulation and intravascular volume. *British Journal of Nursing, 19*(3), 153, 155–159.

Lahm, T., McCaslin, C. A., Wozniak, T. C., et al. (2010). Medical and surgical treatment of acute right ventricular failure. *Journal of the American College of Cardiology, 56*(18), 1435–1446.

Link, M. S., Atkins, D. L., Passman, R. S., et al. (2010). Part 6: Electrical therapies: Automated external defibrillators, defibrillation, cardioversion, and pacing: 2010 American Heart Association Guidelines for Cardiopulmonary Resuscitation and Emergency Cardiovascular Care. *Circulation, 122*(18 Suppl 3), S706–S719.

Martin, B. (2010). *Family presence during resuscitation and invasive procedures.* Retrieved from www.aacn.org/WD/Practice/Docs/PracticeAlerts/Family%20Presence%2004-2010%20final.pdf.

McCance, K. L., & Huether, S. E. (2015). *Pathophysiology. The biologic basis for disease in adults and children* (7th ed.). St. Louis, MO: Elsevier Mosby.

Moorman, L. P. (2010). Implantable cardioverter-defibrillator: Not just another device. *American Nurse Today, 5*(1), 12–14.

Morton, P. G., & Fontaine, D. K. (2012). *Critical care nursing. A holistic approach* (10th ed.). Philadelphia, PA: Lippincott Williams & Wilkins.

Moseley, M. J., Allen, D., & Martell, M. (2010). Electrocardiogram lead selection using critical thinking. *Dimensions of Critical Care Nursing, 29*(6), 253–258.

Ndefo, U. A., Erowele, G. I., Ebiasah, R., & Green, W. (2010). Clevidipine: A new intravenous option for the management of acute hypertension. *American Journal of Health System Pharmacy, 67*(5), 351–360.

Neumar, R. W., Otto, C. W., Link, et al. (2010). Part 8: Adult advanced cardiovascular life support: 2010 American Heart Association guidelines for cardiopulmonary resuscitation and emergency cardiovascular care. *Circulation, 122*(18 Suppl 3), S729–S767.

O'Connor, R. E., Brady, W., Brooks, S. C., et al. (2010). Part 10: Acute coronary syndromes: 2010 American Heart Association guidelines for cardiopulmonary resuscitation and emergency cardiovascular care. *Circulation, 122*(18 Suppl 3), S787–S817.

Pagana, K. D., & Pagana, T. J. (2010). *Mosby's manual of diagnostic and laboratory tests* (4th ed.). St. Louis, MO: Mosby Elsevier.

Palmer, B. (2011). Systematic cardiac rhythm strip analysis. *MEDSURG Nursing, 20*(2), 96–97.

Peberdy, M. A., Callaway, C. W., Neumar, R. W., et al. (2010). Part 9: Post-cardiac arrest care: 2010 American Heart Association guidelines for cardiopulmonary resuscitation and emergency cardiovascular care. *Circulation, 122*(18 Suppl 3), S768–S786.

Polly, D. M., Paciullo, C. A., & Hatfield, C. J. (2011). Management of hypertensive emergency and urgency. *Advanced Emergency Nursing Journal, 33*(2), 127–136.

Roberts, M. (2010). Clinical utility and adverse effects of amiodarone therapy. *AACN Advanced Critical Care, 21*(4), 333–338.

Sandau, K. E., Sendelbach, S., Frederickson, J., & Doran, K. (2010). National survey of cardiologists' standard of practice for continuous ST-segment monitoring. *American Journal of Critical Care, 19*(2), 112–123.

Scheibly, K. (2010). Indications for implantation of cardiac pacemakers. *AACN Advanced Critical Care, 21*(2), 227–232.

Scheibly, K. (2010). Pacemaker timing and electrocardiogram interpretation. *AACN Advanced Critical Care, 21*(4), 386–396.

Scheibly, K. (2010). Systematic assessment of basic pacemaker function. *AACN Advanced Critical Care, 21*(3), 322–328.

Seupaul, R. A., & Wilbur, L. G. (2011). Evidence-based emergency medicine. Does therapeutic hypothermia benefit survivors of cardiac arrest? *Annals of Emergency Medicine, 58*(3), 282–283.

Smithburger, P. L., Kane-Gill, S. L., Nestor, B. L., & Seybert, A. l (2010). Recent advances in the treatment of hypertensive emergencies. *Critical Care Nurse, 30*(5), 24–31.

Tachjian, A., Maria, V., & Jahangir, A. (2010). Use of herbal products and potential interactions in patients with cardiovascular disease. *Journal of the American College of Cardiology, 55*(6), 515–525.

Tomte, O., Draegni, T., Mangschau, A., et al. (2011). A comparison of intravascular and surface cooling techniques in comatose cardiac arrest survivors. *Critical Care Medicine, 39*(3), 443–449.

Travers, A. H., Rea, T. D., Bobrow, B. J., et al. (2010). Part 4: CPR overview: 2010 American Heart Association guidelines for cardiopulmonary resuscitation and emergency cardiovascular care. *Circulation, 122*(18 Suppl 3), S676–S684.

Urden, L., Stacy, K., & Lough, M. (2010). *Critical care nursing: Diagnosis and management* (6th ed.). St. Louis, MO: Mosby Elsevier.

Vadera, R. (2011). Does antihypertensive drug therapy decrease morbidity or mortality in patients with a hypertensive emergency? *Annals Emergency Medicine, 57*(1), 64–65.

Wiegand, D. L. -M. (Ed.). (2011). *AACN procedure manual for critical care* (6th ed.) Philadelphia, PA: Saunders Elsevier.

Yancy, C. W., Jessup, M., Bozkurt, B., Butler, J., Casey, D. E., et al. (2013). ACCF/AHA Practice Guidelines for the Management of Heart Failure. *Circulation, 128*:e240–e327. Retrieve from http://circ.ahajournals.org/content/128/16/e240.short?rss=1&ssource=mfr.

Chapter 4

Afshari, A., Brok, J., Moller, A. M., & Wetterslev, J. (2010A). Aerosolized prostacyclin for acute lung injury (ALI) and acute respiratory distress syndrome (ARDS). *Cochrane Database Systematic Reviews, 8*, CD007733.

Afshari, A., Brok, J., Moller, A. M., & Wetterslev, J. (2010B). Inhaled nitric oxide for acute respiratory distress syndrome (ARDS) and acute lung injury in children and adults. *Cochrane Database Systematic Reviews, 7*, CD002787.

Andrews, P., & Habashi, N. M. (2010). Weaning patients from the mechanical ventilator: The nurse's role. *American Nurse Today, 5*(3), 11–14.

Baird, M. S., & Bethel, S. (2010). *Manual of critical care nursing. Nursing interventions and collaborative management* (6th ed.). St. Louis, MO: Mosby Elsevier.

Baker, K., Barsamian, J., Leone, D., et al. (2013). Routine dyspnea assessment on unit admission. *American Journal of Nursing, 113*(11), 42–49; quiz 50.

Baselski, V., & Klutts, J. S. (2013). Quantitative Cultures of Bronchoscopically Obtained Specimens Should Be Performed for Optimal Management of Ventilator-Associated Pneumonia. *Journal Clinical Microbiology, 51*(3), 740–744. Retrieved from http://jcm.asm.org/content/51/3/740.full. doi: 10.1128/JCM.03383-12.

Barbera, J. A., & Blanco, I. (2009). Pulmonary hypertension in patients with chronic obstructive pulmonary disease: Advances in pathophysiology and management. *Drugs, 69*(9), 1153–1171.

Barnette, L., & Kautz, D. D. (2013). Creative ways to teach arterial blood gas interpretation. *Dimensions of Critical Care Nursing, 32*(2), 84–87.

Bauman, M. (2011). Chest-tube care: The more you know, the easier it gets. *American Nurse Today, 6*(9), 27–32. Retrieved from www.americannursetoday.com/assets/0/434/436/440/8172/8174/8176/8256/1d298438-82c6-439d-8b2e-77ffaf165fca.pdf.

Bauman, M., & Cosgrove, C. (2012). Understanding end-tidal CO_2 monitoring. *American Nurse Today, 7*(11), 12–17.

Bel, E. H., Sousa, A., Fleming, L., et al. (2011). Diagnosis and definition of severe refractory asthma: an international consensus statement from the Innovative Medicine Initiative (IMI). *Thorax, 66*(10), 910–917.

Boka, K. (2014). Pulmonary Embolism Clinical Scoring Systems. *Medscape News and Perspectives.* Retrieved from http://emedicine.medscape.com/article/1918940-overview#showall.

Booker, S., Murff, S., Kitko, L., & Jablonski, R. (2013). Mouth care to reduce ventilator-associated pneumonia. *American Journal of Nursing, 113*(10), 24–30; quiz 31.

Boutou, A. K., Abatzidou, F., Tryfon, S., et al. (2011). Diagnostic accuracy of the rapid shallow breathing index to predict a successful spontaneous breathing trial outcome in mechanically ventilated patients with chronic obstructive pulmonary disease. *Heart & Lung, 40*(2), 105–110.

Campbell, M. L. (2011). Dyspnea. *AACN Adv Crit Care, 22*(3), 257–264.

Carlisle, H. (2014). The case for capnography in patients receiving opioids. *American Nurse Today, 9*(9), 22–27.

Carson, J. L., Carless, P. A., & Hébert, P. C. (2013). Outcomes using lower vs higher hemoglobin thresholds for red blood cell transfusion. *Journal of the American Medical Association, 309*, 83.

Chlan, L., Tracy, M. F., & Grossbach, I. (2011). Achieving quality patient-ventilator management: advancing evidence-based nursing care. *Critical Care Nurse, 31*(6), 46–50.

Collins, T. A. (2013). Packed red blood cell transfusions in critically ill patients. *Critical Care Nurse, 31*(1), 25–34.

Corbridge, S., & Corbridge, T. C. (2010). Asthma in adolescents and adults. *American Journal of Nursing, 110*(5), 28–38; quiz 39–40.

Deutschman, C. S., & Neligan, P. J. (2010). *Evidence-based practice of critical care.* Philadelphia, PA: Saunders Elsevier.

El Khoury, M. Y., Panos, R. J., Ying, J., & Almoosa, K. F. (2010). Value of the PaO: FiO ratio and Rapid Shallow Breathing Index in predicting successful extubation in hypoxemic respiratory failure. *Heart & Lung, 39*(6), 529–536.

El-Khatib, M. F., Zeineldine, S., Ayoub, C., Husari, A., & Bou-Khalil, P. K. (2010). Critical care clinicians' knowledge of evidence-based guidelines for preventing ventilator-associated pneumonia. *American Journal of Critical Care, 19*(3), 272–276.

Elpern, E., Killeen, K., Patel, G., & Senecal, P. A. (2013). The application of intermittent pneumatic compression devices for thromboprophylaxis: An observational study found frequent errors in the application of these mechanical devices in ICUs. *American Journal of Nursing, 113*(4), 30–36; quiz 37. http://dx.doi.org/10.1097/01.NAJ.0000428736.48428.10.

Feider, L. L., Mitchell, P., & Bridges, E. (2010). Oral care practices for orally intubated critically ill adults. *Am J Crit Care, 19*(2), 175–183.

Fohl, A. L., & Regal, R. E. (2011). Proton pump inhibitor-associated pneumonia: Not a breath of fresh air after all? *World Journal of Gastrointestinal Pharmacology and Therapeutics, 2*(3), 17–26. http://dx.doi.org/10.4292/wjgpt.v2.i3.17.

Gin-Sing, W. (2010). Pulmonary arterial hypertension: a multidisciplinary approach to care. *Nursing Standard, 24*(38), 40–47.

Grossbach, I., Chlan, L., & Tracy, M. F. (2011). Overview of mechanical ventilatory support and management of patient- and ventilator-related responses. *Critical Care Nurse, 31*(3), 30–44. http://dx.doi.org/10.4037/ccn2011595.

Humbert, M., Lau, E. M., Montani, D., Jaïs, X., Sitbon, O., & Simonneau, G. (2014). Advances in therapeutic interventions for patients with pulmonary arterial hypertension. *Circulation, 130*(24), 2189–2208. http://dx.doi.org/10.1161/CIRCULATIONAHA.114.006974.

Kearon, C., Akl, E. A., Comerota, A. J., et al. (2012). Antithrombotic therapy for VTE disease: Antithrombotic therapy and prevention of thrombosis, (9th ed.). American College of Chest Physicians Evidence-Based Clinical Practice Guidelines. *Chest, 141*(2 Suppl), e419s–e494s.

Kenny, D. J., & Goodman, P. (2010). Care of the patient with enteral tube feeding: an evidence-based practice protocol. *Nursing Research, 59*(1 Suppl), S22–S31. http://dx.doi.org/10.1097/NNR.0b013e3181c3bfe9.

Kesecioglu, J. (2010). Farewell to exogenous surfactant therapy in acute lung injury/acute respiratory distress syndrome! Or, must we start all over again? *Critical Care Medicine, 38*(7), 1606–1607.

Khalid, I., Doshi, P., & DiGiovine, B. (2010). Early enteral nutrition and outcomes of critically ill patients treated with vasopressors and mechanical ventilation. *American Journal of Critical Care, 19*(3), 261–268.

Kingman, M. S., & Chin, K. (2013). Safety recommendations for administering intravenous prostacyclins in the hospital. *Critical Care Nurse, 33*(5), 32–39. http://dx.doi.org/10.4037/ccn2013608.

Kjonegaard, R., Fields, W., & King, M. L. (2010). Current practice in airway management: A descriptive evaluation. *American Journal of Critical Care, 19*(2), 168–173; quiz 174.

Kollef, M. H., Zilberberg, M. D., Shorr, A. F., et al. (2011). Epidemiology, microbiology and outcomes of healthcare-associated and community-acquired bacteremia: A multicenter cohort study. *Journal of Infection, 62*(2), 130–135.

Laird, P., & Ruppert, S. D. (2011). Acute respiratory distress syndrome—a case study. *Critical Care Nursing Quarterly, 34*(2), 165–174.

Lyerla, F., LeRouge, C., Cooke, D. A., Turpin, D., & Wilson, L. (2010). A nursing clinical decision support system and potential predictors of head-of-bed position for patients receiving mechanical ventilation. *American Journal of Critical Care, 19*(1), 39–47.

Makic, M. B., VonRueden, K. T., Rauen, C. A., & Chadwick, J. (2011). Evidence-based practice habits: Putting more sacred cows out to pasture. *Critical Care Nurse, 31*(2), 38–61; quiz 62.

Martin, G. (2012). *The new definition of ARDS.* Retrieved from www.medscape.com/viewarticle/773257.

Maselli, D. J., & Restrepo, M. I. (2011). Strategies in the prevention of ventilator-associated pneumonia. *Therapeutic Advances in Respiratory Disease, 5*(2), 131–141.

Metheny, N. A., & Frantz, R. A. (2013). Head-of-bed elevation in critically ill patients: A review. *Critical Care Nurse, 33*(3), 53–66; quiz 67.

Morris, L. L., McIntosh, E., & Whitmer, A. (2014). The importance of tracheostomy progression in the intensive care unit. *Critical Care Nurse, 34*(1), 40–48; quiz 50. http://dx.doi.org/10.4037/ccn2014722.

Morris, L. L., Whitmer, A., & McIntosh, E. (2013). Tracheostomy care and complications in the intensive care unit. *Critical Care Nurse, 33*(5), 18–30. http://dx.doi.org/10.4037/ccn2013518.

Penaloza, A., Verschuren, F., Meyer, G., Quentin-Georget, S., Soulie, C., Thys, F., et al. (2013). Comparison of the unstructured clinician gestalt, the Wells Score, and the Revised Geneva Score to estimate pretest probability for suspected pulmonary embolism. *Annals of Emergency Medicine, 62*(2), 117e–124e. Retrieved from www.ncbi.nlm.nih.gov/pubmed/23433653. http://dx.doi.org/10.1016/j.annemergmed.2012.11.002.

Phillips, C. R. (2013). .The Berlin definition: real change or the emperor's new clothes? *Critical Care, 17*(4), 174. http://dx.doi.org/10.1186/cc12761.

Racco, M. (2012). An enteral nutrition protocol to improve efficiency in achieving nutritional goals. *Critical Care Nurse, 32*(4), 72–75. http://dx.doi.org/10.4037/ccn2012625.

Ranieri, V. M., Rubenfeld, G. D., Thompson, B. T., Ferguson, N. D., Caldwell, E., Fan, E., Camporota, L., & Slutsky, A. S. (2012). ARDS Definition Task Force. Acute respiratory distress syndrome: The Berlin Definition. *Journal of the American Medical Association, 307*(23), 2526–2533. http://dx.doi.org/10.1001/jama.2012.5669.

Roark, D. C. (2012). Working toward perfection on the pneumonia core measure. *Journal of Emergency Nursing, 38*(2), 127–129; quiz 199.

Ruiz, C. (2013). Astute assessment saves a patient with PE. *American Nurse Today, 8*(3), 17–18.

Scala, R., Naldi, M., & Maccari, U. (2010). Early fiberoptic bronchoscopy during non-invasive ventilation in patients with decompensated chronic obstructive pulmonary disease due to community-acquired-pneumonia. *Critical Care, 14*(2), R80. http://dx.doi.org/10.1186/cc8993.

Shorr, A. F., Chan, C. M., & Zilberberg, M. D. (2011). Diagnostics and epidemiology in ventilator-associated pneumonia. *Therapeutic Advances in Respiratory Disease, 5*(2), 121–130.

Short, J. (2010). Use of dexmedetomidine for primary sedation in a general intensive care unit. *Critical Care Nurse, 30*(1), 29–38; quiz 39.

Smithburger, P. L., Campbell, S., & Kane-Gill, S. L. (2013). Alteplase treatment of acute pulmonary embolism in the intensive care unit. *Critical Care Nurse, 33*(2), 17–27. http://dx.doi.org/10.4037/ccn2013626.

Staudinger, T., Bojic, A., Holzinger, U., et al. (2010). Continuous lateral rotation therapy to prevent ventilator-associated pneumonia. *Critical Care Medicine, 38*(2), 486–490.

Stewart, M. L. (2014). Interruptions in enteral nutrition delivery in critically ill patients and recommendations for clinical practice. *Critical Care Nurse, 34*(4), 14–21; quiz 22.

Stonecypher, K. (2010). Ventilator-associated pneumonia: The importance of oral care in intubated adults. *Critical Care Nursing Quarterly, 33*(4), 339–347.

Stringham, R., & Shah, N. R. (2010). Pulmonary arterial hypertension: An update on diagnosis and treatment. *American Family Physician, 82*(4), 370–377.

Wang, J., Ma, Y., & Fang, Q. (2013). Extubation with or without spontaneous breathing trial. *Critical Care Nurse, 33*(6), 50–55.

Ward, J. J. (2013). High-flow oxygen administration by nasal cannula for adult and perinatal patients. *Respiratory Care, 58*(1), 98–122. Retrieved from http://rc.rcjournal.com/content/58/1/98.full.pdf+html. doi: 10.4187/respcare.01941.

Williams, J. W., Cox, C. E., Hargett, C. W., et al. (2012). *Noninvasive positive-pressure ventilation (NPPV) for acute respiratory failure.* Agency for Healthcare Research and Quality. Retrieved from www.ncbi.nlm.nih.gov/books/NBK99179/.

Winkelman, C., & Chiang, L. C. (2010). Manual turns in patients receiving mechanical ventilation. *Critical Care Nurse, 30*(4), 36–44.

Woidtke, R. (2013). Adult obstructive sleep apnea: Taking a patient-centered approach. *American Nurse Today, 8*(7), 12–15.

Young, A. C. (2010). Non-invasive ventilation-status quo for status asthmaticus? *Respirology, 15*(4), 585–586.

Zahran, E. M., & El-Razik, A. A. (2011). Tracheal suctioning with verses without saline instillation. *Journal of American Science, 7*(8), 23–32.

Chapter 5

Abay, M. C., Reyes, J. D., Everts, K., & Wisser, J. (2007). Current literature questions the routine use of low-dose dopamine. *AANA Journal, 75*(1), 57–63.

American Association of Critical-Care Nurses. (2010). *Core curriculum for progressive care nursing.* St. Louis, MO: Saunders Elsevier.

Badve, S. V., Hawley, C. M., McDonald, S. P., Mudge, D. W., Rosman, J. B., Brown, F. G., & Johnson, D. W. (2008). Automated and continuous ambulatory peritoneal dialysis have similar outcomes. *Kidney International, 73*(4), 480–488. http://dx.doi.org/10.1038/sj.ki.5002705.

Bagshaw, S. M., Uchino, S., Bellomo, R., Morimatsu, H., Morgera, S., Schetz, M., et al. (2009). Timing of renal replacement therapy and clinical outcomes in critically ill patients with severe acute kidney injury. *Journal of Critical Care, 24*(1), 129–140.

Bellomo, R., Kellum, J. A., & Ronco, C. (2012). Acute kidney injury. *The Lancet, 380*(9857), 1904.

Bentley, M. L., Corwin, H. L., & Dasta, J. (2010). Drug-induced acute kidney injury in the critically ill adult: Recognition and prevention strategies. *Critical Care Medicine, 38*(6 Suppl), S169–S174.

Boyle, M., & Baldwin, I. (2010). Understanding the continuous renal replacement therapy circuit for acute renal failure support: A quality issue in the intensive care unit. *AACN Advanced Critical Care, 21*(4), 367–375.

Chuly, M., & Burns, S. M. (2014). *AACN essentials of progressive care nursing* (3rd ed.). New York, NY: McGraw-Hill.

Dennison, R. D. (2013). *Pass CCRN!* (4th ed.). St. Louis, MO: Elsevier.

Dirkes, S. (2011). Acute kidney injury: Not just acute renal failure anymore? *Critical Care Nurse, 31*(1), 37–49; quiz 50.

Kallenbach, J., Gutch, C. F., Stoner, M. H., & Corea, A. L. (2011). *Review of hemodialysis for nurses and dialysis personnel* (8th ed.). St. Louis, MO: Mosby.

Kraut, J. A., & Xing, S. X. (2011). Approach to the evaluation of a patient with an increased serum osmolal gap and high-anion-gap metabolic acidosis. *American Journal of Kidney Disease, 58*(3), 480–484.

Lane, B. R., Poggio, E. D., Herts, B. R., Novick, A. C., & Campbell, S. S. (2009). Renal function assessment in the era of chronic kidney disease: Renewed emphasis on renal function centered patient care. *The Journal of Urology, 182*(2), 435–444.

Martin, R. K. (2010). Acute kidney injury: Advances in definition, pathophysiology, and diagnosis. *AACN Advanced Critical Care, 21*(4), 350–356.

McCance, K. L., & Huether, S. A. (2013). *Pathophysiology: Biological basis for disease in adults and children* (7th ed.). St. Louis, MO: Elsevier.

Merhaut, S., & Trupp, R. J. (2010). Cardiorenal dysfunction. *AACN Advanced Critical Care, 21*(4), 357–364; quiz 365–356.

Schneider, A. G., Bellomo, R., Bagshaw, S. M., Glassford, N. J., Lo, S., Jun, M., Cass, .A.M., & Gallagher, M. (2013). Choice of renal replacement therapy modality and dialysis dependence after acute kidney injury: A systematic review and meta-analysis. *Intensive Care Medicine, 39*(6), 987–997.

Wiegand, D. L.-M. (Ed.) (2011). *AACN Procedure manual for critical care* (6th ed.). Philadelphia, PA: Saunders.

Chapter 6

Amerine, E. (2007). Get optimum outcomes for acute pancreatitis patients. *Nurse Practitioner, 32*(6), 44–48.

Andreoli, T., Carpenter, C., Griggs, R. C., & Loscalzo, J. (2010). *Cecil essentials of medicine* (8th ed.). St. Louis, MO: Elsevier.

Andris, A. (2010). Pancreatitis: Understanding the disease and implications for care. *AACN Advanced Critical Care, 21*(2), 195–204.

Andris, A. (2010). Pancreatitis: understanding the disease and implications for care. *AACN Advanced Critical Care, 21*(2), 195–204.

Barba, K., Fitzgerald, P., & Wood, S. (2007). Managing peptic ulcer disease. *Nursing 2007, 37*(7) 56hn1-56hn4.

Blei, A. T. (2007). Portal hypertension and its complications. *Current Opinions Gastroenterology, 23*(3), 275–282.

Boundless. (14 Nov. 2014). Hepatic portal circulation. *Boundless Anatomy and Physiology.* Retrieved from www.boundless.com/physiology/textbooks/boundless-anatomy-and-physiology-textbook/the-cardiovascular-system-blood-vessels-19/blood-flow-through-the-body-185/hepatic-portal-circulation-926-5131/.

Bourgault, A. M., & Halm, M. A. (2009). Feeding tube placement in adults: Safe verification method for blindly inserted tubes. *American Journal Critical Care, 18*(1), 73–76.

Bourgault, A. M., Ipe, L., Weaver, J., Swartz, S., & O'Dea, P. J. (2007). Development of evidence-based guidelines and critical care nurses' knowledge of enteral feeding. *Critical Care Nurse, 27*(4), 17–22 25–19; quiz 30.

Bowman, A., Greiner, J. E., Doerschug, K. C., Little, S. B., Bombei, C. L., & Comried, L. M. (2005). Implementation of an evidence-based feeding protocol and aspiration risk reduction algorithm. *Critical Care Nurse Quarterly, 28*(4), 324–333; quiz 334–325.

Brush, K. A. (2007). Abdominal compartment syndrome: The pressure is on. *Nursing, 37*(7), 36–41; quiz 40–31.

Brush, K. A. (2007). Measuring intra-abdominal pressure. *Nursing, 37*(7), 42–44.

Bureau, C., Garcia-Pagan, J. C., Otal, P., Pomier-Layrargues, G., Chabbert, V., Cortez, C., Perreault, P., Peron, J. M., Abraldes, J. G., Bouchard, L., Bilbao, J. I., Bosch, J., Rousseau, H., & Vinel, J. P. (2004). Improved clinical outcome using polytetrafluoroethylene-coated stents for TIPS: results of a randomized study. *Gastroenterology, 126*(2), 469–475.

Cannon-Diehl, M. R. (2010). Emerging issues for the postbariatric surgical patient. *Critical Care Nursing Quarterly, 33*(4), 361–370.

Carroll, J. K., Herrick, B., Gipson, T., & Lee, S. P. (2007). Acute pancreatitis: Diagnosis, prognosis, and treatment. *American Family Physician, 75*(10), 1513–1520.

Cerqueira, R. M., Andrade, L., Correia, M. R., Fernandes, C. D., & Manso, M. C. (2012). Risk factors for in-hospital mortality in United States. *European Journal of Gastroenterology & Hepatology, 24*(5), 551–557. Retrieved from http://journals.lww.com/eurojgh/Abstract/2012/05000/Risk_factors_for_in_hospital_mortality_in.13.aspx. doi:10.1097/MEG.0b013e3283510448.

Chen, L. (2010). A literature review of intensive insulin therapy and mortality in critically ill patients. *Clinical Nurse Specialist, 24*(2), 80–86.

De Waele, J. J., De Laet, I., Kirkpatrick, A. W., & Hoste, E. (2011). Intra-abdominal hypertension and abdominal compartment syndrome. *American Journal Kidney Disease, 57*(1), 159–169.

DeKeyser Ganz, F., Fink, N. F., Raanan, O., Asher, M., Bruttin, M., Nun, M. B., et al. (2009). ICU nurses' oral-care practices and the current best evidence. *Journal Nursing Scholarship, 41*(2), 132–138.

de-Madaria, E. (2014). Fluid therapy in acute pancreatitis—Aggressive or adequate? Time for reappraisal. *Pancreatology, 14*(6), 433–435.

De-Souza, D. A., & Greene, L. J. (2005). Intestinal permeability and systemic infections in critically ill patients: Effect of glutamine. *Critical Care Medicine, 33*(5), 1125–1135.

Devries, J. H. (2010). Glucose variability is associated with intensive care unit mortality. *Critical Care Medicine, 38*(3), 838–842.

Dib, N., Oberti, F., & Cales, P. (2006). Current management of the complications of portal hypertension: variceal bleeding and ascites. *Canadian Medical Association Journal, 174*(10), 1433–1443.

Feinstein, L. B., Holman, R. C., Yorita-Christensen, K. L., Steiner, C. A., & Swerdlow, D. L. (2010). *Trends in hospitalizations for peptic ulcer disease, United States, 1998–2005. Emerging Infectious Disease.* Retrieved from wwwnc.cdc.gov/eid/article/16/9/09-1126.htm. doi:10.3201/eid1609.091126.

Fisher, E. M., & Brown, D. K. (2010). Hepatorenal syndrome: Beyond liver failure. *AACN Advanced Critical Care, 21*(2), 165–186.

Gallagher, J. J. (2010). Intra-abdominal hypertension: Detecting and managing a lethal complication of critical illness. *AACN Advanced Critical Care, 21*(2), 205–219.

Greer, D. (2006). Peptic ulcer disease—Pharmacological treatment. *Hospital Pharmacist, 13,* 245–250.

Heidelbaugh, J. J., & Bruderly, M. (2006). Cirrhosis and chronic liver failure: Part I. Diagnosis and evaluation. *American Family Physician, 74*(5), 756–762.

Heidelbaugh, J. J., & Bruderly, M. (2006). Cirrhosis and chronic liver failure: Part II. Diagnosis and evaluation. *American Family Physician, 74*(5), 767–776.

Holcomb, S. S. (2007). Stopping the destruction of acute pancreatitis. *Nursing, 37*(6), 42–48.

Holzinger, U., Feldbacher, M., Bachlechner, A., Kitzberger, R., Fuhrmann, V., & Madl, C. (2008). Improvement of glucose control in the intensive care unit: An interdisciplinary collaboration study. *American Journal Critical Care, 17*(2), 150–156.

Johnson, T. M., Overgard, E. B., Cohen, A. E., & DiBaise, J. K. (2013). Nutrition assessment and management in advanced liver disease. *Nutrition Clinical Practice, 28*(1), 15–29. Retrieved from http://ncp.sagepub.com/content/28/1/15.long. DOI: 10.1177/0884533612469027.

Jones, D. E. (2008). Pathogenesis of primary biliary cirrhosis. *Postgraduate Medical Journal, 84*(987), 23–33.

Kenny, D. J., & Goodman, P. (2010). Care of the patient with enteral tube feeding: An evidence-based practice protocol. *Nursing Research, 59*(1 Suppl), S22–S31.

Keske, L. A., & Letizia, M. (2010). Clostridium difficile infection: Essential information for nurses. *MEDSURG Nurse, 19*(6), 329–332.

Keys, V. A. (2013). Alcohol withdrawal during hospitalization. *American Journal Nursing, 111*(1), 40–44. Retrieved from www.studymode.com/essays/Alcohol-Withdrawal-During-Hospitalization-1462954.html.

Khalid, I., Doshi, P., & DiGiovine, B. (2010). Early enteral nutrition and outcomes of critically ill patients treated with vasopressors and mechanical ventilation. *American Journal Critical Care, 19*(3), 261–268.

Kimball, E. J., Baraghoshi, G. K., Mone, M. C., Hansen, H. J., Adams, D. M., Alder, S. C., et al. (2009). A comparison of infusion volumes in the measurement of intra-abdominal pressure. *Journal Intensive Care Medicine, 24*(4), 261–268.

Langell, J. T., & Mulvihill, S. J. (2008). Gastrointestinal perforation and the acute abdomen. *Medical Clinics North America, 92*(3), 599–625.

Lantz, M. (2008). Failure to thrive. *Clinical Geriatrics.* Retrieved from http://50.28.4.237/articles/Failure-Thrive?page=0,0.

Larson, A. M. (2010). Diagnosis and management of acute liver failure. *Current Opinion in Gastroenterology, 26*(3), 214–221.

Manuel, A., & Maynard, N. D. (2009). *Nutritional support.* Retrieved from www.medscape.com/viewarticle/703713.

Marchiondo, K. (2010). Acute pancreatitis. *MEDSURG Nursing, 19*(1), 54–55.

Marrero, F., Qadeer, M. A., & Lasher, B. A. (2008). Severe complications of inflammatory bowel disease. *Medical Clinics North America, 92*(3), 671–686.

Mayo-Smith, M. F. (1997 Jul 9). Pharmacological management of alcohol withdrawal. A meta-analysis and evidence-based practice guideline. American Society of Addiction Medicine Working Group on Pharmacological Management of Alcohol Withdrawal. *Journal of the American Medical Association, 278*(2), 144–151.

McCance, K. L., & Huether, S. E. (2006). *Pathophysiology: The biologic basis for disease in adults and children* (5th ed., rev.). St. Louis, MO: Elsevier Mosby.

McClave, S., Chang, W. K., Dhaliwal, R., & Heyland, D. K. (2006). Nutrition support in acute pancreatitis: A systematic review of the literature. *Journal of Parenteral and Enteral Nutrition, 30*(2), 143–156.

McKinley, M. G. (2009). Recognizing and responding to acute liver failure. *Nursing, 39*(3), 38–44; quiz 44–35.

Metheny, N. (2009). Verification of feeding tube placement (blindly inserted). Retrieved from www.aacn.org/WD/Practice/Docs/PracticeAlerts/Verification_of_Feeding_Tube_Placement_05-2005.pdf.

Metheny, N. A. (2006). Preventing respiratory complications of tube feedings: Evidence-based practice. *American Journal Critical Care, 15*(4), 360–369.

Metheny, N. A. (2008). Residual volume measurement should be retained in enteral feeding protocols. *American Journal Critical Care, 17*(1), 62–64.

Metheny, N. A., Clouse, R. E., Chang, Y. H., Stewart, B. J., Oliver, D. A., & Kollef, M. H. (2006). Tracheobronchial aspiration of gastric contents in critically ill tube-fed patients: Frequency, outcomes, and risk factors. *Critical Care Medicine, 34*(4), 1007–1015.

Metheny, N. A., Schallom, L., Oliver, D. A., & Clouse, R. E. (2008). Gastric residual volume and aspiration in critically ill patients receiving gastric feedings. *American Journal Critical Care, 17*(6), 512–519; quiz 520.

Pluta, A., Gutkowski, K., & Hartleb, M. (2010). Coagulopathy in liver diseases. *Advances Medical Science, 55*(1), 16–21.

Radovich, P. (2008). Buying time for patients with acute liver failure. *American Nurse Today, 3*(11), 10–11.

Reising, D. L., & Neal, R. S. (2005). Enteral tube flushing. *American Journal Nursing, 105*(3), 58–63; quiz 63–54.

Riddle, E., Bush, J., Tittle, M., & Dilkhush, D. (2010). Alcohol withdrawal: Development of a standing order set. *Critical Care Nurse, 30*(3), 38–47; quiz 48.

Rylah, B., & Vercueil, A. (2010). Intensive therapy of the patient with liver disease. *British Journal Hospital Medicine (Lond), 71*(7), 377–381.

Sabol, V. K. (2004). Nutrition assessment of the critically ill adult. *AACN Clinical Issues, 15*(4), 595–606.

Sanborn, C. (2009). Controlling blood glucose in hospital patients. *American Nurse Today, 4*(6), 10–12.

Sargent, S. (2007). Hepatic nursing. Pathophysiology and management of hepatic encephalopathy. *British Journal Nursing, 16*(6), 335–339.

Schepers, N. J., Besselink, M. G. H., van Santvoort, H. C., Bakker, O. J., & Bruno, M. J. (2013). Early management of acute pancreatitis. *Best Practice & Research Clinical Gastroenterology, 27*(2013), 727–743.

Schuppan, D., & Afdhal, N. H. (2008). Liver cirrhosis. *Lancet, 371*(9615), 838–851.

Siow, E. (2008). Enteral versus parenteral nutrition for acute pancreatitis. *Critical Care Nurse, 28*(4), 19–25, 27–31; quiz 32.

Smith, M. M. (2010). Emergency: Variceal hemorrhage from esophageal varices associated with alcoholic liver disease. *American Journal Nurse, 110*(2), 32–39; quiz 40–31.

Stacy, K. M. (2014). Gastrointestinal anatomy and physiology. In: L. D. Urden, K. M. Stacy, & M. E. Lough (Eds.), *Thelan's critical care nursing diagnosis and management* (7th ed.). St. Louis, MO: Mosby.

Sullivan, J. T., Sykora, K., Schneiderman, J., Naranjo, C. A., & Sellers, E. M. (1989). Assessment of alcohol withdrawal: The revised clinical institute withdrawal assessment for alcohol scale (CIWA-Ar). *British Journal of Addiction, 84*(11), 1353–1357.

Tenner, S., Baillie, J., DeWitt, J., & Swaroop, S. (2013). Management of acute pancreatitis. *American Journal of Gastroenterology, 108,* 1400–1415.

Trevino, C. (2010). Small bowel obstruction: The art of management. *AACN Advanced Critical Care, 21*(2), 187–194.

Tripathi, D., & Redhead, D. (2006). Transjugular intrahepatic portosystemic stent-shunt: Technical factors and new developments. *European Journal Gastroenterology, 18*(11), 1127–1133.

Twedell, D., Lansing, R., McGuire, J., Palmersheim, P., & Baird, G. (2009). Providing holistic care to bariatric patients. *Journal Continuing Education in Nursing, 40*(10), 438–439.

Wang, S., Feng, X., Li, S., Liu, C., Xu, B., Bai, B., & Zhao, Q. (2014). The ability of current scoring systems in differentiating transient and persistent organ failure in patients with acute pancreatitis. *J Crit Care, 29*(4) 693 e697–611.

Chapter 7

Blair, E. (2014). Insulin A to Z: A guide on different types of insulin. *Joslin Diabetes Guidelines.* Retrieved from http://www.joslin.org/info/insulin_a_to_z_a_guide_on_different_types_of_insulin.html.

Chen, L. (2010). A literature review of intensive insulin therapy and mortality in critically ill patients. *Clinical Nurse Specialist, 24*(2), 80–86.

Cook, A., Laughlin, D., Moore, M., North, D., Wilkins, K., Wong, G., et al. (2009). Differences in glucose values obtained from point-of-care glucose meters and laboratory analysis in critically ill patients. *American Journal of Critical Care, 18*(1), 65–71; quiz 72.

Guthrie, D. W., Guthrie, R. A., Hinnen, D., & Childs, B. P. (2011). It's time to abandon the sliding scale. *Journal of Family Practice, 60*(5), 266–270.

Guyton, A. C., & Hall, J. T. (2011). *Textbook of medical physiology* (12th ed.). Philadelphia, PA: Saunders.

Devries, J. H. (2010). Glucose variability is associated with intensive care unit mortality. *Critical Care Medicine, 38*(3), 838–842.

Holzinger, U., Feldbacher, M., Bachlechner, A., Kitzberger, R., Fuhrmann, V., & Madl, C. (2008). Improvement of glucose control in the intensive care unit: An interdisciplinary collaboration study. *American Journal of Critical Care, 17*(2), 150–156.

Kraut, J. A., & Xing, S. X. (2011). Approach to the evaluation of a patient with an increased serum osmolal gap and high-anion-gap metabolic acidosis. *American Journal of Kidney Diseases, 58*(3), 480–484.

Joslin Diabetes Center. (2014). *Clinical guideline for adults with diabetes.* Retrieved from www.joslin.org/docs/Adult_guideline_-update_thru_10-23-14_2.pdf.

Joslin Guidelines. (2014). *Oral Diabetes Medication Summary Chart.* Retrieved from www.joslin.org/info/oral_diabetes_medications_summary_chart.html.

McCance, K. L., & Huether, S. E. (Eds.). (2013). *Pathophysiology: The biologic basis for disease in adults and children* (6th ed.) St. Louis, MO: Mosby.

National Health Service (NHS). (2011). *National Institute for Health and Care Excellence (NICE). Pathways for diabetes.* Retrieved from http://pathways.nice.org.uk/pathways/diabetes.

McAdams-Jones, D. (2008). Reversing SIADH. *American Nurse Today, 3*(9), 40.

Neithercott, T. (2011). 6 ways to prevent and treat low blood glucose. *Diabetes Forecast, 64*(4), 46–47.

Realsen, J. M., & Chase, H. P. (2011). Recent advances in the prevention of hypoglycemia in type 1 diabetes. *Diabetes Technology & Therapeutics, 13*(12), 1177–1186.

Sanborn, C. (2009). Controlling blood glucose in hospital patients. *American Nurse Today, 4*(6), 10–12.

Savage, M., & Hilton, L. (2010). Managing diabetic ketoacidosis in adults: New national guidance from the JBDS. *Journal of Diabetes Nursing, 14*(6), 220–225.

Shearer, A., Boehmer, M., Closs, M., Dela Rosa, R., Hamilton, J., Horton, K., et al. (2009). Comparison of glucose point-of-care values with laboratory values in critically ill patients. *American Journal of Critical Care, 18*(3), 224–230.

Stunkard, M. E., Pikul, V. T., & Foley, K. (2011). Hyperosmolar hyperglycemic syndrome with rhabdomyolysis. *Clinical Laboratory Science, 24*(1), 8–13.

Sutton, L., & Chapman-Novakofski, K. (2011). Hypoglycemia education needs. *Qualitative Health Research, 21*(9), 1220–1228.

Thompson, R. (2011). Comprehensive case study: Diabetes ketoacidosis. *MEDSURG Nursing, 20*(6), 338–339.

Tsang, Man-Wo (2012). The management of type 2 diabetic patients with hypoglycaemic agents. *ISRN Endocrinology.* http://dx.doi.org/10.5402/2012/478120.

Yang, Y., Salam, Z. H., Ong, B. C., & Yang, K. S. (2011). Respiratory dysfunction in patients with sepsis: Protective effect of diabetes mellitus. *American Journal of Critical Care, 20*(2), e41–e44.

Chapter 8

Becattini, C., Lignani, A., & Agnelli, G. (2010). New anticoagulants for the prevention of venous thromboembolism. *Journal Drug Design and Develop Therapy, 4*, 49–60.

Blaisdell, F. W. (2012). Causes, preventntion, and treatment of intravascular coagulation and disseminated intravascular coagulation. *Journal Trauma and Acute Care Surgery, 72*, 1719–1722.

Cannon-Diehl, M. R. (2010). Transfusion in the critically ill: Does it affect outcome? *Critical Care Nursing Quarterly, 33*(4), 324–338.

Collins, T. A. (2011). Packed red blood cell transfusions in critically ill patients. *Critical Care Nurse, 31*(1), 25–33; quiz 34.

Crowther, M. A., Cook, D. J., Albert, M., Williamson, D., Meade, M., Granton, J., et al. (2010). The 4Ts scoring system for heparin-induced thrombocytopenia in medical-surgical intensive care unit patients. *Journal of Critical Care, 25*(2), 287–293.

Farwell, A. L. (2010). Saving muscle: Evidence-based strategies for reducing door-to-balloon times for ST-segment elevation myocardial infarction patients. *Journal Emergency Nursing, 36*(3), 231–237.

Favaloro, E. J. (2010). Laboratory testing in disseminated intravascular coagulation. *Seminars in Thrombosis and Hemostasis Journal, 36*(4), 458–467.

Ferri, F. F. (2014). *Ferri's clinical advisor: 5 books in one.* Philadelphia, PA: Elsevier/Mosby.

Fletcher, B., & Thalinger, K. K. (2010). Prasugrel as antiplatelet therapy in patients with acute coronary syndromes or undergoing percutaneous coronary intervention. *Critical Care Nurse, 30*(5), 45–54.

George, J. N. (2010). Management of immune thrombocytopenia: Something old, something new. *New England Journal of Medicine, 363*(20), 1959–1961.

Greinacher, A., & Selleng, K. (2010). Thrombocytopenia in the intensive care unit patient. *American Society of Hematology Education Program, 2010*(1), 135–143.

Guyton, A. C., & Hall, J. E. (2010). *Textbook of medical physiology* (12th ed.). Philadelphia, PA: Saunders.

Hammond, B. B. (2010). Four steps to reducing door-to-balloon time. *Journal Emergency Nursing, 36*(3), 217–220.

Hunt, C. W. (2010). Immune thrombocytopenia purpura. *MEDSURG Nursing, 19*(4), 237–239.

Ignatavicius, D. D., & Workman, M. L. (2010). *Medical-surgical nursing: Patient centered collaborative care* (6th ed.). Philadelphia, PA: Elsevier/Saunders.

Iwai, K., Uchino, S., Endo, A., Saito, K., Kase, Y., & Takinami, M. (2010). Prospective external validation of the new scoring system for disseminated intravascular coagulation by Japanese Association for Acute Medicine (JAAM). *Thrombosis Research, 126*(3), 217–221.

Kansagara, D., Dyer, E., Englander, H., Fu, R., Freeman, M., & Kagen, D. (2013). Treatment of anemia in patients with heart disease: A systematic review. *Annals of Internal Medicine, 159*, 746–757.

Kaufman, R. M., Djulbegovic, B., Gernsheimer, T., Kleinman, S., Tinmuth, A. T., Capocelli, K. E., Cipollw, D., Cohn, C. S., Fung, M. K., Grossmann, B. J., Mintz, P. D., O'Malley, B. A., Sesok-Pizzini, D. A., Shander, A., Stack, G. E., Webert, K. E., Weinstein, R., Welch, B. G., Whitman, G. J., Wong, E. C., & Tobian, A. A. (2015). Platelet transfusion: A clinical practice guideline from the AABB. *Annals Internal Medicine, 162*(3), 205–213. Retrieved from http://annals.org/article.aspx?articleID=1930861. doi:10-7326/M14-1589.

Levi, M. (2015). Thrombosis and hemostasis issues in critically ill patients. *Seminars in Thrombosis and Hemostasis, 41*(1), 7–8. http://dx.doi.org/10.1055/s-0035-1544216.

Liebman, H. A., & Pullarkat, V. (2011). Diagnosis and management of immune thrombocytopenia in the era of thrombopoietic mimetics. *American Hematology Society, Hematology Educations Program, 2011*(1), 384–390. Retrieve from http://asheducationbook.hematologylibrary.org/content/2011/1/384.full. doi:10.1182/asheducation-2011.1.384.

Lippi, G., & Cervellin, G. (2010). Disseminated intravascular coagulation in trauma injuries. *Seminars in Thrombosis and Hemostasis, 36*(4), 378–387.

Mayer, B. (2010). Hematologic disorders and oncologic emergencies. In: L. D. Urden, K. M. Stacy, & M. E. Lough (Eds.), *Thelan's critical care nursing* (6th ed.). St. Louis, MO: Elsevier/Mosby.

McCance, K. L., & Huether, S. E. (2013). *Pathophysiology: The biologic basis for disease in adults and children* (7th ed.). St. Louis, MO: Elsevier.

Miller, V., & Hodder, S. (2014). Beneficial impact of antiretroviral therapy on non-AIDS mortality. *AIDS, 28*, 273–274.

Murphy, K. M., Travers, P., & Walport, M. (2011). *Janeway's immunobiology* (8th ed.). New York, NY: Garland.

Owens, A. P., 3rd, & Mackman, N. (2010). Tissue factor and thrombosis: The clot starts here. *Journal of Thrombosis and Haemostasis, 104*(3), 432–439.

Pluta, A., Gutkowski, K., & Hartleb, M. (2010). Coagulopathy in liver diseases. *Advances in Medical Science, 55*(1), 16–21.

Porter, R. S. (Ed.). (2011). *Merck manual of diagnosis and therapy* (19th ed.). Whitehouse Station, NJ: Merck Sharp & Dohme Corporation.

Powers, C. M. (2011). Use of alteplase beyond 3 hours of ischemic stroke onset. *Advanced Emergency Nurse Journal, 33*(1), 65–70.

Priziola, J. L., Smythe, M. A., & Dager, W. E. (2010). Drug-induced thrombocytopenia in critically ill patients. *Critical Care Medicine, 38*(6 Suppl), S145–S154.

Qaseem, A., Humphrey, L. L., Fitterman, N., Starkey, M., & Shekelle, P. (2013). Treatment of anemia in patients with heart disease: A clinical practice guideline from the American College of Physicians. *Annals of Internal Medicine, 159*, 770–779.

Rondina, M. T., Walker, A., & Pendleton, R. C. (2010). Drug-induced thrombocytopenia for the hospitalist physician with a focus on heparin-induced thrombocytopenia. *Hospital Practice, 38*(2), 19–28.

Russell, M., & Suarez, C. (2014). Hematologic disorders and oncologic emergencies. In L. D. Urden, K. M. Stacy, & M. E. Lough (Eds.), *Thelan's critical care nursing* (7th ed.). St. Louis, MO: Elsevier/Mosby.

Sihler, K. C., & Napolitano, L. M. (2010). Complications of massive transfusion. *Chest, 137*(1), 209–220.

Skidmore-Roth, L. (2011). *Mosby's 2011 nursing drug reference* (24th ed.). St. Louis, MO: Elsevier/Mosby.

Thachil, J., Fitzmaurice, D. A., & Toh, C. H. (2010). Appropriate use of D-dimer in hospital patients. *American Journal of Medicine, 123*(1), 17–19.

Thota, S., Kistangari, G., Daw, H., & Spiro, T. (2012). Immune thrombocytopenia in adults: An update. *Cleveland Clinic Journal of Medicine, 79*(9), 641–650. Retrieved from www.ccjm.org/content/79/9/641.full.pdf+html.

Vallerand, A. H., Sanoski, C. A., & Deglin, J. H. (2013). *Davis drug guide for nurses* (13th ed.). Philadelphia, PA: Davis.

Watson, C. J. E., & Dark, J. H., 1 (2012). Organ transplantation: historical perspective and current practice. *British Journal Anaesthia, 108*(suppl 1), i29–i42. Retrieved from http://bja.oxfordjournals.org/content/108/suppl_1/i29.full.pdf+html.

Wilson, B. A., Shannon, M. T., & Shields, K. (2011). *Nurse's drug guide 2011.* Upper Saddle River, NJ: Pearson/Prentice Hall.

Chapter 9

American Association of Critical-Care Nurses. (2010). *Core curriculum for progressive care nursing.* St. Louis, MO: Saunders Elsevier.

Bader, M. K., & Littlejohns, L. R. (Eds.). (2010). *American Association of Neuroscience (AANN) Core curriculum for neuroscience nursing* (5th ed.). St. Louis, MO: Saunders.

Baird, M. S., & Bethel, S. (2010). *Manual of critical care nursing. Nursing interventions and collaborative management* (6th ed.). St. Louis, MO: Mosby Elsevier.

Chuly, M., & Burns, S. M. (2010). *AACN essentials of progressive care nursing* (2nd ed.). New York, NY: McGraw-Hill.

Connolly, Jr., E. S., Rabinstein, A. A., Carhuapoma, J. R., et al. (2012). Guidelines for the management of aneurysmal subarachnoid hemorrhage: A guideline for healthcare professionals from the American Heart Association/American Stroke Association. *Stroke, 43*(6), 1–24.

Deutschman, C. S., & Neligan, P. J. (2010). *Evidence-based practice of critical care.* Philadelphia, PA: Saunders Elsevier.

Goldstein, L. B., Bushnell, C. D., Adams, R. J., et al. (2011). Guidelines for the primary prevention of stroke: A guideline for healthcare professionals from the American Heart Association/American Stroke Association. *Stroke, 42*(2), 517–584.

Guyton, A. C., & Hall, J. E. (2010). *Textbook of medical physiology* (12th ed.). Philadelphia, PA: Saunders.

Harding, A. (2010). Stroke scales you can use. *Journal of Emergency Nursing, 36*(1), 40–52.

Hung, O. L., & Shih, R. D. (2011). Antiepileptic drugs: The old and the new. *Emergency Medicine Clinics of North America, 29*, 141–150.

Hutchinson, P. J., Kolias, A. G., Czosnyka, M., et al. (2013). Intracranial pressure monitoring in severe traumatic brain injury. *BMJ, 346*, f1000. http://dx.doi.org/10.1136/bmj.f1000.

Ignatavicius, D. D., & Workman, M. L. (2010). *Medical-surgical nursing: Patient centered collaborative care* (6th ed.). Philadelphia, PA: Elsevier/Saunders.

Jauch, E. C., Saver, J. L., Adams, H. P., et al. (2013). Guidelines for the early management of patients with acute ischemic stroke: A guideline for healthcare professionals from the American Heart Association/American Stroke Association. *Stroke, 44*(3), 870–947. http://dx.doi.org/10.1161/STR.0b013e318284056a.

Jauch, E. C., Cucchiara, B., Adeoye, O., et al. (2010). Part 11: Adult stroke: 2010 American Heart Association guidelines for cardiopulmonary resuscitation and emergency cardiovascular care. *Circulation, 122*(18 Suppl 3), S818–S828.

Jeffrey, S. (2010). *New AHA/ASA guidelines on management of intracerebral hemorrhage.* Retrieved from www.medscape.com/viewarticle/726066.

McCance, K. L., & Huether, S. E. (2013). *Pathophysiology: The biologic basis for disease in adults and children* (7th ed.). St. Louis, MO: Elsevier.

Morgenstern, L. B., Hemphill, J. C., Anderson, C., Becker, K., Broderick, J. P., Connolly, E. S., Greenberg, S. M., Huang, J. N., Macdonald, R. H., Messé, S. R., Mitchell, P. H., Selim, M., & Tamargo, R. J. (2010). Guidelines for the management of spontaneous intracerebral hemorrhage: a guideline for healthcare professionals from the American Heart Association/American Stroke Association. *Stroke, 41*, 2108–2129.

Pagana, K. D., & Pagana, T. J. (2010). *Mosby's manual of diagnostic and laboratory tests* (4th ed.). St. Louis, MO: Mosby Elsevier.

Pope, J. V., & Edlow, J. A. (2012). Avoiding misdiagnosis in patients with neurological emergencies. *Emergency Medicine International.* Retrieved from www.hindawi.com/journals/emi/2012/949275/cta/, doi: 10.1155/2012/949275.

Powers, C. M. (2011). Use of alteplase beyond 3 hours of ischemic stroke onset. *Advanced Emergency Nursing Journal, 33*(1), 65–70.

Reinhardt, M. R. (2010). Subarachnoid hemorrhage. *J Emerg Nurs, 36*(4), 327–329.

Sacco, R. L., Kasner, S. E., Broderick, J. P., et al. (2013). AHA/ASA expert consensus document: An updated definition of stroke for the 21st century. *Stroke, 44*, 2064–2089. http://dx.doi.org/10.1161/STR.0b013e318296aeca.

Schachter, S. C. (2013). *Types of seizures.* Retrieved from www.epilepsy.com/epilepsy/types_seizures.

Trembly, A. (2010). Stroke care in the 21st century. *Nursing Management, 41*(6), 30–36; quiz 36–37.

Urden, L., Stacy, K., & Lough, M. (2010). *Critical care nursing: Diagnosis and management* (6th ed.). St. Louis, MO: Mosby.

Wiegand, D. L. -M. (Ed.). (2011). *AACN procedure manual for critical care* (6th ed.). Philadelphia, PA: Saunders Elsevier.

Chapter 10

Ahrens, T. (2010). Stroke volume optimization versus central venous pressure in fluid management. *Critical Care Nurse, 30*(2), 71–73.

Angus, D. C., & van der Poll, T. (2013). Severe sepsis and septic shock. *New England Journal Medicine, 369*(9), 840–851.

Arnold, J. J., & Williams, P. M. (2011). Anaphylaxis: Recognition and management. *American Family Physician, 84*(10), 1111–1118.

Association for the Advancement of Wound Care (AAWC). (2010). *Association for the Advancement of Wound Care guideline of pressure ulcer guidelines.* Retrieved from www.guideline.gov/content.aspx?id=24361.

Bockenstedt, T. L., Baker, S. N., Weant, K. A., & Mason, M. A. (2012). Review of vasopressor therapy in the setting of vasodilatory shock. *Advanced Emergency Nursing Journal, 34*(1), 16–23.

Burney, M., Underwood, J., McEvoy, S., Nelson, G., Dzierba, A., Kauari, V., & Chong, D. (2012). Early detection and treatment of severe sepsis in the emergency department: Identifying barriers to implementation of a protocol-based approach. *Journal of Emergency Nursing, 38*(6), 512–517.

Cannon-Diehl, M. R. (2010). Transfusion in the critically ill: Does it affect outcome? *Crit Care Nurs Q, 33*(4), 324–338.

Casserly, B., Read, R., & Levy, M. M. (2011). Hemodynamic monitoring in sepsis. *Critical Care Nursing Clinics of North America, 23*, 149–169.

De Backer, D., Biston, P., Devriendt, J., Madl, C., Chochrad, D., Aldecoa, C., et al. (2010). Comparison of dopamine and norepinephrine in the treatment of shock. *New England Journal of Medicine, 362*(9), 779–789.

Dellinger, R. P., Levy, M. M., Rhodes, A., Annane, D., Gerlach, H., Opal, S. M., Sevransky, J. E., Sprung, C. L., Douglas, I. S., Jaeschke, R., Osborn, T. M., Nunnally, M. E., Townsend, S. R., Reinhart, K., Kleinpell, R. M., Angus, D. C., Deutschman, C. S., Machado, F. R., Rubenfeld, G. D., Webb, S. A., Beale, R. J., Vincent, J. L., & Moreno, R. (2012). Surviving sepsis campaign: International guidelines for management of severe sepsis and septic shock. *Critical Care Medicine, 41*(2), 580–637.

Gustot, T. (2011). Multiple organ failure in sepsis: Prognosis and role of systemic inflammatory response. *Current Opinion Critical Care, 17*(2), 153–159.

Hartog, C. S., Bauer, M., & Reinhart, K. (2011). The efficacy and safety of colloid resuscitation in the critically ill. *Anesthesia & Analgesia, 112*(1), 156–164.

Janis, J. E., & Harrison, B. (2014). Wound healing: Part I. Basic science. *Plastic and Reconstructive Surgery, 133*(2), 199–207.

Jones, B., Higginson, R., & Santos, A. (2010). Critical care: Assessing blood pressure, circulation and intravascular volume. *British Journal of Nursing, 19*(3), 153, 155–159.

Kaur, P., Basu, S., & Kaur, R. (2011). Transfusion protocol in trauma. *Journal of Emergencies, Trauma and Shock, 4*(1), 103–108. Retrieved from www.ncbi.nlm.nih.gov/pmc/articles/PMC3097557/#!po=60.52632011. doi: 10.4103/0974-2700.76844.

Klein, T., & Ramani, G. V. (2012). Assessment and management of cardiogenic shock in the emergency department. *Cardiology Clinics, 30*(4), 651–664.

Kollef, M. H., Zilberberg, M. D., Shorr, A. F., Vo, L., Schein, J., Micek, S. T., et al. (2011). Epidemiology, microbiology and outcomes of healthcare-associated and community-acquired bacteremia: A multicenter cohort study. *Journal of Infection, 62*(2), 130–135.

Levins, T. T. (2010). Shock: Early recognition and management. *Journal of Emergency Nursing, 36*(4), 300–301.

Marik, P. E., Baram, M., & Vahid, B. (2008). Does central venous pressure predict fluid responsiveness? A systematic review of the literature and a tale of seven mares. *Chest, 134*, 172–178.

McAtee, M. E. (2011). Cardiogenic shock. *Critical Care Nursing Clinics of North America, 23*(4), 607–615.

Moore, K. (2011). Managing hemorrhagic shock in trauma: Are we still drowning patients in the field? *Journal of Emergency Nursing, 37*(6), 594–596.

Morrison, C. A., Carrick, M. M., Norman, M. A., Scott, B. G., Welsh, F. J., Tsai, P., Liscum, K. R., Wall, M. J., & Mattox, K. L. (2011). Hypotensive resuscitation strategy reduces transfusion requirements and severe postoperative coagulopathy in trauma patients with hemorrhagic shock: Preliminary results of a randomized controlled trial. *Journal of Trauma, 70*(3), 652–663.

Murphy, P. S., & Evans, G. R. (2012). Advances in wound healing: A review of current wound healing products. *Plastic Surgery International*. Retrieved from www.hindawi.com/journals/psi/2012/190436/cta/.

National Consensus Project for Palliative Care. (2013). *Clinical practice guidelines for palliative care* (3rd ed.). Retrieved from https://www.hpna.org/multimedia/NCP_Clinical_Practice_Guidelines_3rd_Edition.pdf.

NeSmith, E., Weinrich, S., Andrews, J., Medeiros, R., Hawkins, M., Weinrich, M., et al. (2011). Substance use and the systemic inflammatory response syndrome (SIRS) following trauma. *Journal of Trauma Nursing, 18*(2), 79–86.

O'Malley, P. (2010). Vasopressors in septic shock: A possible deadly intervention. *Clin Nurse Spec, 24*(5), 235–237.

Perel, P., & Roberts, I. (2011). Colloids versus crystalloids for fluid resuscitation in critically ill patients. *Cochrane Database Systematic Reviews, 2011*(3), 1–62 CD000567.

Pierrakos, C., & Vincent, J. L. (2010). Sepsis biomarkers: A review. *Critical Care, 14*(1), R15.

Pollack, A., Uriel, N., George, I., Kodali, S., Takayama, H., Naka, Y., et al. (2012). A stepwise progression in the treatment of cardiogenic shock. *Heart & Lung, 41*(5), 500–504.

Sandrock, C. E., & Albertson, T. E. (2010). Controversies in the treatment of sepsis. *Seminars in Respiratory and Critical Care Medicine, 31*(1), 66–78.

Sprung, C. L., Brezls, M., Goodman, S., & Weiss, Y. G. (2011). Corticosteroid therapy for patients in septic shock: Some progress in a difficult decision. *Critical Care Medicine, 39*(3), 571–574.

Turi, S. K., & Von Ah, D. (2013). Implementation of early goal-directed therapy for septic patients in the emergency department: a review of the literature. *Journal of Emergency Nursing, 39*(1), 13–19.

Vanzant, A. M., & Schmelzer, M. (2011). Detecting and treating sepsis in the emergency department. *Journal of Emergency Nursing, 37*(1), 47–54.

Whiteside, M., & Fletcher, A. (2010). Anaphylactic shock: No time to think. *Journal of the Royal College of Physicians Edinburgh, 40*(2), 145–147; quiz 148.

Yarema, T. C., & Yost, S. (2011). Low-dose corticosteroids to treat septic shock: A critical literature review. *Critical Care Nurse, 31*(6), 16–26.

Chapter 11

Alexander, E. (2009). Delirium in the intensive care unit: Medications as risk factors. *Critical Care Nurse, 29*(1), 85–87.

Allen, J., & Alexander, E. (2012). Prevention, recognition, and management of delirium in the intensive care unit. *AACN Advanced Critical Care, 23*(1), 12–13 5-11; quiz.

American Association of Critical-Care Nurses. (2012). Delirium assessment and management. *Critical Care Nurse, 32*(1), 79–82.

American Association of Critical Care Nurses. (2011). *AACN practice alert: Delirium assessment and management*. Retrieved from www.aacn.org/WD/practice/docs/practicealerts/delirium-practice-alert-2011.pdf.

Baker, S. J. (2011). Key words: a prescriptive approach to reducing patient anxiety and improving safety. *Journal of Emergency Nursing, 37*(6), 571–574.

Balas, M. C., Rice, M., Chaperon, C., Smith, H., Disbot, M., & Fuchs, B. (2012). Management of delirium in critically ill older adults. *Critical Care Nurse, 32*(4), 15–26.

Barr, J., Fraser, G. L., Puntillo, K., Ely, E. W., Gelinas, C., Dasta, J. F., et al. (2013). Clinical practice guidelines for the management of pain, agitation, and delirium in adult patients in the intensive care unit: Executive summary. *American Journal of Health-System Pharmacy, 70*, 53–58.

Beck-Little, R., & Catton, G. (2011). Child and adolescent suicide in the United States: a population at risk. *Journal of Emergency Nursing, 37*(6), 587–589.

Brummel, N. E., & Girard, T. D. (2013). Preventing delirium in the intensive care unit. *Crit Care Clin, 29*(1), 51–65.

Brummel, N. E., Vasilevskis, E. E., Han, J. H., Boehm, L., Pun, B. T., & Ely, E. W. (2013). Implementing delirium screening in the ICU: Secrets to success. *Critical Care Medicine, 41*(9), 2196–2208.

Caplan, G. (1970). *Theory and practice of mental health consultation*. New York, NY: Basic Books.

Chevrolet, J. C., & Jolliet, P. (2007). Clinical review: Agitation and delirium in the critically ill – significance and management. *Critical Care, 11*(214). Retrieved from http://ccforum.com/content/11/3/214.

Davidson, J. E. (2009). Family-centered care: Meeting the needs of patients' families and helping families adapt to critical illness. *Critical Care Nurse, 29*(3), 28–34; quiz 35.

Devlin, J. W., Fong, J. J., Howard, E. P., Skrobik, Y., McCoy, N., Yasuda, C., & Marshall, J. (2008). Assessment of delirium in the intensive care unit: Nursing practices and perceptions. *American Journal of Critical Care, 17*(6), 555–565.

Eastes, L. E. (2010). Alcohol withdrawal syndrome in trauma patients: A review. *Journal of Emergency Nursing, 36*(5), 507–509.

Ely, E. W., Margolin, R., Francis, J., May, L., Truman, B., Dittus, R., et al. (2001). Evaluation of delirium in critically ill patients: Validation of the Confusion Assessment Method for the Intensive Care Unit (CAM-ICU). *Critical Care Medicine, 29*(7), 1370–1379.

Environmental Protection Agency. (1974). *Information on levels of environmental noise requisite to protect public health and welfare with an adequate margin of safety*. Retrieved from www.nonoise.org/library/levels74/levels74.htm.

Erikson, E. (1968). *Identity, youth and crisis*. New York, NY: W. W. Norton.

Fawcett, J. (2008). Bipolar disorder: Manic-depressive illness. *Merck Manuals Online*. Retrieved from www.merck.com/mmhe/sec07/ch101/ch101c.html.

Folstein, M. F., Folstein, S. E., & McHugh, P. R. (1975). "Mini-mental state": A practical method for grading the cognitive state of patients for the clinician. *Journal of Psychiatric Research, 12*, 189–198.

Gusmao-Flores, D., Salluh, J. I., Chalhub, R. A., & Quarantini, L. C. (2012). The confusion assessment method for the intensive care unit (CAM-ICU) and intensive care delirium screening checklist (ICDSC) for the diagnosis of delirium: A systematic review and meta-analysis of clinical studies. *Critical Care, 16*(4), R115.

Hamilton, P. M. (2007). *Psychiatric emergencies: Caring for people in crisis*. Retrieved from www.nursingceu.com/courses/358/index_nceu.html.

Henneman, E. A., & Cardin, S. (2002). Family-centered critical care: A practical approach to making it happen. *Critical Care Nurse, 22*(6), 12–19.

Horgas, A., & Miller, L. (2008). Pain assessment in people with dementia. *American Journal of Nursing, 108*(7), 62–70; quiz 71.

Inouye, S., van Dyck, C., Alessi, C., Balkin, S., Siegal, A., & Horwitz, R. (1990). Clarifying confusion: The confusion assessment method. *Annals of Internal Medicine, 113*(12), 941–948.

Joint Commission. (2015). *2015 Comprehensive accreditation manual for hospital*. Oak Brook, IL: author.

Juang, J. (2015). Delirium. In *Merck manual: Professional version*. Retrieved from www.merckmanuals.com/professional/neurologic-disorders/delirium-and-dementia/delirium.

Keys, V. A. (2011). Alcohol withdrawal during hospitalization. *Am J Nurs, 111*(1), 40–44; quiz 45–46.

Khan, B., Zawahiri, M., Campbell, N., Fox, G., Weinstein, E., Nazir, A., Farber, M., Buckley, J., McLullich, A., & Boustani, M. (2012). Delirium in hospitalized patients: Implications of current evidence on clinical practice and future avenues for research—A systematic evidence review. *Journal of Hospital Medicine, 7*(7), 580–588.

Lat, I., McMillian, W., Taylor, S., Janzen, J. M., Papdopoulos, S., Korth, L., et al. (2009). The impact of delirium on clinical outcomes in mechanically ventilated surgical and trauma patients. *Critical Care Medicine, 37*(6), 1898–1905.

Leske, J. (1991). Overview of family needs after critical illness: from assessment to intervention. *AACN Clinical Issues in Critical Care Nursing, 2*(2), 220–229.

Maslow, A. (1968). *Toward a psychology of being* (2nd ed.). Princeton, MA: Van Nostrand.

Matthews, E. E. (2011). Sleep disturbances and fatigue in critically ill patients. *AACN Advanced Critical Care, 22*(3), 204–224.

McAdam, J. L., & Puntillo, K. (2009). Symptoms experienced by family members of patients in intensive care units. *American Journal of Critical Care, 18*(3), 200–209; quiz 210.

McCoy, C., & Johnson, K. (2011). Behavioral emergencies: A closer look. *Journal of Emergency Nursing, 37*(1), 104–108.

Mitchell, M., Chaboyer, W., Burmeister, E., & Foster, M. (2009). Positive effects of a nursing intervention on family-centered care in adult critical care. *American Journal of Critical Care, 18*(6), 543–552; quiz 553.

Neal, A., Twibell, R., Osborne, K., & Harris, D. (2010). Providing family-friendly care—even when stress is high and time is short. *American Nurse Today, 5*(11), 9–12.

Nelson, D. P., & Plost, G. (2009). Registered nurses as family care specialists in the intensive care unit. *Critical Care Nurse, 29*(3), 46–52; quiz 53.

Nelson, J. M. (2010). Recognizing, preventing, and managing delirium in hospital patients. *American Nurse Today, 5*(11), 43–45.

Pun, B. T., & Boehm, L. (2011). Delirium in the intensive care unit: assessment and management. *AACN Advanced Critical Care, 22*(3), 225–237.

Pun, B. T., & Ely, E. W. (2007). The importance of diagnosing and managing ICU delirium. *Chest, 132*(2), 624–636.

Pun, B. T., & Boehm, L. (2011). Delirium in the intensive care unit. *AACN Advanced Critical Care, 22*(3), 225–237.

Rattray, J. E., & Hull, A. M. (2008). Emotional outcome after intensive care: Literature review. *J Adv Nurs, 64*(1), 2–13.

Riddle, E., Bush, J., Tittle, M., & Dilkhush, D. (2010). Alcohol withdrawal: Development of a standing order set. *Critical Care Nurse, 30*(3), 38–47; quiz 48.

Riker, R., Picard, J., & Fraser, G. (1999). Prospective evaluation of the Sedation-Agitation Scale for adult critically ill patients. *Critical Care Medicine, 27*, 1325.

Rushton, C. H. (2007). Respect in critical care: A foundational ethical principle. *AACN Advanced Critical Care, 18*(2), 149–156.

Selye, H. (1976). *Stress in health and disease.* Butterworth: Reading, MA.

Sullivan, J. T., Sykora, K., Schneiderman, J., Naranjo, C. A., & Sellers, E. M. (1989). Assessment of alcohol withdrawal: The revised Clinical Institute Withdrawal Assessment for Alcohol scale (CIWA-AR). *British Journal of Addiction, 84*, 1353–1357.

Truman, B., & Ely, E. (2003). Monitoring delirium in critically ill patients: Using the confusion assessment method for the intensive care unit. *Critical Care Nurse, 23*(2), 25–35.

Urden, L., & Stacy, K. (2013). *Critical care nursing: Diagnosis and management* (7th ed.). Mosby: St. Louis, MO.

Wieseke, A., Bantz, D., & May, D. (2011). What you need to know about bipolar disorder. *American Nurse Today, 6*(7), 8–12.

Yates, W. R. (2009). Anxiety disorders. *Emedicine.* Retrieved from http://emedicine.medscape.com/article/286227-overview.

Dysrhythmias: Etiology, Criteria, Significance, and Management

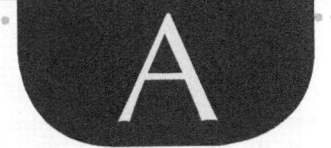

A

NORMAL SINUS RHYTHM

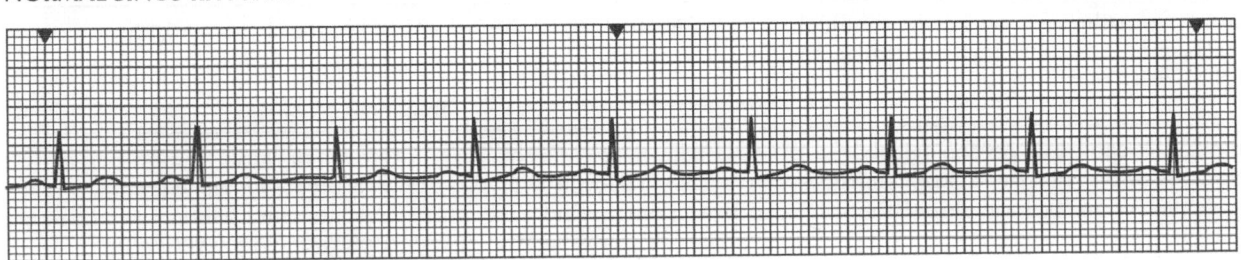

(From Wesley K: *Huszar's basic dysrhythmia and acute coronary syndromes*, ed 4, St. Louis, 2011, Mosby/JEMS.)

Rate	Regularity	P Waves	PR Interval	QRS Duration
60-100/min	Atrial and ventricular rhythms regular	Normal	0.12-0.20 and constant	<0.12

Etiology	Significance	Treatment
Normal	Normal	None

SINUS BRADYCARDIA

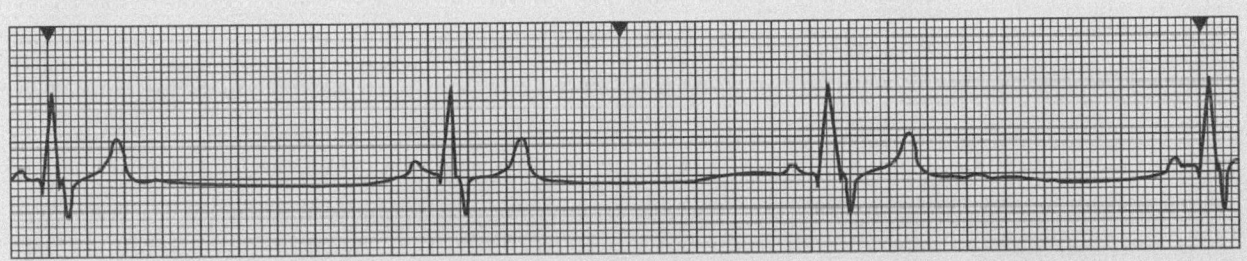

(From Wesley K: *Huszar's basic dysrhythmia and acute coronary syndromes*, ed 4, St. Louis, 2011, Mosby/JEMS.)

Rate	Regularity	P Waves	PR Interval	QRS Duration
<60 beats/min	Atrial and ventricular rhythms regular	Normal	0.12-0.20 and constant	<0.12

Etiology	Significance	Treatment

Athletic heart
• Sleep
• Vagal stimulation
• Myocardial ischemia or infarction
  • Inferior or posterior MI
• Fibrodegenerative changes of the SA node (e.g., sick sinus syndrome)
• Increased ICP
• Hypothermia
• Hypothyroidism
• Neurogenic shock
• Cervical or mediastinal tumor
• Drug effect: digitalis; beta-blockers; calcium channel blockers; opiates
	• Depends on rate
	• If too slow, cardiac output decreases
	  • Clinical manifestations of hypoperfusion may include hypotension, syncope, dyspnea, change in level of consciousness, chest pain, HF, anxiety
	  • Escape beats (e.g., atrial, junctional, ventricular) may occur
		• None if asymptomatic
		• If clinical manifestations of hypoperfusion occur:
		  • Atropine may be used as a temporary treatment in patients who do not have myocardial ischemia
		  • Pacemaker

SINUS TACHYCARDIA

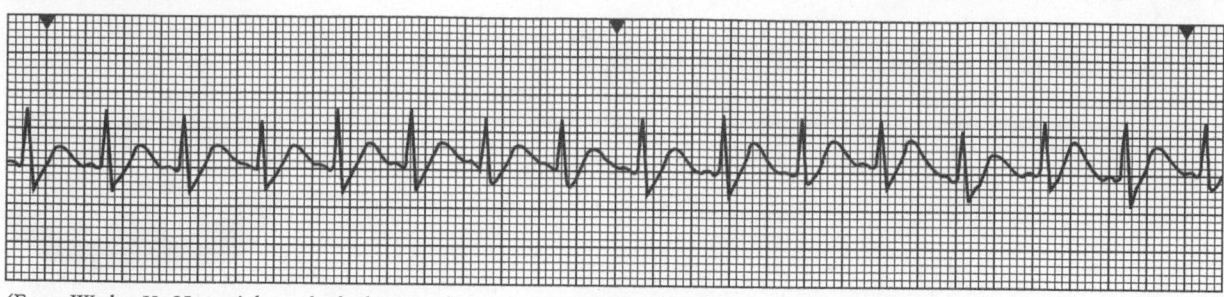

(From Wesley K: *Huszar's basic dysrhythmia and acute coronary syndromes*, ed 4, St. Louis, 2011, Mosby/JEMS.)

Rate	Regularity	P Waves	PR Interval	QRS Duration
>100 beats/min (usually 100-160 beats/min)	Atrial and ventricular rhythms regular	Normal	0.12-0.20 and constant	<0.12

Etiology	Significance	Treatment

• SNS stimulation caused by psychological or physiologic stressors (e.g., stress, fear, anxiety, pain, anger, infection, exercise, dehydration)
• Hypoxia
• Anemia
• Myocardial ischemia or infarction
  • Anterior MI
• Hypovolemia or hypervolemia
• Shock
• Hyperthyroidism
• Heart failure
• Inflammatory heart disease
• Pulmonary embolism
• Fibrodegenerative changes (e.g., sick sinus syndrome with tachy-brady manifestation)
• Drug effect: epinephrine, isoproterenol; dopamine; atropine; caffeine; nicotine; amphetamines; cocaine; alcohol; aminophylline
	• Usually not significant except in patients with heart disease—then may cause angina, MI, HF, or shock	• Treatment of cause
		  • Anxiolytics for anxiety
		  • Analgesics for pain
		  • Antipyretics for fever
		  • Fluids for hypovolemia
		  • Treatment of HF
		  • Avoidance of stimulants
		  • Beta-blockers for hyperthyroidism
		• Usually does not require other treatment but the following may also be used:
		  • Oxygen
		  • Sedation and/or beta-blocker may be used to decrease or block the effects of catecholamines

SINUS DYSRHYTHMIA (also referred to as sinus arrhythmia)

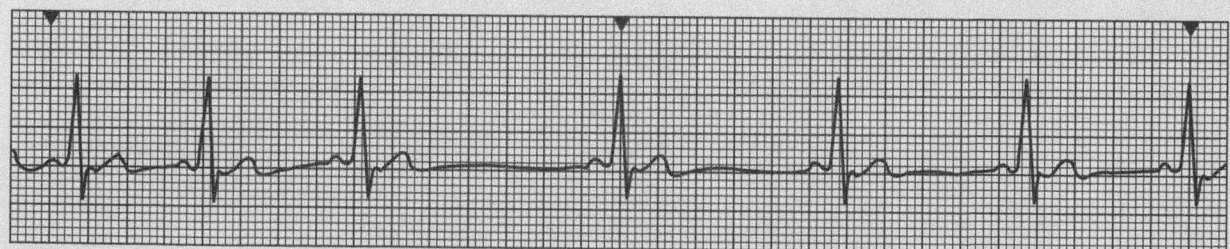

(From Wesley K: *Huszar's basic dysrhythmia and acute coronary syndromes*, ed 4, St. Louis, 2011, Mosby/JEMS.)

Rate	Regularity	P Waves	PR Interval	QRS Duration
Usually 60-100 beats/min but may be slower or faster	Atrial and ventricular rhythms regularly irregular; rate increases with inspiration (so R-R interval shortens) and decreases with expiration (so R-R interval lengthens); difference between shortest and longest R-R intervals <0.12	Normal	0.12-0.20 and usually constant; may vary slightly with rate variation	<0.12

Etiology	Significance	Treatment
• Normal; variation in sympathetic and parasympathetic stimulation during ventilation • In older patients, may indicate sick sinus syndrome • Digitalis toxicity	• Normal variation • May be seen in digitalis toxicity	• None • Discontinuance of digitalis if toxicity is the cause

SINUS BLOCK (i.e., sinus exit block)

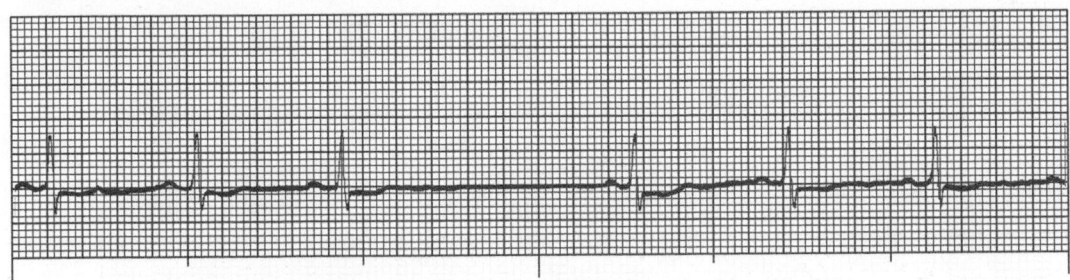

(From Aehlert B: *ECGs made easy*, ed 5, St. Louis, 2013, Elsevier Mosby.)

Rate	Regularity	P Waves	PR Interval	QRS Duration
Dependent on underlying rhythm	Atrial and ventricular rhythms regular with an irregularity; R-R interval at block measures an exact multiple of the normal R-R interval	One or more entire cardiac cycle is absent; P wave absent during block	None during block	QRS absent during block

Etiology	Significance	Treatment
• Fibrodegenerative changes of the sinus node (e.g., sick sinus syndrome) • Ischemia of SA node (e.g., MI) • Vagal stimulation • Carotid sinus hypersensitivity • Inflammatory heart disease (e.g., myocarditis) • Drug toxicity: digitalis, quinidine, procainamide	• Depends on frequency and duration of pauses • If patient loses consciousness (Stokes-Adams attacks), very significant and requires treatment	• Discontinuance of digitalis if toxicity is cause • Atropine • Pacemaker if frequent pauses or long pauses or if patient having syncope (i.e., Stokes-Adams attacks)

SINUS ARREST

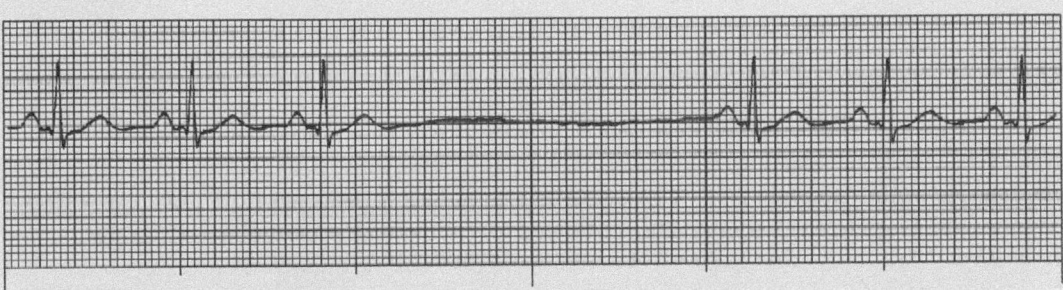

(From Aehlert B: *ECGs made easy*, ed 5, St. Louis, 2013, Elsevier Mosby.)

Rate	Regularity	P Waves	PR Interval	QRS Duration
Dependent on underlying rhythm	Atrial and ventricular rhythms regular with an irregularity (a pause); R-R interval at pause measures more or less than an exact multiple of the normal R-R interval	Indefinite period of time without an entire cardiac cycle; P wave absent during arrest	None during arrest	QRS absent during arrest

Etiology	Significance	Treatment
• Fibrodegenerative changes (e.g., sick sinus syndrome) • Ischemia of SA node (e.g., MI) • Vagal stimulation • Carotid sinus hypersensitivity • Electrolyte imbalance • Drug toxicity: digitalis, beta-blockers	• Depends on frequency and duration of pauses • If patient loses consciousness (Stokes-Adams attacks), considered significant and requires treatment	• Discontinuance of digitalis if toxicity is cause • Atropine • Pacemaker if frequent pauses or long (>3 second) pauses or if patient having Stokes-Adams attacks

PREMATURE ATRIAL CONTRACTION

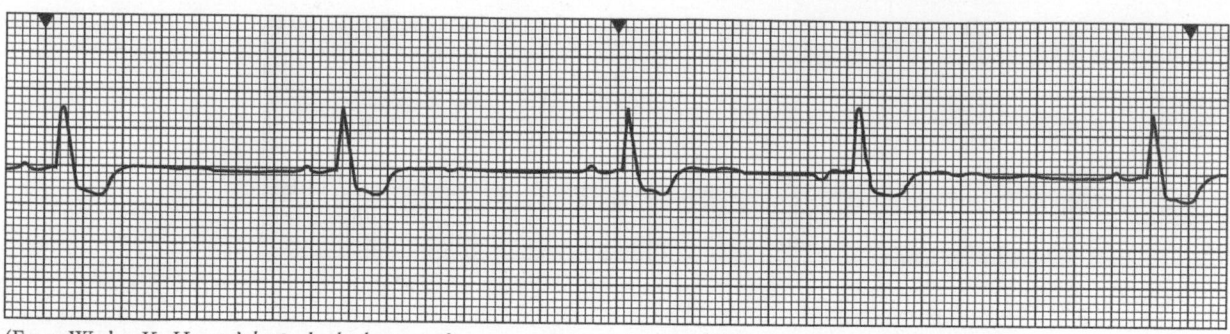

(From Wesley K: *Huszar's basic dysrhythmia and acute coronary syndromes*, ed 4, St. Louis, 2011, Mosby/JEMS.)

Rate	Regularity	P Waves	PR Interval	QRS Duration
Dependent on underlying rhythm	Dependent on underlying rhythm; PAC interrupts underlying rhythm	P wave of this early beat differs from sinus P; the ectopic P wave is early and may be flattened, notched, or lost in preceding T wave	Usually 0.12-0.20 but may be greater than 0.20	<0.12

Etiology	Significance	Treatment
• SNS stimulation caused by psychological or physiologic stressors (e.g., stress, fear, anxiety, pain, anger, infection, exercise, dehydration) • Hypoxia • Myocardial ischemia or infarction • Valvular heart disease (e.g., mitral stenosis; mitral valve prolapse) • Heart failure • Inflammatory heart disease (e.g., myocarditis) • Electrolyte imbalance • Drug effect: caffeine; nicotine; alcohol	• Usually benign but may precede atrial tachycardia, flutter, or fibrillation • Considered significant if >6/min	• Treatment of cause • Usually no treatment necessary; but if frequent, treatment may include digitalis, quinidine, propranolol, beta-blockers, calcium channel blockers, or anxiolytics

WANDERING ATRIAL PACEMAKER

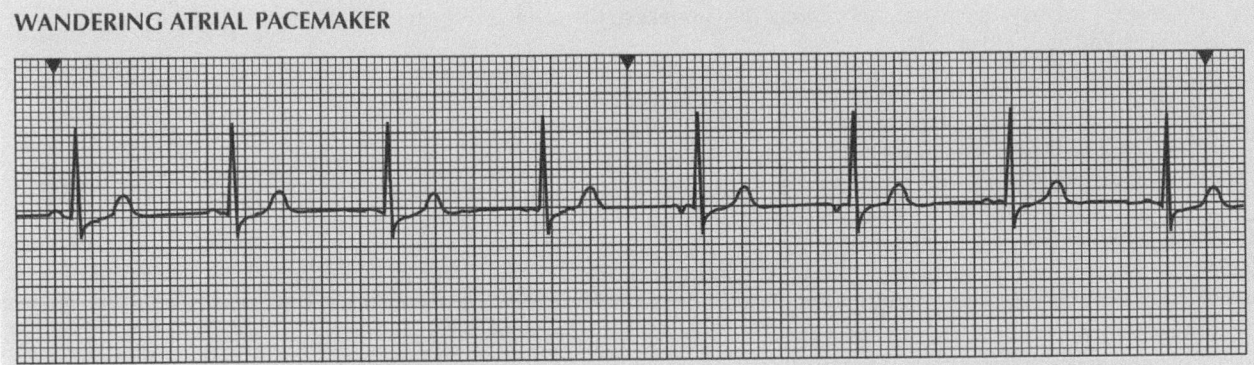

(From Wesley K: *Huszar's basic dysrhythmia and acute coronary syndromes*, ed 4, St. Louis, 2011, Mosby/JEMS.)

Rate	Regularity	P Waves	PR Interval	QRS Duration
Usually 60-100 beats/min	Atrial and ventricular rhythms usually slightly irregular	P waves look different beat to beat; at least 3 different-looking P waves	0.12-0.20 and may vary	<0.12

Etiology	Significance	Treatment
• Vagal stimulation • Sinus bradycardia • Digitalis toxicity	• May represent multiple atrial escape beats	• Usually none needed • Discontinuance of digitalis if toxicity is suspected • Atropine may be used to increase slow sinus rate

SUPRAVENTRICULAR TACHYCARDIA (Supraventricular tachycardia refers to any narrow QRS tachycardia whose focus cannot be definitely identified; the term should be used only when a more definitive diagnosis cannot be made)

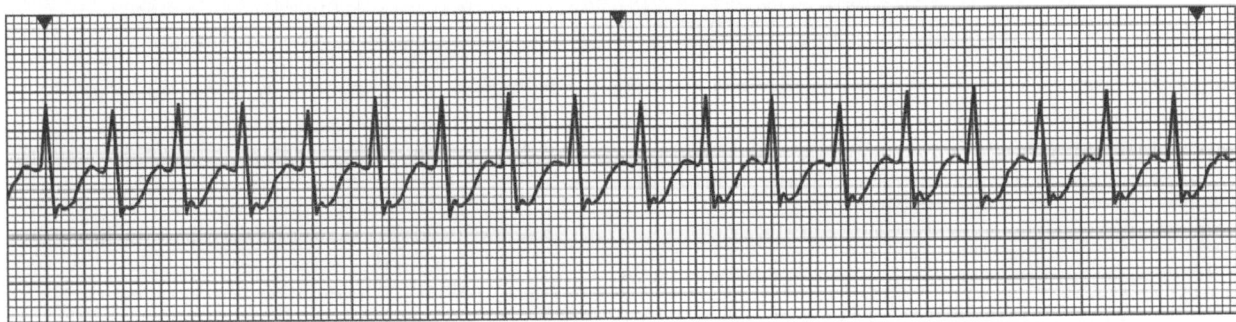

(From Wesley K: *Huszar's basic dysrhythmia and acute coronary syndromes*, ed 4, St. Louis, 2011, Mosby/JEMS.)

Rate	Regularity	P Waves	PR Interval	QRS Duration
>100 beats/min; usually 150-250 beats/min	Atrial and ventricular rhythms regular	P waves are impossible to distinguish; may be lost in QRS or preceding T wave	Cannot measure	<0.12

Etiology	Significance	Treatment
• Depends on whether sinus, atrial, or junctional	• Depends on whether sinus, atrial, or junctional	• Depends on whether sinus, atrial, or junctional

ATRIAL TACHYCARDIA (Paroxysmal atrial tachycardia [PAT] refers to the sudden interruption of sinus rhythm by a rapid ectopic focus—starts and ends abruptly)

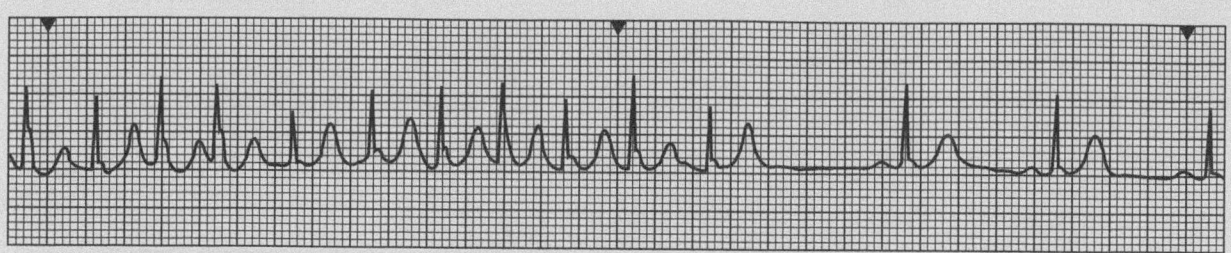

(From Wesley K: *Huszar's basic dysrhythmia and acute coronary syndromes*, ed 4, St. Louis, 2011, Mosby/JEMS.)

Rate	Regularity	P Waves	PR Interval	QRS Duration
150-250/min	Atrial and ventricular rhythms regular	P wave differs from sinus P; may merge with preceding T wave	0.12-0.20	<0.12

Etiology	Significance	Treatment

• SNS stimulation caused by psychological or physiologic stressors (e.g., stress, fear, anxiety, pain, anger, infection, exercise, dehydration)
• Hypoxia
• Myocardial ischemia or infarction
• Valvular heart disease (e.g., mitral valve prolapse)
• Chronic obstructive pulmonary disease
• Hyperthyroidism
• Inflammatory heart disease (e.g., myocarditis)
• Wolff-Parkinson-White syndrome
• Drug effect: caffeine; nicotine; alcohol
• Drug toxicity: digitalis (frequently PAT with block)
	• Patient may experience palpitations and clinical manifestations of hypoperfusion (e.g., hypotension, syncope, chest pain, HF) because diastolic filling time and preload is greatly reduced
	• Myocardial oxygen consumption is increased and myocardial oxygen supply is decreased, so myocardial ischemia may occur or worsen
		• Depends on patient's tolerance, cause, and history of previous attacks
		• Discontinuance of digitalis if toxicity is suspected
		• Initial treatment: vagal stimulation; adenosine; if the rhythm persists, continue with the following:
		  • Calcium channel blockers (e.g., diltiazem [Cardizem], verapamil [Calan])
		  • Beta-blockers
		  • Digoxin if not the cause
		  • Synchronized cardioversion
		• Other considerations
		  • Right atrial pacing
		  • Ablation may be indicated for recurrent AV nodal reentrant tachycardia
		• NOTE: If QRS is wide (e.g., associated with WPW): do NOT use adenosine, beta-blockers, calcium channel blockers, or digoxin; preferred agent is amiodarone; if WPW, ablation is preferred long-term treatment

MULTIFOCAL ATRIAL TACHYCARDIA (also called chaotic atrial rhythm)

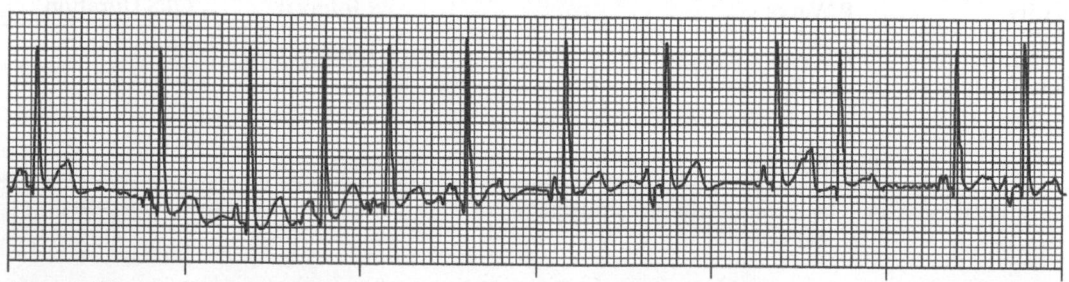

(From Aehlert B: *ECGs made easy*, ed 5, St. Louis, 2013, Elsevier Mosby.)

Rate	Regularity	P Waves	PR Interval	QRS Duration
Usually 100-150 beats/min	Atrial and ventricular rhythms usually slightly irregular	P waves look different beat to beat; at least 3 different-looking P waves	0.12-0.20 and may vary	<0.12

Etiology	Significance	Treatment
• Pulmonary hypertension (e.g., COPD, pulmonary embolism) • Valvular heart disease • Heart failure • Electrolyte imbalance • Drug toxicity: digitalis	• Demonstrates atrial irritability, which may lead to atrial tachycardia, flutter, fibrillation	• Treatment of cause: electrolyte replacement, treatment of heart failure, etc. • Discontinuance of digitalis if toxicity is suspected • If normal LV function: verapamil, beta-blocker, amiodarone, digoxin, flecainide, propafenone • If abnormal LV function: amiodarone, diltiazem, digoxin

ATRIAL FIBRILLATION

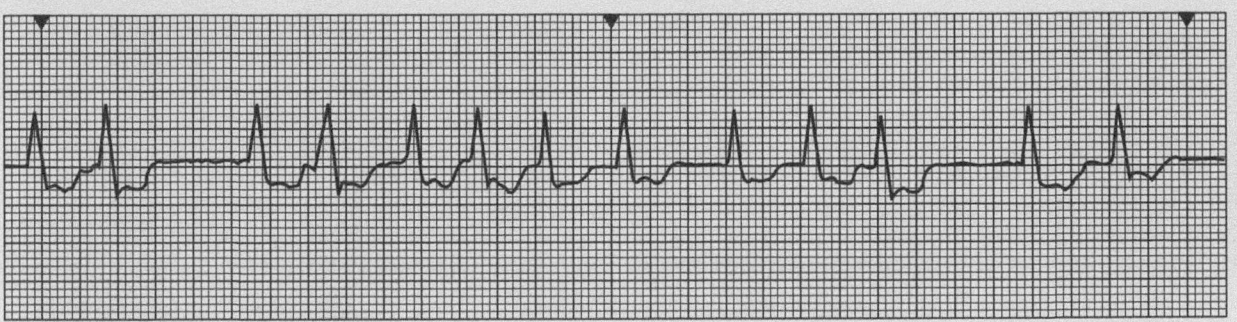

(From Wesley K: *Huszar's basic dysrhythmia and acute coronary syndromes*, ed 4, St. Louis, 2011, Mosby/JEMS.)

Rate	Regularity	P Waves	PR Interval	QRS Duration
Atrial rate >350 beats/min; ventricular rate varies greatly depending on conduction through AV node	Atrial fibrillatory waves irregular; ventricular rhythm irregularly irregular	No true P waves; fibrillatory waves manifested by quivering baseline	No true P waves	<0.12

Etiology	Significance	Treatment
<ul><li>Myocardial ischemia or infarction<ul><li>Especially anterior MI</li></ul></li><li>Valvular heart disease (e.g., mitral or tricuspid stenosis or regurgitation)</li><li>Heart failure</li><li>Cardiomyopathy</li><li>Hyperthyroidism</li><li>Inflammatory heart disease (e.g., pericarditis)</li><li>Hypertension</li><li>Post cardiotomy</li><li>Pulmonary hypertension (e.g., COPD, pulmonary embolism)</li><li>Wolff-Parkinson-White (WPW) syndrome</li><li>Drug effect: alcohol</li></ul>	<ul><li>No effective atrial contraction, so loss of atrial kick</li><li>Mural thrombi formation predisposes to emboli</li><li>Significance varies greatly on rate: may cause clinical manifestations of hypoperfusion (e.g., hypotension, syncope, chest pain, HF)</li></ul>	<ul><li>Normal LV function: beta-blocker or calcium channel blocker for rate control at rest and during exercise; digoxin as a second-line drug (only controls rate at rest)</li><li>Abnormal LV function: digoxin, diltiazem, or amiodarone</li><li>Although no additional treatment is required acutely if rate is controlled (between 60 and 100 beats/min), it is desirable to actually convert the AF to NSR if possible to reduce the risk of stroke and increase ventricular diastolic filling volume and cardiac output (considered rhythm control and maintenance)</li><li>Normal LV function with duration <48 hours: cardioversion or amiodarone, ibutilide, dofetilide, procainamide, disopyramide, flecainide, propafenone, sotalol</li><li>Abnormal LV function of <48 hours duration: cardioversion or amiodarone</li><li>Duration >48 hours duration or unknown duration: anticoagulation with INR between 2 and 3 for 3 weeks followed by cardioversion</li><li>If slow ventricular response rate: atropine or pacemaker may be needed</li><li>Digitalis should be considered as cause of slow ventricular response rate; withhold digitalis if it's the cause</li><li>NOTE: If associated with WPW: do NOT use adenosine, beta-blockers, calcium channel blockers, or digoxin; preferred agent is amiodarone</li><li>Other nonacute considerations</li><li>Overdrive pacing</li><li>Implantable atrial defibrillator</li><li>Ablation or Maze procedure may be performed</li><li>Long-term anticoagulation is needed for chronic AF to prevent mural thrombi and risk for embolic stroke; desirable INR 2 to 3</li></ul>

ATRIAL FLUTTER

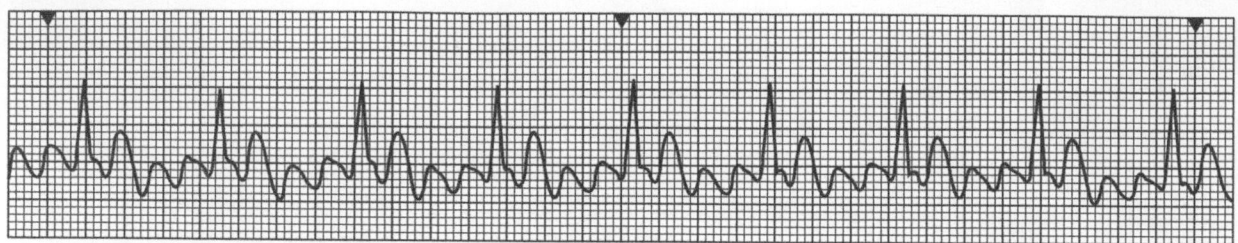

(From Wesley K: *Huszar's basic dysrhythmia and acute coronary syndromes*, ed 4, St. Louis, 2011, Mosby/JEMS.)

Rate	Regularity	P Waves	PR Interval	QRS Duration
Atrial rate approximately 300 beats/min; ventricular rate varies with conduction through the AV node; 2:1 atrial flutter has a ventricular rate of approximately 150 beats/min, 4:1 atrial flutter has a ventricular rate of approximately 75 beats/min	Atrial flutter waves regular; ventricular rhythm (response) usually regular	No true P waves; flutter waves have characteristic sawtooth appearance	No true P waves	<0.12

Etiology	Significance	Treatment
• Myocardial ischemia or infarction • Valvular heart disease • Heart failure • Cardiomyopathy • Hyperthyroidism • Inflammatory heart disease (e.g., pericarditis) • Hypertension • Post cardiotomy • Pulmonary hypertension (e.g., COPD, pulmonary embolus) • Drug effect: alcohol • Drug toxicity: digitalis	• No effectiveness of atrial contraction • Significance varies greatly depending on rate • If rate is very rapid, may cause clinical manifestations of hypoperfusion (e.g., hypotension, syncope, chest pain, HF) because diastolic filling time and preload is greatly reduced	• As for atrial fibrillation • Although adenosine is not indicated for treatment of atrial flutter, it may slow the rhythm enough to recognize the flutter waves • Anticoagulation may be prescribed for atrial flutter, but the risk of mural thrombi and stroke is considered lower than for atrial fibrillation

PREMATURE JUNCTIONAL CONTRACTION

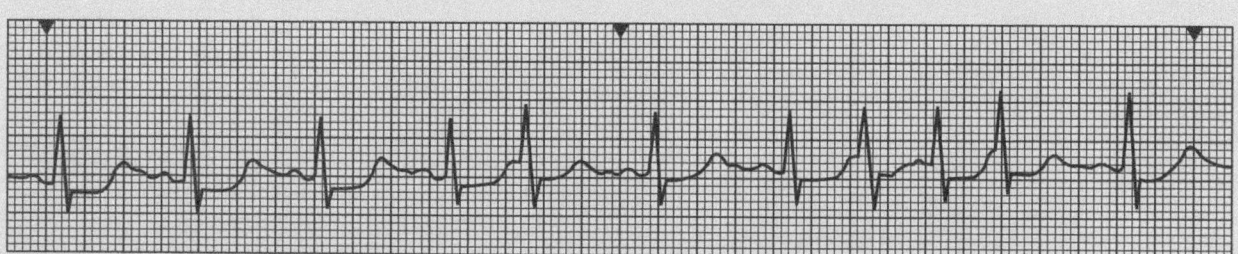

(From Wesley K: *Huszar's basic dysrhythmia and acute coronary syndromes*, ed 4, St. Louis, 2011, Mosby/JEMS.)

Rate	Regularity	P Waves	PR Interval	QRS Duration
Dependent on underlying rhythm	Dependent on underlying rhythm; PJC interrupts underlying rhythm	P wave if visible will be inverted; may be in front of, in, or after the QRS complex	Can be measured only if P wave is in front of QRS; PR will be <0.12 if measurable	<0.12

Etiology	Significance	Treatment
• SNS stimulation caused by psychological or physiologic stressors (e.g., stress, fear, anxiety, pain, anger, infection, exercise, dehydration) • Hypoxia • Myocardial ischemia or infarction. • Especially inferior MI • Valvular heart disease • Heart failure • Electrolyte imbalance • Drug effect: nicotine; caffeine; alcohol • Drug toxicity: digitalis • Also etiology as for PACs	• Usually benign but may predispose to junctional tachycardia if frequent	• Usually none necessary but sedation or beta-blockers may be used • Discontinuance of digitalis if toxicity is cause • Sedation • Beta-blockers

JUNCTIONAL ESCAPE RHYTHM

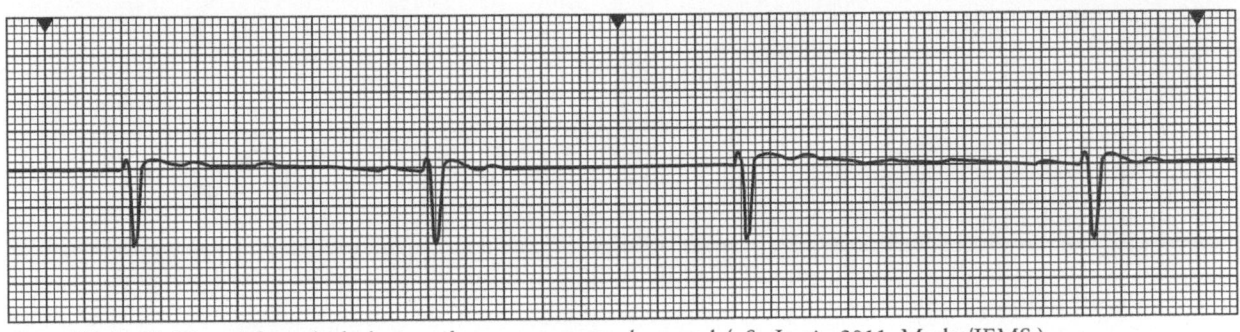

(From Wesley K: *Huszar's basic dysrhythmia and acute coronary syndromes*, ed 4, St. Louis, 2011, Mosby/JEMS.)

Rate	Regularity	P Waves	PR Interval	QRS Duration
40-60 beats/min	Atrial and ventricular rhythms regular	If visible, P wave inverted; may be in front of, in, or after the QRS complex	Can be measured only if P wave is in front of QRS; PR will be <0.12 if measurable	<0.12

Etiology	Significance	Treatment
• Vagal stimulation • SA block • Complete AV block • Myocardial ischemia or infarction • Valvular heart disease • Hypoxia • Post-cardiotomy • Drug toxicity: digitalis	• Protects patient from asystole • Do not suppress	• Note that this is *not* irritability; it is escape, so it is treated by accelerating the sinus node • Atropine • Pacemaker may be needed • Discontinuance of digitalis if digitalis toxicity is cause; it is a frequent cause of this rhythm

ACCLERATED JUNCTIONAL RHYTHM

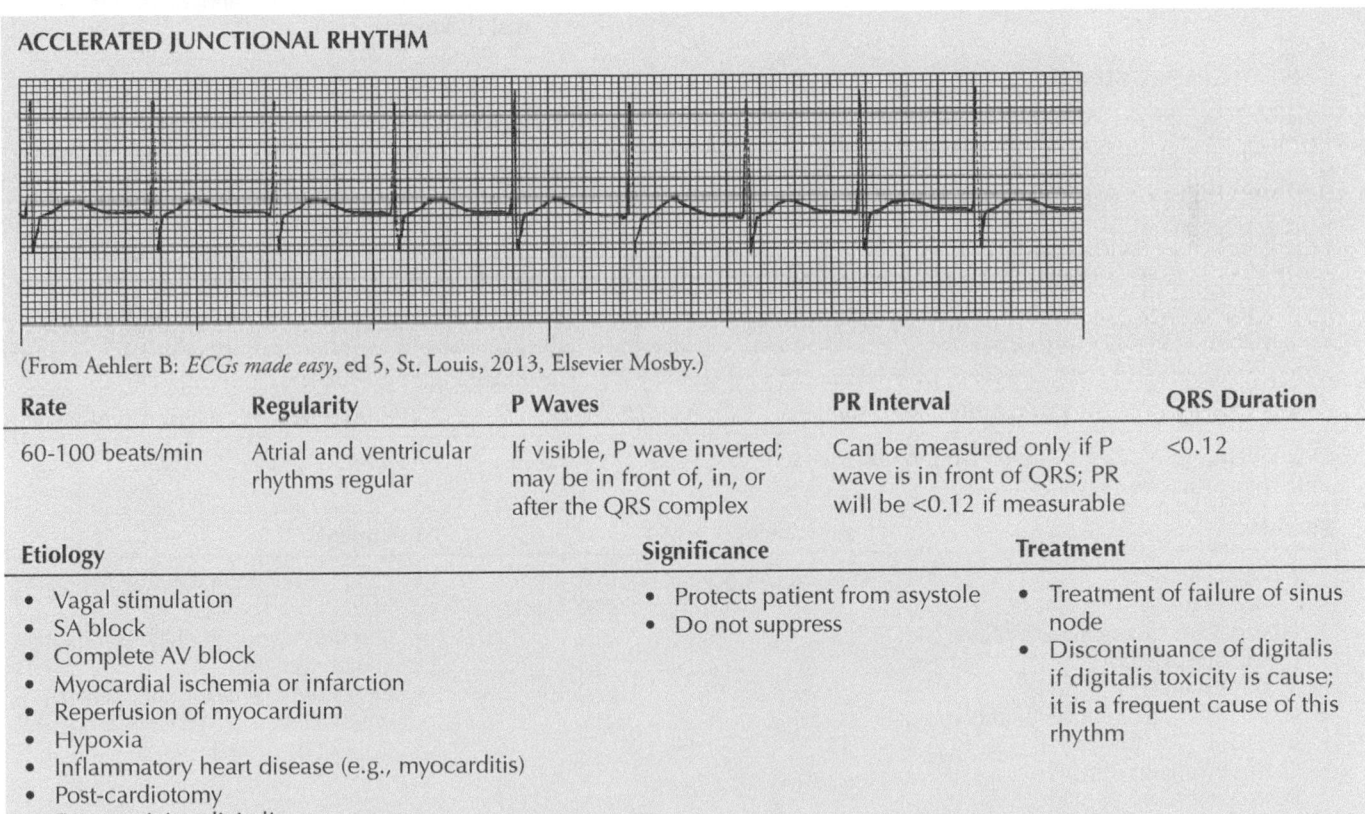

(From Aehlert B: *ECGs made easy*, ed 5, St. Louis, 2013, Elsevier Mosby.)

Rate	Regularity	P Waves	PR Interval	QRS Duration
60-100 beats/min	Atrial and ventricular rhythms regular	If visible, P wave inverted; may be in front of, in, or after the QRS complex	Can be measured only if P wave is in front of QRS; PR will be <0.12 if measurable	<0.12

Etiology	Significance	Treatment
• Vagal stimulation • SA block • Complete AV block • Myocardial ischemia or infarction • Reperfusion of myocardium • Hypoxia • Inflammatory heart disease (e.g., myocarditis) • Post-cardiotomy • Drug toxicity: digitalis	• Protects patient from asystole • Do not suppress	• Treatment of failure of sinus node • Discontinuance of digitalis if digitalis toxicity is cause; it is a frequent cause of this rhythm

JUNCTIONAL TACHYCARDIA

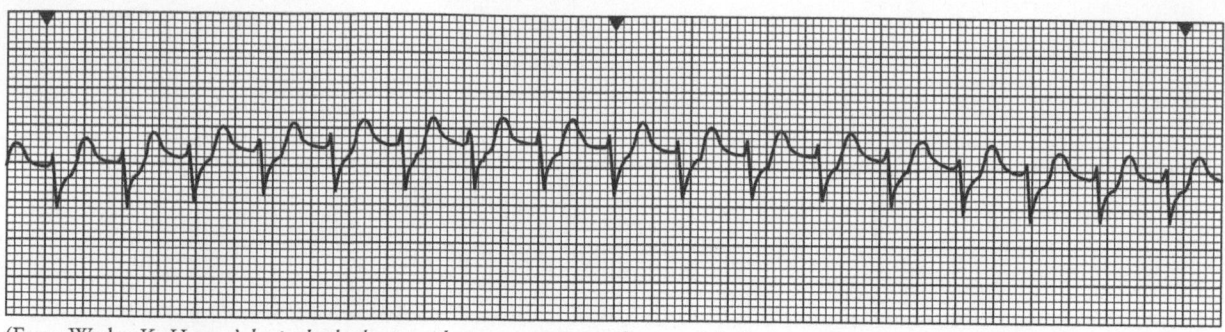

(From Wesley K: *Huszar's basic dysrhythmia and acute coronary syndromes*, ed 4, St. Louis, 2011, Mosby/JEMS.)

Rate	Regularity	P Waves	PR Interval	QRS Duration
>100 beats/min; usually 100-180 beats/min	Atrial and ventricular rhythms regular	If visible, P wave inverted; may be in front of, in, or after the QRS complex	Can be measured only if P wave is in front of QRS; PR will be <0.12 if measurable	<0.12

Etiology	Significance	Treatment
• Myocardial ischemia or infarction • Reperfusion of myocardium • Inflammatory heart disease • Post-cardiotomy • Drug toxicity: digitalis, theophylline	• Usually stops spontaneously and is usually tolerated well	• Treatment of cause • Discontinuance of digitalis if digitalis toxicity is cause • Vagal stimulation • Adenosine • Amiodarone • Beta-blockers or calcium channel blockers if normal LV function

FIRST-DEGREE AV BLOCK

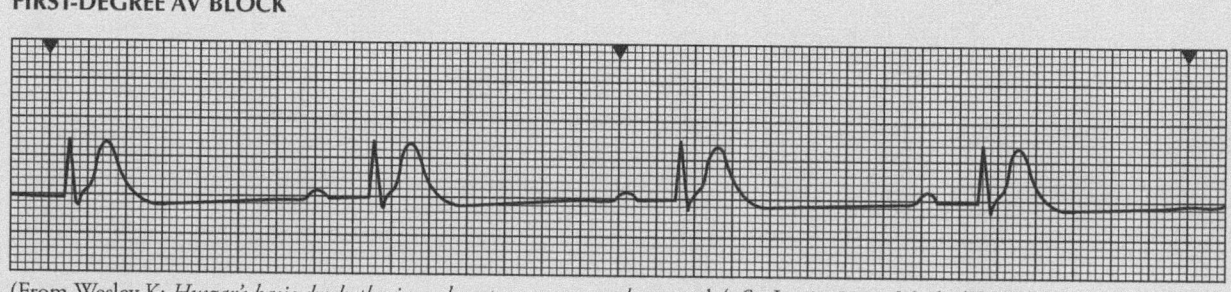

(From Wesley K: *Huszar's basic dysrhythmia and acute coronary syndromes*, ed 4, St. Louis, 2011, Mosby/JEMS.)

Rate	Regularity	P Waves	PR Interval	QRS Duration
Dependent on underlying rhythm	Dependent on underlying rhythm	Normal	>0.20	<0.12

Etiology	Significance	Treatment
• Normal variation • Congenital • Fibrodegenerative changes of the conduction system • Vagal stimulation • Myocardial ischemia or infarction • Myocardial contusion • Cardiomyopathy • Post-cardiotomy • Inflammatory heart disease (e.g., myocarditis) • Electrolyte imbalance • Drug toxicity: digitalis; beta-blockers; calcium channel blockers	• Relatively benign but may progress to second- or third-degree block	• Close observation for progression of block • Discontinuance of digitalis if digitalis toxicity is cause • Drugs or pacemaker not needed unless there is also a sinus bradycardia with hypoperfusion

SECOND DEGREE AV BLOCK TYPE I (previously referred to as Mobitz I; also known as Wenckebach)

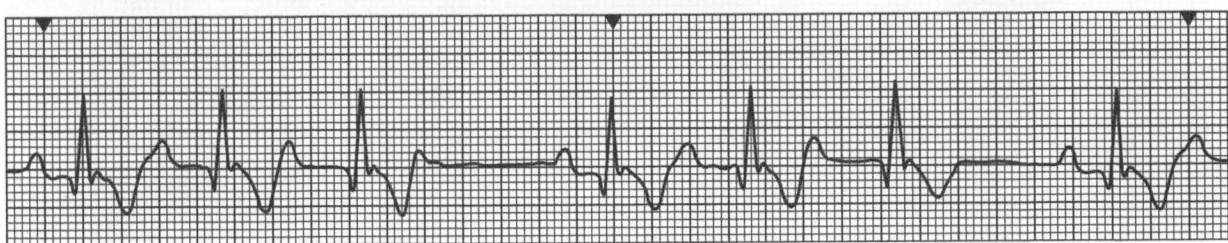

(From Wesley K: *Huszar's basic dysrhythmia and acute coronary syndromes*, ed 4, St. Louis, 2011, Mosby/JEMS.)

Rate	Regularity	P Waves	PR Interval	QRS Duration
Atrial rate dependent on underlying rhythm; ventricular rate dependent on conduction ratio; atrial rate > ventricular rate	Atrial rhythm regular, ventricular rhythm irregular (P-P interval is regular but R-R interval is irregular); groupings identifiable between P waves that were not conducted	Normal, but some P waves not followed by a QRS	Normal PR interval progressively lengthens until a P wave is not followed by a QRS; entire cycle begins again with normal PR interval	<0.12

Etiology	Significance	Treatment
• Fibrodegenerative changes of the conduction system • Myocardial ischemia or infarction • Inferior or posterior MI • Post-cardiotomy • Inflammatory heart disease • Myocardial contusion • Drug toxicity: digitalis; beta-blockers; calcium channel blockers	• Block is at AV node • Occurs more often in Inferior MIs (RCA lesion) • Relatively benign: usually transient, and does not usually progress to complete heart block	• Does not usually require treatment • Close monitoring for progression of block • Discontinuance of digitalis if digitalis toxicity is cause • Transvenous pacemaker or atropine may be used if rate slow and patient symptomatic

SECOND-DEGREE AV BLOCK TYPE II (previously referred to as Mobitz II) (2:1 block is a second-degree block but may be either type I or type II; the QRS width may be helpful in differentiating between the two; if the QRS is of normal width, it is probably type I; if the QRS is 0.12 or greater, it is probably type II)

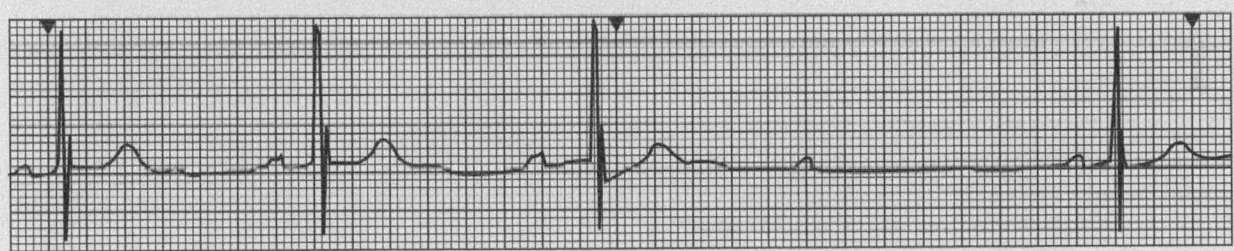

(From Wesley K: *Huszar's basic dysrhythmia and acute coronary syndromes*, ed 4, St. Louis, 2011, Mosby/JEMS.)

Rate	Regularity	P Waves	PR Interval	QRS Duration
Atrial rate dependent on underlying rhythm; ventricular rate dependent on conduction ratio but usually <60 beats/min; atrial rate > ventricular rate	Atrial rhythm regular, ventricular rhythm regular or irregular depending on whether conduction ratio varies or is constant; P-P interval regular, but some R-R intervals may be twice normal	P waves normal, but there are P waves not followed by a QRS without preceding progressive lengthening	Usually 0.12-0.20 of conducted P waves but may be longer; constant for each conducted QRS	0.12 or >

Etiology	Significance	Treatment
• Myocardial ischemia or infarction • Anterior MI • Hypertension • Valvular heart disease • Conduction system fibrosis • Inflammatory heart disease (e.g., myocarditis) • Post-cardiotomy • Myocardial contusion	• Block is at bundle of His, which accounts for the slight widening of the QRS complex • Occurs more often in anterior MIs (LAD lesion) • Ominous as it often progresses to third-degree heart block	• Atropine may be used but is not usually helpful • Transcutaneous or transvenous pacemaker

THIRD-DEGREE (OR COMPLETE) AV BLOCK

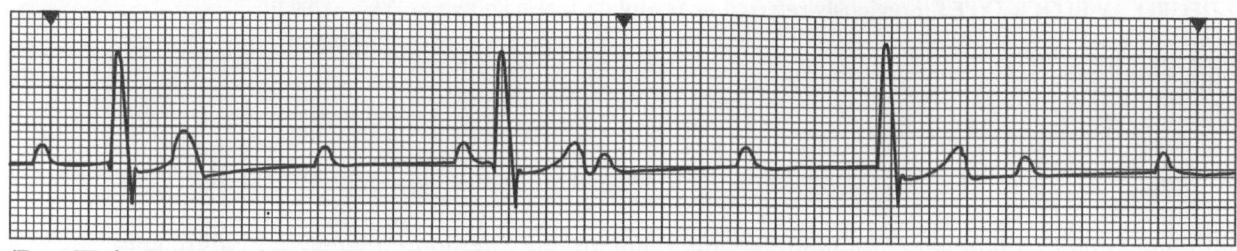

(From Wesley K: *Huszar's basic dysrhythmia and acute coronary syndromes*, ed 4, St. Louis, 2011, Mosby/JEMS.)

Rate	Regularity	P Waves	PR Interval	QRS Duration
Atrial rate dependent on underlying rhythm. Ventricular rate dependent on focus of escape rhythm (40-60 beats/min if escape focus is junctional); (20-40 beats/min if escape focus is ventricular)	Atrial rhythm regular, ventricular rhythm usually regular; P-P interval regular; R-R interval usually regular	Normal but P waves not followed by (associated with) QRS	No consistent PR interval; no relationship between the P waves and the QRS complexes	<0.12 if escape focus is junctional; ≥0.12 if escape focus is ventricular

Etiology	Significance	Treatment

• Myocardial ischemia or infarction
• Conduction system fibrosis
• Inflammatory heart disease
• Post-cardiotomy
• Myocardial contusion
• Hypoxia
• Electrolyte imbalance
• Drug toxicity: digitalis
	• If no escape rhythm is established, the patient has ventricular asystole	• Close observation for clinical manifestations of hypoperfusion if inferior MI with junctional escape rhythm
		• Atropine may be used but is not usually helpful
		• Pacemaker especially if:
		  • Anterior MI
		  • Inferior MI with ventricular escape rhythm

PREMATURE VENTRICULAR CONTRACTION

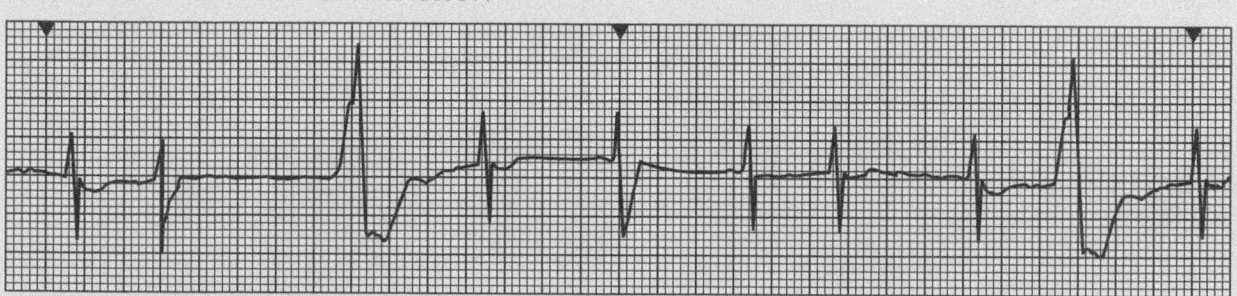

(From Wesley K: *Huszar's basic dysrhythmia and acute coronary syndromes*, ed 4, St. Louis, 2011, Mosby/JEMS.)

Rate	Regularity	P Waves	PR Interval	QRS Duration
Dependent on underlying rhythm	Dependent on underlying rhythm; PVC interrupts underlying rhythm	No associated P wave	No associated P wave; cannot measure PR	0.12 or >; QRS of PVC looks different than normal QRSs

Etiology	Significance	Treatment

• SNS stimulation caused by psychological or physiologic stressors (e.g., stress, fear, anxiety, pain, anger, infection, exercise, dehydration) or adrenergic drugs (e.g., epinephrine, isoproterenol, dopamine)
• Hypoxia
• Acidosis
• Myocardial ischemia or infarction
• Reperfusion of myocardium
• Heart failure
• Cardiomyopathy
• Myocardial contusion
• Ventricular aneurysm
• Valvular heart disease
• Electrolyte imbalance
• Drugs: caffeine, nicotine, alcohol, cocaine
• Drug toxicity: digitalis; aminophylline
	• PVCs of most significance: may predispose to VT or VF
	  • Frequent (>6/min)
	  • Bigeminal
	  • Multifocal
	  • R on T phenomenon
	  • Couplets
	  • Runs of ventricular tachycardia (3 or more PVCs in a row)
	• Pulse amplitude of PVC is reduced due to decreased filling time
		• Treatment of cause (e.g., oxygen, electrolyte replacement, discontinue digitalis)
		• No treatment required if only occasional, unifocal, and does not occur on previous T wave (R on T)
		• If frequent, multifocal, R on T, couplets, or runs of VT or symptomatic: amiodarone, lidocaine, beta-blockers

MONOMORPHIC VENTRICULAR TACHYCARDIA

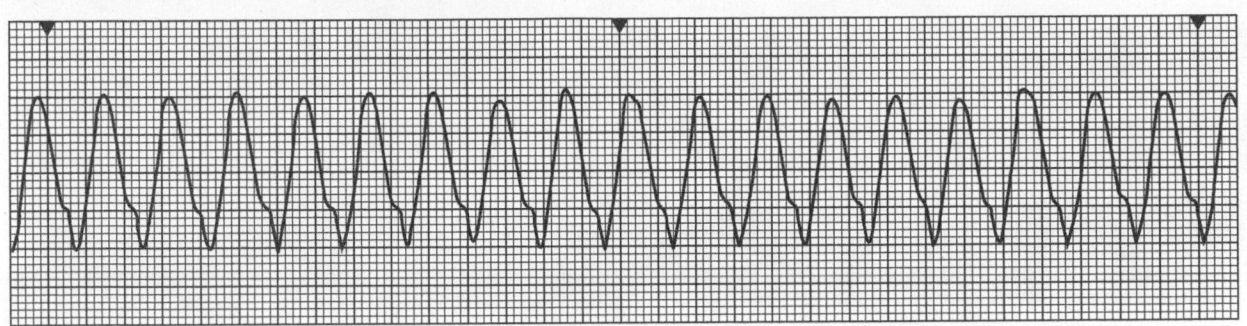

(From Wesley K: *Huszar's basic dysrhythmia and acute coronary syndromes*, ed 4, St. Louis, 2011, Mosby/JEMS.)

Rate	Regularity	P Waves	PR Interval	QRS Duration
100-250 beats/min VT is usually ~150 beats/min; VT at 200-250 beats/min may be called ventricular flutter	Ventricular rhythm usually regular; if dissociated P waves are identifiable, atrial rhythm regular	No associated P waves but may have dissociated P waves scattered through the rhythm	No associated P waves; cannot measure PR	0.12 or >; QRS of VT looks different than normal QRSs

Etiology	Significance	Treatment
• SNS stimulation caused by psychological or physiologic stressors (e.g., stress, fear, anxiety, pain, anger, infection, exercise, dehydration) or adrenergic drugs (e.g., epinephrine, isoproterenol, dopamine) • Hypoxia • Acidosis • Myocardial ischemia or infarction • Reperfusion of myocardium • Cardiomyopathy • Myocardial contusion • Ventricular aneurysm • Valvular heart disease • Post-cardiotomy • R on T PVC • Electrolyte imbalance • Drugs: caffeine, nicotine, alcohol, cocaine • Drug toxicity: digitalis	• Ominous as it may progress to ventricular fibrillation • Symptoms depend on underlying heart disease, rate, and duration of VT • May cause angina, HF, and shock	• Treatment of cause • If normal LV function: procainamide, amiodarone, lidocaine, sotalol • If impaired LV function: amiodarone, lidocaine, cardioversion • If having hypotension, chest pain, or pulmonary edema: immediate sedation and cardioversion • If pulseless: treat as VF (e.g., CPR, defibrillation, vasopressin or epinephrine, amiodarone)

POLYMORPHIC VENTRICULAR TACHYCARDIA (Torsades de pointes if preceded by prolonged QT)

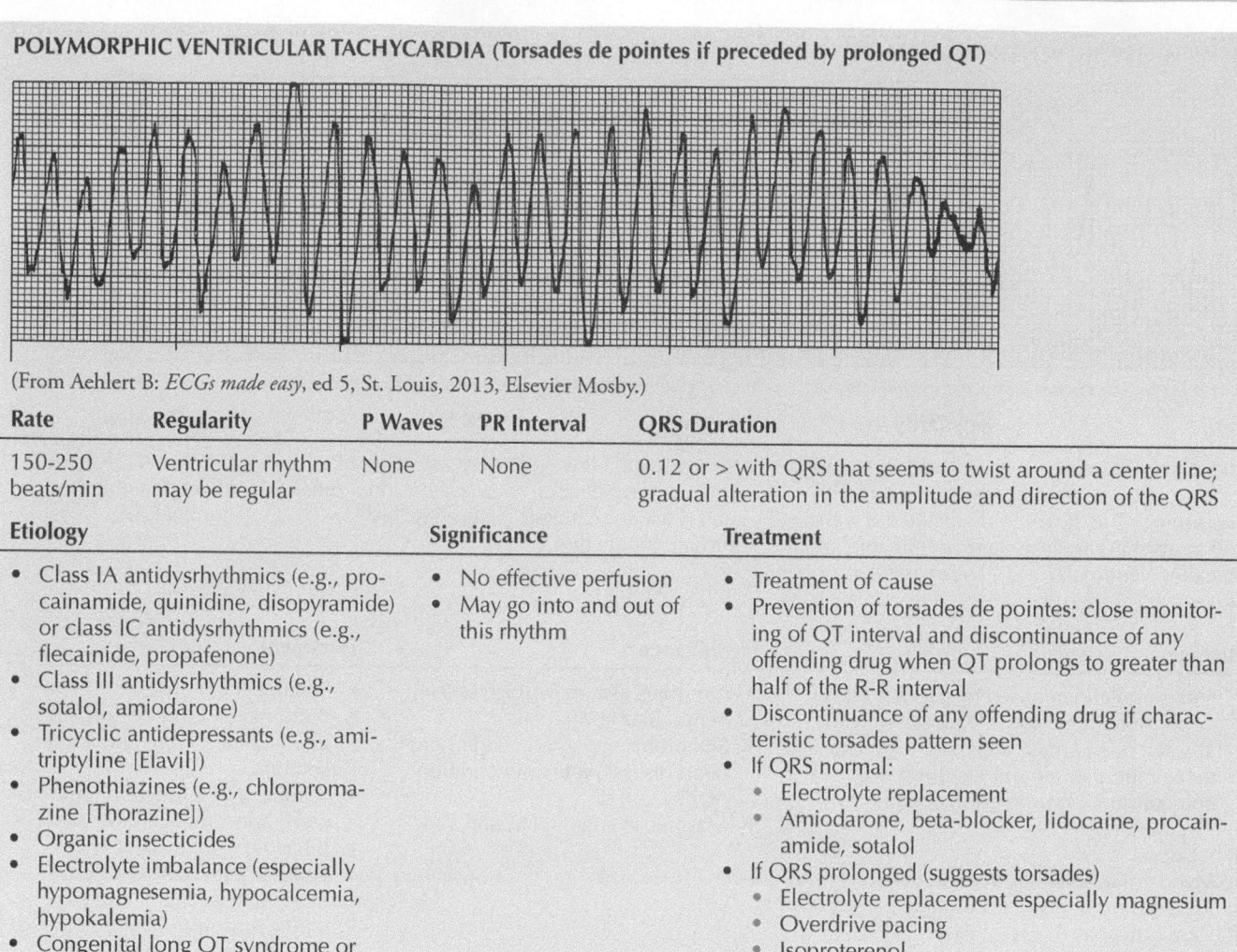

(From Aehlert B: *ECGs made easy*, ed 5, St. Louis, 2013, Elsevier Mosby.)

Rate	Regularity	P Waves	PR Interval	QRS Duration
150-250 beats/min	Ventricular rhythm may be regular	None	None	0.12 or > with QRS that seems to twist around a center line; gradual alteration in the amplitude and direction of the QRS

Etiology	Significance	Treatment
• Class IA antidysrhythmics (e.g., pro-cainamide, quinidine, disopyramide) or class IC antidysrhythmics (e.g., flecainide, propafenone) • Class III antidysrhythmics (e.g., sotalol, amiodarone) • Tricyclic antidepressants (e.g., amitriptyline [Elavil]) • Phenothiazines (e.g., chlorpromazine [Thorazine]) • Organic insecticides • Electrolyte imbalance (especially hypomagnesemia, hypocalcemia, hypokalemia) • Congenital long QT syndrome or Brugada syndrome • Marked bradycardia • Hypothermia • Subarachnoid hemorrhage	• No effective perfusion • May go into and out of this rhythm	• Treatment of cause • Prevention of torsades de pointes: close monitoring of QT interval and discontinuance of any offending drug when QT prolongs to greater than half of the R-R interval • Discontinuance of any offending drug if characteristic torsades pattern seen • If QRS normal: • Electrolyte replacement • Amiodarone, beta-blocker, lidocaine, procainamide, sotalol • If QRS prolonged (suggests torsades) • Electrolyte replacement especially magnesium • Overdrive pacing • Isoproterenol • Phenytoin • Lidocaine • If impaired LV function: amiodarone, lidocaine, cardioversion

VENTRICULAR FIBRILLATION

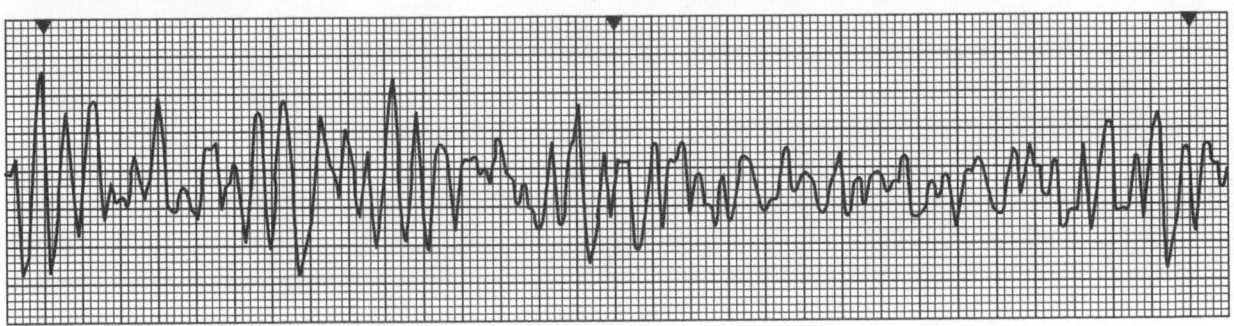

(From Wesley K: *Huszar's basic dysrhythmia and acute coronary syndromes*, ed 4, St. Louis, 2011, Mosby/JEMS.)

Rate	Regularity	P Waves	PR Interval	QRS Duration
None	Irregular; chaotic baseline	None	None	None

Etiology	Significance	Treatment
• SNS stimulation caused by psychological or physiologic stressors (e.g., stress, fear, anxiety, pain, anger, infection, exercise, dehydration) or adrenergic drugs (e.g., epinephrine, isoproterenol, dopamine) • Hypoxia • Myocardial ischemia or infarction • R on T PVC • Electrical shock including microshock • Brugada syndrome (familial) • Drowning • Hypothermia • Drug toxicity: digitalis • Dying heart	• Lethal within 4-6 minutes • No cardiac output • Symptoms include: loss of consciousness, pulse, blood pressure, and ventilation; anoxic seizures	• CPR until defibrillator available and ready then after defibrillation and between successive defibrillation attempts • Immediate defibrillation (150-200 joules [biphasic energy], 360 joules [monophasic energy]) • Vasopressin or epinephrine • Intubation • Antidysrhythmics: amiodarone or lidocaine • Post-resuscitation care

IDIOVENTRICULAR RHYTHM

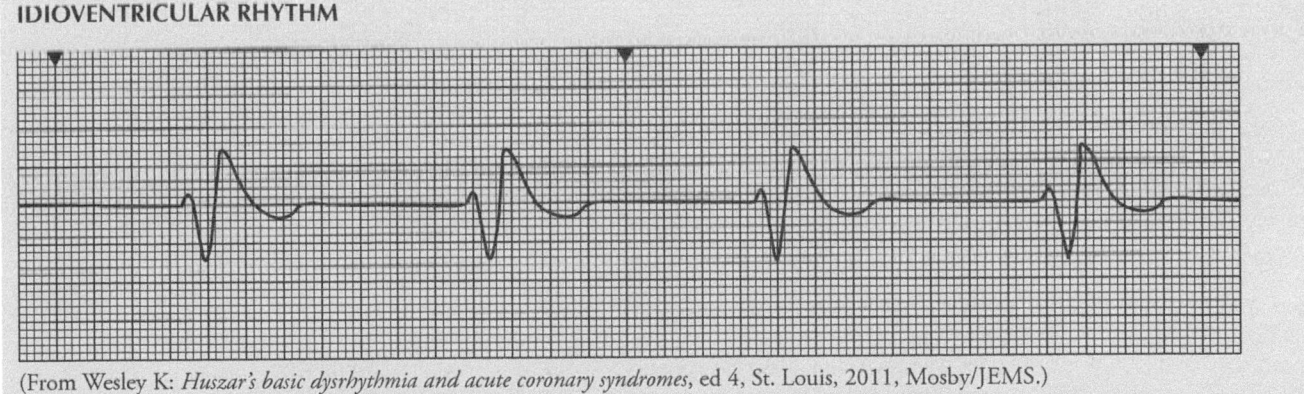

(From Wesley K: *Huszar's basic dysrhythmia and acute coronary syndromes*, ed 4, St. Louis, 2011, Mosby/JEMS.)

Rate	Regularity	P Waves	PR Interval	QRS Duration
20-40 beats/min	Ventricular rhythm usually regular; no atrial activity	None	None	0.12 or >

Etiology	Significance	Treatment
• Vagal stimulation • Failure of higher pacemakers (e.g., ischemia or fibrosis of conduction system) • Myocardial ischemia or infarction • Third-degree AV block • Drug toxicity: digitalis	• Protects the patient from asystole but very unreliable • Do not suppress	• Acceleration of higher pacemakers with atropine • Pacemaker • If pulseless: • CPR • Epinephrine • Pacemaker • Consideration and treatment of causes

ACCELERATED IDIOVENTRICULAR RHYTHM

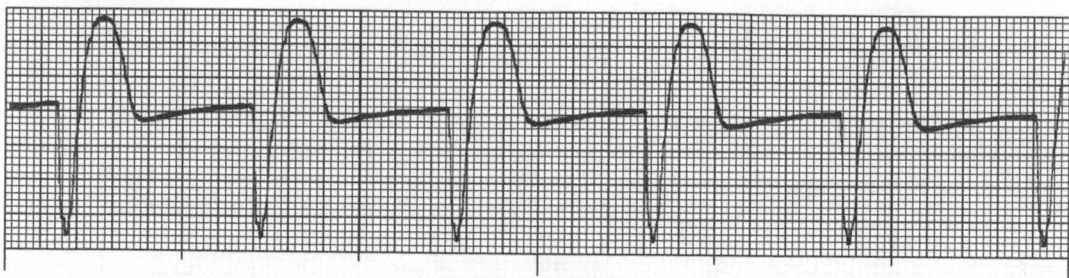

(From Aehlert B: *ECGs made easy*, ed 5, St. Louis, 2013, Elsevier Mosby.)

Rate	Regularity	P Waves	PR Interval	QRS Duration
40-100 beats/min	Ventricular rhythm usually regular; no atrial activity	None	None	0.12 or >

Etiology	Significance	Treatment
• Failure of higher pacemakers (e.g., ischemia or fibrosis of conduction system) • Myocardial ischemia or infarction • Reperfusion of myocardium • Drug toxicity: digitalis	• Protects the patient from asystole but very unreliable • Do not suppress	• Acceleration of higher pacemakers with atropine • Pacemaker

ASYSTOLE

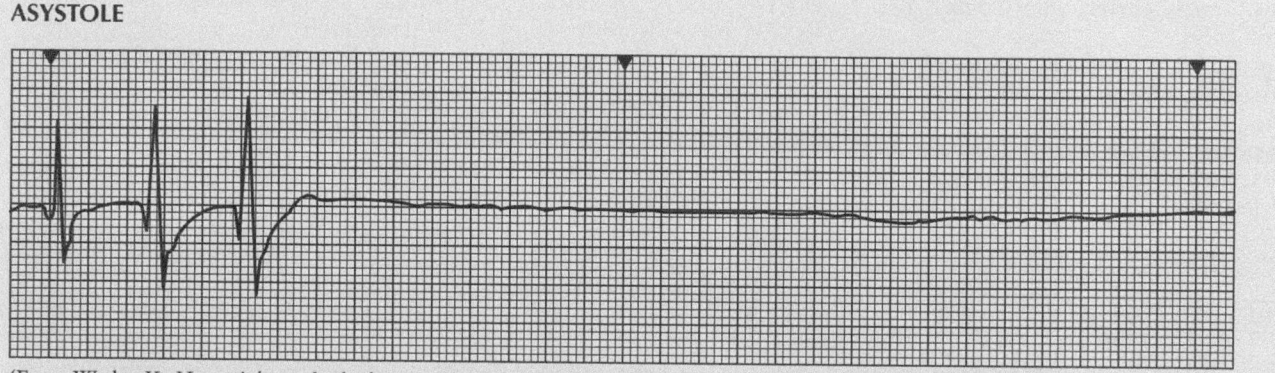

(From Wesley K: *Huszar's basic dysrhythmia and acute coronary syndromes*, ed 4, St. Louis, 2011, Mosby/JEMS.)

Rate	Regularity	P Waves	PR Interval	QRS Duration
None	No atrial or ventricular activity	None	None	None

Etiology	Significance	Treatment

• Vagal stimulation
• Hypoxia
• Acidosis
• Shock
• Myocardial ischemia or infarction
• Third-degree AV block
• Anaphylaxis
• Hypothermia
• Drug overdose
• Dying heart
	• Lethal within 4-6 minutes
	• No cardiac output
	• Symptoms include: loss of consciousness, pulse, blood pressure, and ventilation; anoxic seizures
		• CPR
		• Epinephrine
		• Pacemaker
		• Confirmation of rhythm in second lead to rule out ventricular fibrillation
		• Consideration of causes and treatment accordingly
		  • 5 Hs: hypovolemia. hypoxia, hydrogen ion (acidosis), hyper/hypokalemia, and hypothermia
		  • 5 Ts: tension pneumothorax, tamponade (cardiac), toxins, thrombosis (coronary), and thrombosis (pulmonary)

Hemodynamic Parameters, Methods of Measurement or Calculation, and Normal Values

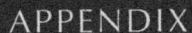

B

Parameter	Method of Measurement or Calculation	Normal
Heart rate (HR)	Measured: Count rate at apex or number of R waves by ECG monitor	60-100 beats/min
Mean arterial pressure (MAP)	Calculated: [BP systolic + (BP diastolic × 2)] ÷ 3 Systolic and diastolic pressures can be obtained by direct (arterial line) or indirect (auscultated using a sphygmomanometer)	70-105 mm Hg (Normal systolic BP is 90-140 mm Hg; normal diastolic BP is 60-90 mm Hg)
Cardiac output (CO)	Measured: Usually by thermodilution technique	4-8 L/min
Cardiac index (CI)	Calculated: CO ÷ by body surface area (BSA)	2.5-4 L/min/m^2
Stroke volume (SV)	Calculated: CO ÷ HR	60-120 mL/beat
Stroke index (SI)	Calculated: SV ÷ BSA	30-65 mL/m^2/beat
Central venous pressure (CVP)	Measured: At the tip of a catheter (frequently multilumen) in the superior vena cava; may be measured with a transducer or a water manometer	2-6 mm Hg (transducer) 3-8 cm H_2O (water manometer)
Right atrial pressure (RAP)	Measured: At the proximal port of the PAC; this port is located in the right atrium	2-6 mm Hg 3-8 cm H_2O
Pulmonary artery pressure (PAP)	Measured: At the distal port of the PAC with the balloon deflated; the tip is located in a pulmonary arteriole	Systolic (PAs): 15-30 mm Hg Diastolic (PAd): 5-15 mm Hg Mean (PAm): 10-20 mm Hg
Pulmonary artery occlusive pressure (PAOP)	Measured: At the distal port of the PAC with the balloon inflated; because right heart pressures are blocked by the inflated balloon, PAOP indirectly reflects left atrial pressure, left ventricular end-diastolic pressure (LVEDP), and left ventricular preload	8-12 mm Hg (Note: Although 8-12 mm Hg is "normal," many patients require a higher pressure [as high as 15-20 mm Hg] to achieve optimal stretch on the myofibrils and optimal preload)
Systemic vascular resistance (SVR)	Calculated: [(MAP − RAP) × 80] ÷ CO	800-1400 dynes/sec/cm^{-5}
Systemic vascular resistance index (SVRI)	Calculated: [(MAP − RAP) × 80] ÷ CI	2000-2400 dynes/sec/cm^{-5}/m^2
Pulmonary vascular resistance (PVR)	Calculated: [(PAm − PAOP) × 80] ÷ CO	100-250 dynes/sec/cm^{-5}
Pulmonary vascular resistance index (PVRI)	Calculated: [(PAm − PAOP) × 80] ÷ CI	225-315 dynes/sec/cm^{-5}/m^2

Continued

Parameter	Method of Measurement or Calculation	Normal
Left ventricular stroke work index (LVSWI)	Calculated: $[SI \times (MAP - PAOP)] \times 0.0136$	45-65 g•m/m^2
Right ventricular stroke work index (RVSWI)	Calculated: $[SI \times (PAm - RAP)] \times 0.0136$	5-12 g•m/m^2
Right ventricular end-diastolic volume (RVEDV)	Measured: By thermodilution method with REF PAC	100-160 mL
Right ventricular end-diastolic volume index (RVEDVI)	Calculated: RVEDV ÷ BSA	60-100 mL/m^2
Right ventricular end-systolic volume (RVESV)	Measured: By thermodilution method with REF PAC	50-100 mL
Right ventricular end-systolic volume index (RVESVI)	Calculated: RVESV ÷ BSA	30-60 mL/m^2
Right ventricular ejection fraction (RVEF)	Measured: By thermodilution method with REF PAC	40%-60%
Arterial oxygen saturation (SaO$_2$)	Measured: By pulse oximetry or by arterial blood gas analysis	95%-100%
Mixed venous oxygen saturation (SvO$_2$)	Measured: By SvO$_2$ port of a fiberoptic oximetric PAC or by mixed venous blood gas analysis	60%-80%
Central venous oxygen saturation (ScvO$_2$)	Measured: By fiberoptic oximetric central venous catheter or by venous blood gas analysis	65%-85%
Arterial oxygen content (CaO$_2$)	Calculated: $1.34 \times Hgb \times SaO_2$	18-20 mL/dL
Venous oxygen content (CvO$_2$)	Calculated: $1.34 \times Hgb \times SvO_2$	12-16 mL/dL
Oxygen delivery (DO$_2$)	Calculated: $CO \times CaO_2 \times 10$	900-1100 mL/min
Oxygen delivery index (DO$_2$I)	Calculated: $CI \times CaO_2 \times 10$	550-650 mL/min/m^2
Oxygen consumption (VO$_2$)	Calculated: $CO \times Hgb \times 13.4 \times (SaO_2 - SvO_2)$	200-300 mL/min
Oxygen consumption index (VO$_2$I)	Calculated: $CI \times Hgb \times 13.4 \times (SaO_2 - SvO_2)$	110-160 mL/min/m^2
Oxygen extraction ratio (O$_2$ER)	Calculated: $CaO_2 - CvO_2/CaO_2$	22%-30%
Oxygen extraction index (O$_2$EI)	Calculated: $SaO_2 - SvO_2/SaO_2$	20%-27%
Coronary artery perfusion pressure (CAPP)	Calculated: Diastolic BP − PAOP	60-80 mm Hg

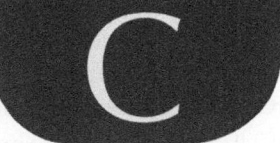
Common Abbreviations and Acronyms Used in Progressive Care Nursing

2,3-DPG	2,3-diphosphoglyceric acid
a	Alveolar
A	Arterial
A-a	Arterial/alveolar (as in A-a gradient)
A_2	Aortic (first) component of S_2
AAA	Abdominal aortic aneurysm
AACN	American Association of Critical-Care Nurses
AAL	Anterior axillary line
ABG	Arterial blood gas
ABI	Ankle-brachial index
AC	Assist-control
ACC	American College of Cardiology
ACE	Angiotensin converting enzyme
ACE	Academic Center for Evidence-Based Practice
ACLS	Advanced cardiac life support
ACS	Acute coronary syndrome
ACT	Activated clotting time
ACTH	Adrenocorticotropic hormone
ADA	American Diabetic Association
ADH	Antidiuretic hormone
ADL	Activities of daily living
ADP	Adenosine diphosphate
AED	Automated external defibrillator
AF	Atrial fibrillation
AGREE	Appraisal of Guidelines for Research and Evaluation
AHA	American Heart Association
AHA	American Hospital Association
AHRQ	Agency for Healthcare Research and Quality
AIDS	Acquired immune deficiency syndrome
AIVR	Accelerated idioventricular rhythm
AKI	Acute kidney injury
ALF	Acute liver failure
ALI	Acute lung injury
ALS	Amyotrophic lateralizing sclerosis
ALT	Alanine aminotransferase
AMP	Applied Measurement Professionals
ANA	American Nurses Association
ANCC	American Nurses Certification Corporation
ANP	Atrial natriuretic peptide
ANS	Autonomic nervous system

AP	Anterior posterior
APA	American Psychiatric Association
APRN	Advanced practice registered nurse
APRV	Airway pressure release ventilation
aPTT	Activated partial thromboplastin time
aPTT	Activated partial prothrombin time
AR	Aortic regurgitation
ARB	Angiotensin receptor blocker
ARDS	Acute respiratory distress syndrome
ARF	Acute respiratory failure
AS	Aortic stenosis
ASA	Acetylsalicylic acid (aspirin)
AST	Aspartate aminotransferase
ATN	Acute tubular necrosis
ATP	Adenosine triphosphate
AV	Atrioventricular
AV	Arteriovenous
AV	Audiovisual
AVM	Arteriovenous malformation
BBB	Bundle branch block
BE	Base excess
BiPAP	Positive airway pressure on both inspiration and expiration
BiVAD	Biventricular assist device
BLS	Basic life support
BM	Bowel movement
BMI	Body mass index
BNP	Brain-type natriuretic peptide
BP	Blood pressure
BPOC	Bar-code point of care
BSA	Body surface area
BSN	Bachelor of science in nursing
BUN	Blood urea nitrogen
C	Celsius (also referred to as centigrade)
CABG	Coronary artery bypass graft
CAD	Coronary artery disease
CaO_2	Oxygen content in arterial blood
CAP	Community-acquired pneumonia
CAPP	Coronary artery perfusion pressure
CASS	Continuous aspiration of subglottic secretions
CAVH	Continuous arteriovenous hemofiltration

CAVHD	Continuous arteriovenous hemodialysis	$D_{50}W$	50% dextrose in water
CBC	Complete blood count	D_5LR	5% dextrose in Lactated Ringer's
CBF	Cerebral blood flow	D_5NS	5% dextrose in normal saline
CCNS	Acute Care/Critical Care Clinical Nurse Specialist	D_5W	5% dextrose in water
CCRN	Certification in Acute/Critical Care Nursing	DAI	Diffuse axonal injury
CCU	Critical care unit or cardiac care unit	dB	decibels
CDC	Center for Disease Control	DBP	Diastolic blood pressure
CEA	Carcinoembryonic antigen	DCA	Directional coronary atherectomy
CHB	Complete heart block	DES	Drug-eluding stent
CHO	Carbohydrate	DHA	Docosahexanoic acid
CHP	Capillary hydrostatic pressure	DI	Diabetes insipidus
CI	Cardiac index	DIC	Disseminated intravascular coagulation
CINAHL	Cumulative Index of Nursing and Allied Health Literature	DKA	Diabetes ketoacidosis
CK	Creatinine kinase	dl	Deciliter
CKD	Chronic kidney disease	DM	Diabetes mellitus
CK-MB	Creatinine kinase-myocardial band	DNA	Deoxyribonucleic acid
CLRT	Continuous lateral rotation therapy	DNR	Do not resuscitate
cm	Centimeter	DO_2	Oxygen delivery to the tissues
CMV	Cytomegalovirus	DO_2I	Delivery of oxygen to the tissue index
CNM	Certified nurse midwife	DT	Delirium tremens
CNML	Certification as Nurse Manager and Leader	DTBT	Door to balloon time
CNS	Central nervous system	DTR	Deep tendon reflexes
CNS	Clinical nurse specialist	DVT	Deep vein thrombosis
CO	Cardiac output	EAB	Extraanatomical bypass
CO_2	Carbon dioxide	EBCT	Electron beam computerized tomography
COLD	Chronic obstructive lung disease	EBP	Evidence-based practice
COP	Colloidal oncotic pressure	ECF	Extracellular fluid
COPD	Chronic obstructive pulmonary disease	ECF-A	Eosinophil chemotactic factor of anaphylaxis
CPAP	Continuous positive airway pressure	ECG	Electrocardiogram (may also be abbreviated EKG)
CPB	Cardiopulmonary bypass	ECMO	Extracorpeal membrane oxygenator
CPG	Clinical practice guideline	ED	Emergency department
CPOE	Computerized provider order entry	EDH	Epidural hematoma
CPP	Cerebral perfusion pressure	EEG	Electroencephalogram
CPR	Cardiopulmonary resuscitation	EF	Ejection fraction
CRH	Corticotropin releasing hormone	ELCA	Excimer laser coronary arthrectomy
CRNA	Certified registered nurse anesthetists	ELISA	Enzyme linked immunosorbent assay
CRRT	Continuous renal replacement therapy	EMG	Electromyogram
CRT	Cardiac resynchronization therapy	EMI	Electromagnetic interference
CSF	Cerebrospinal fluid	EMR	Electronic medical record
CSF	Colony stimulating factor	EMS	Emergency management system
CSW	Cerebral salt wasting	EMTALA	Emergency Medical Treatment and Labor Act
CT	Computerized tomography	ENG	Electronystagmography
cTnI	Cardiac troponin I	EOM	Extraocular movement
cTnT	Cardiac troponin T	EPA	Eicosapentaenoic acid
CVA	Costovertebral angle	EPA	Environmental Protection Agency
CVA	Cerebrovascular accident	EPS	Electrophysiology studies
CvO_2	Oxygen content in venous blood	EPS	Extrapyramidal symptoms
CVP	Central venous pressure	ERCP	Endoscopic retrograde cholangiopancreatography
CVVH	Continuous venovenous hemofiltration	ERV	Expiratory reserve volume
CVVHD	Continuous venovenous hemodialysis	ESR	Eosinophil sedimentation rate
CVVHDF	Continuous venovenous hemodiafiltration	ET	Endotracheal
$D_{10}W$	10% dextrose in water	ETC	Esophageal tracheal Combitube

ETT	Exercise tolerance test		IABP	Intraaortic balloon pump
EVG	Endovascular graft		IBW	Ideal body weight
F	Fahrenheit		IC	Inspiratory capacity
f	Frequency of ventilation		ICD	Implantable cardioverter-defibrillator
FAST	Focused abdominal sonography for trauma		ICH	Intracranial hematoma
FDA	Food and Drug Administration		ICOP	Interstitial colloidal oncotic pressure
FEV	Forced expiratory capacity		ICP	Intracranial pressure
FFP	Fresh frozen plasma		ICS	Intercostal space
FIO_2	Fraction of inspired oxygen		ICU	Intensive care unit
FRC	Functional residual capacity		Ig	Immunoglobulin
FSP	Fibrin split products (also referred to as *fibrin degradation products*)		IHI	Institute for Healthcare Improvement
			IHP	Interstitial hydrostatic pressure
FT_c	Flow time corrected		IHSS	Idiopathic hypertrophic subaortic stenosis
FTT	Failure to thrive		IL	Interleukin
FVC	Forced vital capacity		ILV	Independent lung ventilation
g	Gram		IM	Intramuscular
GABA	Gamma-aminobutyric acid		IMV	Intermittent mandatory ventilation
GALT	Gut associated lymphoid tissue		INH	Isoniazid
GCS	Glasgow coma scale		INR	International normalized ratio
GERD	Gastroesophageal reflux disease		IO	Intraosseous
GFR	Glomerular filtration rate		IOM	Institute of Medicine
GGT	Gamma-glutamyl transferase		IPBH	Intraparenchymal brain hemorrhage
GI	Gastrointestinal		IPPB	Intermittent positive pressure breathing
GP	Glycoprotein		IRA	Infarct-related artery
GU	Genitourinary		IRB	Institutional review board
H^+	Hydrogen ion		IRV	Inspiratory reserve volume
H_2O	Water		IRV	Inverse ratio ventilation
HAP	Hospital-acquired pneumonia		ISMP	Institute for Safe Medication Practices
HAT	Heparin-associated thrombocytopenia		ITP	Idiopathic thrombocytopenia purpura
HBV	Hepatitis B virus		IU	International units
HCAP	Health care–associated pneumonia		IV	Intravenous
HCl	Hydrochloric		IVP	Intravenous pyelogram
HCO_3	Bicarbonate		IVUS	Intravascular ultrasound
Hct	Hematocrit		JCAHO	Joint Commission on Accreditation of Health-care Organizations
HDL	High-density lipoproteins			
HELLP	Hemolysis, elevated liver enzyme levels, and low platelet count (as in HELLP syndrome)		JVD	Jugular venous distention
			kg	Kilogram
			KUB	Kidneys, ureters, bladder (same as flat plate of abdomen)
HF	Heart failure			
Hg	Mercury		KVO	Keep vein open
Hgb	Hemoglobin		L	Liter
HHS	Hyperglycemic hyperosmolar state		LA	Left atria
HIPAA	Health Insurance Portability and Accountability Act		LAAL	Left anterior axillary line
			LAD	Left anterior descending (artery)
HIT	Heparin-induced thrombocytopenia		LAD	Left axis deviation
HIV	Human immunodeficiency virus		LAE	Left atrial enlargement
HLA	Human leukocyte antigen		LAH	Left anterior hemibundle
HME	Heat and moisture exchanger		LAP	Left atrial pressure
HMO	Health maintenance organization		LBB	Left bundle branch
HOB	Head of bed		LBBB	Left bundle branch block
HR	Heart rate		LCA	Left circumflex artery
HRSA	Health Resources and Services Administration		LDH	Lactic dehydrogenase
HRT	Hormone replacement therapy		LDL	Low-density lipoproteins
I:E	Inspiration:expiration		LES	Lower esophageal sphincter

LGL	Lown-Ganong-Levine
LICS	Left intercostal space
LLQ	Left lower quadrant
LMA	Laryngeal mask airway
LMAL	Left midaxillary line
LMCL	Left midclavicular line
LMN	Lower motor neuron
LMWH	Low molecular weight heparin
LOC	Level of consciousness
LP	Lumbar puncture
LPAL	Left posterior axillary line
LPH	Left posterior hemibundle
LPN	Licensed practical nurse (a.k.a. licensed vocational nurse)
LR	Lactated Ringer's
LSB	Left sternal border
LUQ	Left upper quadrant
LV	Left ventricle
LVAD	Left ventricular assist device
LVF	Left ventricular failure
LVH	Left ventricular hypertrophy
LVMI	Left ventricular myocardial infarction
LVSWI	Left ventricular stroke work index
M_1	Mitral (first) component of S_1
mA	Milliampere (unit of measurement for electrical current)
MAL	Midaxillary line
MALT	Mucosal associated lymphoid tissues
MAO	Monoamide oxidase (as in MAO inhibitors)
MAP	Mean arterial pressure
MAP	Multidisciplinary action plan
mcg	Microgram (unit of measurement for weight)
MCH	Mean corpuscular hemoglobin
MCHC	Mean corpuscular hemoglobin concentration
MCL	Midclavicular line
MCL_1	Modified chest lead 1
MCL_6	Modified chest lead 6
MCT	Medium chain triglycerides
MCV	Mean corpuscular volume
MDF	Myocardial depressant factor
M_E	Minute ventilation exhaled
mEq	Milliequivalent (unit of measurement for solutes in solution)
mg	Milligram (unit of measurement for weight)
MI	Myocardial infarction
MIC	Minimum inhibitory concentration
MIDCABG	Minimally-invasive coronary artery bypass graft
min	Minute
MIP	Maximal inspiratory pressure (or force) (also referred to as negative inspiratory pressure [or force])
mL	Milliliter (unit of measurement for volume)
mm	Millimeter (unit of measurement for length)
mm Hg	Millimeters of mercury

MODS	Multiple organ dysfunction syndrome
mOsm/kg	Milliosmoles per kilogram
mOsm/L	Milliosmoles per liter
MR	Mitral regurgitation
MRA	Magnetic resonance angiography
MRS	Magnetic resonance spectroscopy
MRI	Magnetic resonance imaging
MS	Mitral stenosis
MSG	Monosodium glutamate
MSL	Midsternal line
MUGA	Multiple-gated acquisition scan
MV	Mechanical ventilation
MVC	Motor vehicle collision
MVO_2	Myocardial oxygen consumption
MVP	Mitral valve prolapse
MVV	Maximal voluntary ventilation
NASPE	North American Society of Pacing and Electrophysiology
NCLEX	National Council Licensure Examination
NCQA	National Committee for Quality Assurance
NCSBN	National Council of State Boards of Nursing
NDE	Near-death experience
NDNQI	National Database of Nursing Quality Indicators
NG	Nasogastric
NIF	Negative inspiratory force
NIH	National Institutes of Health
NIHSS	National Institutes of Health Stroke Scale
NK	Natural killer
NP	Nurse practitioner
NPO	Nothing by mouth
NPPV	Noninvasive positive pressure ventilation
NPSG	National Patient Safety Goals
NQF	National quality forum
NS	Normal saline
NSAID	Nonsteroidal antiinflammatory drugs
NSR	Normal sinus rhythm
NTG	Nitroglycerin
NTP	Nitroprusside
NYHA	New York Heart Association
O_2	Oxygen
O_2EI	Oxygen extraction index
O_2ER	Oxygen extraction ratio
OCD	Obsessive compulsive disorder
OPB	Ova, parasites, blood
OPCABG	Off-pump coronary artery bypass graft
OPG	Oculoplethysmography
P/F	PaO_2/FIO_2 (as in P/F ratio)
P_2	Pulmonic (second) component of S_2
PA	Pulmonary artery
PA	Posterior anterior
PAC	Pulmonary artery catheter
PAC	Premature atrial contraction

$PaCO_2$	Partial pressure of carbon dioxide in arterial blood
PAd	Pulmonary artery diastolic pressure
PAL	Posterior axillary line
PAm	Pulmonary artery pressure mean
PaO_2	Pressure of oxygen in arterial blood
PAO_2	Pressure of oxygen in alveolar blood
PAOP	Pulmonary artery occlusive pressure (previously referred to as pulmonary capillary wedge pressure or pulmonary artery wedge pressure)
PAP	Pulmonary artery pressure
PAs	Pulmonary artery systolic pressure
PAT	Paroxysmal atrial tachycardia
Pb	Barometric pressure
PC/IRV	Pressure controlled/inverse ratio ventilation
PCA	Patient controlled analgesia
PCCN	Certification in Progressive Care Nursing
PCI	Percutaneous coronary intervention
PCR	Polymerase chain reaction
PCV	Pressure-controlled ventilation
PD	Postural drainage
PDA	Patent ductus arteriosus
PDE	Phosphodiesterase
PDF	Probability density function
PDSA	Plan-Do-Study-Act
PE	Pulmonary embolism
PEA	Pulseless electrical activity
P_ECO_2	Partial pressure of carbon dioxide in exhaled air
PEEP	Positive end-expiratory pressure
PEFR	Peak expiratory flow rate
PEG	Percutaneous endoscopic gastrostomy
PEJ	Percutaneous endoscopic jejunostomy
PET	Positron emission tomography
$P_{et}CO_2$	Partial pressure of carbon dioxide in end-tidal air
PFT	Pulmonary function tests
pH	Hydrogen ion concentration
pHi	Intramucosal pH
PICC	Percutaneously inserted central catheter
PICOT	Problem, intervention, comparison, outcome, timing (i.e., format for a clinical question)
PIP	Peak inspiratory pressure
PJC	Premature junctional contraction
PMI	Point of maximal impulse
PML	Progressive multifocal leukoencephalopathy
PMN	Polymorphonuclear leukocytes
PMR	Papillary muscle rupture
PMR	Progressive muscle relaxation
PND	Paroxysmal nocturnal dyspnea
PNS	Parasympathetic nervous system
PO	Oral
PPD	Purified protein derivative
PPF	Plasma protein fraction
PPI	Proton pump inhibitor
PPN	Peripheral parenteral nutrition
PQRST	Provocation, palliation, quality, quantity, region, radiation, severity, timing (i.e., pain description)
PRCV	Pressure-regulated volume-controlled
PSV	Pressure support ventilation
PSVT	Paroxysmal supraventricular tachycardia
PT	Prothrombin time
PT	Physical therapy
PTCA	Percutaneous transluminal coronary angioplasty
$P_{tc}O_2$	Transcutaneous partial pressure of oxygen
PTMR	Percutaneous transmyocardial revascularization
PTSD	Post-traumatic stress disorder
PTSMA	Percutaneous transluminal septal myocardial ablation
PTU	Propylthiouracil
PV	Peak velocity
PVC	Premature ventricular contraction
PVC	Polyvinyl chloride
PVR	Pulmonary vascular resistance
PVRI	Pulmonary vascular resistance index
Q	Perfusion
QI	Quality improvement
QM	Quality management
QSEN	Quality and Safety Education for Nurses
QT_c	QT interval corrected for rate
RA	Right atrium
RAAL	Right anterior axillary line
RAAS	Renin-angiotensin-aldosterone system
RAD	Right axis deviation
RAE	Right atrial enlargement
RAP	Right atrial pressure
RAS	Reticular activating system
RBB	Right bundle branch
RBBB	Right bundle branch block
RBC	Red blood cell
RCA	Right coronary artery
REF	Right (ventricular) ejection fraction
REM	Rapid eye movement
RHD	Rheumatic heart disease
RICS	Right intercostal space
RIND	Reversible ischemic neurologic deficit
RLQ	Right lower quadrant
RMAL	Right midaxillary line
RMCL	Right midclavicular line
RN	Registered nurse
RNA	Ribonucleic acid
ROM	Range of motion
ROSC	Return of spontaneous circulation
r-PA	Recombinant plasminogen activator

RPAL	Right posterior axillary line	SVV	Stroke volume variability
RQ	Respiratory quotient	T	Temperature
RR	Respiratory rate	T_1	Tricuspid (second) component of S_1
RSB	Right sternal border	TAA	Thoracic aortic aneurysm
RSBI	Rapid shallow breathing index	TB	Tuberculosis
rSO_2	Regional oxygen saturation index	TBI	Toe-brachial index
RSV	Respiratory syncytial virus	TCA	Tricyclic antidepressants
rt-PA	Recombinant tissue plasminogen activator	$TcPO_2$	Transcutaneous carbon dioxide
RUQ	Right upper quadrant	TEC	Transluminal extraction catheter
RV	Right ventricle	TEE	Transesophageal echocardiography
RV	Residual volume	TENS	Transcutaneous electrical nerve stimulation
RVAD	Right ventricular assist device	TIA	Transient ischemic attack
RVF	Right ventricular failure	TIBC	Total iron-binding capacity
RVH	Right ventricular hypertrophy	TIPS	Transjugular intrahepatic portosystemic shunt
RVMI	Right ventricular myocardial infarction	TLC	Total lung capacity
RVSWI	Right ventricular stroke work index	TLC	Total lymphocyte count
RYGB	Roux-Y gastric bypass	TMP/SMX	Trimethoprim/sulfamethoxazole
S_1	The first heart sound	TNA	Total nutrient admixture
S_2	The second heart sound	TNF	Tumor necrosis factor
SA	Sinoatrial	TPN	Total parenteral nutrition
SAED	Semiautomatic external defibrillator	TR	Tricuspid regurgitation
SAH	Subarachnoid hemorrhage	TRH	Thyrotropin releasing hormone
SaO_2	Oxygen saturation of arterial blood	TSH	Thyroid stimulating hormone
SBAR	Situation, Background, Assessment, Recommendation	TTP	Thrombotic thrombocytopenia purpura
SC	Subcutaneous	UAGA	Uniform Anatomical Gift Act
SCI	Spinal cord injury	UAP	Unlicensed assistive personnel
SCUF	Slow continuous ultrafiltration	UES	Upper esophageal sphincter
$S_{cv}O_2$	Oxygen saturation of central venous blood	UFH	Unfractionated heparin
SDH	Subdural hematoma	UMN	Upper motor neuron
SI	Stroke index	UTI	Urinary tract infection
SIADH	Syndrome of inappropriate antidiuretic hormone	V	Ventilation
SIMV	Synchronized intermittent mandatory ventilation	V/Q	Ventilation/perfusion ratio
		V/Q	Ventilation/perfusion
SIRS	Systemic inflammatory response syndrome	V_A	Alveolar minute ventilation
SjO_2	Oxygen saturation of jugular venous blood	VAC	Vacuum assisted closure
		VAD	Ventricular assist device
SK	Streptokinase	VAP	Ventilator-associated pneumonia
SLE	Systemic lupus erythematosus	VAPSV	Volume-assured pressure support ventilation
SNS	Sympathetic nervous system	VBG	Vertical banded gastroplasty
SPECT	Single photon emission computed tomography	VC	Vital capacity
		V_D	Anatomical deadspace
SpO_2	Oxygen saturation in plasma (e.g., pulse oximetry)	V_E	Minute ventilation
		VF	Ventricular fibrillation
SRS-A	Slow reacting substance of anaphylaxis	VILI	Ventilator-induced lung injury
STEMI	ST segment elevation myocardial infarction	VO_2	Oxygen consumption by the tissues
STTI	Sigma Theta Tau International	VO_2I	Consumption of oxygen by the tissue index
SV	Stroke volume	VPR	Volume pressure response
SvO_2	Oxygen saturation of mixed venous blood	VSD	Ventricular septal defect
SVR	Systemic vascular resistance	VT	Ventricular tachycardia
SVRI	Systemic vascular resistance index	V_T	Tidal volume
		WBC	White blood cell
SVT	Supraventricular tachycardia	WPW	Wolff-Parkinson-White syndrome

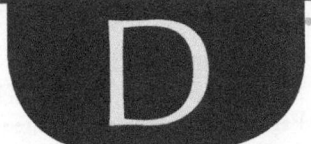

Normal Laboratory Values

BLOOD

Chemistries

Sodium: 136-145 mEq/L
Potassium: 3.5-5.0 mEq/L
Chloride: 96-106 mEq/L
Calcium: 8.5-10.5 mg/dL
Phosphorus: 3.0-4.5 mg/dL
Magnesium: 1.5-2.2 mEq/L or 1.8 to 2.4 mg/dL
CO_2: 23-30 mEq/L
Glucose: 70-110 mEq/L
BUN: 5-20 mg/dL
Creatinine: 0.7-1.5 mg/dL
Uric acid: 3-7 mg/dL
Osmolality: 280-295 mOsm/L
Lactate: 1-2 mmol/L
Ammonia: 15-110 mOsm/dL
Iron: 50-150 mcg/dL
Iron-binding capacity: 250-410 mcg/dL
Carcinoembryonic antigen (CEA): <2 ng/mL
Homocysteine: normal <15 μmol/L
C-reactive protein: normal <1 mg/dL
Brain-type natriuretic peptide (BNP): normal <100 picograms/mL
Bilirubin
    Total: 0.3-1.3 mg/dL
    Direct: 0.1-0.3 mg/dL
    Indirect: 0.1-1.0 mg/dL

Proteins

Total protein: 6-8 g/dL
C-reactive protein: <0.8 mg/dL
Albumin: 3.5-4.5 g/dL
Prealbumin: 15-32 mg/dL
Transferrin: 250-300 mg/dL
Globulin: 2.3-3.5 g/dL
Albumin/globulin ratio (A/G): 1.5/1-2.5/1
Fibrinogen: 200-400 mg/dL or 2-4 g/L

Lipids

Cholesterol: 150-200 mg/dL
Triglycerides: 40-150 mg/dL
Lipoprotein-cholesterol fractionation
    HDL: 29-77 mg/dL
    LDL: 62-130 mg/dL

Enzymes

Total CK: normal 55-170 U/L for males; 30-135 U/L for females
CK-MB: 0-4% of total CK
LDH: 90-200 IU/L
LDH-1: 17%-25% of total LDH
Alanine aminotransferase (ALT): 5-36 units/mL (formerly called SGPT)
Aspartate aminotransferase (AST): 15-45 units/mL (formerly called SGOT)
Gammaglutamyl transferase (GGT): 5-38 IU/L
Alkaline phosphatase: 30-85 IU/L
Amylase: 56-190 IU/L
Lipase: 0-1.5 units/mL

Muscle Proteins

Myoglobin: normal <110 ng/mL
Troponin I: normal <1.5 ng/mL
Troponin T: normal <0.1 ng/mL

Arterial Blood Gases

pH: normal 7.35-7.45
$PaCO_2$: normal 35-45 mm Hg
HCO_3^-: normal 22-26 mEq/L
Base excess: -2 - +2
PaO_2: normal 80->100 mm Hg
SaO_2: > 95%

Hematology

Red blood cells (RBC): $4.4\text{-}5.9 \times 10^6$/mL for males; $3.8\text{-}5.2 \times 10^6$/mL for females; red cell indices include the following:
    Mean corpuscular volume (MCV): 80-100 μm^3
    Mean corpuscular hemoglobin (MCH): 27-31 pg
    Mean corpuscular hemoglobin concentration (MCHC): 32-36 g/dL
Reticulocyte count: 0.5%-1.5% of RBC
Erythrocyte sedimentation rate: normal up to 15 mm/hr for males; up to 20 mm/hr for females
Hematocrit: 40%-52% for males; 35%-47% for females
Hemoglobin: 13-18 g/dL for males; 12-16 g/dL for females
White blood cells (WBC): 3,500-11,000 mm^3
Differential
    Neutrophils: 40%-80%
    Eosinophils: 0%-5%
    Basophils: 0%-2%

Monocytes: 3%-8%

Lymphocytes: 10%-40%

Immune profile

    CD4 cell count: 800 cells/mm^3; varies with age

    CD4/CD8 ratio: helper cells:suppressor/cytotoxic cells
      ratio: 1.8

HIV antibody screening: negative

Clotting Profile

Prothrombin time (PT): 12-15 seconds

Partial thromboplastin time (PTT): 60-70 seconds

Activated partial thromboplastin time (aPTT): 25-38 seconds

Activated clotting time (ACT): 70-120 seconds

International normalized ratio (INR): normal <2.0

Thrombin time: 10-15 seconds

Bleeding time: 1-9.5 minutes

Lee White clotting time: 6-12 minutes

Platelets: 150,000-400,000/mm^3

Fibrinogen: 200-400 mg/dL or 2-4 g/L

Fibrin degradation products (FDPs) (also referred to as fibrin
split products [FSPs]): 0-10 mcg/dL

D-dimer: normal <250 ng/mL

Hormones

Triiodothyronine (T3): 0.2-0.3 mcg/dL

Thyroxine (T4): 6-12 mcg/dL

ACTH: 15-100 pg/mL in AM, 10-50 pg/mL in PM

Cortisol: 6-28 mcg/dL at 8 AM, 4-12 mcg/dL at 4 PM; 2-12
mcg/dL at 8 PM

ADH: 1-5 pg/mL

Toxicology

Alcohol: 0 mg/dL

Dilantin: therapeutic 10-20 mcg/mL

Digoxin: therapeutic 0.5-2.0 ng/mL

Lidocaine: therapeutic 1.5-5.0 mcg/mL

Phenobarbital: therapeutic 10-40 mcg/mL

Theophylline: therapeutic 10-20 ng/dL

URINE

Glucose: negative

Ketones: negative

Protein: 0-8 mg/dL; <150 mg/24-hour urine output

Amylase: 3-21 IU/hour

Bilirubin: negative

Urobilinogen: <1 mg/dL

RBCs: 0-2/low-power field

WBCs: 0-4/low-power field

Hemoglobin/myoglobin: negative

Bilirubin: none

Specific gravity: 1.005-1.030

Osmolality: 50-1200 mOsm/L

Creatinine clearance: 85-135 mL/min

Culture and sensitivity: no bacteria present; if bacteria are
present appropriate antibiotic therapy is identified

pH: 4.0-8.0 with average of 6.0

Spot urine electrolytes

    Sodium: 40-220 mEq/L/day

    Potassium: 25-120 mEq/L/day

    Chloride: 110-250 mEq/day

Hormone metabolites

    17-hydroxycorticosteroids: 4.5-10 mg/24 hours for males,
    2.5-10 mg/24 hours for females

    17-ketosteroids: 8-15 mg/24 hours for males, 6-12 mg/24
    hours for females

STOOL

Fecal occult blood test: negative

Ova, parasites, blood (OPB): negative

Fecal fat: 5 g/24 hour

Urobilinogen: 0-4 mg/day

Culture: Intestinal flora

Assay for *Clostridium difficile* toxin A or B: normal negative;
positive if diarrhea is caused *C. difficile*

Note: Values may vary depending on laboratory.

Formulae Significant to Progressive Care Nursing

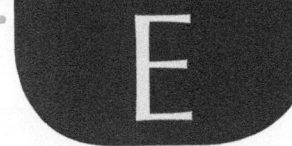

GENERAL

Conversion

To convert pounds to kilograms	1 lb = .45 kg
To convert inches to cm	1 in = 2.54 cm
To convert mm Hg to cm of H_2O	1 mm Hg = 1.36 cm H_2O
To convert Fahrenheit to Celsius	(°F − 32) ÷ 1.8

Drug Administration

To calculate mcg/kg/min if you know the rate of the infusion	$\dfrac{(mcg/mL) \times (mL/hr)}{(60\ min/hour) \times (kg\ of\ body\ weight)}$
To calculate rate in mL/hour if you know the dose in mcg/kg/min	$\dfrac{(dose\ in\ mcg/kg/min) \times (60\ min/hr) \times (kg\ of\ body\ weight)}{mcg/mL\ of\ the\ solution}$
To calculate mg/min if you know the rate of the infusion	$\dfrac{(mg/mL) \times (mL/hr)}{(60\ min/hour)}$
To calculate rate in mL/hour if you know the dose in mg/min	$\dfrac{(dose\ in\ mg/min) \times (60\ min/hr)}{mg/mL\ of\ the\ solution}$
To calculate mcg/min if you know the rate of the infusion	$\dfrac{(mcg/mL) \times (mL/hr)}{(60\ min/hour)}$
To calculate rate in mL/hour if you know the dose in mcg/min	$\dfrac{(dose\ in\ mcg/min) \times (60\ min/hr)}{mcg/mL\ of\ the\ solution}$

CARDIOVASCULAR

Parameter	Method of Calculation	Normal
Mean arterial pressure (MAP)	[BP systolic + (BP diastolic × 2)] ÷ 3	70-105 mm Hg (Normal systolic BP 90-140 mm Hg; normal diastolic BP 60-90 mm Hg)
Coronary artery perfusion pressure (CAPP)	Diastolic BP − PAOP	60-80 mm Hg
Corrected QT (QT_c)	QT ÷ $\sqrt{RR}$	0.35-0.43 seconds

PULMONARY

Parameter	Method of Calculation	Normal
a/A ratio	(PaO_2/PAO_2) Note: PAO_2 is calculated as: FIO_2 (760 − 47) − ($PaCO_2/0.8$) Note: FIO_2: fraction of inspired oxygen (written as a decimal) Pb: barometric pressure (760 mm Hg at sea level, adjust for higher altitudes) $PaCO_2$: arterial carbon dioxide tension 47 is the pressure of water vapor at sea level and is subtracted from barometric pressure; 0.8 is the usual respiratory quotient	normal >0.8 moderately abnormal 0.5-0.8 significantly abnormal 0.25-0.5 critically abnormal <0.25
PaO_2/FIO_2 ratio	$\dfrac{PaO_2}{FIO_2\ (decimal)}$	>300 300 = ~15% shunt 200 = ~20% shunt

Continued

NEUROLOGIC

Parameter	Method of Calculation	Normal
Cerebral perfusion pressure (CPP)	MAP – ICP	60-100 mm Hg

NUTRITION

Parameter	Method of Calculation	Normal
Body mass index (BMI)	Weight (kg)/Ht (m) × Ht (m)	Optimal: 20-25 Obesity: >25 Underweight: <20

FLUID, ELECTROLYTE, ACID-BASE

Parameter	Method of Calculation	Normal
Serum osmolality	$(2 \times Na) + \dfrac{BUN}{2.6} + \dfrac{glucose}{18}$	280-295 mOsm/L
Anion gap	$(Na + K) - (Cl + HCO_3)$ Note: may also use CO_2 content from venous blood for HCO_3	5-15 Note: some formulas omit potassium; if potassium is omitted, normal is 8-12

Index

Pages followed by *b*, *t*, or *f* refer to boxes, tables, or figures, respectively.